PHARMATECTURE™

Minimizing Medications To Maximize Results

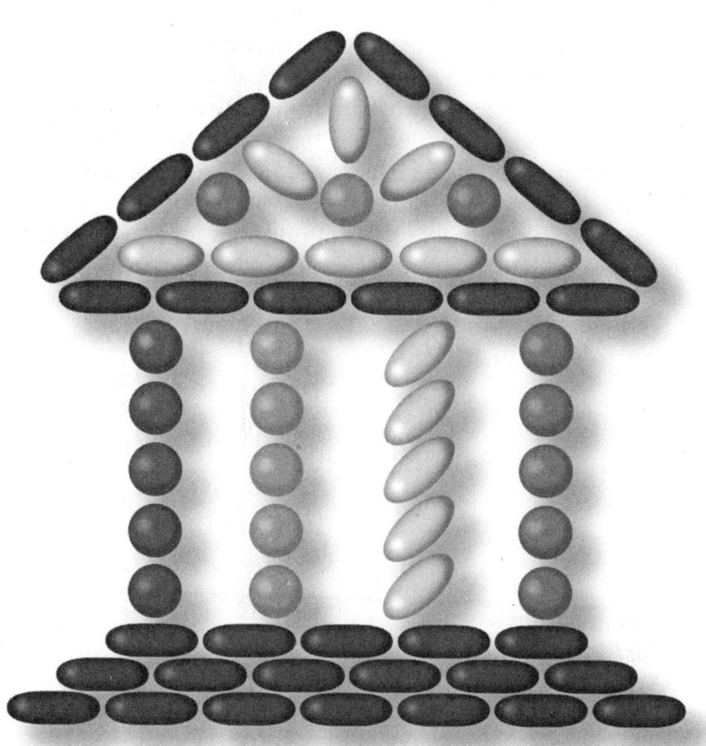

GIDEON BOSKER, MD FACEP

Pharmatecture™: Minimizing Medications To Maximize Results

ISBN 1-57439-047-3

Printed in the United States of America

Published by
Facts and Comparisons
111 West Port Plaza, Suite 300
St. Louis, Missouri 63146-3098
314-216-2100
Toll free customer service 800/223-0054

Dedication

To my patients, who, over the years have taught me both the pearls and pitfalls of drug therapy.

Table of Contents

Preface

In the world of clinical medicine, experience is frequently the best guide. After more than 15 years of evaluating and treating patients who were suffering from the consequences of excessive, inappropriate, or suboptimal drug prescribing, I felt there was a need for a source of practical information that would present a systematic approach for constructing safe and cost-effective drug regimens for the outpatient setting. Against the backdrop of mounting cost-containment pressures that required prescribers to accomplish more with less, this approach would have to address real world issues that balanced institutional needs with those of individual patients and their families. As this drug prescribing system evolved, it became clear to me that its primary objective was to direct physicians and pharmacists toward prescribing approaches that would minimize medications in order to maximize clinical results.

With these issues in clear focus, the second edition of Pharmatecture is intended as a guide for all prescribers—physicians, pharmacists, nurse practitioners, physician assistants—who are faced with the daily challenge of selecting drugs that will meet therapeutic objectives without adversely affecting quality of life. In particular, the strategies in this book are consistent with a new mission statement for choosing medications that encompass *all* of the factors that enter into the equation for drug selection. These considerations include: cost, side effects, compliance, quality assurance, and disease prevention. It also encompasses such risk management issues as drug-drug and drug-disease interactions, smartness and productivity levels of medications, regimen durability, dose stability, duration of therapy, and the relative "noise levels" of medications drugs vs the noise levels of the disease against which they are directed.

If, based on the principles contained in this book, prescribers can improve therapeutic outcomes while maintaining quality-of-life for their patients, Pharmatecture™ will have achieved its purpose.

Gideon Bosker, MD FACEP

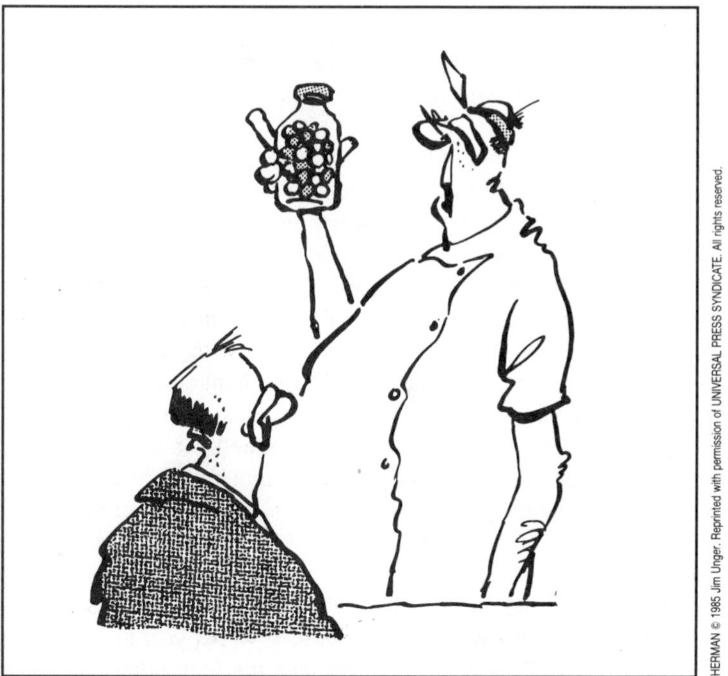

"I'm not sure what these are, but take them for a couple of weeks and let me know how you feel."

Introduction

Better living through pharmacology has become a way of life. When appropriately used and wisely combined, drugs are fundamental to optimizing clinical outcome and maintaining good health. Appropriately prescribed medications keep people alive. They sometimes cure fatal diseases. They make it possible for people to lead more productive, active, pain-free lives.

Stated simply, drugs are some of the most ingenious biomolecular solutions ever devised. That is the good news. The bad news is that a wide array of pharmacological options are available for human use, complicating choices for physicians, and therefore, increasing the risk of polypharmacy and drug interactions.

In light of the importance of drug therapy in clinical disease, constructing safe, cost-effective drug regimens, especially for chronic conditions managed in the outpatient setting, is one of the most important clinical challenges facing health care providers. [1,2,3,4] It should be emphasized that attitudes toward outpatient drug therapy have changed dramatically over the past decade.[5,6,7,8] The mounting pressures of cost containment in health care, the emergence of public policy mandates encouraging out-of-hospital management of both acute and chronic diseases, the financial and clinical hazards associated with polypharmacy, and the introduction of increasingly potent oral agents are just some of the factors inducing physicians and formulary managers to develop innovative pharmacotherapeutic strategies.[7,9,10,11]

In this regard, it should be stressed that the whole issue of drug prescribing is more than just a day-to-day, patient-to-patient clinical activity. It is a public policy issue. There will be increasing pressure during the next decade and beyond to use drugs in the most cost effective manner possible. To achieve these public policy goals—most are clearly aimed at containment of health care expenditures—a new discipline, pharmacoeconomics, has evolved to focus attention on and evaluate total outcome costs associated with different pharmacotherapeutic interventions. In an age characterized by vigilant cost management in health care, the day may come when pharmacists and physicians are restricted in the number of different prescription ingredients permitted for patients. Healthcare maintenance organizations (HMOs), in an attempt to curb drug costs, are likely to introduce capitated pharmacological maintenance programs in which predetermined dollar amounts will be allotted for patients with various medical disorders. For example, depending on the clinical disorder, insurance companies, managed care networks, and HMOs will allocate, let's say, $280 per year for drug treatment of a patient with hypertension, $440 per year to manage the patient with coronary artery disease, $440 to manage the individual with major depression, $580 to manage diabetes mellitus, and so on.

Operating under these stringent fiscal group rules, pharmacists and physicians will be free to choose whatever drugs they please, but the annual drug expenditures will have to conform to the capitated limits established by third-party, government-funded, or HMO payor organizations. This new world order in clinical pharmacotherapeutics has made "necessity the mother of invention" when it comes to drug prescribing and, in turn, is fueling the development of new approaches, such as Pharmatecture™, to guide long-term drug regimen construction.[12,13,14]

Good News, Bad News

Perceptions also are changing about the relative risks and benefits of drug therapy.[15,16,17,18,19] Although clinicians may think of coronary angiograms and surgical interventions as invasive procedures, the fact is, prescribing a drug has the potential for being one of the most invasive acts in which a physician or consulting pharmacists can participate. When used in a systematic, rational manner, drugs have the capacity to reduce morbidity, improve or relieve symptoms, enhance the quality of life, and prolong survival. But there also are other, more problematic aspects to long-term pharmacologic intervention—side effects, financial hardship, and the potential for quality-of-life impairment.

Clinical studies demonstrate that the majority of drugs used in the outpatient environment have the potential for producing adverse effects, including subtle impairments in cognitive, sexual, sleep, and emotional function.[1,12,20] I am reminded of the patient who, during an office visit with his physician, explained, "I feel a lot better since I ran out of those pills you gave me." If a patient takes regular medication for a chronic condition, but endures negative side effects, then something is wrong. Consequently, in the case of many chronic diseases managed in the ambulatory environment, committing a patient to a medication for 5, 10, or 15 years can be characterized as an invasive act, carrying with it all the attendant responsibilities of risk-to-benefit analyses, clinical vigilance, the need for meticulous follow-up, and continuous reevaluation of the need for medication.

Increasingly, how patients *feel* while taking their medications, to what extent a drug preserves quality-of-life, and its negative side effects have become just as important as whether or not a particular medication gets the job done. Put another way, "pill-wise, patient-foolish" approaches to drug therapy no longer are acceptable. More and more, the selection of a drug depends as much on its efficacy as on its ability to maintain the patient's functional status with minimal side effects.

To be sure, the growing number of pharmacotherapeutic choices allows physicians to treat patients more safely, rapidly, and effectively than ever before. Progress, however, also has pitfalls. With increased drug use comes the potential for drug interactions. For example, many drugs that function well in *isolation* of other agents can induce drug interactions when *combined* with other medications. With the dramatic expansion of drug classes and a growing menu of potentially useful pharmacologic interventions, physicians are not only given new opportunities for drug-based management, but also face the increased risk of producing drug-induced side effects, quality-of-life impairment, and interactions.

The Pharmacological Imperative

The pharmacological imperative is upon us: Drugs are playing an increasingly pivotal role in the management of clinical disorders. In turn, as drug therapy succeeds in prolonging life, new conditions emerge that require additional pharmacological palliation. As a result, the number of prescription ingredients in an average drug regimen seems to have swelled dangerously out of control. Considering the recent explosion in the number of useful chemical agents, it is not surprising that polypharmacy is common in the treatment of elderly patients with chronic disease. In searching for an antidote to these trends, drug therapy consultants and physicians have forged new, comprehensive approaches to treatment. Prescribing methods are being developed that take into account all the factors influencing safety, value, efficacy, and cost-effectiveness of long-term drug regimens. Objectives include identifying drugs associated with good medication compliance, galvanizing strategies for optimizing drug selection within drug classes, using drugs in appropriate combinations, improving techniques for detecting drug toxicity and adverse drug reactions, and improving quality of life.

Achieving these goals will not be easy, but one thing is clear: The pharmacological imperative forces physicians to re-examine traditional approaches to drug regimen construction. In the United States, approximately two thirds of all physician visits result in a drug prescription.[1] It has been estimated that a patient visiting a U.S. physician for a specific complaint receives approximately four times more medication than a person with similar complaints in Scotland. Other studies show that up to 60% of physicians prescribe antibiotics to treat the common cold.[1]

The sheer number of pharmacological options creates the need for a simple, clinically applicable, and systematic approach to drug regimen design. There are presently 13,000 prescription drugs available in the United States, and the annual expenditure on prescription drugs is estimated to be in excess of $28 billion. In 1994, physicians generated 2.8 billion prescriptions, or about eight prescriptions for every man, woman, and child in the country. The increase in prescription drug use was accompanied by a corresponding increase in adverse reactions to drugs. It was estimated that between 10% and 15% of all hospitalized patients experience an adverse reaction to a drug at some point during their hospital stay.[6,7,21,22] Other studies show that 25% of all hospital admissions of patients over 65 years of age are associated with, or precipitated by, a drug-related incident.[16,23,24] Although many adverse drug reactions are relatively minor and have predictable occurrences, estimates of adverse reactions serious enough to cause hospitalization range from 0.5% to as high as 8%.[1,25,26,27]

The Information Gap

Not surprisingly, the staggering explosion in our pharmacopoeia has created a profound information and education gap that, to some extent, threatens the safety and quality of pharmacy-based medicine as it is practiced in the contemporary medical environment. For example, by the time a physician completes a three-year residency program, five years have elapsed since his or her course in clinical pharmacology. During this interval, approximately 100 new drugs will become available,[1] and the majority of drugs prescribed will be for agents about which the physicians received no formal education. Against the backdrop of rapidly expanding pharmacologic options, the Health and Public Policy Committee of the American College of Physicians points out that, "After completion of formal medical school and house officer training, there is no exposure to intelligent, informative, and unbiased assessments of drug therapy." This white paper goes on to comment that "the entire [educational] process can be characterized as largely random, incomplete and subject to distortion."[1]

Because drug therapy is the primary defense against common illnesses, more and more the art of clinical pharmacology—as well as the art of medicine, for that matter—has become synonymous with how well and how wisely a drug regimen is constructed. With so many new therapeutic agents tumbling into the pharmacist's and physician's arsenal, however, designing safe, cost-effective, quality-of-life enhancing drug regimens is increasingly problematic. In developing a rational, systematic, hands-on approach to drug regimen construction, several things appear necessary. For one, prescribing drugs *reflexively* must give way to prescribing drugs *selectively*. Moreover, opportunities for reducing overall *pharmacologic* burden—i.e. the number, frequency, and dosage level of medications—must be considered by physicians at every point in the therapeutic decision-making process. State-of-the-art drug prescribing in the contemporary medical environment, as well as in the future, should not only emphasize introducing drugs to normalize test results and objective parameters (i.e., blood pressure control, blood sugar and cholesterol levels, pulmonary function tests, etc.), but should consider quality of life, side effects, compliance, cost, drug-drug interactions, drug-disease interactions, and the ''smartness'' of prescription ingredients, i.e., the number of target organs and clinical endpoints that can be serviced within the context of a *single* prescription ingredient.

In previous decades, physicians were preoccupied simply with "getting the numbers (abnormal laboratory values, physiological parameters, etc.) square" on a piece of paper. In recent years, however, their pharmacotherapeutic mandate has expanded to include maintaining quality-of-life as an essential criterion against which the success of a drug regimen is measured.

Stated simply, we are in the midst of an epidemic of excessive, inappropriate, and suboptional drug prescribing in middle-aged and older Americans.[1,21,23,28] Developing viable solutions to this problem requires us to understand the full scope of the problem. In 1994, North Americans spent $14 billion hospitalizing 265,000 patients for drug-related problems.[1] During this same interval,[9,16,17] it is estimated that $10.5 billion was spent servicing noncompliance-induced disease deterioration. In other words, the health-care sector spent almost $11 billion on drugs, clinical services, and hospitalizations for individuals whose clinical conditions became worse or who developed complications simply because of poor medication compliance. Noncompliance with medications is an issue of special concern, because physicians are able to exert little control over factors influencing noncompliance. Clearly, innovative approaches relying on some combination of patient education reassurance, cost-savings, and reduction of daily dose frequency are required for noncompliant patients.

Pharmatecture™

With these issues in clear focus, the purpose of this book is to provide pharmacists and physicians a hands-on approach to drug regimen construction in the outpatient environment. This new approach called Pharmatecture, is a drug prescribing system that weds pharmacology with architectural concepts to provide a practical, clinically useful strategy for the construction of outpatient drug regimens. Since pharmatecture represents a systematic drug selection system that employs an architectural metaphor to help guide the construction of optimal drug regimens, it can be applied to new regimens as well as to the remodeling, deconstruction, and reconstruction of preexisting polypharmacy combinations. The strategies that underpin the pharmatecture-based approach to drug selection are not only designed to increase patient compliance and reduce side effects, but also to ensure therapeutic efficacy, cost-effective drug selection, and to increase safety of drug prescribing.[27]

[1]American College of Physicians. Improving medical education in therapeutics. Ann Intern Med 1988; 108:145-47.

[2]Colley CA, Lucas LM. Polypharmacy: the cure becomes the disease. (Review) J Gen Intern Med 1993 May; 8(5):278-83.

[3]De Santis G, Harvey KJ, Howard D, Mashford ML, Moulds RF. Improving the quality of antibiotic prescription patterns in general practice. The role of intervention. Med J Aust 1994 April 18; 160(8):502-5.

[4]Kahl A, Blandford DH, Krueger K, Zwick DI. Geriatric education centers address medication issues affecting older adults. Public Health Reports-Hyattsville 1992 Jan-Feb; 107(1):37-47.

[5]Peck CC, Temple R, Collins JM. Understanding consequences of concurrent therapies. JAMA1993 March 24; 269(12):1550-52.

[6]Poulsen RL. Some current factors influencing the prescribing and use of psychiatric drugs. Public Health Reports-Hyattsville 1992 Jan-Feb; 107(1):47-53.

[7]Safavi KT, Hayward RA. Choosing between apples and apples: physicians' choices of prescription drugs that have similar side effects and efficacies. J Gen Intern Med 1992 Jan-Feb; 7(1):32-7.

[8]Wetle T. Age as a risk factor for inadequate treatment. (Editorial) JAMA 1987; 258:516.

[9]Lamy PP. Compliance in long-term care. Geriatrika 1985; 1(8)32.

[10]Peck CC, Temple RJ, Collins JM. Drug interactions: The death pen. (Letter) JAMA 1993 Sept 15; 270(11):1317.

[11]Valentine C. Use computers to detect inappropriate prescriptions. (Letter, Comment) BMJ 1993 July 3; 307(6895):61.

[12]Hux JE, Levinton CM, Naylor CD. Prescribing propensity; influence of life-expectancy gains and drug cost. J Gen Intern Med 1994 April; 9(4);195-201.

[13]Inman W, Pearce G. Prescriber profile and post-marketing surveillance. Lancet 1993 Sept 11; 342(8872):658-61.

[14]Jones JK. Assessing potential risk of drugs: The elusive target. Ann Intern Med 1992 Oct 15; 117(8):691-92.

[15]Belitsos NJ. Overprescribing of benzodiazepine hypnotic drugs in the elderly. (Letter, comment). Am J Med 1991 Sept; 91(3):321.

[16]Bloom JA, Frank JW, Shafir MS, Martiquet P. Potentially undesirable prescribing and drug use among the elderly. Measurable and remediable. Canadian Family Physician 1993 Nov; 39:2337-45.

[17]Burns LR, Denton M, Goldfein S. Warrick L. Morenz B, Sales B. The use of continuous quality improvement methods in the development and dissemination of medical practice guidelines. QRB 1992 Dec; 18(12):434-9.

[18]Grob PR. Antibiotic prescribing practices and patient compliance in the community. (Review) Scand J Infect Dis Suppl 1992; 83:7-14.

[19]Hamilton IJ, Reay LM, Sullivan FM. A survey of general practitioners' attitudes to benzodiazepine overprescribing. Health Bulletin 1990 Nov; 48(6):299-03.

[20]Chinburapa V, Larson LN. The importance of side effects and outcomes in differentiating between prescription drug products. J Clin Pharm Ther 1992 Dec; 17(6):333-42.

[21]Ashburn PE. Polypharmacy in skilled-nursing facilities. (Letter, Comment) Ann Intern Med 1993 April 15; 118(8):649-51.

[22]Swanson PO. Drug treatment of Parkinson's disease: is ''polypharmacy'' best? (Review) J Neurol Neurosurg Psychiatry 1994 April; 57(4):401-3.

[23]Beers MH, Ouslander JG, Fingold SF, Morgenstern H, Ruben DB, Rogers W, Zeffren MJ, Beck JC. Inappropriate medication prescribing in skilled-nursing facilities. Ann Intern Med 1992 Oct 15; 117(8):684-9.

[24]Bliss MR. Prescribing for the elderly. BMJ 1981; 282:203-6.

[25]Huszonek JJ, Dewan MJ, Koss M, Hadoby WJ, Ispahani A. Antidepressant side effects and physician prescribing patterns. Ann Clin Psychiatry 1993 March; 5(1):7-11.

[26]Jordan LK, Jordan LO. Prudent prescribing. Prescribing suggestions for physicians. North Carolina Medical Journal 1992 Nov; 53(11):585-8.

[27]Lamy PP. Adverse drug effects. Clin Geriatr Med 1990; 6:293-305.

[28]Beers MH, Fingold SF, Ouslander JG, Ruben DB, Morgenstern H, Beck JC. Characteristics and quality of prescribing by doctors practicing in nursing homes. J Am Geriatr Soc 1993 Aug; 41(8):802-7.

1

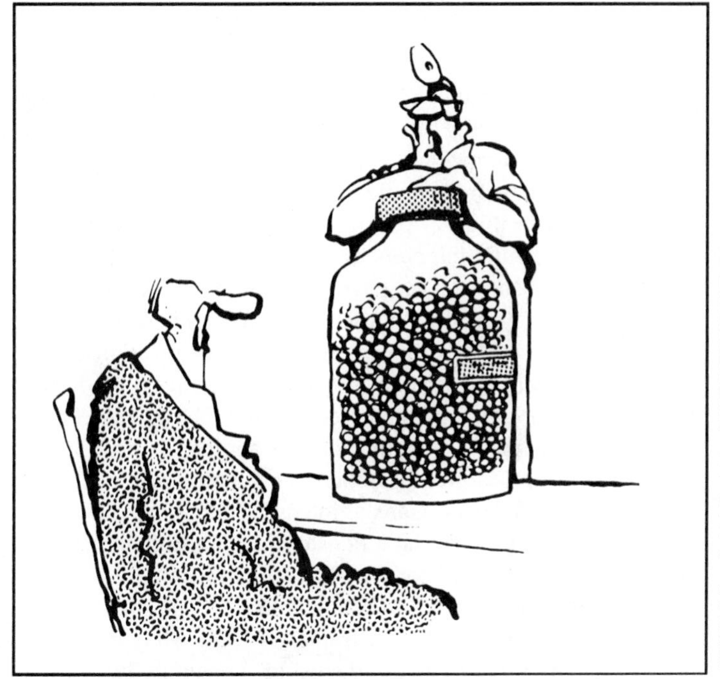

"I hope you're not one of those people who have trouble swallowing pills."

Pharmatecture™
A Systematic Approach to Pharmacologic Assessment and Drug Regimen Design

Pharmatecture™ is a drug prescribing system that melds time-honored architectural principles and concepts used for the construction of three-dimensional structures, with the objectives, strategies, and clinical approaches that comprise the foundations of clinical pharmacology. Put simply, pharmatecture is the science of *designing* drug regimens for the new millennium. Why pharmatecture? Because in much the same way architects design three-dimensional houses and skyscrapers out of glass, steel, and stone, clinicians are in the business of designing "drug houses" for their patients. Not only are the analogies between designing structures for the built landscape and fabricating a chemical environment using prescription ingredients quite striking, but they provide the underpinnings for an approach that can shape, simplify, and streamline drug prescribing in day-to-day clinical practice.

When it comes to constructing drug regimens, pharmacists and physicians mix, match, layer, and combine medications much like architects stitch together diverse building materials to form an integrated composition.[1,2,3] While architects work with granite, wood, glass, stone, and steel, clinicians usually draw on pharmacologic building blocks—i.e., selective serotonin reuptake inhibitors (SSRIs), calcium channel antagonists, prostaglandin inhibitors, statins and beta agonists—for their therapeutic constructions. Consequently, for the purpose of analogy, one can think of pharmacists and physicians, who engage primarily in pharmacotherapeutic interventions as "pharmatects". They are builders of pharmacologic environments or, pharmatecturally speaking, "drug houses," for their patients. By the term "drug house," of course, is meant a pharmacologic environment consisting of one or more prescription medications.

One can think of these drug houses as chemical environments that are both *built* and *maintained* by pharmacists and physicians. For example, when a physician prescribes a beta-blocker for angina, an aspirin a day for secondary prevention of myocardial infarction, a calcium blocker for hypertension, a statin to lower blood cholesterol, an angiotensin converting enzyme (ACE) inhibitor for congestive heart failure, and a nonsteroidal anti-inflammatory drug (NSAID) for arthritis, he or she has constructed a pharmacologic environment in which a patient may have to "live" for many years.[4,5] The final architecture of this drug house—its building blocks, its framework, its safety considerations, its foundation—are the primary determinants of its durability, cost-effectiveness, and patient-friendliness.

Pharmacologic Framework

From a pharmatectural perspective, how safe this drug house is over time, how effectively it meets the patient's functional objectives, and the physician's clinical goals how much it costs, and how good the patient feels living inside that house, are the most important criteria against which the success and durability of a drug regimen can be measured. Clearly, drug houses designed by physicians are not three-dimensional architectural environments but they are quantifiable environments, nevertheless, with the capacity to produce distinct side effect profiles and outcomes.[1,6,7] A drug house can be thought of as a pharmacologically determined milieu, consisting of many different prescription ingredients with active biochemical properties. These building blocks sometimes interact to produce positive results, and sometimes they create negative effects for the patient living within its pharmacologic framework.[8,9] Over time, pharmacologic building blocks may even become obsolete or unsafe. The introduction of better materials (i.e., newer, better medications) may necessitate remodeling a drug house, that is, deconstructing and reconstructing it according to the best materials currently available. In the final analysis, like a work of architecture, a drug house must satisfy specific functional, safety, and quality-of-life objectives.

Interestingly, many of the same criteria against which the success, quality, and suitability of a work of architecture are measured, also apply to pharmacologic environments constructed by practitioners trying to achieve optimal therapeutic outcomes. In addition, the manner in which building materials are chosen in the architectural world is similar to the way pharmacologic building blocks are selected in the therapeutic sphere. For example, architectural works are fabricated from a wide variety of building materials, from glass and plastic to wood and stone. Within budgetary constraints, an architect has the freedom to choose among these options. Extensive catalogues consisting of thousands of different types of building materials—many of them very similar except for slight differences in color, texture, or weight—are consulted to evaluate the desirability of one product over another.

A similar process guides the selection of medications. Physicians consult many different types of references—formulary lists, drug catalogues, clinical monographs, such established resources as *Drug Facts and Comparisons,* as well as software programs—to guide their selection of pharmacologic building blocks. This is a necessary process because all the options within a given drug class are not created equal. There are, in fact, better drugs and worse drugs, with some drugs making better building blocks than others.[10,11,12,13,14] For example, some antihistamines (diphenhydramine) are more likely to cause sedation than others (loratidine), while one H_2 blocker (cimeditine, Tagamet®) may have a greater propensity for causing drug interactions through inhibition of P450 cytochrome oxidase system than another H_2 blocker (famotidine, Pepcid®).[7,15] Moreover, advantages and disadvantages of drugs vary according to their therapeutic class. In some cases, pharmacologic inferiority and superiority may be determined by the risk of drug interactions, in others by compliance patterns, and in other classes, by side effect profiles. For example, some potentially very effective antibiotics (e.g., erythromycin) have a significant incidence of side effects and, therefore, are associated with higher discontinuation rates, making them therapeutically less effective in some patients. To maximize pharmatectural effectiveness, physicians must select among various options in order to determine which pharmacotherapeutic building blocks offer unique advantages in some patients, but might pose a risk in others.

Safe Construction of Drug Regimens

Architecture has been called "the beautiful necessity," a description that underscores the fact that the building arts do not exist for beauty's sake alone. At the very minimum, a work of architecture has to satisfy certain functional criteria. First and foremost among these are safety considerations: No matter what other goals are accomplished, a house must meet certain building codes pertaining to electrical, heating, plumbing, and waste disposal systems. To be sure, once these rudimentary criteria are met, the best works of architecture also function on a spiritual level. Ideally, they please the eye with a well-chosen color, elevate the mood by the way light is apportioned in a space, or excite the imagination with a properly chosen ornament.

Similarly, much like an architectural work, drug houses designed by pharmacists or physicians should address both *safety* and *life quality* issues. First, the risk of producing side effects should be minimized. All organ systems—renal, pulmonary, cardiovascular, neurological, dermatological—should be protected from toxic effects. In addition, drugs used to build a pharmacologic environment should not adversely affect underlying diseases or interact with other medications.[16] Moreover, the safety of a drug should be confirmed in the patient population in whom its use is being contemplated. "Safety first" is a mandate that applies equally to both architecture and pharmatecture. Finally, drug houses also must meet functional objectives and clinical target goals (cholesterol levels, blood pressure, mood normalization).[17,18,19,20,21]

But safety is only the beginning. Once the basic pharmacologic building codes are met, with all organ systems operative, and side effect safety checks completed, the *livability* of a drug house becomes an extremely important pharmatectural issue. If architecture is the beautiful necessity, then pharmatecture can be characterized as the *endurable* necessity. In other words, if patients cannot endure living in their drug houses, the fragile walls of their chemical abode eventually will come tumbling down. Noncompliance will undermine therapeutic results, and new problems will surface that may require patching with still more drugs.[22,23] In the world of pharmatecture, then, livability, affordability, and endurability are of paramount importance. Like great works of architecture, the best-designed drug houses also make their inhabitants feel better, more optimistic about life, and healthier for living within their pharmacological walls.[24,25] These subjective aspects of long-term drug therapy are increasingly important features that should be incorporated into the final therapeutic equation.

Less Is More

There also are important *quantitative* parameters that govern the construction of contemporary drug houses. Like modern architecture, pharmatecture subscribes to the guiding principle that, "Less is more." In other words, the more a physician can achieve in the way of desired clinical effects using the *fewest* number of prescription ingredients, at the *lowest* dosage, for the *shortest* duration permissible, and at *lowest* daily dose frequency, the better off the patient will be. In this regard, studies demonstrate that the risk of scheduling errors, drug toxicity, and drug-related adverse side effects are most closely correlated with the total number of prescription ingredients a patient is taking and the total pill count in the daily drug regimen.[4,8,9,11,24,26,27,28,29,30,31]

Moreover, studies of drug use consistently show a negative relationship between medication compliance and the number of drugs taken by the patient.[1,28,29,31,32,33] Specifically, taking three or more drugs increases the likelihood that the patient will be either deliberately or unknowingly noncompliant. Compliance also tends to decrease with time. For example, patients are more likely to take antibiotics in the first stages of treatment than the later stages, with one study showing that only 8% of patients prescribed a 10-day course of antibiotics were actually taking the medication on the tenth day of therapy.[28,29] With respect to long-term therapy, the percentage of patients who adhere faithfully to treatment plans for hypertension and other chronic diseases rapidly declines after the initial diagnosis and early months of treatment. With respect to daily dose frequency, compliance studies show a decrease in medication compliance with increasing daily dose frequency.[31] Many pitfalls, both financial and clinical, associated with polypharmacy can be minimized by subscribing to the "less is more" approach for drug regimen design.

Foundation Drugs

While architects work within a certain structural framework to ensure sound physical construction, physicians operate within a conceptual framework governed by such issues as comfort, cost, and quality-of-life issues associated with drug therapy. Architects emphasize that a house is only as good as its foundation. And so it is with drug regimens. It is important to identify so-called *foundation drugs,* that is, those agents that will stand the test of time in terms of drug and disease interactions, and that can be used as *monotherapy* for long durations. In other words, to avoid excessive costs and other problems associated with altering drug regimens over time, physicians should prescribe agents that safely allow addition of other drugs, without incurring the risk of drug-drug or drug-disease interactions.[34,35]

These are the broad brush strokes of a drug prescribing system that is designed to promote cost-effective pharmacologic intervention in the outpatient setting. The following sections discuss specific parameters of this system in detail and their implementation in clinical practice.

PHARMATECTURE™: THE SYSTEM IN PRACTICE

For all practical purposes, pharmatecture can be seen as the science of *building* drug regimens. Science, in this case, means using a logical, systematic approach for drug regimen design in the outpatient setting. This is an approach that stresses optimizing drug selection, enhancing patient medication compliance, and streamlining drug regimens, always with an eye toward drug reduction, elimination, simplification, and consolidation (DRESC™). (See Chapter 7)

WINDOWS

Architects pay special attention to windows in their building designs. Physicians also must consider windows—windows of *opportunity* and *vulnerability* as they relate to the selection of individual drugs, and the design of long-term, outpatient drug regimens.

Windows of Vulnerability

One window of vulnerability is noncompliance with medications, which is now recognized as a public health problem. Noncompliance is associated with staggering clinical and economic consequences.[29,36,37,38] For example, Americans now spend almost $11 billion annually servicing poor therapeutic outcomes associated with medication noncompliance.[33,39] Noncompliance-induced disease deterioration has been observed in such chronic conditions as hypertension, seizures, and diabetes mellitis, as well as in acute diseases such as sexually transmitted disorders, especially chlamydial infections. Most studies demonstrate that noncompliance with medications is exacerbated by increasing daily dose frequency, excessive side effects, lack of patient education, and cost of the drug.[40,41,42] Attention to these factors promotes improved medication compliance, and as a result, may yield better therapeutic outcomes. Not surprisingly, the pharmatectural approach to drug prescribing highlights pharmacology-, physician-, and patient-oriented strategies designed to enhance drug compliance.[29,30,31,43]

Inappropriate drug use takes many forms and can produce a wide range of undesirable consequences. Consider the following patient scenarios as glimpses into the window of vulnerability associated with poor medication compliance:

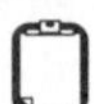

> ***A 62-year-old gentleman*** *with high blood pressure discontinues his medication because its side effects make him feel worse than he does when he is not on medication. His hypertension is no longer in control and he eventually has a stroke leading to prolonged hospitalization, subsequent rehabilitation, and permanent disability.*

Analysis: In this example, the side effects of the antihypertensive drug are more uncomfortable than the disease (silent hypertension). As expected, the patient opts for the "silence" of the disease rather than the excessive "noise level" of the medication. The end result is noncompliance-mediated therapeutic failure, increased morbidity, and poor outcome.

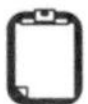

> ***A 35-year old woman*** *suffering from depression stops taking her antidepressant drug because she sees no improvement in her condition after 1 week of drug therapy. She grows more and more depressed and, eventually, her employment is terminated because she is unable to perform her job duties. When asked why she stopped taking her medicine, she indicates she was not aware that the benefits of some antidepressants become apparent only after the drug has been taken for several weeks.*

Analysis: This patient received inadequate education from her physician or pharmacist regarding the relationship between duration of antidepressant therapy and onset of therapeutic benefits. The result is premature discontinuation of drug therapy and exacerbation of symptoms associated with her depression.

> ***A 55-year-old patient*** *taking diuretics and digoxin for congestive heart failure stops taking his potassium supplement because he finds it unpalatable. Eventually, his serum potassium level drops. The potassium deficiency, in combination with the digoxin therapy, produces a poten-*

tially life-threatening heart rhythm disturbance necessitating an emergency department visit and subsequent hospitalization.[36]

Analysis: In this patient, discontinuation of one drug (potassium) potentiates the side effects of another drug (digoxin). This case also illustrates the risk of medication noncompliance and clinical consequences associated with construction of complex (i.e., three or more different prescription ingredients) drug regimens. Lack of patient education might also have played a role. The importance of maintaining potassium levels should have been stressed. Finally, simplification of the drug regimen might have prevented this patient's deterioration caused by a heart rhythm disturbance. In this regard, a combination drug that combines a diuretic with a potassium-sparing drug (e.g., aldactone with hydrochlorothiazide, Aldactazide®; triamterene with hydrochlorothiazide, Maxzide®) would have simplified drug intake, enhanced compliance, and minimized the risk of hypokalemia-induced potentiation of digoxin toxicity.

***An 82-year-old woman** on a fixed income stops taking her anti-anginal medication because she feels she can no longer afford it. Within one week of discontinuing her drug, she experiences increasing frequency of angina and severity of chest discomfort. These symptoms precipitate an emergency department visit and subsequent short-term hospitalization. She is discharged on a less expensive anti-anginal agent. The cost of her hospitalization is $6,543.45.*

Analysis: This case illustrates the potentially devastating consequences of *cost-mediated* medication noncompliance. The irony is that the discontinuation of the drug because of cost considerations resulted in an expensive hospitalization. Although the cost of medications is frequently justified, especially for once-daily drugs with few side effects, for many individuals cost is the bottom line affecting long-term adherence to a therapeutic program. When managing individuals who are extremely sensitive to drug cost, less expensive agents might produce better overall clinical outcomes, even if these drugs have other features (complicated dosing schedule, side effects, etc.) usually associated with poor compliance.[36,38,39,44]

Compliance Problems

Noncompliance is widespread among ambulatory patients, especially the elderly. The extent of noncompliance generally is estimated at about 40%, although some studies place the estimate as a high as 75%.[22,36,45,46] Omission or underuse of medications is the most common form of noncompliance, with some studies reporting that among older persons on long-term therapy, 59% of patients made one or more errors and that 26% made potentially serious errors.[36,39,44] Nearly 66% of the patients who made errors *omitted* prescribed medications. Interestingly, not only was underuse the most prevalent type of noncompliance, but researchers found that many elderly patients who omit drugs do so *deliber-*

ately, primarily because they think they do not need the medication in the dosage prescribed.[47,48] In general, the major reason medications are *underused* is a dissatisfaction with some part of the drug regimen, i.e., with the type, amount, dosage schedule, or side effects. Because of these concerns, patients make adjustments in their drug therapy, often omitting medications to suit their perceived needs.

Patient education plays an important role in promoting medication compliance. Despite laws mandating pharmacists to instruct patients about safe and effective use of new prescriptions, in a Seattle, Washington study, only 44% of those regularly using prescription drugs could recall pharmacists instructing them on use, whereas 80% recalled that their physician had done so.[28,49] Only 52% reported their physician had instructed them about possible side effects, and only 30% reported receiving this information from their pharmacist. The fact is, a large percentage of patients, especially the elderly, lack basic information about their drugs.[33,50,148] They are uninformed about the name and purpose of their prescription drugs, the dosage schedules, as well as the duration of therapy, possible side effects, and adverse consequences. Fortunately, these problems have solutions. While mastery of this basic information does not guarantee compliance, there are numerous studies suggesting it is at least a necessary condition for ensuring compliance.[28,30,44,51,52] It is well-established, for example, that when patients are provided with specific and detailed instructions about their particular drug regimen, compliance improves. Moreover, individualized instruction is effective when the mode of communication is either oral or written.[48,51,53,54,55]

Economic Barriers. Another barrier to compliance is economic: many patients simply cannot afford prescription medications in the quantity called for by prescription directions. In one study of 290 chronically ill patients discharged from a general hospital in Canada, it was found that the financial burden imposed by drug costs was the primary reason given by patients for noncompliance with drug treatment.[53] Examining the relationship between drug expenditures and the rate of noncompliance, the study revealed that the average monthly cost of drugs prescribed for noncompliant patients was almost three times higher than the cost of drugs for those who did comply.[49,55] These studies argue for the importance of taking cost factors into consideration when building drug regimens.[44,47,55,56]

Intelligent Noncompliance. Usually, patient omission of drugs undermines therapeutic efficacy. However, there are situations when omission of drugs or self-administration of lower than prescribed dosages of drugs may actually be beneficial. It may be appropriate for patients with side effects from taking too many drugs, an excessive dose of a single drug, to cut back on their medication intake.[52] This type of behavior is called, "intelligent noncompliance," and is best able to serve the patient's interest when undertaken in *collaboration* with the physician or pharmacist.[52] Intelligent noncompliance requires that open doors of communication are maintained between patient and physician or pharmacist, so that alterations perceived as necessary by the patient are managed within the context of the overall drug regimen.

Noncompliance and Polypharmacy. Pharmatecturally speaking, the journey from the prescription pad to an optimal clinical outcome is oftentimes derailed by poor medication compliance. Selecting the appropriate drug for the appropriate patient is simply not enough to guarantee desirable outcomes. For example, one may prescribe the indicated drug for a condition, but the therapeutic result may be compromised by less-than-optimal medication intake. Of special concern is the observation that *being noncompliant with a medication actually increases the patient's risk of receiving additional, unnecessary drugs.*[36,38,39,48,53]

In other words, noncompliance with medications can be dangerous. Patients who fail to take their medications as prescribed actually *increase* the likelihood that they will become victims of unnecessary polypharmacy. Why? Because when a patient is noncompliant with medication, poor therapeutic results frequently are observed. As a rule, poor results are expressed in patients as abnormal test results. Almost without exception, the way physicians respond to abnormal disease parameters is by: (1) initiating pharmacologic therapy; (2) continuing existing drug therapy but at a higher dose; (3) adding a new drug to the regimen, or; (4) eliminating the drug that is perceived as ineffective and substituting an agent from a different therapeutic class.

Herein lies the pharmacological rub. In so many cases, when poor medication intake produces unsatisfactory results, patients are prescribed additional, unnecessary drugs to correct the problem. Although less is *usually* more when it comes to drug therapy, the opposite is generally true when *patients* decide on their own that they can get by with fewer medication doses than required.

Although drugs are prescribed for many different reasons, abnormal laboratory values or measurable physiological parameters are the primary reasons physicians initiate therapy with prescription drugs. In most situations, unless noncompliance is recognized by the clinician, to normalize these abnormal end points, the physician either increases the dose of the medication the patient already has failed to take appropriately, or even worse, the clinician will add another medication to the drug regimen. This can be the beginning of a cycle in which noncompliance-mediated disease deterioration induces excessive drug prescribing. Thus, noncompliance not only has the potential for fueling polypharmacy, but it is oftentimes associated with cost-ineffective drug prescribing. Generally speaking, then, patient-mediated noncompliance, when accompanied by inadequate medication intake, can produce poor therapeutic outcomes that tend to generate more drugs, almost always to the patient's detriment.

Factors Influencing Compliance. Clearly, noncompliance is an important window of vulnerability when it comes to drug therapy, and interventional strategies designed to improve medication intake are central to the pharmatectural approach. As previously mentioned, many factors influence medication compliance including: patient education, written instructions reinforcing medication intake, cost of the drug, and total pharmacologic burden. Attention to these issues is mandatory for maximizing medication compliance. Studies demonstrate that if patients know the function of the drug prescribed for them, they are far less likely to have another drug added to their regimen (Figure 1-1). No single factor, however, is as important for preserving optimal medication intake as daily dose *frequency.* Many trials have confirmed that both scheduling errors and unnecessary drug additions are significantly reduced when medications are prescribed on a once-daily basis (Figure 1-2).[31,40,42,54,57]

Figure 1-1

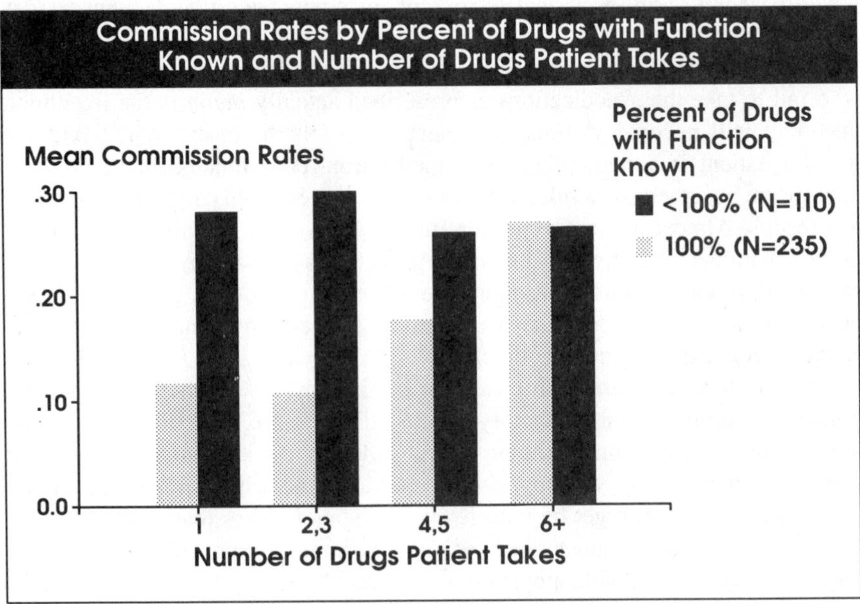

Figure 1-2

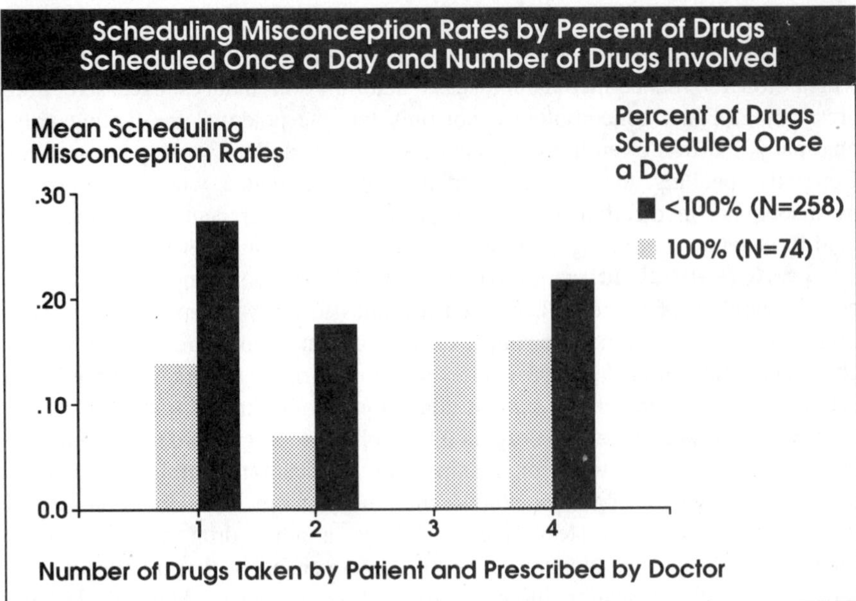

To be sure, the importance of once-daily dosing is much more than a marketing point promulgated by pharmaceutical companies. In fact, there are now "science of compliance" studies demonstrating the undeniable link between daily dose frequency and drug compliance.[31] Eschewing traditional pill counting methods that have characterized previous medication compliance trials, these studies are unique because they rely upon computer microchips to monitor daily medication intake. An accurate chronicle of medication intake is facilitated by microchips that are surreptitiously embedded into the lids of pill bottles. Every time the patient removes the lid to retrieve a pill, the microchip registers, within 15 minutes, the time of day and date the pill bottle is opened. In this manner, a record of pill consumption is recorded without patient input for a 180-day period, at which time the bottles and microchips are collected, and a computer printout of medication intake is generated for evaluation.

The results of these studies are quite fascinating, and confirm that obtaining a realistic assessment of drug intake requires honesty from patients who, as a rule, are either not very forthcoming, or, occasionally, are frankly delusional about their medication intake. In fact, when the results of the microchip data are compared to written questionnaires, on which patients have documented their perceptions of medication compliance, there is a significant divergence between the computer-generated data and questionnaire results. In other words, when it comes to medication compliance, very nice people lie through their teeth. These studies demonstrate in no uncertain terms, first, that medication intake is closely linked to daily dose frequency and, second, that it is unwise to rely upon patient perceptions to make accurate assessments of their medication intake.[22,23,55] Overall, these investigations show that once-daily dosing is associated with a compliance rate of about 92%, twice-daily dosing with compliance rates of about 85%, and three- and four-times daily dosing with rates of about 50% over the long term.[31,43,58,59]

Choosing Once-daily Medications. Based on these and other studies, the most direct pharmatectural approach for addressing the window of vulnerability manifested by poor medication compliance is the use of once-daily medications. Although simplification of dosing schedule is an important strategic maneuver for constructing drug regimens, it should be stressed that once-daily medications represent a *necessary,* but not *sufficient* condition for optimal medication compliance. In other words, simply because a drug can be dosed on a once-daily basis does not give the physician carte blanche for its use. There are, after all, other windows of vulnerability—side effects, drug interaction profiles, cost, etc.—which may require physicians to discriminate among many different medication options dosed on a once-daily basis.

Within each drug class, there are better and worse once-daily preparations and, for each clinical situation an attempt should be made to identify the safest once-daily preparation with the greatest efficacy and fewest side effects.[5] For example, even though flurazepam (Dalmane®) is dosed on a once-daily basis, it has a prolonged, 120 hour half-life, and therefore, is more likely to cause somnolence, falling,[60] and hip fractures than the intermediate-acting, once-daily benzodiazepines which, in general, are safer and associated with fewer, protracted side effects.[12,21,47,61,62] Among the tricyclic antidepressants (TCAs), amitryptiline (Elavil®) can be dosed on a once-daily basis. However, it produces more anticholinergic side effects (dry mouth, sedation, orthostatic hypotension) than such once-daily, selective serotonin reuptake inhibitors (SSRIs) as sertraline (Zoloft®), which demonstrates similar efficacy in the treatment of depression but has a more favorable profile as far as anticholinergic side effects. Even among the once-daily SSRIs, there may be a need for discriminating among the available options.[14,35,63,64,65]

Because cardiovascular drugs are associated with a high incidence of side effects,[34,66,67,68] special vigilance is required when choosing among once-daily medications used to treat heart disease. With respect to calcium channel blockers, verapamil (Calan®) is available as a once-daily preparation, but it is more likely to be associated with sinus bradycardia, congestive heart failure, or conduction inhibition than a calcium blocker such as amlodipine (Norvasc®), which tends not to produce clinically significant adverse effects on the conduction system or myocardial pump function.[7,32,68,69] The important point is that among the compliance-enhancing, once-daily preparations within a drug class, the physician or pharmacist should attempt to identify those agents with the fewest side effects and safest drug interaction profiles.

Patient Education

From a pharmatectural perspective, there are many opportunities for closing the window of vulnerability associated with medication noncompliance.[1,10,21,70,71] Some of these involve selection of medications based on their pharmacologic properties as discussed above. Other approaches must address informational and behavioral needs.[51,53] To be effective in reducing noncompliance, the health care provider must function as teacher, motivator, and persuader. Accurate information about drug intake should be conveyed and the patient must be motivated to take the drugs as instructed. This requires good patient-pharmacist and patient-physician communication. The risk of noncompliance can be reduced by careful labeling of prescriptions. This entails placing both the name and purpose of each drug on the prescription container. Moreover, regimens should be simplified. Each regimen should be examined periodically to ensure that it is the simplest, safest, and most effective therapy currently available. In addition, efforts should be made to titrate medications against treatment response to determine the smallest amount of medication required. Finally, unnecessary medications should be eliminated.

Windows of Opportunity: Smart Drugs

By windows of opportunity is meant the recognition that optimizing drug selection requires identification of so-called "smart drugs". Smart drugs, of course, do not make pharmacists, physicians, or patients smarter, but they do offer an important window of opportunity to reduce a patient's overall pharmacological burden (i.e., the number of different prescription ingredients in the drug regimen), which is an important risk factor for noncompliance, as well as drug-drug and drug-disease interactions.

Smart drugs share many of the properties and advantages associated with "smart bombs", in that they do more with less, and at lower overall cost. Smart bombs, of course, travel precisely to their targets and, therefore, obviate the need for dumping several hundred conventional bombs to accomplish a strategic endpoint. Although smart bombs carry a princely price tag—sometimes costing as much as $600,000—it, nevertheless, is more cost-effective to launch one of these so-called, smart, laser-guided, Sidewinder missiles than it is to send up a B-52 and dump a bunch of "dumb" (conventional) bombs in order to accomplish the same mission.

Like smart bombs, smart drugs also have the capacity to target their action against well-defined endpoints. These smart pharmacologic agents, however, go one step farther, insofar as they can be thought of as smart bombs with multiple warheads. The smartest drugs can hit many targets simultaneously. Specifically, from a pharmatectural point of view, smart drugs are "high productivity" medications that possess the uncanny ability to strike all the necessary clinical endpoints with *one* active prescription ingredient. It is as if they have been designed to: (1) survey a disease landscape and identify the entire cluster of pathophysiological derangements—or, in the case of infectious diseases, anticipate all the co-infecting organisms—that characterize the condition; (2) target many endpoints simultaneously; and (3) service many impaired target-organs associated with the condition, and do so with a *single* pharmacotherapeutic agent.

The specificity and comprehensiveness of targeting afforded by smart drugs *minimizes* dependency on several different drugs to achieve therapeutic end points that once required many agents working in combination. The final result of optimizing drug prescribing through the use of smart drugs is a *reduction in overall pharmacologic burden.* This reduction decreases excessive and unnecessary costs incurred from drug-drug and drug-disease interactions which, studies confirm, are closely tied to the total number of different prescription ingredients in a drug regimen.[15,26,72-75]

Smart Drugs: Patient Specificity

Perhaps more than any other drug class, antibiotics are selected according to their "smartness". To understand the meaning of smartness as it applies to drug therapy, it is helpful to consider the manner in which oral antimicrobials are chosen for the management of infections. In general, when choosing an antibiotic, the physician mentally lists the etiologic organisms most likely to be involved in the infection. Then, whenever possible, an attempt is made to identify a *single* antibiotic that provides antimicrobial activity against *all* the likely offenders. For example, in the case of uncomplicated urinary tract infection, trimethoprim-sulfamethoxazole (Bactrim®) is considered a smart drug, since it will treat the expected species of E. coli and other gram negative organisms usually implicated in such infections. On the other hand, for skin and soft tissue infections, dicloxacillin, azithromycin (Zithromax®) or cephalexin (Keflex®) would represent smart drugs because they cover both streptococcal and staphylococcal species most often implicated in these conditions.

As might be expected, the smartness of a drug *varies* according to the situation. In this regard, it should be stressed that any given antibiotic, statin, antihypertensive, or antidepressant will not, in every patient, *always* be smarter than some other drug to which it is being compared. In other words, in one patient, drug A may be smarter than drug B, but in another case, the converse may be true. Drug smartness, from a pharmatectural perspective, is *patient-specific.* The relative wisdom of any pharmacotherapeutic decision depends upon the medication's suitability for the individual patient—with all the attendant demographic, host, clinical, and environmental factors—in which the drug's use is being considered.

For example, in a non-immunologically compromised, healthy outpatient with a bacterial exacerbation of chronic obstructive pulmonary disease or a community-acquired pneumonia, azithromycin (Zithromax®), levofloxacin (Levaquin®), and trovafloxacin (Trovan®) are smart drugs, because they provide activity against the four principal pathogens—*Streptococcus pneumoniae, Hemophilus influenzae, Moraxella catarrhalis,* and mycoplasma—that are most often implicated in these outpatient infections involving the lung. On the other hand, in a community-acquired pulmonary infection occurring in a patient with AIDS, a drug such as trimethoprim-sulfamethoxazole may represent a smarter choice, because it is active against *Pneumocystis carinii* pneumonia (PCP), a common infectious complication of this disease. In general, selecting antibiotics according to their smartness reduces the risk of pharmacologically reservicing (i.e., retreating) patients and, therefore, represents a cost-effective approach to management of infectious diseases.

From a pharmatectural perspective, identifying smart, high productivity drugs plays a critical role in Total Pharmacotherapeutic Quality Management (TPQM™, see below), an approach designed to pharmacologically service patients with the *fewest* number of drugs at the lowest cost. To achieve this goal, smart drugs must be tailored to individual patient needs. Consider the following illustration: Imagine you are faced with the challenge of constructing a drug regimen for an individual who suffers from all of the following conditions simultaneously: migraine headaches, hereditary familial tremor, angina, and hypertension. Moreover, suppose this patient also requires secondary prevention of myocardial infarction. What would represent a "smart" drug for this particular patient? There are many possibilities and combinations, but, compared to other choices, a beta-blocker would be considered a smart drug because it has the potential capacity to treat all these conditions with a *single* prescription ingredient. In other words, each of the conditions afflicting this patient is potentially improved by a lipophilic beta-blocker such as propranolol. If one had *not* selected the smart drug approach to this patient, the physician might have prescribed sumatriptan for the migraine headache, a benzodiazepine to control the tremors, a calcium blocker for angina, an ACE inhibitor for the high blood pressure, and aspirin plus a beta-blocker to prevent secondary myocardial infarction.[76] This six-story "drug house" would probably incur greater cost, increase the risk of drug reactions and interactions, and, possibly, produce more quality-of-life impairment than the single agent construction. Although this is an exaggerated and very theoretical example, it does emphasize the need for identifying single medications with *multiple sites of action* and/or clinical effects, and, whenever possible, matching such drugs with the appropriate clinical profile.

Additional examples of smart drugs include ACE inhibitors, which have the capacity for simultaneously treating congestive heart failure, hypertension, and protecting the kidney in patients with diabetic renal disease.[47,77-81] Among cardiovascular agents, smart medications include calcium blockers that can offer symptomatic relief in angina and treat high blood pressure, and such peripheral alpha-blockers as doxazosin (Cardura®), which can reduce blood pressure, and provide symptomatic relief in patients with benign prostatic hypertrophy. When it comes to lipid management, the HMG-CoA reductase inhibitor atorvastatin (Lipitor®) is indicated both for reducing LDL cholesterol *and* treating elevated triglyceride levels. Among the psychotropics, heterocyclic antidepressants have the capacity to treat depression, and provide symptomatic relief in patients with diabetic neuropathy.

BUILDING MATERIALS: BETTER CHOICES, WORSE CHOICES

When it comes to designing buildings, architects bear the responsibility for identifying better and worse materials. Much like a physician trying to select the antiarrhythmic agent that is ideally suited for a patient's heart problem, architects are always faced with the challenge of choosing among many different material options for their projects. For example, maple is a hardwood and, therefore, is far better suited than softer woods such as mahogany or fir for the construction of bowling alley lanes or floors for a basketball court. Among the many materials available for a particular architectural purpose, there are superior and inferior choices depending upon functional needs, climate, durability, and safety considerations.

And so it is with pharmacologic options. *The fact is that all drugs within a drug class are not created equal.* There are better and worse choices, with some pharmacologic building blocks clearly offering advantages over others.[10,11] As a rule, physicians select medications according to cost, efficacy, safety, side effect profile, and their own clinical experience.[4,5,13,14,82] In this vein, the pharmatectural approach to outpatient drug construction stresses the importance of distinguishing among chemical agents (i.e., building materials) *within* a drug class, evaluating their similarities and differences, accounting for the nuances, comparing their relative smartness, and then selecting the medication best suited for a particular therapeutic objective in a specific patient subgroup.[17,27,83,84] For example, among the beta-blockers, lipophilic agents such as propranolol (Inderal®) have greater central nervous system (CNS) penetration than hydrophilic beta-blockers such as atenolol (Tenormin®) which, some studies show, may be associated with less fatigue, depression, somnolence, and sexual dysfunction. While atenolol may, in some cases, represent a better choice for the treatment of hypertension, angina, or prevention of myocardial infarction, propranolol is better-suited for the prophylaxis of migraine headaches because of its CNS penetration.

The necessity for distinguishing between better and worse pharmacologic options is especially important in geriatric patients,[20,85,86] in whom side effects, drug interactions, half-life of medications, and functional considerations play a critical role.[6,10,71,87] In the treatment of major depression in the elderly, for example, SSRIs appear to have some advantages over tricyclic antidepressants. Although identifying the best choices between and within drug classes is central to the pharmatectural approach, perhaps, even more important, is arriving at the proper *combination* of better drugs. Since many patients require treatment with multiple medications, the enlightened pharmatect not only selects the best agents *within* a drug class, but takes this process one step further and evaluates a drug's suitability for use in combination with other drugs. Many excellent drugs, for example, function well in *isolation* of other agents[83,90,91,92] but, when combined with other medications, can produce problems. The key is to identify better drugs that can be combined safely and effectively.[9,15,16,74,93]

This is especially true for cardiovascular drugs. For example, although verapamil may provide good blood pressure control with minimal side effects in some older patients, the addition of a beta-blocker to a regimen that includes verapamil may result in symptomatic bradycardia, AV node conduction disturbances, or clinically significant myocardial suppression in a significant minority of *susceptible* older individuals with underlying CHF or pre-existing conduction disturbances. Therefore, other calcium blockers (i.e., amlodipine, felodipine) may be preferable because they usually can be used safely in such patients in combination with other drugs.[69,94]

Similar considerations are important when prescribing antimicrobials. For example, although erythromycin and clarithromycin (Biaxin®) may produce excellent clinical results when used in isolation of other agents, they are more likely to be associated with certain drug interactions than azithromycin (Zithromax®), another antibiotic with similar antimicrobial activity.

As far as less-than-optimal drug combinations are concerned, one potential pitfall is the use of ACE inhibitors in elderly patients with hypertension (Figure 1-3). Although ACE inhibitors frequently are an excellent choice for many older hypertensive patients, it should be noted that many elderly individuals may be taking other agents (potassium-sparing diuretics or NSAIDs) that can interact with this class of antihypertensive. Most important among them, perhaps, are the nonsteroidal anti-inflammatory drugs (NSAIDs), commonly used for management of chronic arthritic conditions. NSAIDs decrease prostaglandin synthesis which, in turn, decreases aldosterone secretion causing a reduction in renal potassium excretion. When ACE inhibitors are added to NSAIDs, one may observe additive suppression of the renin-angiotensin-aldosterone axis, which can produce clinically significant elevations in serum potassium levels.

Figure 1-3 ACE Inhibitor – NSAID Drug Interactions

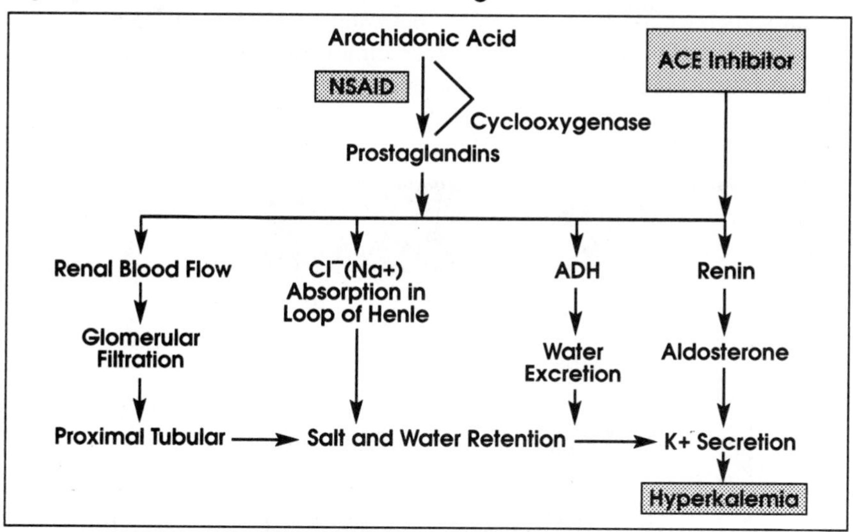

GUIDING PRINCIPLES

Less Is More

For many centuries, the world of architecture was dominated by buildings copiously robed with ornaments, figurines, and decorative embellishments in all shapes and sizes. A prestigious lineage of architectural works, from the Greek Parthenon to Italian Borromini Churches to the Gothic-inspired Woolworth Building in New York City, subscribed to this "more is better" philosophy. In the early 1930s, however, there was a precipitous rebellion against this kind of ornament-rich architecture, and the intellectual driving force behind the Bauhaus movement, Mies Van der Rohe, coined the expression "less is more." With this modernistic pronouncement came a generation of simpler, stylistically straightforward buildings, stripped bare to their essentials, in which function took precedence over frippery, fanciful forms, and figurative flourishes. This was a conceptual revolution that produced such clean, gleaming skyscrapers as the Seagram's Building, Rockefeller Center, and the Empire State Building. Less became more and, in the process, much more was accomplished with far less.

The pharmatectural approach to drug regimen design strongly supports this "less is more" philosophy. (Figure 1-4) When it comes to drug regimens, there oftentimes is beauty in *simplicity*. Pharmacologically speaking, the more that can be achieved using the fewest number of prescription ingredients, at the lowest clinically effective dose, and the lowest daily dose frequency, the better off the patient usually will be. Support for this position comes from many investigations, all of which confirm that the total number of different prescription drugs in a patient's regimen is the single most important determinant of drug interactions.[16,72,93,95] While using fewer drugs at their lowest effective dose is a virtuous goal, accomplishing this in clinical practice is far more problematic.

Figure 1-4

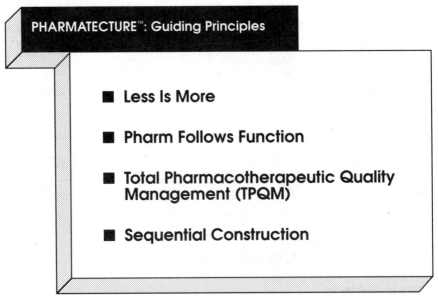

PHARMATECTURE™: Guiding Principles

- **Less Is More**
- **Pharm Follows Function**
- **Total Pharmacotherapeutic Quality Management (TPQM)**
- **Sequential Construction**

Polyphysicians

Achieving therapeutic goals with fewer drugs is especially difficult in older persons, in whom polypharmacy is the norm. Consequently, any approach to reducing pharmacological burden and making good on the "less is more" philosophy must address and moderate the forces that fuel excessive drug prescribing in this population. First, many older patients are afflicted with more than one chronic disease. This fact, coupled with the increased number of hospitalizations that multiple illnesses bring, makes the simultaneous administration of many different medications, frequently prescribed by *different* physicians, commonplace. In this regard, when it comes to excessive drug prescribing, it should be emphasized that the problem of more than one clinician managing the pharmacologic aspects of a patient's disease is at the root of much polypharmacy. In other words, "polyphysicians" are often the precursors to polypharmacy.

Pharmatecture For The Geriatric Patient

Elderly patients in emotional distress often seek medical attention under the pretense of having a physical illness. On occasion, physicians may fail to link the patient's perceived physical complaints with their emotional distress, and instead focus on finding a pharmacotherapeutic solution to address each symptom. Consequently, there is a tendency for physicians to consummate outpatient visits, especially from the elderly, with prescriptions for an analgesic, diuretic, hypnotic, or sedative—all because their underlying depression may have produced somatic complaints. Accordingly, fewer unnecessary medications will be introduced into a drug regimen if physicians can tame a well-documented compulsion to service vague symptoms of unclear etiology with pharmacologic therapy.[11,21,82,91]

Communication. Compounding the problems caused by somatic complaints is the difficulty elderly patients have with communication. Many elderly patients are intimidated by health care professionals and are uncomfortable communicating information about drug-related side effects or the cost of their medications. If physicians do not give patients enough time to express their concerns about drug therapy, create a comfortable climate in which patients can express themselves, and question their own attitudes about what the patient is saying, one or more prescriptions of *questionable* value and safety may be the result. Whenever physicians assess patients' progress from histories provided by caretakers, a special note of caution is necessary. Caretakers may feel frustrated or harrassed by elderly persons with dementia, and may attempt to pressure physicians to prescribe medications that will help restore their sense of control over such patients. The result may be the introduction of an unnecessary medication for symptomatic relief or a psychotropic medication that is potent enough to neutralize the patient.

Suboptimal Medication Patterns. There are other reasons that the "less is more" approach is difficult to implement in the elderly population. Besides the presence of multiple diseases, somatic complaints, and communication problems, the elderly also may receive an excessive number of drugs because of the way they take pharmaceuticals. Although compliance is a major obstacle in many patients, it is a particularly vexing problem in the elderly.[8,22,45,75,85,96] Many elderly patients suffer from diminished hearing, poor vision, and joint disease. These conditions may leave them unable to understand instructions regarding drug intake, make it difficult to swallow large tablets, read labels, and open container lids, especially if they are of the child-proof variety.

Older persons may have cultural attitudes that make taking certain drugs at odds with long-standing beliefs, and others cannot reach the pharmacist or physician because of a lack of transportation. As a result of these problems, a significant percentage of elderly patients do not take medications they need, and this leads to a poor clinical response. Unless noncompliance is recognized as a potential cause of such therapeutic failures, physicians may be prone to *increasing* dosages of *existing* drugs, or worse, prescribe additional medications.[8,97]

Side Effects. The large number of drugs consumed by many older persons, combined with their inability to tolerate the effects of many pharmaceuticals, increases their susceptibility to adverse drug reactions and toxicity.[36,60,64,77,98] This is especially true for gastrointestinal intolerance associated with NSAID use, for CNS depression with benzodiazepines, for anticholinergic effects of diphenhydramine, for the nocturnal cough associated with ACE inhibitors, the depression induced by beta-blockers,[99,100,101] and the somnolence caused by heterocyclic antidepressants. In some cases, physicians may not recognize new symptoms as being due to drug effects, especially if one or more of the problematic drugs was prescribed by *another* physician, or if it is an over-the-counter (OTC) agent.[73] As is the case with poor compliance, physicians may prescribe more drugs to treat the effects of *other* drugs whose side effects are *mistaken* for *disease*-mediated exacerbation of symptoms, rather than drug toxicity.

Appropriateness of Indications. Finally, many elderly patients come to physicians already taking medications that may have been prescribed years earlier *without* adequate indications. Occasionally, a drug may have been introduced into a regimen based on a faulty diagnosis. Unfortunately, the elderly tend to be creatures of habit, clinging to these medications like pharmacologic security blankets and refusing to have them eliminated from their drug lists—or even their dosages reduced—despite the clinical wisdom of such modifications.

There are, however, general principles that make it possible to achieve the pharmatectural objective of "less is more". This requires an emphasis on making *specific* diagnoses, obtaining a meticulous history of drug usage, understanding the pharmacology of drugs, simplifying therapeutic regimens, and identifying drug-induced symptoms. In the end, these approaches will be effective only if the primary drug prescriber communicates openly with consulting physicians who, after only a single encounter with the patient, may have prescribed a drug without a full understanding of the patient's overall clinical picture. Systematic application of these principles will produce less costly, safer, and more manageable drug regimens.

Building a Drug House: Sequential Construction

Architects understand that buildings must follow an ordered sequence of construction. First, the foundation is laid, then the house is framed, then windows are inserted, electrical and plumbing systems installed, and only then, is the finish work begun. The more complicated the house, the more painstaking and specific the sequence of adding these elements. The same is true for drug houses, which also must follow *sequential construction.* What this means is that there are many different options for treating patients and, in general, drug prescribing also should follow a sequential order. From a pharmatectural perspective, this means prescribing as drugs of first choice those agents shown to work most of the time at a reasonable cost while incurring minimal toxicity. Monotherapeutic agents with regimen durability and dose stability are recommended as initial choices, or "foundation" drugs. Only if these medications fail should the next tier of drugs be introduced into the drug regimen. This process continues with the progressive addition of more expensive or toxic medications until therapeutic results are achieved.

There are many diseases for which drug houses are frequently constructed in poor sequence. One common example is the premature use of theophylline for the management of asthma. Although theophylline can be used for the treatment of asthma, it is associated with more side effects and risk of toxicity than other therapeutic options, such as inhaled beta-agonists or inhaled steroids. In patients with mild, intermittent asthma, sequential pharmacologic construction might begin with a trial of an inhaled beta-agonist such as albuterol (Proventil®) on an as-needed basis. If the patient does not seem to be responding to the beta-agonist, the next step is to *teach* the patient once again how to use the inhaler appropriately. Studies show that many patients use inhalers like breath freshener spray or room deodorizers, and poor results may reflect inadequate medication (inhaler) use rather than the failure of the drug. If the patient is adequately instructed and *still* fails therapy, then inhaled steroids should be added as the primary bulwark of defense against exacerbations of acute bronchial asthma. If both inhaled steroids and beta-agonists fail to alleviate symptoms, sequential addition of oral prednisone therapy and/or leuktreine inhibitors can be considered. Sequential construction applies to most chronic diseases, such as congestive heart failure, in which ACE inhibitors are generally used before the addition of digoxin; in esophageal reflux disease, in which H_2-blockers are given a trial prior to using proton pump blockers; and adult onset diabetes mellitus, in which sulfonylureas are used before introduction of metformin or Rezulin.

Sequential construction is an important cost-saving and side effect-sparing maneuver that should be employed when building complicated drug houses in patients who seem to require increasingly intensive therapy to produce therapeutic results.

Pharmatectural Versus Therapeutic Substitution: Critical Real World Distinctions

In an era characterized by intense scrutiny of drug costs,[94,102,103] the concept of therapeutic substitution was introduced to permit pharmacy-based substitution of less expensive, but therapeutically equivalent, pharmacologic alternatives. In general, such substitutions are sanctioned only when bioequivalency is demonstrated between less and more expensive alternatives. (i.e., generic versus trade name drugs), or in the case of two different chemical compounds, when the two drugs are shown to produce virtually equivalent therapeutic results.

From a pharmatectural perspective, drug substitution is an extremely simplistic concept and, what is more worrisome, is associated with the risk of using drugs that *appear* to be interchangeable based on their chemical properties but, in fact, yield very different clinical outcomes in the "real world." To address the potential limitations of adherence to this concept, the pharmatectural perspective on therapeutic substitution accounts for a wide range of parameters—chemical, behavioral, financial, perceptual, toxicological—that influence therapeutic endpoints, and which must be considered when assessing the substitutability of one drug for another.

This approach, called "pharmatectural substitution," acknowledges that many different factors come into play when evaluating whether two drugs are actually substitutable for one another. Pharmatectural substitution stresses that, in the *real world* of pharmacotherapeutic management, one drug can replace another only if they overlap on *all* the following parameters:

- **Smartness.** To ensure equal performance in meeting clinical objectives, the drug being considered as a substitute must be as smart as the drug it will replace. In other words, it must have an equally comprehensive range of indications and provide the same degree of pharmacologic efficacy. For example, two statins may not be substitutable if one (atorvastatin) lowers cholesterol more than another (fluvastatin). Or, two macrolides may not be substitutable if one (azithromycin) provides coverage of *H. influenzae,* but the other (erythromycin) does not.
- **Daily dose frequency.** To ensure comparable compliance, the drug considered as a possible substitute should be dosed on the same daily basis, or *less frequently* than the drug being considered for replacement.
- **Side effect profile.** The drug considered as a possible substitute should have the same or a more advantageous side effect profile as the drug being considered for replacement. For example, diphenhydramine may cause more drowsiness and sedation than loratidine, and therefore, should not be considered substitutable.
- **Drug-drug compatibility.** The drug interaction profile of the drug being considered as a possible substitute should be the same or more desirable than for the drug being considered for replacement.
- **Drug-disease compatibility.** The drug-disease interaction profile of the drug being considered as a possible substitute should be the same or more desirable than for the drug being considered for replacement. One calcium blocker (amlodipine) may have demonstrated safety in patients with stage IV congestive heart failure, whereas other calcium blockers (diltiazem, verapamil) have not had this safety profile confirmed.
- **Cost.** Drugs evaluated for possible exchange must either cost the same, or the potential substitute must cost less than the drug being replaced.

Two drugs are considered candidates for pharmaceutical substitution only if they satisfy *all* the equivalency parameters as outlined above. The importance of satisfying all the aforementioned criteria is easily illustrated. For example, if I have drug A in one hand and drug B in another, and these two agents satisfy all the criteria mentioned, except drug A is dosed *three* times a day and drug B is dosed *once* a day, are these two medications pharmatecturally substitutable? The answer is "Not necessarily." Why? Because the drug dosed three times daily may be subject to compromised compliance, and therefore, may produce therapeutically less satisfactory results than the once-daily medication. If drug A and B are similar in every respect, except drug B produces inhibition of the p-450 cytochrome oxidase system and drug A does not, are these agents pharmatecturally equivalent? Again, the answer is "No," because drug B, especially in a patient with multiple medications has the potential to produce clinically significant drug interactions. If the two agents meet all the aforementioned parameters, but drug A is likely to cause conduction abnormalities in the heart, but drug B has no such liability, are these two agents pharmatecturally or, for that matter, therapeutically, equivalent? Once again, "Probably not," because one may produce exacerbation of an underlying cardiac condition while the other drug is likely free of such complications.

It should be stressed that pharmatectural substitution supports drug substitutions for the purpose of cost savings. But it attempts to ensure that two drugs have identical safety profiles, behave in the same way, and produce equivalent outcomes in actual clinical practice. The key to any drug substitution or comprehensive prescribing system is flexibility, something pharmatecture encourages.

Pharmacology Follows Function

The caveat that pharmacology should follow function, or more simply, "pharm follows function," plays a governing role in the pharmatectural approach to drug regimen design. This concept has broad implications for how pharmacists and physicians should think about building safe, cost-effective drug houses. In fact, from these three simple words issue a prescribing directive that occupies the intellectual nexus point of the entire pharmatecture system: Pharmacologic interventions, rather than simply being pegged to *diseases,* should serve the *functional objectives* and target goals of specific patients and address their unique constellation of conditions. Not surprisingly, virtually all pharmatectural principles either directly or indirectly flow from this caveat.

Many readers, of course, will recognize that this pharmatectural guidepost is inspired by the time-honored architectural mandate, "form follows function."[1] An understanding of how this concept changed the face of modern architecture will help illuminate the strategic importance of applying "pharm follows function" principles to the domain of clinical pharmacology.

Although function has always played an important role in architecture, for many centuries, the final form that buildings took was based as much on ornamental concerns as it was on functional needs. In the early 1900s, however, with the rise of modern architecture, these attitudes changed dramatically, and it was the Chicago architect, Louis Sullivan, who popularized the notion that "form follows function." What this meant, from a practical point of view, was that *functional* objectives now emerged as the major determinants of building design, and they became the primary generators of the final form a house or skyscraper would take. Under this scheme, buildings no longer would be constructed according to styles, the whims of fashion, or time-pegged preferences for one kind of ornamental flourish versus another. Instead, buildings would be shaped almost exclusively according to the functional needs programmed by the architectural work.

Tailoring Therapy. In a similar manner, functional needs and clinical objectives should also predominate in the design of *drug* houses. Extrapolation from numerous clinical trials suggests that the most cost-effective, therapeutically specific, and safest drug regimens are constructed around the principle that pharm follows function. This scheme represents a significant departure from the approaches that have governed prescribing practices in the past. For so long, most drug therapy has been symptom- or disease-oriented. In other words, the clinician identified a disease and then prescribed a drug for that condition. If another disease or symptom surfaced, another drug was added, and before long the patient would be taking several different agents, some of which might be redundant or, even worse, conflict with other drugs in the regimen or exacerbate underlying conditions.

Generally speaking, redundant, excessive, suboptimal, and costly drug houses are a byproduct of poorly integrated medication regimens that are built around disease states, rather than around functional needs and end-organ requirements. The reality is, diseases are characterized by a range of pathophysiological abnormalities, end-organ disturbances, metabolic alterations, and clinical derangements. Regardless of the disease, each patient has a *unique* cluster of these abnormalities, and pharmacologic therapy must follow, or service, the *mix* of symptoms and target organ needs that are specific to that individual.

In short, pharm must follow function. Until recently, this concept was very difficult to apply to clinical practice. Now, however, this approach is very feasible because we are able to characterize, quantify, and analyze many different parameters associated with a disease state, and then generate a composite picture of how these features affect the patient. This permits a better, more tailored fit between drug and patient. In fact, from a pharmatectural perspective, it no longer makes sense, and, therefore, it is not clinically useful to say, "This patient has 'hypertension,' or 'diabetes,' or 'heart disease,' " and then go on to match a drug with the appropriate condition. Sophisticated diagnostic techniques allow a broader and more in-depth characterization of clinical disorders, thus permitting drugs to be chosen that provide a more tailored fit to the patient's functional needs and clinical abnormalities. For example a diabetic with elevated triglycerides *and* LDL levels may be a good candidate for the HMG-CoA reductase inhibitor atorvastatin. Early, adult onset diabetes may be well-controlled with a sulfonylurea, whereas those diabetics with high insulin requirements may benefit from Rezulin. It follows that, because diseases express themselves in *different* ways in *different* individuals, the pharmacologically integrated approach to drug therapy recognizes that every patient with hypertension, depression, or arthritis, is different from all the other patients in a particular group, despite the fact they may carry the same disease label. Consequently, their pharmacologic needs also will be different. The key is to customize.

The Disease Kaleidoscope. The pharm follows function approach to medication prescribing addresses these patient variations and, in the process, suggests a different mechanism for constructing drug regimens. One analogy that is helpful for illustrating how pharm follows function applies to clinical pharmacotherapeutics, is to think of a disease as a kaleidoscope. In this kaleidoscope, the number, shape, and size of the colored glass shards and pieces remain constant. Now think of the colored fragments as different abnormalities associated with a particular disease, such as, say, high blood pressure. In this kaleidoscope of hypertension, imagine red represents renal function, yellow represents left ventricular mass, green represents lipid profile, purple represents cerebrovascular disease, etc. In addition, let's assume the more color a piece transmits, the greater the severity of the problem and vice versa. Now, depending how you turn the tube and how the components fall, they will create a different image, sometimes with one color (disease abnormality) or intensity (severity) predominating, and sometimes with others making a stronger showing.

In other words, each patient exhibits a different face of a particular disease state. In fact, there are as many faces as there are kaleidoscopic arrangements. Accordingly, one individual may have a little bit of this and a lot of that, and another may have a lot of this and little bit of that. For example, one patient with hypertension may have elevated cholesterol, mild kidney dysfunction, a history of a previous heart attack, diastolic hypertension, and diabetes. However, with a slight rotation in the kaleidoscope of hypertension, the colors rearrange themselves and we can see yet another patient—one with primarily systolic blood pressure elevation, no heart or renal problems, and an extremely favorable lipid profile. Drug therapy (the "pharm" component) must address the kaleidoscopic mix of objectives and functional goals. The first patient, for example, may benefit from a drug that is smart enough to prevent renal deterioration, reduce the risk of secondary myocardial infarction, and has a favorable effect on lipid levels, whereas the second patient will benefit most from a drug with established efficacy in *systolic* hypertension.

What this means is that, in a drug prescribing system in which pharm follows function, physicians no longer use drugs primarily to treat symptoms or diseases. They use drugs to treat individual patients! In other words, drug therapy is integrated—it is linked and targeted to the entire complex of issues requiring attention in a specific patient. As strange as this may seem, if you ask the practicing pharmatect what drug he or she would use to treat diabetes, depression, high blood pressure, pneumonia, or virtually any other disorder, he or she could not give you an answer. This is because pharmatects do not focus their attention on diseases, per se, but rather they direct their drug therapy at the kaleidoscopic *mix of disease-generated abnormalities and endpoints* as visualized in the *individual* patient.

This is a much different way of approaching drug therapy than has been traditionally practiced. The physician and pharmacist attuned to pharmatectural principles will tailor drug choices and combinations according to the unique mix of needs for a specific patient. To achieve this goal, physicians and pharmacists, in collaboration with patients, should list and prioritize the *entire constellation* of functional needs, metabolic abnormalities, pathophysiological derangements, symptom-relief objectives, and prevention goals pertaining to the patient's condition. This detailed list of functional and clinical end points will then generate a list of drugs that correct these abnormalities or achieve the target goals enumerated. If pharmatectural principles are applied, this regimen will feature either a single smart drug, or the fewest number of drugs best suited to pharmacologically service the patient's needs. If the diagnoses are accurate and the drugs are carefully prescribed with the patient's specific goals clearly in mind, pharmacology will inevitably follow function. The result will be a cost-effective, clinically targeted drug house in which pharmacologic redundancy is eliminated and clinical outcomes are optimized.

There are numerous clinical examples that testify to the wisdom of this approach. Consider, for example, the myriad therapeutic options available for the treatment of depression. The pharmacopiea includes heterocyclic antidepressants, MAO inhibitors, SSRIs, and other agents. How does one apply the "pharm follows function" concept to help choose among these options? The first step is to identify the functional objectives of the patient. For example, it should be recognized that some patients suffer from insomnia as a result of depression. In these patients, the functional objectives for pharmacologic intervention include not only alleviation of their depressive symptoms (feelings of sadness, crying spells, low self-esteem, etc.) but also management of sleep dysfunction. In this subset of patients, a sedating antidepressant such as trazodone (Desyrel®) taken at bedtime might be better suited to meet the patient's needs.

Similar examples illustrating the importance of linking pharmacology with function can be offered for diabetes, heart failure, and hypertension. For example, the patient who has insulin-dependent diabetes mellitus complicated by proteinuria, high blood pressure, and congestive heart failure will have these functional needs best managed by an ACE inhibitor. On the other hand, a diabetic with hypertension whose physical exertion is limited by angina pectoris precipitated by coronary artery can be serviced by a calcium channel blocker. And finally, the diabetic hypertensive with symptoms of benign prostatic hypertrophy might benefit from a peripheral alpha-blocker such as doxazosin. In every patient, regardless of the disease entity, the most cost-effective, integrated approach to drug therapy will emerge if pharm follows function and if other pharmatectural principles also are applied to the patient's overall therapeutic program.

Total Pharmacotherapeutic Quality Management (TPQM™)

A central aspect of pharmatecture is Total Quality Management (TQM). This is a quality-assurance, maintenance, and improvement process that has been incorporated into a number of disciplines under similar banners, including continuous quality improvement (CQI), continuous quality management, and other variations. From an architectural point of view, TQM is devoted to producing state-of-the-art buildings that combine the durable and visually pleasing materials into structures that meet the ever-expanding—and increasingly complex—range of human and technological needs that contemporary buildings must serve.

Much like the evolving relationship between building materials and architectural design, the relationship between drug therapy and disease states also is in a state of constant flux. In this regard, *new* indications for established drugs are constantly being approved, unexpected drug interactions are reported in post-marketing surveillance studies, and newer agents with less toxicity and expanded indications continually are being introduced. In addition, chronic diseases present an ever-expanding list of associated abnormalities that are either amenable to drug therapy, or, on occasion, even exacerbated by medications once thought to represent drugs of choice.

In the world of pharmatecture, Total Pharmacotherapeutic Quality Management TPQM™ (See Figure 1-5) plays a central role in ensuring that drug regimens and medication choices are periodically reviewed by the physician or pharmacist. Specifically, regimens should be evaluated and reviewed on a regular basis to ensure that: (1) they have kept pace with newer drugs, developments, and therapeutic options as they surface in the pharmaceutical marketplace; (2) they continue to provide the full range of pharmacologic servicing required by the patient; and (3) they still represent the most cost-effective, compliance-enhancing approach to drug therapy for the patient's clinical needs.

Quality Choices. The power of TPQM as an assessment and quality assurance tool is best explained using an historical example. For example, consider a disease such as hypertension which, it is estimated, afflicts as many as 50 million Americans. When it comes to drug therapy, this is just one of many common diseases that has witnessed dramatic changes over the past 20 years. More information is available than ever before to guide clinicians in managing this important public health problem. Unfortunately, this increase in information has made the pharmacotherapeutic choices increasingly complex.

In fact, most of the advances in drug therapy for hypertension can be explained simply by analyzing the shifting emphasis on various clinical aspects and functional end points of this disease. This is where TPQM plays a valuable role in drug therapy. The usefulness of TPQM in building and maintaining state-of-the-art drug houses for common diseases such as hypertension is best illustrated by taking a journey in Jules Verne's time machine. Imagine, for a moment, that we travel back to the year 1980 and find ourselves transported to a doctor's office in St. Louis, Missouri. There, we encounter a family physician who has just recorded an elevated blood pressure reading in a patient and, therefore, is faced

Figure 1-5

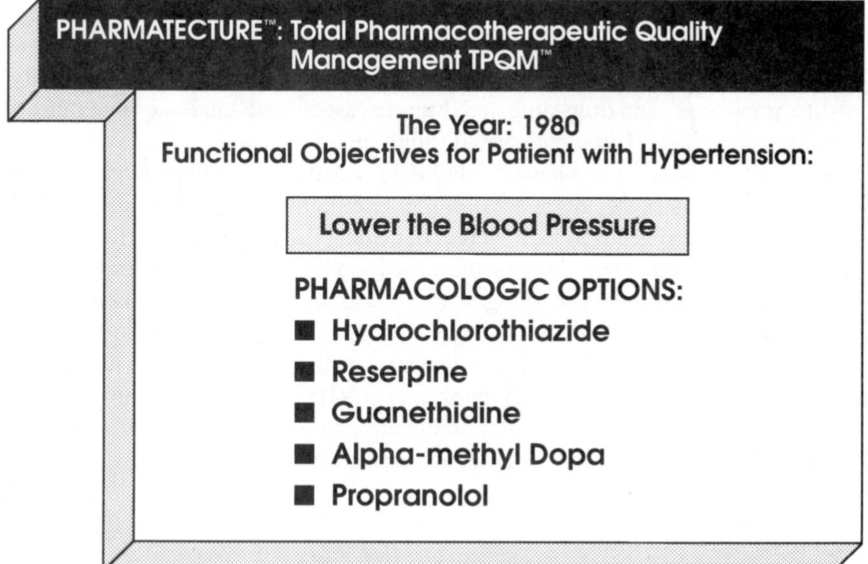

with initiating drug therapy. (Figure 1-5) Let's assume for a moment that the physician is interested in providing TPQM for this patient. To meet this goal, the clinician will ask the following question: "What functional objective(s) am I trying to achieve in this patient?".

Remember, this is 1980! The functional goals for treatment of high blood pressure were limited then. What's more, the full range of therapeutic, functional, preventive, and drug-disease interaction concerns was poorly characterized at this time. In fact, there was only one well-accepted end point in 1980—to lower the diastolic blood pressure to reduce the risk of stroke. In other words, in 1980, applying TPQM in a patient with high blood pressure, required little more than the selection of a drug that would reduce diastolic blood pressure to less than 90 mm Hg. For all practical purposes, this was the primary therapeutic goal physicians had during this era.

Consequently, to achieve TPQM almost two decades ago, physicians felt relatively comfortable selecting from a smorgasbord of medications (reserpine, guanethidine, hydralazine, propranolol, alpha-methyldopa, etc.) to accomplish this end point. These drugs successfully lowered diastolic blood pressure, but they also had the potential to produce a wide range of undesirable side effects, quality-of-life impairments, and drug-disease interactions that, history would eventually show, patients would prefer to live without. Unfortunately, many patients stopped taking their medication. In fact, one can argue that the side effects associated with these agents oftentimes exceeded the discomfort of hypertension, thus producing an epidemic of noncompliance-induced disease deterioration among Americans with hypertension.

Now let's step back in the time machine and journey to the year 2000. We are transported to an ambulatory care clinic, this time in Portland, Oregon. Here, we encounter a consulting pharmacist and physician discussing options for implementing TPQM in a 70-year old man with newly diagnosed high blood pressure. Things are much different now. In the year 2000, when these clinicians ask the same question posed by the family practitioner 20 years ago, "What functional end points are we trying to achieve in a patient with hypertension?" something different happens. A new TPQM readout appears (Figure 1-6) There emerges an expanded constellation of target-organ needs, physiological end points, quality-of-life, preventive, and drug-drug and drug-disease interaction issues that must be considered for TPQM in a patient with high blood pressure.

In other words, to implement TPQM in a patient with hypertension in the year 2000, means satisfying *many different* end points. As in 1980, the diastolic blood pressure still needs to be lowered, but studies also demonstrate that caution should be exercised in not lowering diastolic blood pressure too low, especially in frail, older persons with underlying heart disease. In addition, new classifications stress the importance of managing *systolic* as well as diastolic blood pressure elevations. In addition, TPQM for patients with high blood pressure means recognizing that left ventricular hypertrophy (LVH) is an independent risk factor for morbidity in these patients. Consequently, in persons with this co-morbid finding, drugs proven to reduce LVH are preferred.

Figure 1-6

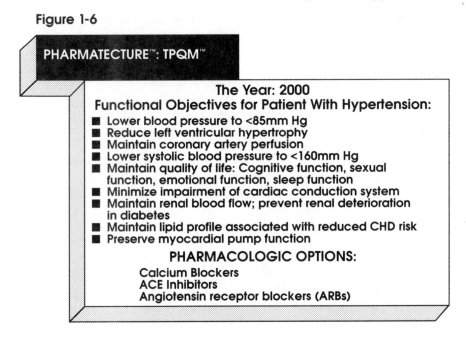

PHARMATECTURE™: TPQM™

The Year: 2000

Functional Objectives for Patient With Hypertension:

- Lower blood pressure to <85mm Hg
- Reduce left ventricular hypertrophy
- Maintain coronary artery perfusion
- Lower systolic blood pressure to <160mm Hg
- Maintain quality of life: Cognitive function, sexual function, emotional function, sleep function
- Minimize impairment of cardiac conduction system
- Maintain renal blood flow; prevent renal deterioration in diabetes
- Maintain lipid profile associated with reduced CHD risk
- Preserve myocardial pump function

PHARMACOLOGIC OPTIONS:

Calcium Blockers
ACE Inhibitors
Angiotensin receptor blockers (ARBs)

In addition, drug therapy for high blood pressure also must take into account other medical conditions. Abnormalities associated with overlapping disease states—ranging from high blood pressure and heart disease to diabetes, kidney disease, and hyperlipidemia—have produced new goals in antihypertensive drug therapy. For example, approximately 40% of patients over the age of 70 who have hypertension also have significant coronary atherosclerosis. Some of these patients may even have coronary artery lesions significant enough to produce silent myocardial ischemia. Hence, the use of antihypertensive agents that can maintain coronary artery perfusion, reduce the risk of recurrent MI, and manage angina should be encouraged, particularly in patients with hypertension and underlying coronary heart disease.[104-109]

Other hypertensive patients, especially those with diabetes, a previous history of myocardial infarction, and/or congestive heart failure, benefit from ACE inhibitors, which improve outcomes in patients with poor heart function. Still other hypertensive patients have conduction system abnormalities, i.e., they are prone to slow heart rates or disturbances in AV node conduction. Hence, prevention-oriented TPQM would include avoiding drugs that are known to impair impulse conduction in the heart. Finally, about 45% of all hypertensive patients have clinically significant elevations in blood lipid levels. When blood cholesterol levels are elevated or HDL/LDL ratios are low, drugs known to maintain neutral lipid profiles and, therefore, reduce coronary heart disease (CHD) risk, are preferable to drug combinations (beta-blocker and thiazide diuretic) that elevate lipid levels.

Although it seems routine now, in 1980, physicians and pharmacists infrequently invoked quality-of-life (maintenance and enhancement) issues as essential functional criteria against which to measure the success of their antihypertensive regimens. New attitudes that argue for inclusion of quality-of-life issues in drug therapy are supported by large-scale investigations.[106,110,111,112,113] Clinical trials in recent years confirmed that drugs used for the treatment of high blood pressure can impair many cognitive, sexual, and neuropsychiatric parameters.[111,114,115] In the 1990s, quality-of-life maintenance became such a popular cause that pharmacists and physicians became increasingly aware of the importance of including these issues as part of the value-added equation for drug therapy of all kinds. As a result, TPQM for the patient with high blood pressure now means prescribing drugs that meet a number of requirements and drawing upon a different set of pharmacologic options. It means identifying those agents best able to service the *full* set of patient needs—physiological, pharmacological, and functional.

This kind of analysis can be applied to many different outpatient conditions. Regardless of the disease, however, one thing is clear. Periodic reviews of drug regimens that stress TPQM will produce better-tolerated drug combinations that incorporate both prevention and outcome-effectiveness into the therapeutic program.

Foundations of a Drug Regimen

In the world of building construction, it is well-accepted that a house or skyscraper is only as good as its *foundation*. It is difficult to expand, remodel, or reconstruct a house with a poor foundation. And so it is with drug regimens. In fact, much of the unnecessary—and, more importantly, avoidable—expenditures fueling drug costs result from the constant reshuffling (adding and subtracting) in polypharmacy drug regimens that is required to keep pharmacologic harmony among different agents. This is called the *pharmacologic "churn factor."* Pharmacologic churning not only incurs direct costs associated with drug discontinuation and initiation, but from adverse drug-related events that produce costly hospitalizations.[36,39,101,116] Most often, these problems arise when pharmacists or physicians initiate long-term drug therapy without considering whether the agent is a good foundation drug, in other words: (a) whether or not it will tend to be *compatible* with the other drugs or diseases that may come into the picture over time, [Please refer to Chapter 3, the Drug-Drug and Drug-Disease Incompatibility Profile (DIP™) System.]; and (b) whether or not the drug maintains its therapeutic efficacy over the long haul.

One of the best criterion for identifying a foundation drug is the "TE Index," or the Toleration-Efficacy Index. The two principal reasons a medication will *fail* to achieve its intended therapeutic goal is: (a) poor toleration, leading to drug discontinuation or poor compliance; and (b) poor efficacy related to suboptimal potency or other intrinsic pharmacological deficiencies. Drugs that have a high TE Index, i.e., that combine confirmation of long-term patient toleration *and* maintenance of potency are well-suited to be foundation drugs.

Figure 1-7

PHARMATECTURE™: Foundation of a Drug Regimen

- **Toleration-Efficacy Index: Durability**
- **Minimal Drug-Drug Incompatibilities**
- **Minimal Drug-Disease Incompatibilities**

Accordingly, the pharmatectural approach to designing drug regimens stresses the importance of identifying and selecting *centerpiece* drugs as initial therapeutic agents. Centerpiece agents, or foundation drugs (Figure 1-7), should be initiated *early* in the natural history of a chronic disease. These medications are characterized as foundation drugs because they are hospitable to the addition of a wide range of prescription ingredients without incurring drug interactions, and because they can be used safely in the setting of complications or comorbid conditions that may arise as a result of—or that frequently accompany—the primary disease. Centerpiece drugs also will have an excellent Toleration-Efficacy Index, thereby minimizing the risk of polypharmacy. The Drug Incompatibility Profile (DIP) system discussed in Chapter 3 provides a practical approach for making drug selections based on some of these principles.

From a pharmatectural perspective, then, the use of foundation drugs represents an important step in safe outcome-effective drug selection. As mentioned, much of the cost associated with long-term drug therapy results from the shuffling of therapeutic agents in order to prevent drug interactions, and from adding medications to poorly performing medications. Consequently, one of the most important aspects of constructing safe, cost-effective, long-term drug regimens is selecting agents on a *proactive* basis. Medications with a low-risk for producing drug-drug or drug-disease interactions and documented long-term efficacy, can serve as a foundation for drug regimens to which additions, alterations, and deletions can be made over time without adversely affecting emerging conditions.

Framework and Safety Considerations

An architectural framework is constructed based on time-honored engineering principles to which the architectural skeleton must adhere. The same is true for pharmatectural constructions, in which compliance, comfort, quality-of-life, and cost-effectiveness constitute important rafters in the framework of all drug regimens. (Figure 1-8) All drug regimens must be designed with this framework in mind.

All works of architecture must pass a *safety inspection.* For example, building codes mandate that electrical, heating and cooling, pollution control, and plumbing systems meet basic standards to ensure safety for human use. Safety is an equally important pharmatectural issue. Many safety considerations (drug interactions, side effect profiles, polypharmacy, etc.) have already been discussed. But at the root of all safe drug prescribing is the mandate for selecting drugs that have low toxicity and then using these drugs at the lowest effective therapeutic dose. These safety considerations, along with compliance, comfort, quality-of-life, and cost-efficacy constitute the full pharmatectural framework for drug regimen construction.

Prevention First

Pharmatecture also stresses the importance of prevention-oriented pharmacology. When indicated, such medications as aspirin, beta-blockers, statins, ACE inhibitors, Vitamin E, and folic acid should be considered for disease prevention. This proactive approach to disease management has the potential to reduce premature onset of acquired conditions—or delay end organ deterioration (renal dysfunction in diabetes, pump failure in heart disease)—and promote significant savings in drug therapy.

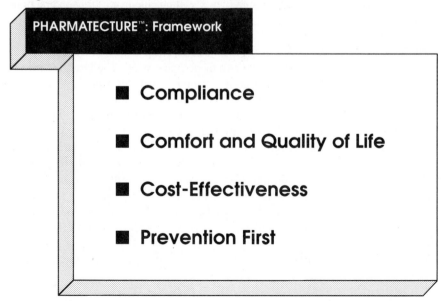

Figure 1-8

- **Compliance**
- **Comfort and Quality of Life**
- **Cost-Effectiveness**
- **Prevention First**

Styles of Pharmatecture

A New York skyline, with its variegated collection of skyscrapers, serves as a vivid testimonial to a wide range of architectural styles. In fact, there may be almost as many styles as there are architects. In the world of drug prescribing, there are also *stylistic* differences in the way pharmacists and physicians select and combine medications. These variations have important therapeutic and policy implications. In fact, the wide range of prescribing styles suggests there is no universally accepted system for designing safe, intelligent, and cost-effective drug regimens. It also emphasizes that physicians have failed to reach a consensus on what the principal goals should be in drug prescribing, and which factors (cost, smartness, side effects, convenience, etc.) are most important.

It is staggering to observe just how different drug prescribing styles are. For example, in most of the symposia on drug prescribing that I have conducted, I present physicians and pharmacists in attendance with a patient case study, and ask them to design what they feel is an appropriate drug regimen. It is remarkable how many different drug houses are constructed for the same patient! Some physicians may build their drug regimen using four prescription drugs, whereas another may prescribe only two drugs. Perhaps, this is the "art" of drug prescribing. No matter what you call it, and regardless of how tenaciously we may cling to our particular style of drug prescribing, there frequently are better—and worse—approaches to drug regimen design. Although a consensus on drug prescribing is difficult to build, we need to move away from traditional drug prescribing approaches toward more contemporary strategies, i.e., those that emphasize simpler, integrated drug regimens that are constructed with an eye towards prevention, enhancing compliance, and minimizing drug interactions.

Kitsch Pharmatecture

The world of architecture is replete with numerous examples of wacky, bombastic, or otherworldly building designs, many of which fall into the category of "Roadside Americana." Architectural critics have dubbed these works, "kitsch architecture," to highlight the fact that they are whimsical, vernacular works. And usually, they are designed by non-architects who defy most of the fundamental principles of good design.

Unfortunately, pharmacists and physicians acknowledge that there is also "Kitsch Pharmatecture." (Figure 1-9) Kitsch pharmatecture refers to those drug additions, deletions, and alterations made by the *patient,* without pharmacist or physician collaboration.

Kitsch pharmatecture can take many different forms. In this regard, OTC drugs may be added to the regimen, medications are exchanged, dosing schedules are altered, and a work of kitsch pharmatecture is created. For example, a patient taking an anti-Parkinsonism drug with anticholinergic properties may go to the pharmacy and purchase diphenhydramine (Benadryl®) for self-treatment of allergy symptoms. The anticholinergic properties from the two drugs in combination may be enough to produce urinary retention. Another patient may be

Figure 1-9

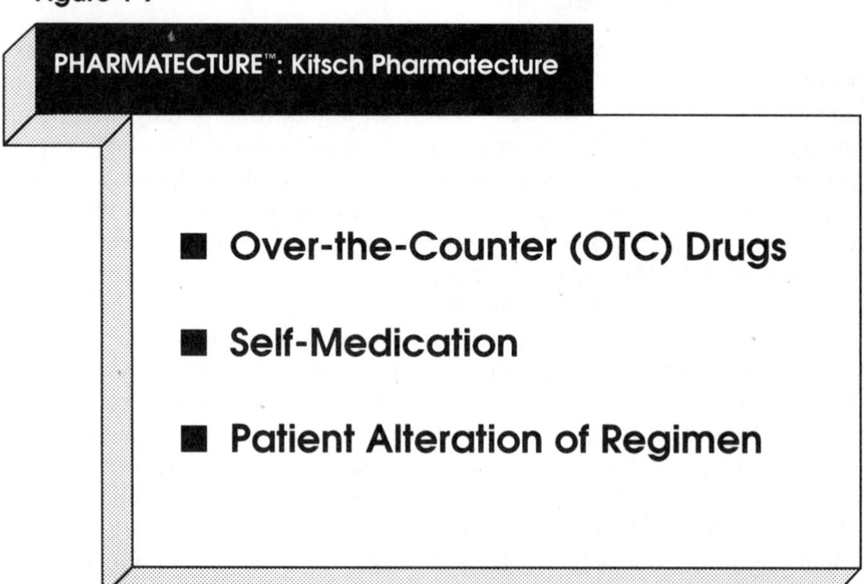

prescribed an NSAID such as nabumetone (Relafen®), and then purchase OTC ibuprofen, failing to understand that the two drugs in combination may produce additive gastrointestinal side effects.

The widespread prevalence of kitsch pharmatecture emphasizes the importance of obtaining comprehensive drug histories from patients. These histories must be meticulous and make a special effort to identify OTC agents that may interfere with the established drug house constructed by the practitioner. Kitsch pharmatecture will become an increasing problem as more prescription agents gain approval for OTC distribution.

Remodeling

Great old buildings frequently don't stand the test of time, unless they have been remodeled to address current needs and stylistic preferences. The same is true for drug houses. The aim of the pharmatecture program is to critically evaluate drug regimens and then, based on good clinical trials, *desconstruct* and *reconstruct* the drug house so it makes use of smart, safe drugs that service all the functional objectives of a particular patient. This deconstruction and reconstruction must be gradual, and is discussed in more detail in the following chapters.

[1]Jordan LK 3d, Jordan LO. Prudent prescribing. Prescribing suggestions for physicians. NC Med J 1992 Nov; 53(11):585-8.

[2]Parrish RH. Understanding physician prescribing behavior. Am J Hosp Pharm 1991 March; 48(3):463.

[3]Reus VI. Rational polypharmacy in the treatment of mood disorders. Ann Clin Psychiatry 1993 June; 5(2):91-100.

[4]Burns LR, Denton M, Goldfein S, Warrick L, Morenz B, Sales B. The use of continuous quality improvement methods in the development and dissemination of medical practice guidelines. QRB 1992 Dec; 18(12):434-9.

[5]Chinburapa V, Larson LN. The importance of side effects and outcomes in differentiating between prescription drug products. J Clin Pharm Ther 1992 Dec; 17(6):333-42.

[6]Kahl A, Blandford DH, Krueger K, Zwick DI. Geriatric education centers address medication issues affecting older adults. Public Health Reports - Hyattsville 1992 Jan-Feb; 107(1):37-47.

[7]Lamy, PP. Adverse drug effects. Clin Geriatr Med 1990; 6:293-305.

[8]Lexchin J. Why are we still poisoning the elderly so often? Canadian Family Physician 1993 Nov; 39:2298-300, 2304-7.

[9]Peck CC, Temple RJ, Collins JM. Drug interactions: The death pen. JAMA 1993 Sept 15; 270(11):1317.

[10]Beers MH, Fingold SF, Ouslander JG, Ruben DB, Morgenstern H, Beck JC. Characteristics and quality of prescribing by doctors practicing in nursing homes. J Am Geriatr Soc 1993 Aug; 41(8);802-7.

[11]Beers MH, Ouslander JG, Fingold SF, Morgenstern H, Ruben DB, Rogers W, Zeffren MJ, Beck JC. Inappropriate medication prescribing in skilled-nursing facilities. Ann Intern Med 1992 Oct 15; 117(8):684-9.

[12]Belitsos NJ. Overprescribing of benzodiazepine hypnotic drugs in the elderly [letter; comment]. Am J Med 1991 Sept; 91(3):321.

[13]Bjornson DC, Rector TS, Daniels CE, Wertheimer AI, Snowdon DA, Litman TJ. Impact of drug-use review program intervention of prescribing after publication of a randomized clinical trial. Am J Hosp Pharm 1990 July; 47(7):1541-6.

[14]Bliss MR. Prescribing for the elderly. BMJ 1981; 282:203-6.

[15]LeSage J. Polypharmacy in geriatric patients. Nurs Clin North Am 1991 June; 26(2):273-90.

[16]Peck CC, Temple R, Collins JM. Understanding consequences of concurrent therapies. JAMA 1993 March 24; 269(12):1550-52.

[17]Thomas DR. "The brown bag" and other approaches to decreasing polypharmacy in the elderly. NC Med J 1991 Nov; 52(11):565-6.

[18]Ungvarski P, Schmidt J. Polypharmacy: dangers of multiple-drug therapy in patients with immunodeficiency virus infection. Home Healthcare Nurse 1993 March-April; 11(2):68-69.

[19]Valentine C. Use computers to detect inappropriate prescription. BMJ 1993 July 3; 307(6895):61.

[20]Bloom JA, Frank JW, Shafir MS, Martiquet P. Potentially undesirable prescribing and drug use among the elderly. Measurable and remediable. Canadian Family Physician 1993 Nov; 39:2337-45.

[21]Brahams D. Benzodiazepine overprescribing: successful initiative in New York State. Lancet 1990 Dec 1; 336(8727):1372-3.

[22]Weintraub M. Compliance in the elderly. Clin Geriatr Med 1990; 6:445-52.

[23]Roth HP, Caron HS. Accuracy of doctor's estimates and patients' statements on adherence to a drug regimen. Clin Pharmacol Ther 1978; 23;361-70.

[24]Oates LN, Scholz MJ, Hoffert MJ. Polypharmacy in a headache center population. Headache 1993 Sept; 33(8):436-8.

[25]Olfson M, Pincus HA, Sabshin M. Pharmacotherapy in outpatient psychiatric practice. Am J Psychiatry 1994 April; 151(4):580-5.

[26]Ashburn PE. Polypharmacy in skilled-nursing facilities. Ann Intern Med 1993 April 15; 118(8):649-50; discussion 650-1.

[27]Collins TM, Zimmerman DR. Programs for monitoring inappropriate prescribing of controlled drugs; evaluation and recommendations. Am J Hosp Pharm 1992 July; 49(7):1765-8.

[28]Beardon PH, McGilchrist MM, McKendrick AD, McDevitt DG, MacDonald TM. Primary noncompliance with prescribed medication in primary care. BMJ 1993 Oct; 307(6908):846-8.

[29]Berg JS, Dischler J, Wagner DJ, Raia JJ, Palmer-Shevlin N. Medication compliance; a healthcare problem. Ann Pharmacother 1993 Sept; 27(9 Suppl):S1-24.

[30]Botelho RJ, Dudrak R. 2d. Home assessment of adherence to long-term medication in the elderly. J Fam Prac 1992 July; 35(1):61-5.

[31]Eisen SA, Miller DK, Woodward RS, Spitznagel E, Przybeck TR. The effect of prescribed daily dose frequency on patient medication compliance. Arch Intern Med 1990 Sept; 150(9):1881-4.

[32]Jones JK. Assessing potential risk of drugs: The elusive target. Ann Intern Med 1992 Oct 15; 117(8):691-692.

[33]Litchman HM. Medication noncompliance: a significant problem and possible strategies. Rhode Island Medicine 1993 Dec; 76(12):608-10.

[34]Lamy PP. A "risk" approach to adverse drug reactions. J Am Geriatr Soc 1988; 36:79.

[35]Larson EB. et al. Adverse drug reactions associated with global cognitive impairment in elderly persons. Ann Intern Med 1987; 107:169-173.

[36]Col N, Franale JE, Kronholm P. The role of medication and adverse drug reactions in hospitalizations of the elderly. Arch Intern Med 1990 April; 150(4):841-5.

[37]Futrell DP. Drug compliance, Are you getting the most out of your medicine? NC Med J 1993 Oct; 54(10):523-4.

[38]Hood JC, Murphy JE. Patient noncompliance can lead to hospital readmissions. Hospitals 1978; 52:79-82, 84.

[39]McNally DL, Wertheimer D. Strategies to reduce the high cost of patient noncompliance. Md Med J 1992 March; 41(3):223-5.

[40]Steiner JF, Robbins LJ, Roth SC, Hammond WS. The effect of prescription size on acquisition of maintenance medications. J Gen Intern Med 1993 June; 8(6):306-10.

[41]Stewart RB, Caranasos GJ. Medication compliance in the elderly. Med Clin North America 1989; 73:1551-1563.

[42]Sclar DA, Chin A, Skaer TL, Okamoto MP, Nakahiro RK, Gill MA. Effect of health education in promoting prescription refill compliance among patients with hypertension. Clin Ther 1991 July-August; 13(4):489-95.

[43]Deyo RA, Inui TS, Sullivan B. Noncompliance with arthritis drugs: magnitude, correlates, and clinical implications. J Rheumatol 1981; 8:931-36.

[44]Conn VS, Taylor SG, Kelley S. Medication regimen complexity and adherence among older adults. Journal of Nursing Scholarship 1991 Winter; 23(4):231-5.

[45]Lamy PP. Compliance in long-term care. Geriatrika 1985; 1(8):32.

[46]Cochrane RA, Mandal AR, Ledger-Scott M, Walker R. Changes in drug treatment after discharge from hospital in geriatric patients. BMJ 1992 Sept 19; 305(6855):694-6.

[47]Anonymous. Prescription drugs and older consumers issued August 10, 1990. Michigan-Medicine 1991 Feb; 90(2):27-31.

[48]Anonymous. Writing prescription instructions. Can Med Assoc J 1991 March 15; 144(6):647-8.

[49]Coleman TJ. Non-redemption of prescriptions. Linked to poor consultation. BMJ 1994 Jan 8; 308(6921):135.

[50]Ito S, Koren G, Einarson TR. Maternal noncompliance with antibiotics during breastfeeding. Ann of Pharmacother 1993 Jan; 27(1):40-2.

[51]Park DC, Morrell RW, Frieske D, Kincaid D. Medication adherence behaviors in older adults; effects of external cognitive supports. Psychology & Aging 1992 June; 7(2):252-6.

[52]Knight JR, Campbell AJ, Williams SM, Clark DW. Knowledgeable noncompliance with prescribed drugs in elderly subjects—a study with particular reference to nonsteroidal antiinflammatory and antidepressant drugs. J Clin Pharm Ther 1991 April; 16(2):131-7.

[53]Macdonald ET, Macdonald JB, Phoenix M. Improving drug compliance after hospital discharge. BMJ 1977: 2:618-621.

[54]Phillips SL, Carr-Lopez SM. Impact of a pharmacist on medication discontinuation in a hospital-based geriatric clinic. Am J Hosp Pharm 1990 May; 47(5):1075-9.

[55]Green LW, Purrell CO, Koop CE, et al. Programs to reduce drug errors in the elderly: direct and indirect evidence from patient education. Improving Medication Compliance, Reston, Va: National Pharm Council, 1985.

[56]Kucukarslan S, Hakim Z, Sullivan D, Taylor S, Grauer D, Haugtvedt C, Zgarrick D. Points to consider about prescription drug prices: an overview of federal policy and pricing studies. Clin Ther 1993 July-Aug; 15(4):726-38.

[57]Skaer TL, Sclar DA, Markowski DJ, Won JK. Effect of value-added utilities on prescription refill compliance and Medicaid health care expenditures—a study of patients with non-insulin dependent diabetes mellitus. J Clin Pharm Ther 1993 Aug; 18(4):295-9.

[58]Jordan LK. 3d., Jordan LO. Prudent prescribing. Prescribing suggestions for physicians. NC Med J 1992 Nov; 53(11):585-8.

[59]Keen PJ. What is the best dosage schedule for patients? J R Soc Med 1991 Nov; 84(11):640-1.

[60]Granek E, et al. Medications and diagnosis in relation to falls in a long-term care facility. J Am Geriatric Soc 1987; 35:505.

[61]Cormack MA, Howells E. Factors linked to the prescribing of benzodiazepines by general practice principals and trainees. Fam Pract 1992 Dec; 9(4):466-71.

[62]Hamilton IJ, Reay LM, Sullivan FM. A survey of general practitioners' attitudes to benzodiazepine overprescribing. Health Bulletin 1990 Nov; 48(6):299-303.

[63]Bauman JH. Kimelblatt BJ. Cimetidine as an inhibitor of drug metabolism: therapeutic implications and review of the literature. Drug Intell Clin Pharm 1982; 16:380.

[64]Greenblatt DJ, Shader RI. Anticholinergics. N Engl J Med 1984; 288(23):1215-1218.

[65]Nesbit F. Noncompliance with psychotropic drug prescriptions. Am J Psychiatry 1994 May; 152(5):783-4.

[66]Halpern MT, Irwin DE, Brown RE, Clouse J, Hatziandreu EJ. Patient adherence to prescribed potassium supplement therapy. Clin Ther 1993 Nov-Dec; 15(6):1133-45; discussion 1120.

[67]Held P. Effects of beta-blockers on ventricular dysfunction after myocardial infarction: tolerability and survival effects. Am J Cardiol 1993 March 25; 71(9):39C-44C.

[68]Johnston D, Duffin D. Drug-patient interactions and their relevance in the treatment of heart failure. Am J Cardiol 1992 Oct 8; 70(10):109C-112C.

[69]Hussar DA. New drugs of 1993. Am Pharm 1994 March; NS34(3):24-47, 51-6; quiz 57-9.

[70]Huszonek JJ, Dewan MJ, Koss M, Hardoby WJ, Ispahani A. Antidepressant side effects and physician prescribing patterns Ann Clin Psychiatry 1993 March ; 5(1):7-11.

[71]Inman W, Pearce G. Prescriber profile and post-marketing surveillance. Lancet 1993 Sept 11; 342(8872):658-61.

[72]Colley CA, Lucas LM. Polypharmacy: the cure becomes the disease. Gen Intern Med 1993 May; 8(5):278-83.

[73]Holden MD. Over-the-counter medications: Do you know what your patients are taking? Postgrad Med 1992 June; 91(8):191-194, 199-200.

[74]Kroenke K, Pinholt EM. Reducing polypharmacy in the elderly. A controlled trial of physician feedback. J Am Geriatr Soc 1990 Jan; 38(1):31-6.

[75]Montamat SC, Cusak B. Overcoming problems with polypharmacy and drug misuse in the elderly. Clin Geriatr Med 1992 Feb; 8(1):143-58.

[76]Frishman WH. Beta-adrenergic blockers as cardioprotective agents. Am J Cardiol 1992 Dec 21; 70(21):21-61.

[77]Downs GE, Linkewich JA, DiPalma JR. Drug interactions in elderly diabetics. Geriatrics 1986; 36(7):45.

[78]Hood, WB, Jr. Role of converting enzyme inhibitors in the treatment of heart failure. J Am Coll Cardiol 1993 Oct; 22(4 Suppl a):154A-157A..

[79]Khosla S, Somberg J. Mild heart failure: why the switch to ACE inhibitors? Geriatrics 1993 Nov; 48(11):47-8, 51-4.

[80]Pfeffer M. Angiotensin converting enzyme inhibition in congestive heart failure: benefit and perspective. Am Heart J 1993 Sept; 126(3 Pt 2):789-93.

[81]Richard C, Thuillez C, Depret J, Auzepy P, Giudicelli JF. Regional hemodynamic effects of perindopril in congestive heart failure. Am Heart J 1993 Sept; 126(3 Pt 2):782-8.

[82]Chinburapa V, Larson LN, Brucks M, Draugalis J, Bootman JL, Puto CP. Physician prescribing decisions: the effects of situational involvement and task complexity on information acquisition and decision making. Soc Sci Med 1993 June; 36(11):1473-82.

[83]De Santis G, Harvey KJ, Howard D, Mashford ML, Moulds RF. Improving the quality of antibiotic prescription patterns in general practice. The role of educational intervention. Med Aust 1994 April 18; 160(8):502-5.

[84]Reveilleau S, Boissel JP, Alamercery Y. Do prescribers know the results of key clinical trials? GEP (Groupe d'etude do la Prescription). Fundam Clin Pharacol 1991; 5(4):265-73.

[85]Davidson W, Molloy DW, Somers G, Bedard M. Relation between physician characteristics and prescribing for elderly people in New Brunswick. Can Med Assoc J 1994 March 15; 150(6):917-21.

[86]Holt WS Jr., Mazzuca SA. Prescribing behaviors of family physicians in the treatment of osteoarthritis. Fam Med 1992 Sept-Oct; 24(7):524-7.

[87]Hux JE, Levinton CM, Naylor CD. Prescribing propensity; influence of life-expectancy gains and drug costs. J Gen Inter Med 1994 April; 9(4):195-201.

[88]Mant A, Saunders NA. Polypharmacy in the elderly. Med J Aust 1990 June 4; 152(11):613.

[89]Stewart RB, Yedinak KC, Ware MR. Polypharmacy in psychiatry: three case studies and methods for prevention. Ann Pharmacother 1992 April; 26(4):529-33.

[90]American college of Physicians Improving medical education in therapeutics. Ann Intern Med 1988; 108:145-147.

[91]Greenblat RM, Hollander H, McMaster JR, Henke CJ. Polypharmacy among patients attending an AIDS clinic: utilization of prescribed, unorthodox, and investigational treatments. J Acquir Immune Defic Syndr 1991; 4(2):136-43.

[92]Meyer TJ, Van Kooten D, Marsh S, Prochazka AV. Reduction of polypharmacy by feedback to clinicians. J Gen Intern Med 1991 March-April: 6(2):133-6.

[93]Lisi DM. Reducing polypharmacy. J Am Geriatr Society 1991 Jan; 39(1):103-5.

[94]Abernathy DR, Andrawis NS. Critical drug interactions: A guide to important examples. Drug Ther 1993; Cot 15-27.

[95]Safavi KT, Hayward RA. Choosing between apples and apples: physicians' choices of prescription drugs that have similar side effects and efficacies. Gen Intern Med 1992 Jan-Feb; 7(1):32-7.

[96]Nolan L, O'Malley K. Prescribing for the elderly. Part II. Prescribing patterns: differences due to age. J Am Geriatr Soc 1988; 36:245-254.

[97]Poulsen RL. Some current factors influencing the prescribing and use of psychiatric drugs. Public Health Reports - Hyattsville 1992 Jan-Feb; 107(1):47-53.

[98]Gilley J. Towards rational prescribing. BMJ 1994 March 19; 308(6931):731-2.

[99]Medications for the elderly. A report of the Royal College of Physicians. J R Coll of Physicians 1984; 18:7-17.

[100]Montamat SC, Cusak BJ, Vestal RE. Management of drug therapy in the elderly. N Engl J Med 1989; 321:303-309.

[101]Pickles H, Fuller S. Prescriptions, adverse reactions, and the elderly. Lancet 1986; 2(8497):40.

[102]Berger MS. A proposal for using generics. Pa Med 1993 May; 96(5)10.

[103]Ellmers SE. Limiting the drugs list. The trouble with generic prescribing. BMJ 1993 June 19; 306(6893):1687.

[104]Ben-Ishay D, Leibel B, Stessman J. Calcium channel blockers in the management of hypertension in the elderly. Am J Med 1986; (81 Suppl 6a)81:30-34.

[105]Abernethy DR, Schwartz JB, Plachetka JR, et al. Comparison in young and elderly patients of pharmacodynamics and disposition of labetalol in systemic hypertension. Am J Cardiol 1987; 60:697-702.

[106]Ahronheim J. Practical pharmacology for older patients; avoiding adverse drug effects. Mt Sinai J Med 1993 Nov; 60(6):497-501.

[107]Amery A, et al. Mortality and morbidity results from the European working party on high blood pressure in the elderly. Lancet 1985; 1:1349-1354.

[108]Amir M, Cristal N, Bar-On D, Loidl A. Does the combination of ACE inhibitor and calcium antagonist control hypertension and improve quality of life? The LOMIR-MCT-IL study experience. Blood Pressure 1994; Suppl 1:40-2.

[109]Ancill RJ, Carlyle WW, Liang RA, Holliday SG. Agitation in the demented elderly: a role for the benzodiazepines?. Int Clin Psychopharmacol 1991 Winter; 6(3):141-6.

[110]Baxter JD. Minimizing the side effects of glucocorticoid therapy. [Review] Adv Intern Med 1990; 35:173-93.

[111]Bulpitt CJ, Fletcher AE. Drug treatment and quality of life in the elderly. [Review] Clin Geriatr Med 1990 May; 6(2):309-17.

[112]Coons SJ, Kaplan RM. Assessing health-related quality of life: application to drug therapy. Clin Ther 1992; 14(6):850-8; discussion 849.

[113]deBoer JB, van Dan FS, Sprangers MA, Frissen PH, Lange JM. Longitudinal study on the Quality of Life of symptomatic HIV-infected patients in a trial of zidovudine versus zidovudine and interferon-alpha. AIDS 1993 July; 7(7):947-53.

[114]Dimenas E, Wallander MA, Svardsudd K, Wiklund I. Aspects of quality of life on treatment with felodipine. Euro J Clin Pharmacol 1991; 40(2):141-7.

[115]Fletcher AE, Battersby C, Adnitt P, Underwood N, Jurgensen HJ, Bulpitt CJ. Quality of life on antihypertensive therapy: a double-blind trial comparing quality of life on pinacidil and nifedipine in combination with a thiazide diuretic. European Pinacidil Study Group. J Cardiovas Pharmaco 1992 July; 20(1):108-14.

[116]Gibaldi M. Prescription drugs and health care reform. Pharmacotherapy 1993 Nov-Dec; 13(6):583-9.

2

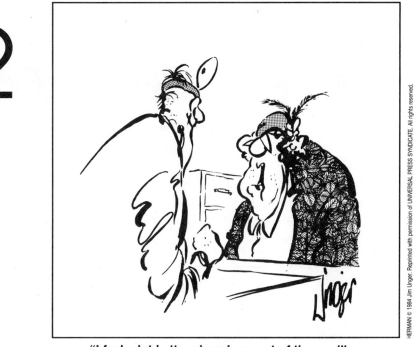

"I feel a lot better since I ran out of those pills you gave me."

Construction of Drug Regimens: Pharmatectural Principles Put Into Practice

The blueprint for drug regimen construction is now in place. The preceding chapter presented, the broad brush strokes for a hands-on approach to designing, building, and maintaining drug regimens. Pitfalls associated with inappropriate drug prescribing were highlighted and general approaches to remodeling regimens were introduced. The purpose of this chapter is more specific—to generate working drawings, that is, to outline specific strategies and drug selection techniques that will optimize therapeutic outcomes and produce more cost-effective drug regimens. While these pharmatectural principles and concepts can be applied to the construction of virtually all outpatient regimens, there are certain patients and specific clinical situations for which this system is especially applicable. (See Figure 2-1) These include individuals treated with polypharmacy regimens, those at high risk for noncompliance[1] and drug-related adverse patient events;[2] the elderly;[3] individuals with conditions and risk factors known to benefit from *prevention*-oriented pharmacotherapeutics; patients on chronic drug therapy;[4] persons prone to excessive or poorly monitored over-the-counter (OTC) drug intake; and those suffering from multiple medical conditions.

Figure 2-1

Patient Candidates For Pharmatectural Intervention
• Patients on polypharmacy • Patients receiving drugs from multiple sources (polyphysicians) • Patients at risk for medication noncompliance • The elderly • Regimens employing drugs with multiple daily dose frequency • Poorly monitored drug intake • Patients at risk for over-the-counter (OTC) drug intake • Regimens with drugs known to produce drug-drug and drug-disease interactions

Many different issues influence the effectiveness, compliance, and tolerability of a drug regimen. As a result, the pharmatectural approach, with its emphasis on the multiple factors that shape drug intake and affect therapeutic results, will almost always pay some therapeutic dividends when designing long-term drug regimens. But the most dramatic impact of this system will be seen in patients who are living in excessive, inappropriate, cost-ineffective, and compliance-compromising pharmacological environments. Consequently, recognizing those patients who will benefit from drug reduction, elimination, simplification, and consolidation (DRESC™ program: Please see Chapter 7) is a critical first step before remodeling of therapeutic regimens can begin.

One of the main purposes of this chapter is to help physicians identify those patients who will benefit most from the system. Strategies are presented for recognizing inferior drug houses, i.e., those pharmacologic environments compromised by drug "rot" (poor drug selection) and poor construction methods (suboptimal regimen design). In addition, approaches to building durable, prevention-oriented drug houses are presented. A step-by-step approach to sequential drug construction is outlined. Because the elderly are at high risk for drug-related complications and excessive pharmacologic burden, troubleshooting pharmacologic environments in this population is emphasized. Finally, medications most likely to cause drug-related side effects are highlighted and approaches to minimizing their toxicity are discussed in detail.

PUTTING PHARMATECTURE TO WORK

Principles Into Practice. Regardless of the patient or pharmacologic dilemma, putting pharmatecture into practice is a challenging—and usually—a therapeutically rewarding process for both patient and prescriber. Moreover, the opportunities are plentiful in this system for creative problem-solving. Pharmatecture, after all, is driven by a patient-specific approach to regimen design, and therefore it promotes flexibility in drug selection and innovative solutions. When pharmatectural intervention is indicated, however, the step-by-step process of pharmacologic assessment, drug selection, and regimen remodeling always should be conducted in a logical and systematic manner.

The pharmatectural process usually begins with a comprehensive review of the patient's current drug regimen. Because effectiveness of drug therapy is influenced by a variety of factors, the medication list is analyzed from several perspectives (See Figure 2-2). For example, special functional needs, prevention-oriented issues, and compliance problems are identified. This is followed by a pharmacologic evaluation of efficacy, cost, risk for drug interactions, potential side effects, and quality-of-life issues. The prescriber should also assess the impact that these medications may have on concomitant disease states. After this information is gathered, the process of sequential deconstruction and reconstruction of the drug regimen begins. Once started, remodeling is always undertaken with special regard for compliance enhancement, cost control, and with an eye towards drug reduction, elimination, simplification and consolidation (DRESC Program; See Chapter 7).

Figure 2-2

Systematic Analysis of Drug House Construction

- Functional needs of patient
- Does pharm follow function?
- Prevention-oriented drug therapy
- Medication compliance survey
- Drug interaction profile
- Side effect profile
- Cost control
- Quality of life maintenance

Sequential Construction: A Three-Phase Process. Pharmatectural modifications are most effectively accomplished within the framework of a *three-step* remodeling process. Whether designing a new drug house or reconstructing an existing regimen, the pharmacist or physician can expect to be building inspector, architect, and general contractor. These roles correspond to three distinct functions—inspection, design, and construction—that comprise a step-by-step approach to sequential drug house reconstruction (See Figure 2-3). Detailed discussions that address drug selection techniques, possible side effects, preventive pharmacology, and design approaches for each phase of pharmatectural reconstruction are presented later in this chapter. Before these specifics are introduced, however, it is helpful to have a rough working sketch of the process that will guide the prescribing practitioner.

Figure 2-3

Sequential Drug House Construction	
Phase I:	Inspection of Drug Regimen
Phase II:	Design Review
Phase III:	Construction or Remodeling

Phase I: Drug Regimen Inspection. A meticulous and comprehensive inspection of the existing drug regimen, combined with an assessment of its suitability for the patient's unique constellation of clinical disorders and behavioral patterns, is a prerequisite to pharmatectural reconstruction. As part of the initial drug regimen evaluation phase, the pharmatect will assume the responsibilities of a building *inspector*. For all practical purposes, this inspection phase is a fact-finding mission that sets the stage for subsequent modifications of the drug regimen. Poor drug choices, unnecessary complexity in the regimen's construction,[5,6] pharmacologic redundancy, compliance-compromising features,[1,7-9] omission of prevention-oriented building blocks, and drug-induced side effects related to the drug regimen are identified. Information suggesting possible noncompliance with medications is carefully reviewed, including detection of subtherapeutic serum drug levels, abnormal clinical parameters (elevated blood pressure, cholesterol levels, and/or blood sugar), and patient admission of erratic drug consumption. Dosage form, preferences, and special administration requirements also should be documented. The patient's existing drug house is examined to ensure that basic safety codes are being met. A review of all the patient's known medications is conducted to confirm that drug dosages, schedules, and interaction profiles are within acceptable guidelines.[10-12]

During this phase, indications for drug use are reconfirmed and potential drug and disease incompatibilities are identified. Comprehensive reference sources, such as *Drug Facts and Comparisons,* should be consulted to help make these evaluations. The inspection phase requires time, patience, and understanding on the part of the physician and pharmacist. A careful history is taken from the patient, and the regimen is screened for possible drug-induced, quality-of-life impairments that might render an agent unsafe to the patient's physical, psychological, sexual, or cognitive health.[13,14,15,16,17,18] An accurate count of pharmacologic building blocks is conducted, noting the number of different active ingredients as well as the total daily pill count. Vigilant and aggressive questioning may be required to determine the full range and patterns of drug intake. If the drug house is comprised of more than *five* pharmacologic building blocks, a polypharmacy warning is issued. When the pharmacologic burden is in this range, the environment is considered to be at very high risk for safety code violations, and options for eliminating excessive building materials should be considered.[19-23]

As building inspector, the physician examines the drug house not only from the perspective of safety, but reviews all aspects of the construction to determine whether sufficient attention was given to patient education and preventive pharmacology.[24] Clearly, polypharmacy increases the likelihood that safety violations (e.g., unneccesary medications, drug interactions, etc.) will be uncovered, and, in turn, opportunities should be explored for reducing drug intake while maintaining therapeutic objectives.[25-28] But the regimen must also be evaluated for the possible *omission* of *prevention-oriented* pharmacologic building blocks that might improve long-term clinical outcomes and reduce the need for further pharmacotherapy. If the patient has risk factors for heart disease, for example, have medications such as statins, beta-blockers, aspirin, and nutritional supplements been considered? The omission of prevention-oriented medication[29-31] is considered to be a flagrant safety violation.[32-36] Other building code violations such as the use of ineffective medications, excessive use of drugs dosed multiple times daily, failure to step-down drug dose for chronic conditions (hypertension, arthritis, asthma, etc.), regimen complexity, duplication of active ingredients, and lack of adequate patient education are also noted.[14] Once identified, possible solutions, alterations, and recommendations are listed that can correct these problems and that will satisfy drug house safety codes.

Phase II: Drug Regimen Design. Once inspection of the drug house is completed and potential problems are identified, strategies for regimen reconstruction are developed. During the second phase of sequential reconstruction, the clinician assumes the role of architect. Findings gleaned from the inspection phase are reviewed, and an overall design plan for the drug house is generated. This scheme incorporates a number of specifications: the total number of different drugs, specific pharmacologic ingredients, advantageous drug combinations, and other features. At this point in the process, the physician or pharmacist weighs the advantages and disadvantages of specific medications and combinations of drugs. Accordingly, decisions are made to *eliminate* specific pharmacologic building blocks and/or to add others. Inevitably, empirical data and value judgements about the desirability of one agent over another will come into play. A careful, comparative assessment of possible side effects is made so that the most user-friendly building materials within each drug class can be incorporated into the pharmacologic environment.

Naturally, drug houses are not constructed in an economic vacuum. Consideration is always given to how much the patient, pharmacy, or institution can afford to spend.[5,37-42] Whenever possible, an attempt is made to consolidate therapy with smart drugs that can perform several functions (i.e., symptom-relief and/or target organ salvage) simultaneously with fewer agents and, therefore, will reduce pharmacologic burden and total drug cost. During this design phase, an overall scheme for the final pharmacologic environment is generated. This includes detailed working drawings that reflect: (a) Reduction in the total number of different drugs that comprise the drug house; (b) a prioritization of preferred agents based on side effect profiles; (c) a plan for preventive pharmacotherapy; and (d) safety of specific drug combinations.

Phase III: Construction of Drug Regimen. During the third phase, the design is translated into a pharmacologic environment. To achieve this goal, the physician and pharmacist play the roles of general contractors. In other words, the design plans are put into practice and the nuts and bolts of constructing a new pharmacologic environment can proceed in earnest. It should be stressed that the process of altering a drug house requires patience. Several visits with the patient are usually required. Patient education, delivery of accurate information, and reassurance are important at this stage. Substitutions, deletions, and consolidations are made incrementally, usually one drug change or substitution per 12-week period, with progress evaluations conducted at 4-week intervals. In the case of progressive, acute, or high-risk conditions, modifications in the regimen may have to be made more rapidly. The step-by-step approach to deconstructing and reconstructing drug regimens (DRESC™ Program) is presented in Chapter 7.

Pharmatecture™: Design and Structure

It should be stressed that when it comes to pharmatectural remodeling, not all drug houses need to be gutted. Some constructions are basically solid and require only minor, cosmetic changes or minimal structural modifications. Not surprisingly, however, patients who live in drug houses that are intrinsically *unstable* are likely to benefit most from the application of this drug prescribing system. As might be expected, primary candidates for a pharmatecture-based approach to drug regimen design include the elderly, patients with chronic diseases on multiple medications, and those individuals on long-term drug therapy in whom quality-of-life and economic issues are of major concern.[16,17,43,44] Pharmatectural approaches to drug prescribing also are especially useful in patients prone to medication noncompliance. Because establishing medication compliance is fundamental to the stability of any drug house, this problem plays a special role in the pharmatecture system and deserves special discussion.

Because pharmatecture promotes medication compliance through simplification, it is essential to identify patients with behavioral, pharmacologic, economic, or therapeutic requirements known to place them at high risk for suboptimal drug intake. These individuals will usually benefit from remodeling approaches. Although pharmatecture can be instrumental in improving therapeutic outcomes in these patients, the full benefits of the system will not be achieved unless the pharmacist or physician also can ensure *adherence* to the drug regimen.

To maximize the usefulness of this prescribing system, it is important to address these issues and to identify specific applications, concerns, and candidates suitable for pharmatecture-based interventions. A number of risk factors, clinical profiles, and therapeutic pitfalls are highlighted below.

Unstable Foundations. The long-term stability and cost-effectiveness of a drug house depends on maintenance of medication compliance. In an era when efficacious drug therapies exist or are being developed at a rapid rate, it is discouraging that one half of patients for whom appropriate medications are prescribed fail to receive full benefit as a result of inadequate adherence to treatment. From a pharmatectural point of view, noncompliance is like having "drug rot," i.e., a house full of termites that are slowly but perceptibly eroding the structural integrity of the construction.

The morbidity and cost of pharmacologically servicing patients who get sicker because of noncompliance-mediated therapeutic failure is staggering. It is now estimated that 125,000 deaths annually can be attributed to noncompliance. This includes individuals with treatable diseases who either fail to take[5,6,53,54] their medications properly, or fail to take them at all. Thousands more are hospitalized or placed in nursing homes, while others are not well enough to work or enjoy recreational activities, simply because of suboptimal compliance patterns with prescribed medications. Overall, the health care system spends $11 billion annually to mop up poor outcomes associated with suboptimal drug intake.[55,56,57]

In fact, the consequences of medication noncompliance have reached epidemic proportions. Many reviews, involving hundreds of methodologically sound studies, have emphasized the magnitude and pervasiveness of this problem. Some have called medication noncompliance the invisible epidemic.[1,45-47] A report in the *National Council of Patient Information & Education* estimates that 1.8 billion prescription medications dispensed annually are not taken correctly. According to these estimates, only one-third of patients take all their prescribed medications, another third take some fraction of their prescription, and the final third do not take *any* of their prescribed drugs.[48-50] Other organizations have corroborated these findings. For example, the National Pharmaceutical Council reports that up to 90% of all outpatients make an error in their drug intake. Add to this the 21% of all patients who (according to a survey by the American Association of Retired Persons) never get their prescription filled. In summary, noncompliance is arguably one of the most important factors undermining clinical outcomes associated with long-term drug therapy.[24,51,52]

Designing For Compliance. From a pharmatectural perspective, ensuring medication compliance is a necessary, but not sufficient, condition for maximizing effectiveness and cost-efficacy of any drug regimen. In this regard, the most important factors influencing medication compliance include: (a) daily dose frequency, (b) cost of the medication, (c) side-effects, and (d) patient education. Depending on the patient, each of these factors will play a *more or less* important role in maintaining medication compliance. The pharmatectural approach to the problem of medication noncompliance is relatively straightforward. For each patient, the pharmacist or physician should attempt to prioritize which factors represent the most *significant* deterrents to drug intake, and then modify those features *first* to improve patient compliance. These patient-specific alterations should be made with the understanding that daily dose frequency is the most important factor influencing drug compliance. Consequently, whenever possible, once-daily medications are preferred building blocks for most drug house foundations[58,59] (See Figure 2-4).

This goal notwithstanding, there are unique considerations that come into play for specific patient groups.[8,46,52,60] Maximizing compliance requires striking the appropriate balance between economic and other aspects of drug therapy. For example, in the case of an indigent or elderly patient on a fixed income, drug acquisition cost may, but will not always, be more important than adverse side effects or dose frequency in determining long-term adherence to a drug regi-

Figure 2-4

Designing For Compliance	
• Once Daily Medications	• Patient Motivation
• Cost Suitable For Patient	• Medication Monitoring
• Written Instructions	• Livability of Drug House
• Pill Bottle Labeling	• Communication

men.[5,57,61] Consequently, the emphasis for selecting pharmacologic building blocks in this subgroup should be on using drugs of *lower cost.* On the other hand, in the case of an affluent individual for whom medication cost is *not* the principal determinant of drug access, other factors are more important. In these individuals, quietly festering side effects, subtle mood alterations, and the inconvenience associated with multiple daily dose frequency are more likely to stand in the way of long-term medication compliance. Consequently, agents that provide value-added benefits in these areas are preferred in these patients.

Just how important cost factors are in determining medication compliance is a fiercely debated issue. Clearly, though, cost is a factor, but the effect of cost on noncompliance will *vary* from patient to patient. When barriers to drug intake are primarily economic, cost should take precedence in drug selection, but when cost factors are *not* the principal concern, the focus should be on drug smartness, convenience, quality-of-life maintenance, and preventive pharmacology. Optimizing selection of pharmacologic building blocks means identifying which drug-related feature—cost, comfort, convenience, dose frequency, possible side effects—is most likely to impair compliance, and then choosing the medication that, based on this prioritization, is the least likely to compromise drug intake. When cost factors are not a concern, maximal compliance is achieved with once-daily preparations that have excellent side effect profiles.[19]

Foundation Maintenance. As far as medication compliance, patient-specific drug selection is only part of the picture. Designing foundations associated with good compliance also depends on a number of more general educational and surveillance factors that are independent of the specific pharmacologic agents chosen. For example, the physician or pharmacist may choose an excellent drug with minimal side effects, but the patient may fail to comply because he or she is unclear of its intended purpose, effectiveness, or potential pitfalls.[52,62,67] Regardless of which drugs are selected, certain strategies are useful in preventing and treating noncompliance, and pharmatecture advocates their implementation. For example, to be effective in maintaining consistent medication intake, particularly in those who have chronic illnesses, the pharmacist or physician must function as teacher, motivator, and persuader. As a teacher, the clinician must use communication skills that ensure the patient understands and can recall the drug-related information that is conveyed. To motivate the patient, the physician should employ strategies designed to attract the patient's attention so that the patient listens to instructions about drug therapy. Finally, even if the patient is motivated to listen to the physician's or pharmacist's message, and even if the message is understood and remembered, the patient will not act on it unless he or she accepts its importance to the therapeutic program.

The pharmacist and physician must also be good persuaders. Specific oral and written communication strategies have been developed that physicians and pharmacists can use to improve medication compliance.[63-65] The purpose of these strategies is to break down barriers to noncompliance. When dealing with multiple drug regimens, physicians can reduce the risk of noncompliance by requesting that, not only the name, but also the purpose of each drug be placed on the prescription container. Labeling of this kind reduces chances for error, especially those errors that are made when there are prescriptions from more than one physician or when prescriptions are filled by many different pharmacists. Careful labeling, of course, requires that the physician be willing to take the time to write the purpose of each drug on the prescription and that the pharmacist be willing to talk to the physician if the instructions are not clear to the patient. Such labeling should be simple, direct, and in terminology easily understood by all patients, regardless of age or educational level; for example, "digoxin—heart pill"; "ampicillin—antibiotic for infection"; and "hydrochlorothiazide—water pill."

Additional benefits accrue from *simplifying* the drug regimen. Physicians and pharmacists should examine each regimen and make sure it is the safest, simplest, and most effective therapy available. An effort should be made to titrate medications against treatment response to determine the *smallest* amount of medication required to achieve therapeutic goals. When it is not feasible to simplify a complex regimen, pharmacists may use a patient profile system to question patients about drug use and to determine whether drugs are being refilled promptly.[9] The format of patient profiles can range from file cards to computer-based systems that are available and represent the optimal approach to compliance monitoring. Prescriptions in such computer systems are filed by name as well as number. The system requirements vary, but the basic components involve a brief history of the patient to determine health status, diagnoses, current drug regimen (including both prescription and nonprescription drugs), dates of drug refills, drug allergies, health insurance coverage, and the names and specialties of physicians writing prescriptions for the patient. By maintaining patient profiles, the pharmacist can also proactively guard against drug-drug and drug-disease interactions that can adversely affect therapeutic results.[66]

When prescribed for long durations, even regimens consisting primarily of once-daily drugs with excellent side effect profiles are prone to noncompliance. Two strategies have been shown to be helpful in this situation. First, the physician or pharmacist may monitor for continued compliance by arranging for the patient to make periodic visits and by performing pill counts. Secondly, the physican can periodically assess the patient's status, carefully review the treatment regimen, and discuss the specifics of the treatment plan at each visit. This kind of meticulous review may also uncover medications with dosages that can be tapered, or other agents that are candidates for discontinuation or reevaluation.

A Failure To Communicate. As already mentioned, patient knowledge about their clinical condition and drug regimens influences compliance. Put simply, patients must both have information and understand recommendations to comply with their drug regimen. This is especially true in the elderly. A considerable amount of noncompliance is involuntary and caused by a disparity between patient and provider understanding. Common errors in medication instruction include the following: (1) prescribing but not discussing medications with the patient, (2) lack of information regarding regimen duration, and (3) incomplete and infrequent written instructions. One study demonstrated that among patients who had a poor understanding of their regimen, only 17% complied with physicians' instructions. By contrast, 60% of patients with accurate information cooperated.[57]

Patients already on long-term therapy, especially the elderly, have a tendency not to communicate problems, side effects, or even financial concerns associated with medication intake. These individuals may perceive, sometimes with good reason, that the pharmacist or physician does not have the time to answer specific questions regarding the drug regimen. As a result, side effects associated with drug intake may get overlooked. In addition, it should be stressed that many older patients matured in an era during which a limited number of therapeutic agents were available for many common medical conditions. These individuals may not realize that a wide variety of therapeutic options are now available as alternatives to the initial medication selected by their pharmacist or physician.

When these perceptions govern attitudes toward drug therapy, individuals may respond very stoically to their regimen, accepting drug-associated side effects as unavoidable. They may be reluctant to question the necessity for their existing medications. Some patients may even fear that if they stop their current medications, there will be few options remaining for therapeutic intervention. Unless told otherwise, patients may even think that drugs dosed many times daily are more effective than medications dosed less frequently. These attitudes can make it difficult for many patients to accept and cooperate with attempts at pharmatectural reconstruction. The elderly, in particular, are known to cling persistently to long-standing drug regimens, viewing them as essential to their survival.

Enhancing medication compliance is part of the pharmatectural approach to drug therapy. In addition to specific manipulations that can be made at the pharmacotherapeutic level (e.g., optimizing drug selections, daily dose frequency alterations, simplification, consolidation, and shortening duration), attention should also be paid to modification of social networks, patient education, and supervision.[8,52,56,57,62] Patient adherence to drug regimens improves with more frequent and direct communication. Specifically, compliance increases when frequency of outpatient visits is increased, home visits are added, patients receive negative feedback about noncompliance, a medication monitor is used, and continuity of care is provided.

Accordingly, pharmacists and physicians should provide each patient with information regarding the risks and benefits of proposed medications. Information about adverse drug effects and the efficacy of proposed treatment should be stressed by the physician and pharmacist. Written instructions should be provided. Eventually, computer-based work stations will facilitate the communication of accurate drug-related information between pharmacist and physician.[67,68]

Intelligent Noncompliance. Although pharmatecture stresses the importance of medication compliance, it also recognizes the necessity for *intelligent noncompliance.* In other words, patients should be encouraged to report and act on side effects that appear to be serious enough to warrant discontinuation or dosage reduction of a drug. Patient-activated drug cessation, however, should *always be communicated* to the physician or pharmacist, without fear of penalty or chastisement; it is important to facilitate communication during the patient encounter. A relationship must be established, usually during the inspection phase, that is conducive to obtaining accurate feedback about the livability of a patient's drug house. Pharmacists and physicians should stress that, in the event the first drug prescribed produces undesirable side effects, other equally effective and, perhaps, more user-friendly agents are available. When necessary, intelligent noncompliance should be used as an option of last resort. Flexibility is the key to pharmatectural adjustments. Channels of communication must remain open between pharmacist, physician, and patient, and the opportunity to answer questions regarding medication intake and side effects should be part of every pharmacist- and physician-patient encounter.

BUILDING INSPECTIONS

Detecting Faulty Constructions And Drug House Safety Checks

A comprehensive and detailed inspection of a patient's drug regimen is a critical component of the pharmatectural process. The purpose of this inspection, which is a prelude to reconstruction, is multifold: (a) to detect "cracks" in the pharmacologic foundation of the drug house (i.e., to identify possible *omission* of drugs that are indicated for disease prevention); (b) to assess the livability of the environment from the patient's perspective (i.e., to evaluate quality-of-life, convenience, and possible side effects); (c) to reconfirm original indications for drug use; (d) to analyze existing pharmacologic building blocks to ensure they still represent good choices for the patient's clinical condition; and (e) to determine whether better, smarter drugs are now available that produce superior results.

Because many issues must be evaluated, the inspection process is multidisciplinary in nature. It includes not only a review of the the regimen itself, but an evaluation of compliance with the regimen, its success (or failure) in producing the desired clinical outcome, and patient response to the pharmacologic environment. Moreover, every inspection should include a survey of the patient's active clinical problem list. So-called "silent" diseases should be noted in case of medication noncompliance.

Not surprisingly, there are almost as many ways to inspect a drug house as there are drugs. A pharmacologic environment can be surveyed directly, or by reviewing secondary sources where the blueprints of the patient's drug house are kept on file. Usually, the pharmacist or physician can sketch the rough outlines of a patient's intended drug regimen by consulting such secondary sources as a computerized pharmacy database (if available), the patient's medical records, and hospital discharge summaries, all of which record pharmacotherapeutic treatment plans. Although such clinical documents provide valuable information, unfortunately, these secondary sources frequently reflect little more than planned therapeutic regimens, and may diverge substantially from the drugs the patient is actually taking. These discrepancies should be noted. Occasionally, changes in drug therapy are not recorded, which can create additional confusion.

Given these pitfalls, there is no substitute for examining the patient's pharmacopoeia in a direct, hands-on fashion in the office or pharmacy. Patients should be encouraged to collect all their medicines, whether prescription or nonprescription, and bring them for evaluation to the physician's office or pharmacy. This information is an important part of the database. Based on a review of written records, a thorough history from the patient, and inspection of the pill bottles provided by the patient, the physician or pharmacist should attempt to reconstruct the patient's current drug regimen and pattern of intake. This approach is effective for discovering multiple sources of prescriptions.

Conducting drug house safety checks is a valuable exercise for all patients on long-term drug therapy. They are especially useful, however, when targeted at individuals at high risk for faulty drug house construction. In this regard, there are a number of risk factors that raise red flags and suggest that safety codes are likely to be violated. Predisposing factors that point to faulty constructions include: (a) polypharmacy; (b) kitsch pharmatecture (patient self-medication or unmonitored alterations in drug consumption; (c) OTC drug use (drug reactions and interactions); (d) complex drug regimens (erratic scheduling, multiple dosing); (e) drug prescribing from multiple physicians; (f) the presence of silent diseases such as hypertension; and (g) *excessive* reliance on *generic* medications (which suggests less pharmacotherapeutically advanced drugs are being used). When one or more of these factors is identified, a drug-by-drug analysis for possible complications is indicated.

Inspecting Every Nook and Cranny. Screening for high-risk prescribing patterns is only part of the process required to uncover violations in pharmatectural safety codes. In this regard, the mere presence of risk factors neither guarantees that violations are present nor that adverse consequences have resulted. And conversely, the absence of risk factors does not ensure that the drug house is in good working order. Consequently, the most fruitful inspections of drug houses cover every nook and cranny, and include a review of the medical records, screening for drug interactions, measurement of serum drug levels when indicated, and detailed interviews with the patient and family members.

A Room by Room Search. Cursory investigations produce unreliable assessments that provide little guidance for drug house reconstruction. Hence, there is no substitute for a "room-by-room" search to uncover drug-related problems. The most productive evaluations result when pharmacists and physicians conduct drug house inspections with the zeal of investigative journalists.

For example, when a patient is asked about the tolerability of a regimen, he may confide to his physician or pharmacist that, "Everything is going fine." Statements of this kind should be interpreted with caution because, if accepted at face value, a host of drug-related problems may be overlooked. It is important to incorporate use of open-ended questions. So often, we hear physicians say that the patient seems to be tolerating his regimen "without any problems." Assessments of this kind can undermine detection of serious flaws in the way the drug house has been designed. Most patients do not possess the information and experience necessary to make associations between drug intake and side effects, and all too frequently, physicians take patients at their word. From a pharmatectural perspective, it is the pharmacist's and physician's responsibility to make these associations and to paint a realistic picture of just how well (or how poorly) the patient is thriving in a drug environment.

Because the patient's initial impression of how things are going may not account for the full range of drug-related problems, it is important to give the patient a closer look and to ask more probing questions. In this regard, the inspection process must be thorough, detailed, and, when necessary, delve into personal habits and behavior patterns. Drug house inspections rely on gathering and comparing information from several different sources: patient impressions of side effects, known associations between drug intake and side effects, medical records, pill bottle inspections, patient perceptions of drug intake, and family members' accounts of the patient's behavioral and sexual patterns.

Finally, the undesirable consequences of inferior drug houses take many different forms. It is not good enough simply to look for the *recognized* hazards of drug therapy, such as adverse drug reactions. Rather, the full spectrum of problems, drug-related difficulties and safety code violations must be considered.

Stairway To Heaven: The Pitfalls of Polypharmacy. Drug houses constructed from *several* pharmacologic building blocks require a thorough inspection because the likelihood of detecting suboptimal drug combinations, unnecessary medications, and drug-induced adverse side effects increases as the number of prescribed drugs increases. For example, compliance is reduced and the risk of adverse drug reactions increased when the drug regimen is complex, of long duration, dependent on an alteration in the patient's lifestyle, inconvenient, or expensive. Put another way, there is value in simplicity. In patients with diabetes or congestive heart failure, for example, medication errors are observed in less than 15% of patients when only one drug is prescribed; increases to 25% when two drugs are taken; and exceeds 35% when five or more drugs are consumed.[19,20,51,69]

Patients consuming *four or more* drugs are at high risk for *noncompliance*-mediated disease deterioration. Consequently, pharmatectural principles stressing drug reduction, elimination, and simplification can yield significant benefits in this patient population. A number of different strategies should be considered in this high-risk group. First, the regimen should be made less complex by reducing the number of different medications required. If a patient is taking nitroglycerin for angina and a diuretic for hypertension, the pharmacist or physician should consider a substitution such as a calcium channel blocker (e.g., amlodipine) that consolidates drug therapy into a single prescription ingredient.

Reduction of complexity can also be accomplished by avoiding the routine prescription of nonessential medication, and avoiding unnecessary doses or variations in scheduling (such as synchronized doses). Complexity can also be modified by prioritizing the regimen, and by minimizing both inconvenience and the risk of forgetting a dose by matching the regimen schedule to the patient's regular daily activities.

Polypharmacy constructions offer many windows of opportunity for pharmatectural intervention, among them, drug modifications, application of smart drug therapy, and regimen reconstruction. The elderly are especially sensitive to both the intended, pharmacologic effects of drugs and their undesirable adverse reactions. Compounding this problem is the fact that they are frequently innocent victims of a bona fide epidemic of excessive drug prescribing. Put simply, increased sensitivity to drug side effects combined with prescription drug overuse is an unsavory combination that can produce an uninhabitable drug house, especially for the elderly.

Of all prescription drugs, 25% are taken by those over 65 years of age, although the group comprises less than 12% of the population. The average older person fills more than twice as many prescriptions as those under age 65.[38] Polypharmacy, variable compliance, and multiple diseases, combined with altered physiologic response, make the elderly especially prone to adverse drug reactions. In addition, studies now confirm that medication errors may be compounded by acute hospitalization.[2,70] A group of internists at Brooke Army Medical Center evaluated the medical records of 417 consecutive patients discharged from the hospital, noted the discharge drugs and doses on leaving, and then reassessed the patients 1 month later with respect to their current medications, schedules, and dosing. They found that 50% of patients appear to make some kind of medication error after discharge from the hospital. Based on this study, acute hospitalization is an additional risk factor for drug house deterioration. Accordingly, pharmacists and physicians should routinely attempt to confirm that drug regimens after hospitalization are maintained as prescribed and that inadvertent deletions, additions, or changes in dose amount or frequency are not made.[2,47,70]

As would be expected, the human and resource costs of adverse drug effects are substantial in patients taking multiple drug regimens. Considerable morbidity in the elderly, such as syncope, falls, and change in mental status are associated with drugs used to treat high blood pressure and central nervous system disorders.[71,72] Adverse side effects must always be suspected in any elderly patient who presents with new symptoms of confusion or worsening of a pre-existing dementia, and in patients with symptoms related to altered cardiovascular homeostasis, including falls, sleepiness, and syncopal episodes.[4,72,73]

Kitsch Pharmatecture: When Patients Remodel. Too many designers can spoil a drug house, especially when one of the designers is the *patient.* In general, designing and building a drug house should be the responsibility of a single individual, usually the patient's primary care physician. However, this physician must work in collaboration with pharmacists and other prescribers as required and should communicate openly with the patient about the rationale for choices and changes in the regimen. Unfortunately, even the most intelligently designed drug house can be undermined by patients who get into the drug house remodeling business and start taking pharmacologic matters into their own hands. When patients get in the habit of building their own pharmacologic environments, the primary prescriber can anticipate a wide range of undesirable consequences, from unexpected drug interactions to life-threatening side effects.

Although patients of all ages have shown a tendency to design their own drug houses,[2,50] the problem of kitsch pharmatecture is especially prevalent in the elderly. First of all, obtaining accurate information regarding medication intake in the elderly is problematic at best. Up to 60% of all drugs taken by the elderly are OTC medications (See Figure 2-5). Frequently, their consumption of nonprescription drugs is not reported to a pharmacist or physician, despite a careful drug history. The seriousness of this problem is shown by studies from London Hospital, which show that even when elderly patients are interviewed with vigilance, up to 40% of patients fail to acknowledge significant intake of OTC medications. Moreover, a greater percentage of patients provide inaccurate information about their compliance patterns with *prescribed* medications.[56,62]

Figure 2-5

Kitsch Pharmatecture: Patients Remodel Their Regimens	
OTC Drugs	
• Cimetidine	• Phenylpropanolamine
• Diphenhydramine	• Salicylates
• NSAIDs	

Consequently, repeated questioning and probing are required to elicit an accurate pharmacological history, and no drug house inspection is complete without a thorough survey of nonprescription drug intake. Many OTC drugs have the potential for exacerbating the toxic effects of prescribed drugs and worsening existing conditions, especially in the elderly. For example, a patient taking oral corticosteroid medication such as prednisone may then self-medicate with an OTC nonsteroidal anti-inflammatory drug (NSAID) such as ibuprofen, increasing the risk of gastric ulceration by four-fold. NSAIDs also have the potential to cause renal deterioration, especially in older patients with heart disease, diabetes, and pre-existing kidney disease. They are among the most widely used OTC drugs in the world, despite having a number of well-known potential side effects.

Indiscriminate use of common analgesics such as aspirin also can lead to unexpected consequences. In the case of salicylates, which are contained in more than 200 OTC compounds, uncontrolled and nondirected use can lead to subtle signs of toxicity, and result in confusion, irritability, tinnitus (although this is not a good warning signal in the elderly, who are likely to have it already), vision disturbances, sweating, nausea, vomiting, and diarrhea. Since many of these symptoms may be inappropriately ascribed to old age, toxicity may be overlooked by both patient and provider.

The antipyretic action of aspirin can also cause subnormal temperatures in the elderly. Elderly patients receiving aspirin sometimes complain of shivering. Combined use of aspirin and other drugs can jeopardize the effectiveness of the thermoregulatory mechanisms and may lead to accidental hypothermia. With respect to drug interactions, unregulated salicylate intake can cause impaired hemostasis, hypoprothombinemia, and gastrointestinal bleeding in patients taking oral anticoagulants. At higher doses, aspirin can displace protein-bound first generation oral hypoglycemics from their binding sites, placing patients at risk for increased hypoglycemia. Although nondirected aspirin intake clearly poses a risk to older patients, it should be stressed that failure to prescribe aspirin for secondary prevention of myocardial infarction is a certifiable sin of *omission.*[30,34,35]

Among drugs whose actions are potentiated by concomitant aspirin intake is methotrexate. Decreased clearance of methotrexate and increased methotrexate toxicity is reported with aspirin doses of greater than 2 g/day. Although not a drug interaction, it should be stressed that aspirin and NSAIDs can also precipitate asthma in patients with asthma, idiosyncratic asthma sensitivity, and nasal polyps or sinusitis. Greater awareness of the potential adverse effects of aspirin, particularly in the elderly, has led to a substantial increase in the use of acetaminophen, which, with its analgesic and antipyretic properties, is often a suitable and desirable substitute.

Other classes of OTC drugs, such as antihistaminic hypnotics, have anticholinergic effects that may precipitate acute confusion or worsen dementia.[74-77] In addition, a number of common allergy/decongestant preparations contain anticholinergic drugs in conjunction with alpha-adrenergic agonists, a combination that can easily precipitate urinary retention or incontinence. Cold remedies containing phenylpropanolamine, a potent peripheral vascoconstrictor, can cause significant elevations in blood pressure, especially when patients self-medicate with quantities that exceed 150 mg of phenylpropanolamine, which is twice the maximum recommended dose. Finally, the availability of OTC cimetidine, which is a known inhibitor of the p-450 cytochrome oxidase system, can produce drug-drug interactions with theophylline and other medications.

Silent Diseases: Drug Houses That Crumble. The purpose of drug house inspections is not only to uncover drugs that are potentially problematic, but to identify diseases that, because of their relatively *silent* and quiescent nature, predispose to poor medication intake over a long duration. Silent diseases, because they produce minimal symptoms, provide less inducement for medication intake. For example, among chronic medical conditions, such relatively silent conditions as hypertension are associated with an unusually high risk of noncompliance. Consider these discouraging observations: up to 50% of patients with hypertension fail to follow referral advice; over 50% fail to follow-up on a long-term basis, and only two-thirds of those who remain under care consume enough medications to adequately control their blood pressure.[78-80]

Overall, only 30% of identified patients with hypertension outside of special care programs are under good control. These findings suggest that the patient with a relatively *silent* condition such as hypertension may value very differently the statistical probability of *future* health benefits from drug therapy relative to the present reality of the inconvenience and side effects associated with prescribed medications. This predisposes the individual to poor medication compliance. Consequently, patients with hypertension, hyperlipidemia, diabetes, and similar chronic conditions, in which the *noise level of the drug tends to be greater than the noise level of the disease,* are ideal candidates for compliance-enhancing approaches.

When inspections uncover the presence of one or more relatively silent diseases, the pharmacist and physician should attempt to assess the noise level of the diseases as well as the noise level of the medications that are used to manage these conditions. The noise level of the disease is defined as the severity of symptoms, changes in daily activity patterns as a result of the disorder, patient perceptions about the risks of not taking medications, and their perceptions about the seriousness of their condition. The noise level of the drug is defined as its side effect profile, cost, convenience of dosing, perceptions about the value of the drug in treating the patient's disorder, and duration of therapy.

When the noise level of the drug is *greater* than the noise level of the disease, patients will have a tendency to take refuge in the silence of the disease rather than tolerate the noise level of the medication. (Figure 2-6) The result is therapeutically significant noncompliance. To avoid this problem, drug reconstructions should attempt to identify medications with noise levels *lower* than the diseases against which they are directed. This will increase the likelihood of maintaining long-term compliance and improve therapeutic outcomes. It follows that for highly symptomatic diseases that are perceived as a significant threat to the patient's well-being, there is more flexibility in selecting pharmacologic building blocks. In general, these individuals are much more likely to tolerate medications that make the disease more bearable, even if their potential side effects or convenience parameters are less than ideal.

Figure 2-6

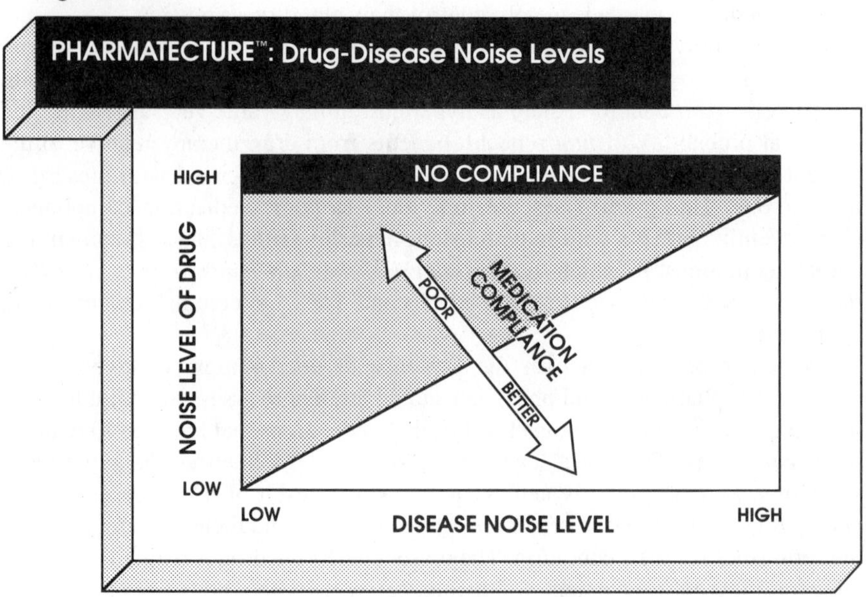

Housecleaning: Frequency and Duration: Drug house inspections should include a medication review that evaluates drugs from the perspective of dosing frequency and duration of therapy, since these are critical factors influencing medication compliance. When patients are committed to long-term therapy, the risk of compromised drug intake is high, and adjustments should be made to minimize the negative impact of chronic therapy. For example, one study found a 30% incidence rate of dosage errors in patients with diabetes for 1 to 5 years, but an 80% dosage error rate in patients who had the disease for 20 years. Even estimates of less-than-perfect compliance for short-term courses dosed four times daily are reported to be as high as 92%, and average about 50% for chronic diseases.[20,58,59] Studies looking at antibiotic intake have shown that only 45% of individuals complete a 10-day course of therapy.

Consequently, compliance issues and pharmatecture-based simplification strategies should be considered for short-term, as well as long-term drug regimens. Patients whose regimens include drugs that are dosed multiple times daily will benefit from pharmatectural modifications. In general, significant compliance-enhancing benefits will be achieved by reducing daily dose frequency of prescribed medications. When available and financially feasible, once-daily medications are almost always preferred. Modifying *duration* of drug therapy usually is more problematic, although many infectious diseases can now be treated successfully with single-dose regimens. Clinically important examples of one-dose therapies include: 2 g of metronidazole (Flagyl®) orally for nonspecific bacterial vaginosis; 1 g of azithromycin (Zithromax®) orally for uncomplicated chlamydial cervicitis and urethritis; and 400 mg cefixime (Suprax®) orally for gonococcal urethritis. (See Chapter 5) Such single-dose herapeutic regimens should be identified and incorporated into clinical practice when appropriate.

Polyphysicians: The Road to Polypharmacy. Inspection of the regimen should not only make note of the medications themselves, but should identify the prescribing sources (physicians, pharmacists, nurse practitioners, etc.). When there is *more* than one prescribing source, the drug house should be carefully scrutinized for medication duplications, drug interactions, and drug-disease incompatibilities. The road to polypharmacy is usually paved with good intentions, but when a number of different subspecialists are involved, the drug house needs a thorough going-over. Because subspecialists frequently focus on just one aspect of the patient's pathophysiological or pharmacologic landscape, drug houses designed by multiple sources are frequently unstable or are built with redundant materials. Polyprescribers are an important risk factor for polypharmacy, and when multiple prescribing sources are identified, drugs in the regimen should be re-evaluated to ensure that they are still indicated and compatible with other agents that might have been added by other sources. Whenever possible, all the building blocks in a patient's drug house should originate from a *single* prescribing source.

Mortgage Payments: Expensive Drug Houses. No drug house inspection is complete without a basic, no-holds barred cost-analysis of the mortgage payments required to service the regimen on a month-to-month basis. When drug houses become too expensive, patients attempt to save money by skipping drug doses, consuming medications only in response to symptomatic deterioration, and failing to fill prescriptions for the more expensive drugs in the regimen. The end result is noncompliance-mediated disease deterioration and, down the road, the necessity for even greater expenditures to mop up therapeutic failures.

Drug costs are an important element of pharmatectural construction. To get a handle on this aspect of building maintenance, a total monthly budget for the existing drug regimen should be generated, and should include a careful cost itemization on a drug-by-drug basis. The patient's, instititution's, or health plan's capacity for maintaining these costs should be evaluated. (If costs are deemed excessive, opportunities for making pharmatectural substitutions should be considered.) However, rarely should drug acquisition cost be the *only* factor in drug house design. In other words, if patients *are* able to afford more effective but expensive agents, these building blocks should be retained in the regimen.

In general, when trimming down mortgage payments for drug houses, budgetary allocations should favor medications used to treat life-threatening conditions such as coronary heart disease, stroke, chronic obstructive pulmonary disease, cardiac arrhythmias, renal disease, and diabetes. From a cost-benefit standpoint, more expensive drugs are justified in these conditions because the risks and costs of poor therapeutic outcome are substantial. On the other hand, when treating diseases that are primarily symptomatic in nature, such as ulcer disease or arthritis, it may be useful to reduce costs by incorporating into the regimens drugs of lower cost that have proven efficacy. As mentioned, symptomatic diseases are characterized by high noise levels, which are a powerful inducement to compliance, regardless of possible side effects.

Shaky Foundations: Building Blocks That Do Not Stand The Test of Time. Some materials simply don't stand the test of time. Drug houses should be inspected for medications that are obsolete and can be replaced by better agents, or are being used beyond their window of therapeutic opportunity. Examples of drugs that have the potential for elimination or substitution in selected patients include dipyridamole (Persantine®), H_2 blockers, NSAIDs, benzodiazepines, misoprostol, theophylline, and many others.[11,12,81-83] (See Chapter 7.)

This Old House: Generic Constructions. From a pharmatectural perspective, old drug houses that feature a *preponderance* of generic pharmacologic building blocks need close examination. A pharmacologic environment of this kind may have been created with cost as the top priority, rather than "if all else is equal, choose the less expensive agent." In many instances, generic drugs are appropriate and effective, e.g., aspirin, atenolol, trimethoprim-sulfa. The proper pharmacologic agent should be chosen first; then determine if it is a multisource drug.

There are two issues: (1) Therapeutic Applicability (Is it the best building material?); and (2) Generic Substitution (Is it the best building material available from several suppliers, and, therefore, is a cost choice available?). Without question, the first issue, therapeutic applicability, should be addressed and answered. Once determined, then investigate if generics are available.

The advantages of the newer (and, usually, single source, more expensive) agents should not be overlooked since improvements in drug delivery systems, reductions in daily dose frequency, improved side effects profiles, or improved antimicrobial coverage may be available and justify increased cost. Any of these advantages may save money in the long-run by increasing compliance and reducing future hospitalizations or therapy.

In summary, a drug house built with a preponderance of generic building blocks deserves close inspection to determine if optimal therapy is being given. Newer therapy may be available that is safer or more effective. However, the reverse also may be true, i.e., that a trade name drug is being appropriately used and that a cheaper equivalent agent is available.

THE PHARMATECTURAL SAFETY CODE

Drug-Related Adverse Patient Events (DRAPEs). No drug house inspection is complete without assessing the risk of incurring drug-related adverse events. The key to making this inspection useful, however, is recognizing the full range of potential pitfalls associated with drug therapy. Detection of drug-related complications is essential because one of the principal objectives of pharmatecture is constructing drug regimens that reduce the risk of (a) adverse side effects, (b) primary drug reactions, and (c) drug interactions in patients on polypharmacy. The ultimate goals are to improve quality of life, maintain work performance, and reduce the unnecessary costs associated with managing medication side effects and drug-induced hospitalizations.

Detecting Drug Rot. Until recently, drug-related adverse consequences were viewed in rather simplistic terms. Traditionally, pharmacists and physicians were on the lookout for run-of-the-mill, adverse drug reactions (ADRs): e.g., diarrhea associated with ampicillin, a rash from a sulfa antibiotic, confusion from cimetidine, or depression after beginning therapy with a beta-blocker. Although these primary drug reactions must be recognized and appropriately managed, there is a wide spectrum of drug-related liabilities that must be considered in order to construct safe, cost-effective drug regimens.[21,51,84,85] To achieve these objectives, pharmatecture focuses on drug-related adverse patient events (DRAPEs), which include any undesired, less than optimal effects of drug therapy.[86,87]

The DRAPE approach is especially useful as a guide to pharmatectural reconstruction because it reflects the *full* spectrum of drug-related difficulties and poor outcomes associated with pharmacotherapy. Accordingly, it includes not only recognized hazards of drug therapy, such as adverse drug reactions, drug interactions, effects of OTC drugs, and potential hazards of combining alcohol with prescribed drugs, but also incorporates less direct problems associated with prescription drug use, such as noncompliance and self-medication.

Accordingly, pharmatectural alterations in a drug regimen should be considered when an inspection uncovers one or more of the following categories of DRAPEs:

- **Primary drug reaction.** Any reaction in a patient that is noxious and unintended and that occurs at doses normally used for prophylaxis, diagnosis, or therapy.

- **Drug interactions.** When two or more drugs, prescription or nonprescription, interact in such a way as to potentiate the adverse side effects of one of the agents.

- **Treatment failure.** A failure to accomplish the goals of treatment because of inadequate or inappropriate drug therapy.

- **Intentional noncompliance.** A failure to accomplish the goals of treatment because of deliberate nonadherence to a therapeutic program:

- **Medication error and scheduling misconception.** A failure to accomplish the goals of treatment because of accidental or unintentional nonadherence to a therapeutic program.

- **Alcohol-related problems.** Interactions between alcohol and prescribed drugs, and problems associated with altered drug intake patterns because of alcohol consumption.

Are There DRAPEs In The House? The prevalence, etiology, and risk of incurring DRAPEs is well studied, especially in older patients. In one large Canadian study evaluating 718 patients taking prescribed drugs and admitted through an emergency department, DRAPEs were identified in 162 (23%) admissions. Many patients had more than one category of DRAPE. Overall, adverse drug reactions represented about one half of all DRAPEs, with 25% of individuals within this group experiencing drug interactions. Intentional noncompliance was identified as a cause for admission in about one quarter of patients, and treatment failure was assigned as the reason in about 34% of patients (See Figure 2-7).[86]

When looking for possible DRAPEs, the following observations will help pharmacists and physicians conduct a systematic review of drug-related problems. First, it should be emphasized that age is not an independent risk factor for DRAPEs. The risk of having a DRAPE is linked to the number of diseases a patient has and the number of drugs being taken. As it happens, older patients are afflicted with more diseases and tend be on more medications; therefore, they are more likely to suffer from DRAPEs. These risk factors have important implications for preventing drug-related problems. Because most diseases are managed but not eliminated, the most effective way to reduce the risk of DRAPEs is by reducing the *number* of different prescription ingredients in the regimen.[66,88-90]

Figure 2-7

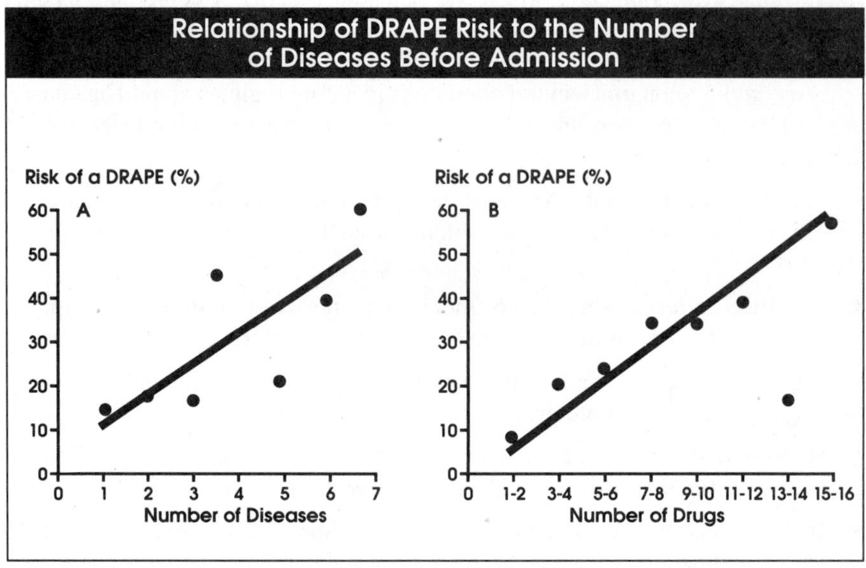

A comprehensive review of systems, signs, and symptoms is fundamental to uncovering DRAPEs (See Figure 2-8). Of special diagnostic importance is the fact that 50% of all DRAPEs affect the cardiovascular system.[82,86,88] Congestive heart failure is the most common DRAPE in this category, affecting nearly 40% of patients with drug-related cardiac problems, followed by angina, hypotension, and atrial fibrillation. The unusually high incidence of DRAPEs affecting the cardiovascular system should be considered a warning. When building regimens to treat hypertension and cardiovascular conditions, special vigilance is required because drug classes used to treat these disorders represent a high-risk category for causing DRAPEs.[91-96]

Figure 2-8

Clinical Manifestations of the 193 Drug-related Adverse Patient Events (DRAPEs)

CLINICAL MANIFESTATIONS	NUMBER	(%)
CARDIOVASCULAR: TOTAL	**103**	**(53%)**
Congestive Heart Failure	41	(21%)
Angina	9	(5%)
Hypotension	8	(4%)
Atrial Fibrillation	7	(4%)
CENTRAL NERVOUS SYSTEM: TOTAL	**68**	**(35%)**
Confusion	16	(8%)
Fatigue/Lethargy	6	(3%)
Dizziness	5	(3%)
Cerebrovascular Accident	5	(3%)
GASTROINTESTINAL: TOTAL	**40**	**(21%)**
Nausea/Vomiting	12	(6%)
Anorexia	6	(3%)
RENAL AND GENITO-URINARY: TOTAL	**36**	**(19%)**
Hypokalemia	10	(5%)
Dehydration	4	(2%)
ENDOCRINE	17	(9%)
RESPIRATORY	15	(8%)
HEMATOLOGICAL	12	(6%)
DERMATOLOGICAL	8	(4%)
OTHER MANIFESTATIONS	16	(8%)

*There were 315 clinical manifestations associated with the 193 DRAPEs; therefore, total is more than 100%.

One third of all DRAPEs affect the central nervous system.[82,86,88] Confusion is the most common manifestation followed by fatigue, lethargy, dizziness, and syncope.[75,97-99] About 60% of these adverse reactions are caused by drugs used to treat neurological disorders, about one third are caused by cardiovascular agents, and the remainder by drugs used to treat other disorders.

About 20% of all DRAPE events are associated with a gastrointestinal problem or a metabolic abnormality. Drugs most often associated with DRAPEs include systemic steroids, digoxin, NSAIDs, calcium blockers, beta-blockers, theophylline, diuretics, and benzodiazepines.[92,100-105]

Figure 2-9

Drugs Most Often Implicated in Drug-related Adverse Patient Event (DRAPEs)

Drug or Drug Group	Incidence in Users	Total Number	Number as ADR*
Systemic Steroids	27%	19	11
Digoxin	22%	38	10
NSAIDS	20%	10	7
Alphamethyldopa	20%	9	1
Calcium Channel Blockers	19%	8	6
Beta-Blockers	18%	18	12
Theophylline	17%	12	0
Furosemide	16%	31	7
Sympathomimetics	14%	10	0
Thiazides	12%	19	10
Benzodiazepines	10%	10	5

*ADR: Adverse Drug Reactions

PHARMATECTURAL TROUBLESHOOTING

Putting The Rafters and Girders Into Place

Because complex factors influence drug intake and therapeutic efficacy in the older patient, pharmatectural surveillance and drug prescribing strategies play a central role in the geriatric age group. Many co-existing issues must be addressed simultaneously and designing a pharmatectural blueprint for these patients can be difficult. One of the problems associated with drug regimen design in the elderly includes deciding whether to prescribe fewer drugs or more drugs.

Unfortunately, the answer to this question is not as straightforward as it may seem. In the previous discussion of DRAPEs, the necessity for reducing pharmacologic burden was stressed. And while this strategy usually is the most prudent course, there is no consistently optimal plan for constructing a drug house, even when it comes to the number of pharmacologic building blocks. Every patient is different, and sometimes the *addition* of a drug, especially if it has prevention-oriented properties, represents the optimal therapeutic strategy.

Pharmacologic Building Blocks—More or Less. One of the principal objectives of this system is to reduce the risks and therapeutic pitfalls associated with both over- and under-prescribing of medications. Excessive drug prescribing is one of the principal causes of DRAPEs. Medications frequently are used without adequate indications. Common examples include dipyridamole (Persantine®), theophylline (Theo-Dur®), cimetidine (Tagamet®), triazolam (Halcion®), digoxin (Lanoxin®),[103] alprazolam (Xanax®) and pentoxyphylline (Trental®). In other cases, drugs are maintained in the regimen long *after* their window of therapeutic opportunity has closed. Nonsteroidal anti-inflammatory drugs (NSAIDs), sedative-hypnotics, and narcotic analgesics are common offenders. On the other hand, there are very useful and, occasionally, relatively inexpensive drugs—e.g., aspirin, estrogen, calcium, pneumococcal vaccine (Pneumovax®), beta-blockers, and warfarin—with well-documented, prevention-oriented benefits that, frequently, are inappropriately *omitted* from the therapeutic regimen.

Pharmatecturally speaking, the *exclusion* of prevention-oriented, health-maintaining pharmacologic building blocks from a drug house can compromise its structural integrity and long-term durability. Pharmacologic *underservicing* may result from a number of factors. For example, the physician or pharmacist may fail to identify patients whose risk factors and clinical history mandate the need for a *prevention*-oriented medication. Sometimes, patients are put on appropriate prevention-oriented drugs (antihypertensives or statins) but at doses insufficient to achieve target goals. And even when such patients are identified, the pharmatect may be unaware of the role, existence, appropriate dose, or benefits of specific drugs for these conditions. Finally, underservicing can result from patient noncompliance.

With these issues in mind, evaluating patients for possible benefits associated with *prevention-oriented* drug therapy plays an important role in Total Pharmacotherapeutic Quality Management (TPQM™). Implementing TPQM means surveying drug houses to ensure that clinically indicated, prevention-oriented pharmacologic building blocks are in place. This pharmatectural strategy can improve clinical outcomes, delay progression of many chronic diseases, and reduce overall drug costs. In this regard, it should be stressed that the failure to implement prevention-oriented drug therapies—e.g., aspirin for prevention of myocardial reinfarction, stroke, and for thromboembolism prophylaxis associated with chronic atrial fibrillation; statins for prevention of MI and stroke; dietary calcium supplementation or alendronate for prevention of osteoporosis; estrogen replacement therapy for cardioprotection; beta-blockers for prevention of reinfarction; vitamin E or folic acid to prevent coronary artery disease; and angiotensin converting enzyme (ACE) inhibitors to delay progression of diabetic renal disease—may actually *increase* long-term pharmacologic expenditures.

Consequently, a systematic approach to solid foundation-building is the most practical way to ensure the durability and reduce long-term maintenance costs of drug houses for patients with chronic disease.

Building Codes For Preventive Maintenance. A significant percentage of patients have chronic diseases that can deteriorate if pharmacologically underserviced. From a pharmatectural point of view, these patients can be seen as having structural defects in the foundations of their drug houses and are at high risk for incurring increased drug-related expenditures over the long term. A cycle occurs in which more costly agents (thrombolytics, heparin, erythropoietin, intravenous antibiotics, etc.) and procedural interventions (angioplasty, surgical repair of hip fractures, rehabilitation) are used to treat acute illnesses (stroke, myocardial infarction, pneumonia, renal disease, hip fractures, etc.) that might have been delayed, or avoided entirely, with less costly, prevention-oriented pharmacotherapy. As you might expect, balancing sins of commission (drug overuse) with sins of omission (drug underuse) is a formidable challenge and an important component of the pharmatectural approach to drug house design.

Total outcome costs associated with pharmacotherapy can be reduced not only by eliminating unnecessary drugs, but by including agents that are useful in disease prevention. Of course, the financial and clinical toll of *excessive* drug prescribing is readily apparent—more drugs mean greater cost, increased risk for drug interactions, and noncompliance-mediated therapeutic failures. Although the liabilities of under-prescribing are far more subtle to detect, they are every bit as devastating, both financially and clinically. In this regard, pharmatecture advocates a prevention-oriented, quality assurance check-up to ensure that pharmacologic rafters and girders are in place to prevent premature disease deterioration. Specific therapeutic approaches to reducing long-term pharmacologic maintenance costs are discussed in the next section.

Preventive Pharmacology: Designing a Solid Foundation

Building a solid infrastructure for drug houses inhabited by patients with chronic diseases is an important pharmatectural objective (See Figure 2-10). To ensure the structural integrity of pharmacologic environments constructed for these patients and to reduce long-term costs, the following medications with prevention-oriented properties should be considered for possible inclusion in the drug regimens of appropriate patient subgroups.

Calcium Supplementation for Osteoporosis. The picture has finally solidified for the role of calcium in preventing postmenopausal osteoporosis. Until recently, the optimal treatment for prevention of osteoporosis was fiercely debated. Estrogen replacement therapy has been shown effective in preventing the rapid loss of bone that accompanies the early postmenopausal years.[106] Calcium supplementation also retards postmenopausal bone loss, especially in older women (who have a slower rate of bone loss than women in their immediate postmenopausal years). One important study[107] of modest calcium

Figure 2-10

Prevention-Oriented Drug Therapy
• Calcium supplementation
• Statins for heart disease
• Estrogen replacement therapy (ERT)
• Atredonale for osteoporosis
• Aspirin prophylaxis and myocardial infarction
• Estrogen for prevention of Parkinson's dementia?
• Evista for osteoporosis
• Warfarin and stroke
• Tamoxifen for breast cancer
• Beta-Blockers for cardioprotection
• Pneumococcal vaccine
• NSAIDs for Alzheimer's disease?
• ACE inhibitors for CHF and diabetes
• Estrogen for Alzheimer's disease?
• Misoprostol and NSAID-induced GI tract ulceration
• Vitamin D for osteoporosis

supplementation in women taking less than 400 mg of dietary calcium per day showed significant benefit in slowing osteoporosis. However, the broader question is the efficacy of calcium supplementation in normal women who are not deficient in dietary calcium. In other words, should supplemental calcium therapy be a structural component of every drug house occupied by a postmenopausal woman?[108] The answer is probably, "Yes."

Australian investigators have shed important new light on this question. In a study designed to evaluate the benefits of providing an additional 1000 mg/day of supplemental calcium to postmenopausal women who were already consuming an average of 750 mg/day of dietary calcium, results indicated that the rate of bone loss density was reduced by 43% in those taking the calcium supplement compared to controls. In the femur the rate of loss was reduced by 35%, and bone loss was eliminated in the trunk. These benefits were not influenced by the amount of dietary calcium, and they were sustained for 2 years following entry into the study.[107-110]

The pharmatectural implications of this study are clear. To prevent premature bone loss, drug houses for postmenopausal women should include at least 1500 mg of calcium per day (diet plus supplements). Those who do not get sufficient exposure to sunlight should also include a vitamin D supplement (400 to 800 U/day). In a recent study of 290 patients consecutively admitted to the general medical ward of Massachusetts General Hospital, 57% of patients had deficient vitamin D levels. Twenty-two percent were severely deficient, suggesting this deficiency is an alarming public health problem. At present, it appears that calcium and vitamin D supplementation alone are sufficient to halt the rapid reduction in bone mass that characterizes early menopause. For this reason, hormonal replacement therapy with estrogen (see below) is, at present, the foundation of treatment for prevention of osteoporosis during the first 3 to 5 years of menopause.[107,111]

Estrogen Replacement Therapy (ERT): Osteoporosis, Alzheimer's Disease, and Cardioprotection. Estrogen replacement therapy (ERT) should be a foundation building block for virtually all drug houses constructed on behalf of postmenopausal women. The appropriate role and method for ERT still remains somewhat controversial in clinical practice, but the evidence supporting its routine use has rapidly mounted in recent years.[106,112-114] On the beneficial side, ERT significantly reduces the rate of postmenopausal bone loss, thereby decreasing the number of hip fractures related to osteoporosis by as much as 60%. Evista also has been approved to prevent osteoporosis. Furthermore, although conflicting results are reported, the consensus of existing epidemiologic data strongly suggests that ERT can reduce the risk of ischemic heart disease in postmenopausal women by as much as 40% to 50%, as long as estrogen therapy is started at the onset of menopause, and *prior* to the development of heart disease. A recent study, in which postmenopausal women *with* heart disease started on estrogen had a *higher* incidence of recurrent myocardial infarction than those not started on estrogen, has prompted a more cautious assessment of the effectiveness and timing of ERT. On the downside, although again results conflict, epidemiologic data suggests that ERT may increase the risk of breast cancer in postmenopausal women; a recent study suggested the increase in risk may be as high as 30%.[114] Other studies fail to confirm the link between ERT and breast cancer. There is also evidence to suggest that estrogen users develop better differentiated tumors; and, that mortality data support the contention that accelerated growth of a pre-existing tumor and detection/surveillance bias are influencing the results of positive observational studies linking estrogen to increased risk of breast cancer. Furthermore, there is clear evidence that ERT increases the risk of endometrial cancer sixfold, although this increase can largely be prevented by the concomitant use of progestins.[106,114]

Proponents of ERT argue, however, that even if the rates of endometrial and breast cancer are increased, these detrimental effects are largely outweighed by the substantial beneficial effects ERT has on osteoporosis, cardiovascular disease, and, perhaps, stroke. There is also early data to suggest that the onset of Alzheimer's disease may be delayed by estrogen. A recent study also suggests estrogen use was associated with a marginally lower risk of dementia in women with Parkinson's disease. Nevertheless, concerns about the more immediate potential increases in cancer compared to the long-term protective effects on cardiovascular disorders and osteoporosis has deterred many patients and clinicians from initiating ERT. In addition, the inconvenience of the resumption in menstrual bleeding that sometimes occurs with combined estrogen-progestin treatment, and the subsequent increased cancer surveillance procedures (endometrial biopsy) also tend to discourage patients from using ERT.

Despite these barriers to ERT, and because cardiovascular disease is the leading cause of death in women, ERT is important for postmenopausal women. The most compelling evidence for including ERT as an essential part of the drug house in postmenopausal women comes from the Harvard Medical School and Harvard School of Public Health, Nurses Health Study, initiated in 1976. In 1985, this research group reported a beneficial effect of ERT in reducing cardiovascular disease, based on 4 years of follow-up examination in 48,470 women. More recently, the 10-year follow-up data were reported and are equally impressive.[114] Overall, the risk for current users of estrogen, adjusted for age and other risk factors, was reduced by approximately 50% in comparison to women who never used estrogen. The risk was reduced in women who experienced either natural or surgical menopause. These benefits were also present in a subgroup of patients otherwise at low risk for cardiovascular disease.

Even when patients with diabetes, hypertension, hypercholesterolemia, smoking, or obesity were excluded, ERT conferred a 47% reduction in study end points, which include nonfatal myocardial infarction, fatal and nonfatal stroke, total cardiovascular mortality, and deaths from all causes.[114] The degree of protection associated with estrogen use did not differ based on the duration of estrogen therapy, independent of the patient's age. The only effect of dosage noted was an apparent increase in risk for coronary disease among women using more than 1.25 mg/d estrogen.

Although estrogen replacement therapy in postmenopausal women has been shown to reduce the risk of osteoporosis and coronary heart disease, the effects of estrogen on the risk of stroke is somewhat more controversial, but evidence is mounting that it is protective against this disease as well.[112] In addition, data regarding estrogen-progestin combinations and stroke risk are rather limited. This is an important issue because stroke is one of the leading causes of death in the elderly population, as well as a major cause of disability and morbidity. To clarify these issues, and to further solidify the benefits of ERT, a group from Harvard and the University of Upsala in Sweden evaluated 23,008 women, who were followed over a 6-year period. Depending on the form of estrogen used, the results demonstrated a 25% to 40% overall reduction in first-time strokes. Of special interest is the fact that concomitant use of progestational agents that minimize the risk of endometrial cancer did not seem to counter the benefits of estrogen on stroke risk.[112]

Based on these two studies[107,112] evaluating the risks and benefits of ERT, the following therapeutic approach appears pharmatecturally sound. Virtually all postmenopausal women should be considered candidates for ERT; the final decision should be made by the patient and her physician after weighing all relevant medical and nonmedical (e.g., fear of breast cancer) risks for that individual. A history of breast cancer or other estrogen-sensitive malignancy should be the primary consideration used to evaluate inclusion of estrogen in the drug regimen of a postmenopausal woman. When these risk factors are absent, but one or more risk factors for cardiovascular disease are present, ERT is almost always indicated. The potential risk of initiating ERT in women who already have heart disease also needs to be clarified. A recent study suggests initiation of estrogen in postmenopausal women with a history of myocardial infarction may actually increase the risk of MI recurrence. In women who have had a hysterectomy, the benefits of ERT generally outweigh the risks because there is no risk of endometrial cancer or recurrence of menstrual bleeding. These women should be treated with unopposed estrogen at a daily dose of 0.625 mg conjugated estrogen (Premarin®) or an equivalent oral or transdermal preparation.

In women without hysterectomy, progestins should be added to the drug house to minimize the risk of endometrial cancer. The addition of progestin is important because, as recent studies demonstrate, cardiovascular protection is conferred even when progestin is added to the standard dose of conjugated estrogen. The potential blunting by progestin of beneficial effects on lipid levels associated with estrogen use do not seem to have a major impact on clinical cardiovascular goals. Hence, combination therapy will both provide cardioprotection and decrease risk of endometrial cancer. The standard recommended cyclical estrogen/progestin regimen (0.625 mg conjugated estrogen days 1 to 25 each month, along with 10 mg medroxyprogesterone) frequently results in withdrawal bleeding, which can affect long-term compliance. The use of continuous low-dose progesterone (2.5 mg per day medroxyprogesterone) along with estrogen use can greatly reduce the frequency of bleeding and thereby improve tolerability of ERT. Doses greater than 1.25 mg of conjugated estrogen (or its equivalent) should be avoided. Finally, once a decision to institute estrogen therapy is made, it should be started as soon as possible after the onset of menopause.

Estrogen Agonists/Antagonists: Preventing Breast Cancer. Although their role is not precisely defined, studies suggest that tamoxifen and raloxifene (Evista) can prevent breast cancer. The Tamoxifen Preventive Trial initiated in the U.S. in 1992 followed women at increased risk for breast cancer. Early in 1998, after about four years of follow-up, the study was unblinded because there were 45% fewer cases of breast cancer in the group treated with 20 mg tamoxifen daily. These favorable breast cancer outcomes were not without risk. There was a 2.4-fold increase in postmenopausal endometrial cancer, a 2.8-fold increase in pulmonary embolism, and a 1.6-fold increase in venous thromboembolism. As far as the estrogen agonist/antagonist raloxifene, short-term studies reported at the 1998 meeting of the American Society of Clinical Oncologists showed a 54% overall reduction in all invasive breast tumors at the end of 33 months among 7,705 women treated with raloxifene for osteoporosis. Long-term clinical data will be needed to identify the subgroup of women most likely to benefit from raloxifene prophylaxis.

Raloxifene (Evista) was approved by the FDA in December of 1997, and marked the introduction of a new class of hormones known as selective estrogen reception modulators (SERM). Approved for the prevention of bone wasting (osteoporosis), raloxifene has been the subject of intense investigation because these agents have the capacity to stimulate estrogen receptors in some tissues, while blocking the effects of estrogen stimulation in other tissues. In this regard, raloxifene has estrogen-like effects on bones and cholesterol levels, but does not appear to stimulate, and may even act as an "antiestrogen" in breast and uterine tissues.

Currently, this drug is approved for prevention of bone wasting in postmenopausal women, and is very effective for this indication. The usual dose is 60 mg daily without regard to meals, and supplemental vitamin D and calcium is recommended if dietary intake is inadequate. The daily cost of the drug is about $1.90, which is about five times the cost of Premarin.

The decision to use raloxifene versus standard estrogen therapy (Premarin) must be individualized on a patient-by-patient basis. There are clinically significant differences between the estrogen and estrogen agonists/antagonists that should be considered before making a therapeutic decision. First, although raloxifene shows promise for cardiovascular protection and osteoporosis, long-term outcomes are not presently known; studies are presently underway to settle some of these issues. Hormone replacement with estrogen has been around for many years and has been shown to be safe and effective—and much less expensive.

The proven and postulated benefits of estrogen replacement, including prevention of osteoporosis, heart disease, and possibly, Alzheimer's Disease, are in stark contrast to the unknown effect of raloxifene on these diseases. Estrogen has also been shown to prevent heart disease after coronary artery bypass surgery. Even in the case of bone wasting, the increase in bone mineral density with raloxifene did not seem as impressive as it is for 0.625 mg of Premarin. And while we expect raloxifene to protect against breast cancer (like another SERM, tamoxifen), this is not yet proven.

The potential disadvantages of raloxifene should be mentioned. This drug can worsen post-menopausal symptoms such as hot flashes, vaginal dryness, and decreased sexual desire. Based on this data, raloxifene should be seen as an alternative to estrogen for the prevention of osteoporosis, and viewed as an option for women afraid of or unable to take estrogen.

Aspirin: Prevention of Stroke and Heart Disease. There's nothing like having an aspirin in the house. Although aspirin therapy can cause undesirable side effects (gastric ulceration, gastrointestinal bleeding), it is now clear that, in low doses, salicyclates confer protection from many serious conditions, including recurrent myocardial infarction, embolic stroke associated with chronic atrial fibrillation (in patients who are not candidates for warfarin therapy), colon cancer and ischemic stroke.[32,33,35] These conditions are so prevalent, especially among the elderly—and the necessity for their prevention so urgent—that few individuals in this age group will fail to benefit from inclusion of low-dose aspirin in their drug regimens.[30,31,35,115,116]

Although adjusted-dose warfarin is the standard for stroke prevention in patients with non-valvular atrial fibrillation (AF), such patients are a heterogeneous group with widely variable stroke rates within subgroups. The Stroke Prevention in AF (SPAF) III study prospectively studied low-risk AF patients—i.e., those lacking thromboembolic risk factors—and assessed their thromboembolic event rate on 325 mg aspirin per day. Low-risk outpatients with AF were defined based on absence of four factors: (1) recent heart failure or reduced LV function;

(2) systolic BP < 160 mm Hg; (3) previous thromboembolism; or (4) females older than 75. Although patients developed risk factors at a rate of 6% per year, the primary event rate on aspirin was 2% per year, and disabling strokes occurred at less than 1% per year in low-risk AF patients on 325 mg/day of aspirin. A history of hypertension increased the observed stroke rate to 4% per year, as did age, which increased the stroke rate to 1.7% per year. The major bleeding rate was 0.5% per year, and almost all were gastrointestinal bleeds.

The study suggests patients can be divided into three risk groups: (1) a low-risk group (embolic event rate 1%) with no hypertension, no LV dysfunction, no prior embolic events and no women >75 years of age; (2) an intermediate risk group (stroke rate 3-4% per year) with hypertension; and (3) a high-risk group with two or more of the risks cited above. The high risk group clearly benefits from adjusted-dose warfarin therapy (see below), as do patients with valvular disease and other indications for warfarin. The low-risk group can be treated with aspirin 325 mg/day alone; whether aspirin alone is sufficient for the intermediate risk group is not known, although most experts would lean toward warfarin for this group. Overall, it appears that the group of AF outpatients who achieve adequate thromboembolic prophylaxis with aspirin alone is growing.

When considering aspirin prophylaxis, it should be stressed that, depending on the condition for which protection is being contemplated, different doses of aspirin are required. For prevention of recurrent myocardial infarction, 80 mg aspirin orally each day (or, alternatively, 160 mg orally every other day) has been shown to substantially decrease adverse cardiovascular events. In the absence of contraindications, this dose of aspirin should be used in all patients who have sustained a myocardial infarction. The role of aspirin in *primary* prevention of heart attacks is less clear, although data points in the direction of using low-dose aspirin for primary prevention of myocardial infarction in all male patients over 45 who have at least one coronary risk factor and no contraindications to aspirin use. Currently, most consensus panels recommend low-dose aspirin for men > 45 years of age, diabetics, individuals with a family history of polyposis of the colon, and, of course, all individuals with evidence of coronary or cerebrovascular disease. The value of aspirin for primary prevention in elderly women is not confirmed. A smaller Dutch TIA Trial Study Group has compared two doses of aspirin (30 mg vs. 283 mg) in patients after a transient ischemic attack (TIA) or minor stroke and found that extremely low doses (i.e., 30 mg) can be effective for stroke prevention.[32,34,35]

Aspirin is shown to reduce the risks of death from vascular causes, stroke, and nonfatal myocardial infarction in patients with a previous stroke or TIAs. The need for stroke prevention in elderly patients with history of TIA or stroke is especially pressing, since the annual risk for a serious vascular event is about 10% per year. The Dutch group followed 2,000 elderly patients for about 2.6 years and found that low-dose aspirin (30 mg) equaled standard dose (283 mg) aspirin in ability to prevent death from vascular causes, nonfatal stroke, and nonfatal myocardial infarction. The incidence of major bleeding complications was reduced only slightly, compared with patients taking 283 mg/day, whereas the incidence of minor bleeding complications was reduced by almost 50%.

Based on these studies, there should almost always be an aspirin in the drug house. From a pharmatectural perspective, aspirin is an important foundation drug in all older patients who have had a previous stroke, myocardial infarction, or TIA. The question remains, exactly how much aspirin is enough to acheive prevention, yet minimize side effects. At present, aspirin doses should be tailored to the specific patient. When secondary prevention of stroke or TIA is the objective, the 30 mg dose is also justified based on results of the aforementioned Dutch Trial. When prevention of recurrent myocardial infarction is the goal, the accepted dose of 80 mg aspirin/day is appropriate. When aspirin therapy is being considered to prevent stroke in patients with chronic atrial fibrillation, higher doses (325 mg/day) are recommended.[117] (For additional information, see Chapter 4, Section on Clinical Guidelines for Antithrombotic Therapy.)

Stroke Prevention and Warfarin (Coumadin®). It should be stressed that stroke prevention in chronic atrial fibrillation is best managed with low-dose warfarin (Coumadin®) therapy, which produces a 74% reduction in systemic and cerebrovascular embolization over 1 year compared with placebo. However, occasionally patients are poor candidates for warfarin, and aspirin should be considered as a substitute. When prevention of stroke associated with chronic atrial fibrillation is the goal, the only dose of aspirin shown to be consistently protective is 325 mg/day.[31,117,118]

Individuals with atrial fibrillation who are ideally suited for warfarin prophylaxis include those without a history of gastric or peptic ulcer disease, patients who are not at risk for traumatic injuries due to falls, patients with no previous history of hemorrhagic stroke, individuals with well-controlled blood pressure, and persons who are likely to be compliant with their medications and participate responsibly in long-term follow-up care. Warfarin should be administered at a dose sufficient to achieve an INR of 2.0 to 3.0. Warfarin doses producing longer INRs do not significantly improve thromboembolic prophylaxis in patients with chronic atrial fibrillation. In addition, the best benefit-to-risk ratios for warfarin use are reported in elderly patients with documented heart disease and left ventricular impairment. The use of warfarin in younger individuals who have intermittent or lone atrial fibrillation, but no coronary artery disease, is controversial. Those patients who, because of their risk and/or compliance profiles, are unsuitable candidates for warfarin prophylaxis in atrial fibrillation, may benefit from aspirin prophylaxis (325 mg aspirin/day), which has been shown to reduce the rate of systemic and cerebral embolization by about 49% per year. It should be stressed that in eligible patients either warfarin or aspirin should be selected for thromboembolic prophylaxis, and that, as a rule, the two agents should not be used in combination unless the increased risk of gastrointestinal hemorrhage is justified (e.g., recurrent thromboembolic events during adequate warfarin therapy).[33,34] Also clear is the fact that *high-risk* AF patients clearly benefit more from warfarin than aspirin therapy.

Beta-Blockers for Prevention of Myocardial Reinfarction. It is well-known that some patients do not tolerate beta-blocker therapy and, therefore, are at greater risk for experiencing myriad side effects associated with this drug class, including depression, cardiosuppression, conduction disturbances, and bradycardia. For these reasons, many older patients simply are never even considered to be candidates for long-term, prevention-oriented therapy with this drug—a pattern of underuse that is emphasized in medical and pharmacological literature.[29,36] This is unfortunate, because in older patients, including diabetics, with coronary heart disease, the potential side effects of the drug are outweighed by the proven benefits associated with reduction of arrhythmias and recurrent myocardial infarction.[70,119,120]

Beta-blockers have been shown to reduce blood pressure, lower heart rate, and decrease threshold for ventricular arrhythmias, which appears to explain their documented efficacy in reducing mortality and sudden death following myocardial infarction. Initiation of intravenous beta-blocker therapy (when not contraindicated) shortly after myocardial infarction and then continuing long-term outpatient beta-blocker therapy will reduce cardiovascular mortality by 22% to 27% over a 2-year period.[36] Consequently, beta-blockers should be considered a fundamental building block in the drug regimens of *all* patients who have myocardial infarction, have no contraindications to the drug's use, and who demonstrate a willingness to tolerate this agent's potential side effects. With respect to drug choice and dose, atenolol (Tenormin®) 25 mg to 50 mg/day, is an acceptable initial dose for secondary prevention in coronary heart disease.

CHOLESTEROL-REDUCING AGENTS

According to the Framingham Heart Study, the prevalence of coronary artery disease in the diabetic patient is about twice that in the general Population. Although the increased susceptibility to heart disease is almost certainly related in part to impaired glucose homeostasis, the patient with NIDDM is also susceptible to abnormalities in the lipoprotein metabolism that include increases in plasma VLDL triglycerides and VLDL and LDL cholesterol, and decreases in HDL cholesterol. Based on epidemiologic studies in the general population, there is evidence to suggest that pharmacologic and dietary interventions that achieve beneficial effects on plasma lipid levels (i.e., reduction in serum LDL and VLDL cholesterol and elevation of HDL cholesterol) may decrease the risk of coronary heart disease in patients with NIDDM.

According to available data, an average reduction in total cholesterol levels of 26%, as observed with lovastatin therapy, should reduce the risk of coronary heart disease by about 50%. This reduction in risk should put patients with NIDDM at about the same baseline risk for heart disease as the general population.

The relative importance of multiple factors that place patients with NIDDM at increased risk for heart disease is not precisely known. Nevertheless, reduction of elevated plasma cholesterol and triglyceride levels with dietary or pharmacologic intervention is advisable in diabetic patients with risk factors for coronary artery disease.

Unfortunately, despite the potential life-prolonging effects of lipid-lowering medications, compliance with this therapeutic class is less than optimal. In a study evaluating 7,287 Medicaid enrollees (82% women) in New Jersey, patients failed to fill lipid-lowering drug prescriptions for about 40% of the study year. In addition, patients were more likely to comply with statins than with cholestyramine (prescriptions filled 64% vs. 36% of the days of the year). As might be expected, individuals with hypertension, diabetes, or coronary artery disease were more likely to persist with the medication.

Guidelines for Screening and Treatment of Hypercholesterolemia

Hypercholesterolemia remains one of the leading risk factors for coronary heart disease (CHD), affecting over 20% of the population. Effective means for its detection and treatment are available, but many unresolved issues remain, including whom to screen, what to screen for, whom to treat, and what is the best approach to treatment. Several years ago the National Institutes of Health established the Expert Panel on the Detection, Evaluation, and Treatment of High Blood Cholesterol in Adults. This consensus panel established the National Cholesterol Education Program and has just issued its Second Report, which addresses many of the basic questions related to screening and treatment of hypercholesterolemia.

In formulating its Second Report,[60] the panel considered the expanding body of new data that has become available since its First Report in 1988. The basic approach to screening is reasserted, namely that a non-fasting cholesterol be obtained every 5 years in adults 20 years of age and older. Added to this position is the recommendation that an HDL cholesterol be obtained at the same time, provided the means are available for its accurate detection. This addition of an HDL cholesterol determination is based on recognition of the emerging importance of a low HDL cholesterol (<35 mg/dl) as an independent risk factor for coronary disease. The use of total CHD risk as the basis for management decision continues to be recommended and reemphasized. A gradient of risk is identified and based in part on CHD risk factors in addition to degree of LDL cholesterol elevation, which continues to be the predominant determinant of CHD risk due to hypercholesterolemia. Hypercholesterolemic patients with established CHD or another form of atherosclerotic disease (peripheral arterial insufficiency, symptomatic carotid artery disease) are assigned to the highest category of risk. Those with 2 major CHD risk factors (smoking, hypertension, diabetes, family history of premature CHD, male sex, age >45 in men and >55 in women, low HDL cholesterol) but no established CHD are in the next highest risk category. Those with hypercholesterolemia and less than 2 major risk factors are in the last of the increased risk categories.

Management decisions are based predominantly on this risk assessment and can be summarized in the following table adopted from the Second Report:

Patient Category	Initial LDL Level (mg/dl)	LDL Goal (mg/dl)
DIETARY THERAPY		
No CHD, <2 risk factors	>160	<160
No CHD, >2 risk factors	>130	<130
With CHD	>100	<100
ADD DRUG TREATMENT		
No CHD, <2 risk factors	>190	<160
No CHD, >2 risk factors	>160	<130
With CHD	>130	<100

Also addressed was the finding of an increase in non-cardiac deaths among those treated with lipid-lowering medication but not among those treated with diet alone. The reasons for this finding are unknown at present. The increase nullifies the reductions achieved in cardiac deaths and caused the panel to recommend delaying use of drug therapy in most young persons and pre-menopausal women who are at otherwise low CHD risk.

The panel recommended more attention be given to recognition and treatment of low HDL cholesterol because of its role as a major CHD risk factor. Finally, the benefits of exercise and weight reduction are emphasized and urged as important complements to a dietary program.

The Second Report goes a long way toward correcting some of the deficiencies of the first, particularly the inattention to the potential importance of HDL cholesterol, exercise, and weight reduction. The panel's special contribution of basing management recommendations on total CHD risk and not just degree of lipid abnormality is strengthened and made even more clinically useful. Finally, the recognition of a potential risk associated with use of pharmacologic therapy is an important caution—one that should encourage more emphasis on non-pharmacologic efforts, especially in young, lower risk persons. However, pharmacologic therapy remains very important in very-high-risk persons, such as those with established CHD. Their reduction in CHD risk with use of drug therapy far exceeds the observed increase in risk of noncardiac deaths.

Following release of the NCEP guidelines, many new studies provide a robust and persuasive database supporting LDL cholesterol-lowering in the large majority of patients with CAD or normal subjects with mild or moderate dyslipidemia—with or without other CAD risk factors. The Air Force/Texas Coronary Atherosclerosis Study (AF/TEXCAPS) enrolled 6,605 healthy individuals (15% women) who were free of clinical CAD and randomized to lovastatin or placebo. The subjects had an average total and LDL cholesterol, and below average HDL cholesterol. At 5.2 years of average follow-up, lovastatin reduced the risk of fatal or nonfatal MI by 40%, and unstable angina by 32%. In addition, treatment with the statin reduced the need for revascularization by one-third and the risk for both cardiovascular and coronary events by one-fourth. The target LDL-C level was 110 mg/dl, less than that recommended by NCEP target goals in individuals with 2 or more coronary risk factors.

Along with 4S, CARE, and LIPID trials, AFCAP/TEXCAPS confirms that lipid lowering is effective in the elderly and is at least as beneficial in women as in men. In addition to cardiovascular events, these studies also point to LDL cholesterol lowering as effective for lowering risk of cerebrovascular disease in individuals free of this condition prior to entry. AFCAP/TEXCAPS also suggest that individuals at highest risk—diabetics, smokers, and hypertensives—have the greatest proportional benefits associated with LDL cholesterol reduction.

Pneumococcal Vaccine for Prevention of Complications and Severity of Pneumonia. Some prevention-oriented building blocks (e.g., aspirin, estrogen) are used on a daily basis, and can be viewed as a permanent part of a patient's drug house. In contrast, other agents, such as the polyvalent pneumococcal vaccine (Pneumovax®), are introduced in the pharmacologic environment every six years to provide seasonal reinforcement for prevention of complications of high-risk diseases, such as pneumonia. Based on recent studies evaluating the efficacy of the vaccine in selected populations, it seems prudent to recommend vaccination of all elderly individuals with a high-risk condition (e.g., coronary heart disease, diabetes, congestive heart failure, pulmonary disease, alcoholism, rheumatoid arthritis, stroke, chronic hepatic disease, and renal insufficiency) that places them at high risk for complications of pneumococcal pneumonia and associated infectious complications.[121] Patients with severe liver or kidney disease, or with AIDS, require more frequent vaccination.

ACE Inhibitors to Prevent MI and Congestive Heart Failure. Many older patients suffer from cardiovascular disease and, consequently, live in drug houses that reflect chronic therapy directed at preventing recurrence and/or deterioration of heart-related conditions. In this vein, the rationale for including aspirin, estrogen, and/or beta-blockers as part of the permanent foundation for selected patients has been discussed in detail above. The role of vitamin E, folic acid, and statins also should be considered. ACE inhibitors should be used for their preventive properties in patients with heart disease. Initially, ACE inhibitors were introduced for management of hypertension. However, studies also confirm their usefulness in prolonging longevity and decreasing morbidity (including the need for hospitalization) in patients who have symptomatic congestive heart failure (CHF) and for improving their exercise tolerance and functional status. Accordingly, this drug class has become the mainstay of patients with early, symptomatic CHF, especially when it is part of a regimen that also includes digoxin and diuretics.[122-124]

The role of these agents in *asymptomatic* patients is less clear. However, recent trials now confirm that ACE inhibitors such as enalapril and captopril may play an equally important therapeutic and prevention-oriented role in patients with *asymptomatic* left-ventricular dysfunction following myocardial infarction. In particular, the evidence confirms that long-term administration of captopril (25 mg to 50 mg by mouth three times daily) is associated with a reduction in morbidity and mortality from major cardiovascular events. The ISIS IV trial, in fact, suggests that ACE inhibitors probably have cardioprotective effects in patients who have had MI, even in the *absence* of left ventricular dysfunction. The reduction in re-infarction was potentiated in the subgroup treated with a combination of ACE inhibitors and nitrates. In an attempt to evaluate the possible cardioprotective effects of ACE inhibitors in diabetics, GISSI-3 investigators retrospectively analyzed their data with respect to a history of diabetes and insulin use. In GISSI-3, suspected acute MI patients were randomized to lisinopril with or without nitrates within 24 hours following MI. They found ACEI treatment decreased mortality at six weeks from 12% in the no therapy group to 9%. The 30% mortality reduction with lisinopril in the diabetic group was much greater than the 5% reduction observed in non-diabetics. The study suggests ACE inhibitor use post-MI may affect outcomes in the diabetic patient. In addition, when ranipril (up to 20 mg/d) was compared to HCTZ (up to 50 mg/d), superior regression of LV hypertrophy was observed.

Based on these studies, then, it is reasonable to prescribe ACE inhibitors for patients who have ejection fractions lower than 0.40, asymptomatic LV dysfunction, and perhaps, *all* individuals, following MI. Benefits are observed when ACE inhibition is instituted within 3 to 16 days after myocardial infarction and are independent of the advantages conferred by use of beta-blockers and aspirin, as discussed above—who are recovering from a myocardial infarction. When ACE inhibitors are indicated, it is essential to prescribe sufficiently high doses of the drug, i.e., doses higher than those used to treat hypertension and which have been shown to prolong survival in patients with CHF.

ACE Inhibitors for Prevention of Diabetic Renal Disease. ACE inhibitors (i.e., captopril, enalapril) also should be considered essential pharmacologic building blocks for type II normotensive diabetics with microalbuminuria and *normal* renal function. Although the exact mechanism of the beneficial effects of ACE inhibitors on preservation of renal function is unclear, it most likely relates, at least in part, to the ability of these drugs to dilate the efferent arteriole of the glomerulus, decrease intraglomerular capillary pressure, and reduce capillary membrane permeability.[123-125]

Most of the evidence regarding the benefits of ACE inhibitors on preserving renal function in diabetics have accrued from studies primarily involving patients with type I diabetes. Although approximately 40% of type I diabetics eventually develop nephropathy compared with 20% of type II patients, there are 10 times as many patients with type II disease as there are with type I. Consequently, the absolute number of patients with end-stage renal disease with type II diabetes far exceeds those with type I.

That ACE inhibitors help slow the progression of nephropathy in type II diabetes is confirmed by a very carefully conducted Israeli study that demonstrated amelioration of proteinuria and preservation of renal function in normotensive patients with type II diabetes. This relatively long trial consisted of type II diabetics whose blood pressure was normal at entry and was controlled as necessary during the study. Normotensive patients were given enalapril 10 mg/day. Every 3 to 4 months over a period of 5 years, blood glucose, creatinine, electrolytes, glycosylated hemoglobin, and 24-hour urine protein excretion were determined. During the course of the study, if elevated blood pressure (systolic blood pressure > 145 mm Hg or diastolic blood pressure > 95 mm Hg) was detected on two separate occasions (i.e., enalapril *alone* was not able to control blood pressure), treatment with long-acting nifedipine (Procardia XL®) was instititued. Over the study period, albuminuria essentially remained stable in the enalapril group, while increasing significantly in patients on placebo. Renal function declined by only 1% in the enalapril group, whereas in the placebo group renal function steadily deteriorated by 13% overall between the initial evaluation and 5-year follow-up.[125] This study provides compelling evidence for inclusion of ACE inhibitors to prevent renal disease in patients who have had type II diabetes for a period of less than 10 years and who demonstrate microalbuminuria.[125]

Tight blood pressure control is clearly the most effective means of slowing the progression of nephropathy in diabetic patients with hypertension and renal insufficiency. ACE inhibitors have become important agents for these patients because they have the most consistent effects on reducing proteinuria and preserving renal function in this population. It may still be premature to prescribe this drug uniformly to all patients with type II diabetes, at least until longer-term trials using more precise measurements of renal function are available. Nevertheless, ACE inhibitors are probably justified routinely in type I diabetics, in whom microalbuminuria and a positive family history for cardiovascular disease or hypertension or both are known to be risk factors for nephropathy. In patients with type II diabetes, only microalbuminuria was shown to predict nephropathy and increased morbidity associated with renal deterioration. Based on recent studies, then, it seems justified to consider the routine, prophylactic use of low-dose ACE inhibitors (e.g., enalapril 10 mg every day) in patients with type II diabetes and microalbuminuria, even in the *absence* of hypertension. When hypertension is present with microalbuminuria, ACE inhibitors can be considered smart drugs because they service two target organs (peripheral vasculature and kidneys) with a single prescription ingredient. This prevention-oriented approach to drug house construction is likely to reduce the long-term costs of servicing renal deterioration and related complications associated with this common clinical disorder.

Finally, it should be pointed out that about 50% of patients on an ACE inhibitor for hypertension may have their hypertension control attenuated by an aspirin dose of 300 mg ASA/day, regardless of the severity of their hypertension. A 100 mg ASA/day regimen does not appear to counteract the vasodilatory dose of ACE inhibitors.

Misoprostol (Cytotec®) and Omeprazole (Prilosec®) for Prevention of NSAID-Induced Peptic Ulceration. Although necessary for many older patients with severe osteoarthritis, chronic use of NSAIDs may compromise the safety of geriatric drug regimens. Not surprisingly, one of the most controversial areas in the area of preventive pharmacologic maintenance concerns the use of misoprostol in countering the adverse gastrointestinal effects of NSAIDs. The debate as to whether and when misoprostol should be used to prevent NSAID-induced gastrointestinal hemorrhage continues. This is a very important issue because NSAIDs are widely used, the associated risks are significant, and the cost of prevention could be staggering. Almost 100 million prescriptions are written annually in the United States for NSAIDs, exposing about 8% of the population to its side effect risks and complications, which are estimated to cost $3.9 billion per year for the arthritic population alone.[83,126,127]

Although NSAIDs are associated with a wide range of problems that include gastrointestinal tract bleeding, renal dysfunction, and central nervous system changes, this important drug class is highly effective in reducing pain, minimizing functional impairment, and improving quality of life for several million elderly individuals with chronic osteoarthritis and other inflammatory disorders. As a result, balancing the therapeutic properties of NSAIDs against their potential liabilities is an important clinical issue.

Not surprisingly, most attempts at reducing the risk of NSAID-mediated gastrointestinal tract hemorrhage focused on prophylaxis against the development of gastric erosions and ulceration. Many pharmacists and physicians recommend traditional antiulcer therapies, such as histamine-2 receptor antagonists, antacids, and sucralfate, even though these drugs are not effective in preventing ulcerations, nor are they approved by the FDA for this purpose. A more aggressive approach advocates the use of misoprostol, a synthetic prostaglandin E1 analogue that reduces the risk of NSAID-induced ulcers, and perhaps their complications. At issue is its efficacy in patients on long-term NSAID therapy.

The debate surrounding misoprostol use for prevention is especially fierce, and in response to an aggressive marketing campaign launched by the drug's manufacturer, clinicians are divided. One group, which responds with great sensitivity to medico-legal concerns, advocates universal prophylaxis with misoprostol in all elderly patients who are committed to long-term therapy with NSAIDs for primary prevention of gastrointestinal tract hemorrhage. Another faction recommends misoprostol prophylaxis in all patients with a history of "gastric symptoms or complaints" and in all patients 60 years and older requiring chronic NSAID therapy. Still another group suggests that misoprostol use should be limited to a select population of patients who have had radiographically or endoscopically proven gastric or peptic ulceration (secondary prevention). Still another group offers this consensus: the risk of gastrointestinal tract hemorrhage in those patients with a previous history of bleeding gastric ulcer is so great that the more prudent course is to avoid NSAIDs altogether and consider other forms of therapy.

Two recent, related studies (called the OMNIUM and ASTRONAUT studies) have examined the effects of a variety of regimens on ulcers related to nonsteroidal anti-inflammatory drugs (NSAIDs). In the first study, 935 older individuals on chronic NSAID therapy—who had ulcers or 10 or more erosions—were treated with omeprazole 20 or 40 mg daily, or misoprostol 200 mcg daily and evaluated at six months. Investigators found that the overall rates of successful treatment of ulcers, erosions, and symptoms associated with NSAIDs were similar for the two doses of omeprazole and for misoprostol. Therapy with omeprazole was associated with a lower rate of relapse than misoprostol and was better tolerated. In the second study, 541 patients who *required* continuous treatment with NSAIDs, and who also had ulcers or erosions, were randomly assigned to either omeprazole 20 or 40 mg daily or ranitidine 150 mg orally bid for 4-8 weeks. The initial treatment response was better with both doses of omeprazole rather than ranitidine, with a 79-80% success rate on the proton blocker and a 63% success rate in those on ranitidine.

These large, well conducted studies shed valuable light on how to prevent NSAID-related gastrointestinal complications. First, acid-suppressing drugs are effective in healing NSAID-related ulcers and erosions, in relieving NSAID-related symptoms, and preventing NSAID-related pathology following initial healing if the drugs are continued. Second, the proton pump inhibitor, omeprazole, in a dose of 20-40 mg daily, is more effective than ranitidine in healing NSAID ulcers. And third, although initial healing rates for misoprostol and omeprazole were similar, omeprazole was more effective in the prevention of relapse and was better tolerated. Based on these studies, it appears as if the proton pump blocker omeprazole is the agent of choice for patients with NSAID-related upper GI erosions or ulcerations and who require long-term NSAID therapy.

Based on landmark studies trying to evaluate this issue, omeprazole or misoprostol is cost-effective and pharmatecturally justifiable in patients who absolutely require NSAID therapy for their condition and who also have a documented history of gastrointestinal ulceration, erosions, or hemorrhage.[104,127,128] They probably should not be used for *routine* prophylactic use in patients whose only risk factor is age. Finally, it must be emphasized that the use of NSAIDs in any patient with a previous history of gastrointestinal tract hemorrhage or ulceration carries a risk that, even with misoprostol prophylaxis, is formidable enough to warrant consideration of therapeutic options other than NSAIDs.[126]

Preventive maintenance is required for all drug houses in which NSAIDs are used as a building material in order to prevent complications associated with this therapeutic class. Based on many studies evaluating the risk, prevention, and epidemiology of NSAID-induced gastrointestinal tract hemorrhage, the following recommendations should be incorporated into drug house construction and surveillance practices: (1) Because there is a significant association between increasing doses of NSAIDs and the risk of developing peptic ulcer disease and complications requiring hospitalization, pharmacists and physicians are advised to use the lowest dose of NSAID possible to achieve acceptable functional status and pain control in patients with osteoarthritic disorders; (2) because the risk for developing NSAID-induced complications is observed during the first 30 days of drug therapy, patients should be followed very carefully during this vulnerable period. The presence of gastrointestinal complaints, weakness, melena, or other symptoms referrable to the gastrointestinal tract or cardiovascular system necessitate immediate follow-up; and (3) monitoring for occult blood is strongly recommended in older patients requiring standard or greater doses of NSAIDs.[129,130]

When It's Time To Remodel: Designer Drug Houses

Once a prevention-oriented foundation is in place, adverse drug events and side effects have been minimized, and routine safety checks are completed, it is time to evaluate the structural integrity of the drug house. This means taking into consideration both the level of craftsmanship and choice of *specific* materials, and a drug-by-drug evaluation of the pharmacological environment. Indications, schedules, and dosages for specific agents and classes of drugs that are commonly misused should be assessed. In this regard, cardiovascular agents, antidepressants, sedative-hypnotics, and antipsychotic drugs deserve the greatest scrutiny. Based on such parameters as safety, half-life, and smartness, there are generally better and worse building blocks within each drug class, and there are inferior and superior remodeling strategies. Oftentimes, it is preferrable to educate and evaluate, rather than medicate.

Home Is Where The Heart Is: Designing Cardiovascular Drug Houses

Drugs with cardiovascular effects must be used with special care, especially in the older age group, in which one-half of all DRAPEs are associated with medications used to treat coronary artery disease, high blood pressure, and congestive heart failure. The pitfalls associated with cardiovascular drugs come in many different forms. For example, digoxin half-life may increase by 40% in normal elderly patients, and even levels of digoxin in the therapeutic range may produce nonspecific symptoms (such as anorexia or changes in mental status) normally attributed to chronic illness. Elderly hypertensive patients have impaired homeostatic mechanisms and are prone to postural hypotension. Diuretics can produce hypokalemia, hypovolemia, fatigue, and hypotension, especially in combination with potent vasodilators and anticholinergic antidepressants. The cost-savings associated with using diuretic agents or beta-blockers as initial therapy in hypertension must be weighed against the possibility of quality-of-life disturbances which, although usually not life-threatening, can be irksome and irritating over the long term. Other antihypertensive agents, such as ACE inhibitors, can cause cough, especially in elderly females. Use of angiotensin receptor blockers (losartan, etc.) may ameliorate this problem. Among the calcium channel blockers, verapamil should be noted for its propensity to cause bradycardia, conduction disturbances, and myocardial suppression, especially when used in the elderly who are taking high doses of beta-blockers. In general, vigilance is required when selecting drugs used to treat cardiovascular disorders. Special design considerations with respect to prescribing for cardiovascular conditions apply to a number of therapeutic agents and drug classes, which are discussed below.[3,91,92,94,131,132]

Digoxin: Cost-Effective Maintenance. For no single drug is the application of TPQM™ more important than it is for the time-honored cardiac glycoside, digoxin (Lanoxin®). Digoxin is the sixth most commonly prescribed drug in the United States, it has a long and distinguished history that dates to antiquity, and yet, debate still rages concerning its appropriate use for long-term therapy of cardiovascular conditions. Because of its widespread use and narrow toxic/therapeutic ratio, many pharmacists and physicians have started questioning indiscriminate digoxin use in the outpatient setting and are attempting to identify more precisely those patients most likely to benefit from its long-term use. Although a number of studies have questioned the appropriateness of digoxin therapy for patients with congestive heart failure, as well as its relative efficacy compared to ACE inhibitors, most experts still agree that at least one of the following indications must be met to justify inclusion of digoxin in the regimen of patients with cardiovascular disease: (1) control of rapid ventricular rate in patients with chronic atrial fibrillation; (2) improvement of myocardial performance in patients with congestive heart failure associated with left ventricular systolic dysfunction[133] or (3) as an add-on medication for patients who are already taking maximal doses of an ACE inhibitor for treatment of CHF.

As a rule, prescribing digoxin to patients with rapid ventricular rates precipitated by atrial fibrillation is usually straightforward and rarely poses a clinical dilemma. When chronic atrial fibrillation is present, and attempts at pharmacologic or electrical cardioversion are unsuccessful, digoxin is indicated for rate control. Lower doses (0.125 mg digoxin daily) should be tried first to achieve rate control and should be increased only if lower doses are unsuccessful. Although digoxin should be used in patients with atrial fibrillation and a rapid ventricular rate, the drug regimen should also include either coumadin or aspirin to prevent thromboembolic complications as indiciated.

If the use of digoxin in atrial fibrillation is rather straightforward, selecting patients with ventricular systolic dysfunction, or those patients with congestive heart failure who are appropriate candidates for digoxin therapy, is much more problematic. The fact is, digoxin is still *overused* to treat congestive heart failure. Interestingly, digoxin is overused in this patient population not because it isn't useful for the management of congestive heart failure—it is extremely effective for the symptomatic treatment of systolic dysfunction—but because congestive heart failure is *overdiagnosed* in the *outpatient* setting. Studies suggest that up to 42% of patients presently receiving digoxin are taking the drug for questionable reasons and that digoxin can be discontinued in these individuals without compromising their clinical status.[35] Further, a significant number of elderly patients have diastolic dysfunction, which is more appropriately treated with ACE inhibitors.

Because digoxin is a widely prescribed agent, the pharmaco-economic and clinical consequences of inappropriate prescribing can be significant. To determine what clinical criteria must be satisfied to justify cost-effective use of digoxin in patients with normal sinus rhythm, a Veterans Administration Hospital Study in San Francisco evaluated 242 patients in order to identify potential pitfalls associated with digoxin use. To reduce the risk of unnecessary prescribing for this drug, they attempted to determine whether noninvasive testing (i.e., echocardiography) is indicated in outpatients to establish the diagnosis of congestive heart failure. In this investigation, patients with documented atrial fibrillation and confirmed left ventricular systolic dysfunction (ejection fraction less than 45%)

were classified appropriate candidates for digoxin therapy. With respect to establishing guidelines for digoxin use, the two most important observations were: (1) the finding that 18% of patients receiving digoxin for congestive heart failure and normal sinus rhythm had *preserved* systolic function; and (2) the finding that detection of an S3 gallop on physical examination was neither specific nor sensitive for decreased ejection fraction.

Based on these findings, it was concluded that the major problem associated with excessive use of digoxin in this population is the *difficulty of assessing left ventricular systolic dysfunction.* Because a substantial percentage of patients with normal sinus rhythm are at risk of being inaccurately diagnosed as having systolic dysfunction, and consequently being started on digoxin therapy, the investigators recommended that all patients in whom digoxin therapy is contemplated undergo noninvasive left ventricular assessment to ensure that appropriate criteria are met for institution of digoxin therapy. This investigation is important from a pharmaco-economic standpoint because it identifies a subset of patients (i.e., those with normal sinus rhythm) who, in the absence of noninvasive echocardiographic studies, are at especially high risk for being inaccurately diagnosed as having systolic ventricular dysfunction.[133-136] Even more important, perhaps, is the fact that echocardiographic assessment can provide valuable information that enhances patient management, suggest clinical conditions not appreciated on physical examination, and spare a large number of patients the unnecessary risks and subtle toxic effects of long-term digoxin therapy.[134-136]

At present, patients who are in normal sinus rhythm and are taking digoxin should be evaluated for the possibility of digoxin discontinuation. Noninvasive assessment of cardiac function is the best method for evaluating a patient's suitability for digoxin cessation. In this regard, if echocardiographic assessment demonstrates normal left ventricular systolic function, and the patient is not taking an ACE inhibitor, the dose of digoxin can be gradually decreased. The patient's progress should be monitored every 2 weeks to ensure that clinical deterioration does not result from the drug's discontinuation.

Digoxin and ACE Inhibitors. Whether digoxin can, or should, be discontinued in patients already taking an ACE inhibitor is another matter altogether. Although digoxin has been the traditional choice for treatment of congestive heart failure, in recent years ACE inhibitors have been shown to improve clinical status and survival in patients with congestive heart failure. As more patients are being treated with ACE inhibitors, an important question is whether the use of ACE inhibitors obviates the need for digoxin therapy. In other words, can digoxin be eliminated from a regimen that contains an ACE inhibitor? This is an important issue from a pharmatectural perspective because it suggests an opportunity to streamline drug therapy in patients with cardiovascular conditions.

To answer this question, a multi-center group conducted a study[103] on the effect of withdrawing digoxin from patients with chronic congestive heart failure. The patients had class II or III heart failure, with a left ventricular ejection fraction of less than 35%, and were clinically stable on a program of digoxin, diuretics, and ACE inhibitors. Heart failure worsened severely enough in 23 of the 93 patients randomized to withdrawal of digoxin to warrant their dropping out of the study, compared to 4 of the 85 patients who continued to receive the cardiac glycoside. The risk of increasing the severity of heart failure was six times greater in the group in whom digoxin was discontinued. Similar deteriorations in quality of life, ejection fraction, heart rate, and body weight were also noted. Of interest, many of the changes did not occur until several *weeks* after discontinuing digoxin therapy.[103]

What this study demonstrates is that discontinuing digoxin in patients *known* to have congestive heart failure, even if they are on an ACE inhibitor, is a potentially treacherous plan of action. For patients with chronic congestive heart failure who have systolic dysfunction and an ejection fraction less than 35%, digoxin can be an important component of the medical regimen. Patients responding favorably to a program of digoxin, diuretics, and ACE inhibitors should not have their digoxin withdrawn because there is a significant risk of functional deterioration. Given the proven efficacy of ACE inhibitors in diastolic ventricular dysfunction, their relatively well-tolerated side effect profile, and their improvement of survival in patients with congestive heart failure, many pharmacists and physicians advocate that initial therapy for congestive heart failure include this drug class. In a study evaluating 7500 patients with confirmed CHF on digoxin, it was found that digoxin did *not* improve overall survival, but it did reduce the number of exacerbations of CHF, the number of emergency department visits, and days of hospitalization required for management of CHF.

The Pressure Is On: Designing Regimens For Antihypertensive Therapy. Optimal therapy for high blood pressure remains an extremely controversial issue. As recently as 15 years ago, state-of-the-art management of patients who had mild to moderate elevations in blood pressure and who required drug therapy for their disease was relatively simple, and consisted of merely selecting an agent that would lower diastolic blood pressure to a range between 80 and 90 mm Hg. Because the primary emphasis was on lowering diastolic blood pressure, with minimal concern for other metabolic, renal, cardiovascular, and quality-of-life parameters associated with hypertension, it is not surprising that pharmacists and physicians prescribed reserpine, guanethidine, hydralazine, alphamethyldopa, hydrochlorothiazide, and propranolol.

In 1993, the Fifth Report of the Joint National Committee on Detection, Evaluation, and Treatment of High Blood Pressure (JNC V) attempted to set standards based on a consensus analysis of leaders in the field and contributed to progress in the primary prevention and control of high blood pressure. The JNC V Report introduced recommendations that appear to be motivated primarily by drug acquisition cost issues, rather than by concerns for quality of life, compliance maintenance, comprehensive pharmacologic servicing, smart drug therapy, and reduction in total outcome costs accruing from preventive pharmacologic maintenance. With respect to initial monotherapy for high blood pressure, JNC V argued that because beta-blockers and diuretics are the only classes of drugs shown to reduce cardiovascular morbidity and mortality in controlled clinical trials, these two classes of drugs are preferred for initial drug therapy. The alternative drugs—calcium antagonists, ACE inhibitors, and alpha-one receptor blockers—are equally effective in reducing blood pressure. However, the report argued that, although these alternative drugs have potentially important benefits, they have not been used in long-term controlled clinical trials to demonstrate their efficacy in reducing morbidity and mortality and, therefore, should be reserved for special indications, or when diuretics or beta-blockers are unacceptable or ineffective.

The JNC VI report released in 1998 reconsidered the role of ACE inhibitors and calcium blockers, and upgraded their status to "first line" agents for pharmacological management of hypertension. Calcium channel blockers among them, dihydropyridines such as amlodipine—were identified as suitable for elderly patients with systolic hypertension. Initial antihypertensive therapy with ACE inhibitors should be considered especially in diabetic patients. The expansion of first line agents endorsed by JNV VI is consistent with pharmatectural approaches to medication prescribing in heart disease. This strategy is designed to account for all the "real world" factors that go into the equation for drug selection. These "real world" factors include not only underlying associated conditions, but the cost of drug, the compliance profile, side effects, drug-drug incompatibility, drug-disease incompatibility, regimen durability, the smartness of a medication, and dose stability.

Cardiovascular Therapy: Optimizing Clinical Success Profiles

In general, cardiovascular drugs associated with optimal clinical success profiles will satisfy the following parameters: (1) they will demonstrate *regimen durability,* i.e., they can be used as monotherapy over the long term with a low probability of discontinuation because of side effects, and without the necessity for add-on drugs; (2) the agent will have *cardiokindness,* i.e., it will not have negative inotropic effects, it will not adversely affect the conduction system, it will not cause bradycardia or tachycardia, and it will not produce adverse metabolic effects; and (3) the agent will have dose stability, i.e., it will achieve its therapeutic objectives over the long term at the original starting dose, thereby reducing the toxicity and cost increases associated with higher dose ranges.

Regimen Durability. Treatment of hypertension and cardiovascular disease is a long-term affair. Drugs must be evaluated not only by their capacity to produce short-term results in clinical trials, but according to their capacity for "standing the test of time" as *monotherapy* over the long haul. These drugs represent a *cost-effective* choice because expenditures associated with having to introduce pharmacologic reinforcements—i.e. "add-on" drugs—into the regimen can be prevented. In addition, the long-term use of a *single* agent also is associated with a decreased risk of drug-drug and drug-disease interactions.

Psychoactive Drugs

Psychoactive drugs are often a vital part of medical therapy in the elderly. Unfortunately, they also pose unique problems. The benzodiazepine sedative-hypnotic drugs exemplify a group of drugs that have similar therapeutic effects but vary considerably in their pharmacokinetic properties in the elderly. While death due to overdose with benzodiazepines is rare, these drugs can cause excessive sedation, lethargy, short-term memory impairment, falls, and a decrease in attention and reaction time in the elderly.

Sedatives and Hypnotics: Avoid Safety Violations. Although a recent consensus panel of the National Institutes of Health discouraged the use of hypnotics for chronic insomnia, benzodiazepines may be appropriate for short-term therapy of anxiety or insomnia associated with specific situations.[141] If this class of drug is used, it should be stressed that long-acting agents such as flurazepam hydrochloride (Dalmane®) with a half-life of 150 hours—as well as diazepam (Valium®) and chlordiazepoxide (Librium®)—should be avoided in the geriatric patient. A rational approach would be to consider nonpharmacologic therapies first. If this proves unsuccessful, and a benzodiazepine must be used, those agents with relatively short half-lives such as lorazepam (Ativan®, 12 hour half-life) and temazepam (Restoril®, 10-hour half-life) are preferred.[142-147]

There is considerable debate regarding the safe use of triazolam in older patients, in whom such drug-related side effects as short-term memory loss, addiction potential, and confusion are reported. Triazolam is one of the most widely prescribed hypnotics in the United States. Its relatively short serum half-life reduces the risks of daytime and cumulative sedation compared with longer acting hypnotics such as flurazepam. However, behavioral disturbances and impairment of memory have been reported, with particular concern for the elderly who seem to be more sensitive to the medication. The mechanism and severity of susceptibility to the adverse effects of triazolam remain incompletely defined and the subject of considerable research.[145]

A study at the New England Medical Center in Boston,[100] however, clarified a number of prescribing and pharmacokinetic issues regarding triazolam use in the elderly. Using both 0.125 mg and 0.25 mg doses of the drug, elderly subjects manifested higher serum levels than did younger participants because of a 50% reduction in drug clearance. Degree of sedation and psychomotor retardation were greater in the elderly and paralleled increases in serum triazolam levels.

Post-marketing surveillance studies, which showed many potential problems with triazolam, are widely publicized. These side effects were more frequent at the initial recommended dose of triazolam (i.e., 0.5 mg to 0.75 mg by mouth at bedtime) although, they can also occur with lower doses of the drug. Inasmuch as the dosing range for triazolam has been modified considerably since the drug was introduced into the market, new prescribing practices are possible. When used at the currently recommended dose range of 0.0625 to 0.125 mg triazolam orally, this sedative-hypnotic is well-tolerated and has a side effect profile similar to other short- and intermediate-acting benzodiazepines. The issue of an idiosyncratic behavioral disturbance triggered by triazolam remains a concern, and the literature must still be followed carefully for more details about its occurrence and identifying patients at risk.

Despite the short-term value of intermediate- and short-acting benzodiazepines, these drugs are still overused and inappropriately prescribed for many individuals in the geriatric age group. From a pharmatectural perspective, reduction and/or elimination of benzodiazepine use in the elderly is a remodeling priority. When it comes to insomnia, it is oftentimes preferable to evaluate rather than medicate the patient. Reduction in hypnotic use can be facilitated by characterizing suboptimal prescribing patterns and diagnostic pitfalls associated with overuse of these agents for patients with insomnia.

A study performed by Jerry Avorn at Harvard Medical School has shed light on the diagnostic, assessment, and prescribing patterns that underpin excessive hypnotic use in the elderly.[102] Using an interview format, the study compared the decision-making process of 500 primary care physicians and 300 nurse practitioners when managing a hypothetical 77-year-old patient with insomnia. In this study, fewer than half of all physicians asked for any information about the patient's sleep pattern, and less than one quarter inquired about the patient's evening caffeine consumption. Furthermore, two thirds of physicians recommended the use of a hypnotic, most often triazolam, followed by flurazepam.

Approximately one in three adults in the United States has some trouble sleeping during a given year. Patients clamor for sedatives as sleep aids. Despite the pressures to prescribe, insomnia should always be regarded as a symptom rather than a diagnosis. In some cases, insomnia may be a manifestation of depression, which is appropriately treated with antidepressants. A basic but thorough history to elucidate underlying medical or psychological illnesses, sleep apnea syndrome, or behavioral patterns that may be responsible for the sleep disturbance is essential for proper diagnosis and therapy. Initially, nonpharmacologic approaches to insomnia should be tried in most patients.

Up The Down Staircase: Minding The Drug House

"Why should I take my Elavil?" a depressed patient protested to me 15 years ago. "These drugs make me feel worse than my disease." And she was right. For many years, medications used to treat neuropsychiatric conditions were anything but user-friendly. Although they worked, patients frequently paid a steep price in side effects and risking dangerous drug interactions.

For many, taking these drugs was a worse ordeal than the disease itself. In some cases, side effects were so disrupting to quality-of-life many people let their mood disorders go untreated. Many sought "refuge" in the symptoms of their disease, rather than tolerate the side effects of the medications. Put simply, the potential benefits of these pills didn't justify the known risks and downsides, especially for those with mood disorders of mild to moderate severity.

In the past 20 years, all of this has all changed, especially for the treatment of depression. Finally, psychiatric medications are available that have relatively low "noise levels"—that is, they have minimal side effects, are convenient to take, and produce fewer symptoms than the disease itself. The end result: people actually want to stay on medications for long periods.

The greatest advances have been made for treatment of depression, (Prozac, Zoloft, Paxil), schizophrenia [risperidone (Risperdal), olanzapine (Zyprexa)], and obsessive-compulsive disorders [paroxetine (Paxil), sertraline (Zoloft)]. These pills have improved quality-of-life in people suffering from psychiatric disease.

Such drugs as Prozac (Fluoxetine), Zoloft (sertraline), and Ambien (zolpidem tartrate) have become household words among patients.

The reasons for the evolution are quite clear. The threshold for using these drugs has been lowered to limbo levels by a new class of antidepressants known as selective serotonin reuptake inhibitors (SSRIs).

The signs of depression are unmistakable and the toll on personal and business life potentially devastating. Sadness, crying spells, excessive sleeping or eating, declining libido, and withdrawal—these are the telltale signs and symptoms of depression. Drug therapy is required for most individuals with depressive symptoms that are severe enough to compromise work, sleep patterns, or social activities. One of the most important questions surrounding the use of SSRIs is: Are these drugs overused? Maybe, but maybe not. Better living through chemistry does not, and should not, play favorites. What is so different about the hundreds of thousands of people with a chemical "make-up" that predisposes them to high cholesterol levels taking drugs to reduce their risk for heart disease, from those with a "chemical" predisposition for depression taking SSRIs to reduce their risk for a lifetime of psyche-scorching melancholy? Probably, there is very little difference.

Are antidepressants being used appropriately? Or, have these medications become such a permanent part of our personal—and now, collective—pharmacology that we've lost sight of which mood swings are serious enough to be treated with drugs, and which ones are a normal part of life and should simply be left alone, without pharmacological tweaking. Have the SSRIs become "quick fixes?" Many experts would say, "Yes, these drugs are ubiquitous and overused, and we have lost perspective." They would argue we have taken the path of least resistance by pressing pills into service for every minor psycho-perturbation that ails us.

There are no easy answers, but the fact is, these medications are probably underused. Deciding when to use these medications can be difficult. After all, depression doesn't begin at one serotonin level and suddenly disappear at another. To a great extent, a patient's suitability for antidepressant therapy depends on whether the relationship between friction-causing events in the external world (divorce, disappointment, disability, and death) and the neurotransmitters that make up their internal chemistry, produces symptoms that are disabling enough to get in the way of life's "normal" functions. Each patient exists somewhere on the spectrum between light and dark, between life-blinding joy and joy-blinding sadness. For the millions of people in the mid-range, who fall somewhere on the morose-to-mania spectrum between the suicidal tendencies of Nicholas Cage in *Leaving Las Vegas*, and the "What me Worry?" smiling face of Mad Man Alfred E. Neuman, the need for antidepressant therapy is based on hard clinical criteria.

From a practical perspective, pharmacology must follow functional needs. And specifically, the need to function, day in and day out. Symptoms of depression include sadness, low self-esteem, lethargy, feelings of worthlessness, difficulty sleeping, sudden weight changes, crying spells, difficulty concentrating, asocial behavior, extreme agitation, and withdrawal. Ask your patients the following questions. Are you sleeping well enough? Are you sad too much of the time? Do you have recurrent feelings of worthlessness, guilt, or low self-esteem? Have your eating patterns changed to the point of gaining or losing an excessive amount of weight? Have you stopped having fun or wanting to have fun? Has your sex drive changed dramatically? Have you lost your sex drive?

Although frequently the need for antidepressants is very clear, in many situations it is not. Ultimately, the decision to start an SSRI antidepressant should be made using established criteria and measurement tools that predict successful outcomes with drug-based therapy.

Selective Serotonin Reuptake Inhibitors (SSRIs): High Productivity Medications For Depression and Other Related Mood Disorders

From a pharmatectural perspective, the underuse of pharmacotherapeutic agents to treat neuropsychiatric illness has been underscored by data presented in *The Global Burden of Disease* (Christopher, J. L., and Lopez, Alan D). Calling attention to the "unseen burden of psychiatric disease," data in this summary presented to the World Health Organization demonstrate clearly that disability plays a central role in determining the overall health status of a population. Yet that role has, until now, been almost invisible to public health. The leading causes of disability are shown to be substantially different from the leading causes of death, thus casting serious doubt on the practice of judging a population's health from its mortality statistics alone.

Most significantly, the study shows that the burden of psychiatric conditions has been heavily underestimated, and that failure to treat this broad spectrum of illnesses has quality of life—and potentially—economic consequences related to worker productivity. Of the ten leading causes of disability worldwide in 1990, measured in years lived with a disability, five were *psychiatric* conditions: unipolar depression, alcohol use, bipolar affective disorder (manic depression), schizophrenia, and obsessive-compulsive disorder. Unipolar depression alone was responsible for more than one in every ten years of life lived with a disability worldwide. Altogether, psychiatric and neurologic conditions accounted for 28% per all disability-related time lost, compared with 1.4% of all deaths and 1.1% of years of life lost. The predominance of these conditions is by no means restricted to the rich countries, although their burden is highest in the established market economies.

Despite increasing recognition of the efficacy of drug-based interventions for psychiatric disease, this modality is still relatively underused. Strategies that enhance detection of patient subgroups eligible for pharmacological therapies are essential. In this regard, one of the major advances in pharmacotherapeutic management of mood disorders is evidence-based confirmation that selective serotonin reuptake inhibitors (SSRIs) have the capacity to produce positive clinical outcomes not only in depression, but in a wide range of related mood disorders, including obsessive-compulsive disorder (OCD), panic disorder, seasonal affective disorder (SAD), dysthymia, and other related conditions. This class of medications is also being studied for its effectiveness for treatment of depression that is associated with specific age, situational or disease-mediated triggers: post myocardial depression, post-partum depression, childhood depression, depression associated with Alzheimer's disease, as well as other patient subgroups.

Among the SSRIs, sertraline (Zoloft®), fluoxetine (Prozac®), and paroxetine (Paxil®) have been widely evaluated for their effectiveness in a wide range of psychiatric disorders. Although there are differences among drugs in this class, each of these SSRIs is effective for its approved indication(s), and it may be difficult to categorically recommend one agent over the other for all patient subgroups. However, because sertraline has been studied extensively and is approved for three distinct psychiatric disorders (depression, OCD, and panic disorder), it provides a comprehensive model for identifying clinical syndromes, symptom complexes, and targeting variant conditions in which SSRIs have been evaluated and found to be potentially useful.

The efficacy of sertraline in major depression has been demonstrated in results of studies enrolling a total of more than 12,000 patients. The efficacy of this SSRI is superior to that of placebo in the treatment of major depression, as measured on recognized depression rating scales, and there is no antidepressant dose-response. Moreover, in double-blind studies, sertraline is at least as effective as the tricyclic antidepressants (TCAs) in the treatment of major depression, and is associated with fewer side effects. Sertraline also has comparable efficacy to fluoxetine in double-blind studies in the treatment of major depression.

Sertraline is effective in moderate and severe depression, and in cases where anxiety, insomnia, or melancholia associated with depression have been identified as predominant symptoms. Double-blind studies in the treatment of pure dysthymia have shown sertraline to have superior efficacy to placebo and equivalent efficacy to imipramine, but with better tolerability than the TCA. Finally, preliminary data suggest that sertraline may also have efficacy in other depressive disorders, such as seasonal affective disorder, premenstrual dysphoric disorder, postpartum depression, and atypical depression. Studies are currently under way to evaluate the role of SSRIs in these conditions.

The benefits of sertraline as a treatment for depression has been established in two placebo-controlled studies in adult outpatients meeting DSM-III criteria for major depression. The first was an 8-week study with flexible dosing of sertraline in a range of 50 to 200 mg/day; the mean dose for completers was 145 mg/day. The second was a 6-week fixed-dose study, including sertraline doses of 50, 100, and 200 mg/day. Overall, these studies demonstrated sertraline to be superior to placebo on the Hamilton Depression Rating Scale and the Clinical Global Impression Severity and Improvement scales. Study 2 was not readily interpretable regarding a dose response relationship for effectiveness.

The third study involved depressed outpatients who had responded by the end of an initial 8-week open treatment phase on sertraline 50 to 200 mg/day. These patients (n=295) were randomized to continuation for 44 weeks on double-blind sertraline 50 to 200 mg/day or placebo. A statistically significant lower relapse rate was observed for patients taking sertraline compared to those on placebo. The mean dose for completers was 70 mg/day. Analyses for gender effects on outcome did not suggest any differential responsiveness on the basis of sex.

Targeting Patients and Syndromes that Are Appropriate for SSRI Therapy

Identifying patient subgroups that can benefit from SSRI therapy is essential for maximizing clinical outcomes. The following sections provide therapeutic trigger points that physicians and pharmacists should consider for possible initiation of an SSRI-based treatment program.

Depression. A major depressive episode implies a prominent and relatively persistent depressed or dysphoric mood that usually interferes with daily functioning (nearly every day for at least 2 weeks); it should include at least 4 of the following 8 symptoms: change in appetite, change in sleep, psychomotor agitation or retardation, loss of interest in usual activities or decrease in sexual drive, increased fatigue, feelings of guilt or worthlessness, slowed thinking or impaired concentration, and a suicide attempt or suicidal ideation.

Sertraline hydrochloride is indicated for the treatment of depression. Its efficacy in the treatment of a major depressive episode was established in six to eight week controlled trials of outpatients whose diagnoses corresponded most closely to the DSM-III category of major depressive disorder. The efficacy of sertraline in maintaining an antidepressant response for up to 44 weeks following 8 weeks of open-label acute treatment (52 weeks total) was demonstrated in a placebo-controlled trial. The usefulness of the drug in patients receiving sertraline for extended periods should be re-evaluated periodically.

It is generally agreed that acute episodes of depression require several months or longer of sustained pharmacologic therapy. Whether the dose of antidepressant needed to induce remission is identical to the dose needed to maintain or sustain euthymia is unknown. Systematic evaluation of sertraline has shown that its antidepressant efficacy is maintained for periods of up to 44 weeks following 8 weeks of open-label acute treatment (52 weeks total) at a dose of 50 to 200 mg/day (mean dose of 70 mg/day).

Anxiety and Depression. Although some forms of anxiety and certain affective disorders appear to be distinct entities, it has been increasingly recognized that anxiety and depression frequently co-exist in the same patient. In fact, the lifetime prevalence of anxiety disorders in chronic major depression has been reported to be high, with panic disorder (7.9%), general anxiety disorder (11.2%) and social phobia (15.8%) occurring most frequently in combination with depression. Not only are overlapping syndromes common, but patients with co-existing depression and anxiety tend to have a more serious prognosis, with one study sample of more than 300 patients showing a clear relationship between the presence of anxiety symptoms and the severity of depressive illness. As a result of these associations, clinicians should evaluate anxiety as a possible treatment trigger for initiation of SSRI therapy if it has been determined that the anxiety is part of a symptom complex that satisfies the diagnostic criteria for depression, OCD, or panic disorder.

In the past, many clinicians held the opinion that the presence of prominent anxiety symptoms required the use of sedating antidepressants, such as a TCAs, or even benzodiazepines. However, the SSRIs, which are recognized as being less sedating than TCAs, have been shown to relieve symptoms of anxiety in patients with major depression. This is not entirely unexpected, as a relationship between anxiety symptoms and serotonin has been documented in previous studies.

Dysthymia. Dysthymia is a subchronic or chronic depressive condition characterized by less severity than major depression. It is defined in DSM-IV as a persistently depressed mood, or a loss of pleasure for at least 2 years, but of insufficient severity to warrant a diagnosis of major depression. Field studies suggest that the prevalence rates for dysthymia range between 1% and 9%. Dysthymia shares diagnostic criteria with major depression, anxiety disorders and personality disorders, making its differentiation from these conditions difficult. As there is considerable overlap between major depression and dysthymia, the term "pure dysthymia" is used to distinguish individuals with dysthymia who do not develop major depression or other psychiatric conditions. However, about 50% all dysthymic patients simultaneously fulfill the diagnostic criteria for major depression and are described as having "double depression." Studies in these patients have shown that, while the majority recover from the major depressive disorder, less than 50% have recovered from the underlying dysthymia 2 years later.

Despite evidence from controlled trials suggesting that antidepressant medication is effective in a substantial proportion of dysthymic patients, this condition has been under-diagnosed and under-treated. Because dysthymia is associated with considerable impairment of social functioning and warrants aggressive pharmacotherapy, there is no evidence to support the practice of using lower doses of antidepressant medication in dysthymia. Achieving an adequate dosage of medication in dysthymia can, however, be a challenge as patients tend to be less willing than those with severe major depression to tolerate side-effects. The SSRIs, with their favorable side-effect profile, have potential for the successful long-term management of this disorder.

Seasonal Affective Disorder (SAD). This is a well-characterized syndrome in which individuals suffer annual episodes of depression, the onset of which usually occurs at the same time every year—typically in the autumn or early winter. The depressive episodes are often characterized by atypical features such as increased appetite, weight gain, morning fatigue and hypersomnia. Conventional heterocyclic antidepressants are associated with anticholinergic-related side-effects that may exacerbate these symptoms (i.e., drowsiness) and, therefore, may be expected to be poorly tolerated by SAD patients. Light therapy appears to be effective in the short-term treatment of patients with SAD, although it can be time consuming and inconvenient.

Premenstrual Dysphoric Disorder (PDD). Premenstrual dysphoric disorder is the new diagnostic label for late luteal phase dysphoric disorder (LLPDD) and may be considered as a more severe form of premenstrual syndrome (PMS). It is classified as a "Depressive Disorder, Not Otherwise Specified" in DSM-IV. Premenstrual dysphoric disorder is characterized by irritability, mood swings, anxiety, depression, impaired concentration, alterations in sleep and appetite, as well as various physical symptoms (e.g., fluid retention, breast tenderness). These symptoms occur in the premenstrual phase only, resolving shortly after the onset of menstruation.

Despite a clear link between PDD and depression, as evidenced by symptom overlap and the likelihood of women with PDD to subsequently develop major depression, relatively few placebo-controlled trials of antidepressants in this disorder have been performed. Among those tested in double-blind trials, agents with specificity for enhancement of serotonergic function, including sertraline and fluoxetine, have clearly demonstrated efficacy. These findings support the proposed role of serotonergic hypoactivity in the pathogenesis of PDD.

Atypical Depression. Atypical depression falls under the DSM-IV classification of "Depressive Disorder Not Otherwise Specified,"which includes those depressive disorders that do not meet all of the criteria for a specific mood disorder. Its clinical presentation differs from that of Major Depressive Disorder in that it is associated with hypersomnia rather than insomnia; hyperphagia rather than anorexia; psychomotor agitation rather than retardation; and anxious or irritable mood rather than dysphoria. Interpersonal hypersensitivity and leaden fatigue are also characteristic. Atypical depression may be misdiagnosed as a personality disorder due to the presence of long-standing irritability and hostility. Tricyclic antidepressant therapy has been suggested to be less effective than the SSRIs for patients whose depression is marked by hyperphagia, hypersomnia, and high mood reactivity.

Depression in the Elderly. Depression in the elderly can cause significant morbidity and has been associated with delayed recovery from hip fractures and proposed as a predisposing factor for acute myocardial infarction. Unfortunately, the disease is under-recognized and under-treated in the geriatric population. In this regard, sertraline demonstrates at least equivalent efficacy to the tricyclic antidepressants (TCAs) in double-blind studies in elderly patients with depression. It also appears to have a significantly greater effect than the TCA nortriptyline in quality of life assessments in elderly patients, and appears to be of comparable efficacy to fluoxetine in the depressed elderly. Sertraline has been shown in a large primary-care study to have similar efficacy in elderly and younger depressed patients.

From a practical clinical perspective, the pharmacokinetics of sertraline permit once-daily dosing, which is likely to aid compliance in the elderly. The pharmacokinetics of sertraline (in contrast to other selective serotonin reuptake inhibitors (SSRIs) such as paroxetine and fluoxetine) are similar in the elderly to those in younger patients, so dosage adjustment is not necessary in older patients. The side-effect profile of sertraline also is favorable for use in elderly. It lacks significant anticholinergic and cardiac effects; does not impair cognitive function; and may be associated with a lower risk of drug interactions, compared with the TCAs and other SSRIs. Sertraline has been shown to be a slightly weaker inhibitor of important cytochrome P450 isoenzymes than some other selective serotonin reuptake inhibitors, and to have a relatively low potential for pharmacokinetic drug interactions mediated by these mechanisms.

Obsessive-Compulsive Disorder (OCD). Obsessive-compulsive disorder (OCD) is characterized by excessive ritualization of routine activities, recurrent disturbing thoughts (obsessions) or chronic fixation with meaningless tasks or activities (compulsions), such as hand-washing, excessive neatness, arranging objects in a line, that interfere with normal daily function. People with this condition are frequently "paralyzed" by these rituals and obsessions, and desperately need help. Medications may normalize behavior patterns in people afflicted with this problem, thereby, improving quality of life and productivity, as well as promoting participation in useful, life-enhancing activities.

The SSRIs are now considered by most experts to be the initial drugs of choice for the treatment of obsessive-compulsive disorder (OCD). In this regard, large studies involving nearly 600 patients have demonstrated that sertraline is superior to placebo in the treatment of obsessive-compulsive disorder (OCD). In patients with OCD, therapeutic benefits are generally seen from 2 to 3 weeks after the start of sertraline treatment, with further ongoing improvements during the course of 12 weeks of treatment.

Sertraline does not appear to exhibit a dose-response relationship in OCD, i.e., doses of 50 to 220 mg/day have been effective. Therefore, 50 mg/day is the recommended starting dose, which is likely to be effective in the majority of OCD patients. A long-term study has shown that the improvements in the symptoms of OCD are maintained for up to 2 years with continued sertraline therapy. The drug appears to be well tolerated in both short- and long-term treatment of OCD, with one study demonstrating significantly superior tolerability to clomipramine.

Because OCD frequently is diagnosed in the pediatric age group, evaluation of SSRI safety and efficacy in this population is essential. The efficacy of sertraline for the treatment of obsessive-compulsive disorder was demonstrated in a 12-week, multicenter, placebo-controlled study with 187 outpatients between the ages of 6 and 17 (the effectiveness of sertraline in pediatric patients with depression or panic disorder has not been systematically evaluated). The adverse event profile observed in pediatric OCD patients was generally similar to that observed in adult studies with sertraline. As with other SSRIs, decreased appetite and weight loss have been observed. Consequently, regular monitoring of weight and growth is recommended if treatment of a child with an SSRI is to be continued long term. Safety and effectiveness in pediatric patients below the age of 6 have not been established.

Panic Disorder. Sertraline is indicated for the treatment of panic disorder with or without agoraphobia as defined in DSM-IV. The efficacy of sertraline was established in three 10 to 12 week trials in panic disorder patients whose diagnoses corresponded to the DSM-III-R category of panic disorder.

Panic disorder is characterized by the occurrence of unexpected panic attacks, worry about the implications or consequences of the attacks, or a significant change in behavior related to the attacks. Panic disorder (DSM-IV) is characterized by recurrent unexpected panic attacks, i.e., a discrete period of intense fear or discomfort in which four (or more) of the following symptoms develop abruptly and reach a peak within 10 minutes: (1) palpitations, pounding heart, or accelerated heart rate; (2) sweating; (3) trembling or shaking; (4)

sensations of shortness of breath or smothering; (5) feeling of choking; (6) chest pain or discomfort; (7) nausea or abdominal distress; (8) feeling dizzy, unsteady, lightheaded, or faint; (9) derealization (feelings of unreality) or depersonalization (being detached from oneself); (10) fear of losing control; (11) fear of dying; (12) paresthesias; (13) chills or hot flushes.

Preventing Relapse and Recurrence of Depression: Guidelines for Duration of Therapy

Compounding the underuse of SSRIs in depression and other conditions for which they are indicated is the lack of consensus regarding duration of therapy and criteria for drug discontinuation. To clarify these issues, the World Health Organization (WHO), the International Committee for Advancement of Neurology and Psychiatry (ICNAP), and the American Psychiatric Organization (APA) have generated recommendations for duration of antidepressant treatment. Although they differ in their specifics, all three position statements concur, in general terms and philosophy, that antidepressant therapy should be maintained until resolution of the depressive episode is confirmed, and that recurrences should be treated aggressively with a low threshold for chronic maintenance therapy.

The WHO consensus statement urges that antidepressant therapy be continued for at least 6 months after full recovery from depression. Once clinically stable, antidepressant medication should be discontinued gradually and the patient seen about 3 weeks after cessation of all antidepressants, at which point neuropsychiatric status should be evaluated. If well, the patient should be assessed subsequently at 2-month intervals for up to 6 months. Long-term prophylactic treatment is recommended for patients who have experienced more than one severe episode of depressive illness, especially if one or more episodes have occurred in the previous 5 years. One option for long-term treatment in such cases is the use of an antidepressant to which the patient is known to have responded.

The American Psychiatric Association Practice Guideline for Major Depressive Disorder in Adults suggests that patients with a first episode of major depression, who have responded to an antidepressant agent, should be maintained on a full therapeutic dose of that medication for at least 16 to 20 weeks *after* initial remission. For those patients with recurrent unipolar depression of sufficient severity and frequency, it is recommended that maintenance therapy be continued for a prolonged period, in some cases indefinitely.

The International Committee for the Advancement of Neuroscience and Psychiatry consensus report states that, to consolidate the acute response to antidepressant therapy, treatment should be continued for 4 to 6 months after symptom resolution. In cases of recurrent episodes of depression (defined as two major depressive episodes in 5 years, or three previous episodes), there is evidence that long-term treatment with some antidepressants reduces the risk of new episodes of depression. This protective effect is maintained for at least 5 years, as long as antidepressant therapy is maintained at full dosage. If prophylactic treatment is indicated, it should probably be continued indefinitely.

In a one-year study, sertraline has been shown to significantly reduce both the rate of relapse of the primary depressive episode and the rate of recurrence of new episodes in comparison with placebo. Compared with imipramine (Tofranil), sertraline appears to produce significantly greater improvement in depressive symptoms during long-term treatment.

In the case of depression and obsessive-compulsive disorder, sertraline treatment should be administered at a dose of 50 mg/day. For panic disorder in adults, treatment should be initiated with a dose of 25 mg/day. After one week, the dose should be increased to 50 mg/day. While a relationship between dose and effect has not been established for depression, OCD, or panic disorder, patients were dosed in a range of 50 to 200 mg/day in the clinical trials demonstrating the effectiveness of sertraline for these indications. Consequently, a dose of 50 mg, administered once daily, is recommended as the initial dose. Patients not responding to a 50 mg dose may benefit from the dose increases up to a maximum of 200 mg/day. Given the 24-hour elimination half-life of this SSRI, dose changes should not occur at intervals of less than 1 week. The medication should be administered once daily, either in the morning or evening. For managing children and adolescents with OCD, treatment should be initiated with a dose of 25 mg once daily in children (ages 6 to 12) and at a dose of 50 mg once daily in adolescents (ages 13 to 17).

Drug-Drug Interactions. Patients on SSRI therapy should be considered at risk for possible drug-drug interaction. In two separate in vivo interaction studies, sertraline was co-administered with cytochrome P450 3A4 substrates or carbamazepine (Tegretol), under steady-state conditions. The results of these studies demonstrated the sertraline co-administration did not increase plasma concentrations of carbamazepine. These data suggest that sertraline's extent of inhibition of P450 3A4 activity is not likely to be of clinical significance.

Many SSRIs (including sertraline) and other antidepressants, inhibit the biochemical activity of the drug metabolizing isoenzyme cytochrome P450 2D6 and, therefore, may increase the plasma concentrations of co-administered drugs that are metabolized by P450 2D6. The drugs for which this potential interaction is of greatest concern are those metabolized primarily by 2D6 and which have a narrow therapeutic index, i.e., the tricyclic antidepressants and the Type 1C antiarrhythmics propafenone (Rythmol) and flecainide (Tambocor). The extent to which this interaction is an important clinical problem depends on the extent of the inhibition of P450 2D6 by the antidepressant and the therapeutic index of the co-administered drug.

There is variability among the antidepressants in the extent of clinically important 2D6 inhibition, and in fact, sertraline at lower doses, has a less prominent inhibitory effect on 2D6 than some other antidepressants in the class. Nevertheless, even sertraline has the potential for clinically important 2D6 inhibition. Consequently, concomitant use of a drug metabolized by P450 2D6 with sertraline may require lower doses than usually prescribed for the other drug.

Furthermore, whenever this SSRI is withdrawn from co-therapy, an increased dose of the co-administered drug may be required.

Concomitant use in patients taking monoamine oxidase inhibitors (MAOIs) is *contraindicated.* Cases of serious, sometimes fatal, reactions have been reported in patients receiving sertraline in combination with a monoamine oxidase inhibitor (MAOI). Symptoms of a drug interaction between an SSRI and an MAOI include: hyperthermia, rigidity, myoclonus, autonomic instability with possible rapid fluctuations of vital signs, mental status changes that include confusion, irritability, and extreme agitation progressing to delirium and coma. These reactions have also been reported in patients who have recently discontinued an SSRI and have been started on an MAOI. Some cases presented with features resembling neuroleptic malignant syndrome. Therefore, sertraline and other SSRIs should not be used in combination with an MAOI, or within 14 days of discontinuing treatment with an MAOI. Similarly, at least 14 days should be allowed after stopping.

Adverse Effects. Drug-related adverse effects occur with all SSRIs, and can involve the following: CNS: insomnia, somnolence, nervousness, anxiety, dizziness, tremor; Cardiovascular: palpitations, vasodilation, pain; GI: nausea, diarrhea, dry mouth, anorexia, constipation, dyspepsia; Musculoskeletal: myalgia, arthralgia; Respiratory: yawning; Skin: sweating, rash; Special senses: vision disturbances/blurred vision, taste change; GU: sexual dysfunction, abnormal ejaculation; Body as a whole: headache; asthenia; abdominal pain, flu-like symptoms.

When drug therapy is needed for an affective disorder such as depression, antidepressants can provide dramatic improvements in quality-of-life, mood, sleep behavior, cognitive function, and pain perception for many patients. In fact, numerous studies confirm that depression is under-diagnosed and antidepressants may actually be underused. The fact is, when used appropriately, this drug class occupies a unique position in the geriatric pharmacopoeia.[148,149]

Antidepressants. From a pharmatectural point of view, antidepressants give pharmacists and physicians the opportunity to *consolidate* many different drugs into a single active agent that is capable of pharmacologically servicing a wide range of symptoms. In particular, they are useful for simplifying and reconstructing the foundations of drug regimens oriented toward management of insomnia, somatization disorders, chronic pain, and recurrent panic attacks. With respect to reduction of pharmacologic burden, these agents are smart drugs that can (a) provide sedation to induce sleep in patients with chronic insomnia; (b) treat depression; (c) reduce the frequency of panic attacks; (d) manage pain associated with diabetic mononeuropathy; (e) treat anxiety associated with panic disorder; and (f) treat obsessive-compulsive disorder (OCD). Despite the potential advantages of low-dose antidepressant therapy, care is needed in selecting the most appropriate agent and dose schedule.[150-152]

Antipsychotics: A Sane Approach To Drug Selection. The antipsychotic/neuroleptic drugs, which are useful in the management of behavioral and psychiatric disorders, have similar pharmacokinetic and antipsychotic properties. However, their hypotensive, anticholinergic, and extrapyramidal side effects vary substantially. For example, drugs such as haloperidol (Haldol®) and trifluoperazine (Stelazine®) should be avoided in patients in whom induction of extrapyramidal side effects would be especially worrisome, e.g., those with gait disorders and Parkinson's disease. On the other hand, in patients with postural hypotension, gait instability, or patients with conduction disorders, drugs such as chlorpromazine (Thorazine®) and thioridazine (Mellaril®) are not recommended, because of their propensity to cause sedation, hypotension, and anticholinergic toxicity.[145,153,154] In general, this category of drugs should be given only to severely behaviorally disturbed, elderly patients or patients previously stabilized on neuroleptics who are at risk of harm to themselves or others; moreover, a clear therapeutic end point must be closely monitored.[146,155,156]

The House That Pharmatecture Built

The working drawings for drug house construction are now in place. Specific strategies are outlined for drug selection, compliance enhancement, and construction of prevention-oriented drug houses. Patient groups at high risk for inhabiting or creating suboptimal drug houses have been highlighted. In particular, strategies for conducting a thorough drug house inspection have been discussed in detail and the importance of identifying and characterizing the full spectrum of DRAPEs before pharmatectural reconstruction is stressed. From a pharmatectural perspective, the safest and most durable drug houses are the product of a systematic, three-phase process consisting of drug house inspection, design, and reconstruction. When consistent with pharmatectural guidelines, this process will produce cost-effective pharmacologic constructions associated with optimal therapeutic outcomes and quality-of-life maintenance.

[1]Berg JS, Dischler J, Wagner DJ, Raia JJ, Palmer-Shevlin N. Medication compliance; a healthcare problem. Ann Pharmacother 1993 Sept; 27(9 Suppl):S1-24.

[2]Col N, Fanale JE, Kronholm P. The role of medication noncompliance and adverse drug reactions in hospitalizations of the elderly. Arch Intern Med 1990 April;150(4):841-5.

[3]Riegger GA. Lessons from recent randomized controlled trials for the management of congestive heart failure. Am J Cardiol 1993 June 24;71(17):38E-40E.

[4]Pickles H, Fuller S. Prescriptions, adverse reactions, and the elderly. Lancet 1986;2(8497):40.

[5]Steiner JF, Robbins LJ, Roth SC, Hammond WS. The effect of prescription size on acquisition of maintenance medications. J Gen Intern Med 1993 June;8(6):306-10.

[6]Stewart RB, Caranasos GJ. Medication compliance in the elderly. Med Clin North Am 1989;73:1551-63.

[7]Beardon PH, McGilchrist MM, McKendrick AD, McDevitt DG, MacDonald TM. Primary noncompliance with prescribed medication in primary care. BMJ 1993 Oct 2;307(6908):846-8.

[8]Botelho RJ, Dudrak R 2d. Home assessment of adherence to long-term medication in the elderly. J Fam Prac 1992 July;35(1):61-5.

[9]Hamilton RA, Bricland LL. Use of prescription-refill records to assess patient compliance. Am J Hosp Pharm 1992 July;49(7):1691-6.

[10]Beers MH, Fingold SF, Ouslander JG, Ruben DB, Morgenstern H, Beck JC. Characteristics and quality of prescribing by doctors practicing in nursing homes. J Am Geriatr Soc 1993 Aug;41(8):802-7.

[11]Beers MH, Ouslander JG, Fingold SF, Morgenstern H, Ruben DB, Rogers W, Zeffren MJ, Beck JC. Inappropriate medication prescribing in skilled-nursing facilities. Ann Intern Med 1992 Oct 15;117(8):684-9.

[12]Beers MH, Ouslander JG, Rollingeer I, Reuben DB, Brooks J, Beck JC. Explicit criteria for determining inappropriate medication use in nursing home residents. [Review] Arch Intern Med 1991 Sept;151(9):1825-32.

[13]Nolan L, O'Malley K. Adverse effects of antidepressants in the elderly. [Review] Drugs Aging 1992 Sept-Oct; 2(5):450-8.

[14]Willcox SM, Himmelstein DU, Woolhander S. Inappropriate drug prescribing for the community-dwelling elderly. JAMA 1994 July 27;272(4):292-6.

[15]Abernethy DR, Schwartz JB, Plachetka JR, et al. Comparison in young and elderly patients of pharmacodynamics and disposition of labetalol in systemic hypertension. Am J Cardiol 1987;60:697-702.

[16]Amir M, Cristal N, Bar-On D, Loidl A. Does the combination of ACE inhibitor and calcium antagonist control hypertension and improve quality of life? The LOMIR-MCT-IL study experience. Blood Press 1994;Suppl 1:40-2.

[17]Bulpitt CJ, Fletcher AE. Drug treatment and quality of life in the elderly. [Review] Clin Geriatr Med 1990 May;6(2):309-17.

[18]Coons SJ, Kaplan RM. Assessing health-related quality of life: application to drug therapy. Clin Ther 1992;14(6):850-8; discussion 849.

[19]Conn VS, Taylor SG, Kelley S. Medication regimen complexity and adherence among older adults. Image J Nurs Sch 1991 Winter;23(4):231-5.

[20]Downs GE, Linkewich JA, DiPalma JR. Drug interactions in elderly diabetics. Geriatrics 1986;36(7):45.

[21]Lamy PP. A "risk" approach to adverse drug reactions. J Am Geriatr Soc 1988;36:79.

[22]May FE, Stewart B, Cluff LE. Drug interactions and multiple drug administrations. Clin Pharmacol Ther 1970;2:705.

[23]Ouslander JG. Drug therapy in the elderly. Ann Intern Med 1981;95:711-22.

[24]Knight JR, Campbell AJ, Williams SM, Clark DW. Knowledgeable noncompliance with prescribed drugs in elderly subjects—a study with particular reference to nonsteroidal antiinflammatory and antidepressant drugs. J Clin Pharm Ther 1991 April;16(2):131-7.

[25]Ballenger JC. Medication discontinuation in panic disorder. J Clin Psychiatry 1992 March;53 Suppl:26-31.

[26]Ballenger JC, Pecknold J, Rickels K, Sellers EM. Medication discontinuation in panic disorder. J Clin Psychiatry 1993 Oct;54 Suppl:15-21; discussion 22-4.

[27]Dichter MA. Deciding to discontinue antiepileptic mediation. Hosp Pract (Off Ed) 1992 Oct 30;27(10A):16, 21-2.

[28]Gherpelli JK, Kok F, dal Forno S, Elkis LC, Lefevre BH, Diament AJ. Discontinuing medication in epileptic children: a study of risk factors related to recurrence. Epilepsia 1992 July-Aug; 33(4):681-6.

[29]Held P. Effects of beta-blockers on ventricular dysfunction after myocardial infarction: tolerability and survival effects. Am J Cardiol 1993 March 25;71(9):39C-44C.

[30]Hennekens CH, Jonas MA, Buring JE. The benefits of aspirin in acute myocardial infarction. Still a well-kept secret in the United States. Arch Intern Med 1994 Jan 10;154(1):37-9.

[31]Kanter MC, Sherman DG. Strategies for preventing stroke. Curr Opin Neurol Neurosurg 1993 Feb;6(1):60-5.

[32]Barnett HJ. Aspirin in stroke prevention. An overview. Stroke 1990 Dec;21(12 Suppl):IV40-3.

[33]Bower S, Sandercock P. Antiplatelet and anticoagulant therapy. Curr Opin Neurol Neurosur 1993 Feb;6(1):55-9.

[34]Couch JR. Antiplatelet therapy in the treatment of cerebrovascular disease. Clin Cardiol 1993 Oct;16(10):703-10.

[35]Dalen JE, Goldberg RJ. Prophylactic aspirin and the elderly population. Clin Geriat Med 1992 Feb;8(1):119-26.

[36]Frishman WH. Beta-adrenergic blockers as cardioprotective agents. Am J Cardiol 1992 Dec 21;70(21):21-61.

[37]Anonymous. Clinton team works with drug companies to expand access, restrict costs. Am J Hosp Pharm 1993 March;50(3):388, 391.

[38]Anonymous. Prescription drugs and older consumers. Report of the Governor's task force on prescription drugs and older consumers issued August 10, 1990. Mich Med 1991 Feb;90(2):27-31.

[39]Cooling H. Non-redemption of prescriptions. Homeless people miss out on prescribed treatment. BMJ 1994 Jan 8;308(6921):135-6.

[40]Gibaldi M. Prescription drugs and health care reform. Pharmacotherapy 1993 Nov-Dec; 13(6):583-9.

[41]Kucukarslan S, Hakim Z, Sullivan D, Taylor S, Grauer D, Haugtvedt C, Zgarrick D. Points to consider about prescription drug prices: an overview of federal policy and pricing studies. Clin Ther 1993 July-Aug;15(4):726-38.

[42]Shulkin DJ, Giardino AP, Freenock TF, Jr., Henriksen DS, Richman C, Friedlander MS, Pandelidis SM, Heywood TJ. Generic versus brand name drug prescribing by resident physicians in Pennsylvania. Am J Hosp Pharm 1992 March;49(3):625-6.

[43]Ahronheim J. Practical pharmacology for older patients; avoiding adverse drug effects. Mt Sinai J Med 1993 Nov;60(6):497-501.

[44]Bailey RA, Ashcraft NA. Pharmacist-physician drug fair for educating physicians in cost-effective prescribing. Am J Hosp Pharm 1993 Oct;50(10):2088-9.

[45]Berger MS. A proposal for using generics. Pa Med 1993 May;96(5):10.

[46]Emrys-Jones G. Dispensing in general practice. Dispensing improves compliance. BMJ 1993 June 26;306(6894):1749.

[47]Macdonald ET, Macdonald JB, Phoenix M. Improving drug compliance after hospital discharge. BMJ 1977;2:618-621.

[48]Coleman TJ. Non-redemption of prescriptions. Linked to poor consultation. BMJ 1994 Jan 8;308(6921):135.

[49]Futrell DP. Drug compliance. Are you getting the most out of your medicine? N C Med J 1993 Oct;54(10):523-4.

[50]Ito S, Koren G, Einarson TR. Maternal noncompliance with antibiotics during breastfeeding. Ann Pharmacother 1993 Jan;27(1):40-2.

[51]Deyo RA, Inui TS, Sullivan B. Noncompliance with arthritis drugs: magnitude, correlates, and clinical implications. J Rheumatol 1981;8:931-6.

[52]Litchman HM. Medication noncompliance: a significant problem and possible strategies. R I Med 1993 Dec;76(12):608-10.

[53]Skaer TL, Sclar DA, Markowski DJ, Won JK. Effect of value-added utilities on prescription refill compliance and Medicaid health care expenditures—a study of patients with non-insulin dependent diabetes mellitus. J Clin Pharm Ther 1993 Aug;18(4):295-9.

[54]Tilson HH. Social policy and drug safety. Clin Geriatr Med 1987;2(1):165.

[55]McEvoy G. American hospital formulary service drug information. Bethesda, Md: American Society of Hospital Pharmacists, 1985;12-13.

[56]McNally DL, Wertheimer D. Strategies to reduce the high cost of patient noncompliance. M Med J 1992 March;41(3):223-5.

[57]Phillips SL, Carr-Lopez SM. Impact of a pharmacist on medication discontinuation in a hospital-based geriatric clinic. Am J Hosp Pharmacy 1990 May;47(5):1075-9.

[58]Eisen SA, Miller DK, Woodward RS, Spitznagel E, Przybeck TR. The effect of prescribed daily dose frequency on patient medication compliance. Arch Intern Med 1990 Sept;150(9):1881-4.

[59]Keen PJ. What is the best dosage schedule for patients? J R Soc Med 1991 Nov;84(11):640-1.

[60]Anonymous. Writing prescription instructions. Can Med Assoc J 1991 March 15;144(6):647-8.

[61]Sclar DA, Chin A, Skaer TL, Okamoto MP, Nakahiro RK, Gill MA. Effect of health education in promoting prescription refill compliance among patients with hypertension. Clin Ther 1991 July-Aug;13(4):489-95.

[62]Park DC, Morrell RW, Frieske D, Kincaid D. Medication adherence behaviors in older adults; effects of external cognitive supports. Psychol Aging 1992 June;7(2):252-6.

[63]Green LW, Purrell CO, Koop CE, et al. Programs to reduce drug errors in the elderly: direct and indirect evidence from patient education. In: Improving medication compliance. Reston, Va: National Pharm Council, 1985.

[64]Kahl A, Blandford DH, Krueger K, Zwick DI. Geriatric education centers address medication issues affecting older adults. Public Health Rep 1992 Jan-Feb;107(1):37-47.

[65]Roth HP, Caron HS. Accuracy of doctor's estimates and patients' statements on adherence to a drug regimen. Clin Pharm Ther 1978;23:361-370.

[66]Abernathy DR, Andrawis NS. Critical drug interactions: A guide to important examples. Drug Ther 1993;Cot 15-27.

[67]Fox GN. Drug interactions software programs. J Fam Pract 1991;33(3):273-80.

[68]Valentine C. Use computers to detect inappropriate prescriptions. BMJ 1993 July 3;307(6895):61.

[69]Johnston D, Duffin D. Drug-patient interactions and their relevance in the treatment of heart failure. Am J Cardiol 1992 Oct 8;70(10):109C-12C.

[70]Cochrane RA, Mandal AR, Ledger-Scott M, Walker R. Changes in drug treatment after discharge from hospital in geriatric patients. BMJ 1992 Sept 19;305(6855):694-6.

[71]Granek E, et al. Medications and diagnosis in relation to falls in a long-term care facility. J Am Geriatr Soc 1987;35:505.

[72]Larson EB, et al. Adverse drug reactions associated with global cognitive impairment in elderly persons. Ann Intern Med 1987;107:169-73.

[73]Nolan L, O'Malley K. Prescribing for the elderly I. Sensitivity of the elderly to adverse drug reactions. J Am Geriatr Soc 1988;36:142-49.

[74]Greenblatt DJ, Shader RI. Anticholinergics. N Engl J Med 1984;288(23):1215-18.

[75]Blazer DG, Federspiel CF, Ray WA, et al. The risk of anticholinergic toxicity in the elderly: a study of prescribing practices in two populations. J Gerontol 1983;38:31-5.

[76]Chan CH, Ruskiewicz RJ. Anticholinergic side effects of trazodone combined with another pharmacologic agent [letter]. Am J Psychiatry 1990 April;147(4):533.

[77]Jue SG, Vestal RE. Adverse drug reactions in the elderly: a critical review. Medicine in Old Age-Clinical Pharmacology and Drug Therapy, London, 1985.

[78]Burris JF. Hypertension management in the elderly. [Review] Heart Disease Stroke 1994 March-April;3(2):77-83.

[79]Flack JM, Woolley A, Esunge P, Grimm RH. A rational approach to hypertension treatment in the older patient. [Review] Geriatrics 1992 Nov;47(11):24-8,33-8.

[80]Furguson RP, Wetle T, Dubitzky D, Winsemius D. Relative importance to elderly patients of effectiveness, adverse effects, convenience and cost of antihypertensive medications. A pilot study. Drugs Aging 1994 Jan;4(1):56-62.

[81]Girgis L, Brooks P. Nonsteroidal anti-inflammatory drugs. Differential use in older patient. [Review] Drugs Aging 1994 Feb;4(2):101-12.

[82]Lamy PP. The elderly and drug interactions. J Am Geriatr Soc 1986;34:586-92.

[83]Anonymous. Drugs for treatment of peptic ulcers. Med Lett Drugs Ther 1991 Nov 29;33(858):111-4.

[84]Gilley J. Towards rational prescribing. BMJ 1994 March 19;308(6931):731-2.

[85]Hood JC, Murphy JE. Patient noncompliance can lead to hospital readmissions. Hospitals 1978; 52:79-82, 84.

[86]Jahnigen D, Cooper D, LaForce M. Adverse events among hospitalized elderly patients. J Am Geriatr Soc 1988;36:65-72.

[87]Black AJ, Somers K. Drug-related illness resulting in hospital admission. J R Coll Physicians Lond 1989;18:40-4.

[88]Beers MH, Storrie M, Lee G. Potential adverse drug interactions in the emergency room. An issue in the quality of care. Ann Intern Med 1990 Jan 1;112(1):61-4.

[89]Brodie MJ, Feely J. Adverse drug reactions. BMJ 1988;296:845-9.

[90]Gosney M, Tallis RL. Prescription of contraindicated and interacting drugs in elderly patients admitted to the hospital. Lancet 1984;2:564-7.

[91]Psaty BM, Koepsell TD, et al. The relative risk of incident coronary heart disease associated with recently stopping the use of beta-blockers. JAMA 1990;263.

[92]Wassertheil-Smoller S, Blaufox DM, et al. Effect of antihypertensives on sexual function and quality of life: The TAIM study. Ann Intern Med 1991;114:613-20.

[93]Testa MA, Anderson RB, Nackley JF, et al. Quality of life and antihypertensive therapy in men: A comparison of captopril with enalapril. N Engl J Med 1993;328:907.

[94]Hine LK, Laird NM, et al. Meta-analysis of empirical long-term antiarrhythmic therapy after myocardial infarction. JAMA 1989;262:3037-40.

[95]Landfeld CS, Goldman L. Major bleeding in outpatients treated with warfarin: incidence and prediction by factors known at the start of oupatient therapy. 1989;87:144-52; Landefeld CS, Rosenblatt MW, Goldman L. Bleeding in outpatients treated with warfarin: relation to prothrombin time and important remediable lesions. Am J Med 1989;87:153-9.

[96]Warram JH, Laffel LMB, et al. Excess mortality associated with diuretic therapy in diabetes mellitus. Arch Intern Med 1991;151:1350-6.

[97]Callahan AM, Fava M, Rosenbaus JF. Drug interactions in psychopharmacology. [Review] Psychiatr Clin North Am 1993 Sept;16(3):647-71.

[98]Ciraulo DA, Shader RI. Fluoxetine drug-drug interactions. II. [Review] J Clin Psychopharmacol 1990 June;10(3):213-7.

[99]Larson EB, Kukull WA, Buchner D, et al. Adverse drug reactions associated with global cognitive impairment in elderly persons. Ann Intern Med 1987;107:169-73.

[100]Greenblatt DJ, Harmatz JS, et al. Sensitivity to triazolam in the elderly. N Engl J Med 1991;324;1691-8.

[101]Sessler CN. Theophylline toxicity: clinical features of 116 cases. Am J Med 1990;88:567-76.

[102]Everitt DE, Avorn J, Baker MW. Clinical decision-making in the evaluation and treatment of insomnia. Am J Med 1990;89:357-62.

[103]Packer M, Gheorghiade M, Young JB, et al. Withdrawal of digoxin from patients with chronic congestive heart failure treated with angiotensin converting enzyme inhibitors. N Engl J Med 1993;329:1-7.

[104]Walt RP. Misoprostol for the treatment of peptic ulcer and antiinflammatory drug-induced gastroduodenal ulceration. N Engl J Med 1992;327:1575.

[105]Lann RF, et al. Low-dose prednisone induces rapid reversible axial bone loss in patients with rheumatoid arthritis. Ann Intern Med 1993;119:963-8.

[106]Felson DT, Ahang Y, Hannan MT, et al. The effect of postmenopausal therapy on bone density in elderly women. N Engl J Med 1993;329:1141.

[107]Dawson-Hughes B, Dallal GE, Krall EA, et al. A controlled trial of the effect of calcium supplementation on bone density in postmenopausal women. N Engl J Med 1990;323:878-83.

[108]Reid IR, Ames RW, Gamble GD, et al. Effect of calcium supplementation on bone loss in postmenopausal women. N Engl J Med 1993;328:460-4.

[109]Aloia JF, Vaswni A, Yeh JK, et al. Calcium supplementation with and without hormone replacement therapy to prevent postmenopausal bone loss. Ann Intern Med 1994;120:97.

[110]Tilyard MW, et al. Treatment of postmenopausal osteoporosis with calcitriol or calcium. N Engl J Med 1992;326(6):357-62.

[111]Dawson-Hughes B, Dallal GE, Krall EA, et al. Effect of vitamin D supplementation on wintertime and overall bone loss in healthy postmenopausal women. Ann Intern Med 1991;115:505-12.

[112]Falkeborn M, et al. Hormone replacement therapy and the risk of stroke. Arch Intern Med 1993;153:1201-9.

[113]Prince RL, Smith M, Dick IM, et al. Prevention of postmenopausal osteoporosis: A comparative study of exercise, calcium supplementation, and hormone replacement therapy. N Engl J Med 1991;325:1189-95.

[114]Stampfer MJ, et al. Postmenopausal estrogen therapy and cardiovascular disease. N Engl J Med 1991;325:11.

[115]McAnally LE, Corn CR, Hamilton SF. Aspirin for the prevention of vascular death in women. Ann Pharmacother 1992 Dec;26(12):1530-4.

[116]Winther K, Husted SE, Vissinger H. Low dose acetylsalicylic acid in the antithrombotic treatment of patients with stable angina pectoris and acute coronary syndromes (unstable angina pectoris and acute myocardial infarction). Pharmacol Toxicol 1994 March;74(3):141-7.

[117]Stroke Prevention in Atrial Fibrillation Study Group. Preliminary report of the stroke prevention in atrial fibrillation study. N Engl J Med 1990;322:863-8.

[118]Nelson E. Current use of antiplatelet drugs in stroke syndromes in the USA. Ann N Y Acad Sci 1990;598:368-75.

[119]Singh BN. Advantages of beta blockers versus antiarrhythmic agents and calcium antagonists in secondary prevention after myocardial infarction. Am J Cardiol 1990 Sept 25;66(9):9C-20C.

[120]Gurwitz JH, Goldberg RJ, Chen Z, Gore JM, Alpert JS. Beta-blocker therapy in acute myocardial infarction: evidence for underutilization in the elderly. Am J Med 1992 Dec;93(6):605-10.

[121]Sims RV, Steinmann WC, et al. The clinical effectiveness of pneumococcal vaccine in the elderly. Ann Intern Med 1988;108:653-7.

[122]Hood WB, Jr. Role of converting enzyme inhibitors in the treatment of heart failure. J Am Coll Cardiol 1993 Oct;22(4 Suppl a):154A-7A.

[123]Lewis EJ, Huniskcer LG, Bain RP, et al. The effect of angiotensin converting enzyme inhibition on diabetic nephropathy. N Engl J Med 1993;329:1456.

[124]Zucchelli P, et al. Long-term comparison between captopril and nifedipine in the progression of renal insufficiency. Kidney Int 1992;42:452.

[125]Ravid M, Savin H, Jutrin I, et al. Long-term stabilizing effect of angiotensin converting enzyme inhibition on plasma creatinine and on proteinuria in normotensive type II diabetic patients. Ann Intern Med 1993;188:577.

[126]Bardham KD, Bjarnason I, Scott DL, Griffin WM, Fenn GC, Shield MJ, Morant SV. The prevention and healing of acute non-steroidal anti-inflammatory drug-associated gastroduodenal mucosal damage by misoprostol. Br J Rheumatol 1993 Nov;32(11):990-5.

[127]Gabriel SE, Campion ME, O'Fallon WM. A cost-utility analysis of misoprostol prophylaxis for rheumatoid arthritis patients receiving nonsteroidal anti-inflammatory drugs. Arthritis Rheum 1994 Mar;37(3):333-41.

[128]Graham DY, White RH, Moreland LW, Schubert TT, Katz R, Jaszewski R, Tindall E, Triadafilopoulos G, Stromatt SC, Teoh LS. Duodenal and gastric ulcer prevention with misprostol in arthritis patients taking NSAIDs. Misoprostol Study Group. Ann Intern Med 1993 Aug 15;119(4):257-62.

[129]Stalnikowicz R, Rachmilewitz D. NSAID-induced gastroduodenal damage: is prevention needed? A review and metaanalysis. J Clin Gastroenterol 1993 Oct;17(3):238-43.

[130]Walt RP. Misoprostol for the treatment of peptic ulcer and anti-inflammatory drug-induced gastroduodenal ulceration [Review]. N Engl J Med 1992 Nov 26;327(22):1575-80.

[131]Alderman MH, et al. Treatment-induced blood pressure reduction and the risk of myocardial infarction. JAMA 1989;7:262.

[132]Akhtar M, Breithardt G, Camm AJ, Coumel P, Janse MJ, Lazzara R, Myerberg RJ, Schwartz PJ, Waldo AL, Wellens HJ, et al. CAST and beyond. Implications of the Cardiac Arrhythmia Suppression Trial. Task Force of the Working Group on Arrhythmias of the European Society of Cardiology. [Review]. Circulation 1990 Mar;81(3):1123-7.

[133]Alegro S, Fenster PE, Marcus FI. Digitalis therapy in the elderly. Geriatrics 1985;38:98.

[134]Dall JLC. Maintenance of digoxin in elderly patients BMJ 1970;2:702.

[135]Forman DE, Coletta D, Kenny D, Kosowsky BD, Stoukides J, Rohrer M, Pastore JO. Clinical issues related to discontinuing digoxin therapy in elderly nursing home patients. Arch Intern Med 1991 Nov;151(11):2194-8.

[136]Stults BM. Digoxin use in the elderly. J Am Geriatr Soc 1985;30(3):158.

[137]Ben-Ishay D, Leibel B, Stessman J. Calcium channel blockers in the management of hypertension in the elderly. Am J Med 1986;81(Suppl 6a):30-4.

[138]Fisher ML, Lamey PP. Special considerations in the use of antihypertensive agents in the elderly patient with coexisting disease. Geriatr Med Today 1987;6(11):47.

[139]Avanzini F, Alli C, Bettelli G, Corso R, Colombo F, Mariotti G, Radice M, Torri V, Tognoni G. Antihypertensive efficacy and tolerability of different drug regimens in isolated systolic hypertension in the elderly. Eur Heart J 1994 Feb;15(2):206-12.

[140]SHEP Cooperative Research Group. Prevention of stroke by antihypertensive drug treatment in older persons with isolated systolic hypertension. JAMA 1991;265:3255-65.

[141]Wysowski DK, Baum C. Outpatient use of prescription sedative-hypnotic drugs in the United States, 1970 through 1989. Arch Intern Med 1991 Sept;151(9):1779-83.

[142]Rickels, Schweizer, et al. Long-term therapeutic use of benzodiazepines: Part I, effects of abrupt discontinuation; Part II, effects of gradual taper. Arch Gen Psychiatry 1990;47:899-915.

[143]Anonymous. Anti-anxiety drug usage in the United States, 1989. Statistical Bulletin-Metropolitan Insurance Companies 1991 Jan-Mar;72(1):18-27.

[144]Gilbert A, Owen N, Innes JM, Sansom L. Trial of an intervention to reduce chronic benzodiazepine use among residents of aged-care accommodation. Aust N Z J Med 1993 Aug;23(4):343-7.

[145]Rothschild AJ. Disinhibition, amnestic reactions, and other adverse reactions secondary to triazolam: a review of the literature [Review]. J Clin Psychiatry 1992 Dec; 53 Suppl:69-79.

[146]Suck JA. Psychotropic drug practice in nursing homes. J Am Geriatr Soc 1988;36:409-18.

[147]Swanteck SS, Grossberg GT, Neppe VM, Doubek WG, Martin T, Bender JE. The use of carbamazepine to treat benzodiazepine withdrawal in a geriatric population. J Geriatr Psychiatry Neurol 1991 April-June;4(2):106-9.

[148]Aguglia E, Casacchi GB, et al. Double blinded study of the efficacy and safety of sertraline versus fluoxetine in major depression. Int Clin Psychopharmacol 1994;8:197-202.

[149]Max MB, Lynch SA, Muir J, et al. Effects of desipramine, amitriptyline and fluoxetine on pain in diabetic neuropathy. N Engl J Med 1992;326:1250.

[150]Heston LL, Garrard J, Makris L, Kane RL, Cooper S, Dunham T, Zelterman D. Inadequate treatment of depressed nursing home elderly. J Am Geriatr Soc 1992 Nov;40(11):1117-22.

[151]Katon W., von Korff M, Lin E, Bush T, Ormel J. Adequacy and duration of antidepressant treatment in primary care. Med Care 1992 Jan;30(1):67-76.

[152]Keller MB, et al. Treatment received by depressed patients. JAMA 1982;248(15):1848.

[153]Ray WA, Taylor JA, Meador KG, Lichtenstein MJ, Griffin MR, Fought R, Adams ML, Blazer DG. Reducing antipsychotic drug use in nursing homes. A controlled trial of provider education. Arch Intern Med 1993 Mar 22;153(6):713-21.

[154]Rovner BW, Edelman BA, Cox MP, Shmuely Y. The impact of antipsychotic drug regulations on psychotropic prescribing practices in nursing homes. Am J Psychiatry 1992 Oct;149(10):1390-2.

[155]Semla TP, Pall AK, Poddig B, Brauner DJ. Effect of the Omnibus Reconciliation Act 1987 on antipsychotic prescribing in nursing home residents. Am Geriatr Soc 1994 June;42(6):648-52.

[156]Shorr RI, Fought RL, Ray WA. Changes in antipsychotic drug use in nursing homes during implementaion of the OBRA-87 regulations. JAMA 1994 Feb 2;271(5):358-62.

3

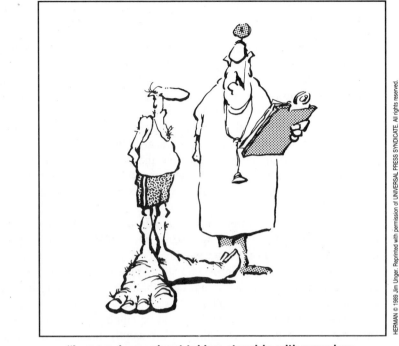

"I warned you about taking steroids with your low blood pressure.'

The Drug and Disease Incompatibility Profile (DIP™) System: Mixing and Matching Pharmacologic Building Blocks

Perhaps it goes without saying that when prescribing drugs, safety comes first.[1-3] Despite the growing recognition that drug reactions and interactions are the nemesis of polypharmacy regimens, few systematic approaches address this problem in a direct manner.[4] The DIP™ system (Drug and Disease Incompatibility Profiles) represents one important solution to these prescribing concerns. Playing a pivotal role in the construction of safe and durable drug houses, the DIP® system is a visually-based, easy-to-use, outpatient practice-oriented drug selection system that pharmacists and clinicians can use to help select commonly used medications based on drug incompatibility profiles.

Identifying centerpiece drugs that are hospitable to the addition of other agents and that do not adversely affect the patient are fundamental clinical and pharmacological priorities. In fact, when it comes to drug interactions, there is a spectrum of pharmacologic issues that must be considered to ensure that drug houses meet pharmatectural safety codes. For example, some drug interactions are very common[5-7] (e.g., the lipid-elevating effects of combining thiazide diuretics and beta-blockers), but their clinical consequences are usually not life-threatening, produce few symptoms, are easily managed, transient, and well-tolerated. However, in other situations, the statistical risk of incurring a drug interaction may be very low (e.g., cardiac arrhythmias produced by the combination of erythromycin and astemizole but the drug-related consequences may be life-threatening.[8,9] Both types of interactions represent potential building code violations, and must be addressed by any system offering guidance for drug selection.[10]

Although there is a tremendous amount of information available regarding drug-drug interactions and drug-disease compatibility profiles, much of it is difficult to access and interpret quickly.[1,2,11,12] This is unfortunate because, in most cases, time is important when making pharmacologic manipulations. Most pharmacists and physicians do not have the time to scan long lists of potential drug-drug and drug-disease interactions for every patient encounter. Even computer-based evaluations and reviews can be cumbersome. The decision to add, combine, or substitute medications is frequently made on the spot, within a limited time framework. Accordingly, prescribing practitioners need a quick approach that weighs the relative risks of combining commonly used pharmacologic building blocks and which also provides quick cross-referencing designed to minimize the other complications of drug therapy.

THE DIP™ SYSTEM

Visually based and stratified according to the relative risk of incurring adverse interactions, the DIP™ system uses a Red-Yellow-Green (i.e., Stop, Caution, Go) drug selection scheme oriented around pie diagrams. Because this pharmatectural approach is based on a color-coded warning system for drug interactions, rather than on a narrative description, the pharmacist or physician can obtain an *instantaneous* reading of potential drug incompatibility profiles. The DIP® system for drug selection is designed to be practical and easy to use. To enhance its day-to-day usefulness, the system emphasizes commonly used drugs. Accordingly, the system incorporates and presents information for a wide range of drug classes including antidepressants, nonsteroidal anti-inflammatory drugs (NSAIDs), corticosteroids, H2 blockers, theophylline, beta-agonists, and oral antibiotics, as well as antihypertensive, antianginal, congestive heart failure-ameliorating, and cardioprotective agents.

With respect to cardiovascular medications, the DIP system provides drug-drug and drug-disease incompatibility profiles for those agents in widest use including, beta-blockers, diuretics, peripheral alpha blockers, ACE inhibitors, calcium blockers, and centrally acting agonists. These drugs deserve special attention because, from a pharmatectural point of view, cardiovascular medications—even those within the same class—can vary in their side effects and drug interactions. These variations can be clinically important because these agents frequently are used in many different combinations and in patients who are at high risk for incurring drug-related problems. As a result, these medications must be distinguished from one another in terms of their drug-drug and drug-disease incompatibility profiles. To address these concerns the DIP system evaluates the suitability of specific cardiovascular agents based on drug-drug as well as drug-disease compatibilities.[3]

One of the purposes of the DIP system is to clarify such distinctions in order to optimize drug selection within and between pharmacologic classes. In addition, the patient's underlying disease landscape also must be considered. To enhance its practical value, the DIP system also evaluates pharmacologic suitability against the backdrop of those diseases most commonly afflicting middle-aged and older Americans (e.g., coronary artery disease, lipid disorders, arthritis, diabetes, congestive heart failure, chronic obstructive pulmonary disease, depression, etc.), as well as against the agents (e.g., beta-blockers, beta-agonists, lipid-lowering agents, calcium blockers, peripheral alpha blockers, nonsteroidal anti-inflammatory drugs, antidepressants, etc.) most likely to be encountered in this patient population.[13-17]

In essence, then, this pharmatectural strategy for optimizing drug selection represents a comprehensive distillation of information gleaned from clinical trials reported in the pharmacologic and medical literature. It also reflects opinions published in expert consensus reports in which the desirability of using different agents for patients on certain drug regimens or with specific disease-cum-risk profiles has been carefully analyzed.[18-21]

GENERAL PRINCIPLES

The DIP system plays a pivotal role in pharmactectural decision-making and should be used to complement a number of other design strategies that are applied to drug house construction. Regardless of which agent or drug class is selected in a given patient or subgroup, adherence to the following drug prescribing principles will help ensure maximal patient compliance and pharmacotherapeutic efficacy: (1) whenever possible, once-a-day drug therapy should be attempted because patient compliance is enhanced significantly by reducing frequency of dosing; (2) adverse side effects must be monitored vigilantly and alterations or substitutions made accordingly; (3) drugs in which the potential for drug-drug interactions are minimized are generally preferrable to those associated with one or more possible interactions; (4) drugs should be used only if clinical efficacy has been proven in rigorous scientific studies; (5) drugs shown to improve quality-of-life and minimize functional impairment should be chosen over drugs known to compromise quality of life; and (6) supplementary written instructions to guide patients in their drug use and alert them to potential side effects should be provided because this approach has been shown to enhance patient compliance and overall satisfaction with the therapeutic regimen.

The DIP™ System Color Scheme

For the sake of simplicity, ease of interpretation, and rapid drug analysis, the DIP system is *color*-based. In this regard, the specific stoplight-scheme colors appearing in DIP profiles are subject to the following interpretations.

Red Designation. Red signifies extreme *caution.* Generally speaking, although there may be unusual exceptions to this rule, the color red in the drug DIP profile suggests that two drugs should never, or rarely, be employed in combination. And when red appears in the *disease* DIP profile, the drug will almost always adversely affect the underlying disease, and should be avoided in patients who have this clinical disorder.

The red designation, however, is given for a number of different situations and can mean several different things. When this color appears in a drug-incompatibility profile, it indicates the primary drug under consideration has a significant probability of being incompatible (i.e., serious drug interactions are likely to occur) with the other drug in the patient's pre-existing pharmacologic landscape. For example, indomethacin (Indocin®) has a high likelihood for producing hemorrhagic, gastric erosions and, therefore, should not be used with oral anticoagulants, a class of agents which increases bleeding time. Consequently, the drug DIP profile for indomethacin indicates a red color for the pie slice associated with anticoagulant therapy.

It should be emphasized that the red classification also appears when the potential consequences of a drug-drug interaction are severe, even though the probability of its occurrence is very *low.* In other words, low probability, life-threatening reactions also elicit a red DIP designation. For example, the interaction between erythromycin and digoxin is not very common, but erythromycin has the capacity to elevate serum digoxin levels and produce cardiotoxicity, a potentially serious drug-related complication in approximately 10% of patients. Consequently, a red color appears for the erythromycin-digoxin interaction.[6,22]

In the case of pie diagrams devoted to disease incompatibility profiles, the color red indicates the agent has a significant likelihood of worsening the natural history of a common, associated complication of the underlying disease. The red color is used both in situations in which the drug-disease interaction is very common (NSAIDs and peptic ulcer disease) and symptomatically disturbing to the patient, as well as in cases in which the drug-disease interaction is rather uncommon (e.g., amitriptyline-induced cardiac arrhythmias), but has potentially serious clinical consequences.[12,23-25]

Yellow Designation. The color yellow signifies that caution and careful evaluation are required before adding the drug under consideration to the exisiting regimen. From a pharmatectural point of view, yellow represents a permissible DIP selection. By no means does a yellow pie slice exclude the use of the drug in combination with the drugs or diseases generating this color. But it does mean there may be better options available (i.e., green designations). Specifically, yellow suggests the drug under consideration usually can be used with safety in conjunction with the drug with which it is being matched. In a significant minority of patients, however, the drug may be either (a) incompatible with the exisiting drug, or (b) another drug combination is preferrable (i.e., a green light combination). For example, NSAIDs usually can be used safely in combination with ACE inhibitors, but in some patients NSAIDs, presumably through prostaglandin inhibition, may compromise the antihypertensive effects of captopril or cause hyperkalemia.[13,17,26,27] Hence, a yellow color is used to suggest caution and the need to reconsider the use of these two agents in combination.[28]

With respect to disease incompatibility profiles, the color yellow suggests that, although the drug can often be used in patients who have this underlying disease, some degree of caution is generally required because the drug may exacerbate the disease, or increase the likelihood of precipitating complications. For example, although digoxin is an excellent choice to treat patients with heart failure caused by left ventricular systolic dysfunction, older patients with advanced congestive heart failure are also more sensitive to potential *toxicity* of digitalis preparations, and therefore, are more likely to experience rhythm disturbances when the drug is used in this setting. Consequently, a yellow pie is used to indicate there is a small, but potentially significant, risk of using digoxin in this patient subgroup.[29,30]

Green Designation. DIP profile pie slices that carry the green color designation represent *optimal* drug-drug and drug-disease combinations. Green pie slices in the drug DIP profile indicate the agent under consideration is almost always compatible with the pre-existing drug. With respect to the DIP profile for drug-disease interactions, green indicates that the newly introduced drug usually will *not* compromise the natural history of, or produce complications associated with, the underlying disease. Almost without exception, drug-drug and drug-disease matchings that are represented by green pie slices represent optimal pharmacologic management with respect to drug-drug and drug-disease interactions.

Using DIP™ Profiles: Risk, Color, and Compatibility

To maximize its clinical utility, the DIP system uses a "stoplight" color scheme to indicate the relative desirability—or unsuitability—of introducing a specific drug into the regimen of a patient who already is taking one or more other agents, and who has one or more commonly encountered clinical disorders. Consequently, each drug analyzed in the DIP system has two pie diagram profiles: (1) A Drug-Drug Incompatibility Profile and; (2) A Drug-Disease Incompatibility Profile. When contemplating the addition of a drug to a patient's existing *regimen,* the pharmacist or physician should consult *both* DIP profiles.

Two-phase Pharmatectural Evaluation

Step 1: First, consult the drug incompatibility profile (DIP) for the specific drug (i.e., amitriptyline, azithromycin, famotidine) that is being considered for addition to the patient's regimen. The name of the principal drug under evaluation appears in a blue box at the top of each figure. Cross check this drug against the twelve other *commonly* used drugs appearing in the DIP profile. If the drug-drug DIP profile (i.e., the appropriate pie slice) indicates the drug that is being contemplated for inclusion in the drug house is *compatible* with other medications in the regimen with respect to drug-*drug* interactions (i.e., the safety of combined use is confirmed by the presence of a "green" pie, which is optimal—although a "yellow" pie is sometimes acceptable), then proceed to Step 2 (below).

Step 2: During this phase, the drug's suitability with respect to drug-*disease* compatibility is evaluated using the disease DIP profile. If the drug-disease DIP profile demonstrates that the drug under consideration for addition has a low (green) or moderate (yellow) risk for adversely affecting any underlying conditions, then it can be added to the regimen with relative safety. Note: When a yellow color appears in a DIP profile, careful consideration is warranted (see below). Finally, other factors will always come into play and should be considered before a final drug selection is made.

THE DIP™ SYSTEM GUIDE: PROFILES INTO PRACTICE

The drug incompatibility profiles that appear in this chapter incorporate the drug classes and specific agents most often employed in primary care; the disease incompatibility profiles consider the use of these medications against the backdrop of those acute and chronic medical disorders most often managed in the outpatient environment. When using the DIP system, please refer to the color plates of specific DIP profiles appearing in a separate section within this chapter. The following sections provide detailed explanations for why certain drug-drug and drug-disease combinations carry red, yellow, or green designations.

Antidepressants

Amitriptyline (Elavil®), Doxepin HCl (Sinequan®). Because they are relatively inexpensive, tricyclic antidepressants (TCAs), such as amitriptyline and doxepin, are still widely used, despite numerous studies showing that serotonin selective reuptake inhibitors (SSRIs) may, in some patient groups, produce a superior risk: benefit profile for the treatment of depression.[40] There are a number of adverse side effects associated with conventional TCAs, including anticholinergic side effects[31] (dry mouth, urinary retention, visual disturbances, confusion), extrapyramidal movement disorders, disturbances in cognition, and cardiovascular side effects. The cardiovascular profile of TCAs is complex.[32] TCAs and their metabolites are highly concentrated in the myocardium, explaining the vulnerability of the heart to TCA toxicity. For example, TCAs are capable of interfering with heart rate, rhythm, and contractility. Conventional TCAs possess a type Ia antiarrhythmic profile.

In patients predisposed to cardiovascular disease, therapeutic vigilance is recommended when using TCAs. When the concentration of parent TCA and metabolites exceeds 1000 ng/ml, the risk of cardiovascular toxicity is greatly enhanced. Because of its frequency and potential severity, TCA-induced postural hypotension is another drug-related adverse effect of special concern. Although the mechanism of postural hypotension is not fully understood, blockade of the alpha-adrenergic receptor is the most plausible explanation.[25,33]

Amitriptyline Drug Incompatibility Profile (Tricyclic Antidepressants) (DIP 3-1). In light of these pharmacologic properties, the Drug Incompatibility Profile for amitriptyline and doxepin reveals red warning designations for combined use of these TCAs with alcohol, monoamine oxidase inhibitors (MAOIs) sympathomimetic amines, and antiarrhythmic agents such as quinidine and procainamide. Concurrent use with alcohol is not recommended because TCAs, especially in higher doses, can cause cognitive impairment and sedation, both of which are exacerbated by alcohol intake. There are also studies showing that the combined use of amitriptyline and alcohol can cause additive euphoria, leading to alcohol abuse. Based on these potential interactions, the combined use of TCAs and alcohol should be avoided whenever possible.[6,7,34]

The pharmacologic effects of TCAs such as desipramine and imipramine may be potentiated by the concomitant use of quinidine, which reduces clearance of these antidepressant medications. Although these effects have not been demonstrated specifically with amitriptyline or doxepin, a red warning, nevertheless, is issued. As a group, the combined use of TCAs and Type Ia antiarrhythmic agents has the potential for producing serious adverse effects on cardiac conduction.[7,32]

When TCAs are used in combination with sympathomimetic amines (epinephrine, norepinephrine, phenylephrine, methylphenidate), clinical disturbances such as hypertension and, in rare circumstances, hypertensive crisis may result. These effects are mediated by inhibition of norepinephrine uptake at presynaptic neurons. Because the consequences of acute hypertension can be severe, especially in the elderly, a red warning designation is given for the combined use of these medications. The use of MAOIs in conjunction with TCAs requires extreme therapeutic vigilance. Although these two agents have been used in combination, there are multiple case reports documenting significant adverse consequences when these medications are used together.[1,6,7] A number of deleterious effects are described, including confusion, hyperexcitability, delirium, coma, hyperpyrexia, convulsions, flushing, headache, and death. If, for some reason, an MAOI and TCA must be used together, the combination is better tolerated when the drugs are started together. When switching from one class to another, a drug-free interval of at least 1 week is recommended when changing from a TCA to an MAOI, and a 2-week drug-free interval is recommended when changing from an MAOI to a TCA. In general, concurrent use is not recommended.[7,35]

A number of drug interactions, although not life-threatening, carry *yellow* DIP® classifications. The anticholinergic side effects associated with TCAs can be exacerbated by combined use with other drugs producing anticholinergic symptoms. These drugs or drug classes include antihistamines (diphenhydramine, Benadryl®), muscle relaxants, antipsychotics, anti-Parkinson agents with atropine-like side effects, and scopolamine-containing antidiarrheal agents. The use of cimetidine with TCAs also requires caution because significant anticholinergic side effects (dry mouth, urinary retention, blurred vision, etc.) are produced by cimetidine-mediated elevations in blood TCA serum levels.[22,36-38]

Finally, caution is warranted for combined use of benzodiazepines and TCAs, especially in patients who require maintenance of motor function related to occupational activities. Because both benzodiazepines and TCAs have sedating properties, increased impairment of skills related to driving are observed when these two classes are used in combination.

Amitriptyline Disease Incompatibility Profile (DIP 3-1). For all practical purposes, TCA use is not encouraged in pregnant patients and in individuals with known life-threatening cardiac arrhythmias. Because high doses of TCAs can prolong conduction times, produce arrhythmias, and stimulate sinus tachycardia, this class should be used with great caution in patients[11] with severe coronary artery disease. Orthostatic hypotension may occur in patients with decreased left ventricular function, justifying a yellow classification in individuals suffering from congestive heart failure. Although the mechanism is unclear, both elevated and decreased blood sugar levels have been reported with TCA use, which suggests cautious use in patients with diabetes mellitus.[7]

Because elderly patients are more susceptible to orthostatic hypotension, coronary artery disease, and cardiac arrhythmias, TCAs should be used cautiously in this population. Confusion caused by TCAs is a well-documented side effect in the elderly. Moreover, because elderly patients with arthritis are encouraged to walk, remain active, and exercise their joints, the potential sedating properties of TCAs may be undesirable. Hence, a yellow designation is given for the combined use of TCAs in patients with chronic arthritis.[39,40]

Seizure thresholds can be reduced by TCA use, a finding that dictates cautious use of these agents in patients with a documented seizure disorder or EEG abnormalities. The drug should be used with caution in patients with renal impairment. TCAs also may produce a range of gastrointestinal symptoms, from epigastric distress and cramps to nausea and vomiting. Consequently, selective use in patients with pre-existing ulcer disease is recommended. Finally, the possibility of suicide in depressed patients must always be considered. Although TCAs are used to treat depression, depressed patients should *not* have access to large quantities of the drug. The yellow classification for combining TCAs with depression alludes to this precautionary prescribing practice, which may help reduce the risk of suicide through TCA ingestion. The warning classification and pharmacologic considerations discussed in this section on TCAs (amitriptyline, doxepin) also apply to desipramine. Additional considerations are discussed in the sections below.

The yellow classification for concomitant antihistamine use is downgraded to a red designation because of the potentially severe anticholinergic reaction between desipramine and cyproheptadine. The aggravation of depression that is observed with the combined use of fluoxetine and desipramine also warrants a similar downgrading to a red designation. All other drug interactions are similar to those seen with amitriptyline. Refer to the previous section for an explanation of potential problems associated with use of various TCA-drug combinations.

The disease incompatibility profiles for desipramine would be similar to those generated for amitriptyline. A detailed discussion and explanation of classifications for these drug-disease combinations can be found in the previous section, Amitriptyline-Disease DIP Profiles.

Trazodone (Desyrel®) (DIP 3-2). Trazodone is a commonly used antidepressant, although its precise mechanism of action is not fully understood.

ANTIDEPRESSANTS

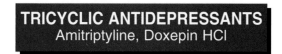

TRICYCLIC ANTIDEPRESSANTS
Amitriptyline, Doxepin HCl

DRUG Incompatibility Profile

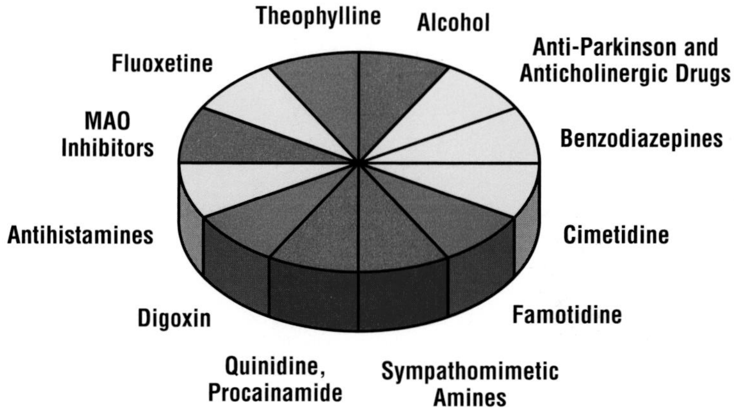

DISEASE Incompatibility Profile

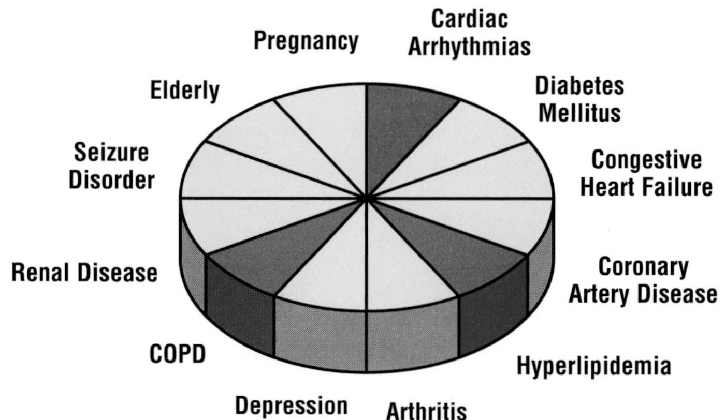

ANTIDEPRESSANTS

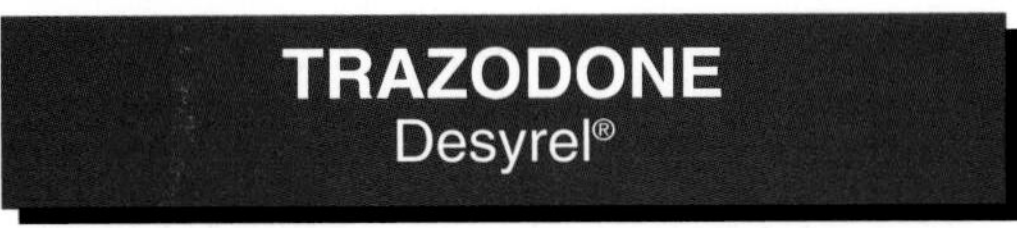

DRUG Incompatibility Profile

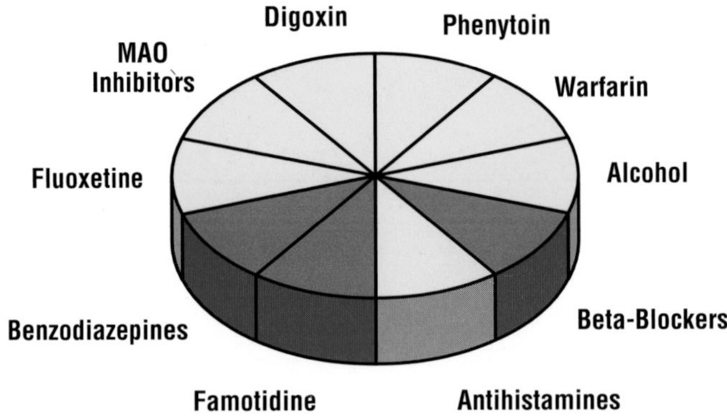

DISEASE Incompatibility Profile

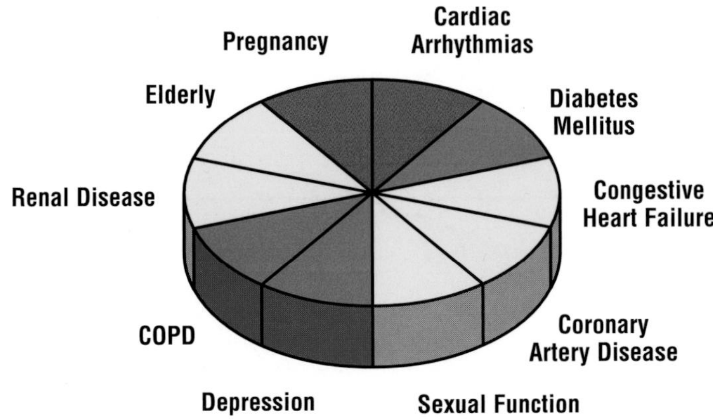

ANTIDEPRESSANTS

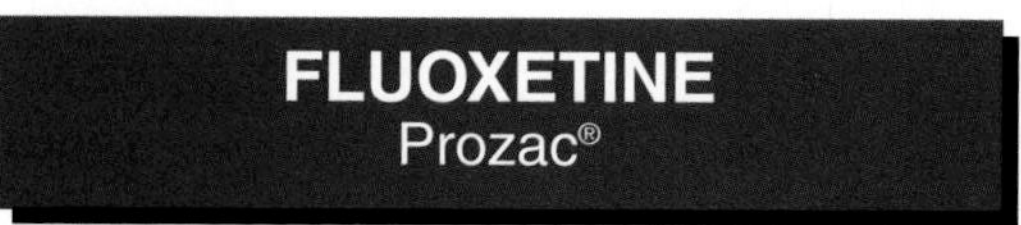

DRUG Incompatibility Profile

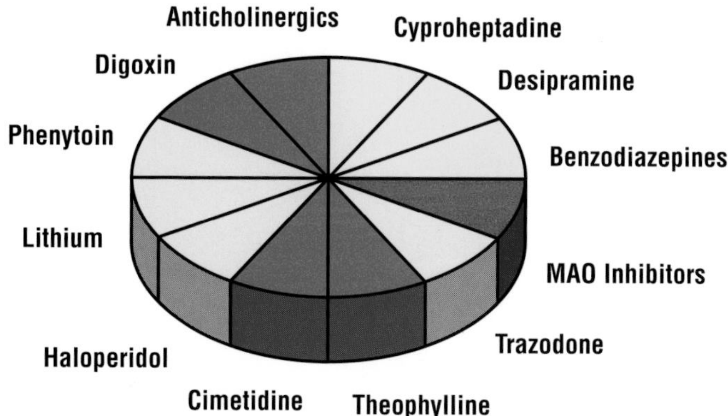

DISEASE Incompatibility Profile

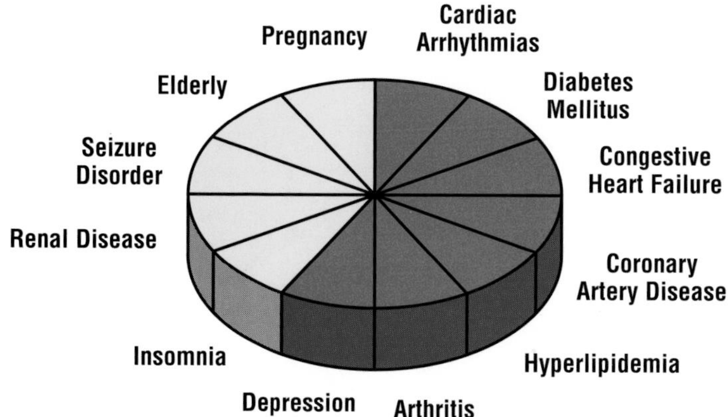

ANTIDEPRESSANTS

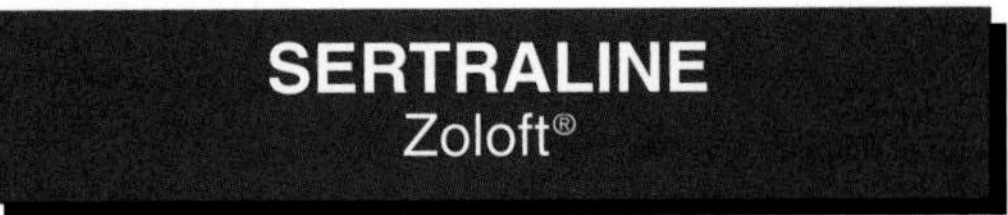

DRUG Incompatibility Profile

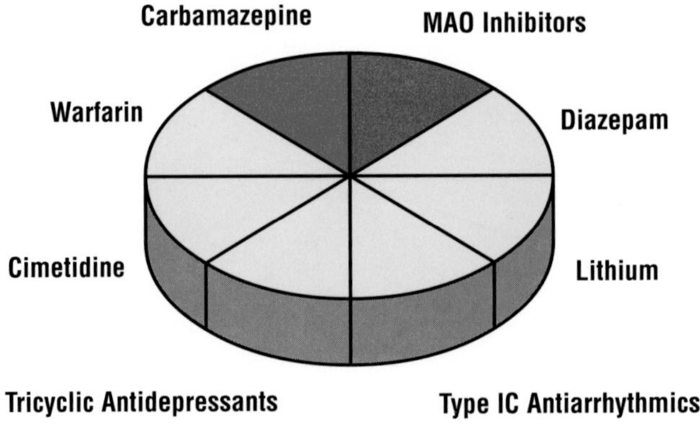

DISEASE Incompatibility Profile

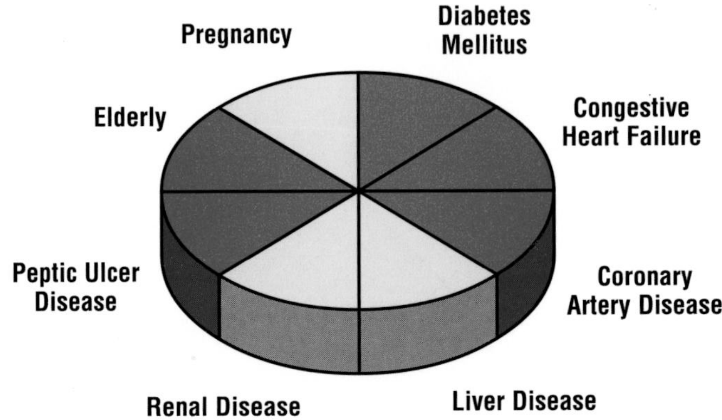

ANTIDEPRESSANTS

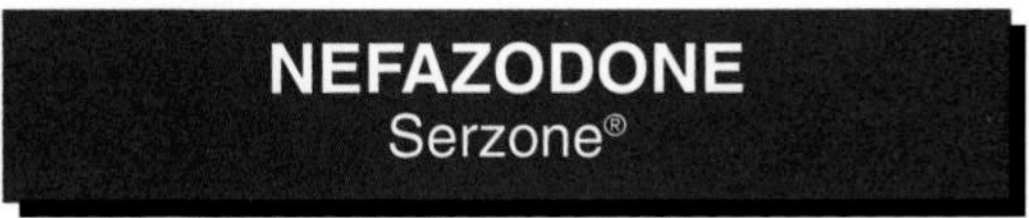

DRUG Incompatibility Profile

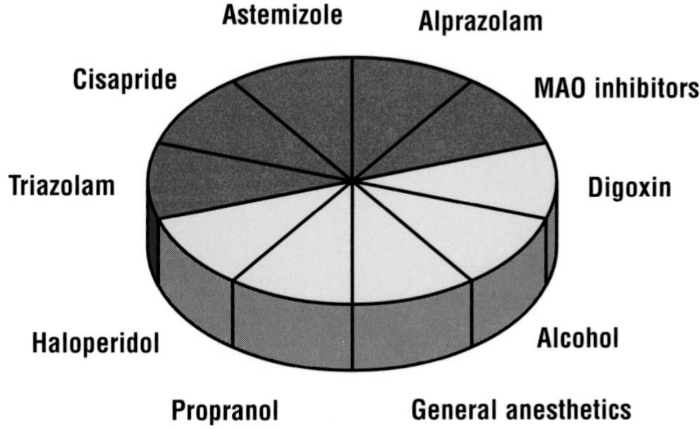

DISEASE Incompatibility Profile

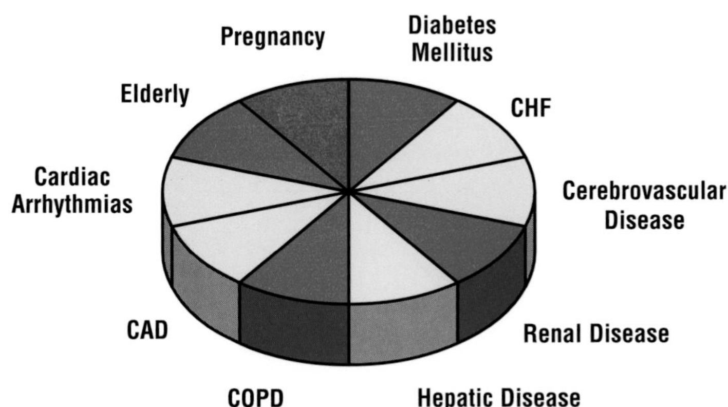

MEDICATIONS FOR ALZHEIMER'S DISEASE

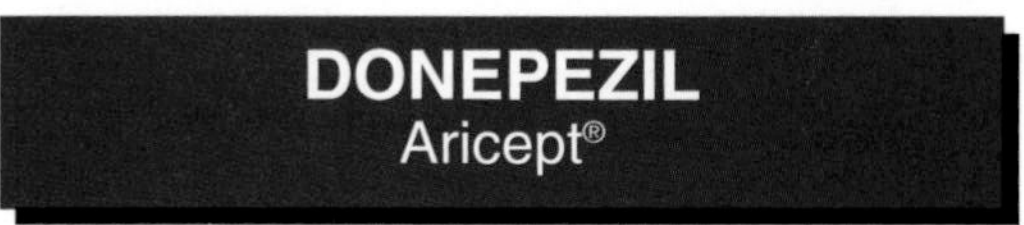

DRUG Incompatibility Profile

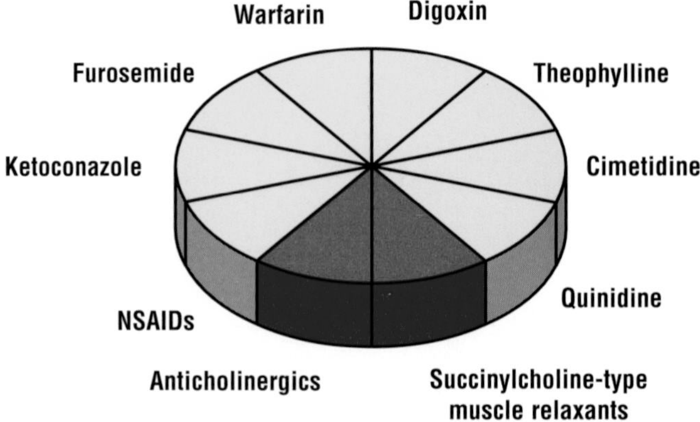

DISEASE Incompatibility Profile

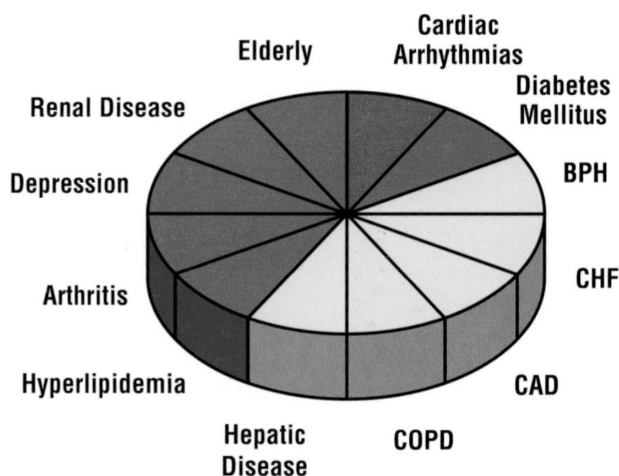

BIPHOSPHANATES

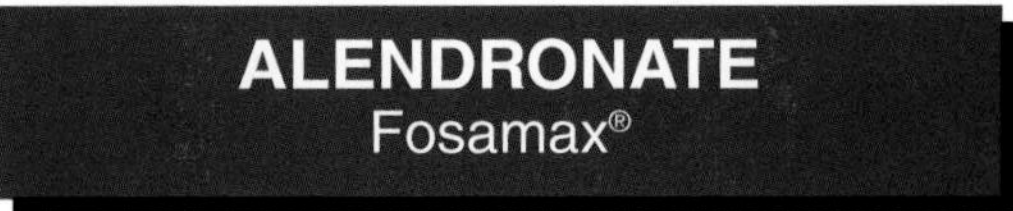

DRUG Incompatibility Profile

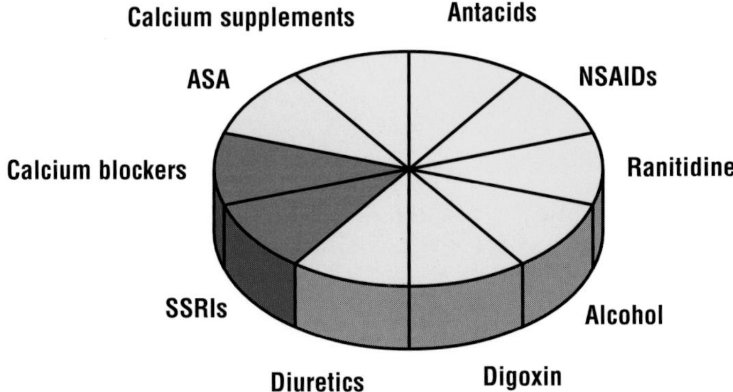

DISEASE Incompatibility Profile

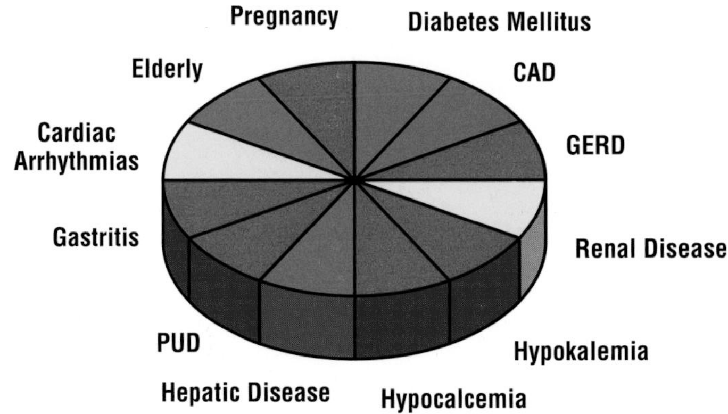

IMPOTENCE MEDICATIONS

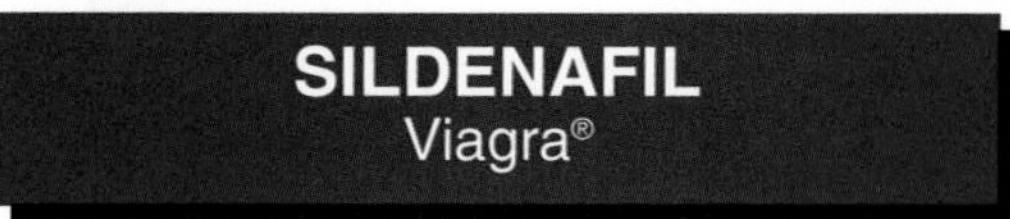

DRUG Incompatibility Profile

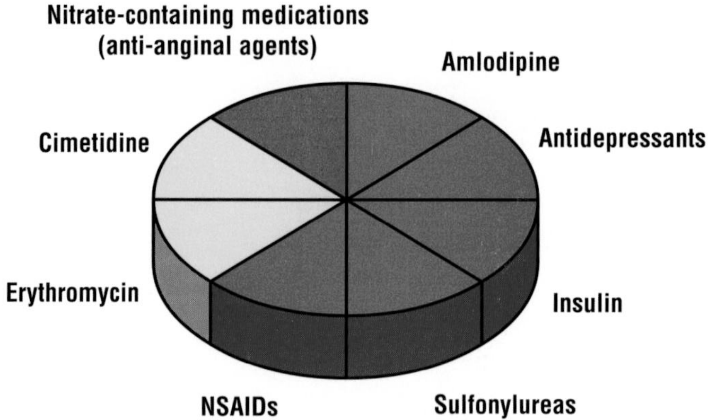

DISEASE Incompatibility Profile

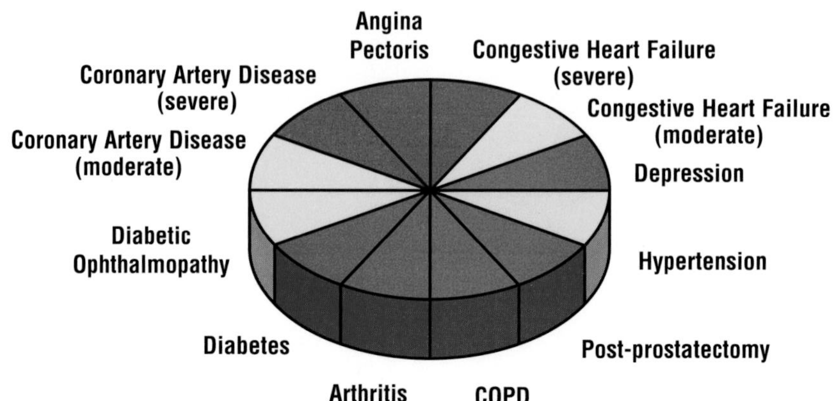

ANTI-INFLAMMATORY AGENTS

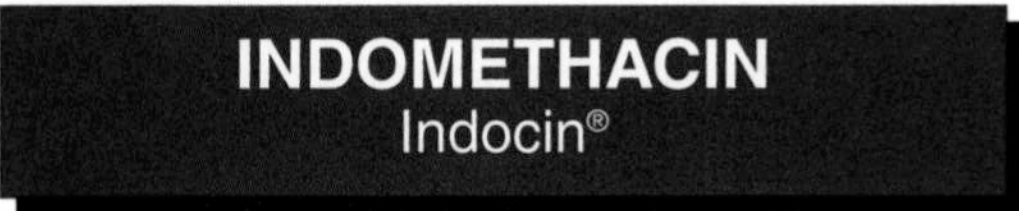

DRUG Incompatibility Profile

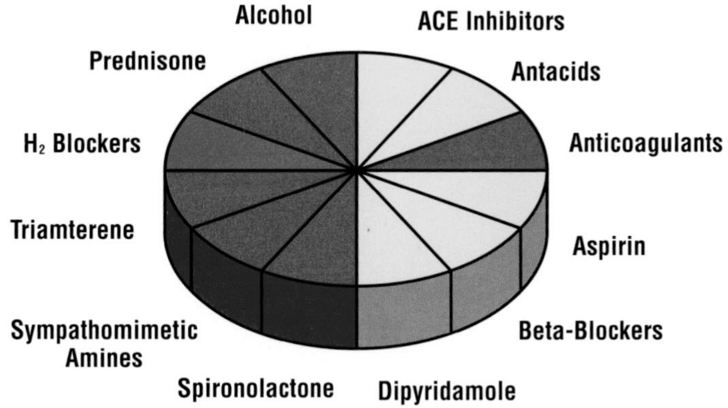

DISEASE Incompatibility Profile

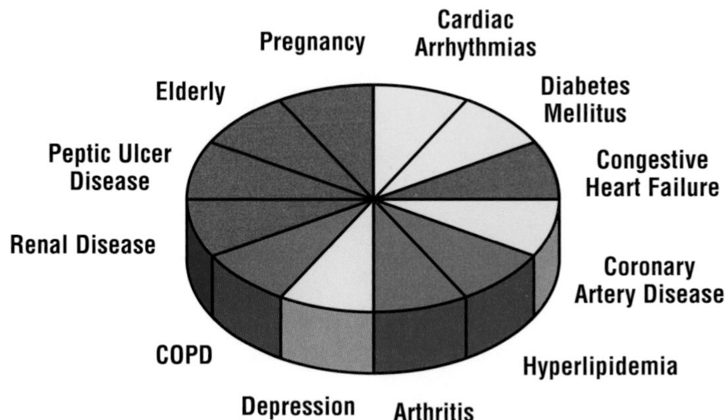

ANTI-INFLAMMATORY AGENTS

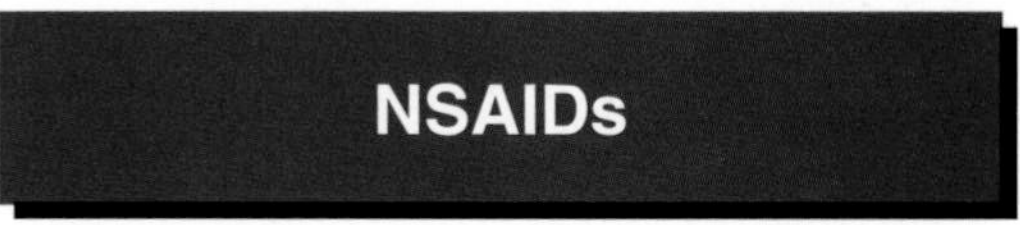

DRUG Incompatibility Profile

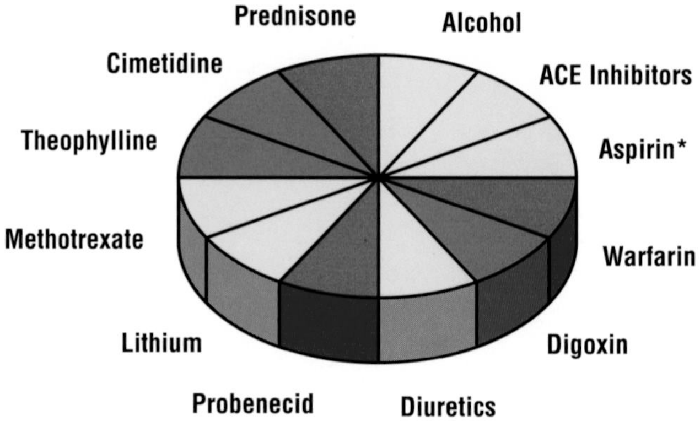

DISEASE Incompatibility Profile

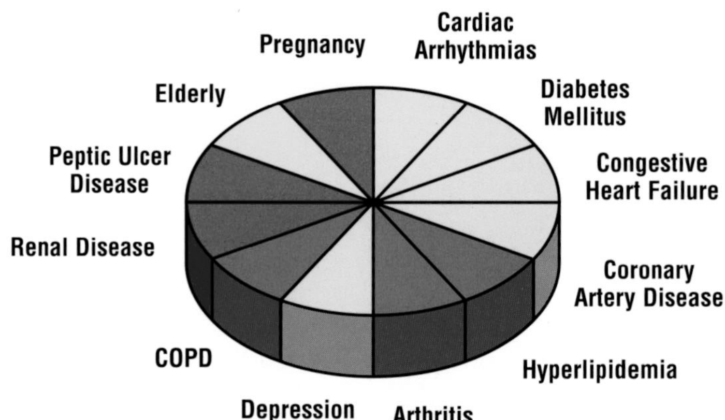

*Aspirin is contraindicated with Ketorolac.

CORTICOSTEROIDS

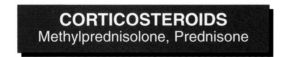

CORTICOSTEROIDS
Methylprednisolone, Prednisone

DRUG Incompatibility Profile

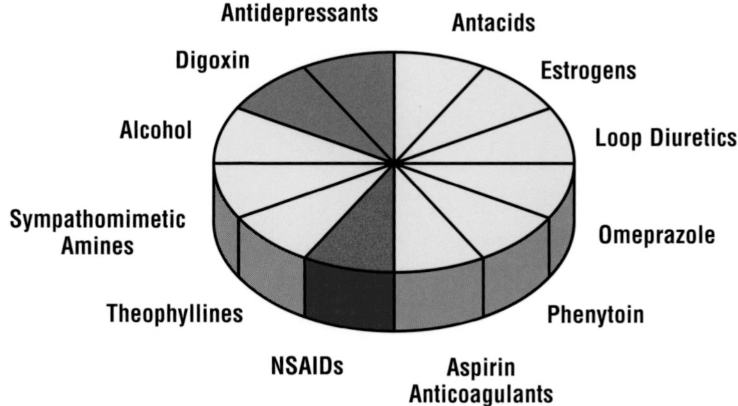

DISEASE Incompatibility Profile

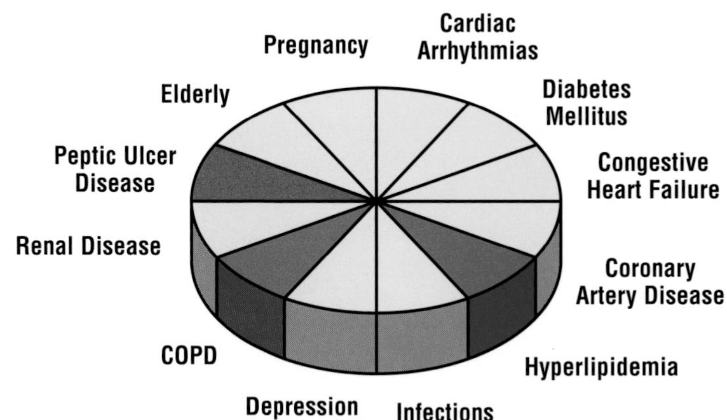

ANTI-PLATELET DRUGS

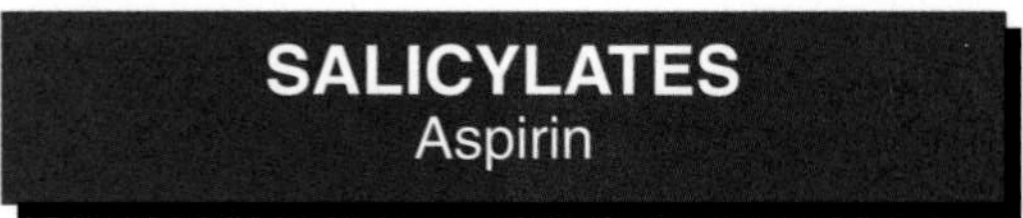

DRUG Incompatibility Profile

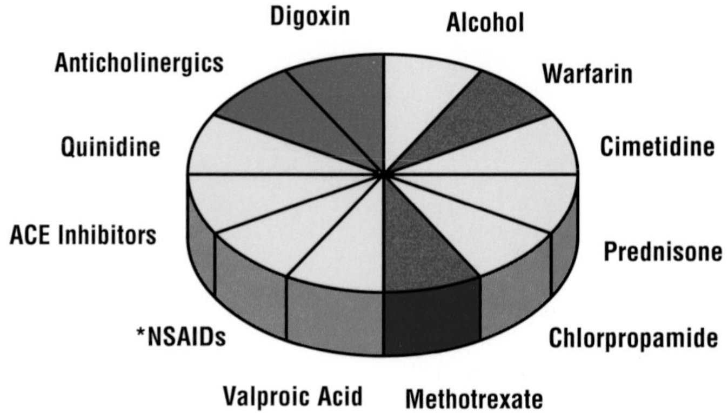

DISEASE Incompatibility Profile

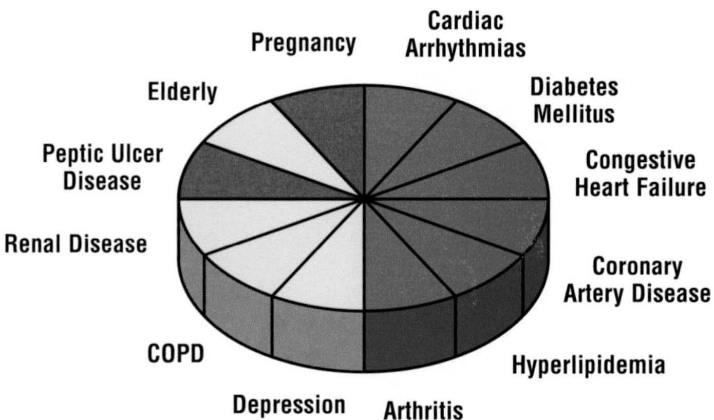

*Except for Ketorolac, which should be red.

LEUKOTRIENE RECEPTOR ANTAGONISTS

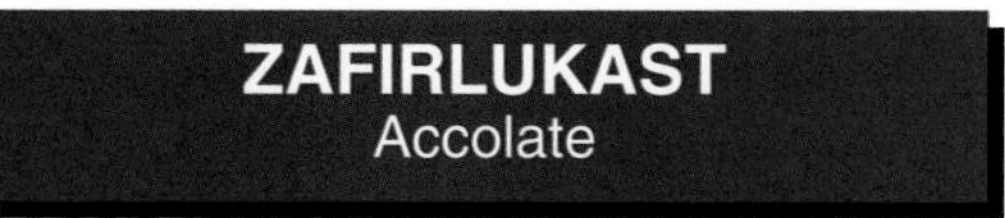

DRUG Incompatibility Profile

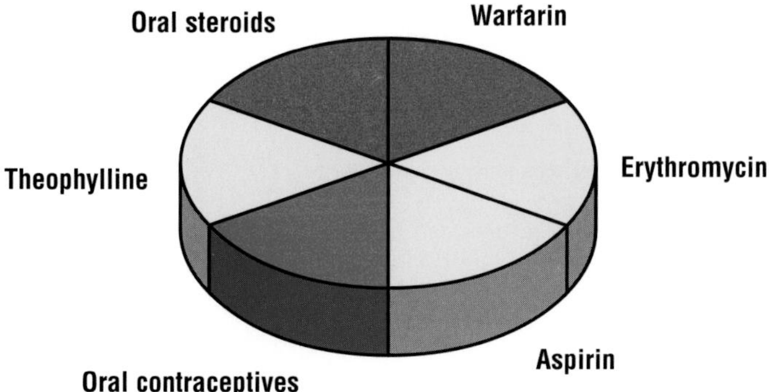

DISEASE Incompatibility Profile

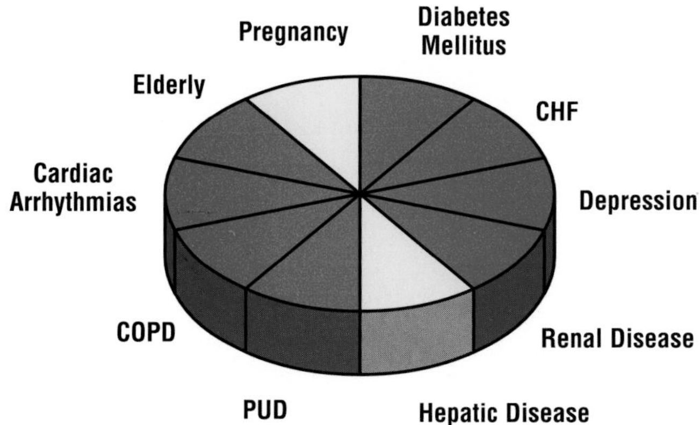

ANTI-CANCER AGENTS

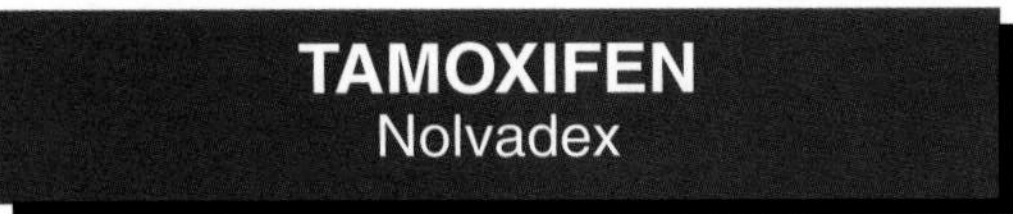

DRUG Incompatibility Profile

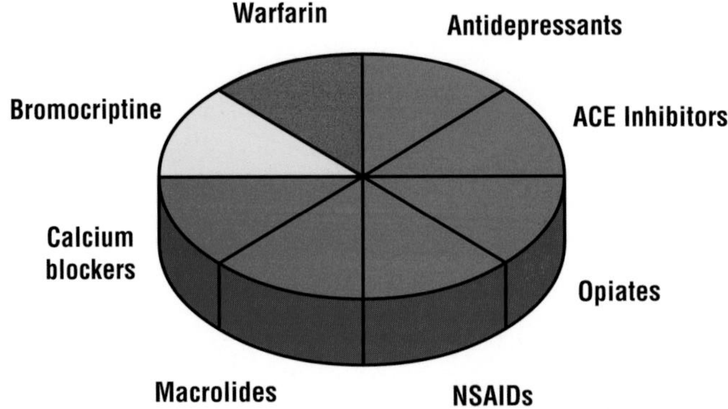

DISEASE Incompatibility Profile

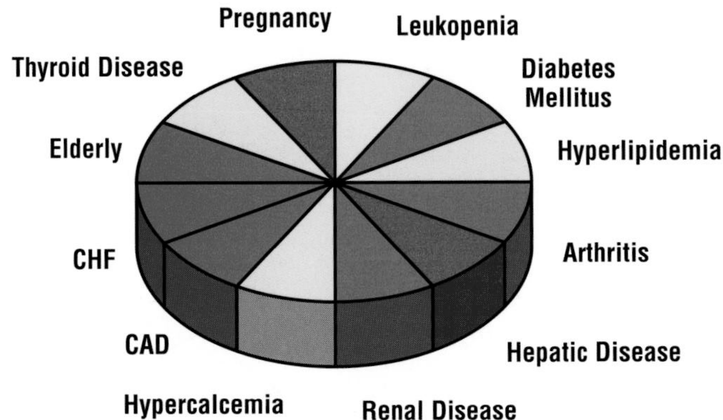

ANTICOAGULANTS

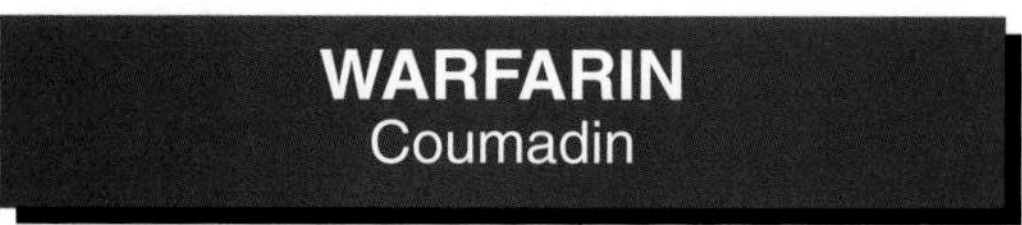

DRUG Incompatibility Profile

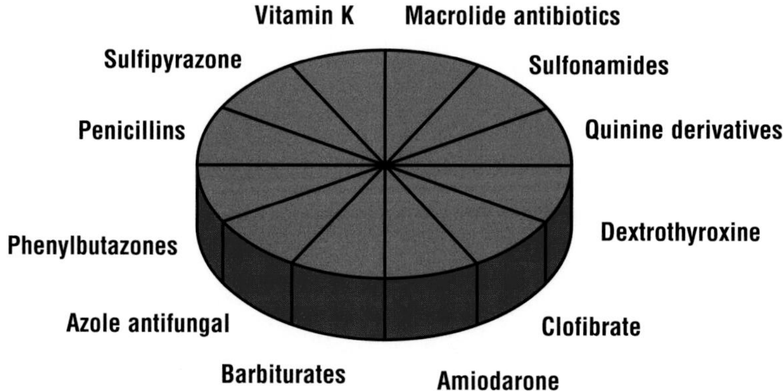

DISEASE Incompatibility Profile

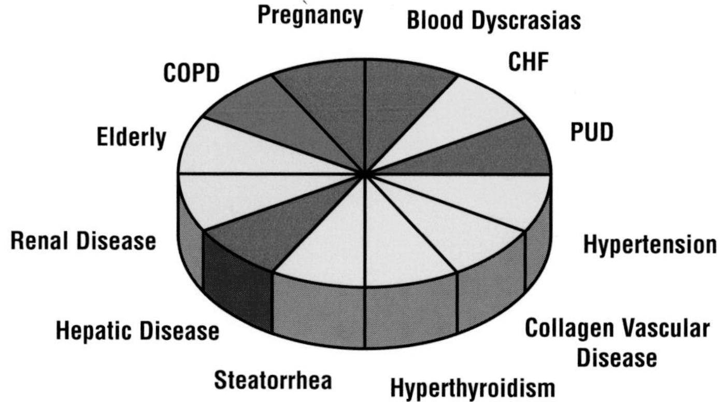

H_2-ANTAGONISTS

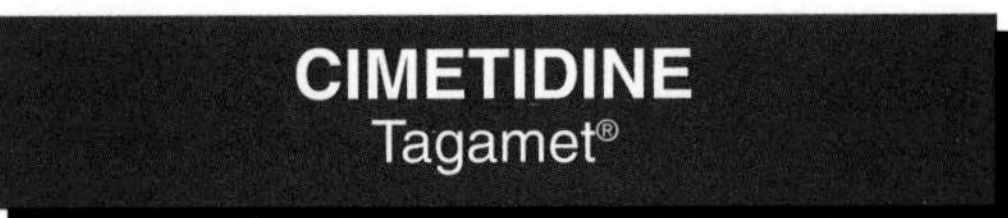

DRUG Incompatibility Profile

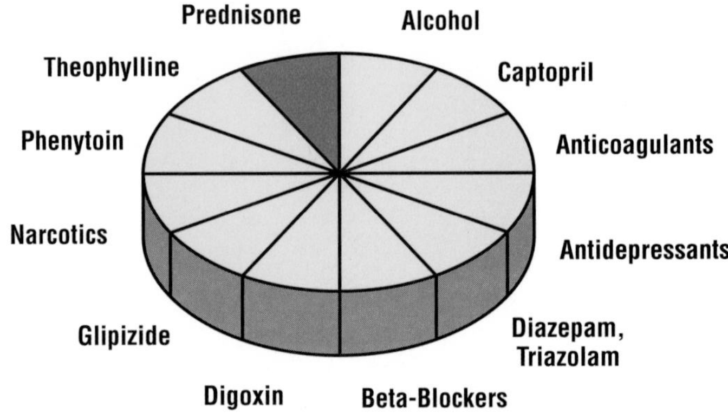

DISEASE Incompatibility Profile

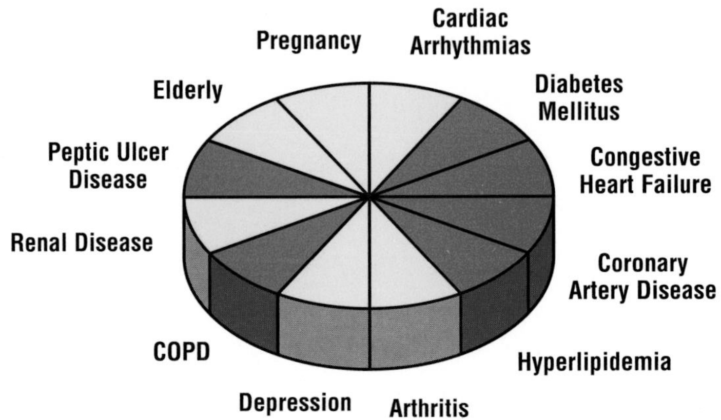

H_2-ANTAGONISTS

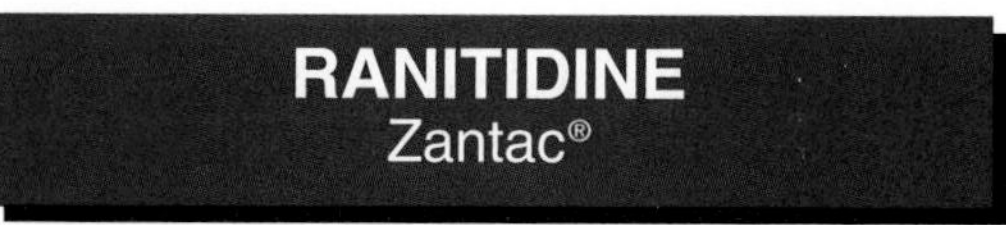

DRUG Incompatibility Profile

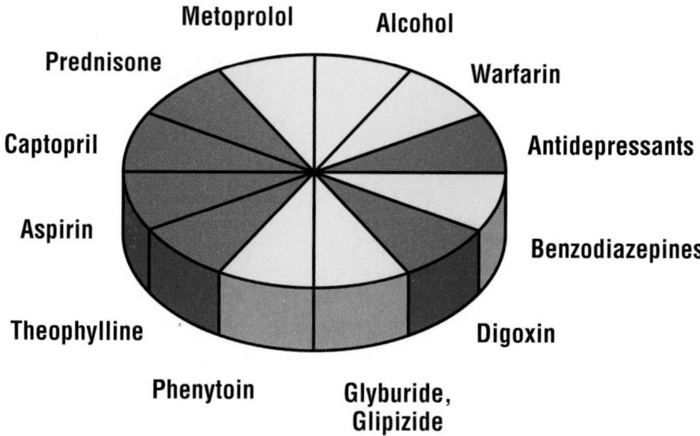

DISEASE Incompatibility Profile

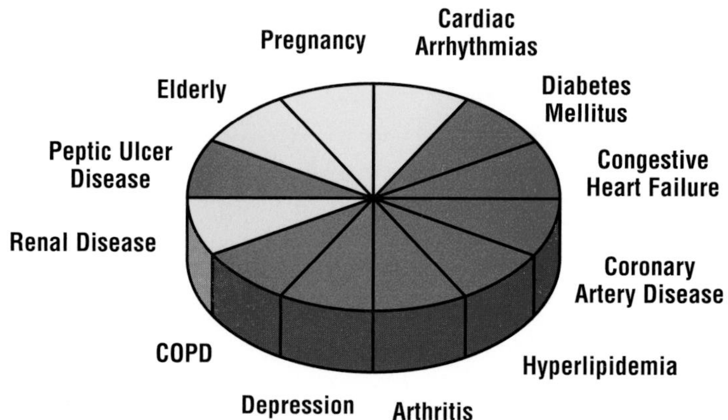

PROTON PUMP BLOCKERS

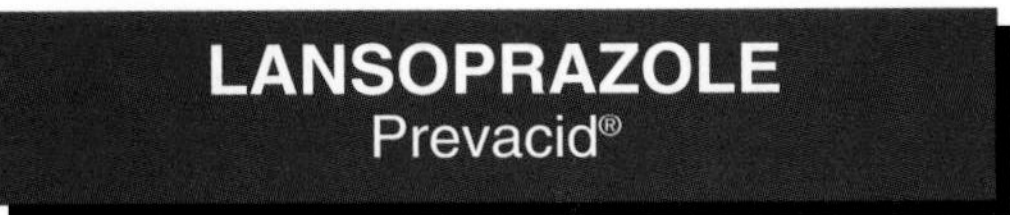

DRUG Incompatibility Profile

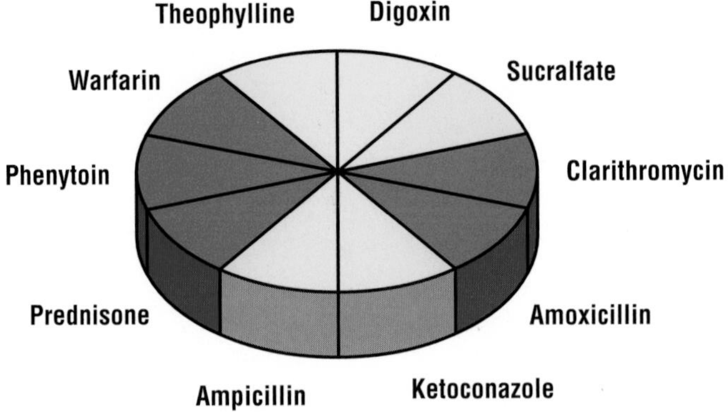

DISEASE Incompatibility Profile

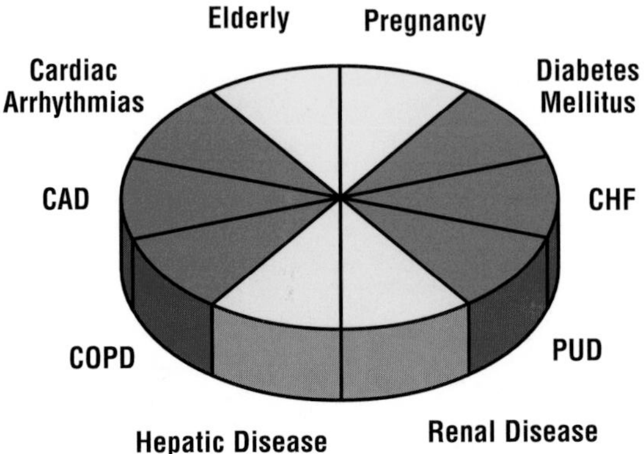

PROTON PUMP BLOCKERS

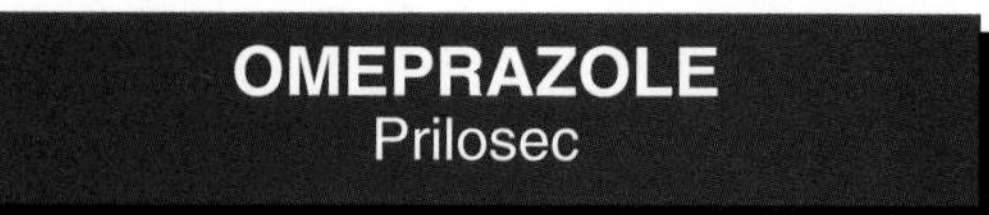

DRUG Incompatibility Profile

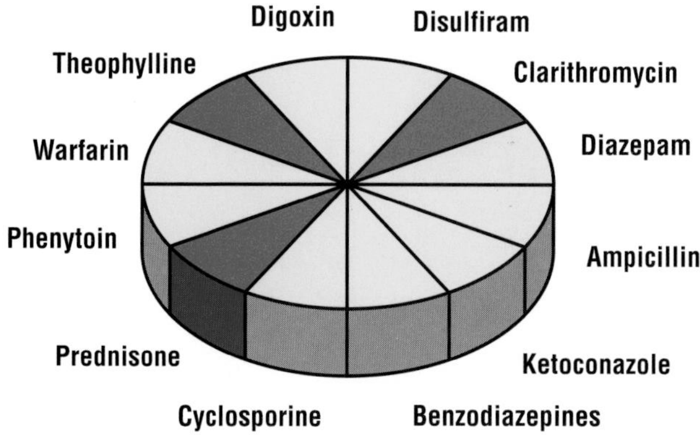

DISEASE Incompatibility Profile

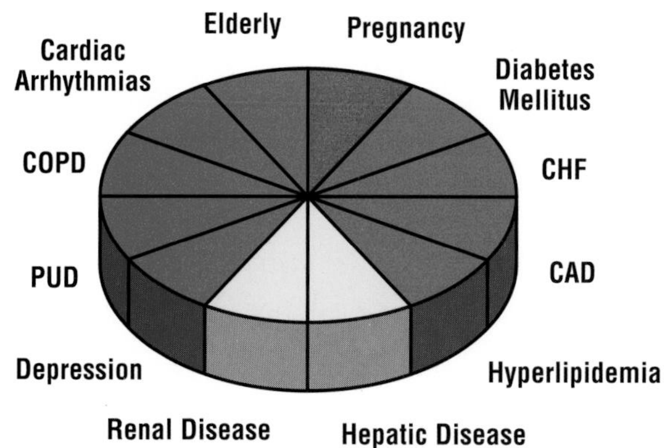

SEDATIVES/ANXIOLYTICS

BENZODIAZEPINES

DRUG Incompatibility Profile

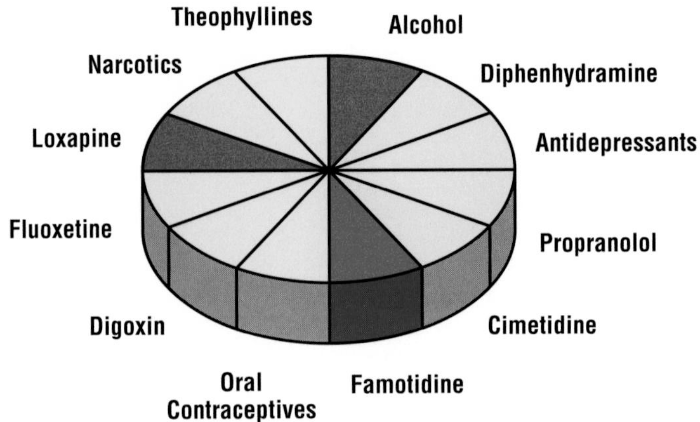

DISEASE Incompatibility Profile

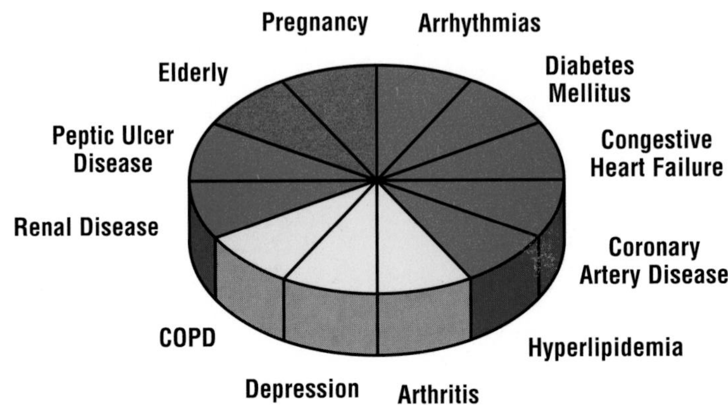

BRONCHODILATORS

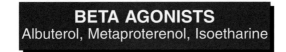

BETA AGONISTS
Albuterol, Metaproterenol, Isoetharine

DRUG Incompatibility Profile

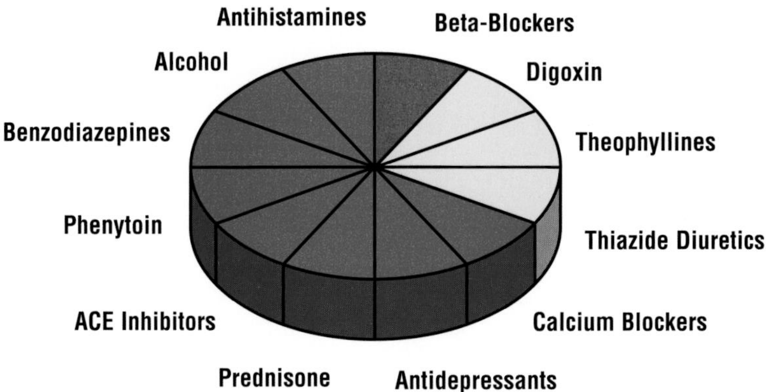

DISEASE Incompatibility Profile

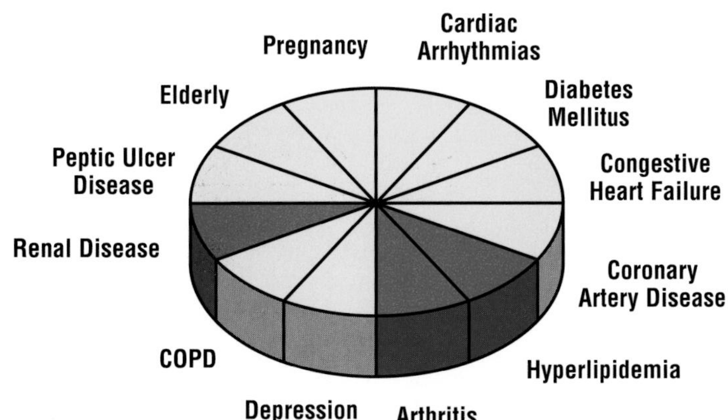

BRONCHODILATORS

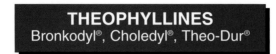

THEOPHYLLINES
Bronkodyl®, Choledyl®, Theo-Dur®

DRUG Incompatibility Profile

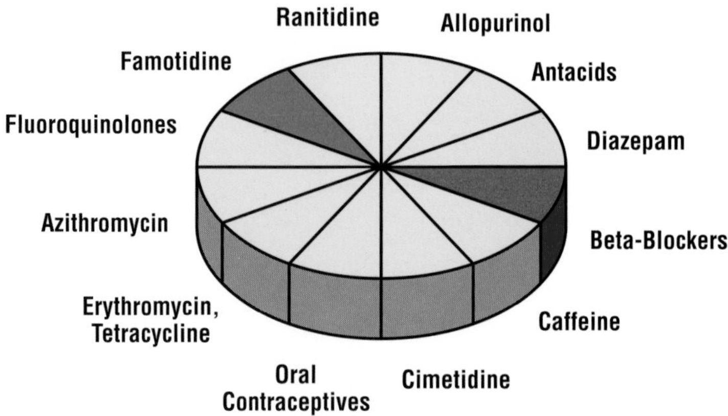

DISEASE Incompatibility Profile

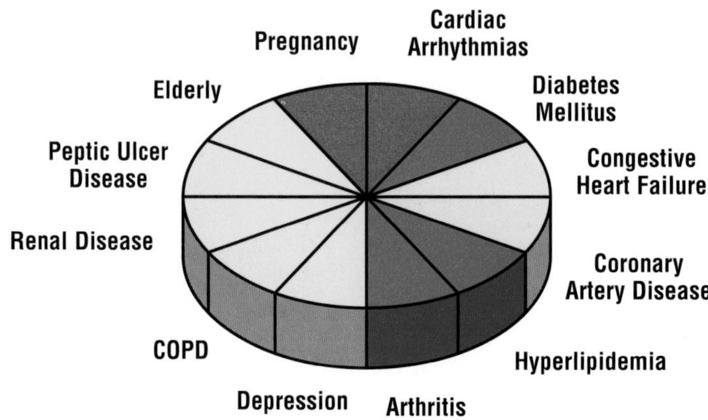

ANTIHISTAMINES

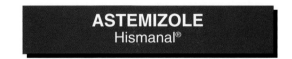

ASTEMIZOLE
Hismanal®

DRUG Incompatibility Profile

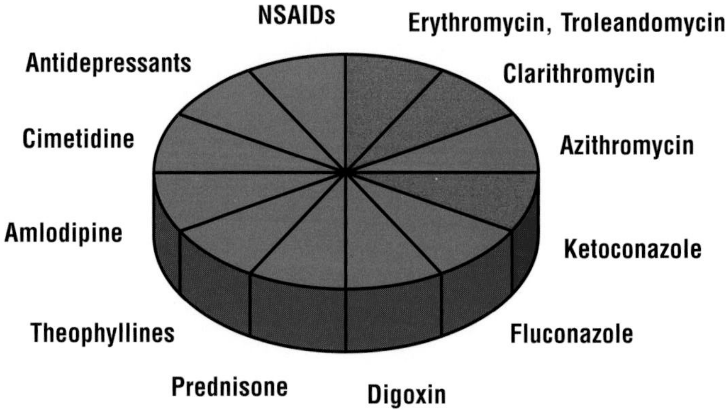

DISEASE Incompatibility Profile

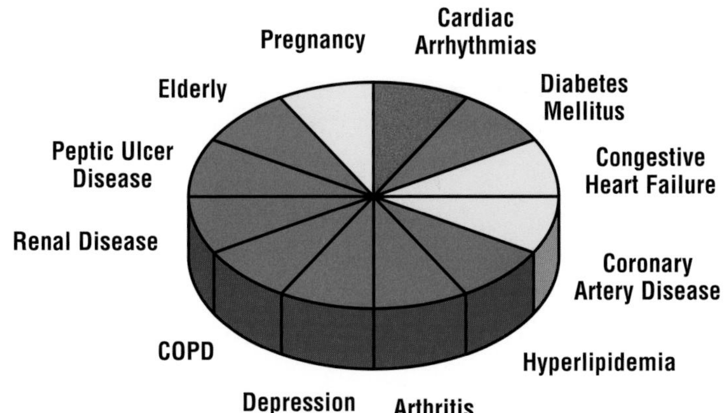

ANTIHISTAMINES

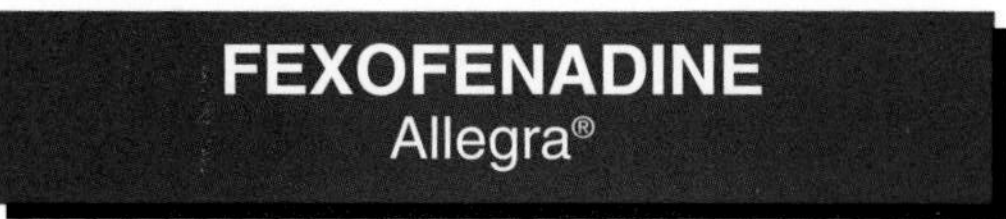

DRUG Incompatibility Profile

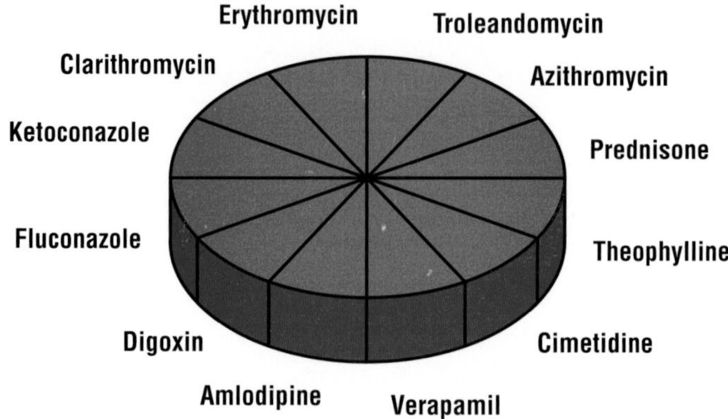

DISEASE Incompatibility Profile

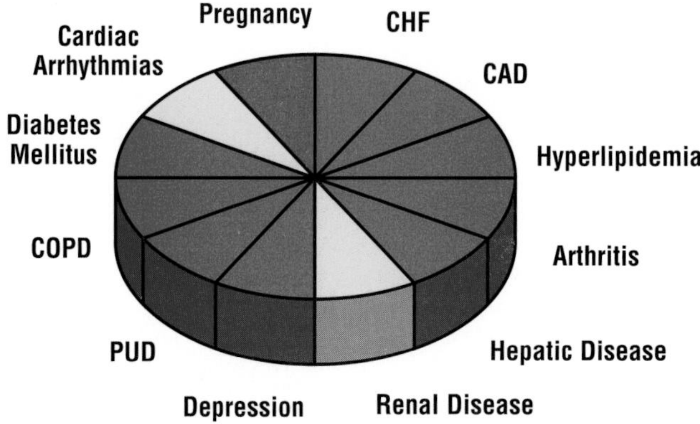

ANTIHISTAMINES

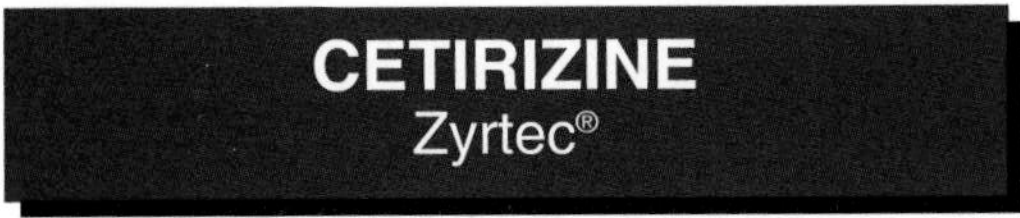

DRUG Incompatibility Profile

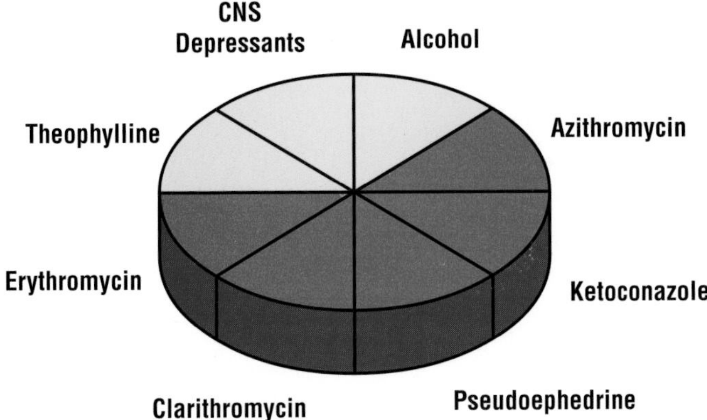

DISEASE Incompatibility Profile

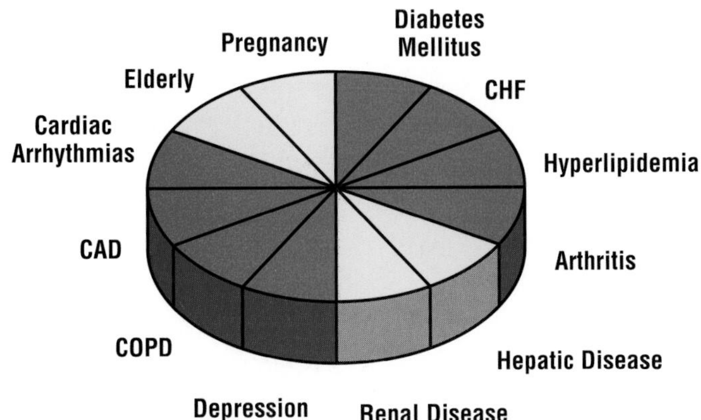

ANTIHISTAMINES

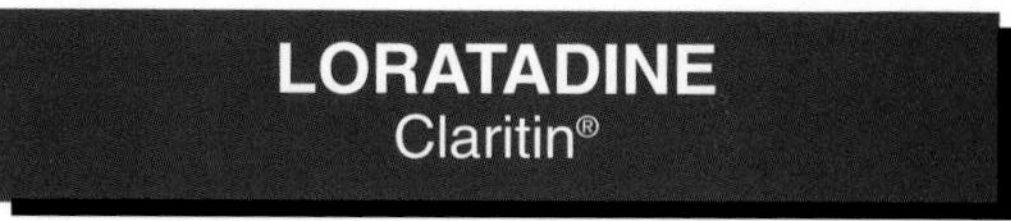

DRUG Incompatibility Profile

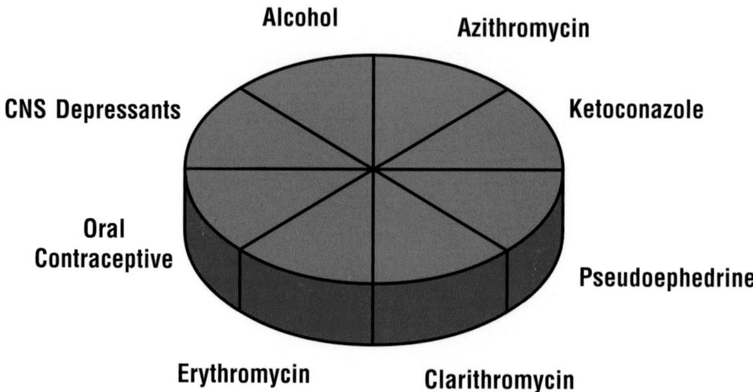

DISEASE Incompatibility Profile

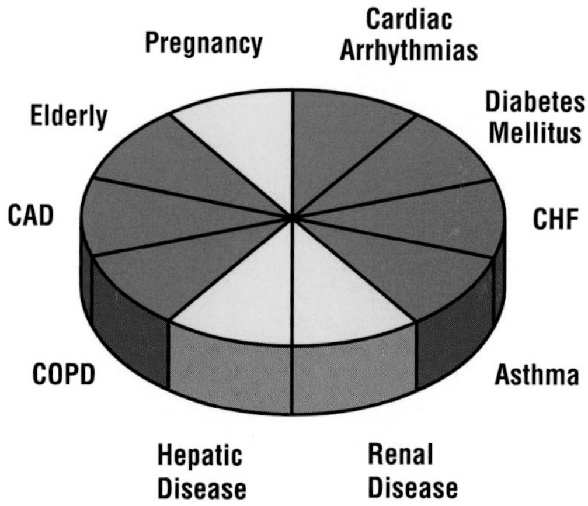

ANTIHISTAMINES

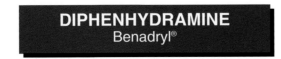

DIPHENHYDRAMINE
Benadryl®

DRUG Incompatibility Profile

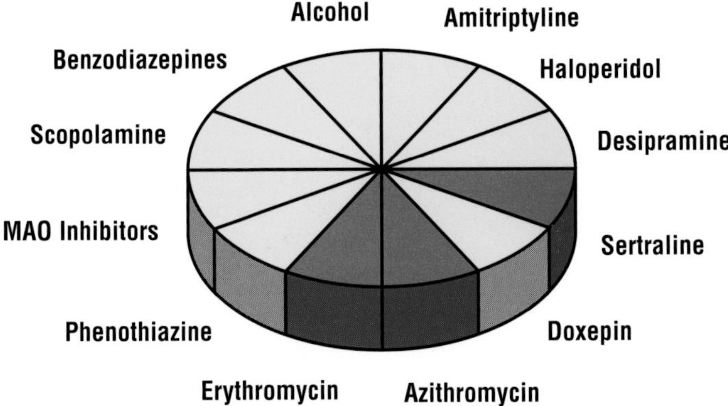

DISEASE Incompatibility Profile

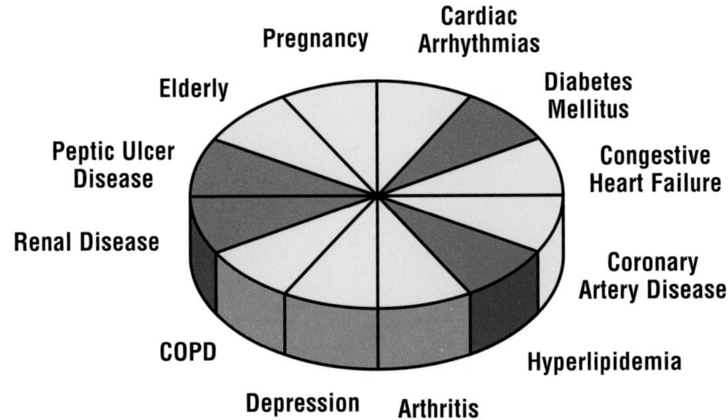

ANTIBIOTICS

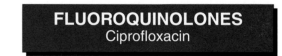

FLUOROQUINOLONES
Ciprofloxacin

DRUG Incompatibility Profile

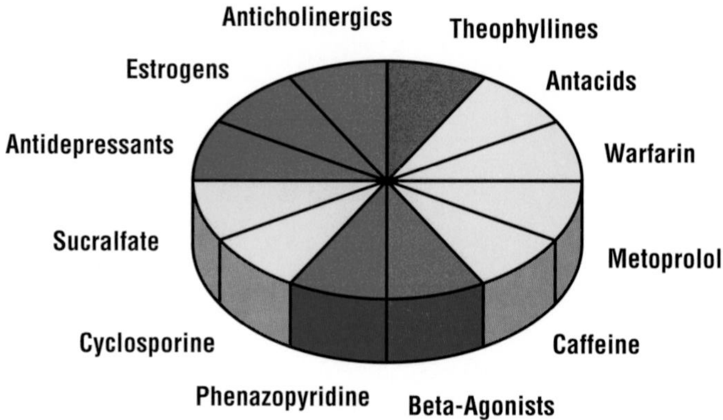

DISEASE Incompatibility Profile

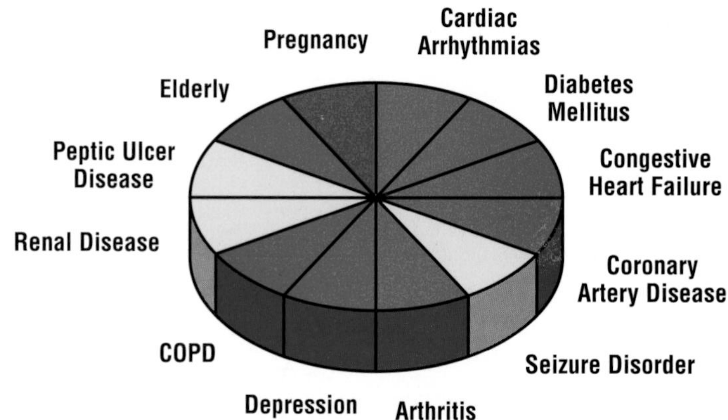

ANTIBIOTICS

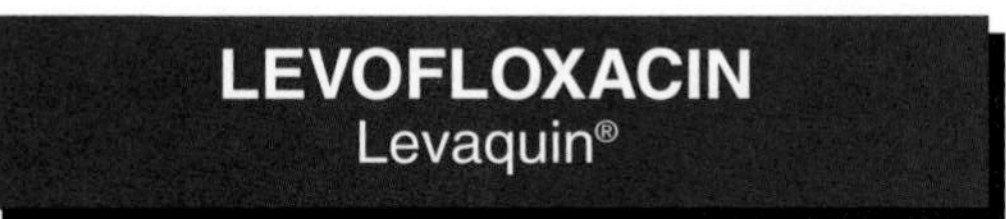

DRUG Incompatibility Profile

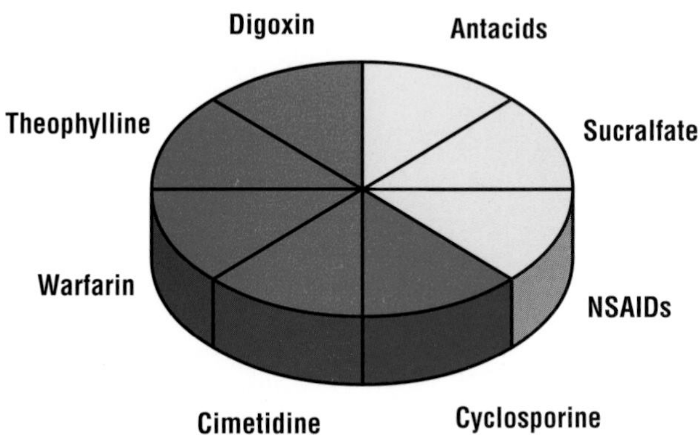

DISEASE Incompatibility Profile

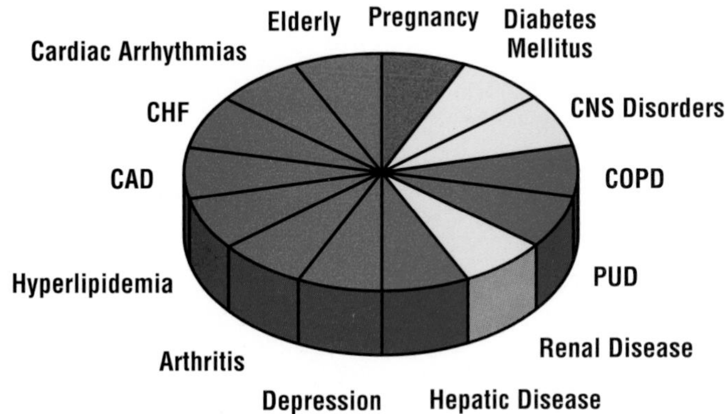

ANTIBIOTICS

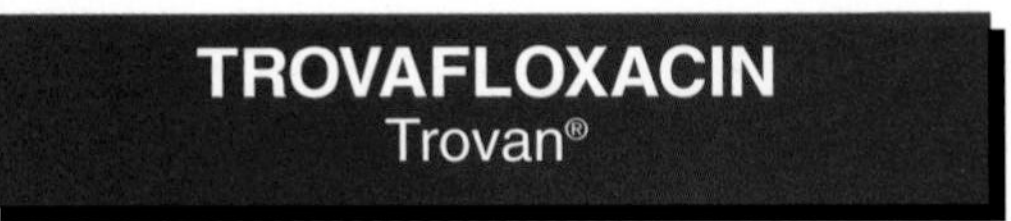

DRUG Incompatibility Profile

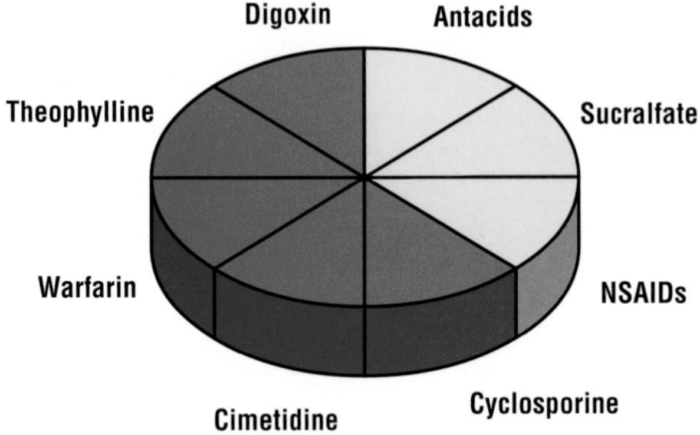

DISEASE Incompatibility Profile

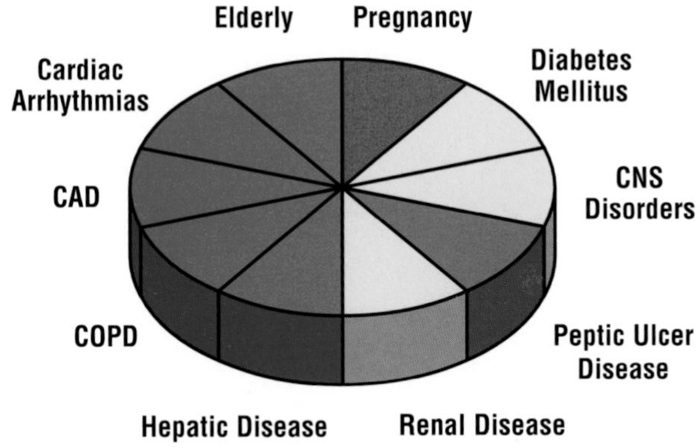

ANTIBIOTICS

ERYTHROMYCIN
Erythrocin®

DRUG Incompatibility Profile

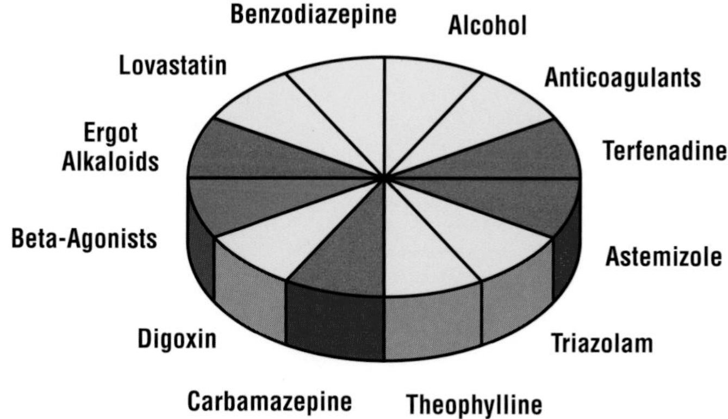

DISEASE Incompatibility Profile

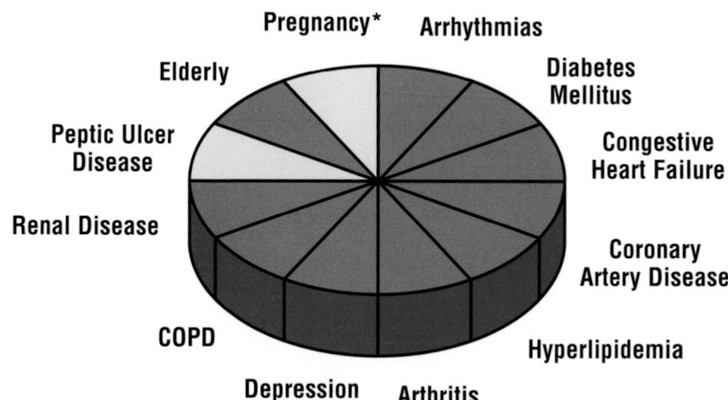

*Clarithromycin should be red and should not be used unless there is no alternative.

ANTIBIOTICS

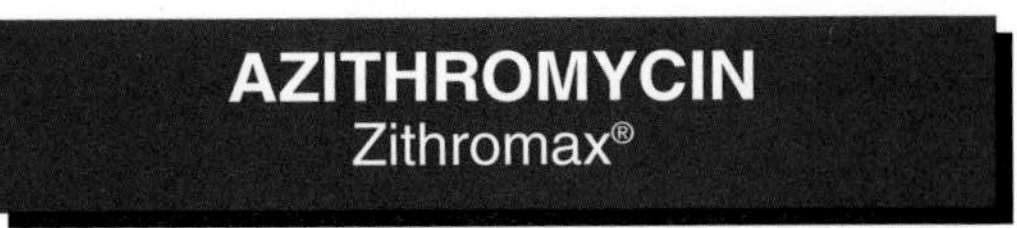

DRUG Incompatibility Profile

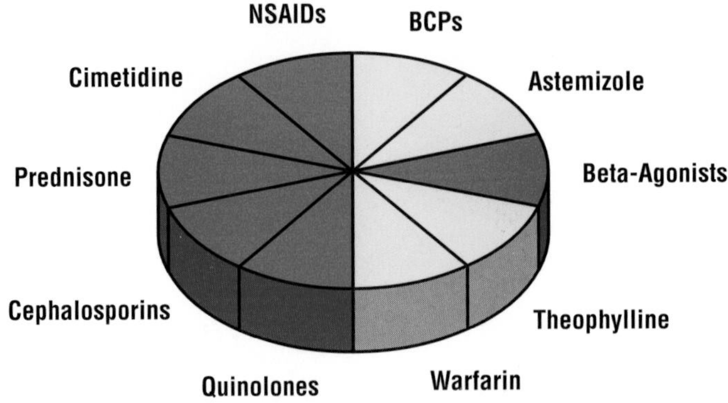

DISEASE Incompatibility Profile

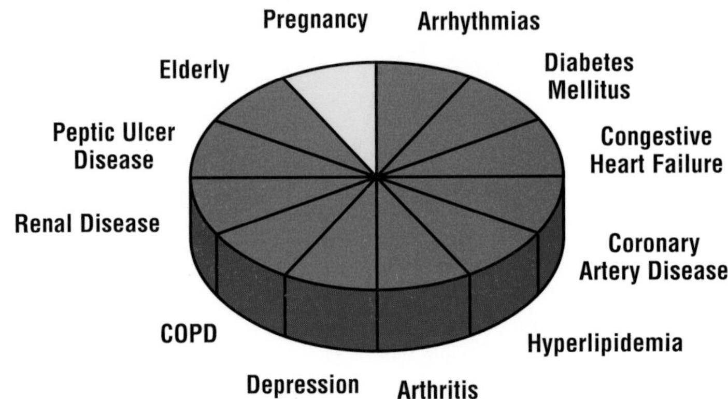

ORAL HYPOGLYCEMICS

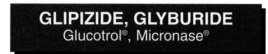

GLIPIZIDE, GLYBURIDE
Glucotrol®, Micronase®

DRUG Incompatibility Profile

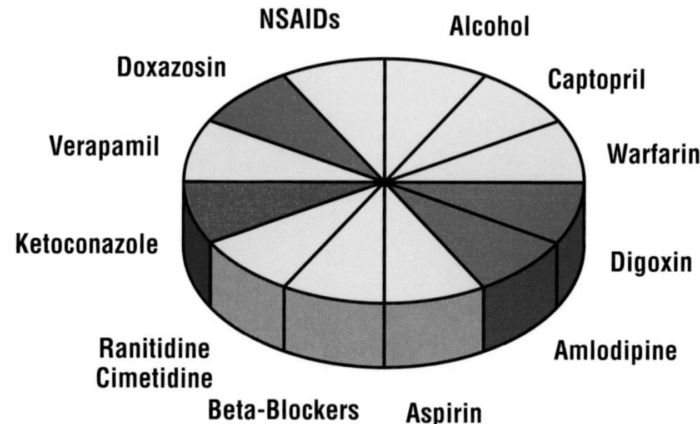

DISEASE Incompatibility Profile

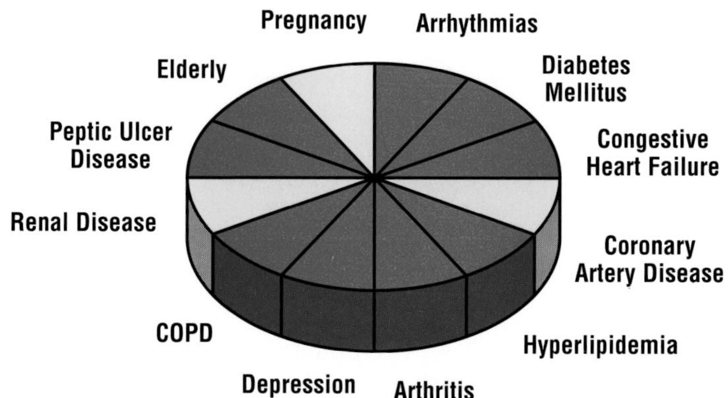

ORAL HYPOGLYCEMIC AGENTS

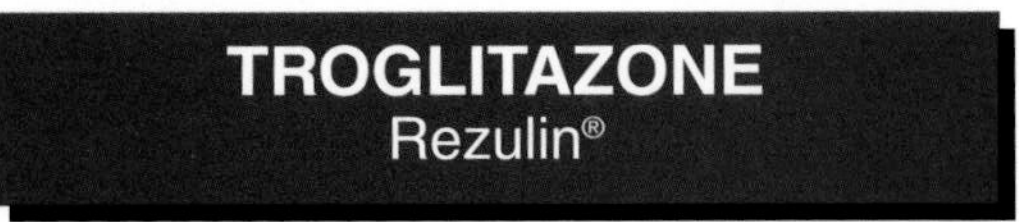

DRUG Incompatibility Profile

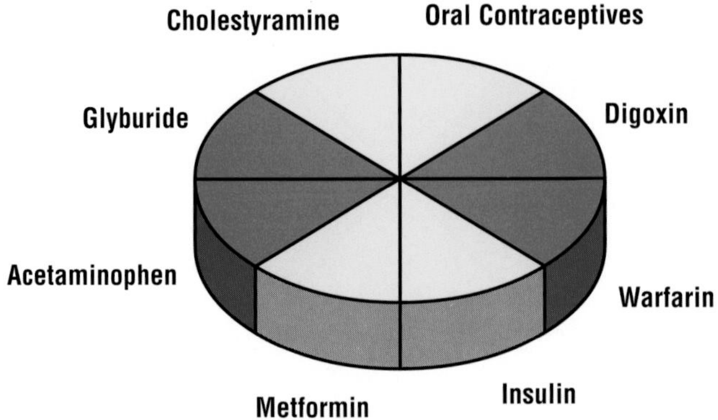

DISEASE Incompatibility Profile

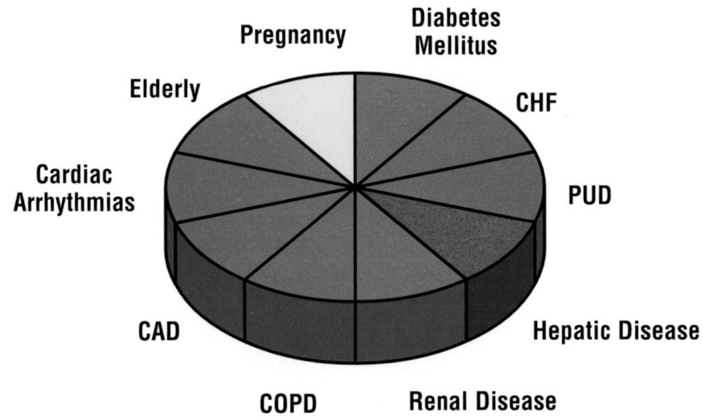

ORAL HYPOGLYCEMIC AGENTS

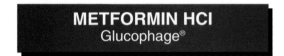

METFORMIN HCI
Glucophage®

DRUG Incompatibility Profile

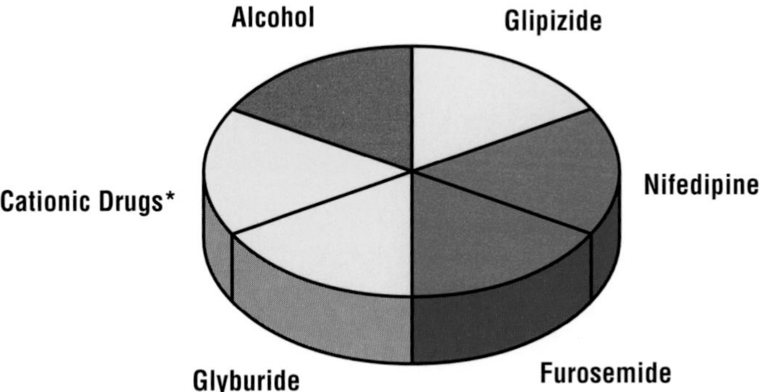

*amilioride, digoxin, morphine, procainamide, quinidine, quinine, ranitidine, triamterene, trimethoprim, and vancomycin

DISEASE Incompatibility Profile

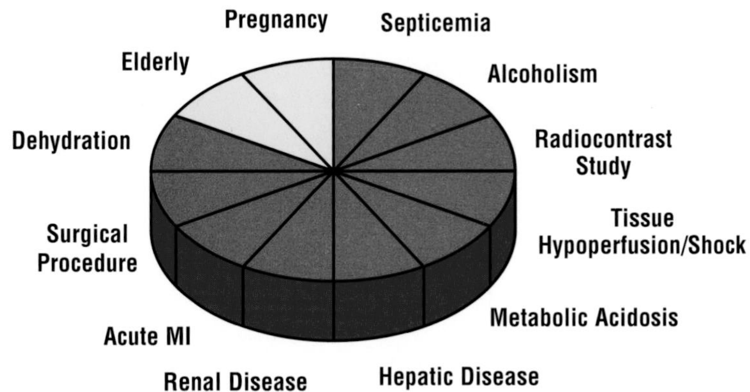

LIPID - LOWERING DRUGS

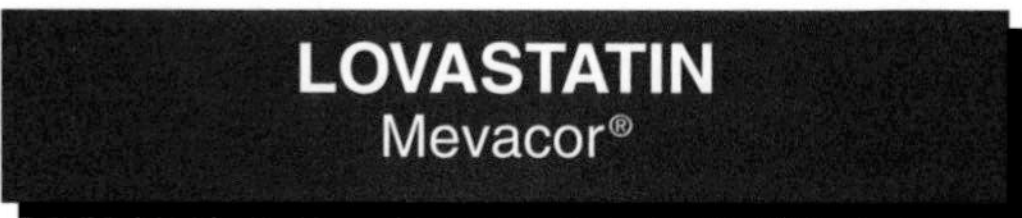

DRUG Incompatibility Profile

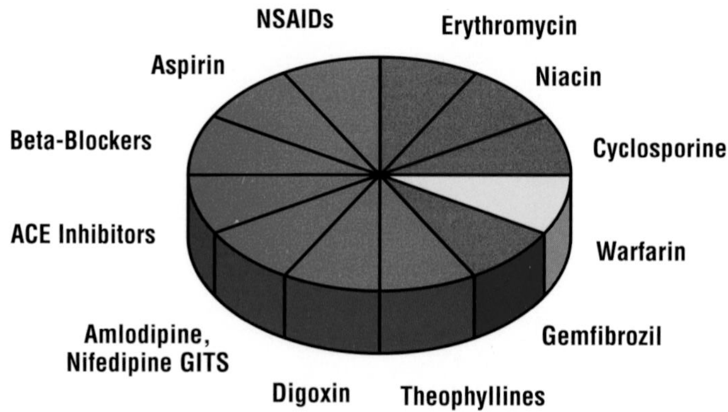

DISEASE Incompatibility Profile

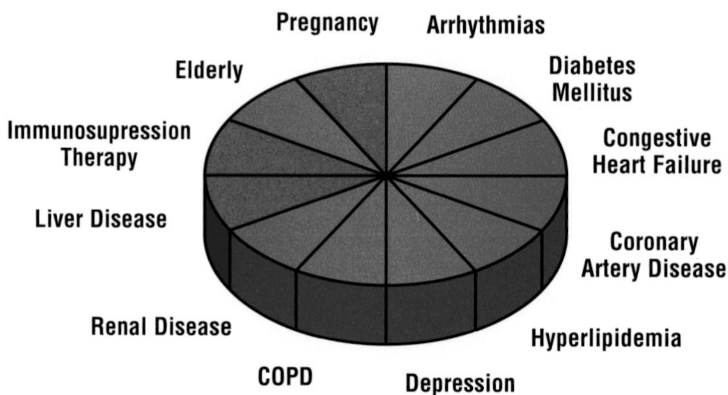

LIPID-LOWERING DRUGS

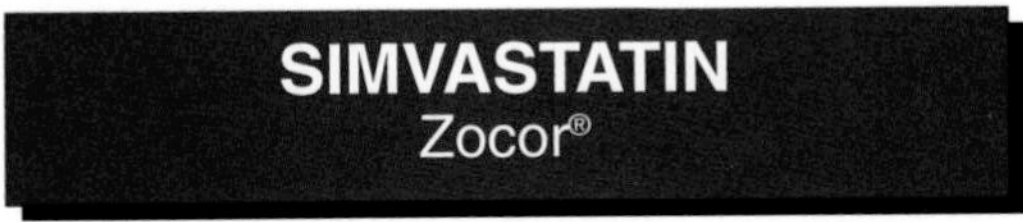

DRUG Incompatibility Profile

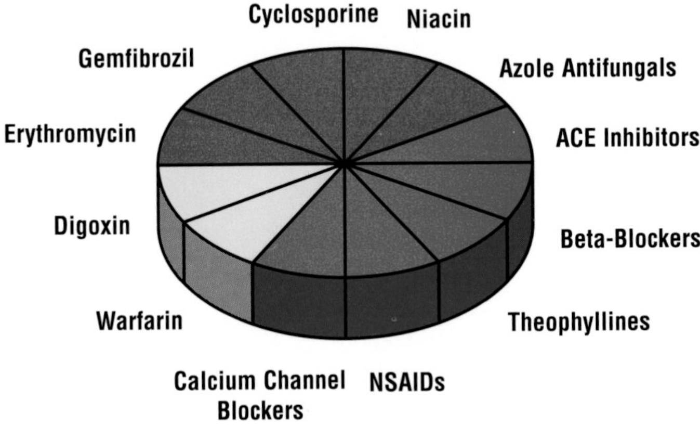

DISEASE Incompatibility Profile

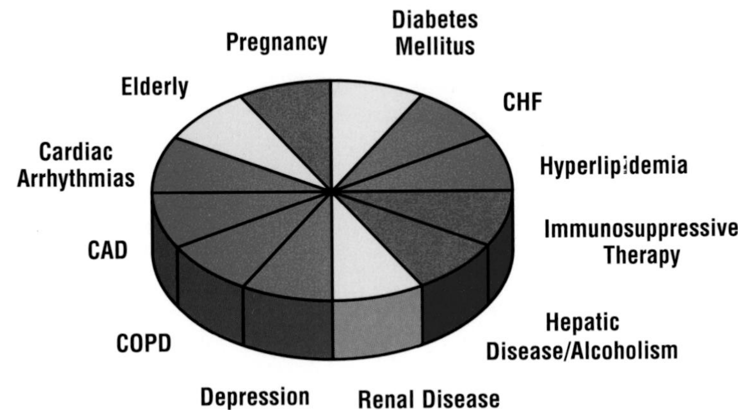

LIPID-LOWERING DRUGS

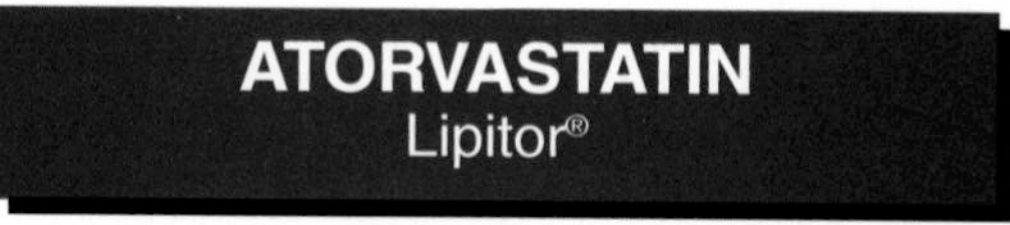

DRUG Incompatibility Profile

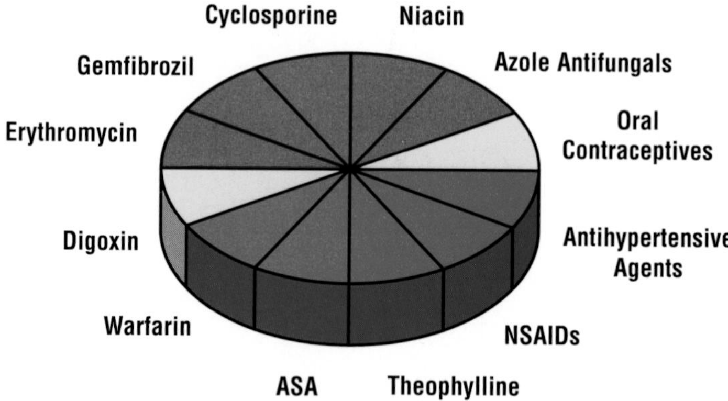

DISEASE Incompatibility Profile

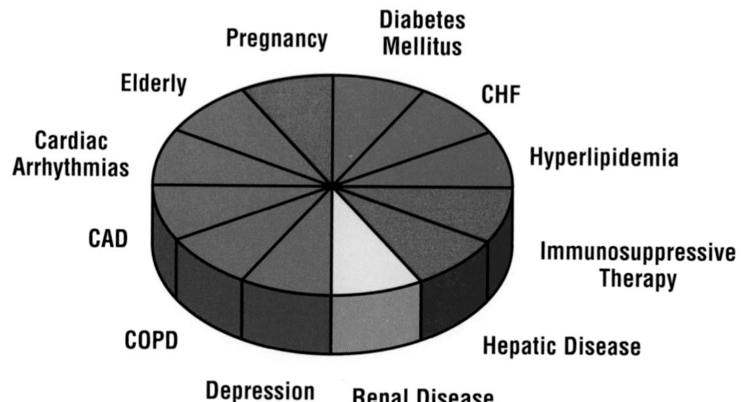

LIPID - LOWERING DRUGS

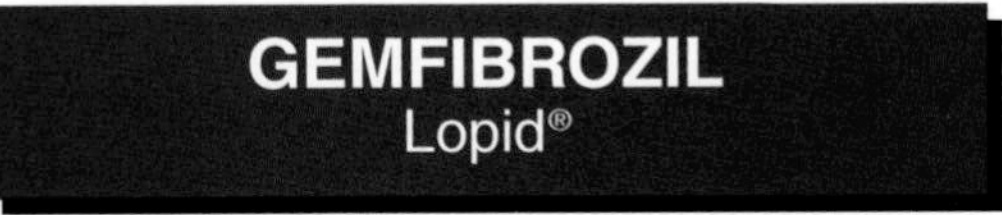

DRUG Incompatibility Profile

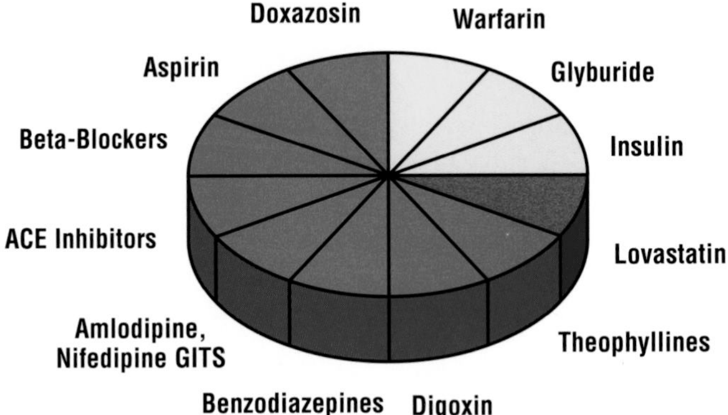

DISEASE Incompatibility Profile

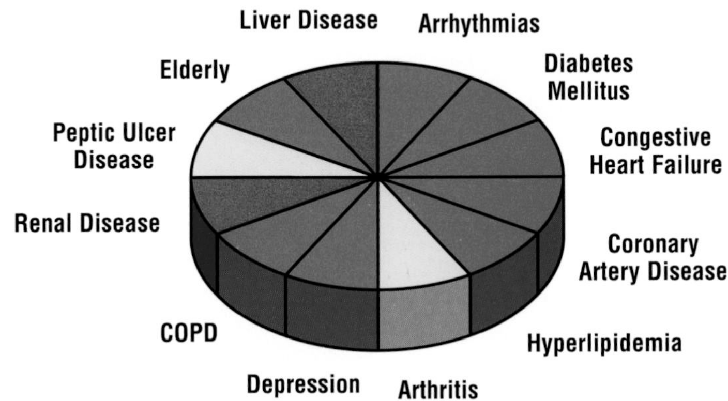

DIURETICS

THIAZIDE DIURETICS
(Hydrochlorothiazide)

DRUG Incompatibility Profile

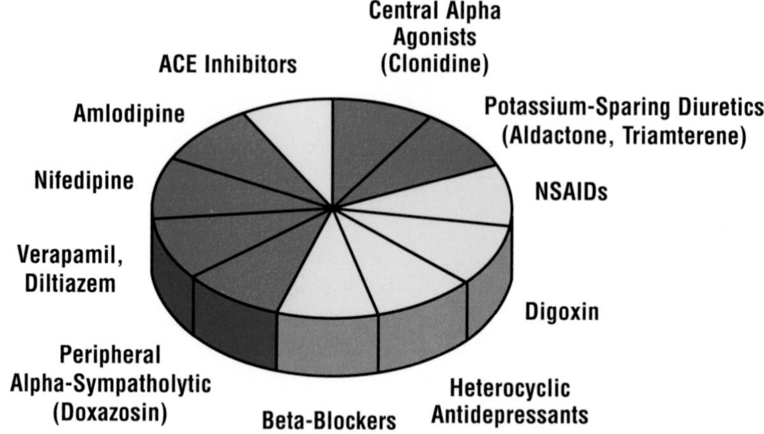

DISEASE Incompatibility Profile

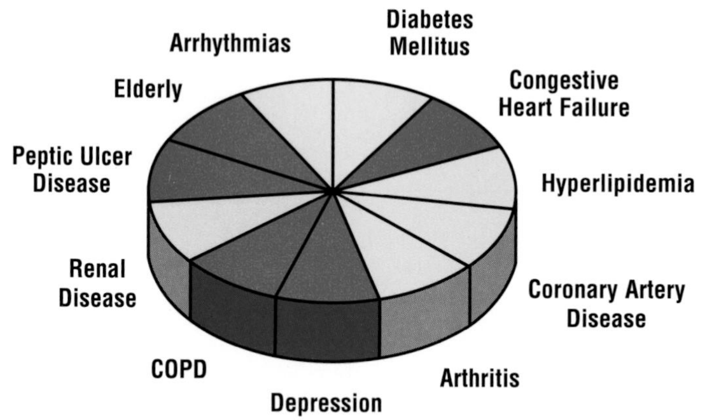

BETA-BLOCKERS

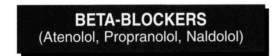

BETA-BLOCKERS
(Atenolol, Propranolol, Naldolol)

DRUG Incompatibility Profile

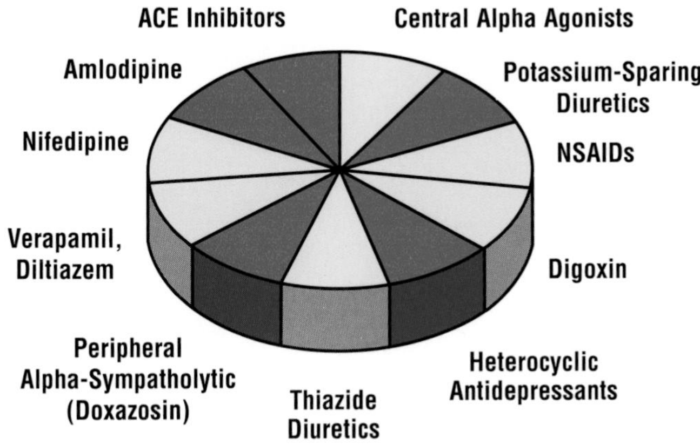

DISEASE Incompatibility Profile

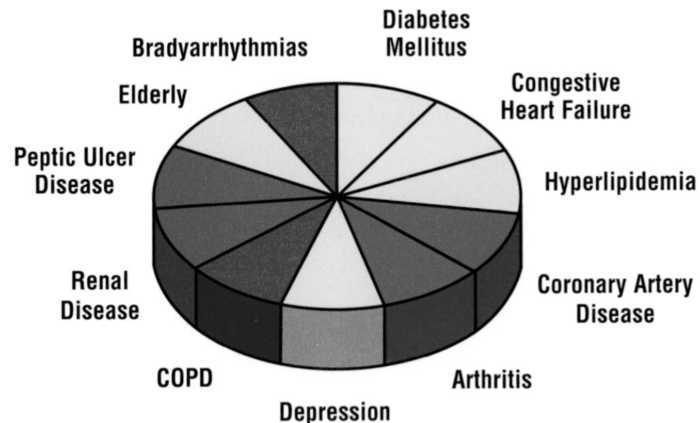

ACE INHIBITORS

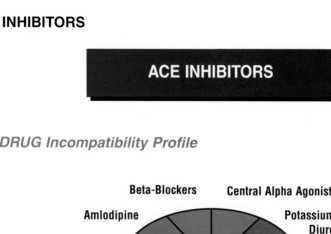

DRUG Incompatibility Profile

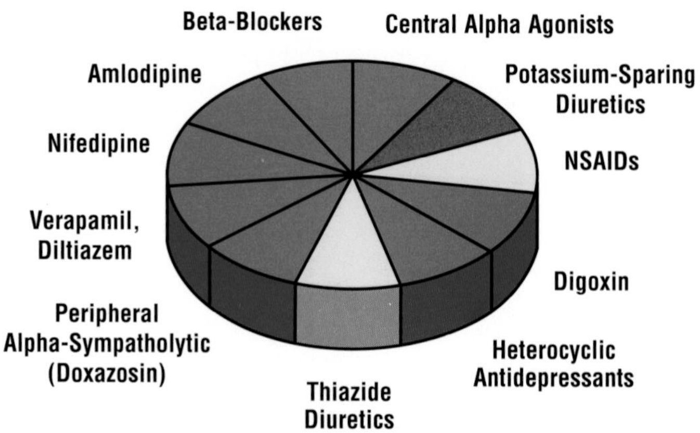

DISEASE Incompatibility Profile

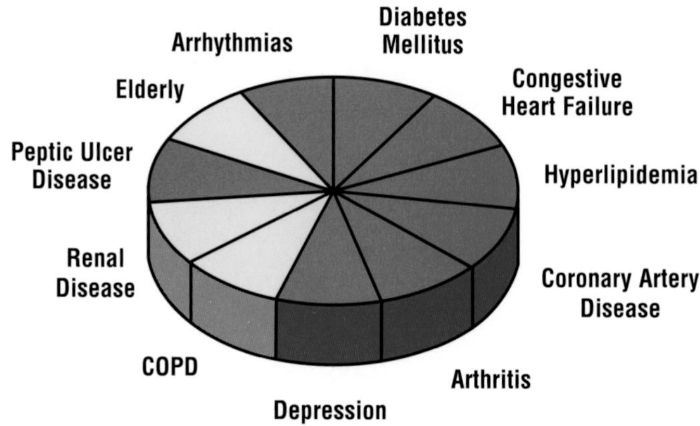

ANGIOTENSIN II RECEPTOR ANTAGONISTS

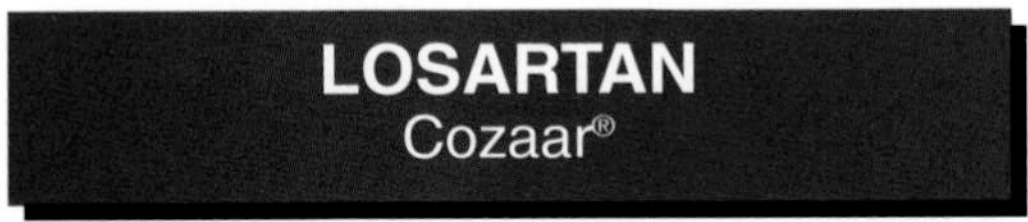

DRUG Incompatibility Profile

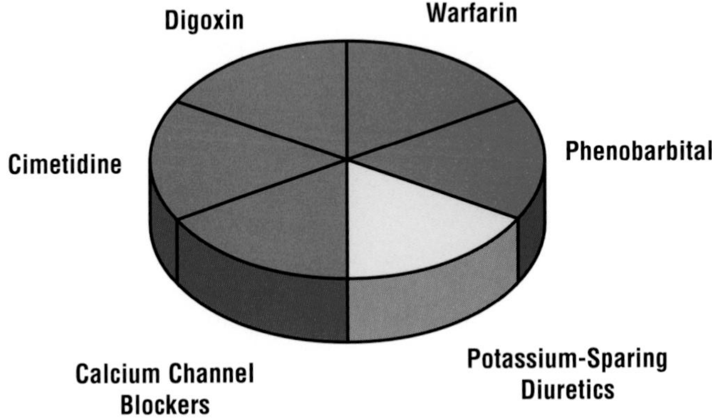

DISEASE Incompatibility Profile

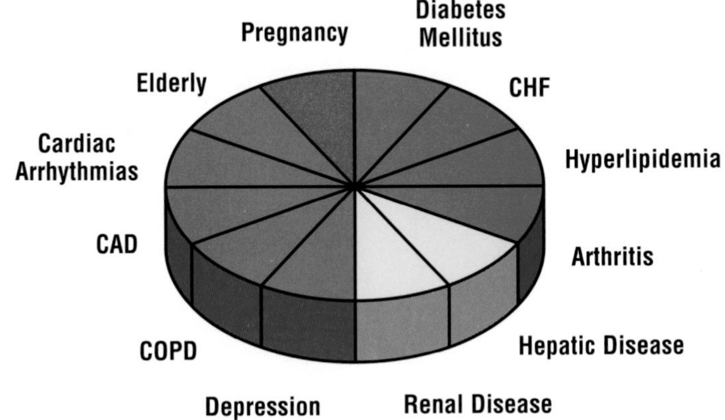

ALPHA-SYMPATHOLYTIC

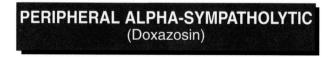

PERIPHERAL ALPHA-SYMPATHOLYTIC
(Doxazosin)

DRUG Incompatibility Profile

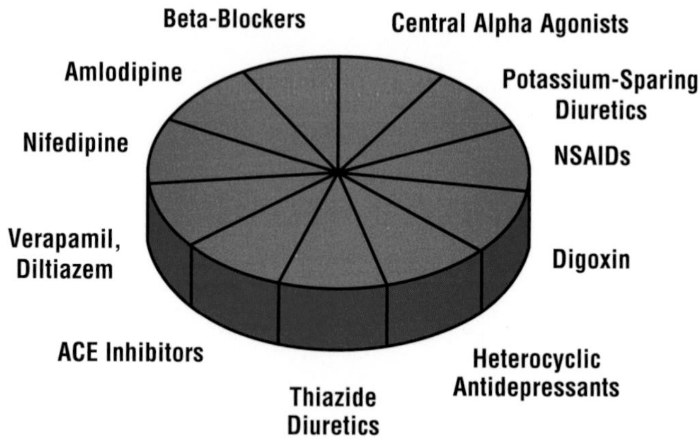

DISEASE Incompatibility Profile

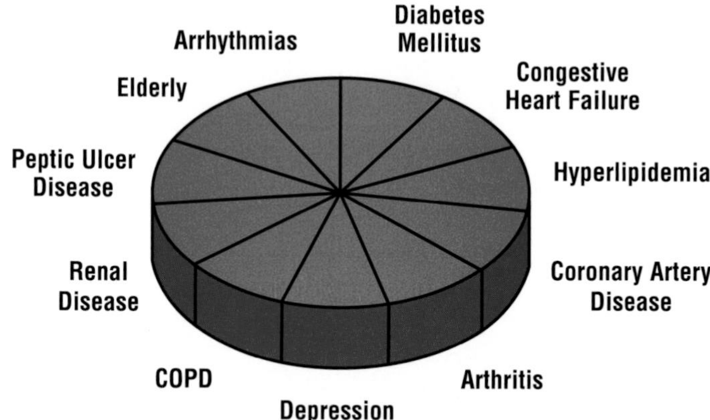

CALCIUM CHANNEL BLOCKERS
(Diltiazem, Verapamil)

DRUG Incompatibility Profile

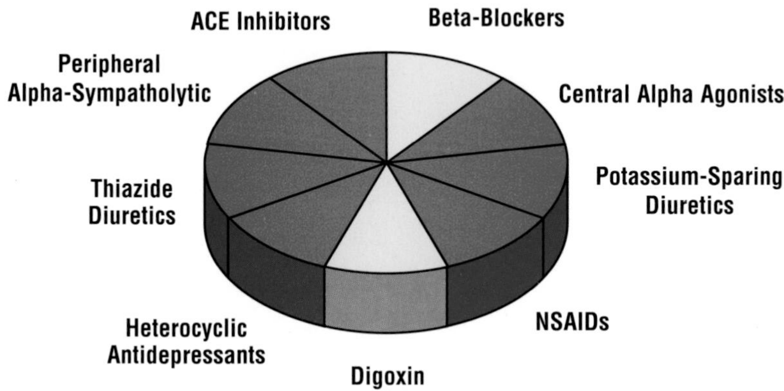

DISEASE Incompatibility Profile

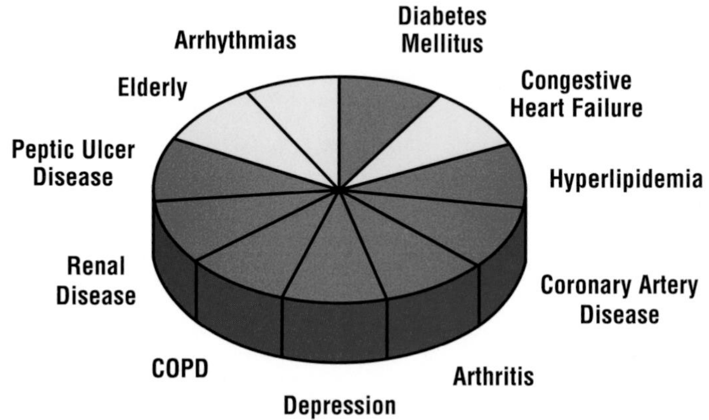

CALCIUM CHANNEL BLOCKERS
(Nifedipine)

DRUG Incompatibility Profile

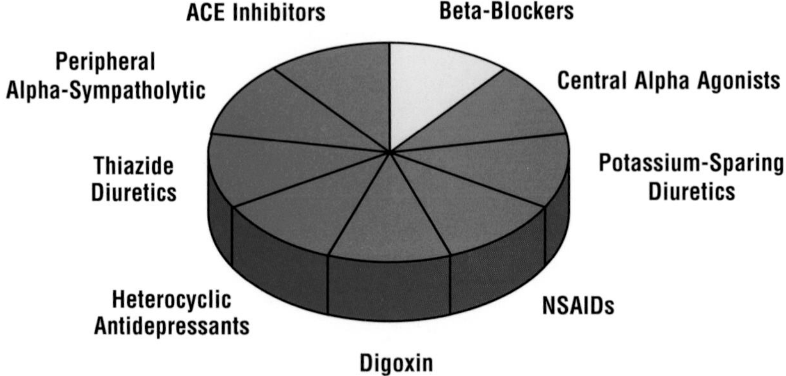

DISEASE Incompatibility Profile

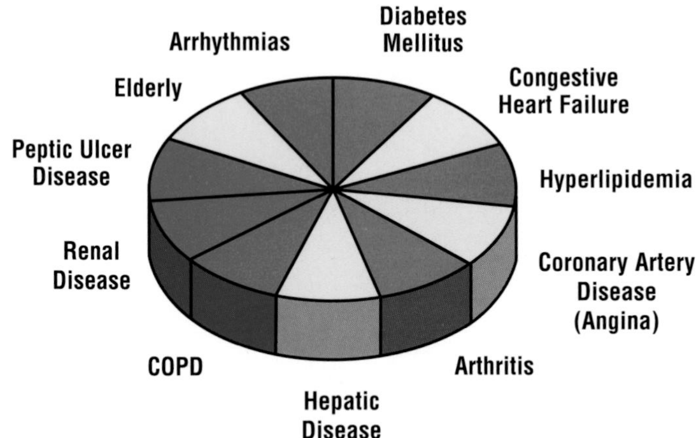

CALCIUM CHANNEL BLOCKER
(Amlodipine, Norvasc®)

DRUG Incompatibility Profile

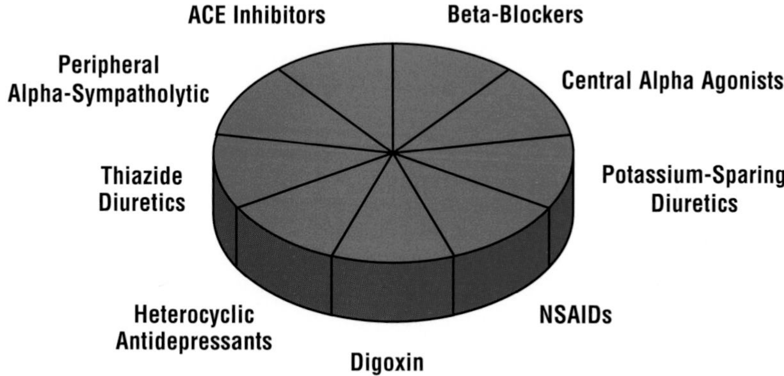

DISEASE Incompatibility Profile

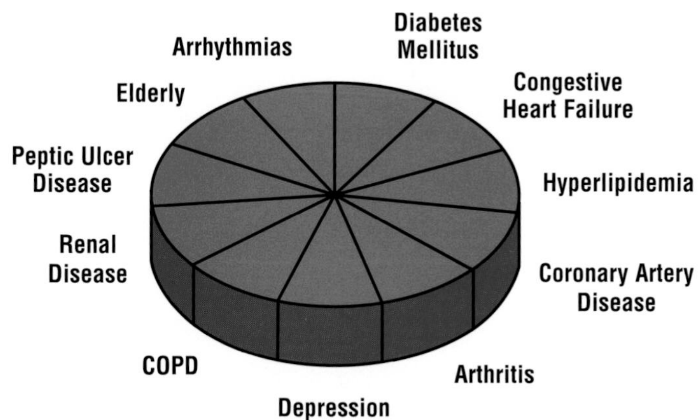

INOTROPIC AGENTS

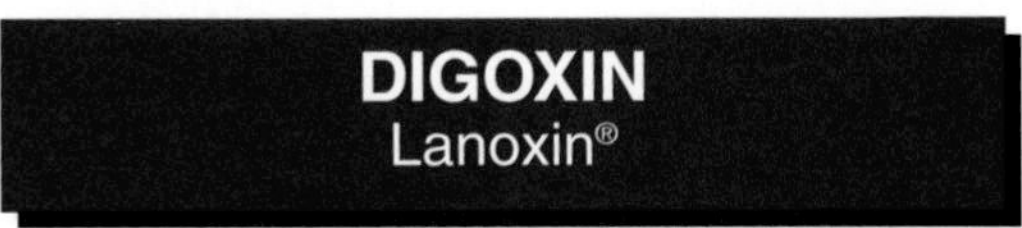

DRUG Incompatibility Profile

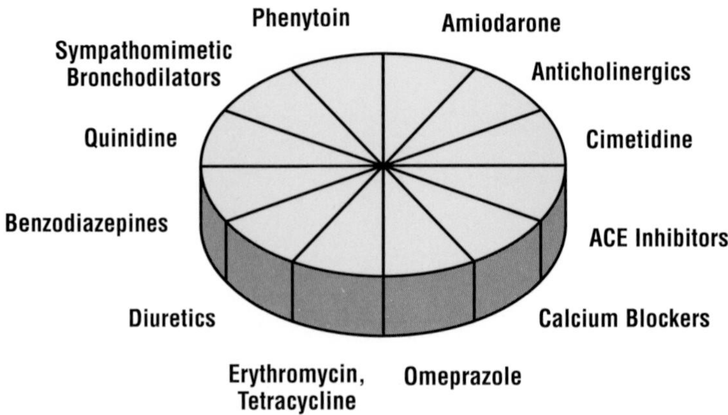

DISEASE Incompatibility Profile

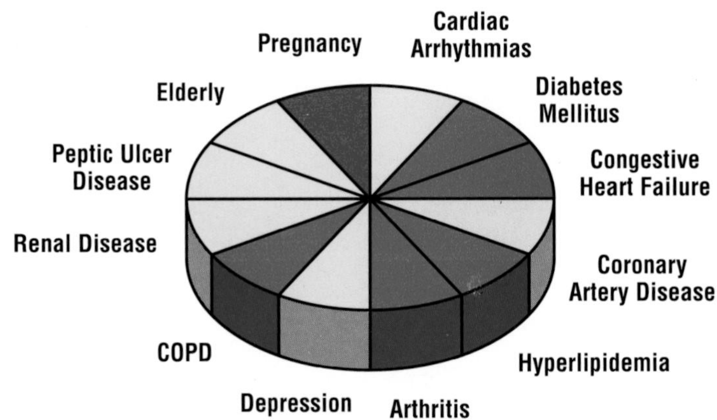

It is not a monoamine oxidase inhibitor, it does not stimulate the CNS, and in animals, it selectively inhibits serotonin uptake. With respect to onset of action, one-half of outpatients responding to trazodone have a significant therapeutic response by the end of the first week of treatment. Three-fourths of responders demonstrate a therapeutic effect by the second week of therapy. As far as drug and disease interactions, trazodone has less anticholinergic toxicity than TCAs, allowing some drugs (e.g., antihistamines, benzodiazepines) to be upgraded to a green designation. On the other hand, there are certain underlying conditions (sexual dysfunction) in which, compared to TCAs, more cautious use is appropriate.[6,7,32]

Trazodone Drug Incompatibility Profile (DIP 3-2). In general, trazodone is less sedating than most TCAs.[41] Although it can cause drowsiness, it can be used in conjunction with alcohol with some degree of caution. Although it is not known how frequently interactions between MAOIs and trazodone occur, a yellow designation admonishes the pharmacist and physician to be aware of possible interactions between these drug classes. Increased phenytoin (Dilantin®) toxicity can be observed with concomitant trazodone therapy, and a yellow cautionary classification is given to create awareness of this possible interaction. Trazodone toxicity may be potentiated by concurrent use with fluoxetine.[41,47] The most common side effect observed in these patients is increased sedation; caution also is recommended before use with diphenhydramine. Although the interaction between trazodone and warfarin (Coumadin®) is apparently rare, there is a report suggesting that trazodone may reduce the anticoagulant effect of warfarin. Most other commonly used drugs, including NSAIDs, beta-blockers, benzodiazepines, and famotidine can be used in conjunction with trazodone with little risk of adverse interactions. These combinations are given green designations.[1,6,7,12,32,34,35]

Trazodone Disease Incompatibility Profile (DIP 3-2). Many of the same warnings discussed in the section on TCAs also apply to trazodone. It should not be used in pregnancy, and its use is strongly discouraged in this patient subgroup. The risk of using trazodone in patients with severe coronary artery disease appears to be greatest during the initial recovery phase of myocardial infarction. Clinical studies and post-marketing surveillance reports indicate that trazodone may be arrhythmogenic in some patients with preexisting cardiac disease, producing a wide spectrum of disturbances, ranging from PVCs and ventricular bigeminy to short runs of ventricular tachycardia.[32] Occasional reports of sinus bradycardia, shortness of breath, and syncope also have surfaced, suggesting caution (i.e., yellow designation) in patients with known congestive heart failure. The drug's propensity to cause priapism is well-documented, and as a result, it should be used cautiously in men with a previous history of sexual dysfunction, especially those with a history of prolonged or inappropriate erections.

Selective Serotonin Reuptake Inhibitors (SSRIs).

This class of antidepressants represents an important advance in the pharmacotherapy of major depression. The SSRIs are comparable in efficacy to the TCAs, but they produce less sedation, are not known to produce adverse cardiac events in therapeutic doses, and carry a category B pregnancy classification. Moreover, the mode of action and side effect profiles associated with SSRIs are different from those seen with TCAs. The DIP® designations for this class of antidepressants reflect these differences.[7,14]

Fluoxetine Drug Incompatibility Profile (DIP 3-3). Although no solid clinical data is presently available to confirm or exclude the possibility of adverse effects from the combined use of MAOIs and fluoxetine, it seems prudent to avoid concomitant use until this issue is settled.[42,43] It is known, however, that depression is aggravated from the combined use of fluoxetine and desipramine, and that fluoxetine's antidepressant effects are reduced by the concomitant use of the antihistamine cyproheptadine. Trazodone toxicity, manifested by excessive sedation, can be precipitated by the introduction of fluoxetine.[41,44] These interactions justify yellow designations. Lithium toxicity is potentiated by the addition of fluoxetine, an observation that necessitates cautious use of these drugs in combination, along with careful monitoring of lithium levels. Fluoxetine, on rare occasions, may produce phenytoin toxicity. Among other commonly used CNS drugs, benzodiazepines such as alprazolam and diazepam interact (i.e., decreased metabolism) with fluoxetine, and may produce excessive drowsiness and sedation. Finally, the combined use of haloperidol and fluoxetine is associated with increased extrapyramidal symptoms, including one possible case of tardive dyskinesia.[6,7,45-48]

Fluoxetine Disease Incompatibility Profile (DIP 3-3). Fluoxetine can produce agitation, insomnia, and anxiety in a significant minority of patients.[44,49] Hence, cautious use is suggested in patients who have insomnia and in elderly patients with sleep or eating disorders. Although this drug rarely produces seizures,[50] careful use in this patient population is recommended. Careful monitoring is required with chronic use of fluoxetine in patients with significant renal impairment.

Sertraline (Zoloft®) (DIP 3-4). Sertraline is an SSRI (selective serotonin reuptake inhibitor) indicated for the treatment of depression, obsessive-compulsive disorder (OCD), and panic attack, including anxiety associated with panic attack. Although it has a favorable drug interaction profile when compared to other drugs in its class, certain precautions should be noted. Cases of serious—and sometimes fatal—reactions have been reported in patients receiving sertraline (sertraline hydrochloride) in combination with a monoamine oxidase inhibitor (MAOI). Symptoms resulting from a drug interaction between an SSRI and a MAOI may include the following: hyperthermia, rigidity, myoclonus, autonomic instability with possible rapid fluctuations of vital signs, mental status changes that include confusion, irritability, and extreme agitation progressing to delirium and coma.

These reactions also have been reported in patients who have recently discontinued an SSRI and have been started on an MAOI. Some cases presented with features resembling neuroleptic malignant syndrome. Therefore, sertraline should not be used in combination with an MAOI, or within 14 days of discontinuing treatment with an MAOI. Similarly, at least 14 days should be allowed after stopping. To alert the clinician of this important drug interaction, a red designation is assigned to the MAOI class.

The clinical significance of other drug interactions is less well characterized, but deserves attention. Because it is tightly bound to plasma proteins, the administration of sertraline hydrochloride to a patient taking another drug that is tightly bound to protein (eg, warfarin, digitoxin) may cause a shift in plasma concentrations potentially resulting in an adverse effect. Conversely, adverse effects may result from displacement of protein bound sertraline by other tightly bound drugs.

In a study comparing prothrombin time following dosing with warfarin (0.75 mg/kg) before and after 21 days of dosing with either sertraline (50-200 mg/day) or placebo, there was a mean increase in prothrombin time of 8% relative to baseline for sertraline compared to a 1% decrease for placebo ($p < 0.02$). The clinical significance of this change is unknown. Accordingly, prothrombin time should be carefully monitored when sertraline therapy is initiated or stopped.

With respect to cimetidine, in a study assessing disposition of sertraline (100 mg) on the second of 8 days of cimetidine administration (800 mg/day), there were significant increases in sertraline mean AUC (50%), Cmax (24%) and half-life (26%) compared to the placebo group. The clinical significance of these changes are unknown.

Some CNS active drugs also may be affected by sertraline. In a study comparing the disposition of intravenously administered diazepam before and after 21 days of dosing with either sertraline (50 to 200 mg/day escalating dose) or placebo, there was a 32% decrease relative to baseline in diazepam clearance for the sertraline group compared to a 19% decrease relative to baseline for the placebo group ($p < 0.03$). Once again, the clinical significance of these changes has not been precisely elucidated and is not fully known. In a placebo-controlled trial in healthy volunteers, the administration of two doses of sertraline did not significantly alter steady-state lithium levels or the renal clearance of lithium. Nonetheless, at this time, it is recommended that plasma lithium levels be monitored following initiation of sertraline therapy with appropriate adjustments to the lithium dose.

There is limited controlled experience regarding the optimal timing of switching from other antidepressants to sertraline. Care and prudent medical judgment should be exercised when switching, particularly from long-acting agents. The duration of an appropriate washout period that should intervene before switching from one selective serotonin reuptake inhibitor (SSRI) to another has not been established.

In two separate in vivo interaction studies, sertraline was co-administered with cytochrome P450 3A4 substrates, terfenadine or carbamazepine, under steady-state conditions. The results of these studies demonstrated the sertraline co-administration did not increase plasma concentrations of terfenadine or carbamazepine. These data suggest that sertraline's extent of inhibition of P450 3A4 activity is not likely to be of clinical significance.

Many antidepressants (eg, the SSRIs, including sertraline, and most tricyclic antidepressants) inhibit the biochemical activity of the drug metabolizing isozyme cytochrome P450 2D6 (debrisoquin hydroxylase), and may increase the plasma concentrations of co-administered drugs that are metabolized by P450 2D6. The drugs for which this potential interaction is of greatest concern are those metabolized primarily by 2D6 and which have a narrow therapeutic index (eg, the tricyclic antidepressants and the Type 1C antiarrhythmics propafenone and flecainide). The extent to which this interaction is an important clinical problem depends on the extent of the inhibition of P450 2D6 by the antidepressant and the therapeutic index of the co-administered drug.

There is variability among the antidepressants in the extent of clinically important 2D6 inhibition, and in fact, sertraline, at lower doses has a less prominent inhibitory effect on 2D6 than some other medications in the SSRI class. Nevertheless, even sertraline has the potential for clinically important 2D6 inhibition. Consequently, concomitant use of a drug metabolized by P450 2D6 with sertraline may require lower doses than usually prescribed for the other drug. Furthermore, whenever sertraline is withdrawn from co-therapy, an increased dose of the co-administered drug may be required.

Sertraline Disease Incompatibility Profile (DIP 3-4). Sertraline has a Category B pregnancy rating. Lower doses should be used in patients with severe renal and hepatic impairment.

Nefazodone (Serzone®) Drug Incompatibility Profile (DIP 3-5). Drugs that may potentially interact adversely when taken in combination with nefazodone include MAOIs, nonsedating antihistamines (astemizole), benzodiazepines, digoxin, haloperidol, and propranolol. Coadministration of astemizole or cisapride with nefazodone is contraindicated. Nefazodone causes a significant increase in triazolam (and other triazolobenzodiazepines) plasma level when the two drugs are taken together. Because nefazodone is an inhibitor of serotonin (and epinepherine) reuptake, it should not be used in combination with any MAOI, or within 14 days of discontinuing treatment with an MAOI. At least 1 week should be allowed after stopping nefazodone before starting MAOI.

Alcohol should be avoided while taking nefazodone because of its CNS depressing effect. Although little is known about the potential for interactions between nefazodone and general anesthetics, it is recommended that prior to elective surgery, nefazodone should be discontinued for a long as feasible. When taken together, nefazodone increases plasma level of digoxin. Caution should be taken with concurrent use of these two agents. In general, caution is indicated when nefazodone is used in combination with any drugs known to be metabolized by the IIIA4 isozyme.

Nefazodone Disease Incompatibility Profile (DIP 3-5). Nefazodone is indicated for depression. It carries Pregnancy Category C and should not be used in pregnant women. Nefazodone should be used with extreme caution in patients with a history of cardiac arrhythmias, MI, unstable heart disease, or CNS disorders. Dosage adjustment may be necessary in patients with hepatic impairment. Because postural hypotension has been reported, nefazodone should be used with caution in patients with conditions—cerebrovascular and cardiovascular disease—that could be exacerbated by hypotension, as well as in individuals with conditions that predispose them to hypotension. Because sinus bradycardia has been observed in patients treated with nefazodone, cautious use is advised in patients with heart disease and sinoatrial node dysfunction.

Donepezil (Aricept®) Drug Incompatibility Profile (DIP 3-6). Because of donepezil's mechanism of action, it should be used with caution in combination with anticholinergic medications since it has the potential to interfere with the activity of anticholinergic medications (red warning). Also, as a cholinesterase inhibitor, it is likely to exaggerate the effects of succinylcholine-type muscle relaxants used during anesthesia. For this reason, a red designation is used. Donepezil is metabolized by the CYP 450 isoenzyme 2D6 and 3A4, and therefore, may affect actions of other medications metabolized through these pathways.

Drugs that may be affected when used concurrently with donepezil include ketoconazole and quinidine. A yellow profile is indicated because studies show that ketoconazole and quinidine inhibit donepezil metabolism in vitro.

Although the clinical significance of these interactions has not yet been determined, clinicians should be aware of a possible interaction. Other drugs that may be affected by donepezil include NSAIDs, furosemide, digoxin, warfarin, theophylline, and cimetidine.

Donepezil Disease Incompatibility Profile (DIP 3-6). Donepezil (Apricept) is indicated for treatment of mild to moderate dementia of the Alzheimer's type. Because of donepezil's pharmacological actions as a cholinesterase inhibitor, it may have vagotonic effects on heart rate (eg, bradycardia). The potential for this action may be particularly important in patients with "sick sinus syndrome" or other supraventricular cardiac conduction conditions. Syncopal episodes have been reported in association with the use of donepezil. Based on the potential to produce bradycardia, a red designation has been issued for cardiac arrhythmias. Specifically, a yellow, cautionary note is indicated for CHF and CAD, inasmuch as these conditions may be associated with bradycardic syndromes.

In addition, as a cholinesterase inhibitor, donepezil may be expected to increase gastric acid secretion due to increased cholinergic activity. Although the precise clinical implications of this action have not been fully elucidated, a yellow warning has been issued for patients with peptic ulcer disease, including erosive esophagitis. Patients predisposed to acid-related gastric disorders should be monitored for occult gastrointestinal bleeding. At the higher (10mg) dose, donepezil can cause diarrhea, nausea, and vomiting. If these symptoms are severe or disabling, dosage reduction is indicated.

Based on the same pharmacological action, a yellow warning is indicated for patients with benign prostatic hypertrophy (BPH) and chronic obstructive pulmonary disease (COPD). Cholinomimetics may cause bladder outflow obstruction, and cholinesterase inhibitors should be prescribed cautiously for patients with a history of asthma or COPD. Donepezil clearance is decreased by 20% in patients with hepatic disease, therefore a yellow warning is indicated. The incidence of transaminase elevations is higher in females. The drug can be used safely in patients with renal disease.

Alendronate (Fosamax®) Drug Incompatibility Profile (DIP 3-7). Alendronate's bioavailability is greatly reduced when it is taken with food. Accordingly, patients should be instructed to take alendronate with only plain water first thing upon arising for at least 30 minutes before consuming the first food, beverage or medication of the day. Drugs that may interact with alendronate include ranitidine, calcium supplements, antacids, and aspirin.

Since aspirin and NSAIDs are associated with gastrointestinal irritation, caution should be used during concomitant use of any of these drugs with alendronate. Other medications—digoxin, diuretics, etc.—that may be exquisitely sensitive to electrolyte changes such as hypocalcemia or hypokalemia should be monitored more closely when used concurrently with alendronate.

Alendronate Disease Incompatibility Profile (DIP 3-7). Alendronate, a biphosphanate, is a highly selective and potent inhibitor of bone resorption. It is indicated for treatment and prevention of osteoporosis in women, and Paget's disease of the bone. Alendronate carried a pregnancy category rate C and should not be given to breastfeeding mothers.

Among its most important side effects is local irritation of the upper gastrointestinal mucosa. As a result, patients with known upper gastrointestinal disease, especially acid-related disorders, should exercise some caution with this drug. In this regard, esophagitis, esophageal ulcers, and esophageal erosions have been reported in patient receiving alendronate. Consequently, caution is required by a number of patient subgroups including those with gastritis, gastroesophageal reflux disease (GERD), peptic ulcer disease (PUD), NSAID-associated gastropathy, and chronic alcohol intake.

Physicians should be alert to signs or symptoms that signal esophageal reaction, and patients who experience such symptoms should be instructed to discontinue alendronate and seek medical attention. Specifically, patients should be instructed to discontinue alendronate if they develop dysphagia, odynophagia, or retrosternal pain. It appears as if the severity, and perhaps, the likelihood of adverse esophageal experiences is increased in those who lie down within 30 minutes of taking the medication, in those who fail to take the drug in combination with a full (6-8 oz) glass of water, and in those who continue alendronate after noting symptoms of esophageal distress.

Appropriate and prudent use of alendronate requires consumption of the drug at least 30 minutes before the first food, beverage, or medication of the day, with plain water only. Other beverages (including mineral water) may lessen the drug's absorption. After the drug is taken, the patient should avoid lying down for at least 30 minutes.

In addition, alendronate is not recommended for patients with renal insufficiency (CrCl < 35mL/min) due to animal studies that show that increased quantities of the drug are present in plasma, kidney, spleen, and tibia of rats with kidney failure. Because of alendronate's pharmacological mechanism of action, hypocalcemia must be corrected before initiating therapy. Hypocalcemia is a contraindication to the drug's use. Because occasional reports of such electrolyte derangements as hypocalcemia, hypokalemia, hypomagnesemia, and hypophosphatemia have occurred, close monitoring of patients with cardiac arrhythmias or electrolyte-sensitive cardiac or renal function appears reasonable.

Impotence Medications

Sildenafil (Viagra) Drug Incompatibility Profile (DIP 3-8). First and foremost, sildenafil (Viagra) should never be prescribed (or taken) in combination with any medications containing nitrates, nitrites, dintrates, or nitroglycerin. Most of these medications are used to treat chest pain associated with angina, and include the following: Nitro-Bid, Imdur, Nitroguard, amyl nitrite, nitroglycerin, Nitrocine, Nitrol ointment, Nitrostat, Nitrolingual spray, Sorbitrate, Deponit, Dilarate SR, Isordil, Monoket, Nitrolingual, Transderm-Nitro, and many others. The combination of sildenafil plus these medications can cause serious reductions in blood pressure that have the potential to be life-threatening. Erythromycin and cimetidine, and other potent inhibitors of the p450 cytochrome oxidase system may cause transient elevations in blood sildenafil levels, and these effects should be considered.

Sildenafil (Viagra®) Disease Incompatibility Profile (DIP 3-8). Sildenafil (Viagra®) has been shown in clinical trials to improve sexual performance in clinically diagnosed impotent men. In studies involving more than 3000 impotent men, 35% to 80% of those who took the drug reported improved sexual performance, while only 20% of those in the placebo (inactive pill) group cited improvement. Men who were diagnosed with impotence and who improved on this medication include those with a wide range of problems: psychogenic impotence; post-prostatectomy; diabetes; spinal cord injury, and other groups. The drug enhances the smooth muscle relaxant effects of nitric oxide, a substance that is normally released in response to sexual stimulation. Smooth muscle relaxation allows blood to enter the penis and produce an erection.

Sildenafil is a safe and effective drug for the treatment of male impotence if used in the appropriate patient population, and if proper attention is paid to possible drug interactions, especially with nitrates. Even though the manufacturer has warned physicians of possible side effects and, especially the danger of prescribing this drug in combination with nitroglycerin-like medications, many of these warnings were initially drowned out by the sheer volume of media coverage.

At the time that this book went to press, a number of deaths in patients who had been taking sildenafil have been reported. Although some deaths appear to have been the result of drug interaction between sildenafil and nitrates (a combination that can cause potentially life-threatening hypotension) others occurred in individuals who were *not* taking nitrates concurrently. The precise cause of death in this (non nitrate-consuming) group has not been fully explained. Moreover, whether or not there was a direct cause and effect between sildenafil and some or all of these adverse outcomes also is not conclusively proven, since a number of problems occurred in elderly, somewhat frail individuals with underlying cardiac disease.

The fact is, a certain percentage of individuals with heart disease suffer adverse consequences from ischemia-inducing activities such as sexual function, even in the *absence* of impotence-rectifying medications such as sildenafil. Consequently, the statistical challenge of confirming or refuting a cause and effect relationship between a drug such as sildenafil and cardiac events in this population is a formidable undertaking. Nevertheless, it seems prudent based on what is known, or what is speculated, at this point in time to consider the potential relationship between intense aerobic activity associated with sexual activity facilitated by sildenafil and the possible susceptibility that some individuals—in particular, those with severe underlying heart disease—might have to sex-related exertion.

The prevailing prescribing philosophy for use of this medication is using common sense. Sildenafil is commonly prescribed for middle-aged and older individuals because this is the population most likely to suffer from erectile dysfunction (ED). Although it can be used in individuals with and without heart disease, it should not be used in individuals with angina pectoris, since these individuals may, at some point in the natural history of their disease—either acutely or subacutely—require nitrate therapy for alleviation of cardiac pain.

Moreover, it appears reasonable to recommend cautious use in people, especially the elderly, with *advanced* heart disease. Because sexual intercourse requires physical exertion, and because this exertion can, in some patients, produce heart symptoms such as angina, shortness of breath, or palpitations, sildenafil should be used cautiously in people who are borderline compensated as far as their cardiac status is concerned. Hence, red warning designations are issued for patients with advanced coronary artery disease, and for those with history of severe, chronic congestive heart failure. From a practical point of view, many of these patients will not have the physical-cum-aerobic stamina to engage in sexual activity, and they should not be "induced" into this lifestyle option by the availability of an impotence drug, especially if they are not engaging in sexual activity at the time use of the drug is being contemplated. In other words, individuals with severe heart disease who have *not* had sexual activity for a prolonged period of time (months to years) should not be started on sildenafil to "jumpstart" their sex life. From what can be surmised at this point in time, the risks may outweigh the potential benefits in this vulnerable group, in whom the stresses of new onset sexual activity cannot be adequately tested.

In elderly individuals who have severe heart disease (arrhythmias, coronary heart disease, and/or severe CHF) but who nevertheless *are* continuing to have sexual activity they characterize as compromised by erectile dysfunction—but with no apparent adverse cardiac effects—the use of sildenafil as impotence therapy would have to be considered highly controversial. There are no published data showing how this potentially vulnerable group might respond from a safety perspective. It is conceivable that sildenafil would produce no problems in a significant percentage of severe heart disease/sexual performers, but it can also be argued that conversion of a marginal, irregular sexual performer into an adequate, regular or high intensity sexual performer could increase oxygen demand sufficiently to alter cardiac status. Although there may be a small group of patients with this profile in whom sildenafil would be appropriate, the overwhelming percentage of these patients, even if they are having sexual activity, should be discouraged from taking a drug that has the potential to dramatically increase metabolic demands of an already marginal cardiovascular system.

Individuals with mild to moderate coronary heart disease are suitable candidates for sildenafil, as long as the following criteria are met: (a) angina, life-threatening arrhythmias, and exercise-induced congestive heart failure are not part of the clinical picture; (b) the patient has demonstrated he can tolerate physical exercise that is as stressful as sexual activity; and (c) the patient is physically active and has good aerobic exercise tolerance while performing daily activities. When sildenafil is used in this group of patients, it is reasonable to start with the lowest dose (25 mg) and gradually increase the dose as needed and as tolerated. Elderly patients without heart disease who are otherwise physically active, have good aerobic exercise tolerance, and are able to tolerate the physical exertion of sexual activity without problems, are excellent candidates for this drug. The drug can be used in patients with well-controlled high blood pressure, as long as they are not taking nitrate-containing compounds. Individuals who develop angina at any point during sildenafil treatment should be taken off the drug.

There is some speculation but no data that because sildenafil transiently inhibits the 5-phosphodiesterase system in the eye, that the drug may be potentially harmful in diabetic patients with opthalmopathy. Further studies are necessary to shed light on this suggestion, and at present, diabetes is not a contraindication to the drug's use.

Finally, although sildenafil is safe and effective when used in the appropriate patient, there are side effects that need to be considered. The side effects are related to the dose of the drug—mildest and less frequent at the 25 mg dose and more frequent at the 100 mg dose—and include headaches (up to 16% of patients), flushing (10%), indigestion (7%), nasal congestion (4%), and visual disturbances/blue coloration (3%).

Anti-Inflammatory Agents

Indomethacin (Indocin®) (DIP 3-9). Anti-inflammatory drugs are associated with a wide range of side effects and drug interactions.[6,7,13,18,32,51] Among all NSAIDs, indomethacin probably has the greatest propensity for producing serious drug and disease interactions. Although it can be a useful anti-inflammatory agent in many conditions, including gout and pericarditis, it has a limited role in the pharmatectural approach to long-term therapeutic management of chronic disorders. The significant number of red and yellow DIP designations explains why this drug should be used with therapeutic vigilance.

Indomethacin Drug Incompatibility Profile (DIP 3-9). Because indomethacin can produce gastric erosions, ulcerations, and clinically significant hemorrhage, strong cautionary warnings (red designations) are justified for the combined use of indomethacin with any of the following drugs: alcohol, aspirin, NSAIDs, corticosteroids, and anticoagulants. Because indomethacin is a potent inhibitor of prostaglandin synthesis, it may alter intrarenal hemodynamics, and can precipitate renal failure in patients on triamterene and spironolactone. Consequently, concurrent use with these drugs should be avoided. Although rarely reported, severe hypertension can result from the combined use of phenylpropanolamine with indomethacin. Until more is known about the potential occurrence of this drug interaction, concurrent use is best avoided.[1,6,7]

Even when used alone, ACE inhibitors can produce hyperkalemia and renal deterioration in a small subset of patients. Not surprisingly, NSAIDs such as indomethacin can potentiate these adverse effects. For example, impaired renal function and renal failure can result from the combined use of captopril and indomethacin. Therefore, extreme caution or avoidance of concurrent administration is strongly recommended. A yellow designation is appropriate for these potential drug interactions. Antacids decrease absorption of indomethacin, causing a reduction in its clinical effect. In addition, indomethacin can produce coronary vasoconstriction, blunt the antianginal effects of beta-blockers, and decrease the hypotensive effects of beta-blockers, all of which justify a yellow warning before using these agents together for extended periods in patients with hypertension or severe coronary artery disease. Indomethacin can be used safely with H2-blockers.

Indomethacin Disease Incompatibility Profile (DIP 3-9). The elderly, as well as patients with a history of peptic ulcer disease, renal dysfunction, or congestive heart failure are poor candidates for chronic indomethacin therapy, which can produce fluid retention, congestive heart failure, deterioration of renal function, gastrointestinal bleeding, dizziness, and confusion. Accordingly, red DIP designations warn against the use of this agent in patients who have these underlying conditions. Because many NSAIDs, including aspirin and indomethacin, can produce CNS side effects, including depression, a yellow warning designation appears in the pie slice in this DIP diagram. The capacity of indomethacin to inhibit the antianginal properties of beta-blockers justifies cautious use in the setting of angina and severe coronary artery disease. Finally, indomethacin can produce changes in glucose metabolism, suggesting that its use in diabetic patients should be closely monitored.

Nonsteroidal Anti-Inflammatory Drugs (NSAIDs) (DIP 3-10). Many of the same precautions that are highlighted for use of indomethacin also apply to the use of other NSAIDs such as ibuprofen, naproxen, and others. In general, the aforementioned NSAIDs are better tolerated than indomethacin and, as a result, many of the red designations are upgraded to cautionary yellow categories for NSAID drug interactions. There are also some important differences between indomethacin and the other classes of NSAIDs, and these differences are reflected in the incompatibility profiles discussed below. Finally, it should be noted that nearly all NSAID-mediated toxicities are *dose*-related and that reducing the risk for drug-related adverse events can usually be accomplished through decreases in drug dosage.

NSAID Drug Incompatibility Profile (DIP 3-10). The adverse gastrointestinal side effects of NSAIDs are well-known. Consequently, their concurrent use with corticosteroids (i.e., prednisone) and warfarin is discouraged. It should be emphasized that when prednisone is used in conjunction with NSAIDs, the risk of severe gastrointestinal bleeding is increased fourfold. Hence, the concomitant use of these two agents requires strong clinical justification, and whenever possible, alternative therapies should be explored. Because of the significant risk for gastrointestinal tract hemorrhage, the use of anticoagulants is often best avoided in patients on NSAID therapy.[1,7,13,32,52]

Strong cautionary (yellow) classifications apply to the use of NSAIDs with aspirin (additive gastrointestinal toxicity), potential for ACE inhibitors (renal deterioration), alcohol (additive gastrointestinal toxicity), and diuretics (potentiation of NSAID-induced renal failure). Methotrexate-NSAID interactions require special mention. Although the mechanism of this drug interaction is not known, reduced renal clearance is suspected. Several NSAIDs cause severe toxic reactions or delayed methotrexate renal clearance. Renal failure and other clinical effects are observed, prompting experts to recommend that nonsteroidal drugs should be stopped 2 to 3 days before intitiating methotrexate therapy, especially in the elderly and patients with impaired renal function. Most NSAIDs increase lithium serum levels, an interaction that can be significant and is preventable with careful monitoring of lithium levels. Finally, hypoglycemia occurs when NSAIDs are combined with tolbutamide, an interaction that results from displacement of the tolbutamide from protein binding sites.

NSAID Disease Incompatibility Profile (DIP 3-10). Most of the NSAIDs are given a category B classification for use in pregnancy. Two agents, mefenamic acid and tolmetin are classified category C. Because these agents can inhibit prostaglandin synthesis and produce adverse effects on the fetus, a red designation (i.e., avoidance, if possible) is issued for the use of NSAIDs in pregnancy. Elderly patients are at higher risk for incurring NSAID-induced central nervous system, renal, GI and cardiovascular side effects; consequently, caution and a careful review of the past medical history is advised before initiating therapy with NSAIDs in the older patient.[53] NSAIDs, especially indomethacin, can aggravate depression, mandating cautious use in this subgroup.[54,55] NSAIDs can cause fluid retention and edema, thereby aggravating symptoms of congestive heart failure. Patients with coronary artery disease are at higher risk for developing renal deterioration from NSAID therapy, and as a result, a cautionary yellow designation is applied to this potential drug-disease interaction. Patients with decreased cardiac output and decreased renal blood flow are especially at risk. Finally, NSAIDs can cause disturbances in glucose metabolism and electrolyte elimination, two features that demand prudent administration in patients with cardiac arrhythmias and diabetes.[1,6,18,24,32,56,57]

Corticosteroids (Prednisone, Methylprednisolone) (DIP 3-11). Corticosteroids can produce salutory effects and symptomatic improvement in a number of inflammatory disorders. Despite their proven efficacy, agents from this class must be used cautiously because these drugs also have the capacity for producing a wide range of adverse drug interactions. The drug and disease incompatibility profiles for these agents highlight the most significant clinical concerns when concurrent use is being considered.[58]

Corticosteroid Drug Incompatibility Profile (DIP 3-11). As discussed in a previous section, the concurrent use of NSAIDs and corticosteroids should be avoided when possible because the risk of producing gastrointestinal tract hemorrhage increases dramatically when these two drug classes are used in combination. A red DIP designation warns against this potentially problematic drug combination.

Yellow DIP designations alert pharmacists and physicians to a number of potential drug interactions. For example, many antacids, except those containing a low dose of aluminum phosphate, can interfere with oral corticosteroid absorption, thereby reducing its therapeutic efficacy. Because the combination of corticosteroids and loop diuretics can lead to increased renal potassium losses, careful monitoring of serum potassium concentrations is recommended. Concurrent use of corticosteroids with alcohol, aspirin, and anticoagulants is sometimes unavoidable, although clinicians should be aware of the adverse gastrointestinal effects that can result from these drug combinations. Omeprazole decreases the clinical effects of corticosteroids through a mechanism that is not yet understood. Phenytoin can produce a decrease in corticosteroid effect through increased metabolism. Although the clinical significance of theophylline and sympathomimetic amine-corticosteroid interactions is not well-established, concurrent use should be considered only with careful monitoring of theophylline serum concentrations.

Corticosteroid Disease Incompatibility Profile (DIP 3-11). Corticosteroids can compromise the natural history of many common clinical disorders, which explains why warning designations (red and yellow DIP pie slices) appear for so many conditions. Perhaps the risk of gastrointestinal tract hemorrhage is the most important adverse effect. In this vein, the presence of active peptic ulcer disease virtually contraindicates the use of corticosteroids.[59]

Because corticosteroids can produce alterations in glucose metabolism, predispose to infections, cause neuropsychiatric symptoms (including psychosis), induce fluid retention, and lead to electrolyte disturbances, the use of drugs such as prednisone requires caution in a number of common disorders including diabetes, depression, congestive heart failure, hypertension, coronary artery disease, and renal failure. Many complications can be prevented by using the lowest possible steroid dose necessary to achieve therapeutic effects and by monitoring parameters (e.g., serum potassium, blood glucose) associated with corticosteroid effects.

Aspirin (Salicylates) (DIP 3-12). Widely available and used for their analgesic, anti-inflammatory, cardioprotective, and antirheumatic effects, salicylates are associated with a number of clinically important adverse drug interactions.[6,7,18,24,51,52]

Aspirin Drug Incompatibility Profile (DIP 3-12). The interaction between salicylates and methotrexate is not conclusively confirmed, but the evidence is strong enough to produce a red (i.e., extreme caution,[6,7] avoid concurrent use if possible) designation for their combined use. Either through decreased clearance or reduction in methotrexate protein binding, salicylates can potentiate methotrexate toxicity. Although human data is retrospective and anecdotal, close patient monitoring is mandatory when these agents are used concurrently.

Clearly, the propensity for salicylates to produce gastric erosions and ulceration usually contraindicates their use in combination with anticoagulants. However, there is a subset of individuals with coronary heart disease, a history of myocardial infarction, and thromboembolic disorders who would benefit from the combined use of anticoagulants and salicylate-mediated antiplatelet properties. Studies confirming that low-dose salicylate therapy (i.e., 80 mg orally daily) is sufficient to achieve therapeutic results makes the concurrent use of warfarin-like drugs more attractive. As yet, however, there are no prospective studies demonstrating the degree of safety of this drug interaction. Consequently, a red designation is used for all salicylate-warfarin combinations. (Except as noted, the DIP profiles in this section do not refer to *low-dose* salicylate therapy.)

A number of drug interactions requiring moderate caution are highlighted with yellow DIP pie slices. The risk of gastrointestinal tract hemorrhage is exacerbated by the concomitant use of alcohol, corticosteroids, or NSAIDs with aspirin. In general, concurrent use of aspirin and NSAIDs is to be discouraged. However, elderly patients with a history of both myocardial infarction and osteoarthritis may benefit from low-dose salicylate therapy for cardioprotection and NSAID therapy for symptomatic improvement of their inflammatory disorder. In such cases, the two agents can be used concurrently, but only with careful clinical monitoring. Although the clinical significance of the quinidine-aspirin interaction is not known, there is some suggestion that these two agents have additive antiplatelet effects and, as a result, can significantly increase bleeding time.[6,7] Concurrent use is recommended only with careful clinical surveillance.

A yellow warning designation is used for concurrent use of cimetidine and aspirin because there is a risk of salicylate toxicity as a result of decreased metabolism. Salicylates can displace chlorpropamide from protein binding sites, increasing their effective serum concentration and, in some cases, producing hypoglycemia. High-dose aspirin therapy may also produce hypoglycemic effects. Displacement of valproate from serum binding sites by salicylates can produce valproate toxicity. This reaction encourages the use of alternative analgesic or antipyretic drugs in patients on valproate. Finally, the inhibition of prostaglandin synthesis mediated by salicylates may be responsible for producing a reduction in antihypertensive effects of captopril therapy.

Leukotriene Receptor Antagonists

Zafirlukast (Accolate®) Drug Incompatibility Profile (DIP 3-13). Because of its inhibition of cytochrome P450 enzymes, zafirlukast should be used cautiously with drugs known to be metabolized by the 2C9 and 3A4 isoenzyme. These include aspirin, erythromycin, terfenadine, and theophylline, all of which may affect zafirlukast levels. Coadministration of zafirlukast with warfarin results in a significant increase in prothrombin time. Accordingly, patients on oral warfarin anticoagulant therapy and zafirlukast should have their PT time monitored closely and anticoagulant dose adjusted accordingly.

Bioavailability of zafirlukast may be decreased when taken with food. Accordingly, patients should be instructed to take their dose at least 1 hour before or 2 hours after meals. When coadministered with erythromycin, zafirlukast bioavailability is decreased by approximately 40%. Coadministration of zafirlukast and theophylline does not affect theophylline plasma level but decreases zafirlukast plasma level by about 30%.

Zafirlukast Disease Incompatibility Profile (DIP 3-13). A selective and competitive leukotriene receptor antagonist, zafirlukast is indicated for prophylaxis and chronic treatment of asthma in adults and children 12 years of age and older. It carries a pregnancy category B rating. This drug may increase one or more liver enzymes during therapy; however, the clinical significance of these elevations is unknown. The drug inhibits the cytochrome P450 CYP3A4 and CYP2C9 isoenzymes. Because of the potential for tumorgenicity shown for zafirlukast in mouse and rat studies and the enhanced sensitivity of neonatal rats and dogs to the adverse effects of zafirlukast, the drug should not be administered to mothers who are breastfeeding.

Anti-Cancer Agents

Tamoxifen (Nolvadex®) Drug Incompatibility Profile (DIP 3-14). When tamoxifen is used in combination with coumarin-type anticoagulants, drug interactions may occur. Where such co-administration exists, careful monitoring of the patient's prothrombin time (PT) is recommended. Concomitant use of bromocriptine and tamoxifen have been shown to elevate tamoxifen serum level.

Tamoxifen Disease Incompatibility Profile (DIP 3-14). A nonsteroidal agent with potent antiestrogenic properties, tamoxifen (Nolvadex) has been shown to reduce the rate of recurrence and death from breast cancer among a wide range of women. Despite its potential benefits, the drug is prescribed for far too few patients. What is clear is that tamoxifen is underprescribed in women with breast cancer, and could save an additional 20,000 lives worldwide if prescribed for more women. Patients with breast cancer should be considered candidates for this medication, and be evaluated accordingly. From a clinical decision-making perspective, the overwhelming majority of women with breast cancer will benefit from this drug.

The finding that tamoxifen has the capacity not only to prevent recurrence of breast cancer but that it can prevent this malignancy in women at high risk for the disease has important implications for women of all ages. Contrary to what many doctors had believed, tamoxifen benefits breast cancer patients of all ages, not just those who have gone through menopause. The drug is effective whether the cancer is localized to the breast or has spread to axillary lymph nodes. The drug also is effective whether the cancer is removed surgically (lumpectomy or mastectomy), or treated with radiation or chemotherapy drugs. A new finding is that the drug also is effective in women whose tumors were negative for estrogen receptors.

The benefits of treating women with breast cancer with tamoxifen outweighs any risk in endometrial cancer, which is often curable if caught early. It also carries a small risk of causing potentially fatal clots to the lung. Over a period of 10 years, however, it is estimated that tamoxifen can prevent 80 deaths due to breast cancer per 1000 women taking tamoxifen for a period of five years, but may cause 2 deaths per 1000 women due to uterine cancer and one death from pulmonary embolism.

Finally, whether tamoxifen's benefits outweigh the risks for *protecting* high risk women against breast cancer remains uncertain. The National Cancer Institute stopped a study on the preventive effects of the drug, more than a year early, after initial results showed it reduced the incidence of first time breast cancer by more than 45%. Given these impressive results, tamoxifen's benefits will likely extend to younger women with breast cancer, as well as those at high risk who are likely to benefit from prevention.

Tamoxifen carries a pregnancy category rating of D. It may cause fetal harm when administered to a pregnant woman. There have been cases of hyperlipidemia reported that are associated with the use of tamoxifen. Periodic monitoring of plasma triglycerides and cholesterol may be indicated in patients with pre-existing hyperlipidemia, inasmuch as the drug has caused hyperlipidemia in a very small percentage of patients. Complete blood counts (including platelet counts) should be used to monitor patients, especially those with pre-existing leukopenia or thrombocytopenia. Liver function tests also are advisable because tamoxifen is associated with changes in liver enzyme levels and, on rare occasions, fatty liver, cholestasis, hepatitis, and hepatic necrosis. Caution should be taken when tamoxifen is used in patients with hepatic insufficiency.

During post-marketing surveillance, T4 elevations were reported for a few postmenopausal women. These elevations were not accompanied by clinical hyperthyroidism. However, patients who have hyperthyroid problems (or who are taking thyroid supplements) should be monitored closely. Hypercalcemia has occurred in some patients with metastatic breast cancer within a few weeks of starting therapy with tamoxifen.

Anticoagulants

Warfarin (Coumadin®) Drug Incompatibility Profiles (DIP 3-15). Warfarin is a narrow therapeutic index drug. Because the potential consequence of warfarin-mediated hemorrhage can range from mild to life-threatening, a red warning designation has been used for all potential warfarin drug-drug interactions. Although widely used, warfarin has been shown to interact with numerous drugs. When warfarin is taken concurrently with macrolide antibiotics, vitamin K, sulfipyrazone, sulfonamides, quinine derivatives, penicillins, phenylbutazones, dextrothyroxine, clofibrate, azole antifungals, barbiturates, amiodarone, or androgen, anticoagulant activity of warfarin will be enhanced and the risk of hemorrhage may be increased. Concurrent use of warfarin with these medications requires careful monitoring of the patient's PT or INR.

Warfarin Disease Incompatibility Profile (DIP 3-15). Used as a anticoagulant to prevent thromboembolism in selected patients at risk for stroke or heart disease, warfarin carries a pregnancy category X rating. It is contraindicated in women who are or may become pregnant because the drug passes through the placental barrier and may cause fatal hemorrhage to the fetus in utero. Furthermore, there have been reports of birth malformations in children born to mothers who have been treated with warfarin during pregnancy.

Hepatic dysfunction can potentiate the response to warfarin through impaired synthesis of clotting factors and decreased metabolism of warfarin. Many other factors may influence response of the patient to warfarin. The following factors, alone or in combination, may be responsible for an increased PT/INR response: blood dyscrasias, cancer, collagen vascular disease, CHF, diarrhea, elevated temperature, hyperthyroidism, poor nutritional state, steatorrhea, vitamin K deficiency. Other conditions, among them, edema, hereditary coumarin resistance, hyperlipidemia, hypothyroidism, and nephrotic syndrome may decrease PT/INR.

It should be noted that specific patient subgroups may demonstrate special sensitivity to warfarin and are subject to an increased risk of hemorrhage, especially if the PT or INR values exceed the therapeutic range. These high-risk groups include: the elderly, debilitated, females, history of stroke, previous episode of gastrointestinal hemorrhage, serious comorbid condition (recent MI, renal insufficiency, severe anemia), atrial fibrillation, trauma, prolonged dietary or nutritional deficiencies, inflammatory bowel disease, postpartum period, and active tuberculosis.

Histamine (H2)-Receptor Antagonists

H2-blockers are used for the treatment of peptic ulcer disease. All four of the currently approved agents—cimetidine, ranitidine, famotidine, and nizatidine—are efficacious, easily taken, and well-tolerated. From the perspective of medication compliance, all four drugs can be taken once a day at bedtime: 800 mg of cimetidine, 300 mg of ranitidine, 40 mg of famotidine, and 300 mg of nizatidine. The potency of these recommended doses is about equal.

Because renal excretion is the major route of elimination of H2-blockers, patients with renal insufficiency should receive reduced doses of agents with dose-related toxicity, e.g., cimetidine. In general, there is little to recommend one H2-blocker over another. There are some subtle but clinically relevant differences, however, that argue for preferential use of one agent over another in specific patient subgroups. All the H2-blockers can produce central nervous symptoms, such as headache and mental confusion. Cimetidine, and to a lesser extent, ranitidine, bind to hepatic cytochrome p-450 microsomal enzymes and may inhibit the catabolism of many drugs metabolized by this system.

These interactions are highlighted in the DIP pie diagrams. Oftentimes, these interactions are *not* clinically significant, with the possible exception of a few drugs that have narrow therapeutic to toxic ratios, such as theophylline, phenytoin, and some anticoagulants, such as warfarin. Despite the infrequency of serious adverse drug interactions, levels of theophylline and phenytoin and prothrombin times (in the case of warfarin), should be more carefully monitored if cimetidine is used in conjunction with these drugs. Alternately, another H2-blocker such as famotidine can be used to avoid the risk of these interactions.

Recently, all the H2-blockers, with the exception of famotidine, were shown to inhibit gastric alcohol dehydrogenase, an enzyme in the stomach that plays an important role in the first-pass metabolism of oral alcohol. Inhibition of this enzyme by H2-blockers may result in more absorption of oral alcohol, higher blood levels, and greater susceptibility to alcohol toxicity.

These and other distinguishing features are highlighted in the drug and disease incompatibility profiles for the three most commonly used H2-blockers—cimetidine, ranitidine, and famotidine.

Cimetidine (Tagamet®) Drug Incompatibilty Profile (DIP 3-16). Most of the potential adverse drug interactions associated with cimitedine carry a yellow designation. For example, the clinical significance of the increased alcohol effect produced by cimetidine-mediated inhibition of acetaldehyde in ALDH-1 deficiency is not known, but patients should be warned that they may experience a greater degree of alcohol intoxication when cimetidine is added to their drug regimen. Rarely, the combined use of cimetidine and captopril produces severe neuropathies in patients with renal impairment. The majority of other interactions result from cimetidine-induced inhibition of the hepatic cytochrome p-450 microsomal enzyme system. In this regard, anticoagulants, phenytoin, antidepressants, benzodiazepines, and theophylline must be monitored for toxic side effects when used in conjunction with cimetidine.[60] The clinical effects of beta-blockers and glipizide also should be monitored if this H2-blocker is added to the medication regimen. Concomitant use of cimetidine and narcotics should be avoided, especially in dialysis patients and in individuals with respiratory depression. The clinical significance of a digoxin-cimetidine interaction is questionable, but digoxin concentrations should be routinely evaluated to avoid possible elevations and toxic effects.[1,6,36,61-63]

Cimetidine Disease Incompatibility Profile (DIP 3-16). Cimetidine can be used with a relative degree of safety in most common clinical disorders, but there are some important drug-disease interactions noted in the DIP figures. Cimetidine carries a category B pregnancy rating. Elderly patients are more likely to have renal impairment and central nervous system disorders. Accordingly, cimetidine should be used with some degree of caution in this population. A wide range of reversible central nervous system effects are produced by this H2-blocker, including confusion, agitation, depression, anxiety, and psychosis. Therefore, some degree of caution is required in patients who have pre-exisiting neuropsychiatric disorders, including depression. Rapid intravenous administration of cimetidine can produce cardiac arrhythmias and hypotension. Because cimetidine can affect the serum levels of many antiarrhythmic agents, a cautionary yellow designation is included for use in patients with cardiac rhythm disturbances. Because most arthritic patients are taking either narcotics or

NSAIDs, both of which can cause central nervous system side effects, the addition of cimetidine, with its propensity for causing confusion, should be monitored closely.[36,62,64]

Ranitidine (Zantac®) Drug Incompatibility Profile (DIP 3-17). Because ranitidine binds to the p-450 cytochrome oxidase system with *weak* affinity, it can produce some of the drug interactions associated with cimetidine use. In general, however, these interactions are not clinically significant, although on rare occasions, they may be. The effects of alcohol, metoprolol, anticoagulants, oral hypoglycemics, benzodiazepines, and phenytoin may all be potentiated by concurrent ranitidine administration. The clinical significance of these interactions is not yet established, but prudence requires calling attention to their possible occurrence.[6,7,35,62]

Ranitidine Disease Incompatibility Profile (DIP 3-17). Because elderly patients often have reduced renal function, ranitidine use should be monitored in this group. Older patients should also be evaluated for possible central nervous system side effects associated with ranitidine use.[65] Bradycardia, tachycardia, and PVCs are seen with rapid intravenous administration of this H2-blocker.[37] A yellow designation is issued to alert the clinician of this possible side effect.[50,66]

Proton Pump Blockers

Lansoprazole (Prevacid®) Drug Incompatibility Profile (DIP 3-18). Lansoprazole is metabolized through the cytochrome P450 system, specifically through CYP3A and CYP2C19. However, lansoprazole does not have clinically significant interactions with other drugs metabolized by the cytochrome P450, such as warfarin, indomethacin, ibuprofen, phenytoin, propranolol, prednisone, diazepam, clarithromycin, or terfenadine. Concurrent use of lansoprazole and theophylline will cause a minor increase in theophylline clearance; therefore, patients who are taking theophylline may need additional titration of their theophylline dosage when lansoprazole is started (or stopped).

Lansoprazole causes a profound and long-lasting inhibition of gastric acid secretion, and therefore, it may interfere with the absorption of drugs for which gastric pH is an important determinant of bioavailability. These drugs include digoxin, ampicillin esters, ketoconazole, and iron salts.

Lansoprazole Disease Incompatibility Profile (DIP 3-18). Lansoprazole is indicated for short-term (up to four weeks) treatment for healing and symptomatic relief of active duodenal ulcer, and for short term (up to 8 weeks) treatment of all grades of erosive esophagitis. The drug carries a pregnancy category B rating and can be used in pregnant woman with caution. Caution should be taken when Prevacid is given to renal impaired patients. Dosage adjustment/reduction may be necessary in patients with hepatic impairment. The clearance of lansoprazole is decreased in the elderly. The initial dosing regimen need not be altered, but subsequent doses > 30 mg/day should not be administered unless additional gastric suppression is needed.

Omeprazole (Prilosec®) Drug Incompatibility Profile (DIP 3-19). Omeprazole is metabolized through the cytochrome P450. It can prolong the elimination of diazepam, warfarin, and phenytoin. Omeprazole also interacts with other drugs metabolized by the P450 system such as cyclosporine, disulfiram, and benzodiazepines. However, no interactions have been identified with theophylline or propranolol.

Omeprazole causes a profound and long-lasting inhibition of gastric acid secretion, therefore, it may interfere with the absorption of drugs where gastric pH is an important determinant of bioavailability, such as digoxin, ampicillin esters, ketoconazole, and iron salts.

Omeprazole Disease Incompatibility Profile (DIP 3-19). Omeprazole is indicated for treatment of active duodenal ulcer, gastroesophageal reflux disease (GERD), and pathological hypersecretory conditions such as Zollinger-Ellison syndrome. It carries a pregnancy category C rating and should not be given to pregnant women. Caution should be taken when Prilosec is given to renal impaired patients. Dosage adjustment/reduction may be necessary in patients with hepatic impairment.

Benzodiazepines

Benzodiazepines are frequently used to relieve short-term anxiety in middle-aged and older patients.[67] Although all these agents—flurazepam, diazepam, chlordiazepoxide, alprazolam,[68] temazepam, oxazepam, etc.—produce central nervous system effects,[69] those agents with a longer half-life tend to be more problematic, especially in the elderly. Somnolence, confusion, and depression are the most common presenting symptoms of anxiolytic toxicity associated with long-acting benzodiazepines. A number of drug-drug interactions also deserve attention, especially those with agents such as narcotics, alcohol, and diphenhydramine, all of which have the capacity for potentiating central nervous system and respiratory depression associated with benzodiazepine use.[70-74]

Benzodiazepine Drug Incompatibility Profile (DIP 3-20). The use of alcohol with anxiolytics should be strongly discouraged because even small amounts of alcohol may impair driving ability in patients taking benzodiazepines. Because the effects of benzodiazepines and alcohol may be additive, a red (avoid concurrent use) designation is used. Several case reports describe a syndrome of hypotension, stupor, and respiratory distress from the combined use of loxapine and lorazepam. Accordingly, these two agents probably should not be used simultaneously.[6,7]

Yellow classifications are used to indicate a number of interactions in which benzodiazepine toxicity is potentiated by concomitant administration of another drug. For example, propranolol and metoprolol may be associated with increased diazepam and clorazepate toxicity. These combinations can be avoided by use of hydrophilic beta-blockers. When beta-blockers and benzodiazepines *must* be used in combination, the concurrent use of hydrophilic beta-blockers such as atenolol and lorazepam is recommended as an alternative. Drugs that are known to produce central nervous system depression or sedation (i.e., narcotics, sedating antihistamines, antidepressants, etc.) should be used cautiously with benzodiazepines. Even fluoxetine, although it is nonsedating, may cause increased impairment of skills related to driving when used with diazepam or alprazolam as a result of decreased clearance.[6,7,35]

Theophylline produces a decrease in diazepam's sedative effects, probably because of adenosine receptor blockade. In general, concurrent use is not recommended.

Benzodiazepine Disease Incompatibility Profile (DIP 3-20). Long-acting benzodiazepines can produce confusion, respiratory depression,[75] disorientation, hallucinations, and falls in the elderly. Consequently, their use in this population should be avoided if possible. Benzodiazepines should not be used in pregnancy. Finally, benzodiazepines should be used only with caution in conditions requiring mobility (arthritis), mental alertness (depression), and respiratory motivation (chronic obstructive pulmonary disease).[71-73]

Sympathomimetic Bronchodilators

Sympathomimetic bronchodilators are used to produce bronchodilation. This is accomplished by relieving reversible bronchospasm through relaxation of bronchiole smooth muscles in such conditions as asthma, bronchitis, emphysema, or bronchiectasis. The relative selectivity of action of beta-agonists is the principal determinant of clinical usefulness and can predict the most likely side effects. The beta-2 selective agents provide the greatest benefits with minimal side effects. Because sympathomimetics with α-agonist properties can produce a number of actions, from pressor effects and nasal decongestion to bronchial dilation and increased myocardial contractility, these drugs should be administered with caution to individuals with unstable vasomotor systems, hypertension, hyperthyroidism, diabetes, prostatic hypertrophy, or a history of seizures. Cautious use is also recommended in elderly patients, in psychoneurotic individuals (who may have a tendency to overuse these drugs), and in patients with long-standing bronchial asthma who have developed degenerative heart disease.

Although generally safe in healthy individuals and well-tolerated, sympathomimetics can cause nervousness, restlessness, and sleeplessness. The presence of these symptoms requires dose reduction. Occasionally, patients develop severe paradoxical airway resistance with repeated, excessive use of inhalants. The precise cause for this is unknown, but when this is observed, the drug should be withdrawn immediately and alternative therapy instituted.

Beta-Agonist (Albuterol, Metaproterenol, Isoetharine) Drug Incompatibility Profile (DIP 3-21). A red warning designation is given for the combined use of beta-blockers and beta-agonists. Beta-blockers antagonize the effects of sympathomimetics, and concurrent use is counterproductive. Moreover, the introduction of a beta-blocker into the drug regimen of a patient with bronchospastic pulmonary disease can produce severe clinical consequences.

A yellow warning for concurrent use of theophylline and beta-agonists reflects the observation that, in children, terbutaline and albuterol may actually decrease theophylline effect by increasing the metabolism of the drug. Theophylline concentrations should be monitored in patients receiving an inhaled beta-agonist in conjunction with oral theophylline. Digoxin toxicity has been observed in patients on digoxin who were administered oral or intravenous albuterol. The precipitating factor may be hypokalemia, or sensitization of the heart by sympathomimetics to digoxin-induced cardiac arrhythmias. Finally, the hypokalemic effects of thiazide diuretics may be potentiated by concomitant use of albuterol.[76]

Beta-Agonist Disease Incompatibility Profile (DIP 3-21). Controlled and moderate intake of sympathomimetic agents is generally safe. However, when use of these agents is chronic and excessive, a number of adverse clinical effects may be observed, especially in patients with underlying central nervous system disorders, cardiovascular disease, asthma, and endocrine disorders.[77] Consequently, a number of yellow warning designations appear in the drug incompatibility profile for albuterol, metaproterenol, and isoetharine. Because beta sympathomimetics are potent central nervous system stimulants and can cause stimulation, restlessness, apprehension, anxiety, and fear, these drugs should be administered with caution to individuals suffering from depression, panic attacks, and anxiety disorders. In addition, beta-agonists are associated with palpitations, changes in blood pressure (elevation and depression), tachycardia, arrhythmias, chest discomfort, PVCs (rare), and other cardiac symptoms. Ephedrine, in particular, can precipitate hypertensive episodes severe enough to cause intracranial hemorrhage, and can induce angina in patients with acute coronary insufficiency.

Accordingly, sympathomimetics should be used with caution in patients with a history of coronary artery disease, congestive heart failure, cardiac arrhythmias, and stroke. Because the elderly are at high risk for having these underlying conditions, a yellow designation is issued for beta-agonist use in this age group. Large doses of intravenous albuterol can aggravate preexisting diabetes mellitus; the role of inhaled albuterol is unknown, but insulin or oral hypoglycemic requirements should be carefully monitored in diabetic patients taking oral sympathomimetics. Most of these agents carry a category C pregnancy classification, and should be avoided in this patient subgroup.

Because beta-agonists can produce heartburn and nausea, their use in patients with peptic ulcer disease should be monitored. Finally, on occasion, inhalants can stimulate bronchospasm and coughing in patients with chronic obstructive pulmonary disease. Accordingly, the possibility of paradoxical deterioration of patients with underlying lung disease should be considered.

Theophyllines

Theophylline compounds (Theo-Dur®, Bronkodyl®, Choledyl®, etc.) are used to provide symptomatic relief and for prevention of reversible bronchospasm associated with chronic bronchitis, asthma, and emphysema. Excessive dosage of the drug can produce serious toxicity, which increases at serum levels > 20 mcg/ml (toxic effects are seen in 75% of patients with serum levels > 25 mcg/ml).[78] Decreased clearance of theophylline is common in the elderly, in patients with liver dysfunction, and in individuals taking medications that inhibit the p-450 hepatic cytochrome oxidase system. Because the therapeutic to toxic ratio is extremely narrow with theophylline, and because the cardiovascular and neurologic side effects of this drug can produce serious clinical consequences, careful monitoring is recommended in a number of patient subgroups, especially in individuals on long-term drug therapy. These concerns are reflected in the drug and disease incompatibility profiles for these agents.[1,6,7,32]

Theophylline Drug Incompatibility Profile (DIP 3-22). A red warning is issued for the combined use of beta-blockers and theophylline,[79] first because beta-blockers should be avoided in asthmatics, and second, because propranolol can decrease theophylline metabolism, thereby producing toxic effects.

Caution is advised when combining theophylline with antacids, as absorption of the bronchodilator may be increased. Allopurinol can produce theophylline toxicity through decreased metabolism. Because cimetidine is a potent inhibitor of the p-450 cytochrome oxidase system, concurrent use of this antiulcer agent can elevate theophylline levels, especially in the elderly and in patients with impaired hepatic function. Ranitidine is a weak binder to the P-450 system and also carries a yellow warning designation, although the risk of inducing theophylline toxicity is extremely rare with this H2-blocker. Famotidine carries a green designation because it has no clinically significant p-450 binding. Theophylline concentrations should be monitored in patients taking cimetidine and ranitidine, as well as in individuals taking oral contraceptives, erythromycin, tetracycline, and flouroquinolones.[80-83] Azithromycin may, in some cases, affect theophylline levels and is given a yellow designation. Finally, some of the stimulatory effects of theophylline can be exacerbated by caffeine.

Theophylline Disease Incompatibility Profile (DIP 3-22). Theophylline use is not recommended in pregnancy (category C classification) or in patients with severe coronary artery disease associated with cardiac arrhythmias. Theophylline can cause dysrhythmias or worsen preexisting arrhythmias. Consequently, any change in rhythm or significant change in heart rate warrants determination of theophylline serum levels.

Because the drug can produce serious cardiac arrhythmias, it should be used with caution in patients with congestive heart failure, a condition that may prolong theophylline half-life and is associated with arrhythmogenesis. Theophylline can produce local gastric irritation and abdominal pain, symptoms that dictate cautious use in patients with peptic ulcer disease. Patients with depression should be warned that theophylline can cause central nervous system disturbances, especially irritability, headache, insomnia, and depression. Patients with chronic obstructive pulmonary disease should be advised that theophylline may cause tachypnea and can increase respiratory rate. The elderly, in general, are more susceptible to theophylline toxicity and show decreased metabolism of the drug.[78]

Antihistamines

Generally speaking, antihistamines are remarkably safe considering their widespread use. The principal concern with these agents involves the arrhythmogenic properties of terfenadine and astemizole when used in combination with drugs (e.g., erythromycin, clarithromycin, troleandomycin) that impair metabolism of these antihistaminic agents. In contrast, diphenhydramine drug and disease incompatibilities reflect this agent's anticholinergic and sedating side effects. These concerns are highlighted in the drug and disease incompatibility profiles discussed below.

Astemizole Drug Incompatibility Profile (DIP 3-23). Many of the same warnings issued for cardiac arrhythmias resulting from combined use of terfenadine with various antibiotics and antifungal agents also apply to astemizole. The principal concern with astemizole is the possibility of producing life-threatening cardiac arrhythmias. The potential clinical consequences of decreasing metabolism of astemizole with concurrent use of such drugs as erythromycin, clarithromycin, and ketoconazole must be recognized. As a result, concurrent use of these medications with astemizole should be avoided in all situations. There are no reported adverse reactions from the combination of fluconazole and astemizole.

Astemizole Disease Incompatibility Profile (DIP 3-23). Red warning designations accompany the drug-disease pie slices indicating risk of using astemizole in patients with cardiac arrhythmias. Yellow designations are used for associated cardiac conditions such as congestive heart failure and coronary artery disease. Use of astemizole in pregnancy is not recommended.

Fexofenadine (Allegra®) Drug Incompatibility Profile (DIP 3-24). Unlike terfenadine, fexofenadine (Allegra) can be safely used in combination with erythromycin, clarithromycin, ketoconazole and troleandomycin. The concurrent use of these drugs with fexofenadine does not cause prolongation of QTc interval.

Fexofenadine Disease Incompatibility Profile (DIP 3-24). Fexofenadine (Allegra) should not be used in pregnant women since it carries a pregnancy category C. Although no prolongation of QTc intervals has been observed in human or animal studies, caution is reasonable when using fexofenadine in patients with cardiac arrhythmias. Alteration of dosage may be needed in patients with decrreased renal function.

Cetirizine Drug Incompatibility Profile (DIP 3-25). Cetirizine is a human metabolite of hydroxyzine. Hydroxyzine is a CNS depressant agent. Although cetirizine does *not* show significant cerebral H1 receptors binding capacity, it should be used with caution in combination with alcohol or any CNS depressants such as narcotics or barbiturates. In studies comparing cetirizine to placebo, patients report sedation, drowsiness, or related symptoms in 8% of those taking placebo, and in about 14% of those taking cetirizine. When avoiding CNS sedation is a *principal* priority in choosing an antihistamine (i.e., elderly), these factors may need to be considered. Theophylline decreases clearance of cetirizine, but the clinical significance of this is not known.

Cetirizine (Zyrtec®) Disease Incompatibility Profile (DIP 3-25). Cetirizine (Zyrtec) carries a pregnancy category B and, therefore, can be used in pregnant women with *caution.* Dose adjustment may be needed in patients with renal and hepatic impairment.

Loratadine (Claritin®) Drug Incompatibility Profile (DIP 3-26). There are no clinically significant drug interactions with loratadine reported at present time.

Loratadine Disease Incompatibility Profile (DIP 3-26). Loratadine (Claritin) carries a pregnancy category B and can be used in pregnant women with caution. Dose adjustment of loratadine may be needed in patients with renal and hepatic impairment.

Diphenhydramine Drug Incompatibility Profile (DIP 3-27). Diphenhydramine can produce clinically significant anticholinergic side effects, central nervous system sedation, impairment of motor function, and urinary retention. Cautious use is advised, especially in the elderly, who may be taking other drugs producing similar side effects. These effects can be exacerbated when this antihistamine is combined with other anticholinergic medications including desipramine, anti-Parkinson drugs, haloperidol, amitriptyline, scopolamine, and phenothiazines. Hallucinations can occur from the combined use of MAOIs and cyproheptadine, although the mechanism is not clear. Caution is recommended for concurrent use of diphenhydramine and central nervous system depressants including alcohol, benzodiazepines, narcotics, antianxiety agents, and barbiturates.[86,88,89]

Diphenhydramine Disease Incompatibility Profile (DIP 3-27). The central nervous system sedating effects of diphenhydramine can be clinically significant, especially in elderly patients and in individuals consuming other anticholinergic drugs. Accordingly, dosage reduction is the prudent approach in patients over the age of 65, especially men with documented prostatic hypertrophy or symptoms suggestive of prostatism. Use of diphenhydramine in depression is recommended with extreme caution only because lassitude, confusion, insomnia, irritability, and nervousness can occur. The sedative effects of diphenhydramine may be undesirable in patients with arthritis, who should be encouraged to walk and maintain normal physical activity if possible. Because diphenhydramine can produce a number of adverse cardiovascular effects, from tachycardia and palpitations to electrocardiographic changes (widening QRS complex) and hypotension, caution is advised when this antihistamine is used in patients with cardiac arrhythmias, coronary artery disease, and congestive heart failure. When the sedating properties of diphenhydramine are likely to present problems, use of a low-sedating agent such as loratidine or cetirizine is recommended.

Antibiotics

Fluoroquinolones (Ciprofloxacin, Norfloxacin) Drug Incompatibility Profile (DIP 3-28). Fluoroquinolones are widely used for outpatient management of such common infections as pyelonephritis, prostatitis, and skin infections. Despite their routine use, a number of drug incompatibilities are worth bearing in mind. Theophylline toxicity may be seen with ciprofloxacin and norfloxacin, and this interaction may be potentiated by the concomitant use of cimetidine. At present, there is some data to suggest that ofloxacin and meflox-acin may not produce this theophylline interaction. Nevertheless, a red DIP® warning designation is used to alert pharmacists and physicians of this possible drug interaction. Interestingly, caffeine toxicity may be observed with concurrent enoxacin and ciprofloxacin administration, a finding that suggests large caffeine intake should be avoided in patients taking this class of antibiotics.

Antacids should not be used with fluoroquinolones because decreased antibiotic effects occur with concurrent use of aluminum, magnesium, and calcium-containing antacids. If the patient must take antacids, they should be taken 2 hours after or 6 hours before administration of a fluoroquinolone antibiotic. A yellow warning is used for anticoagulants[90,91] because increased warfarin effects has been reported from the concurrent use of ciprofloxacin and norfloxacin. The possibility of metoprolol toxicity should be monitored in patients taking ciprofloxacin. Renal status should be monitored in patients taking cyclosporine in conjunction with either ciprofloxacin or norfloxacin. Dosage reduction may be required to avoid nephrotoxicity. Concomitant administration of sucralfate may result in reduced ciprofloxacin or norfloxacin effect.

Fluoroquinolones Disease Incompatibility Profile (DIP 3-28). These agents carry a category C pregnancy rating and should not be used in pregnant women. Alteration of drug dosage may be required in patients with renal impairment. Central nervous system stimulation may occur with ciprofloxacin, and other quinolones, which may lead to tremor, restlessness, confusion, and on very rare occasions, to hallucinations and grand mal seizures. Because of these possible side effects, fluoroquinolones should be used with caution in patients with preexisting central nervous system disorders, including severe cerebrovascular disease and epilepsy. A yellow warning designation is issued for fluoroquinolone use in patients with peptic ulcer disease because the drug can cause abdominal pain and nausea. In addition, many patients with peptic ulcer disease may be taking antacids, which are known to interfere with the absorption of this antibiotic.

Levofloxacin (Levaquin®) Drug Incompatibility Profile (DIP 3-29). Unlike such fluoroquinolones as ciprofloxacin and norfloxacin, levoflox-acin does not affect theophylline or warfarin plasma levels. Also, levofloxacin does not alter cyclosporine level. While chelation by divalent cations is less marked than with other quinolones, concurrent use of aluminum, magnesium, and calcium containing antacids as well as sucrafate, with levofloxacin should be avoided. If the patient must take antacids or sucralfate, they should be taken at least 2 hours before or 2 hours after levofloxacin administration. The concomitant administration of an NSAID with quinolones, including levofloxacin, may increase the risk of CNS stimulation and convulsive seizure, and therefore, this combination should be avoided or used with caution.

Levofloxacin Disease Incompatibility Profile (DIP 3-29). Levofloxacin (Levaquin) carries a pregnancy category C and hence should not be used in pregnant women. Dosage adjustment may be required in patients with renal impairment. As with other quinolones, levofloxacin should be used with caution in any patient with a known or suspected CNS disorder since these drugs may predispose to seizures or lower the seizure threshold. A yellow warning designation is for levofloxacin use in the diabetic patient because the drug can cause disturbances of blood glucose, including symptomatic hyper- and hypoglycemia.

Trovafloxacin (Trovan®) Drug Incompatibility Profile (DIP 3-30). Unlike the first generation fluoroquinolones such as ciprofloxacin and norfloxacin, trovafloxacin does not affect theophylline or warfarin plasma levels. In addition, trovafloxacin does not alter cyclosporine levels. While chelation by divalent cations is less marked than with other quinolones, concurrent use of aluminum, magnesium, and calcium-containing antacids and sucralfate with trovafloxacin should be avoided. If the patient must take antacids or sucralfate, they should be taken at least 2 hours before or 2 hours after trovafloxacin administration. The concomitant administration of a NSAID with a quinolone, including trovafloxacin may increase the risk of CNS stimulation and convulsive seizures, and therefore, concomitant use of these drugs should be avoided or used with caution.

Trovafloxacin Disease Incompatibility Profile (DIP 3-30). A fluorquinolone antibiotic, trovafloxacin carries a pregnancy category C and should not be used in pregnant women. Dosage adjustment may be required in patients with renal impairment. As with other quinolones, trovafloxacin should be used with caution in any patient with a known or suspected CNS disorder that may predispose to seizures or lower the seizure threshold. A yellow warning designation is used for trovafloxacin use in diabetic patients because the drug can cause disturbance of blood glucose, including symptomatic hyper- and hypoglycemia.

Erythromycin Drug Incompatibility Profile (DIP 3-31). The most important drug interactions associated with erythromycin include avoidance of concurrent use with terfenadine, astemizole, carbamazepine, and ergot alkaloids. The potentiation of terfenadine- and astemizole-induced cardiac arrhythmias was discussed in a previous section. Carbamazepine toxicity can be precipitated by concurrent erythromycin therapy, which causes a decrease in carbamazepine metabolism. Ergot alkaloid toxicity can be potentiated by erythromycin, and concurrent use is not recommeded.

Yellow warning designations are used for the combined use of erythromycin and benzodiazepines (i.e., triazolam and midazolam) because increased toxicity is observed as a result of decreased metabolism. The risk of erythromycin-induced elevations of serum theophylline concentration was emphasized in a previous section. Alcohol use should be discouraged during erythromycin therapy, because erythromycin absorption may be reduced. A single report of lovastatin-induced rhabdomyolysis was reported in a patient taking erythromycin. Finally, increased bleeding times are observed in patients who take this antibiotic and oral anticoagulants in combination.

Many of the drug interactions cited for erythromycin also apply to clarithromycin.

Erythromycin Disease Incompatibility Profile (DIP 3-31). Erythromycin can be administered with relative safety in most patients. Because of its propensity to cause gastric distress and abdominal cramping, it should be used with caution in patients with gastrointestinal disorders. It carries a category B rating for pregnancy. It may be used in these patients if no other alternatives are available.[1,6,12,32,92]

Azithromycin Drug Incompatibility Profile (DIP 3-32). Azithromycin has an excellent drug incompatibility profile. It appears as if it can be used in conjunction with astemizole and theophylline, but a yellow designation is given as a precaution. A cautionary yellow designation is issued for use in patients taking oral contraceptives; absorption of oral contraceptives may be decreased by concurrrent administration of azithromycin.[1,6,92] Azithromycin may elevate PT time in patients on warfarin, and monitoring is required.

Azithromycin Disease Incompatibility Profile (DIP 3-32). Azithromycin can be used without the risk of adversely affecting the symptoms of most commonly encountered medical disorders. Although it carries a category B pregnancy rating, this antibiotic is the drug of choice for pregnant women with chlamydia cervicitis.

Oral Hypoglycemic Agents (Sulfonylureas: glipizide, glyburide)

The risk of producing hypoglycemia must always be considered in patients taking chronic oral sulfonyurea therapy. Many other drugs can interact with these agents and produce clinically significant adverse effects. These are highlighted in the drug and disease incompatibility profiles discussed below.

Oral Hypoglycemic Drug Incompatibility Profile (Glipizide, Glyburide) (DIP 3-33). Through an unknown mechanism, miconazole can produce severe hypoglycemia, so a red warning designation against concurrent use appears in the profile.

A yellow warning designation is used for concurrent use of alcohol and sulfonylureas. Patients taking these drugs should be counseled to avoid consumption of large amounts of alcohol, which can potentiate or prolong the hypoglycemic effects of both glipizide and glyburide. On very rare occasions, the increase in insulin sensitivity produced by captopril therapy may cause blood glucose reductions when used in combination with high doses of oral hypoglycemic agents. Both blood sugar levels and prothrombin time should be closely monitored in patients taking warfarin and oral hypoglycemic agents concurrently; increased hypoglycemic effects and increased dicumarol effects may be seen from combined use of these agents.

Beta-blockers should be used with caution in diabetic patients taking oral hypoglycemic agents because (1) beta-blocker receptor blockade can mask the tachycardia and tremor caused by hypoglycemia; and (2) beta-blockers may cause a decreased hypoglycemic effect, possibly as a result of decreased insulin release. NSAIDs can displace first-generation (chlorpropamide) hypoglycemics from their binding sites, causing hypoglycemia, but this is not a problem with second generation agents such as glipizide and glyburide. Finally, verapamil may produce an increased hypoglycemic effect in conjunction with these agents and blood sugar should be monitored.[93]

Oral Hypoglycemic Disease Incompatibility Profile (DIP 3-33). Because insulin requirements frequently diminish in patients with progressive renal parenchymal destruction, individuals with renal impairment are at higher risk for developing spontaneous hypoglycemia, especially when taking oral hypoglycemic agents. Careful monitoring of blood glucose concentrations is warranted in this patient population.

Troglitazone (Rezulin®) Drug Incompatibility Profile (DIP 3-34). In premenopausal anovulatory patients, troglitazone treatment may result in resumption of ovulation. These patients may be at risk for pregnancy. Also, concurrent use of troglitazone with an oral contraceptive containing ethinyl estradiol and norethindrone reduces plasma concentrations of both, which could result in loss of contraceptive efficacy. A higher dose of oral contraceptive or an alternative method of contraception should be considered.

Concomitant administration of cholestyramine with troglitazone results in a 70% reduction of troglitazone absorption; accordingly, coadministration of troglitazone and cholestyramine is not recommended. Even though no information is available on the use of troglitazone with metformin and insulin, troglitazone may reduce insulin and metformin requirements. By increasing insulin receptor sensitivity, troglitazone may produce hypoglycemia. Consequently, patients should be closely monitored when these drugs are combined.

Troglitazone Disease Incompatibility Profile (DIP 3-34). Troglitazone is indicated for Type II diabetes, especially in patients who are on insulin therapy, and whose hyperglycemia (HBA_{1C} level > 8.5%) is inadequately controlled despite insulin therapy of > 30 units/day given as multiple doses. It has a category B pregnancy rating. Dosage adjustment is not necessary in patients with renal dysfunction. Troglitazone should be used with caution in patients with hepatic disease. Very rare reports of death associated with liver failure have been reported in patients taking troglitazone. Consequently, the drug should be avoided in patients with abnormal liver function studies, and if elevated transaminase levels occur during therapy, the drug should be discontinued.

Metformin (Glucophage®) Drug Incompatibility Profile (DIP 3-35). Alcohol is known to potentiate the effect of metformin on lactate metabolism. Therefore, patients on metformin should be warned against excessive alcohol intake. Cationic drugs that are eliminated by renal tubular secretion may have the potential for interaction with metformin by competing for common renal tubular transport systems. Caution should be taken when there is concomitant administration of metformin with these drugs.

Concurrent administration of metformin and sulfonylureas (or adding metformin to a drug in this class) may require a dosage reduction of sulfonylureas. When metformin is used in combination with sulfonylurea therapy, the risk of hypoglycemia associated with sulfonylureas continues and may be increased.

Appropriate precautions, including monitoring and dose adjustment, should be taken.

Metformin Disease Incompatibility Profile (DIP 3-35). Metformin is an orgal hypoglycemic drug indicated for the treatment of non-insulin dependent diabetes mellitus (NIDDM). It carries a pregnancy category B rating. Lactic acidosis is a rare—but potentially fatal—metabolic complication that can occur due to metformin accumulation during treatment. Safe use of the drug can be enhanced by identifying high risk subgroups. Studies had shown that lactic acidosis has occurred primarily in diabetic patients with significant renal insufficiency. The risk of lactic acidosis increases with the degree of renal dysfunction and the patient's age. The drug should not be used in patients with renal disease as suggested by creatinine levels > 1.5 mg/dl (males), > 1.4 mg/dl (females) or a markedly abnormal creatinine clearance. Patients with hepatic disease should avoid taking Glucophage because impaired hepatic function may significantly limit the ability to clear lactate.

Any condition that increases the likelihood of tissue hypoperfusion—and therefore, lactic acid accumulation—or renal dysfunction should prompt at least temporary discontinuation of metformin. Situations or conditions that should deter use of this medication include severe CHF, hypotension, recurrent sepsis, and dehydration.

Lipid-Lowering Drugs

Lovastatin Drug Incompatibility Profile (DIP 3-36). Lovastatin is a cholesterol-lowering agent that inhibits HMG-CoA reductase, the enzyme which catalyzes the conversion of HMG-CoA to mevalonate, an early step in the biosynthetic pathway for cholesterol. The most worrisome drug-related side effects concern the development of myalgia, transient mild elevations in creatine phosphokinase levels, and in rare cases, rhabdomyolysis with its serious nephrotoxic sequelae. This life-threatening complication is observed most often in cardiac transplant patients taking immunosuppressive therapy with cyclosporine. Other drugs associated with lovastatin-mediated myopathy include gemfibrozil, nicotinic acid, and erythromycin, all of which carry DIP warning designations. In general, these agents should not be used concurrently with lovastatin. Finally, bleeding and prolonged prothrombin times are reported as a result of combined lovastatin and anticoagulant therapy.

Lovastatin Disease Incompatibility Profile (DIP 3-36). Lovastatin is contraindicated in pregnancy. Extreme caution is required when used in patients with liver disease and in those undergoing immunosuppression therapy.

Simvastatin (Zocor®) Drug Incompatibility Profile (DIP 3-37). Cyclosporine, gemfibrozil, erythromycin, niacin, and azole (i.e., itraconazole) antifungal agents should not be used concurrently with simvastatin since these combinations increase the potential for simvastatin-mediated myopathy. These warnings also apply to other HMG-Co A reductase inhibitors. In rare cases, rhabdomyolysis has been associated with concomitant administration of these drugs. Simvastatin slightly elevates digoxin plasma concentration. Hence, patients taking digoxin should be monitored appropriately when simvastatin is initiated. Finally, bleeding and prolonged prothrombin times have been reported as a result of combined simvastatin and anticoagulant therapy.

Simvastatin Disease Incompatibility Profile (DIP 3-37). Simvastatin (Zocor) is indicated for lowering total serum and LDL cholesterol levels and has been shown to lower risk of death from recurrent myocardial infarction. It carries a pregnancy category X and should not be used in pregnant women.

When used in patients with pre-existing renal insufficiency, usually as a consequence of long-standing diabetes, simvastatin and has been associated with a risk of developing rhabdomyolysis. The precise clinical significance of this drug-disease interaction is not fully elucidated. Always monitor patients for symptoms and laboratory manifestations of myalgias and myopathy. Patients with these conditions should be monitored very closely while under simvastatin therapy. Patients should be advised to report any muscle tenderness or weakness and CPK levels should be measured.

Extreme caution also is required when simvastatin is used in patients with liver disease, in chronic alcoholism, and in those undergoing immunosuppressive therapy. As a general rule for maximizing safety in all patients taking HMG-CoA reductase inhibitors such as simvastatin, liver function tests should be performed before initiating therapy, at 6 and 12 weeks after initiation of therapy, following dose elevation, and periodically (6 month intervals) thereafter. If transaminase levels continue to rise, especially if they rise to levels three times normal, the drug should be discontinued.

Atorvastatin (Lipitor®) Drug Incompatibility Profile (DIP 3-38). As a general rule, cyclosporine, gemfibrozil, erythromycin, niacin and azole antifungal (itraconazole) agents should not be used concurrently with atorvastatin since there is a potential for atorvastatin-mediated myopathy, and in rare cases, rhabdomyolysis has been associated with concomitant administration of these drugs. These drug-drug interactions apply to the HMG-Co A reductase class as a whole.

Atorvastatin slightly elevates digoxin plasma concentration. The precise clinical significance of this interaction has not been fully elucidated. However, to maximize safety, especially in elderly patients who are likely to have a narrow toxic-to-therapeutic ratio and are taking digoxin in combination with atorvastatin, digoxin levels should be monitored as necessary when atorvastatin is initiated. Levels should be drawn when therapy is initiated, and at 2 to 4 weeks following the first dose. Clinical judgement should dictate the importance of following this interaction.

Coadministration of atorvastatin and oral contraceptives has been shown to increase norethindrone and estradiol plasma levels. These increases should be considered when selecting an oral contraceptive in a woman taking atorvastatin. Finally, unlike some other HMG-Co A reductase inhibitors, atorvastatin has no clinically significant effect on prothrombin time when administered to patients receiving chronic warfarin treatment.

Atorvastatin Disease Incompatibility Profile (DIP 3-38). Atorvastatin (Lipitor) is indicated for lower total and LDL serum cholesterol levels in patients who have failed other (dietary and lifestyle) measures aimed at lipid reduction. It also is indicated for reduction of serum triglyceride levels. It carries a pregnancy category X and should not be used in pregnant women. Extreme caution is required when atorvastatin is used in patients with liver disease and in those undergoing immunosuppressive therapy. Always monitor patients for clinical symptoms and laboratory manifestations suggestive of myalgias and myopathy. Patients with these conditions should be followed very closely while under atorvastatin therapy. Patients should be advised to report any muscle tenderness or weakness and CPK levels should be measured when appropriate.

Caution also is required when atorvastatin is used in patients with liver disease, in individuals suffering from chronic alcoholism, and in those undergoing immunosuppressive therapy. As a general rule for maximizing safety in all patients taking HMG-CoA reductase inhibitors such as atorvastatin, liver function tests should be performed before initiating therapy, at 6 and 12 weeks after initiation of therapy, following dose elevation, and periodically (at least every 6 month intervals) thereafter. If transaminase levels continue to rise, especially if they rise to levels three times normal, the drug should be discontinued. Persistent low level elevations also may prompt discontinuation. The likelihood of encountering liver abnormalities with atorvastatin is dose dependent, and increases significantly at the 40 mg and 80 mg/day dosage ranges.

Gemfibrozil Drug Incompatibility Profile (DIP 3-39). As mentioned in the previous section, avoid concurrent use of gemfibrozil and lovastatin therapy. In unusual cases, warfarin effects can be potentiated by the concurrent use of gemfibrozil. Hypoglycemia is observed in patients taking gemfibrozil and glyburide concurrently. In diabetic patients managed with insulin, hypoglycemic effects may be attenuated by concomitant use of gemfibrozil.

Gemfibrozil Disease Incompatibility Profile (DIP 3-39). Gemfibrozil carries a category B pregnancy classification. It is associated with a high incidence of dyspepsia, making its use in patients with gastrointestinal disorders, including ulcer disease, potentially problematic. This drug can also produce myopathy, arthralgias, painful extremities, and other arthritic symptoms. Accordingly, arthritic patients should be observed for possible deterioration of musculoskeletal symptoms after initiation of gemfibrozil therapy.

The DIP™ System In Cardiovascular Drug Prescribing

The use of the DIP system for cardiovascular disease and hypertension must be considered against the backdrop of many drug interactions and comorbid conditions that characterize the clinical spectrum of heart disease. Over the past decade, the pharmacotherapeutic landscape for the treatment of hypertension has witnessed major tectonic shifts. With more than 40 million Americans currently suffering from elevated blood pressure, and an additional 8 million persons inflicted with either congestive heart failure or chronic angina pectoris, selection of antihypertensive and cardioprotective agents is a major clinical priority for primary care practitioners. However, choosing among specific agents from myriad drug classes—some of which correct one clinical parameter (e.g., blood pressure, chest pain) while deleteriously altering another (e.g., lipid levels, heart rate)—is an increasingly problematic and challenging aspect of pharmacotherapy for cardiovascular disorders.

To a great extent, difficulties in drug prescribing arise because agents with varying pharmacologic effects are frequently added to a preexisting drug regimen, a maneuver which may produce one or more drug interactions. The resulting interactions may be helpful or harmful to the patient, depending on clinical circumstances. Patients taking cardiovascular drug therapy may have other diseases, such as lipid disorders, diabetes, and arthritis, which can be adversely affected by the addition of a new drug to the pharmacologic landscape. Finally, for patients with hypertension, congestive heart failure, or coronary artery disease, it should be stressed that optimal intervention not only requires amelioration of the primary clinical derangement, but careful attention to prevention-oriented pharmacotherapy.

Selection of Cardiovascular Drugs: DIP™ Considerations

A wide variety of agents are available to treat cardiovascular disorders, creating new challenges for practitioners. Optimal pharmacotherapeutic management is becoming less a matter of treating abnormal test results or disabling symptoms and now includes treating a spectrum of coexisting conditions and reducing the patient's overall coronary heart disease risk profile.

An approach aimed at optimizing as many clinical variables as possible requires that: (1) drug interactions are minimized; (2) newly introduced agents do not compromise therapy of associated underlying conditions; (3) drug therapy that successfully treats one abnormality (e.g., hypertension) also will positively affect, or has a neutral affect on, other cardiovascular risk factors; and (4) the newly introduced drug does not impair a patient's functional status, but rather, improves quality of life.

Given the multiple considerations that come into play for an individual patient, pharmacologic intervention for cardiovascular disease can be a formidable task. A drug selection system based on drug and disease incompatibility profiles can guide practitioners through a labyrinthine pharmacologic landscape that, for hypertension and coexistent conditions, has become increasingly complex. In recent years, for example, physicians have been deluged by newly approved pharmaceuticals for the primary treatment of hypertension. With the wide spectrum and proven efficacy of so many agents, optimal antihypertensive therapy requires more than merely selecting a drug that will adequately control diastolic and systolic blood pressure. Ideally, an agent or regimen should be selected that is associated with: (1) high patient compliance; (2) a low incidence of adverse drug reactions and interactions; (3) positive effects on modifiable cardiac risk factors; and (4) preservation or enhancement of quality of life, including cognitive and sexual function.

Aside from DIP considerations, much of the controversy concerning optimal initial antihypertensive therapy revolved around the issue of whether old standbys such as thiazide diuretics and beta-blockers should be replaced with newer drugs such as once-a-day calcium blockers, peripheral alpha-1 blockers, and ACE inhibitors. The issue has fueled fierce debate. In 1989, hydrochlorothiazide was the most frequently dispensed pharmaceutical drug in America, with over 70 million prescriptions filled. The efficacy of hydrochlorothiazide and its acceptable cost to most patients has made this drug a favorite for treatment of essential hypertension. However, recent studies report that up to 70% of patients with elevated blood pressure have elevated serum lipids, prompting experts to raise questions about the wisdom of using diuretics as initial agents of choice for the management of patients with essential hypertension.[94]

One disturbing observation is that although thiazide-based pharmacotherapy for hypertension decreases the incidence of stroke, congestive heart failure, and onset of hypertension-induced nephropathy, no controlled clinical trials have convincingly demonstrated a significant reduction in the rate of myocardial infarction in middle-aged men and women. To explain this apparent paradox (i.e., the lack of effect of antihypertensive therapy on myocardial infarction) some have suggested that the adverse metabolic effects of thiazide diuretics counteract the potential end-organ salvage promoted by blood pressure reduction. Based on what is known about risk factors and coronary artery disease, it can be argued that the impaired glucose tolerance, hyperinsulinemia, lipid abnormalities, hypokalemia, and hyperuricemia induced by thiazide diuretics might contribute significantly to the progression of atherosclerosis or might place *selected* individuals at increased risk for arrhythmias, especially hypertensive patients with underlying coronary artery disease or left ventricular hypertrophy. The issue, however, is far from settled.

Although the precise impact of these metabolic factors is still a matter of speculation, thiazide diuretics have had their image tarnished by numerous investigations painting them as metabolic spoilers.[94-97] Although it is not yet time to abandon thiazide diuretics, the effects that antihypertensive drugs have on blood lipid profiles, platelet aggregation, endothelial vasoreactivity, and insulin sensitivity (i.e., metabolic and hematological parameters that are of paramount importance for cardiopreventive drug therapy) are increasingly important factors in choosing specific therapeutic agents for patients at high risk for coronary artery disease.

In an attempt to clarify some of these issues, investigators participating in the "Treatment of Mild Hypertension Study (TOMHS),"[98,99] the most important and comprehensive recent trial of its kind, have reported on the association between blood lipids and a wide range of commonly used antihypertensive drug classes. In this randomized, placebo-controlled, double-blind clinical trial that followed several hundred patients for 24 months, blood lipid changes associated with five active drugs and a placebo were evaluated. The active drug classes included a selective beta-1 blocker with intrinsic sympathomimetic activity (acebutolol), a calcium channel blocker (amlodipine), a diuretic (chlorthalidone), an alpha-1 blocker (doxazosin) and an ACE inhibitor (enalapril).

The variable effects of these agents on cardiac risk factors and quality of life were analyzed over the study period. Chlorthalidone raised total serum cholesterol level 3 mg% at 12 months from baseline in the study group and 9% more than the placebo group, which had a reduction of almost 6 mg/dl. Other agents had reductions similar to or slightly greater than the placebo, with the peripheral alpha-blocker doxazosin producing the greatest drop (12.9 mg/dl) in total serum cholesterol among the active treatment groups.

With respect to serum triglyceride levels, acebutolol, chlorthalidone and enalapril produced reductions less than the placebo group, whereas doxazosin produced the most dramatic reductions (37.7 mg/dl) as well as the highest HDL/Total Cholesterol ratio after 24 months of therapy. In this study, as in others, the calcium channel blocker had a neutral effect on blood lipids.

Newer trials in progress increasingly focus on generating data that will help practitioners to select cardiovascular agents according to CHD risk, inter-drug compatibility and quality of life measurements. The DIP system discussed below organizes findings from recent clinical studies into a drug prescribing scheme that takes into account both CHD and pharmacologic risk factors as they influence drug use in the contemporary outpatient environment.

DIP™ Profiles For Specific Cardiovascular Agents

With respect to the complex group of cardiovascular drugs, the DIP system includes those classes of antihypertensive, antianginal, CHF-ameliorating, and cardioprotective agents which are in widest use (beta-blockers, diuretics, peripheral alpha blockers, ACE inhibitors, calcium blockers, and centrally acting agonists) and then evaluates them based on drug and disease compatibilities. Frequently, drugs within a given class have unique properties, some of which suggest windows of opportunity or, conversely, windows of vulnerability as far as clinical outcomes are concerned. One of the purposes of the DIP system is to clarify such distinctions in order to optimize drug selection within and between pharmacologic classes.

To enhance its usefulness, the DIP system also evaluates pharmacologic suitability against the backdrop of those diseases most commonly encountered in middle-aged and older Americans (e.g., coronary artery disease, lipid disorders, arthritis, diabetes, congestive heart failure, depression) as well as against the pharmacologic landscape of agents most likely to be encountered in this patient population. This strategy for optimizing drug selection represents a comprehensive distillation of information gleaned from clinical trials reported in the current medical literature. It also reflects opinions published in expert consensus reports in which the desirability of using different classes of antihypertensives and cardiovascular agents for patients on certain drug regimens or with specific disease risks are carefully analyzed.[6,76,100-104]

Thiazide Diuretics Drug Incompatibility Profile (DIP 3-40). Hydrochlorothiazide is an antihypertensive agent that is also effective in the treatment of congestive heart failure. However, caution is required when it is used in combination with digoxin, NSAIDs, and ACE inhibitors. Thiazide diuretics can cause hypokalemia, an electrolyte disturbance that can potentiate digoxin-induced arrhythmias.[105] Monitoring and maintenance of potassium levels is imperative in patients taking thiazide diuretics and concomitant digoxin therapy; many experts now recommend *empiric* potassium supplementation in all patients taking thiazides in combination with digoxin. NSAIDs can precipitate renal dysfunction, especially in the elderly and other individuals with diminished renal perfusion or a reduced glomerular filtration rate. The combined use of an NSAID and thiazide diuretics can place such patients at greater risk for a drug-related adverse patient event. In susceptible patients (e.g., the elderly, those with preexisting renal disease, individuals with diabetes mellitus) the renal complications associated with ACE inhibitors, as well as hypotensive effects, are potentiated by the simultaneous use of a thiazide diuretic.

Thiazide Diuretics Disease Incompatibility Profile (DIP 3-40). With respect to disease incompatibility profiles, thiazide diuretics are associated with a number of potential incompatibilities that may affect their desirability in specific patient subgroups.[95,96,106] These agents are known to impair glucose tolerance, elevate blood insulin levels (due to impairment of insulin-mediated glucose disposal), and increase total serum cholesterol and triglyceride levels. As a result, patients with either insulin or non-insulin dependent diabetes mellitus (NIDDM), individuals with hyperlipoproteinemias, and patients with two or more risk factors for coronary artery disease (CAD), may not be the best candidates for thiazide therapy when other options are available.[97]

Beta-Blocker Drug Incompatibility Profile (DIP 3-41). Beta-blockers were once considered flagship drugs for the monotherapy of elevated blood pressure, despite such well-documented side effects as depression, impotence, and sleep disturbances reported with their long-term use.[107,108] Because of the rapid evolution of antihypertensive drugs that have fewer side effects and which are better suited for CHD risk factor reduction, the use of beta-blockers as monotherapy for lowering blood pressure has waned in relative importance compared to other drug classes. As a result of their capacity to cause drug and disease interactions, they have been recast primarily as agents of choice for the *secondary prevention of myocardial infarction* and as cotherapeutic agents (i.e., in combination with nitrates and/or calcium blockers) for the medical management of angina.

Beta-blockers can reduce both resting and exercise-mediated increases in heart rate. Attenuation of exercise capacity may be undesirable in individuals who wish to pursue nonpharmacologic therapy (exercise, weight reduction, etc.) for blood pressure reduction. The negative chronotropic effects also can be problematic in older patients taking other sinoatrial node suppressing agents such as verapamil or diltiazem. Consequently, caution is always recommended when combining these two drug classes, especially in the elderly, in patients with underlying conduction disease, and in those with marginal left ventricular function. Moreover, hepatic metabolism of the lipophilic beta-blockers propranolol and metoprolol may be affected by coadministration of verapamil and diltiazem. Although in most patients the clinical significance of this effect is minimal, clinicians should be aware of the potential for increased cardiodepressant activity when combining beta-blockers with either verapamil or diltiazem.

Fortunately, beta-blockers are almost always compatible with amlodipine. Consequently, therapy of patients with angina and hypertension who already are on a beta-blocker, is appropriate with amlodipine.[109]

Patients who are on digoxin therapy for inotropic enhancement of left ventricular function may undergo clinical deterioration with the addition of high doses of myocardial suppressant agents such as beta-blockers. On the other hand, *low* dose beta-blocker therapy in patients with CHF is generally safe, and in some cases may be beneficial. Beta-blockers, in high doses, usually are contraindicated in patients with overt heart failure. Even the presence of digoxin in the patient's drug regimen should suggest caution regarding addition of drugs from the beta-blocker class, inasmuch as these patients may have been taking digoxin for improvement of left ventricular function. Finally, reports show that such CNS-penetrating, lipophilic beta-blockers as propranolol can, in some patients, cause depression. Consequently, patients already taking antidepressants for management of psychiatric disorders may respond more favorably to other antihypertensives.

Beta-Blocker Disease Incompatibility Profile (DIP 3-41). With respect to its drug-disease incompatibility profile, beta-blockers in high doses are generally contraindicated in individuals with clinically apparent congestive heart failure and in patients with bronchospastic chronic obstructive pulmonary disease. Because perception of the peripheral manifestations of hypoglycemia is blunted in diabetic patients on beta-blockers, this class of drugs should be used cautiously in this subgroup. Finally, for reasons discussed earlier, beta-blockers may exacerbate clinical depression and hyperlipoproteinemias, thus necessitating caution when used in these patient populations.

ACE Inhibitors Drug Incompatibility Profile (DIP 3-42). For the most part, ACE inhibitors have acceptable clinical profiles as far as drug interactions and compatibility with underlying diseases. However, this class, in selected cases, can cause some problematic drug and disease interactions. Because ACE inhibitors inhibit production of angiotensin II, and thereby decrease aldosterone synthesis, they can cause potassium retention. On occasion, the resulting electrolyte disturbance can be clinically significant. Consequently, the combination of an ACE inhibitor with a potassium-sparing diuretic or potassium-containing salt substitutes (e.g., triamterene, amiloride) is generally not recommended without careful monitoring of the patient.[110]

NSAIDs inhibit cyclooxygenase production, which decreases synthesis of prostaglandins, alters intrarenal hemodynamics, and indirectly leads to suppression of aldosterone secretion. This increases the potential for potassium retention, especially in hyperreninemic patients. As a result, the combination of an ACE inhibitor plus an NSAID is potentially problematic in elderly patients, in diabetics, and in others with diminished renal function. Moreover, because both agents independently have the capacity for causing renal dysfunction, clinicians should avoid, or exercise caution with these two drug classes in combination, especially if other effective agents (e.g., calcium blockers, peripheral alpha-1 blockers) are clinically acceptable.

ACE Inhibitors Disease Incompatibility Profile (DIP 3-42). With respect to drug-disease interactions, a number of clinically important profiles recently surfaced that deserve attention. Although ACE inhibitors are not contraindicated in patients with chronic obstructive pulmonary disease, in smokers, or in others with chronic cardiopulmonary conditions, a recent study analyzing 209 outpatients provides convincing evidence that the incidence of cough associated with enalapril is significantly underestimated and that as many as 10% of patients actually stop the drug within the first several weeks due to the severity of tussive symptoms. Moreover, an additional 15% of patients experience enalapril-mediated cough that is clinically apparent but not severe enough to warrant drug cessation. Other ACE inhibitors have also been associated with cough. In light of these findings, clinicians should be aware of the potential difficulties in distinguishing ACE inhibitor-induced cough from symptoms associated with underlying cardiopulmonary disease. When cough is a recurrent symptom in a given patient, to avoid possible confusion with drug-mediated side effects, selection of another blood pressure-lowering drug may be the prudent therapeutic course.

ACE inhibitors can reduce proteinuria associated with diabetic glomerulosclerosis by decreasing efferent, postglomerular arteriolar resistance. This potential advantage may be offset by the fact that diabetics who already have renal impairment are probably at higher risk for developing increased renal dysfunction with ACE inhibitors. Finally, because patients with chronic arthritic disorders frequently require therapy with anti-inflammatory drugs that are known to affect renal hemodynamics, ACE inhibitors should be used with caution in this vulnerable subgroup.

Angiotension Receptor Antagonists

Losartan (Cozaar®) Drug Incompatibility Profile (DIP 3-43). There are no known clinically significant drug interactions with losartan at the present time. Clinicians may wish to monitor potassium levels in hyporeninemic/hypoaldosteronemic patients who are taking a potassium-sparing diuretic in combination with losartan.

Losartan Disease Incompatibility Profile (DIP 3-43). Losartan is indicated for the treatment of hypertension, either alone or in combination with other antihypertensive agents. When used in pregnancy during the second and third trimester, losartan can cause injury and even death to the developing fetus. For this reason, losartan should not be given to pregnant women. Dosage adjustment may be needed in patients with renal impairment, those who are volume-depleted, and in patients with hepatic impairment. In patients who depend upon activity of the renin-angiotension-aldosterone system, treatment with ACE inhibitors has been associated with oliguria and progressive azotemia and, rarely, with acute renal failure. Losartan would be expected to behave similarly in this high risk group of patients, especially those with bilateral or unilateral renal artery stenosis.

Peripheral Alpha-Blockers Drug and Disease Incompatibility Profiles (DIP 3-44). In an attempt to identify a blood pressure lowering agent that does not impair exercise performance, is associated with minimal interdrug toxicity, and that produces appreciable improvements in coronary heart disease risk, there has been a resurgence of interest in peripheral alpha sympatholytic agents, of which doxazosin is an example. In particular, this peripheral alpha-1-blocker offers a unique window of opportunity for the management of hypertension because: (1) there are no clinically significant drug incompatibilities, which means peripheral alpha-1-blockers can be safely used in conjunction with a wide variety of agents commonly encountered in patients with coronary heart disease risk factors (calcium blockers, beta-blockers, oral hypoglycemics, etc.); and (2) at present, there are no known drug-disease incompatibilities, (i.e., peripheral alpha-blockers such as doxazosin do not compromise therapy of or adversely affect the natural history of diseases that frequently co-exist with atherosclerosis, diabetes, or hypertension).

Calcium Channel Blockers

Any analysis of calcium channel blockers must begin with the following caveat: *Calcium channel blockers are not created equally.* And neither, for that matter, are most drugs within a so-called "drug class." But the differences among calcium blockers are so significant, that prudent selection of these agents requires a detailed understanding of their specific pharmacokinetic features and, in particular, their effects on cardiac function. In this regard, it should be stressed that, although effective for the treatment of hypertension, the calcium blockers verapamil (Calan® SR) and diltiazem (Cardizem® CD) both have the potential for producing negative inotropic effects (i.e., impairment of myocardial pump function and, in vulnerable patients, congestive heart failure), sinoatrial node slowing (bradycardia), and conduction disturbances (AV node conduction block).

Because of their negative inotropic effects, propensity for producing or exacerbating conduction disturbances, and the risk of producing bradycardia (especially when used concurrently in patients taking cardioprotective beta-blockers, in the elderly, and in those with known brady-tachy syndrome), most experts agree that verapamil and diltiazem should be used cautiously in patients predisposed to CHF and bradyarrhythmias. Patients, however, who have *both* high blood pressure *and* supraventricular tachycardia (SVT), represent a subgroup in which these agents *can* play an important (i.e., dual) therapeutic role. With respect to non-cardiac side effects, verapamil is associated with constipation in up to 20% of patients.

From a practical clinical perspective, the overwhelming majority of patients with hypertension do not require therapy for SVT, and therefore, are better served (from both a safety and therapeutic perspective) with once-daily calcium channel blockers that do not clinically suppress myocardial contractility, that do *not* adversely effect conduction system, and that do *not* slow heart rate. These "first-line" calcium blockers are members of the dihydropyridine class.

Even among the dihydropyridines, however, there are significant differences suggesting some agents within this group are preferrable to others. For example, because isradipine is given on a twice-daily basis, it may not have as good medication compliance as that observed with the once-daily dihydropyridines. With respect to side effects, felodipine is associated with peripheral edema in up to 10% to 30% of patients and can produce side effects such as flushing and headache. Nifedipine GITS is associated with peripheral edema in about 9% to 12% of patients on the 60 mg/d dose; it has minimal negative inotropic effects.

Amlodipine is approved for treatment of both high blood pressure and angina, has a unique cardio-friendliness profile. It produces no significant clinical impairment of myocardial pump function, no clinically significant adverse effect on conduction system (including the SA and AV node), does not significantly increase or decrease heart rate, and can be used safely in combination with beta-blockers. Moreover, because amlodipine has been shown *not* to adversely affect clinical outcomes in patients with congestive heart failure (NYHA functional classes II-IV, PRAISE Trial), and has no known clinically significant drug-drug or drug-disease interactions, this agent has emerged as a calcium blocker of choice in patients with hypertension and impaired myocardial pump function.

Finally, although selection of a calcium channel blocker will depend upon specific patient needs, comorbid conditions (diabetes, congestive heart failure, supraventricular tachycardia, etc.), the fact is, treatment of hypertension almost always is a long-term affair. Consequently, anti-hypertensive drugs must be evaluated not only according to their capacity for achieving short-term results in clinical trials but according to their capacity for "standing the test of time" as *monotherapy* over the long haul—i.e., many years after onset of therapy—in a real world environment. This feature, called "regimen durability," has been assessed in the case of at least one calcium blocker in the "Treatment of Mild Hypertension Study (TOMHS, JAMA, August 1993)."

The TOMHS demonstrated that about 82% of patients started on the calcium blocker amlodipine achieve blood pressure-lowering goals on *monotherapy* (i.e., using only this agent) *four years down the road.* This *regimen durability* advantage associated with amlodipine has important clinical and cost implications, because it suggests that, although the initial cost of calcium blockers is greater than beta-blockers or diuretics, expenditures associated with having to introduce pharmacologic reinforcements—i.e., "add-on" drugs—into the antihypertensive regimen may, to some degree, be prevented with drugs that have regimen durability.

Regardless of the agent, blood pressure control is central to the prevention of cardiovascular disease and stroke. A long-term NIH study (ALLHAT) enrolling 40,000 patients using several different classes of antihypertensive medications is presently under way in order to help refine antihypertensive drug choices according to clinical outcomes.

Rapid Access Guidelines: Calcium Channel Blockers

The following guidelines are recommended as a prudent and sensible approach to the use of calcium blockers in the contemporary clinical setting: **(1)** Primary care practitioners should continue to use calcium blockers for approved indications, paying special attention to avoid hypotension as a side effect. **(2)**

Physicians should avoid using calcium channel blockers for non-approved indications. **(3)** Physicians should avoid short-acting calcium blockers. **(4)** As a drug class, calcium channel blockers are *not* indicated, and therefore, should not presently be used in the setting of *acute* coronary ischemia, unstable angina, or for secondary prevention of myocardial infarction. Initiation of calcium channel blocker therapy in the peri- or early post-infarction period should be avoided whenever possible. **(5)** Short-acting *nifedipine capsules* and diltiazem preparations have few, if any, clinical indications for which other, better-tolerated drugs are not available. Hence, their use should be avoided whenever possible. **(6)** Patients with or without ischemic heart disease who are taking *short-acting* nifedipine capsules for the treatment of hypertension or chronic stable angina should be switched to a long half-life calcium blocker. **(7)** Patients with new onset hypertension who do not require verapamil or diltiazem for atrial or ventricular rate control and who are appropriate candidates for calcium blocker therapy should be started on a long half-life calcium blocker such as amlodipine for reasons cited above. **(8)** Patients who are taking and tolerating long-acting calcium blockers verapamil or diltiazem for the treatment supraventricular tachycardia should remain on their medications. **(9)** Except when heart rate control is an issue, the overall trend in calcium blocker prescribing should be *away* from long- or short-acting agents that may produce either myocardial suppression (verapamil and diltiazem) or precipitous vasodilatation (nifedipine capsules) and toward once-daily agents (amlodipine) with a gradual onset of action that also have been shown from a clinically significant perspective *not* to suppress myocardial pump function, adversely affect cardiac conduction, or cause precipitous changes in heart rate or blood pressure.

Verapamil and Diltiazem Drug Incompatibility Profile (DIP 3-45). Although lacking cardioprotective properties, the calcium blockers verapamil and diltiazem are effective antihypertensive and antianginal agents. These two calcium blockers should be used with caution in combination with beta-blockers.[102,109,111] In this regard, symptomatic bradyarrhythmias, AV node conduction disturbances, and clinically significant cardiosuppression are more likely to occur when these calcium blockers are used together in the frail elderly, in patients with impaired left ventricular function, and in those with bradytachycardia. Moreover, verapamil and diltiazem should be titrated carefully in patients who are taking digoxin for control of symptoms precipitated by congestive heart failure. In such patients, the cardiosuppressive effects of calcium blockers must be monitored, as well as serum digoxin levels, which studies show can be elevated with coadministration of verapamil or diltiazem.

Verapamil and Diltiazem Disease Incompatibility Profile (DIP 3-45). With respect to drug-disease incompatibility profiles, the calcium blockers are relatively free of contraindications. Congestive heart failure is a relative contraindication for the use of verapamil, while use of diltiazem is not desirable in patients with significant AV node conduction disease in combination with left ventricular failure. With respect to the cardioprotective effects of diltiazem, a randomized investigation of 2,466 patients from 38 North American hospitals demonstrated that in myocardial infarction patients with radiographic or clinical findings of congestive heart failure or an ejection fraction less than 35%, long-term diltiazem therapy (average dose, 180 mg/d) was associated with a significantly increased number of adverse cardiac events (hazard ratio, 1:41), including reinfarction and mortality from other cardiac causes. These findings are supported by a recent study that shows calcium channel blockers, in general, are unlikely to reduce the rate of initial or recurrent infarction, limit infarct size, or reduce overall mortality rates.[112]

Nifedipine Drug and Disease Incompatibility Profiles (DIP 3-46). Nifedipine (sustained release *long-acting;* Procardia XL or Adalat CC) is a once-daily calcium channel blocker that can be coadministered with the majority of pharmacologic agents used to treat cardiovascular diseases. There is a potential for an interaction between nifedipine and beta-blockers; CHF developed rarely from this combination. Because of its negative inotropic effect, however, it should be used with caution in patients with severe congestive heart failure, especially the elderly, in whom hypotensive effects may be more pronounced. Occasional patients have reported increased frequency, duration, or severity of angina on starting nifedipine or during dosage increases.

Amlodipine Drug and Disease Incompatibility Profiles (Calcium Channel Blocker) (DIP 3-47). Amlodipine is a once-daily calcium blocker that is effective for the treatment of hypertension as well as angina pectoris. It has no clinically significant effects on the SA or AV node and, therefore, can be used safely in combination with beta-blockers. The absence of known clinically significant drug interactions makes the agent especially useful in individuals whose drug regimens are comprised of many different pharmacologic building blocks. Of special importance is the finding that amlodipine does not adversely affect clinical outcome in patients with New York Heart Association stage II, III, or IV functional class congestive heart failure. Consequently, within the class of calcium blockers, amlodipine offers a unique window of opportunity for management of patients with impaired cardiac function who also require concurrent therapy for treatment of hypertension or angina.

Digoxin Drug Incompatibility Profile (DIP 3-48). Digoxin is characterized by a narrow toxic-to-therapeutic ratio, and consequently digoxin levels should be closely monitored in all patients. Special vigilance is required when patients are concurrently taking medications that affect cardiac conduction, electrolyte levels, arrhythmogensis threshold, drug metabolism, and renal function. Consequently, yellow warning designations appear for such drugs as amiodarone, cimetidine, ACE inhibitors, calcium blockers, diuretics, quinidine, bronchodilators, and phenytoin. Caution is also advised for anticholinergic drugs (possible increased digoxin absorption), antibiotics (possible decreased gut metabolism with erthromycin), benzodiazepines (decreased renal excretion), and omperazole (possible increased absorption). Although the precise clinical significance of all these interactions is not fully understood, cautious administration and monitoring of digoxin effects and side-effects is warranted, especially in patients with coronary heart disease and a history of cardiac arrhythmias or conduction disturbances.

Digoxin Disease Incompatibility Profile (DIP 3-48). Digoxin can safely be used in a wide range of patients, including those with hyperlipidemia, arthritis, diabetes, and COPD. It should not be used in pregnant women. Cautionary use is warranted in elderly patients, in patients with gastrointestinal disorders, renal disease, arrythmias, severe CAD, and depression. Because manifestations of digoxin toxicity may include gastric distress and CNS changes, use of this medication should be more carefully monitored in patients with these symptoms.

Pharmatectural Implications of DIP™ System for Heart Disease

At present, comprehensive management of patients with hypertension, diabetes, lipid disorders, or coronary artery disease requires a systematic analysis of drug and disease compatability profiles. When such an analysis is combined with efforts to reduce cardiovascular risk factors, drug prescribing strategies emerge that suggest practical approaches for optimizing selection of specific agents.

[1]Abernathy DR, Andrawis NS. Critical drug interactions: A guide to important examples. Drug Therapy 1993: Cot 15-27.

[2]Alderman J. Drug interactions: the death pen. [Letter] JAMA 1993 Sept 15; 270(11):1316.

[3]FDA Drug Experience Monthly Bulletin: Reports of Suspected Incidents of Adverse Reactions to Drugs. Rockville, Md. US Food and Drug Administration, Bureau of Medicine 1987:87.

[4]Beers MH, Storrie M, Lee G. Potential adverse drug interactions in the emergency room. An issue in the quality of care. Ann Intern Med 1990 Jan 1; 112(1):61-64.

[5]Lamy PP. The elderly and drug interactions. J Am Geriatr Soc 1986;34:586-592.

[6]Mehta M, ed. PDR Guide to Drug Interactions, Side Effects, Indications. Medical Economics Company, 1994.

[7]Rizack MA, Hillman CDM. The Medical Letter Handbook of Adverse Drug Reactions, 1994.

[8]Biglin KE, Faraon MS, Constance TD, Lieh-Lai M. Drug-induced torsades de pointes: a possible interaction of terfenadine and erythromycin [Letter]. Ann Pharmacother 1994 Feb;28(2):282.

[9]Herings RM, Stricker BH, Leufkens HG, Bakker A, Sturmans F, Urquhart J. Public health problems and the rapid estimation of the size of the population at risk. Torsades de pointes and the use of terfenadine and astemizole in The Netherlands. Pharm World Sci 1993 Oct 15;15(5):212-8.

[10]Melmon KL, Morrelli HF, Hoffman BB, et al. eds. Clinical pharmacology: basic principles in therapeutics. 3rd ed. McGraw-Hill 1992:1073-83.

[11]Amodio-Groton M, Currier J. HIV drug interactions. AIDS Clin Care 1991 April;4(4):25-29.

[12]Brodie MJ, Feely J. Adverse drug reactions. BMJ 1988;296:845-9.

[13]Girgis L, Brooks P. Nonsteroidal anti-inflammatory drugs. Differential use in older patients [Review]. Drugs Aging 1994 Feb;4(2):101-12.

[14]Goff DC, Baldessarini RJ. Drug interactions with antipsychotic agents [Review]. J Clin Psychopharmacol 1993 Feb;13(1):57-67.

[15]Gosney M, Tallis RL. Prescription of contraindicated and interacting drugs in elderly patients admitted to hospital. Lancet 1984;2:564-7.

[16]Hamilton RA, Gordon T. Incidence and cost of hospital admissions secondary to drug interactions involving theophylline. Ann Pharmacother 1992 Dec;26(12):1507-11.

[17]Hodsman GP, Johnston CI. Angiotensin converting enzyme inhibitors: drug interactions. Hypertension 1987;5:1-6.

[18]Houston MC. Nonsteroidal anti-inflammatory drugs and antihypertensives [Review]. Am J Med 1991 May 17;90(5A):425-79.

[19]Jue SG, Vestal RE. Adverse drug reactions in the elderly: a critical review. Medicine in Old Age-Clinical Pharmacology and Drug Therapy London, 1985.

[20]Kramer MS, et al. An algorithm for the operational assessment of adverse drug reactions. I. Background, description, and instructions for use. II Demonstration of reproducibility and validity. JAMA 1979;242(7):623-33.

[21]Larson EB, Kukull WA, Buchner D, et al. Adverse drug reactions associated with global cognitive impairment in elderly persons. Ann Intern Med 1987;107:169-73.

[22]Hansten PD. Drug Interactions 1985; ed 5.

[23]Buchan IE, Bird HA. Drug interactions in arthritic patients. Ann Rheum Dis 1991 Oct; 50(10):680-1.

[24]Johnson AG, Seideman P, Day RO. Adverse drug interactions with nonsteroidal anti-inflammatory drugs (NSAIDs). Recognition, management and avoidance [Review]. Drug Saf 1993 Feb;8(2):99-127.

[25]Nolan L, O Malley K. Adverse effects of antidepressants in the elderly [Review]. Drugs Aging 1992 Sept-Oct;2(5):450-8.

[26]Cannon-Babb ML, Schwartz AB. Drug-induced hyperkalemia. Hosp Pract 1986;21(9A):99-107, 111, 114-27.

[27]Hawkins MM, Seelig CB. A case of acute renal failure induced by the co-administration of NSAIDs and captopril. N C Med J 1990 June;51(6):291-2.

[28]Seeling CB, Maloley PA, Campbell JR. Nephrotoxicity associated with concomitant ACE inhibitor and NSAID therapy. South Med J 1990 Oct;83(10):1144-8.

[29]Alegro S, Fenster PE, Marcus FI. Digitalis therapy in the elderly. Geriatrics 1983;38:98.

[30]Dall JLC. Maintenance digoxin in elderly patients. BJM 1970;2:702.

[31]Blazer DG, Federspiel CF, Ray WA, et al. The risk of anticholinergic toxicity in the elderly: a study of prescribing practices in two populations. J Gerontol 1983;38:31-35.

[32]Callahan AM, Fava M, Rosenbaum JF. Drug interactions in psychopharmacology [Review]. Psychiatr Clin North Am 1993 Sept;16(3):647-71.

[33]Garner EM, Kelly MW, Thompson DF. Tricyclic antidepressant withdrawal syndrome [Review]. Ann Pharmacother 1993 Sept;27(9):1068-72.

[34]May FE, Stewart RB, Cluff LE. Drug interactions and multiple drug administration. Clin Pharmacol Ther 1977;22:322-8.

[35]Wright JM. Drug interactions. Clinical Pharmacology: Basic Principles in Therapeutics. 3rd ed 1992;1012-21.

[36]Jenike MA. Cimetidine in elderly patients; review of uses and risks. J Am Geriatr Soc 1987;30(3):170.

[37]Segal R, Russell WL, Oh T, Ben-Joseph R. Use of I.V. cimetidine, ranitidine, and famotidine in 40 hospitals. Am J Hosp Pharm 1993 Oct; 50(10):2077-81.

[38]Shinn AF. Clinical relevance of cimetidine drug interactions [Review]. Drug Saf 1992 Jul-Aug;7(4):245-67.

[39]Peabody CA, Whiteford HA, Hollister LW. Antidepressants with elderly. J Am Geriatr Soc 1986;34:869-74.

[40]Glassman AH, Roose SP. Risks of antidepressants in the elderly: tricyclic antidepressants and arrhythmia-revising risks. [Review] Gerontology 1994; 40 Supp 1:15-20.

[41]Chan CH, Ruskiewicz RJ. Anticholinergic side effects of trazodone combined with another pharmacologic agent [Letter]. Am J Psychiatry 1990 April;147(4):533.

[42]Beasley CM Jr, Masica DN, Heiligenstein JH, Wheadon DE, Zerbe RL. Possible monoamine oxidase inhibitor-serotonin uptake inhibitor interaction: fluoxetine clinical data and preclinical findings [Review]. J Clin Psychopharmcol 1993 Oct;13(5):312-20.

[43]Ciraulo DA, Shader RI. Fluoxetine drug-drug interactions. II [Review]. J Clin Psychopharmacol 1990 June;10(3):213-7.

[44]Ciraulo DA, Shader RI. Fluoxetine drug-drug interactions: I. Antidepressants and antipsychotics [Review]. J Clin Psychopharmacol 1990 Feb;10(1):48-50.

[45]Levinson ML, Lipsy RJ, Fuller DK. Adverse effects and drug interactions associated with fluoxetine therapy [see comments] [Review]. DICP 1991 June;25(6):657-61.

[46]Messiha FS. Fluoxetine: adverse effects and drug-drug interactions [Review]. J Toxicol Clin Toxicol 1993;31(4):603-30.

[47]Suchowersky O, deVries J. Possible interactions between deprenyl and prozac [letter]. Can J Neurol Sci 1990 Aug;17(3):352-3.

[48]Walley T, Pirmohamed M, Proudlove C, Maxwell D. Interaction of metoprolol and fluoxetine [Letter]. Lancet 1993 Apr 10;341(8850):967-8.

[49]Coplan JD, Gorman JM. Detectable levels of fluoxetine metabolites after discontinuation; an unexpected serotonin syndrome [Letter]. Am J Psychiatry 1993 May;150(5):837.

[50]Bauer LA, Black D, Gensler A. Procainamide-cimetidine drug interaction in elderly male patients. J Am Geriatr Soc 1990 April;38(4):467-9.

[51]Klein WA, Krevsky B, Klepper L, Ljubich P, Niewiarowski TJ, Rothstein KO, Dabezies MA, Fisher RS. Nonsteroidal anti-inflammatory drugs and upper gastrointestinal hemorrhage in an urban hospital. Dig Dis Sci 1993 Nov;38(11):2049-55.

[52]Karsh J. Adverse reactions and interactions with aspirin. Considerations in the treatment of the elderly patient [Review]. Drug Saf 1990 Sept-Oct;5(5):317-27.

[53]Laine L. NSAID-induced gastroduodenal injury: what's the score? Gastroenterology 1991 Aug;101(2):555-7.

[54]Lamy PP. A consideration of NSAID use in the elderly. Geriatr Med Today 1988;7(4):30.

[55]Lamy PP. Renal effects of nonsteroidal anti-inflammatory drugs. Heightened risk to the elderly? J Am Geriatr Soc 1986;34:361-7.

[56]Sager DS, Bennett RM. Individualizing the risk/benefit ratio of NSAIDs in older patients [Review]. Geriatrics 1992 Aug;47(8):24-31.

[57]Shorr RI, Ray WA, Daugherty JR, Griffin MR. Concurrent use of nonsteroidal anti-inflammatory drugs and oral anticoagulants places elderly persons at high risk for hemorrhagic peptic ulcer disease. Arch Intern Med 1993 July 26;153(14):1665-70.

[58]Baxter JD. Minimizing the side effects of glucocorticoid therapy [Review]. Adv Intern Med 1990; 35:173-93.

[59]Piper JM, Ray WA, Daugherty JR, Griffin MR. Corticosteroid use and peptic ulcer disease: role of nonsteroidal anti-inflammatory drugs. Ann Intern Med 1991 May 1;114(9):735-40.

[60]Fraser IM, Buttoo KM, Walker SE, Stewart JH, Babul N. Effects of cimetidine and ranitidine on the pharmacokinetics of a chronotherapeutically formulated once-daily theophylline preparation (Uniphyl). Clin Ther 1993 Mar-Apr;15(2):383-93.

[61]Hansten PD. Overview of the safety profile of the H2-receptor antagonists. DICP 1990 Nov; 24(11 Suppl):S38-41.

[62]Tse CS, Iagmin P. Phenytoin and ranitidine interaction [Letter]. Ann Intern Med 1994 May 15;120(10):892-3.

[63]Wormsley KG. Safety profile of ranitidine. A review. Drugs 1993 Dec;46(6):976-85.

[64]Anonymous. Drugs for treatment of peptic ulcers. Med Lett Drugs Ther 1991 Nov 29;33(858):111-4.

[65]Stocky A. Ranitidine and depression [Review]. Aust N Z J Psychiatry 1991 Sept;25(3):415-8.

[66]Ben-Joseph R, Segal R, Russell WL. Risk for adverse events among patients receiving intravenous histamine2-receptor antagonist. Ann Pharmacother 1993 Dec;27(12):1532-7.

[67]Tollefson GD. Adverse drug reaction/interactions in maintenance therapy [Review]. J Clin Psychiatry 1993 Aug;54 Suppl:48-58; discussion 59-60.

[68]Evans RL, Nelson MV, Melethil S, Townsend R, Hornstra RK, Smith RB. Evaluation of the interaction of lithium and alprazolam. J Clin Psychopharmacol 1990 Oct;10(5):355-9.

[69]Sullivan JT, Sellers EM. Detoxification for triazolam physical dependence. J Clin Psychopharmacol 1992 Apr;12(2):124-7.

[70]Closser MH. Benzodiazepines and the elderly. A review of potential problems [Review]. J Subst Abuse Treat 1991;8(1-2):35-41.

[71]Dilsaver SC. Withdrawal phenomena associated with antidepressant and antipsychotic agents [Review]. Drug Saf 1994 Feb;10(2):103-14.

[72]File SE, Andrew N. Benzodiazepine withdrawal: behavioral pharmacology and neurochemical changes [Review]. Biochem Soc Symp 1993;59:97-106.

[73]Greenblatt DJ, Miller LG, Shader RI. Benzodiazepine discontinuation syndromes [Review]. J Psychiatr Res 1990;24 Suppl 2:73-9.

[74]Wysowski DK, Baum C. Outpatient use of prescription sedative-hypnotic drugs in the United States, 1970 through 1989. Arch Intern Med 1991 Sept;151(9):1779-83.

[75]Longe RL. Triazolam dose in older patients [Letter]. J Am Geriatr Soc 1992 Jan; 40(1):103-4.

[76]Lipworth BJ, McDevitt DG, Struthers AD. Hypokalemic and ECG sequelae of combined beta-agonist/diuretic therapy. Protection by conventional doses of spironolactone but not triamterene. Chest 1990 Oct;98(4):811-5.

[77]Ernst P, Habbick B, Suissa S, Hemmelgarn B, Cockcroft D, Buist AS, Horwitz RI, McNutt M, Spitzer WO. Is the association between inhaled beta-agonist use and life-threatening asthma because of confounding by severity? Am Rev Respir Dis 1993 July;1489(1):75-9.

[78]Sessler CN. Theophylline toxicity: clinical features of 116 cases. Am J Med 1990;88:567-76.

[79]Jankel CA, McMillan JA, Martin BC. Effect of drug interactions on outcomes of patients receiving warfarin or theophylline. Am J Hosp Pharm 1994 Mar 1;51(5):661-6.

[80]Grasela TH Jr., Dreis MW. An evaluation of the quinolone-theophylline interaction using the Food and Drug Administration spontaneous reporting system. Arch Intern Med 1992 Mar;152(3):617-21.

[81]Richardson JP. Theophylline toxicity associated with the administration of ciprofloxacin in a nursing home patient. J Am Geriat Soc 1990 Mar;38(3):236-8.

[82]Rockwood RP, Embardo LS. Theophylline ciprofloxacin, erythromycin: a potentially harmful regimen [Letter]. Ann Pharmacother 1993 May;27(5):651-2.

[83]Spivey JM, Laughlin PH, Goss TF, Nix DE. Theophylline toxicity secondary to ciprofloxacin administration. Ann Emerg Med 1991 Oct;20(10):1131-4.

[84]Crane JK, Shih HT. Syncope and cardiac arrhythmia due to an interaction between itraconazole and terfenadine. Am J Med 1993 Oct;95(4):445-6.

[85]Hirschfeld S, Jarosinski P. Drug interaction of terfenadine and carbamazepine [Letter]. Ann Intern Med 1993 June 1;118(11):907-8.

[86]Rice VJ, Snyder HL. The effects of Benadryl and Hismanal on mood, physiological measures, antihistamine detection, and subjective symptoms. Aviat Space Environ Med 1993 Aug;64(8):717-25.

[87]Swims MP. Potential terfenadine-fluoxetine interaction [Letter]. Ann Pharmacother 1993 Nov; 27(11):1404-5.

[88]Kranzelok EP, Anderson GM, Mirik M. Massive diphenhydramine overdose resulting in death. Ann Emerg Med 1982;11(4):212.

[89]Marquardt D. Antihistamines and the heart. West J Med 1993 June;158(6):613-4.

[90]Kamada AK. Possible interaction between ciprofloxacin and warfarin. DICP 1990 Jan;24(1):27-8.

[91]Renzi R, Finkbeiner S. Ciprofloxacin interaction with sodium warfarin: a potentially dangerous side effect. Am J Emerg Med 1991 Nov;9(6):551-2.

[92]Michocki RJ, Lamy PP. A "risk" approach to adverse drug reactions J Am Geriatr Soc 1988; 36:79-81.

[93]Sugarman JR. Hypoglycemia associated hospitalizations in a population with a high prevalence of non-insulin-dependent diabetes mellitus. Diabetes Res Clin Pract 1991 Nov;14(2):139-47.

[94]McVeigh G, Galloway D, Johnston D. The case for low dose diuretics in hypertension: comparison of low and conventional doses of cyclopenthiazide. BMJ 1988;297:95-98.

[95]Kaplan NM. How bad are diuretic-induced hypokalemia and hypercholesterolemia? Arch Intern Med 1989 Dec;149:2649.

[96]Freis ED. Critique of the clinical importance of diuretic-induced hypokalemia and elevated cholesterol level. Arch Intern Med 1989 Dec;149:264-2647.

[97]Warram JH, Laffel LMB, et al. Excess mortality associated with diuretic therapy in diabetes mellitus. Arch Intern Med 1991;151:1350-6.

[98]Anonymous. The effects of nonpharmacologic interventions on blood pressure of persons with high normal levels. Results of the Trials of Hypertension Prevention, Phase I [published erratum appears in JAMA May 6, 1992 267(17):2330] [see comment]. JAMA 1992 Mar 4; 267(9):1213-20.

[99]Whitcroft IA, Thomas JM, Rawsthrone A, Wilkinson N, Thompson H. Effects of alpha and beta adrenoceptor blocking drugs and ACE inhibitors on long term glucose and lipid control in hypertensive non-insulin dependent diabetics. Horm Metab Res Suppl 1990; 22:42-6.

[100]Perks D, Fisher GC. Esmolol and clonidine—a possible interaction [Letter]. Anaesthesia 1992 June;47(6):533-4.

[101]Sagie A, Strasberg B, Kusnieck J, Sclarovsky S. Symptomatic bradycardia induced by the combination of oral diltiazem and beta blockers [see comments]. Clin Cardiol 1991 Apr; 14(4):314-6.

[102]Fisher ML, Lamey PP. Special considerations in the use of antihypertensive agents in the elderly patient with coexisting disease. Geriatr Med Today 1987;6(11):47.

[103]Amery A, et al. Mortality and morbidity results from the European working party on high blood pressure in the elderly. Lancet 1985;1:1349-1354.

[104]Amir M, Cristal N, Bar-On D, Loidl A. Does the combination of ACE inhibitor and calcium antagonist control hypertension and improve quality of life? The LOMIR-MCT-IL study experience. Blood Press 1994;Suppl 1:40-2.

[105]Levy DW, Lye M. Diuretics and potassium in the elderly. J R Coll Physicians Lond 1987;21(2):148.

[106]Hollifield JW, Slaton PE. Thiazide diuretics, hypokalemia, and cardiac arrhythmias. Acta Med Scand 1981;647(suppl):67.

[107]LaPalio L, Schork A, Glasser S, Tifft C. Safety and efficacy of metoprolol in the treatment of hypertension in the elderly. J Am Geriatr Soc 1992 Apr;40(4):354-8.

[108]Wassertheil-Smoller S, Blaufox DM, et al. Effect of antihypertensives on sexual function and quality of life: The TAIM study. Ann Intern Med 1991;114:613-20.

[109]Ben-Ishay D, Leibel B, Stessman J. Calcium channel blockers in the management of hypertension in the elderly. Am J Med 1986;81 (Suppl 6a):30-4.

[110]Lee HC, Pettinger WA. Diuretics potentiate the angiotensin converting-enzyme inhibitor-associated acute renal dysfunction [Letter]. Clin Nephrol 1992 Oct;38(4):236-7.

[111]Arstall MA, Beltrame JF, Mohan P, Wuttke RD, Esterman AJ, Horowitz JD. Incidence of adverse events during treatment with verapamil for suspected acute myocardial infarction. Am J Cardiol 1992 Dec 15;70(20):1611-2.

[112]Held PH, Yusuf S, Furberg CD. Calcium channel blockers in acute myocardial infarction and unstable angina: an overview. Br Med J 1989;299:1187-92.

4

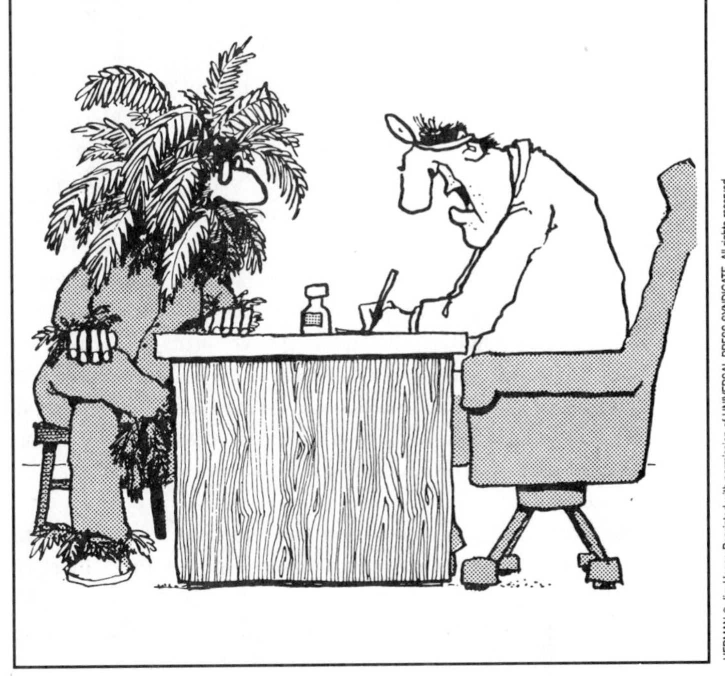

"We'll take you off the vitamins for a couple of days."

Building An Outcome-Effective Drug Regimen: Pearls and Pitfalls

The problems associated with inappropriate,[1,2] suboptimal,[3-5] and excessive drug prescribing[6] in middle aged and older Americans are more than everyday clinical issues. They have become a public health problem.[7-11] In fact, nearly every physician and pharmacist is challenged by the need to recognize and react to the pitfalls of polypharmacy.

For example, consider the following 72-year-old female patient who is taking a number of different medications: albuterol, beclomethasone inhaler, lorazepam, sertraline, aspirin, omeprazole, digoxin, atorvastatin, and enalapril. Clearly, this is a veritable pharmacopoeia of drugs, and it may not even include any over-the-counter medications the patient is taking without physician knowledge or approval.

Several questions immediately come to mind. Is this 72-year-old woman really taking all of these medications? Is she able to keep them all straight? How does she find the time to do anything other than take her medications? How many physicians are prescribing these drugs? Are any of these agents causing or contributing to her present symptoms and clinical deterioration? What drug interactions might explain her chief symptoms of fatigue and lightheadedness? Are some of these medications inappropriate for an elderly patient? Have any of these drugs been used beyond their accepted duration limits? Should these assorted agents be taken together? Why is she taking so many different drugs? Can any of these medications be discontinued without adversely affecting her clinical status?

Polypharmacy is a common problem, and, perhaps, nowhere are its manifestations more visible—and potentially more life-threatening—than in the elderly.[11,14,15] In particular, the risk of polypharmacy increases with the patient's age, the number of diseases with which an individual is afflicted, and the number of different physicians simultaneously providing care for the patient. Although it is hard to lay the blame for polypharmacy on any single factor, the fact is, two-thirds of all physician visits result in a prescription,[6,8] many of which may be unnecessary.

The pressures producing this epidemic of excessive drug prescribing in middle-aged and older Americans are well known. First, there is a perception that modern medicine ought to provide a cure for every symptom or complaint. Patients often expect a drug for everything that ails them, and physicians or pharmacists are often guilty of fostering this expectation. After all, it is much easier and less time consuming to write a prescription than to educate and reassure patients that all they need is a little "tincture of time."

Polypharmacy is not only a risk factor for medication noncompliance, but it increases the risk of drug reactions and interactions, which can range in severity from minimal to life-threatening. With these clinical and pharmacologic concerns in mind, the purpose of this chapter is to discuss and characterize the multiple factors contributing to polypharmacy. This section also reviews and outlines strategies for identifying drug-related adverse patient events (DRAPEs) and for responding to the pitfalls associated with the so-called "Brown Bag Syndrome," a reference to a patient's collection of prescription drugs brought to the physician or pharmacist in a brown paper bag.

DECIPHERING THE BROWN BAG

When a patient who is taking multiple medications presents to the physician or pharmacist with a new sign, symptom, or deterioration of a previously stable chronic condition, complications associated with polypharmacy must be considered. Fortunately, a meticulous medication history can frequently uncover problems associated with complex medication regimens. These include medication noncompliance-mediated therapeutic failures,[16-21] recent addition of drugs known to produce side effects,[22] drug interactions,[23,24] self-medication with a potentially toxic agent,[25] precipitous withdrawal of drugs resulting in an exacerbation of symptoms[26-28] or clinical deterioration.[29-31] The goal of the physician or pharmacist is to recognize these pitfalls of polypharmacy,[28,32] document them, notify the patient's primary physician of potential problems, and, if a new drug must be added as a part of management, to select an agent that will reduce the patient's risk of future drug interactions.

The danger signs of polypharmacy are obvious to the experienced practitioner and pharmacist: too many drugs, too many pills, dosages that are too high, too many prescribers, and too many high-risk medications (i.e., medications with a narrow therapeutic index, agents with steep dose-response relationships, and drugs known to inhibit or induce hepatic enzymes). In addition, four types of patients warrant special attention because of their increased risk of incurring DRAPEs. At particular risk are the critically ill, the elderly, patients with AIDS, and substance abusers. There is some controversy as to whether AIDS is an independent risk factor for drug interactions. In the elderly, the case is quite clear. A number of studies suggest the incidence of drug interactions and inappropriate prescribing practices is increased in the geriatric population.[1,3,7] A landmark study recently demonstrated that about 25% of all Americans over 65 years of age were taking at least one medication deemed to be inappropriate by a panel of national experts.[11]

Patients with AIDS have a higher incidence of toxic reactions to medications than other subgroups treated with similar drugs.[33] These individuals frequently consume five to six different medications daily, including antiretroviral drugs, as well as a number of antibiotic or antifungal agents that are used for prophylaxis against opportunistic infections. AIDS patients with advanced disease are especially susceptible to the toxic effects of their complicated drug houses. Although the precise reasons for this increased sensitivity to drug-related side effects are not fully understood, it may be that HIV-infected individuals tend to take multiple medications for long periods and also have multiorgan system compromise.[33] Finally, such commonly abused drugs as alcohol and stimulants contribute to clinically significant drug interactions, and therefore, substance abuse patients should be screened carefully for the consumption of prescription drugs that are known to potentiate adverse effects.

CLEANING UP THE BROWN BAG

Streamlining drug regimens, deleting problematic agents, and performing clinically advantageous drug substitutions or deletions in the patient's drug regimen ideally should fall within the province of a *single* physician. Nevertheless, all practitioners and pharmacists involved in the patient's care can help in recognizing and rectifying clinical problems and complications associated with polypharmacy. The job begins with a meticulous documentation of all drugs, including prescription, OTC, and recreational drugs being taken by the patient. In addition, an attempt should be made to confirm the dose and frequency of each medication. Correlating clinical deterioration with medication noncompliance or potential drug toxicity is an integral part of this screening process. Special attention should be paid to the recent addition, deletion, or substitution of medications, since such alterations may explain changes in the patient's clinical status. The physician may be able to pinpoint a pharmacologic basis for the patient's clinical deterioration, but more often than not, an association between medication intake and clinical status will be difficult to establish.[15]

Even when a direct link cannot be found between drug intake and patient symptoms, the physician or pharmacist can still perform an extremely valuable function by screening the drugs assembled in the "brown bag" for possible toxicity or inappropriate use.[34] The medication list should always be thoroughly evaluated for the following pitfalls: (1) possible inclusion of unnecessary prescription drugs;[6,35] (2) inclusion of medications that have been prescribed at doses much higher—or lower—than usually required to achieve clinical results;[36] (3) inclusion of drugs that are considered unsuitable or that should be avoided in the elderly;[7,11,24] either because their side effect profile is problematic[2,37] or because other agents with equal therapeutic efficacy, but less toxicity, are available;[3,38] (4) drugs that may be suitable for elimination because of inappropriate or questionable initial indications for their clinical use;[39-42] (5) drugs that may be unnecessary because usage exceeds usual duration limits;[32,43] and (6) drugs that should be avoided because of their propensity to cause drug interactions.

Although the pharmacist or physician may not be able to act on his or her findings during the first patient encounter, clinical impressions regarding polypharmacy should be documented in the patient's chart and communicated to the primary care physician or appropriate specialist. Finally, judicious screening and consultation with authoritative sources before prescribing additional medications will help minimize the adverse consequences of polypharmacy.

BROWN BAG VICTIMS

The pitfalls associated with inappropriate prescribing in middle aged and older adults can be life-threatening. Consider the following case: An 83-year-old white female was brought to the emergency department complaining of bilateral leg cramps, shortness of breath, generalized weakness, and inability to walk for the past 12 hours. The patient had heart disease, high blood pressure, and osteoarthritis, but no history of intrinsic renal disease. On physical examination, the patient was weak and short of breath. She was alert and oriented and able to move all of her extremities. Her cardiovascular examination revealed an irregular rhythm with an S3 gallop. Pulmonary examination revealed bilateral inspiratory rales. Her abdominal examination was normal, and her EKG showed a new, diffusely widened QRS complex. The laboratory examination revealed a BUN concentration of 48, the potassium level was 7.3, and blood glucose was 132 mg. The remainder of the electrolytes were within normal limits. The chest x-ray showed mild congestive heart failure.

The patient's medication list included the following:

(1) insulin, 20 units NPH, 8 regular subq q.a.m.,
(2) amitriptyline, 50 mg PO q.h.s.,
(3) quinidine, 300 mg PO q.i.d.,
(4) isosorbide dinitrate, 20 mg PO t.i.d.,
(5) captopril, 12.5 mg PO b.i.d.,
(6) furosemide, 40 mg PO q.daily,
(7) digoxin, 0.125 mg PO q.daily,
(8) thyroid, two grain q.daily PO,

(9) dipyridamole, 50 mg PO b.i.d.,
(10) aspirin, 325 mg PO q.daily,
(11) calcium, 250 mg PO b.i.d. and
(12) ibuprofen, 400 mg PO t.i.d.

Of special note is that the ibuprofen was started *four days prior to admission.*

This case study illustrates the potential clinical deterioration that can result from drug interactions and polypharmacy. This patient had a number of drug-related adverse reactions, some of which were life-threatening. The newly widened QRS complex, which indicates a serious conduction system abnormality, can result from toxicity associated with three of the medications she was taking. These possibilities include: quinidine, digoxin, and amitriptyline. Hyperkalemia can also be a contributing factor. The most likely precipitating factor that led to this cascade of drug-drug and drug-disease interactions, however, was the introduction of ibuprofen, a nonsteroidal anti-inflammatory drug (NSAID), which precipitated this patient's acute renal deterioration and led to accumulation of quinidine, digoxin, and hyperkalemia.

Most physicians and pharmacists are aware that you cannot take an 83-year-old woman who has 30% reduction in renal function because of her age alone, renal hypoperfusion secondary to congestive cardiomyopathy, diabetic renal disease, is taking multiple drugs affecting kidney function, and then add an NSAID without incurring possible drug/drug or drug/disease interactions. In fact, it is well known that the risk of inducing renal dysfunction with NSAIDs is increased in the elderly, in patients with coronary artery disease, in diabetics, and in patients who are taking diuretics.

What about the patient's acute hyperkalemia? There are a number of possible causes, including: (1) ACE inhibitor-induced inhibition of renin angiotensin and resulting potassium retention; (2) NSAID-mediated inhibition of aldosterone secretion, resulting in hyperkalemia caused by decreased potassium excretion; and (3) possible insulin deficiency. Complicating this patient's renal deterioration and acute hyperkalemia is furosemide-induced prerenal azotemia, which is exacerbated by renal hypoperfusion associated with low cardiac output. In addition, it is important to emphasize that this patient had a high likelihood of having digoxin toxicity. Not only is digoxin excreted through the kidneys, but the patient also was taking quinidine, which is known to inhibit renal excretion of digoxin. In addition, the ibuprofen-induced renal failure contributed to elevated serum digoxin and quinidine levels.

This case is a dramatic illustration of the risks for incurring drug interactions with commonly used medications, such as NSAIDs, ACE inhibitors, digoxin, and antidepressants. The impaired cardiac conduction, renal deterioration, and hyperkalemia—as well as the possible quinidine, digoxin, and amitriptyline toxicities—reflect a life-threatening cascade of interactions and reactions caused by the addition of a single agent to a patient's drug regimen. Pharmacologic management of this patient required a number of steps to both decrease the effects of potentially toxic agents and to correct metabolic abnormalities. Clearly, all of the involved medications should be stopped. The hyperkalemia is best treated by an insulin-glucose infusion and administration of sodium bicarbonate to lower serum potassium level and mitigate the toxic effects of quinidine and amitriptyline. Although use of calcium gluconate is possible for the treatment of hyperkalemia, this patient's likelihood of digoxin toxicity precludes the use of calcium, unless absolutely necessary.

All of these strategies were employed, and within 12 hours of treatment, the patient's QRS complex returned to normal, and renal function improved dramatically.

In addition to the acute, life-threatening drug interaction resulting from the NSAID, it also is important to note that many other agents in this drug house may have been inappropriate for patients in this age group or had questionable indications at best. For example, this elderly patient was taking amitriptyline, which can produce potent anticholinergic side effects, including urinary retention, blurry vision, dry mouth, sedation, confusion, and orthostatic hypotension. A careful examination of the indications for amitriptyline suggested that the patient would be more appropriately treated with a selective serotonin reuptake inhibitor (SSRI). Reevaluation of quinidine therapy also is mandatory. Patients with atrial fibrillation and congestive heart failure who take quinidine for cardioversion have a mortality rate that is twice that observed in patients who are treated with digoxin solely for the purpose of ventricular rate control and continue in atrial fibrillation. In other words, although quinidine may successfully cardiovert the patient and maintain normal sinus rhythm, the patient is also more likely to suffer adverse consequences on quinidine, presumably because of its proarrhythmogenic properties. Therefore, the use of quinidine in this patient requires careful reexamination. Captopril, which is prescribed three times per day, also requires review. Dipyridamole (Persantine®) is probably unnecessary in this patient because aspirin alone will provide adequate anti-platelet effects.

EVALUATION OF MEDICATION COMPLIANCE

Strategies for drug reduction, elimination, simplification, and consolidation, (The DRESC® Program, Chapter 5) are designed to prevent violation of pharmatectural safety codes that can lead to life-threatening drug interactions. From a pharmatectural perspective, drug house deconstruction and reconstruction should not proceed before verifying the patient's pattern of medication compliance.[20,45,46,47] Poor medication compliance is a multifaceted problem that can: (1) prevent effective treatment of a clinical condition; (2) compromise the natural history of a disease; (3) cause additional unnecessary prescriptions to be added in order to compensate for subtherapeutic drug levels and inadequate clinical effects; (4) induce patients to self-medicate with OTC drugs or make alterations in their drug regimens; and (5) precipitate drug-induced side effects.

Defining the relationship between compliance and daily dose frequency is complicated because most published studies use the pill count method for verifying compliance.[21] Results of studies using this methodology must be interpreted with caution because subjects may provide false information about drug intake or little information is provided about the day or time of dose interval. Consequently, the need for clinical trials elucidating factors that enhance or compromise medication compliance has never been greater. Medication compliance is frequently imperfect, and partial compliance with prescribed regimens is difficult to diagnose.[48] Suboptimal medication intake can lead to additional hospitalizations caused by therapeutic failure. In short, major gaps in taking cardiovascular drugs can predispose patients to fluctuating drug concentrations and to withdrawal phenomena.

The Science of Compliance

To evaluate the precise relationship between daily dose frequency and medication compliance, a team of investigators from Washington University School of Medicine and St. Louis University School of Medicine undertook a study[49] designed to investigate the relationship between prescribed daily dose frequency for antihypertensive medications and patient compliance by analyzing the compliance data obtained from unique pill containers that electronically record the date and time of medication removal. When medication compliance was calculated as a simple ratio (number of pill doses removed/number of doses prescribed) times 100, mean patient compliance was higher in the once-daily (96%) and twice-daily (93%) dose regimens than in the three-times daily regimen with which compliance was only 83.8%. More detailed insight into compliance, however, was obtained by examining drug-intake behavior according to a definition in which compliance was measured by the number of days during which the patients took the correct number of prescribed doses within a 24-hour period. Using this more refined index of medication compliance, investigators found that for patients on a once, twice, or thrice daily antihypertensive medication dose regimen, the prescribed number of doses was taken on 83.6%, 74.9%, and 59% of days, respectively.

Based on this study's design, it is clear that if dose frequency decreases from three times to once daily, medication compliance improves by about 42%. Dramatic improvements in drug intake can be made simply by decreasing the daily dose frequency. The clinical implications of these findings are clear. For the purposes of long-term therapy, medication compliance is best assured when patients are prescribed once-daily medications, and any program designed to simplify the drug regimen should take this factor into account.[50,51]

Despite considerable data to the contrary,[21,49] many physicians and pharmacists believe that they can successfully recognize and interpret deviations in medication consumption. However, few practitioners are able to recognize gaps in medication taking. An important study performed at Stanford University[52,53] attempted to identify major gaps in medication-taking behavior and factors that predispose patients to cardiovascular morbidity and mortality because of inadequate medication consumption. In this study, which enrolled 33 patients with cardiovascular conditions, medication intake was evaluated for drug regimens consisting of fewer than six prescription medications. Using electronic surveillance of pill bottle access, these investigators determined that medication-taking gaps of greater than two times the prescribed dosing interval occurred in about 48% of patients. In addition, patient's dosing patterns often produced uncovered intervals ranging from 3 to 25 days with doubtful pharmacologic effectiveness. These lapses in drug intake were underestimated by the patients and not recognized by their treating physicians. Major treatment gaps occurred frequently, even in carefully selected ambulatory populations, and generally escaped detection. These compliance patterns and gaps may contribute to reported excesses of cardiovascular morbidity and mortality in patients who require cardiovascular drug intake to maintain clinical stability.

The degree to which patients, even those with serious cardiovascular diseases, deviated markedly from the prescription was dramatic. The largest single group in this study consisted of near-optimal compliers, which accounted for about 50% to 60% of the total population. These patients were convinced about the value of treatment and are effective in maintaining dose frequency within acceptable limits. The second group, totalling 30% to 40% of ambulatory patients, could be considered partial compliers. These individuals accepted the principle of treatment but failed to adhere with sufficient consistency to avoid clinical problems. Their most common deviation from adequate medication intake was dose omission. Prolonged dosing gaps clearly carry risks of suboptimal clinical benefit, withdrawal or rebound phenomena, and unnecessary and inappropriate escalation of the regimen. The final group, comprising up to 10% of patients, were noncompliers. Even if their intentions were excellent, execution remained poor. Some patients may take medications especially well just before seeing their physicians, confounding the clinical assessment. Consequently, any attempt at streamlining and simplifying drug regimens must be made on the assumption that physicians and pharmacists, even when familiar with their patients, are unable to identify major deviations in medication-taking behavior.[52,53] The fact is, dose omissions are particularly difficult to detect.

Generally speaking, satisfactory adherence to a drug regimen should never be assumed, since potentially important gaps may occur in up to 40% of outpatients. Regular inquiries about obstacles to full compliance should take place at each visit in nonconfrontational ways, seeking solutions rather than fault-finding. Whenever reasonable, longer-acting preparations are preferred to blunt the impact of gaps in medication taking. On occasion, electronic monitoring may prove useful for selected patients when therapeutic goals remain elusive despite apparent adherence to medication compliance.

In summary, any attempts at drug reduction, elimination, simplification, or consolidation must be based on an adequate knowledge of the patient's medication intake patterns. If there is evidence to suggest that a patient is noncompliant with a drug regimen, measures should be taken to simplify the drug regimen and establish a pattern of regular medication intake. On the other hand, if the patient is compliant with the regimen, measures aimed primarily at consolidation of drug therapy are more appropriate.

DRUG HOUSE DEMOLITION: THE ART OF DISCONTINUING MEDICATIONS

There is now a substantial body of evidence[54,55] suggesting that many medications can be discontinued without adversely affecting clinical outcomes.[29,36,56-58] Much of this data comes from studies that evaluate the effect of antipsychotic medication withdrawal in elderly nursing home residents.[10,13,32,58] The implementation of the Nursing Home Reform Amendments of 1987[10,59,60] (Omnibus Reconciliation Act-87) sought to narrowly restrict the use of antipsychotic medications in nursing home patients, invigorating the debate concerning appropriate use of medications in long-term care facilities. It is well known that the primary use of antipsychotic medications is for the treatment of behavioral manifestations of dementia (see Table 4-1). Although there is substantial clinical experience that antipsychotic drugs can calm acutely agitated patients, their effectiveness and appropriateness for long-term management of chronic behavior problems are less well defined.[61] After all, the adverse effects of antipsychotic drugs include tardive dyskinesia and other movement disorders, dystonia, peripheral and central anticholinergic toxicity, impaired alertness, postural hypotension, social withdrawal, and an association with an increased risk of falls and hip fractures. In light of these findings, the OBRA-87 regulations attempt to restrict antipsychotic medication use in dementia to those behaviors that are dangerous to the patient or others, that interfere with the provision of adequate care, or impair resident function.[10,59,60]

Nonpharmacologic Measures. These guidelines also require a trial of nonpharmacologic therapy to control behavior problems, as well as a trial of gradual dose reduction in patients who remain stable over a period of time. Although one study[32] found a 36% decrease in prescriptions for neuroleptic drugs without apparent adverse affects, other experts argue that regulations encouraging withdrawal of antipsychotic medications can have inadvertent negative effects.[32] Some of these concerns are reinforced by the effects of an educational program that encouraged reduction of antipsychotic drug use in nursing home residents.[58] When compared with baseline antipsychotic medication users in control nursing homes, those in the homes in which education for medication reduction was provided had an 18% reduction in antipsychotic medication use, but no increase in behavior problems and less deterioration in short-term memory. However, these patients did have increased reports of depressive symptoms, which led to speculation that anti-psychotic drugs might have been inappropriately discontinued. Most recent studies show that antipsychotic medications, such as benzodiazepines, cyclic antidepressants, and nonbenzodiazepine hypnotic/anxiolytic drugs, with careful clinical monitoring, can be reduced or discontinued in selected nursing home residents without adverse consequences.[2,32,62-64]

Table 4-1

Antipsychotic Medications					
Category and Drug	**Sedative Potency**	**Anticholinergic Potency**	**Orthostatic Hypotensive Potency**	**Extrapyramidal Potency**	**Equivalent Dosage (mg)**
Aliphatic					
Chlorpromazine	High	Moderate	High	Low	100
Triflupromazine	High	Moderate	High	Moderate	30
Piperidines					
Mesoridazine	Moderate	Moderate	Moderate	Moderate	50
Thioridazine	High	High	High	Low	95
Piperazines					
Acetophenazine	Low	Low	Low	Moderate	15
Fluphenazine	Moderate	Low	Low	High	2
Perphenazine	Low	Low	Low	High	8
Trifluperazine	Moderate	Low	Low	High	5
Aliphatics					
Chlorprothixene	High	High	High	Low	75
Piperzines					
Thiothixene	Low	Low	Low	High	5

Table 4-1

Antipsychotic Medications — cont'd.					
Category and Drug	**Sedative Potency**	**Anticholinergic Potency**	**Orthostatic Hypotensive Potency**	**Extrapyramidal Potency**	**Equivalent Dosage (mg)**
Dibenzodiazepines					
Loxapine	Moderate	Moderate	Moderate	High	10
Clozapine	High	High	High	Very low	100
Butyrophenones					
Droperidol	Low	Low	Low	High	1
Haloperidol	Low	Low	Low	High	2
Indolones					
Molindone	Moderate	Moderate	Low	High	10
Diphenylbutylpiperidines					
Pimozide	Low	Low	Low	High	1

Miscellaneous Thioxanthenes Phenothiazines

Neuropsychiatric Medications. One study conducted in 12 community nursing homes that participated in a randomized, controlled trial of an educational program[32] designed to reduce antipsychotic medication use, found that the frequency of behavior problems did not increase in those residents who had their antipsychotic drugs discontinued. In fact, for these residents, psychiatric symptoms *decreased* by 21%. Residents who had their drug discontinued had no deterioration in any of the measures of psychological or behavioral function. Psychiatric and behavioral improvement was most pronounced in those residents who were *not* using other psychotropic drugs. When compared with those nursing home residents remaining on drugs, residents with antipsychotic medications discontinued had no general increase in the frequency of behavior problems; nor was there an increase in specific types of behaviors such as aggression, hostility, and psychotic symptoms, that might be most likely to deteriorate after medication withdrawal. In fact, patients in whom antipsychotic drugs were discontinued had a marked improvement in many psychiatric parameters; moreover, there was no deterioration in any of several other measures of resident functions.[27,28,41]

With careful clinical observation, discontinuation of neuropsychiatric medications can be successfully conducted in both the outpatient setting and in community skilled-care facilities. Numerous studies[3,32,58] suggest that, given the availability of alternative behavioral management techniques, antipsychotics and other psychotropic medications can be successfully discontinued in a large subset of these nursing home patients.[32] These studies provide support to trials of selective withdrawal in long-term care settings.[64] Nevertheless, it is still difficult to identify those specific patients in whom withdrawal is most likely to succeed. Most educational programs aimed at decreasing antipsychotic drug use *exclude* patients with a history of psychosis or substantial violence. These guidelines are also present in OBRA-87. In general, however, drug withdrawal is more likely to be successful in nursing home residents receiving *lower* antipsychotic drug doses, as well as those not using other psychotropic drugs.

Adverse Drug Withdrawal Events (ADWE's). In addition to benzodiazepines,[30,65] antidepressants, and antipsychotics, other drug classes including antihypertensive medications[66,67] can be withdrawn or have their dosages reduced in a significant percentage of patients without adverse clinical consequences.[36,38,43,55,68] Unfortunately, few studies have systematically evaluated the risk of broad-based drug reduction programs. In part, identifying the hazards of drug discontinuation is limited by the lack of accepted, explicit, standardized criteria that can be applied to determine the probability that an adverse clinical event is related to drug discontinuation. Nevertheless, recent studies[32] performed in a Veteran's Hospital attempted to develop and standardize criteria that might link adverse drug withdrawal events (ADWEs) to drug discontinuation. In this study evaluating 62 patients who had 94 ADWEs, it was found that the majority of such events were probably related to drug discontinuation (62%). Most ADWEs were minor (72%); one was associated with hospitalization for myocardial infarction, and none were associated with death. All ADWEs were recurrences of the condition for which the drug was prescribed. Most ADWEs (80%) were associated with three classes of drugs: cardiovascular, CNS, and gastrointestinal. Of all ADWEs, 32% were cardiovascular in nature, with recurrence of hypertension accounting for 11%, exacerbation of heart failure 9%, recurrence of angina 5%, and myocardial infarction 1%. Eleven percent of ADWEs affected the central nervous system, including seizures (7%), hallucinations (2%), and dyskinesia (2%). Four gastrointestinal hemorrhages occurred, but none required hospitalization.

The frequency with which medications required reinstitution varied widely. For example, ranitidine was reinstituted in 17% of cases, haloperidol in 20% of patients, and theophylline in 25% of patients discontinued from the drug. Phenytoin was reinstituted in 30%, digoxin in 40%, and furosemide in 72%. Overall, 60% of all discontinued drugs were not reinstituted. These findings lend support to the idea that drug reduction programs may be successful and have acceptable risks. In this regard, digoxin, furosemide, and ranitidine were those agents most commonly associated with an ADWE of major severity; and, therefore, if discontinued, these patients require careful monitoring.[69,70] It also should be stressed that careful clinical protocols should be followed when withdrawing drugs such as benzodiazepines, theophylline, antidepressants, beta-adrenergic blockers, and many other agents, since discontinuation can be followed by serious physiologic withdrawal symptoms.[26,29-31,42,71]

MEDICATION WITHDRAWAL AND DOSE REDUCTION: WINDOWS OF OPPORTUNITY AND VULNERABILITY.

Antihypertensive Medications

There are as many as 50 million Americans with elevated blood pressure (systolic blood pressure of 160 mm Hg or greater and/or diastolic blood pressure of 85 mm Hg or greater) who are taking antihypertensive medication.[66] Although the majority of these individuals need pharmacologic intervention for their elevated blood pressure, a significant percentage of patients can probably be treated with nonpharmacologic means.[66,68,72,73] The goal of treating hypertensive patients is to prevent morbidity, target organ disease, and mortality associated with high blood pressure, and to control the patient's blood pressure by the least intrusive means possible. Lifestyle modifications, such as weight reduction, increased physical activity, and moderation of dietary sodium and alcohol intake, are used as definitive or adjunctive therapies for the treatment of hypertension. Accordingly, physicians and pharmacists should vigorously encourage their patients to adopt these lifestyle modifications in the hope that medication usage can either be eliminated or reduced in selected individuals.

Nonpharmacologic methods also offer some hope for disease prevention, and they also can modify other risk factors for premature cardiovascular disease. It should be emphasized that the capacity of lifestyle modifications to reduce morbidity or mortality in patients with hypertension is not conclusively documented. However, because of their ability to improve the overall cardiovascular risk profile, lifestyle modification interventions, when properly used, offer multiple benefits at little cost and with minimal risk. Even when these changes are not adequate in themselves to control high blood pressure, they may help reduce the number and dosage requirements of medications needed to manage hypertension. Lifestyle modifications are especially helpful in the large percentage of hypertensive patients who have additional risk factors for premature cardiovascular disease, such as hyperlipidemia or diabetes.[67]

A comprehensive *medicate and modify* approach to managing risk factors offers the best opportunity for reducing death from heart disease. Lifestyle modifications that can improve hypertension control include weight loss, limitation of alcohol intake, aerobic exercise, and reduction of sodium intake. Cessation of cigarette smoking, although not directly associated with a reduction in blood pressure, is strongly advocated since, along with hypertension and hyperlipidemia, it represents one of the major risk factors for coronary artery disease.

Weight Reduction. Weight reduction alone will reduce blood pressure in a large proportion of hypertensive individuals who are more than 10% above ideal weight. A reduction in blood pressure usually occurs early during a weight loss program, often with a weight loss as little as ten pounds. Moreover, weight reduction in overweight, hypertensive patients enhances the blood pressure-lowering effect of concurrent antihypertensive agents and can significantly reduce concomitant cardiovascular risk factors. Therefore, all hypertensive patients who are above their ideal weight should initially be placed on an individualized weight reduction program involving caloric restriction and regular physical activity.

Alcohol Intake. Excessive alcohol intake also can raise blood pressure and cause resistance to antihypertensive therapy. Therefore, a detailed history of current alcohol consumption should be elicited in all patients in whom pharmacologic therapy is being contemplated. In general, hypertensive patients who drink alcoholic beverages should be counseled to limit their daily intake to one ounce of ethanol (two ounces of 100-proof whiskey, eight ounces of wine, or 24 ounces of beer a day). Significant hypertension may develop during withdrawal from heavy alcohol consumption, but the pressor effect of alcohol withdrawal reverses a few days after alcohol consumption is reduced. Minimal to moderate alcohol consumption may reduce the risk of coronary heart disease.

Physical Activity. Regular aerobic physical activity, adequate to achieve at least a moderate level of physical fitness, may be beneficial for both prevention and treatment of hypertension. Physical activity can also enhance weight loss and functional health status, and reduce the risk of cardiovascular disease and overall mortality. Sedentary and unfit normotensive individuals have a 20% to 50% increased risk of developing hypertension when compared with their more active and physically fit peers.

Regular aerobic physical activity can reduce *systolic* blood pressure in hypertensive patients by approximately 10 mm Hg. Effective lowering of blood pressure can be achieved with only moderately intense physical activity. Therefore, physical activity need not be complicated or expensive; for most sedentary patients, such moderate activity as 30 to 45 minutes of brisk walking three to five times weekly is beneficial. When such a program is adopted by the patient, it may be possible to reduce dosages of antihypertensive medications.

Diet. Epidemiologic observations and clinical trials also support an association between dietary sodium intake and blood pressure. A number of therapeutic trials[67] have documented a reduction of blood pressure in response to reduced sodium intake. African-Americans, older people, and patients with hypertension are generally more sensitive to changes in dietary sodium chloride. Because the average consumption of sodium is in excess of 150 mmol/day, moderate dietary sodium chloride reduction to a level of < 100 mmol/day (approximately < 6 grams of sodium chloride or < 2.3 grams of sodium per day) is recommended. With appropriate counseling, this is an achievable diet. In fact, blood pressure may be completely controlled by this degree of sodium chloride restriction in patients with borderline or mild hypertension; in those patients who still need drug therapy, the medication requirements may be decreased.

A high dietary potassium intake also may protect against developing hypertension, and potassium deficiency may increase blood pressure and induce ventricular ectopy. Therefore, normal plasma concentrations of potassium should be maintained, preferably through food sources. If hypokalemia occurs during diuretic therapy, additional potassium may be needed from potassium-containing salt substitutes, potassium supplements, or use of a potassium-sparing diuretic. In many, but not all epidemiologic studies, there is an inverse association between dietary calcium and blood pressure. Calcium deficiency is associated with an increased prevalence of hypertension, and a low calcium intake may amplify the effects of a high sodium intake on blood pressure. An increase in dietary calcium intake may lower blood pressure in some patients with hypertension, but the overall effect is minimal, and there is no way to predict which patients will benefit. Therefore, there is currently no rationale for recommending calcium supplements in excess of the recommended daily allowance.[74-77]

Step-Down Therapy. In patients with *mild* hypertension, these lifestyle modifications should be attempted *prior* to initiation of pharmacologic therapy. However, if an inadequate response is observed *after* an attempt to implement these lifestyle modifications, pharmacologic therapy is indicated. Sound patient treatment includes attempts to decrease the dosage or number of antihypertensive drugs while maintaining lifestyle modifications.[74] In general, complete cessation of an antihypertensive treatment program is usually not indicated. However, after blood pressure is effectively controlled for one year and at least four doctor visits, it may be possible to reduce antihypertensive drug therapy in a deliberate, slow, and progressive manner.[75,76] Caution is advised in patients with a history of coronary artery disease, angina, or arrhythmias. Step-down therapy is especially successful in patients who are also following lifestyle modifications, and a higher percentage of these patients maintain normal blood pressure levels with less, or no medication. Patients whose drugs are discontinued should have regular follow-up, because blood pressure usually rises again to hypertensive levels. In these patients, hypertension can recur, sometimes months or years after discontinuation, especially in the absence of sustained improvements in lifestyle activities known to facilitate nonpharmacologic management.[77]

Digoxin

A number of clinical studies suggest that digoxin is an over-used medication.[39,70] Although it is clear that many individuals are started on digoxin therapy without adequate clinical indications it is inappropriate to discontinue digoxin in patients who require this medication for maintenance of their cardiovascular status.[78] Based on recent studies, specific criteria for digoxin discontinuation are now available.[70,79] Most patients who are on digoxin therapy, who are in normal sinus rhythm, and who have echocardiographic evidence of *normal* systemic ventricular function, probably can have digoxin safely discontinued from their regimen. It should be stressed that discontinuation should be incremental, gradual, and carefully monitored. Patients who have normal systolic ventricular function, but who are taking digoxin for ventricular rate control in the setting of chronic atrial fibrillation, *should not* have digoxin discontinued. The effectiveness of digoxin for maintaining ventricular rate control in patients with supraventricular tachyarrhythmias such as chronic atrial fibrillation is well established. Its role in preventing recurrent episodes of paroxysmal supraventricular tachycardia, however, is less certain.

Digoxin should *not* be discontinued in patients who have documented congestive heart failure.[79] For patients who have congestive heart failure, normal sinus rhythm, systolic dysfunction, and an ejection fraction < 35%, digoxin is an important component of the medical regimen. In addition, patients responding favorably to a program of digoxin, diuretics, and ACE inhibitors should not have their digoxin withdrawn, because there is significant risk of cardiovascular deterioration. There are insufficient data at present comparing the relative benefits and adverse effects of digoxin and ACE inhibitors in chronic congestive heart failure to determine which drug to use first—an important clinical decision. However, digoxin is effective in patients with chronic, stable mild-to-moderate heart failure and most studies documenting a beneficial effect of ACE inhibitors on survival in patients with heart failure used ACE inhibitors in conjunction with a stable regimen of digoxin and diuretics. There is strong evidence of the clinical efficacy of digoxin in patients with normal sinus rhythm and this degree of congestive heart failure. Specifically, withdrawal of digoxin in patients with mild congestive heart failure results in a significant worsening of exercise performance and an increased incidence of, and a decreased time to, treatment failure.

Consequently, digoxin discontinuation is recommended only in patients who have normal sinus rhythm and echocardiographic confirmation of normal systolic ventricular function. When these two variables coexist, gradual and incremental discontinuation of digoxin is indicated but only with careful clinical observation.

Antiarrhythmic Medications

Although mortality from cardiovascular disease decreased over the last 10 years, sudden cardiac death remains a medical problem of epidemic proportion. It is presently estimated that over 250,000 persons die suddenly each year in the United States, and most of these deaths are believed to be a consequence of ventricular tachyarrhythmias.[80,81] The majority of patients who experience sudden death have coronary artery disease, often with prior myocardial infarction. Attempts to reduce sudden cardiovascular mortality have focused on the use of antiarrhythmic agents designed to suppress potentially lethal arrhythmias.[82] In particular, the Cardiac Arrhythmia Suppression Trial (CAST) was designed as a multicenter, randomized, placebo-controlled trial to test the hypothesis that in patients with prior myocardial infarction, the suppression of ventricular premature depolarization improves survival.[80,81] Because ventricular ectopy is an important risk factor for cardiac arrest in patients with a history of myocardial infarction, it was believed by many that drugs that suppress ventricular ectopy would prevent ventricular tachyarrhythmia-based cardiac arrest.[83]

Historically, the oral drugs most frequently used to suppress ventricular ectopy were the type IA antiarrhythmics such as quinidine, procainamide, and disopyramide. The trial was designed to determine whether these type IA agents or the newer agents encainide, flecainide, and moricizine could reduce the risk of sudden cardiac death in patients at high risk because of previous myocardial infarction and the presence of ventricular ectopy. Patients whose arrhythmia was suppressed by encainide, flecainide, or moricizine were randomly assigned to placebo or active drug treatment. The study demonstrated that patients randomly assigned to active treatment with antiarrhythmic agent experienced a 2.5-fold increase in mortality (encainide and flecainide), or no survival benefit (moricizine), compared with those randomly assigned to placebo.[81,82,84] These results show association between the ability of the type I antiarrhythmic agents to suppress ventricular ectopy and their ability to produce sudden cardiac death after acute myocardial infarction.[85] The study also showed the inadequacy of ventricular ectopy suppression as a marker for prevention of sudden cardiac death. Based on the CAST trial, drugs such as encainide, flecainide, and moricizine should not be used for non life-threatening ventricular tachyarrhythmias.[39,80-82,86-88]

The recently completed conventional-versus-amiodarone drug evaluation study (CASCADE Study) suggests that the CAST results may not be generalizable to other antiarrhythmic drugs.[82] In this secondary prevention trial, patients with out-of-hospital ventricular fibrillation not occurring during an acute Q-wave myocardial infarction were studied. Patients were randomly assigned to empiric treatment with amiodarone or to treatment with other antiarrhythmic drugs (including flecainide and moricizine, which were used in the CAST trial, and eight other antiarrhythmic agents). Ventricular fibrillation, syncope-associated defibrillated discharge, and cardiac death occurred less frequently in the amiodarone-treated group. Based on this study, patients with previously documented out-of-hospital ventricular fibrillation may have improved survival rates with the use of amiodarone, although this is still controversial.[89]

Guidelines for Drug Therapy in Patients With Ventricular Arrhythmias

Few clinical decisions in outpatients with heart disease require as much thought and critical analysis. Stated simply, the indications for and approach to drug therapy for patients with ventricular arrhythmias is one of the most controversial and misunderstood areas in clinical cardiology. The problem is especially common for primary care practitioners, who encounter many older patients with and without ischemic heart disease who demonstrate ventricular premature complexes (VPCs) or short runs of ventricular tachycardia (VT) on a routine electrocardiogram or during ambulatory Holter monitoring. From a therapeutic perspective, the critical decision is to determine which patient subgroups will benefit from antiarrhythmic therapy, which patients require invasive intervention with automatic implantable cardioverter-defribrillators (AICD), and which patients simply ought to be followed with no pharmacotherapeutic intervention whatsoever. These are important issues, given the fact that many studies (CAST) have shown that some pharmacologic interventions (Type IA antiarrhythmic agents) used for management of ventricular arrhythmias may be associated with increased mortality. These findings have reframed our approaches to drug therapy for this patient population.

The following section reviews the prognosis and management of ventricular arrhythmias (VA) in patients with and without heart disease. Recommendations and guidelines are based on extraction of pertinent articles obtained from a computer-assisted search of the English literature contained in a MEDLINE database, followed by a manual search of the bibliographies of relevant articles. The emphasis is on studies involving older persons and all articles were reviewed and analyzed in depth. These treatment approaches are recommended in specific subgroups, according to the prognosis, risk of treatment, and benefits of therapy.

Patients With No Heart Disease. First, it should be stressed that, in the studies reviewed, in patients with no clinical evidence of heart disease the presence of VPCs, nonsustained ventricular arrhythmias (VA), or complex ventricular arrhythmias (VA) were not associated with an increased incidence of new coronary events at a two-year follow-up. In addition, they were not associated with an increased incidence of primary ventricular fibrillation or sudden cardiac death. Because nonsustained VT or complex VA are not associated with increased mortality in older persons who have no clinical evidence of heart disease—defined, for all the analyses in this review as the presence of myocardial ischemia, history of myocardial infarction, or left ventricular hypertrophy (LVH)—this review recommends no antiarrhythmic drug treatment of asymptomatic nonsustained VT, VPCs, or complex VA in older persons *without* heart disease.

Class I Antiarrhythmic Drugs. Based on the results of The Cardiac Arrhythmia Suppression Trial (CAST) I, type 1 anti-arrhythmics generally are not recommended for the treatment of VT or complex VA in older or younger patients, even those with heart disease. Similarly, because investigators in the CAST II trial indicated that the use of the antiarrhythmic morcizine may be not only ineffective or harmful, this agent is not recommended for nonsustained VT, VPCs, or complex VA in older or younger persons without heart disease. Based on a meta-analysis of four randomized trials evaluating quinidine, flecainide, mexilitene, tocainide, and propafenone, there was an increased risk of mortality in patients treated with quinidine as compared to patients treated with the other antiarrhythmic agents. In contrast to findings with the aforementioned drugs, one important study demonstrated a decreased incidence of death and recurrent cardiac arrest in patients treated with beta-blockers versus no antiarrhythmic drug.

Based on cumulative data, the use of any class I antiarrhythmic agent usually is not recommended for the treatment of VT or complex VA in older or younger patients with heart disease. However, the use of *beta-blockers* is recommended for treatment of patients resuscitated from prehospital cardiac arrest attributable to ventricular fibrillation.

Calcium Channel Blockers. Calcium channel blockers are of no proven value in the management of patients with ventricular arrhythmias and, therefore, are not recommended for this patient population.

Beta-Blockers. In the majority of clinical trials analyzed, beta-blockers were associated with a reduction in cardiac ischemia, mortality, and risk of ventricular fibrillation in patients complex VA and myocardial infarction. Based on these studies, beta-blockers are recommended for treatment of both older and younger patients with VT or complex VA associated with ischemic or nonischemic heart disease, provided there are no contraindications to beta-blocker therapy.

Amiodarone. Although amiodarone is very effective in suppressing VT and complex VA, the incidence of adverse effects of amiodarone approaches 90% after 5 years of therapy. In one large trial, the incidence of pulmonary toxicity was 10% at 2 years. Based on available studies, amiodarone use in the setting of complex VA or VT should be reserved for patients with life-threatening ventricular tachyarrhythmias in older or younger patients who cannot tolerate or who do not respond to beta-blockers, and are not suitable candidates for implantable cardio-defibrillators.

Angiotensin-Converting Enzyme Inhibitors. Although ACE inhibitors do not possess antiarrhythmic properties, per se, these agents have been shown to produce a significant reduction in complex VA in patients with congestive heart failure (CHF). On the basis of limited available data, ACE inhibitors are reasonable adjunctive agents in patients with VT or complex VA associated with congestive heart failure. Combined use with a beta-blocker may produce additional benefits in older or younger patients with asymptomatic LV systolic dysfunction plus ventricular arrhythmias.

Invasive Intervention. Patients who have life-threatening recurrent VT or ventricular fibrillation that is resistant to antiarrhythmic drugs require invasive intervention which may include: coronary artery bypass graft surgery, aneurysmectomy or infarctectomy, and endocardial resection with or without adjunctive cryoblation based on activation mapping in the operating room. Although these procedures have their place in a small subset of individuals, the automatic implantable cardio-defibrillator (ACID) is currently accepted as the most effective treatment for patients with life-threatening VT or ventricular fibrillation (VF). Based on available studies, ACID is recommended in older or younger patients who have medically refractory sustained VT or VF.

Based on a review of more than 70 studies evaluating the prognosis and effectiveness of management options in patients with ventricular arrhythmias, guidelines are offered that maximize outcomes while reducing risk. These therapeutic approaches, when indicated, include the following principles: (1) patients without heart disease who have non-lifethreatening VA should not be treated with antiarrhythmic drugs; (2) Class I antiarrhythmic drugs should not be used to treat complex VA in older patients with ischemic or nonischemic heart disease, if there are no contraindications to beta-blocker therapy, which is preferred; (3) amiodarone should be reserved for life-threatening VA in older persons who are not responsive to or who cannot tolerate beta-blocker therapy; (4) ACE inhibitors should be part of an antiarrhythmic regimen for patients with VA that is associated with CHF; and (5) patients who have life-threatening VA (including sustained VT or VF) are best managed with automatic implantable cardiodefibrillator (ACID).

The comparative outcome-effectiveness of antiarrhythmic drug therapy was evaluated in the Antiarrhythmics vs. Implantable Defibrillators (AVID) study. Patients who had been resuscitated from the following three types of arrhythmias were eligible for enrollment: VF; sustained VT with syncope; or sustained VT with a left ventricular ejection fraction of 40% or less, and hypotension. Among the 509 patients assigned to antiarrhythmic drug therapy, 356 were started on amiodarone (average maintenance dose 389 mg/day for three months). The study showed mortality was *lower* in the implantable cardio-defibrillator (ICD) group, with a 30% decrease in death rate in the ICD group at a three-year endpoint. The data in the AVID study clearly shows that an ICD should be the *first* consideration in survivors of serious sustained ventricular arrhythmias. However, antiarrythmic drugs and ICDs should not be considered mutually exclusive forms of therapy. Even among ICD recipients, 25% eventually received additional drug therapy.

Finally, underlying causes of complex VA should always be treated, whenever possible. In this regard, treatment of digitalis, toxicity, electrolyte disturbances, left ventricular dysfunction, myocardial ischemia, or hypoxia may help reduce or abolish ventricular arrhythmias. With respect to lifestyle, nonpharmacologic measures, patients should be counseled to avoid alcohol and cigarette smoking.[142]

In general, indications for the use of all antiarrhythmic agents in patients with known coronary artery disease always should be reevaluated.[88] Even patients who are taking quinidine therapy for pharmacologic cardioversion of atrial fibrillation may require reassessment, based on recent studies showing that mortality rates are increased in some patients taking this antiarrhythmic agent.[90] Consultation with a cardiologist is required prior to adjustment of dose or discontinuation of antiarrhythmic therapy.[87,91,92]

Aspirin

Aspirin has become a bulwark of defense for the prevention of coronary artery disease, transient ischemic attacks, and embolic stroke associated with chronic atrial fibrillation (when anticoagulation with warfarin is contraindicated).[93,94] Despite the widespread use of aspirin to prevent both cardiovascular and cerebrovascular conditions, the precise dosage of aspirin required in each condition is still highly controversial.[95,96] In the case of secondary prevention of myocardial infarction, however, 80 mg of aspirin per day, or 160 mg of aspirin every other day, is sufficient for prevention of recurrent myocardial infarction. Generally speaking, patients who are taking aspirin therapy exclusively for the secondary prevention of myocardial infarction should be maintained on no more than 80 mg of aspirin per day. As a rule, higher doses are not required, and patients can be rapidly tapered to a lower dose, which has the advantage of decreased gastrointestinal side effects. However, recent studies suggest that a "booster" weekend dose of aspirin (i.e., a 325 mg dose on Saturday and Sunday every *other* weekend) can augment the cardioprotective effects of 80 mg of aspirin daily. Based on this data, it is recommended that booster doses, as described, accompany long-term aspirin therapy.

The appropriate dose of aspirin for the prevention of transient ischemic attacks and stroke, however, is still debated.[93-96] Nevertheless, it is clear that when stroke prevention is studied in the setting of chronic, nonrheumatic atrial fibrillation, patients who receive 325 mg/day of aspirin have a 42% reduction in ischemic stroke and systemic embolism, as compared with placebo. However, those patients who receive only 75 mg/day of aspirin have a smaller and *insignificant* (16%) reduction in cerebrovascular events. This study suggests that patients who, for one reason or another, are not appropriate candidates for warfarin therapy (which is the drug of choice for the prevention of embolic infarction in older patients with chronic atrial fibrillation and coronary heart disease), should be treated with at least 325 mg of aspirin a day.[95,96]

Although many investigations in the United Kingdom suggest that as much as 1,200 mg per day of aspirin may be required to prevent transient ischemic attacks or minor stroke, there is also evidence reported by the Swedish Aspirin Low-Dose Trial (SALT) that patients who take only 75 mg of aspirin per day will have a significant reduction in stroke and death compared to the placebo group.[95] Moreover, a Dutch study compared low dose (283 mg/day) and very low dose aspirin therapy (30 mg per day). In this very well-designed trial, there were no significant differences in the primary end points of vascular deaths, stroke, and myocardial infarction when the two dosage regimens were compared.[95,96] This study suggests that in patients with a history of aspirin intolerance, gastric erosions, ulcer disease, or gastrointestinal hemorrhage, and who also require stroke prevention, a 30 mg/day aspirin dose may provide significant clinical benefits, while reducing the risks of aspirin-induced side effects. However, it should be stressed that findings suggesting that aspirin doses of 325 mg or less are successful in preventing stroke are not universal. Further circumstantial evidence concerning low- and high-dose aspirin therapy is available from carotid endarterectomy studies, which demonstrate that doses as high as 1000 to 1500 mg of aspirin per day may be required to reduce stroke incidence and deaths. At present, the precise dose of aspirin required to prevent cerebrovascular events in patients with normal sinus rhythm is not known.[94-96]

Specifically, no study of patients with cerebrovascular disease has established that an aspirin dosage of 325 mg/day or less is better or even comparable with 975 mg or more. It is possible that lower doses are effective but are not as effective as higher doses. Based on this data, reduction of aspirin dose should be limited to those conditions in which lower doses are demonstrated to be efficacious, including patients who require aspirin therapy for prevention of myocardial infarction.

Indications, Dosages, and Clinical Guidelines for Antithrombotic Therapy in The Outpatient Setting

Antithrombotic therapy is the primary bulwark of defense for patients with thromboembolic diseases of the arterial and nervous circulatory systems. With so many clinical trials, reviews, and consensus reports recently published, it has been extremely difficult for practitioners to stay current with recommendations for the more than thirty clinical conditions for which antithrombotic therapy has proven effective. To provide practicing clinicians a universal and standardized approach to drug therapy for patients with thromboembolic diseases, the third American College of Chest Physicians Consensus Conference on Antithrombotic Therapy convened in order to set forth state-of-the-art guidelines for these disorders. Although many of these guidelines address issues related to in-hospital treatment, prophylaxis, and management of thromboembolic disorders, the following guidelines, which are distilled from this landmark report, focus on indications and strategies for use of antithrombotic agents—aspirin, warfarin, ticlodipine, enoxaprin, and dipyridamole—in the *outpatient* setting.[143]

Antiplatelet Agents: General Recommendations. Aspirin is indicated for long-term management of patients with stable angina, unstable angina, transient cerebral ischemia, acute myocardial infarction, thrombotic stroke, and peripheral arterial disease. A dose of 160 to 325 mg/day should be used for all indications, except in patients with cerebrovascular disease, in whom a dose of 160 to 325 mg/day is effective, but in whom higher doses (975 mg/day) may prove to be even *more* effective. The advantages versus risks of these higher doses for prevention of stroke remains a controversial point.

In contrast to previous guidelines urging that aspirin prophylaxis primarily directed at prevention of *recurrent* myocardial infarction, current guidelines suggest that aspirin be used as both *primary* and secondary prophylaxis in asymptomatic men and women who are older than 50 years of age in order to prevent myocardial infarction. Aspirin is also indicated in patients with chronic atrial fibrillation in whom warfarin therapy is contraindicated. Although extreme caution is required when aspirin and warfarin are used in combination, studies suggest patients with mechanical heart valves *at high risk* for systemic embolism be treated with a combination of warfarin (maintaining INR between 2.5 and 3.5) and low-dose aspirin. In general, ticlodipine is reserved for use in patients with allergy to aspirin or aspirin intolerance and in patients who develop recurrent thromboembolism despite aspirin therapy.

Venous Thromboembolism. Although treatment is highly individualized, in patients with deep venous thrombosis or pulmonary embolism, long-term anticoagulant therapy should be continued with warfarin for at least 3 months in order to prolong the PT to an INR of 2.0 to 3.0. Patients with recurrent venous thrombosis should be treated indefinitely, as should patients with AT III deficiency. Symptomatic, isolated calf vein thrombosis should be treated with anticoagulation for 3 months. The role of enoxaprin (Lovenox®) and other low molecular weight heparins (LMWH) is discussed below.

Atrial Fibrillation. Long-term oral warfarin therapy (INR 1.5 to 2.0) is recommended for patients with atrial fibrillation (AF) who are eligible to receive anticoagulation therapy. Anticoagulation is presently not recommended for patients who are younger than 60 years of age who have no associated cardiovascular disease (i.e., "lone AF"). Patients with AF who are poor candidates for anticoagulation therapy should be treated with aspirin at a dosage of 325 mg/day.

It is strongly recommended that warfarin therapy be given for 3 weeks before elective cardioversion of patients who have been in AF for more than 2 days and be continued until normal sinus rhythm has been maintained for 4 weeks. In contrast, antithrombotic therapy is *not* recommended for cardioversion of atrial flutter or supraventricular tachycardia or for cardioversion of patients who have been in AF for not more than 2 days, unless other risk factors for systemic embolism are present.

Valvular Heart Disease. Patients with a history of rheumatic mitral valve disease who have either a history of systemic embolism or paroxysmal or chronic AF, should be treated with long-term warfarin therapy in doses sufficient to achieve an INR of 2.0 to 3.0. This antithrombotic approach is also recommended for patients with rheumatic mitral valve disease and normal sinus rhythm if the left atrial diameter is in excess of 5.5 cm. If systemic embolism occurs despite adequate warfarin therapy, the addition of 160 mg to 325 mg aspirin/day should be considered. Because of the risks attending concurrent use of aspirin and warfarin, these patients should be carefully monitored. In patients with recurrent embolism who are unable to take aspirin, or who are deemed inappropriate candidates for *concurrent* aspirin and warfarin therapy, an alternative strategy would be to increase the warfarin dose sufficient to prolong the PT to an INR of 2.5 to 3.5.

Long-term antithrombotic therapy is *not* recommended for patients with mitral valve prolapse who have not experienced systemic embolism, unexplained TIAs, or AF. Those who have manifested signs of TIAs should be treated with long-term aspirin therapy at a dose of 325 to 975 mg/day. Those with documented systemic embolism—and paroxysmal or chronic AF—should be treated with long-term warfarin therapy (INR, 2.0 to 3.0).

Prosthetic Heart Valves. All patients with mechanical prosthetic heart valves should receive long-term anticoagulation therapy with warfarin (INR, 2.5 to 3.5). Aspirin (100 mg/day) offers additional protection when added to warfarin, but with an increased risk of bleeding. Dypyridamole (400 mg/day) may be added to warfarin for additional protection.

Post-Myocardial Infarction. Following acute myocardial infarction, aspirin (80 to 160 mg/day) is recommended for long-term therapy in preference to warfarin because of aspirin's simplicity, safety, and low-cost. It should be stressed that long-term warfarin therapy is recommended in clinical settings associated with increased embolic risk (duration, 1 to 3 months following acute myocardial infarction complicated by severe left ventricular dysfunction, congestive heart failure, previous emboli, or two-dimensional echo evidence of mural thrombi; duration indefinite in patients with AF). Dipyridamole is *not* recommended for survivors of acute MI.

Chronic Coronary Artery Disease. All patients with clinical or laboratory evidence of chronic coronary artery disease (angina, angiographic confirmation, etc.) should receive oral aspirin therapy (160 to 325 mg/day) indefinitely. The indications for primary prevention of MI have been clarified by the consensus conference and are as follows: all patients older than 50 years of age who are free of contraindications to aspirin should be considered for primary prevention with aspirin doses of 180 to 325 mg/day. The benefits of this strategy increase with advancing age and, most likely, with the presence of diabetes mellitus, systolic or diastolic hypertension, cigarette smoking, and lack of exercise. In contrast, the routine use of aspirin for primary prevention of coronary heart disease is *not* recommended for individuals who are younger than 50 years of age, *unless* they have a history of MI, stroke, diabetes, or TIA.

Patients With Coronary Bypass Grafts. Aspirin alone is recommended to reduce the incidence of saphenous vein bypass graft closure. The aspirin dose shown to be beneficial in graft patency is 325 mg/day or higher. One study has shown that dypyridamole therapy (225 mg/day) in addition to aspirin is more effective than aspirin (150 mg/day) therapy alone. Although the duration of benefits seen with aspirin therapy is uncertain, one-year of therapy is currently recommended. For patients who are allergic to aspirin, ticlodipine (250 mg twice daily) has been shown to be effective in one study if started 48 hours after surgery, and may be considered an alternative.

Coronary Angioplasty. Long-term aspirin therapy (160 to 325 mg/day) is recommended in patients following angioplasty, primarily because of its effects on coronary heart disease. Its effect on recurrent stenosis, per se, has not been clarified and is inconsistent.

Peripheral Vascular Disease. Although it is uncertain whether aspirin alone or aspirin with dipyridamole will modify the natural history or clinical course of patients with peripheral vascular disease, because these patients are at high risk for cardiovascular events (stroke and myocardial infarction), they should be given lifelong aspirin therapy (160 to 325 mg/day) in the absence of contraindications. Long-term anticoagulation with warfarin with or without aspirin should *not* be used routinely after femoropopliteal bypass and other vascular reconstructions.

Cerebrovascular Disease. Following carotid endarterectomy, aspirin (325 to 650 mg twice daily) should be given to prevent continuing TIAs and stroke. Although the optimal approach to patients with symptomatic carotid stenosis is uncertain, all patients with asymptomatic carotid disease should be treated with aspirin whether or not they undergo endarterectomy. This recommendation extends to all patients with asymptomatic bruits as well as individuals with TIAs and a history of minor ischemic strokes, where aspirin has been established to be effective in doses ranging from as low as 30 mg/day (TIAs) to 1300 mg/day. While many experts recommend 325 mg/day of aspirin, other authorities believe that higher doses, i.e., 975 to 1300 mg/day confer greater benefit. Although studies suggest ticlodipine is more effective than aspirin in the setting of cerebrovascular disease, it is also more toxic, and, therefore, ticlodipine is recommended for patients who are intolerant to aspirin and those who experience recurrent ischemic events during aspirin therapy.

Clinical Monitoring. Most clinicians agree that oral anticoagulation for venous thromboembolism or atrial fibrillation should be monitored with the goal of maintaining a prothrombin time (PT) 1.3 to 1.5 times control; in patients with mechanical heart valves the PT should be maintained at 1.5 to 2.0 times control. It has become increasingly clear that recommendations such as these are not generalizable and may lead to significant errors in clinical practice, since laboratories throughout North America use different thromboplastin reagents when determining PT valves. The sensitivity of these reagents varies widely and can be measured by the international sensitivity index (ISI). Therefore a PT of 15 at one laboratory might be equivalent to a PT of 24 at another. In order to circumvent this difficulty the INR (International Normalized Ratio) was developed. The INR equals the ratio of patient to control PT taken to the power of the ISI for the particular thromboplastin reagent used. Use of the INR eliminates uncertainty involved in monitoring oral anticoagulation. Unfortunately, most laboratories report only prothrombin times, and clinical decisions based on the PT or ratio of patient to control PT are only accurate when the sensitivity of the thromboplastin reagent is in a narrow range (ISI: 2.2 to 2.6).[144,145]

ISI	**LESS INTENSIVE ANTICOAGULATION** (e.g., DVT, PE, atrial fib., tissue heart valve) **INR 2.0-3.0**		**MORE INTENSIVE ANTICOAGULATION** (e.g., Cardiogenic embolus, Mechanical heart valve) **INR 3.0-4.5**	
	Protime (secs)	**PT ratio** patient/ control	**Protime** (secs)	**PT ratio** patient/ control
1.2	21-30	1.8-2.5	30-42	2.5-3.5
1.4-1.6	20-24	1.6-2.0	26-30	2.2-2.6
1.8-2.0	18-21	1.5-1.7	22-25	1.8-2.1
2.2-2.4	16-19	1.4-1.6	20-22.5	1.6-1.9
2.6-2.8	15.5-18	1.3-1.5	18-21	1.5-1.7

The INR is the most reliable guide in the management of patients receiving warfarin. The therapeutic goal in patients with deep venous thrombosis (DVT), pulmonary embolus (PE), atrial fibrillation, and tissue heart valves is an INR from 2.0 to 3.0. In patients with mechanical heart valves or a cardiogenic embolus the INR should be maintained in a higher range, i.e., 3.0 to 4.5. When dealing with referral laboratories that do not report INRs, anticoagulation can be properly managed through knowledge of the international sensitivity index (ISI) of the thromboplastin reagent that particular lab is currently using. If the ISI falls between 2.2 and 2.6, traditional recommendations are valid. If not, the following chart can be referred to. Choose the row corresponding to the ISI that your lab is using, and underline the adjacent therapeutic goals in order to safely and effectively anticoagulate your patients.

Beware the laboratory that cannot provide you with the ISI of the reagents they use. If they are not willing to correct this shortcoming, a laboratory that is more up-to-date would better serve your patients.[144,145]

Thromboembolic Prophylaxis with Low Molecular Weight Heparin (LMWH)

From a pharmatectural and outcome-effectiveness perspective, the availability of low molecular weight heparins provides an opportunity to manage clinically serious thromboembolic conditions on an outpatient, in-home basis while reducing monitoring and human resource costs associated with prophylaxis of deep venous thromboembolism (DVT). Low molecular weight heparins (LMWHs) have been available for use in the United States since 1993, when enoxaparin was approved by the FDA. Dalteparin was approved by the FDA in 1994.[146] Both are indicated for use in the prophylaxis of deep vein thrombosis (DVT) in patients undergoing surgical procedures. This section will review current indications, treatment protocols, and benefit-to-risk considerations for managing patients at risk for DVT with anti-thromboembolic agents that permit more cost-effective management in the out-of-hospital setting.

LMWH Heparin: Enoxaparin Sodium (Lovenox®). With respect to LMWHs, perhaps the greatest clinical experience, as well as the most studies, available for agents approved for use in the United States, has been accumulated with enoxaparin sodium. Enoxaparin is indicated for the prevention of deep vein thrombosis (DVT), which may predispose to the development of pulmonary embolism. Currently, the principle use of this medication is for patients who are undergoing hip replacement and other orthopedic surgical procedures involving the lower extremities. Prophylaxis with enoxaparin is provided during and following hospitalization. Other candidates suitable for enoxaparin therapy include individuals undergoing knee replacement surgery as well as patients who have had abdominal surgery and are at risk for thromboembolic complications. From a patient selection perspective, those at risk include patients who are more than 40 years of age, obese, those undergoing surgery under general anesthesia lasting longer than 30 minutes, or who have additional risk factors such as malignancy or a history of deep vein thrombosis or pulmonary embolism.

Enoxaparin also is indicated for the prevention of ischemic complications of unstable angina and non-Q-wave myocardial infarction when concurrently administered with aspirin.

Although safety and efficacy of enoxaparin and other LMWHs have been established in numerous studies,[147-151] certain precautions regarding use of LMWHs should be noted. Enoxaparin is contraindicated in patients with active major bleeding, in patients with thrombocytopenia associated with a positive *in vitro* test for anti-platelet antibody in the presence of enoxaparin sodium, or in patients with hypersensitivity to enoxaparin sodium. Moreover, patients with known hypersensitivity to heparin or pork products should not be treated with LMWH.

In addition, enoxaparin should be used with extreme caution in patients with a history of heparin-induced thrombocytopenia. Thrombocytopenia of any degree should be monitored closely, as this occurs at a rate of 0.5% to 2%, depending on the procedure. These rates do not differ significantly from those reported with heparin use. Like other anticoagulants, it should be used with caution in conditions with increased risk of hemorrhage, such as bacterial endocarditis, congenital or acquired bleeding disorders, active ulcerative and angiodysplastic gastrointestinal disease, hemorrhage stroke, shortly after brain, spinal, or ophthalmologic surgery, or in patients treated concomitantly with platelet inhibitors.

Cases of epidural or spinal hematomas have been reported with the associated use of enoxaparin and spinal/epidural anesthesia or spinal puncture resulting in long-term or permanent paralysis. Since 1993, as part of an ongoing Safety Surveillance, there have been more than 49 reports of epidural or spinal hematoma formation with concurrent use of enoxaparin and spinal/epidural anesthesia or spinal puncture. The risk of these events is higher with the use of postoperative indwelling epidural catheters, or by the concomitant use of additional drugs affecting hemostasis such as nonsteroidal anti-inflammatory drugs (NSAIDs). When neuraxial anesthesia (epidural/spinal anesthesia) or spinal puncture is employed, patients anticoagulated or scheduled to be anticoagulated with low molecular weight heparins or heparinoids for prevention of thromboembolic complications are at risk of developing an epidural or spinal hematoma, which can result in long-term or permanent paralysis.

The rise of these events is increased by the use of indwelling epidural catheters for administration of analgesia or by the concomitant use of drugs affecting hemostasis such as NSAIDs, platelet inhibitors, and other anticoagulants. The risk also appears to be increased by traumatic or repeated epidural or spinal puncture. Institutions should develop protocols and quality assurance procedures that can minimize the risk of this complication. Accordingly, patients should be frequently monitored for signs and symptoms of neurological impairment. If neurologic compromise is noted, urgent treatment is necessary. Elderly patients and patients with renal insufficiency may show delayed elimination of enoxaparin. Enoxaparin should be used with care in these patients. If thromboembolic events occur despite enoxaparin prophylaxis, enoxaparin should be discontinued and appropriate therapy initiated.

Dosage Considerations. Dosing considerations play an important role in the convenience of providing thromboembolic prophylaxis. In patients undergoing hip or knee replacement surgery, the recommended dose of enoxaparin injection is 30 mg every 12 hours administered by subcutaneous (sc) injection. Provided that post-surgical hemostasis has been established, the initial dose should be given 12 to 24 hours post-operatively. Up to 14 days administration (average duration 7 to 10 days) of enoxaparin 30 mg every 12 hours has been well tolerated in controlled clinical trials. For hip replacement surgery, a dose of 40 mg once daily sc given initially 12 hours prior to surgery may be considered. Following the initial phase of thromboprophylaxis in hip replacement surgery patients (enoxaparin 30 mg every 12 hours or 40 mg once daily), continued prophylaxis with enoxaparin 40 mg once daily administered by sc injection for 3 weeks is recommended. In patients undergoing abdominal surgery who are at risk for thromboembolic complications, the recommended dose is 40 mg once daily administered by sc injection with the initial dose given 2 hours prior to surgery. The usual duration of administration is 7 to 10 days; up to 12 days administration has been well tolerated in clinical trials.

Some institutions have gained wide experience with enoxaparin prophylaxis of DVT following hip and knee replacement surgery. To enhance the benefit/risk ratio of enoxaparin for post-operative DVT prophylaxis, these institutions have customized dosing administration according to weight, age, and risk factors and have also provided education protocols for patient use in the outpatient setting. In this regard, The Arthritis Institute of Houston, with protocol management under the direction of James Muntz, MD has developed a weight-based and host hemorrhagic risk factor-based protocol for using the LMWH enoxaparin as the foundation drug for post-operative prophylaxis. This protocol provides a comprehensive risk-management sensitive approach to maximizing cost-savings that accrue from out-of-hospital management of DVT prophylaxis with LMWH.

Post-Operative Antithrombotic Therapy Protocol

Thigh high TED hose on both legs day of surgery or on post-op day 1: plantar pneumatic compression device apply in PACU bilateral lower extremities except when walking.

-Anticoagulation orders:

Enoxaparin ___ mg SQ q 12h; administer 1st dose at ___

1. Discharge Planner to set up drug delivery, reimbursement & in-home nursing (optional)
2. Give the patient a *Lovenox Discharge Kit* (include video, guide, and patient education; teach to self-inject).
   - A. For patient less than 90 lbs, decrease enoxaparin dose to 30 mg sub q 24 hours.
   - B. If patient is 280 lbs or higher, increase enoxaparin dose to 30 mg sub q 8 hrs.
   - C. If serum creatinine is 2.0 or higher, decrease enoxaparin to 30 mg sub q 24 hrs.

D. If platelet count drops to one-half the admission level or less than 100,000, then notify doctor of possibility of discontinuing the low molecular weight heparin.

E. If patient is on enoxaparin, do not check INR or PTT.

F. For revision total hip or total knee arthroplasty, consider holding enoxaparin until at least 24 or 36 hours postop after surgeon/internist is comfortable with adequate hemostasis at surgical site.

If there is concern regarding increasing swelling at surgical site while on antithrombotic therapy, notify physician regarding whether or not to continue anticoagulation.

Coumadin ___ mg po qd x 2 nights, then as ordered.

At discharge PT/INR on Monday and Thursday for 4 weeks. Call results to physician for 4 weeks (target INR is 2.0 to 3.0 if possible)

- Protime INR Post-op Day -1 -3 -4
- Other ______________________________
- Enteric coated aspirin 325 mg qhs starting night of surgery.

Arterial Thromboembolic Prophylaxis. In patients with unstable angina or non-Q-wave myocardial infarction, the recommended dose of enoxaparin is 1 mg/kg administered sc every 12 hours in conjunction with oral aspirin therapy (100 to 325 mg/day). Treatment with enoxaparin should be prescribed for a minimum of 2 days and continued until clinical stabilization. The usual duration of treatment is 2 to 8 days. To minimize the risk of bleeding following vascular instrumentation during the treatment of unstable angina, physicians should adhere precisely to the intervals recommended between doses. The vascular access sheath for instrumentation should remain in place for 6 to 8 hours following a dose of enoxaparin. The next scheduled dose should be given no sooner than 6 to 8 hours after sheath removal. The site of the procedure should be observed for signs of bleeding or hematoma formation.

Monitoring. Periodic complete blood counts, including platelet count and stool occult blood tests, are recommended during the course of treatment with LMWHs. When administered at recommended prophylaxis doses, routine coagulation tests such as Prothrombin Time (PT) and Activated Partial Thromboplastin time (aPTT) are relatively insensitive measures of drug activity and, therefore, unsuitable for monitoring. Anti-Factor Xa may be used to monitor the anticoagulant effect of enoxaparin in patients with significant renal impairment. If during LMWH therapy abnormal coagulation parameters of bleeding should occur, anti-Factor Xa levels may be used to monitor anticoagulant effects.

Drug Interactions. Unless needed, agents that may enhance the risk of hemorrhage should be discontinued prior to initiation of enoxaprin therapy. These agents include medications such as: anticoagulants, platelet inhibitors including acetylsalicylic acid, salicylates, NSAIDs (including ketorolac tromethamine), dipyridamole, or sulfinpyrazone. If co-administration is essential, conduct close clinical and laboratory monitoring.

Elevations of Serum Aminotransferases. Asymptomatic increases in aspartate (AST [SGOT]) and alanine (ALT [SGPT]) aminotransferase levels greater than three times the upper limit of normal of the laboratory reference range have been reported in up to 3.9% and 5.5% of patients, respectively, during treatment with enoxaparin sodium injection. Similar significant increases in aminotransferase levels have also been observed in patients and healthy volunteers treated with heparin and other low molecular weight heparins. Such elevations are fully reversible and are rarely associated with increases in bilirubin. Since aminotransferase determinations are important in the differential diagnosis of myocardial infarction, liver disease, and pulmonary emboli, elevations that might be caused by LMWHs should be interpreted with caution.

Medication-Based Paradigm Shifts in Drug Utilization: Thromboembolic Prophylaxis and Treatment with Low Molecular Weight Heparin (LMWHs)

The use of LMWH antithrombotic agents for management of documented DVT presents some unique cost advantages. Deep-vein thrombosis (DVT) is a recognized clinical problem in Western countries, with an estimated annual incidence of 1 per 1,000 inhabitants. The morbidity and mortality of DVT is likely to grow as the population ages and requires surgical procedures (hip and knee replacements) and hospitalizations that predispose them to DVT. The current DVT rate implies that each year approximately 250,000 Americans need to be hospitalized for 5 to 10 days of IV heparin therapy.[152] The standard treatment for DVT is the constant infusion of heparin with the goal of maintaining the activated partial thromboplastin time (aPTT) within a desired therapeutic range. Warfarin is initiated concomitantly with the regimen and maintained as the sole anticoagulant once an International Normalization Ratio (INR) of 2 to 3 is achieved. This therapy is continued for 3 months or longer, depending on the underlying etiology of the thrombotic event. Recently, LMWHs have been studied rigorously as new pharmacologic modalities for treating DVT. Although not yet approved for treatment of DVT, these agents have been investigated in clinical trials evaluating their usefulness for this condition.

LMWHs have better bioavailability, a longer half-life, and more predictable anticoagulant activity than unfractionated heparin. Developed in the late 1970s, they were observed to have a significant inhibitory effect on factors Xa and IIa, as well as provide a lower risk of bleeding than standard heparin.[153] Currently, there are 6 LMWH preparations approved for clinical use in Europe and 2 (enoxaparin and dalteparin) approved for the *prevention* of DVT/pulmonary embolism (PE) in the United States. Each of these LMWHs has a different molecular weight, anti-Xa to anti-IIa activity, rate of plasma clearance, and recommended dosage.[154]

The evaluation of LMWH in the management of thromboembolic disease has been directed primarily toward the degree of venographically proved clot reduction and the confirmation of symptomatic recurrent thrombosis. In one study, investigators compared enoxaparin at 1 mg/kg, sc, every 12 hours, with standard heparin adjusted for a therapeutic aPTT of 1.5 to 2.5 of baseline. Bilateral lower-extremity venography was performed in all patients upon entry and repeated on day 10 of the protocol. The size of the thrombus was assessed qualitatively and quantitatively to demonstrate therapeutic efficacy. Perfusion lung scanning was performed in all patients within 48 hours of study entry and repeated if symptoms or signs of PE developed. Repeat venography revealed that one (1.5%) of 67 patients receiving enoxaparin had extension of the initial DVT compared with 5 (7.5%) of 67 patients who received standard heparin. None of the patients in the enoxaparin-treated group had PE, compared with 2 patients in the standard heparin group. There were no major bleeding problems in either of the two groups.

Other studies[147-151,155] as well as two recent meta-analyses of randomized trials comparing LMWHs agents with heparin concluded that LMWHs administered sc in fixed doses adjusted for body weight and without laboratory monitoring were more effective and safer than standard heparin infusion in the management of acute DVT.[150,151] The LMWHs proved to be safer and more effective than standard heparin in treating hospitalized patients who had acute DVT.

From a pharmacoeconomic perspective, one of the primary objectives of LMWH is establishing the effectiveness, safety, and user-friendliness of this drug for managing DVT in the outpatient setting. To assess this issue, in one study, 500 patients with acute proximal DVT were randomized in an open-label study to either enoxaparin, 1 mg/kg, subcutaneously, every 12 hours, or a constant infusion of standard heparin. The patients were categorized into three groups: (a) outpatients who were not admitted; (b) patients who had DVT who were admitted at night or on weekends and who, for logistic reasons, could not be enrolled in this study immediately; and (c) patients who were hospitalized for other reasons, such as surgery, and in whom DVT was diagnosed subsequently. Of the 247 enoxaparin-treated patients, 149 were outpatients, 76 were hospitalized for 48 hours, and 22 were treated in the hospital. All 253 standard heparin patients, except for two, were managed in the hospital

The principle outcomes of this study were the symptomatic recurrence of venous thromboembolism and bleeding during the period of administration of the study medications or within 48 hours after the completion of therapy. Symptomatic recurrent thromboembolism occurred in 13 (5.3%) of 247 enoxaparin-treated patients and 17 (6.7%) of 253 standard heparin-treated patients. A breakdown of the recurrent events revealed DVT in 11 (4.4%) of 247 patients in the enoxaparin group and 15 (5.9%) of 253 patients in the standard heparin group. Two patients in the standard heparin group had fatal PE on the day of randomization and day 6 of the protocol respectively. Major bleeding complications occurred during the first 7 days of the study in five (2%) of the patients treated with enoxaparin and three (1.1%) of the patients managed with standard heparin. Two episodes of bleeding in the enoxaparin group were fatal; one patient had a subdural hematoma after a fall and the other had associated thrombocytopenia due to chemotherapy and radiation, and bled from an esophageal cancer.

Based on results of these studies, LMWHs have been shown to be safe and more effective in preventing recurrent thrombotic events when compared with the more precise heparin dosing schedules. Moreover, studies evaluating home treatment of DVT suggest that LMWHs administered sc, without laboratory monitoring, in a dose determined by body weight, will likely shift the management of DVT from the inpatient setting to home. LMWHs are still awaiting FDA approval for treatment of this disorder. As these agents await approval for out-of-hospital management of venous thrombosis, a number of institutions have developed inclusionary and exclusionary protocols for patient assignment to LMWH treatment protocols. The following approach developed by the Jefferson Hospital (Philadelphia) Antithrombotic Therapy Service presents a risk-averse algorithm for identifying patients who are suitable for this treatment pathway:

Inclusion Criteria

1. Positive diagnosis of DVT by Doppler Ultrasound or venography.	_____Y	_____N

Exclusion Criteria

1. Unable to provide informed consent	_____Y	_____N
2. Geographic inaccessibility	_____Y	_____N
3. Potential for medication noncompliance	_____Y	_____N
4. Unable to support cost of drug	_____Y	_____N
5. Pregnancy	_____Y	_____N
6. Hereditary or acquired thrombotic disorders	_____Y	_____N
7. Hereditary bleeding disorders	_____Y	_____N
8. Active bleeding (PUD < 6 wk, GI, GU)	_____Y	_____N
9. Concomitant medical problems (Acute CHF, estimated creatinine clearance <30 mL/min, increased LFTs)	_____Y	_____N
10. Suspected pulmonary embolism	_____Y	_____N

Outcome Analysis and Implementation Strategies. Traditionally, patients with established DVT have been hospitalized immediately after diagnosis so that they can receive a continuous IV infusion of unfractionated heparin (UFH).[156] Bed rest is often instituted at the time of diagnosis, along with application of heat to and elevation of the affected limb.[157] Walking is allowed as pain and swelling subside. One to two weeks of hospitalization is common and included 5 to 10 days of UFH treatment in the hospital and institution of oral anticoagulation therapy after 2 to 7 days. Hospitalization has been considered necessary by some because of the risk of fatal pulmonary embolism (PE); however, fatal PE is now considered extremely unlikely during the initial treatment of DVT.[158] For the most part, hospitalization was required primarily for monitoring heparin therapy with laboratory tests and adjusting the heparin dosage in patients who have no major risk factors for bleeding thrombosis.

The emergence of LMWH as a treatment alternative makes initial treatment of uncomplicated DVT in the home setting rather than the hospital a possibility. Among the advantages of this approach would be fewer hospital admissions, increased patient comfort, and decreased overall costs. A disadvantage is that patients would have to be evaluated carefully to identify those who would be more safely treated in the hospital. In addition, much of the responsibility for treatment would be shifted from the medical personnel to the patient and family, requiring self-administration of anticoagulants, self-monitoring for safety and efficacy, and compliance with clinic appointments for dosage adjustments of oral anticoagulants.

From a pharmatectural perspective, the advantage of LMWHs are clear. Because of the lack of effect of LMWHs on thrombin, as well as the improved bioavailability, there is little interpatient or intrapatient variability in response to a given dose.[159,160] Thus, LMWHs can be given in a dose specific for body weight, without the laboratory testing and dosage adjustment customary for UFH. In addition, LMWHs are all effective on a once-daily or twice-daily schedule of sc injection.[159,160]

From these individual studies, it is clear that LMWHs are safe and effective in the treatment of DVT; however, these trials did not support a clear therapeutic advantage of LMWHs over UFH for this indication. In a majority of the studies, there was no significant difference between the preparations in the rate of symptomatic recurrence of thrombosis, the number of bleeding events, or the occurrence of clinically relevant thrombocytopenia. It should be stressed, however, that several meta-analyses published before the outpatient trials were available have shown results more in favor of LMWHs. One analysis did not indicate a significant difference in rates of symptomatic recurrence or adverse events, but there were trends suggesting superiority of LMWHs.[161] Two other analyses indicated significant differences in favor of LMWHs in both safety and efficacy.[150,151]

It is important to note that outcome measures have been assessed for different periods in various trials; in those reviewed here, patients were assessed only during initial treatment with heparin in one study,[164] to the end of maintenance treatment with warfarin in another,[165] and beyond maintenance treatment in two others.[166,167] Also, although all four LMWH preparations have been studied and reported to be safe and effective in the treatment of DVT, it is not clear that they are equivalent. Furthermore, patients in a majority of these studies could have been treated with UFH for up to 48 hours before therapy with an LMWH began. It is unclear how initial treatment with UFH might affect the results. It is possible that true differences do exist in favor of LMWHs but that they are too small to be seen in individual studies of that they are specific to certain preparations. From all current data, it must be concluded that LMWHs are safe and effective treatments of DVT. Further study will be necessary to discern whether any small, but potentially important, differences in safety and efficacy exist.

Pharmacoeconomic Issues. Even assuming therapeutic equivalency between UFH and LMWH, these pharmacotherapeutic strategies must be compared for convenience and cost. Enoxaparin can be administered sc, and patients or their caregivers can be taught this technique. No laboratory test monitoring is necessary during treatment with an LMWH. Injections need to be given only once or twice daily. From these practical standpoints, LMWH has a clear advantage. However, if patients consistently require rehospitalization because of severe or recurrent DVT symptoms, and there is no indication they do when managed with enoxaparin, these benefits may be outweighed by other outcome costs.

From a pharmatectural perspective, the cost analysis comparing medications must be based on total outcome costs in order to guide drug selection. In the thromboembolic model, the average wholesale price (AWP) of heparin sodium 30,000 units in 0.45% sodium chloride injection (an average daily dose) is $23.85. The AWP of enoxaparin sodium 1 mg/kg twice daily is $75.41 per day (based on a body weight of 70 kg).[168] If drug acquisition costs alone drive therapy choices (assuming clinical outcomes are equal), UFH may be preferable. However, from the TPQM (Total Pharmacotherapeutic Quality Management) perspective, institutions should include personnel time and other costs when evaluating the cost-effectiveness of therapy.[169] If hospitalized patients with DVT are to be treated safely, effectively, and at the lowest possible cost, careful analysis of *all* costs will be necessary to determine the appropriate drug choice in individual institutions. While the acquisition cost of LMWHs is greater than UFH, the savings realized by not using hospital facilities could be far higher.

Overall treatment costs are best analyzed through pharmacoeconomic modeling. Consideration of issues such as the perspective from which analysis is viewed, which costs are included (i.e., direct versus indirect costs), and the type and level of reimbursement are vital to thorough cost analysis and often take on a different importance in one medical setting than another. Thus, cost comparisons must be individualized. Suggestions for items to be included in such a cost comparison can be found in the list below. When it is financially advantageous to treat DVT at home, LMWHs should be considered a potential first-line therapy in selected patients with a new diagnosis of DVT who could benefit from being treated in the outpatient environment.

Total Outcome Cost Comparison of DVT* Treatments between Hospital and Home Settings

Hospital Treatment	Home-Based Treatment
Preparation of IV solution	Preparation of LMWH syringes
Maintaining IV access	Patient education on self-administration and monitoring of LMWH therapy
Infusion-pump use	Periodic telephone calls from (or clinic visits with) treatment team
Laboratory monitoring of aPTT (time and materials)	Visiting-nurse services
Nurse or physician time for UFH dosage adjustment	Education of patient on use and monitoring of warfarin (time and materials)
Hospital room charges	
Education of patient on use and monitoring of warfarin (time and materials)	

Monitoring of PT and INR (blood sampling, evaluation, and dosage adjustment)	Monitoring of Patient and INR (blood sampling, evaluation, and dosage adjustment)
Treatment of bleeding or thrombotic complications	Treatment of bleeding or thrombotic complications

(*) DVT = deep vein thrombosis, LMWH = low molecular weight heparin, aPTT = activated partial thromboplastin time, UFH = unfractionated heparin, PT = prothrombin time, INR = International Normalized Ratio.

LMWHs Home-Based Treatment of DVT. As discussed, paradigm shifts in medication usage should be undertaken conservatively until more experience is gained with LMWHs. Initial treatment of DVT at home should follow a protocol in which all aspects of the treatment are clearly defined. This treatment protocol should be written in advance by a team of medical professionals experienced in the treatment of DVT. The protocol should include criteria for patient selection, drug selection, patient and caregiver education, monitoring, and LMWH dose preparation. Each medical facility choosing to begin treating patients with DVT at home will need to develop a protocol that fits its own practice patterns.

In particular, criteria must be developed to identify patients who qualify for home-based treatment of DVT. Most studies evaluating LMWH for outpatient therapy where excluded patients with a high risk of bleeding (malignant hypertension, peptic ulcer disease, recent surgery, known bleeding disorders, thrombocytopenia, high risk of falling), a high risk of recurrent thrombosis (previous CVT, pregnancy), and suspected PE. In addition, patients who lived a long distance from follow-up medical care, who were unable to care for themselves or did not have a competent caregiver in residence, and who were simply too ill to stay at home were not considered candidates for home-based treatment of DVT. Patients had to be willing to participate in their care, including self-administration of medications and follow-up for warfarin dosage adjustment when necessary. With these strict guidelines for patient selection, about 22% to 58% of patients screened in various studies were considered eligible for home-based treatment of DVT.

After a diagnosis of DVT is confirmed and it is determined that the patient is a good candidate for home-based treatment, the patient must be started on an LMWH immediately. As more experience is gained with these drugs, the optimal choice must be made on the basis of ease of administration, cost, and, most important, the treatment team's conclusions about the safety and efficacy of each drug based on the available data.

The patient or caregiver must be taught to administer the medication, monitor for adverse reactions and efficacy, and perform any other self-care deemed necessary (such as bed rest, leg elevation, and use of compression stockings). The patient or caregiver must know what steps to take in the event of a complication. Instruction should begin immediately after diagnosis and can be provided by a nurse, a pharmacist, or both. Written instructions should also be provided.

Monitoring in home-based treatment of DVT with LMWHs should include compliance, subcutaneous injection technique, local adverse effects from the injections, signs of bleeding, signs of recurrent thrombosis, and initiation and monitoring of warfarin therapy. Much of this monitoring can be done by the visiting nurse, who should see the patient daily during the initial treatment period of five to nine days. It may also be useful for a nurse, a pharmacist, or a physician from the treatment team to telephone the patient or caregiver periodically to ensure that treatment is going as planned and that there are no complications.

An LMWH should be administered for at least 5 days and warfarin can be started on the same day as the LMWH or the day after.[156] Blood should be drawn daily to monitor the prothrombin time for the first few days[165]; the International Normalized Ration (INR) should be between 2.0 and 3.0 for two consecutive days before the LMWH is stopped.[156,165,167]

Institutional Experience with Outpatient LMWH Protocols. From a pharmatectural point of view, the ultimate test of adopting new LMWH treatment protocols remains in clinical studies that are set up to evaluate all the parameters and treatment outcomes that go into the equation for drug selection. At Burnaby Hospital, a 515-bed university-affiliated primary and secondary care center in Canada, patient recruitment for clinical trials since 1994 have included the use of low molecular weight heparins (LMWHs) for the prophylaxis of venous thromboembolism. The hospital has established a standardized IV heparin protocol and a pharmacy warfarin dosing service to optimize drug therapy and improve patient care.

They conducted a retrospective evaluation of deep venous thrombosis (DVT) and pulmonary embolism (PE) treatment at the center for a 12-month period between October 1994 and September 1995. During this period, there were 60,000 visits to the emergency department with 108 patients admitted for confirmed diagnosis of DVT or PE during the study period. Risk factors for mortality were clearly identified. It was concluded that 40% of patients with a primary diagnosis of DVT could be treated safely on an outpatient basis with LMWH therapy, and would save more than 250 hospital days per year, or $200,000 per year.

In May 1996, a pilot study of the Outpatient DVT Treatment Program, one of the first of its kind in Canada, was initiated. From Monday to Friday, 8 hours per day, patients were screened and enrolled in the 5-day program which included twice-daily visits to the Medical Day Unit for sc LMWH therapy, INR lab monitoring, and oral warfarin therapy, titrated by the pharmacy Warfarin Dosing Service. Patients received daily medications and health counseling by the nursing and pharmacy staffs. Once discharged from the program, patients were managed by their own family physician. Follow up was continued by telephone for a period of 3 months or until warfarin therapy was discontinued. The program was strongly supported by patients, physicians, nurses, pharmacists, laboratory staff, and administration. Data collection, clinical analysis, and patient recruitment are ongoing, but the most recent data suggest significant cost savings.

Dipyridamole

Attempts to maintain patency of carotid vessels in patients who undergo carotid endarterectomy focus on the use of aspirin and dipyridamole (Persantine®), which is widely administered to patients having mechanical vascular procedures in hopes of reducing the risk of subsequent vascular restenosis. Despite the widespread practice of using dipyridamole to prevent stroke and to prevent carotid artery restenosis following surgery, its value and efficacy have never been formally substantiated in these patient populations. Given the significant cost of dipyridamole and the potential gastric toxicity of aspirin, it is important to establish the role of these agents in preventing stroke and restenosis in patients undergoing endarterectomy. The most comprehensive studies evaluating this issue confirm that restenosis after carotid endarterectomy is not prevented by aspirin and dipyridamole therapy.[97] Consequently, patients who undergo carotid endarterectomy should have dipyridamole eliminated from their perioperative and postoperative management.

On the other hand, because long-term aspirin therapy reduces the risk of nonfatal myocardial infarction, stroke, and vascular mortality in patients with symptomatic coronary, peripheral, or cerebral atherosclerotic vascular disease, aspirin should be useful for patients with stenotic carotid vascular disease as well. The ideal dose of aspirin that should be used to prevent carotid restenosis is not determined, but a range of 30 to 325 mg of aspirin per day seems justified. As for the role of dipyridamole therapy in preventing cerebral thrombotic infarction, there are presently no studies that show that this agent plays any significant role in reducing the risk of cerebrovascular disease.[97,98] Therefore, dipyridamole can be considered for elimination in virtually all patients who are taking the medication exclusively for the secondary prevention of atherothrombotic cerebral infarction. Individuals who are taking dipyridamole in combination with warfarin to prevent thrombus formation associated with cardiac valve replacements should be maintained on this agent pending further studies.[99]

Nitrates

Nitrates are central to the treatment of chronic stable angina pectoris. They are the oldest and, perhaps, most reliable form of antianginal therapy. These agents are effective in all forms of angina (classic, variant, mixed), and are relatively low in cost. Moreover, they are helpful in reducing preload and congestive symptoms, and they are available in a variety of preparations, routes of administration, and dosages. Longer acting oral and transdermal nitrates are widely used to provide angina prophylaxis. However, their ability to deliver long-acting, continuous nitrate therapy is associated with the rapid development of tolerance (defined as a decrease in magnitude and duration of effects despite constant or increased dose and plasma concentration).

Because of tolerance, more intermittent dosing of longer acting nitrates (i.e., isosorbide dinitrate orally three times daily in an asymmetrical schedule, or removal of nitrate patches for 12 hours at night time) to provide a nitrate-free interval is standard practice. While this strategy does reduce the development of tolerance, sometimes there is an increase in anginal episodes during periods of low nitrate levels. The relative inconvenience of using nitrate preparations prompted many experts to recommend their discontinuation in favor of using calcium channel blockers or beta adrenergic receptor antagonists to treat anginal episodes. Recent studies, however, suggest that older nitrate preparations can be discontinued in favor of isosorbide-5-mononitrate (e.g., ISMO®, Monoket®), the major active metabolite of isosorbide dinitrate; it is approved for clinical use in the United States in a regimen of 20 mg twice per day, given 7 hours apart. Similar agents are also available.

Recent studies have suggested that isosorbide mononitrate provides long-acting prophylactic antianginal therapy without the development of either nitrate tolerance, increased rebound angina attacks, or reduced efficacy at the end of its duration of action. Furthermore, this preparation is more convenient due to its twice daily dosing.

Nitrates are clearly important agents for the medical therapy of angina. Many nitrate formulations give clinicians the opportunity to use them in several ways to manage angina. All patients with angina should carry a rapidly acting, short duration preparation, such as nitroglycerin tablets for sublingual use, or a nitroglycerin spray, to alleviate acute anginal attacks. They can also be used before specific activities known to induce angina, such as walking uphill and sexual intercourse. Nitrates should never be used in combination with the male impotence drug sildenafil (Viagra®).

Medications For Asthma

Although the use of theophylline to treat bronchospastic pulmonary disease and asthma decreased significantly over the past several years, studies suggest that theophylline is still an overused medication. Physicians and pharmacists encounter many patients on theophylline therapy in whom the dose can be reduced, or eliminated entirely.[54] It should be stressed that theophylline toxicity can be a serious and life-threatening problem. One study evaluating theophylline overdose in 249 consecutive patients referred to the Massachusetts Poison Control Center attempted to identify risk factors for major toxicity associated with this medication.[100] Major toxicity occurred in 62 patients and caused death in 13. It is important to note that 37% of the patients with theophylline toxicity were inadvertently overmedicated while receiving *long-term* theophylline therapy. Major toxicity was more common in this group than in those with acute (presumably intentional) overdosage. Moreover, the study showed that peak level is the most important risk factor for major toxicity in acute overdosage, and advancing age was the most critical factor in chronic overdosage.[101,102]

In an important subset of older patients who are receiving theophylline therapy for management of chronic asthma, toxicity can be both inadvertent and serious. Up to 20% of such patients receiving long-term theophylline therapy may have at least some toxic manifestations.[100] In fact, the longstanding controversy over the appropriateness of theophylline use has centered not only on the question of its effectiveness when compared with other more modern drugs, but also its narrow therapeutic range.

Currently, it seems clear that theophylline should not be a first-line drug for treatment of mild, intermittent asthma because acute exacerbations of asthmatic reactions are most effectively managed by more powerful and rapidly acting beta-2 agonists. Moreover, chronic suppression of inflammatory mediators of the late asthmatic reaction is best achieved by administration of inhaled steroids. Increasingly, the value of leukotriene inhibitors—zafirlukast (Accolate), montelukast (Singulair), etc.—is being recognized. It appears that these agents have the capacity to reduce oral steroid requirements in patients with moderate-to-severe asthma. Currently, montelukast is the only leukotriene modifier that is dosed once daily, and the only drug in this class FDA approved for use in patients less than 12 years of age. In contrast to zileuton and zafirlukast, montelukast does not interact with warfarin. Montelukast and other leukotriene modifiers are used primarily as corticosteroid-sparing drugs, and currently are recommended as alternatives to low-dose inhaled steroids or cromolyn or nedocromil in mild to persistent asthma. In particular, montelukast permits significant tapering of inhaled steroids in patients requiring moderate to high doses of steroids. When *systemic* steroids are being tapered, caution and close monitoring are recommended. Side effects most often reported with montelukast include headache (18%), influenza (4.2%), and abdominal pain (2.9%). The incidences, however, were not significantly different than with placebo.

In more severe asthma, however, there may be an increasing role for the use of theophylline that is supported by a handful of studies. Particularly in patients with nocturnal complaints, long-term theophylline therapy has a clear role in the alleviation of disease symptoms. Despite the lack of evidence that theophylline provides bronchodilator advantages in the acute setting, there is some evidence showing that hospitalized patients will benefit from early administration of the drug. Clearly, because advancing age increases the likelihood of toxicity from this agent, theophylline should be used with extreme care in elderly patients and should be accompanied by frequent measurements of blood levels (even in the apparently stable patient).

It seems reasonable to consider discontinuation of theophylline therapy in those asthma patients who have *not* been given an adequate trial of beta-2 agonists or inhaled corticosteroid therapy. If a patient presents on theophylline treatment but has no previous history of taking beta-2 agonists or corticosteroids for treatment of asthma, these therapeutic options should be evaluated before continuation of long-term therapy with theophylline. There are, however, some subgroups which seem to benefit from theophylline therapy, including patients who need diaphragmatic stimulation, patients with sleep apnea, and some patients with nocturnal asthma. For most other patients with asthma, however, attempts at discontinuing the medication are justified, especially in older patients in whom toxicity is more common.

Corticosteroids

Because of the wide range of potential side effects that result from chronic therapy with corticosteroids, these agents should be used very judiciously in patients with rheumatoid arthritis and other chronic inflammatory disorders. Low-dose (≤ 10 mg per day prednisone) treatment with steroids is widely used in patients with rheumatoid arthritis, often to induce potent anti-inflammatory effects and symptomatic relief until other anti-inflammatory agents have a chance to work. The incidence and severity of side effects of low-dose steroid therapy are controversial, and many clinicians and pharmacists feel that the positive effects of steroids on the inflammatory process outweigh the risks when used on a short-term basis. An area of particular concern is the effect of steroids on bone mass, as it is widely known that chronic steroid therapy is a powerful inducer of osteoporosis.[103,104] Most trials examining these effects are nonrandomized and, therefore, are subject to selection bias and confounding factors because rheumatoid arthritis itself is a risk factor for bone loss. Furthermore, it is known that the negative influences of steroids on bone mass are more pronounced in the first few months of therapy, so that longitudinal studies that look at bone mass in the chronic phase of therapy may underestimate the effects of these agents on bone.

The major conclusion of a recent study suggests that even low-dose, short-term corticosteroid therapy can cause a significant decrease in bone mineral density that is only partially reversible.[103] Accordingly, it is imperative that steroids be used at the lowest dosages and for the shortest periods of time possible. A common and reasonable approach is to use steroids until other inflammatory agents have a chance to work. However, these medications may require several months before significant impact is noted—well within the timeframe for significant loss in bone mineral density to be induced by prednisone. Recognizing this, preventive strategies to help minimize the degree of bone loss while patients are on steroids are important. However, there is relatively little evidence that documents exactly what treatments are most effective as preventive interventions in this setting. Until there is such evidence, therapeutic approaches that are effective in other situations, such as estrogen replacement, calcium supplements, vitamin D, and calcitonin may be considered. Measurement of bone density during and following steroid therapy in patients with rheumatoid arthritis can help guide the degree and intensity of these various therapies.

When using steroids to manage *acute* inflammatory conditions, it is clear that rapid, short-term tapering courses of steroids are as effective as longer dose reduction measures occurring over several weeks. Specifically, with regard to asthma, patients can be tapered over a period of 3 to 7 days following an acute exacerbation. There is no justification for prolonged tapering over a several week period. Finally, in those patients who are taking long-term steroid therapy, every attempt should be made to reduce the dose to less than 10 mg per day, to avoid suppression of the hypothalamic-pituitary adrenal axis.[103]

Antidepressants

The indications and criteria for discontinuing antidepressant drug therapy are controversial.[105-107] First, most depressive disorders extend over a lifetime, and for the majority of patients, the risk for future episodes of depression increases as the number of past episodes increases.[108,109] Moreover, the length of the well interval between episodes becomes progressively shorter with each new episode. Those individuals who are older at the onset of their depression have a higher probability of relapse during future years if not maintained on treatment. As the number of episodes increases and the patient becomes older, severity also often intensifies, treatment response to conventional antidepressants may diminish or even disappear, and the potentially destructive behavioral consequences of the disorder progressively worsen.[5] This deteriorating lifetime pattern can be modified in many, if not most patients, since antidepressants are effective in preventing most future episodes of depression and preserving quality of life.

With the introduction of selective serotonin reuptake inhibitor (SSRIs), patterns of antidepressant use have changed dramatically. More and more, this class of antidepressants is being used to treat panic disorders, premenstrual dysphoria syndrome, obsessive-compulsive disorders, chronic anxiety associated with panic disorders, as well as seasonal affective disorder (SAD). In addition, it is frequently difficult to determine which patients have a depressive illness that requires long-term maintenance therapy and which patients can be discontinued from their antidepressant medication once their situational crisis resolves. Nevertheless, specific recommendations can be given regarding maintenance versus discontinuation of long-term antidepressant therapy.

Maintenance. Lifetime pharmacologic maintenance usually will be required for patients who are 50 years of age or older when they experience their first episode of depression. Maintenance therapy also appears to be justified in those patients who are 40 years of age or older with two or more prior episodes of depression and for those with three or more prior episodes, regardless of their age.[108,109] Maintenance dosages need to be comparable to established treatment dosages until it is proven that lower doses are effective. When an antidepressant is selected for long-term treatment, strong consideration should be given to the agent's side effect profile (see Table 4-2), since compliance is essential for success. Rapidly accumulating data indicate that the prevailing treatment philosophy for those with major depression probably should *not* shift toward discontinuation of treatment. However, if medications must be discontinued for those at high risk, dosage should be tapered over a prolonged period, patients should be monitored closely, relapses should be expected, and nonpharmacologic treatments such as psychotherapy and phototherapy should be considered, as indicated.

For patients taking antidepressant medication for a situational crisis or anxiety-related symptoms, medication discontinuation is probably more justifiable. It must be emphasized that the pharmacologic consequences of stopping an antidepressant medication may be equal to or greater than those associated with administering it.[31] Discontinuing a medication that is taken for a prolonged period is not an innocuous action. Even SSRIs can produce a withdrawal syndrome characterized by mood-related and neurological symptoms. Nevertheless, despite known risks, clinical or personal reasons sometimes lead to a decision to discontinue antidepressant therapy.

Discontinuation. When discontinuation is possible, how should it be accomplished? Ideally, the schedule for cessation should be gradual. Treatment should be tapered over several weeks, or perhaps, a few months. Data are not available to firmly substantiate that this more gradual reduction strategy is more effective in preventing relapse for most antidepressant medications, but we do know about risks associated with rapid discontinuation, and we have considerable knowledge about the rate of change for receptors and other neurobiological functions following administration and discontinuation of centrally active agents. These clinical and neurobiologic observations suggest that the brain requires months rather than days or weeks to adjust to the changes associated with stopping a medication. For tricyclic or heterocyclic agents, a simple strategy is to reduce the dosage by 25% *every 3 months.* For drugs with a longer half-life and a standardized dosing regimen, such as fluoxetine, this reduction is accomplished by taking the pill at a reduced frequency every quarter, such as every other day, then every third day, and so on, or by switching to lower dosage forms or liquid products and continuing daily administration, and then reducing the dosage by 25% every 3 months. Patients generally tolerate these reduced regimens. The use of a daily diary helps maintain compliance. To assist patients in remaining on course, a withdrawal calendar should be prepared and given to patients and families with clear instructions. It is also important to continue other treatments that are proven valuable, such as interpersonal therapy, phototherapy, or other modalities.

Table 4-2

Antidepressant Medications							
	Category and Drug	Sedative Potency	Anti-cholinergic Potency	Orthostatic Hypotensive Potency	Cardiac Arrhythmogenic Potential	Target Dosage (mg/day)	Dosage Range (mg/day)
Tricyclics	Tertiary amines						
	Amitriptyline	High	Very high	High	Yes	150-200	75-300
	Clomipramine	High	High	High	Yes	150-200	75-250
	Doxepin	High	Moderate	Moderate	Yes	150-200	75-300
	Imipramine	Moderate	Moderate	High	Yes	150-200	75-300
	Trimipramine	High	Moderate	Moderate	Yes	150-200	75-300
	Secondary amines						
	Desipramine	Low	Low	Moderate	Yes	150-200	75-300
	Nortriptyline	Low	Low	Lowest of the tricyclics	Yes	75-100	40-150
	Protriptyline	Low	High	Low	Yes	30	15-60
Related Polycyclics	Amoxapine	Low	Low	Moderate	Yes	150-200	75-300
	Maprotiline	Moderate	Low	Moderate	Yes	150-200	75-200
Atypical Agents	Bupropion	Low	Very low	Very low	Low	300	200-450
	Fluoxetine	Low	Very low	Very low	Low	20	5-80
	Sertraline	Low	Very low	Very low	Low	100-150	50-200
	Trazodone	High	Very low	High	Low	400	50-600

Tricyclic antidepressants with anticholinergic potency require special mention when planning discontinuation of treatment, since receptor regulatory changes occur in patients who are taking medications that block muscarinic receptors for a sustained period. If a tricyclic antidepressant is stopped suddenly, a transient but significant cholinergic supersensitivity will develop in many patients.[28,31] Patients may complain of somatic distress, gastrointestinal symptoms, disturbed sleep patterns that include excessive and vivid dreaming or nightmares, or patients may report frequent awakening and insomnia. Psychomotor disruptions, agitation, anxiety, and activation may also occur. This antidepressant withdrawal syndrome has been described in detail, and many of these anticholinergic withdrawal symptoms are indistinguishable from the symptom profile experienced by patients relapsing into depression. This is another important reason for planning a gradual discontinuation of medications whenever possible, especially when tricyclic antidepressants are being used. As mentioned, patients who are taking SSRIs also require gradual discontinuation from their medication. It is preferable to be cautious and taper these agents gradually to prevent precipitation of a major depressive episode, and to reduce symptoms that may accompany withdrawal.

In summary, recurrent episodes of depression across a lifetime are an unfortunate but predictable characteristic of this affective disorder. The consequences of multiple episodes of depression are almost always debilitating and, on occasion, may even be fatal. Therefore, recurrences should be prevented whenever possible. Maintenance treatment with antidepressant medications is effective in most patients, if dosages are at adequate treatment levels. Individuals with multiple prior episodes of depression, especially if they are elderly and if prior episodes were severe, are at especially high risk for relapse if medications are discontinued. As a result, maintenance regimens at treatment dosage levels probably should be the norm for many or most patients with depressive mood disorders.

Since age at onset and the number of prior episodes both may predict risk of subsequent episodes, a workable formula is that anyone age 50 or more at onset of their first episode, age 40 or more at onset with two or more episodes, or any age with three or more episodes, probably should be considered a candidate for maintenance. If medication discontinuation is absolutely essential, despite known risks, it should be performed gradually, with close monitoring, ongoing use of nonpharmacologic treatments, if possible, and with a strategic plan for prompt intervention if the anticipated relapse occurs.[42,43,48,49]

Benzodiazepines

Benzodiazepine drugs such as alprazolam are widely used for the treatment of anxiety panic disorders. There is considerable debate, as well as negative perceptions, shared by health professionals, pharmacists, patients, lay public, and the media regarding the syndrome associated with benzodiazepine discontinuation. Clearly, there is a need to determine the optimal time for discontinuing these medications, the appropriate reasons for doing so, how discontinuation should be accomplished, and expected outcomes.[65] Recent studies suggest that the majority of patients taking benzodiazepines (see Table 4-3), when slowly tapered, are able to discontinue these agents without a great deal of trouble, particularly after *short-term therapy.*[30] Patients treated with long-term therapy at higher therapeutic doses tend to experience greater difficulty with discontinuation.[27,110] However, if patients are appropriately and adequately prepared, and discontinuation efforts follow a slow and gradual tapering schedule, discontinuation symptoms, if they occur, tend to be transient, mild to moderate in severity, and are generally tolerable by the average patient.

Panic Disorder. Definitive evidence is not yet available regarding the optimal length of treatment for panic disorders, although one recent study documented that 8 months of treatment led to greater improvement than 2 months of therapy, which is certainly in keeping with the experience of most physicians. Another study compared short-term versus extended maintenance treatment in panic disorder patients treated with imipramine and demonstrated that the group who received 12 months of maintenance therapy, following 6 months of acute treatment, had significantly less relapse at follow-up than did the group who received only 6 months of acute treatment.[111]

After 6 to 18 months of effective pharmacotherapy of panic disorder, most physicians attempt to taper and discontinue medications.[112,113] Although one might question discontinuing treatment that proved effective and allowed the patient to return to a near-normal level of functioning, the expense and potential side effects associated with these medications usually will justify an attempt at discontinuation in the majority of cases. Moreover, once the patient has maintained maximal improvement for at least 6 months and has reestablished his or her previous state of functioning and confidence, there are several reasons for reassessing the need for continued treatment.

The most compelling case for discontinuation is that treatment may no longer be necessary.[114] Also, problematic side effects, the wish to conceive, unexpected pregnancy, or emergence of alcohol or drug abuse are all valid reasons for attempting to discontinue effective treatment. Other, less important but equally understandable reasons include the expense and inconvenience involved in taking benzodiazepines or tricyclic antidepressants several times a day and issues of self-esteem. Consequently, the decision to discontinue benzodiazepines, for whatever the reason, should be a mutual one between patient and physician, and the patient should be reassured that in most cases discontinuation can be accomplished without significant adverse consequences. In this regard, it is critical that the medication be tapered slowly and gradually; this minimizes the severity of withdrawal symptoms that may occur with discontinuation. The patient should also be reassured that he or she may experience some anxiety symptoms, but that for most, these will resolve within 1 to 3 weeks. The patient should also be reassured that if it is determined that pharmacologic treatment is required, the medication can be reinstated.

Table 4-3

Benzodiazepines			
Drug	**Equivalent Dosage (mg)**	**Rate of Onset after Oral Dose**	**Half-life (hr)***
Alprazolam	0.5	Intermediate	6-20
Chlordiazepoxide	10.0	Intermediate	30-100
Clonazepam	0.25	Intermediate	18-50
Clorazepate	7.5	Rapid	30-100
Diazepam	5.0	Rapid	30-100
Estazolam	2.0	Intermediate	10-24
Flurazepam	30.0	Rapid to intermediate	50-160
Halazepam	20.0	Intermediate to slow	30-100
Lorazepam	1.0	Intermediate	10-20
Midazolam	—	Intermediate	2-3
Oxazepam	15.0	Intermediate to slow	8-12
Prazepam	10.0	Slow	30-100
Quazepam	15.0	Rapid to intermediate	50-160
Temazepam	30.0	Intermediate	8-20
Triazolam	0.25	Intermediate	1.5-5.0

*The elimination half-life represents the total for all active metabolites; the elderly tend to have the longer half-lives in the range reported.

Timing. Timing is also critical when considering discontinuation, which should be initiated at a relatively unstressful time in the patient's life. For example, the physician should not consider discontinuation for a student when exams are scheduled. Similarly, it would be inappropriate to begin tapering medication for the executive when he has an important presentation pending or a critical business trip to make.

A number of different outcomes are observed when benzodiazepines are discontinued. The first and, obviously, most desirable result is that the patient remains asymptomatic following benzodiazepine discontinuation. Realistically, however, many patients experience transient withdrawal symptoms or rebound panic, both of which generally resolve within 1 to 3 weeks after complete discontinuation of the drug. Present studies suggest that the extent of relapse varies widely from patient to patient but that about 30% to 45% of patients with panic attacks remain well after discontinuation of their therapy.[115]

As mentioned earlier, patient education and reassurance are critical to successful discontinuation of these agents. If patients *know* to expect withdrawal symptoms during discontinuation, they are usually better able to tolerate the symptoms. Studies show that at least some withdrawal symptoms occur in as many as 35% to 90% of patients discontinued from drugs such as alprazolam.[115,116] Given this outcome, the patient should be reassured that if symptoms occur, they are not life-threatening, are generally mild to moderate, and should resolve within a few days or weeks. Again, the patient should understand and agree that tapering will be accomplished slowly, with gradual decreases in dosage to minimize any return of symptoms.

Tapering. The time frame within which discontinuation of benzodiazepines is completed is probably the most important factor in the success of this process. When alprazolam is discontinued rapidly after 8 weeks of acute treatment, 35% of patients experienced rebound panic and withdrawal symptoms; rebound panic can be especially frightening to the patient, since it often occurs with more intensity than the original panic episode.

Unfortunately, much of the clinical data available on discontinuation of benzodiazepines reflects outcomes and symptoms following relatively rapid discontinuation of the drug.[27,30] However, there are some studies that compare rapid versus gradual discontinuation. In general, when benzodiazepines were discontinued abruptly, patients experienced more symptoms than when the drug was discontinued gradually. In one study, 44% of patients suffered recurrent anxiety after abruptly discontinuing compared to none of those in the gradually tapered group.[115] A preponderance of studies suggests that the incidence and severity of withdrawal symptoms can be greatly reduced by slower tapering schedules.[27] Specifically, most patients can discontinue benzodiazepines with few problems if the medication is tapered slowly over a 2 to 4 month period. Finally, discontinuation of benzodiazepine treatment should be discussed in detail with the patient at the beginning of treatment.[111] The patient should be reassured that severe withdrawal symptoms, or exacerbation of psychological symptoms will be managed as required. If the patient is educated about the potential outcomes associated with discontinuation and has adequate support from physician and pharmacist, withdrawal is accomplished with little problem.[65,110]

ANTICONVULSANTS

No definitive rules can be established regarding the discontinuation of anticonvulsant therapy. While some patients have prolonged or permanent remissions of their seizures, it is difficult to predict who will relapse. There are, however, some useful prognostic indicators in children. Slow withdrawal from medication may be considered in patients with idiopathic seizures who are seizure-free for two or more years. The same factors that predict recurrence after a single seizure suggest that the patient will have a relapse off medication. However, even with an electroencephalogram with elliptical activity, the patient may wish to try stopping treatment, so long as the seizure-free period is at least 2 years.[57,58,69]

Phenytoin: Optimal Use

Phenytoin (Dilantin®) is an anticonvulsant medication widely used in the treatment of generalized seizure disorders as well as other forms of epilepsy. It can be used as either ongoing therapy for patients with well established seizure disorders or as prophylaxis in individuals at risk for seizures following neurosurgery, head trauma, or stroke. When used properly, phenytoin is generally safe and highly efficacious but it has a number of properties that can make clinical use complicated.[145] Phenytoin metabolism is non-linear (not directly related to dose and serum concentration) within the therapeutic range. The enzyme system for phenytoin becomes saturated at relatively low plasma concentrations resulting in a progressive *decrease* in the rate of elimination as the dosage is increased. Therefore, after saturation of the enzyme system, a small increase in dosage leads to a large increase in serum phenytoin concentration. Another factor complicating phenytoin dosing is the large individual variation in the disposition of the drug in patients taking the same dosage, so that there can be as much as a fifty fold difference in plasma concentration among individuals taking the drug. Finally, phenytoin has significant interactions with numerous other commonly used medications and its disposition can be affected by variations in serum albumin levels.

Therapeutic Levels. In patients who suffer frequent, recurrent epileptic seizures, a definite reduction in the number of seizures, or the virtual elimination of convulsions, is a well-defined endpoint by which to measure the therapeutic efficacy of phenytoin. In those individuals who have infrequent seizures or are taking phenytoin on a prophylactic basis, the plasma phenytoin concentration is generally the most sensible surrogate marker for assessing a therapeutic response. Unfortunately, there is some uncertainty regarding the optimal plasma concentration for phenytoin. Longitudinal studies have demonstrated that improved seizure control can be achieved for patients with epilepsy when plasma phenytoin concentration exceeds 40 μmol/l. Most of the subjects in these trials had relatively severe seizure disorders, and other studies have suggested that seizure control may be achieved with lower plasma phenytoin concentrations. The overall consensus, however, is that optimal seizure control can be accomplished without toxicity when phenytoin plasma concentration is in the range of 40-80 μmol/l (10-20 μg/ml; 1 μmol/l = 0.25 μg/ml).

The risk for toxicity increases dramatically above 80 μmol/l and is nearly universal above 100 μmol/l. The earliest sign of phenytoin toxicity is usually nystagmus (often seen at levels of 80-120 μmol/l), followed by ataxia (120-160 μmol/l) and mental status changes (>160 μmol/l). Toxicity can develop very insidiously, however, and signs and symptoms may be difficult to distinguish from other neurological diseases, especially in those with underlying neurological disorders or pre-existing cerebellar dysfunction. There is less correlation between plasma concentration and some potential long-term adverse effects of phenytoin. These effects include gingival hyperplasia, acne, hirsutism, coarsening of facial features, folate deficiency and vitamin D deficiency. These manifestations are probably related to the duration of therapy as well as plasma phenytoin concentration.

All methods used to measure phenytoin plasma concentration reflect total concentration, which includes both protein-bound and unbound phenytoin components. In patients with chronic renal or hepatic disease, those in the last trimester of pregnancy, neonates, and individuals taking drugs such as sodium valproate, plasma protein binding can be reduced so that the total phenytoin concentration may greatly underestimate the concentration of unbound, pharmacologically active medication. It is important to recognize these situations, although it is usually not possible to directly estimate the degree of impairment of binding of phenytoin to plasma proteins. Since about 10% of phenytoin is usually unbound in the plasma and the therapeutic range for phenytoin concentration is considered 40-80 μmol/l, a therapeutic range for free (unbound) phenytoin concentration of 4-9 μmol/l has been suggested.

Drug Interactions. A host of commonly used medications can interact with phenytoin and may affect its metabolism. They include: Cimetidine (Tagamet®), amiodarone (Cordarone®), allopurinol (Zyloprim®), chlorpromazine (Thorazine®), imipramine (Tofranil®), isoniazid, metronidazole (Flagyl®), omeprazole (Prilosec®), thioridazine (Mellaril®), and sulfonamides. These medications inhibit phenytoin metabolism and may cause an increase in plasma concentration and heightened risk of toxicity. Sodium valproate inhibits phenytoin metabolism but also displaces phenytoin from protein binding sites. These effects counteract each other, making it difficult to predict and interpret phenytoin concentrations in patients also taking valproate. Acute hepatitis also impairs the liver's ability to metabolize phenytoin, which also can increase the risk for toxicity.

Carbamazepine (Tegretol®) and rifampin stimulate hepatic metabolism of phenytoin, which reduces phenytoin concentration and increases the potential for breakthrough seizures. Folic acid also increases phenytoin clearance by an unknown mechanism, thereby lowering plasma concentration. At the same time, long-term treatment with phenytoin can result in folate deficiency, which when treated with folic acid could lower plasma phenytoin concentration and lead to breakthrough seizures.

Monitoring. Phenytoin is an intergral medication for treatment of seizure disorders and for prophylaxis of seizures in patients following neurosurgery, head trauma, and stroke. Clinicians need to be familiar with its unusual pharmacokinetic properties in order to insure its safe and effective use and to interpret and utilize measurements of plasma concentrations appropriately. Plasma concentration should not be checked unless a steady state has been reached. Generally speaking, this does not occur until three to four weeks after the initiation of treatment. An exception to this principle is if the plasma concentration is being checked because of suspected toxicity, in which case a steady state concentration is unnecessary. Clinical judgement must always be used in conjunction with plasma concentrations. If seizure control is adequate, dosage adjustment is often not necessary, even if the plasma concentration is below the "therapeutic" range. Similarly, if suspicion of phenytoin toxicity is present, reduction of the dosage is appropriate even if the plasma level is below the "toxic" range.

Once a steady state concentration has been achieved, the timing of blood samples to check plasma concentration is unimportant since phenytoin has a rather long half-life and diurnal variation is small even with once daily dosing. Some general guidelines for phenytoin dosage adjustment to achieve desirable levels are as follows: (1) if the plasma concentration is below 20 μmol/l, increase daily dose by 100 mg; (2) if plasma concentration is 20-60 μmol/l, daily dose should be increased by no more than 50 mg; (3) if plasma concentration is above 60 μmol/l, increase daily dose by 25 mg. Finally, clinicians should recognize that many common medications affect phenytoin metabolism and can alter plasma concentration. Moreover, clinical situations also may affect serum protein levels and, therefore, potentially raise the level of unbound plasma phenytoin.

Seizure Management

Nearly 10% of patients who live to 80 years of age will experience a seizure at some point in their life. Most of these patients can be appropriately managed by primary care physicians. It is essential, therefore, for clinicians to be familiar with current concepts in the classification, diagnosis and treatment of seizure disorders.

Seizures can occur secondary to acute processes such as meningitis or hypoxia, but in many instances, normal individuals have a single seizure for which no cause is found. If these idiopathic seizures recur, the patient is said to have epilepsy. Seizures can be partial (originating from a single focus) or generalized at their onset. Examples of partial seizures include simple partial seizures, in which focal motor activity occurs without loss of consciousness, and complex partial (temporal lobe) seizures, in which the patient may act out automatisms but is actually unconscious. Generalized seizures most often encountered in general practice are tonic-clonic (grand mal) and absence (petit mal) seizures. It can often be difficult to clinically distinguish partial seizures which secondarily generalize from true generalized seizures.

The diagnosis of a seizure disorder is made on clinical grounds. Electroencephalography (EEG) is most useful when it is obtained during an event. The interpretation of an interictal EEG is much more difficult because only 30 to 50% of seizure patients have an abnormal EEG at any given time. Furthermore, a small percent of healthy individuals have EEG findings consistent with epilepsy yet never experience a seizure. Interictal EEG is more sensitive when it is performed repeatedly, or when the patient is either sleep-deprived or sleeping during the study. Magnetic resonance imaging (MRI) is also useful in the evaluation of a patient with a seizure disorder. MRI is more sensitive than CT in identifying lesions related to epilepsy, especially if coronal views are obtained. Several medications including ciprofloxacin, theophylline and tricyclic antidepressants can cause generalized seizures (especially in overdose). More commonly, seizures occur secondary to withdrawal from alcohol or sedative medications such as benzodiazepines (e.g., alprazolam-Xanax®).

Evaluation of the patient with a first seizure should focus on ruling out acute etiologies including hypoglycemia, hypoxia, electrolyte abnormalities, alcohol or medication withdrawal and liver or kidney dysfunction. In selected patients, a urine drug screen can be useful. Lumbar puncture need not be performed unless there is clinical evidence of meningitis or encephalitis. A CT scan or MRI should be performed in virtually all patients greater than 18 years of age, and in younger patients with partial seizures or other evidence of a focal neurologic process. Radiologic studies need not be obtained immediately unless the patient is obtunded, or has suffered an acute brain injury, such as a stroke or subdural hematoma. Hospitalization is not required after a first seizure if the patient is alert during a period of observation, and there is a friend or family member who can drive the patient home and stay with them for at least 24 hours. Specific plans for follow-up are essential if such an approach is taken. It is not necessary to begin anti-epileptic drug treatment after a first seizure unless recurrent seizures are highly likely (as in patients with acute brain injury, or a strong family history of epilepsy).

Drug Therapy. Treatment after a single seizure is controversial. The 12 month recurrence rate of an untreated seizure is 16 to 62%, and this rate is increased if the patient has a focal brain injury, a positive interictal EEG, or a family history of epilepsy. The recurrence rate in treated patients is 25 to 41%, and 30% of patients will experience side effects severe enough to warrant discontinuation of the medication. There is no evidence that early initiation of drug therapy improves the natural history of epilepsy. Monotherapy achieves adequate seizure control with tolerable side effects in roughly 50% of patients. Of those who fail, 60% will respond to another single agent. Only a small minority of patients will experience improved control on combination therapy. Dosage should be based on clinical control of seizures and the occurrence of side effects. Some patients will require drug concentrations above the therapeutic range for control, and others will experience toxic effects when drug concentration is in the "therapeutic range." Drug levels are most useful in confirming compliance, evaluating symptoms that might be drug induced, and managing patients who are pregnant or have liver or renal dysfunction.

In adults, most seizures which clinically appear to be generalized are actually partial seizures with secondary generalization. The presence of an aura or focal event at the onset of a generalized seizure suggests the diagnosis of partial seizure with secondary generalization, but an EEG may be necessary to make this distinction. Carbamazepine (Tegretol®) and phenytoin (Dilantin®) are the agents of first choice for partial seizures, whether or not they become secondarily generalized. Carbamazepine is preferable in young women who will wish to avoid facial coarsening and hirsutism (as well as the teratogenic effects) associated with phenytoin. Valproate (Depakene®) is the most effective agent for true generalized seizures. Starting these medications at low doses and gradually increasing them often minimizes side effects. If the initial agent is not effective, another single agent should be tried since combination therapy is rarely superior to properly chosen monotherapy.

If seizures continue to recur after 3 months of treatment, or if there is an associated, progressive neurologic syndrome, a neurologic consultation is advisable. All patients with refractory seizures should undergo MRI scanning, since some epileptic foci can be surgically resected. Refractory symptoms should also prompt the physician to reconsider the diagnosis, since other disorders including pseudoseizure, migraine, narcolepsy, vasovagal attack, arrhythmia, panic disorder and hyperventilation can mimic seizures.

H_2 Receptor Antagonists

H_2 blockers are among the most popular drugs for the treatment of peptic ulcer disease. All four of the currently approved agents—cimetidine, ranitidine, famotidine, and nizatidine—are effective, easily taken, and generally well-tolerated (see Table 4-4). These agents competitively block the histamine H_2 receptor of the acid-producing parietal cells, and thus render the cells less responsive, not only to histamine stimulation but also to the stimulation of acetylcholine and gastrin because of postreceptor interactions. The efficacy of these medications is about equal, and there is little to recommend one H_2 blocker over another, although there are some differences in cost, and cimetidine is more likely to produce drug interactions due to its ability to inhibit the P-450 cytochrome oxidase system.[117,118] All of them can occasionally produce central nervous system symptoms, such as headache and mental confusion. When used long-term and in high doses, as in the treatment of hypersecretory states, cimetidine sometimes causes reversible gynecomastia and impotence. However, omeprazole, rather than an H_2 blocker, is probably the drug of choice today in the treatment of the Zollinger-Ellison syndrome. As mentioned, cimetidine, and to a much lesser extent, ranitidine, bind to hepatic cytochrome P-450 microsomal enzymes and may inhibit the catabolism of many drugs metabolized by this system. This interaction, however, is not usually significant clinically, except in older patients on polypharmacy who are taking drugs that have narrow therapeutic-to-toxic ratios, most notable among them, theophylline, phenytoin, and warfarin. Despite the infrequency of serious adverse drug reactions, levels of theophylline and phenytoin and prothrombin times should be monitored more carefully if cimetidine is used in conjunction with these drugs. On the other hand, another H_2 blocker such as famotidine can be used instead and, therefore, reduce the drug-monitoring costs associated with long-term cimetidine therapy.

Table 4-4

Dosage Schedule for H_2-Receptor Antagonists

Indication	Cimetidine	Ranitidine*	Famotidine
ACUTE OR RECURRENT PEPTIC DISEASE	400 mg po, bid or 800 mg po, hs	150 mg bid or 300 mg po, hs	20 mg po, bid or 40 mg po, hs
SEVERELY ILL PATIENTS	37.5 mg/hr IV (continuous infusion)	6-12 mg/hr IV (continuous infusion)	1.7 mg/hr IV (continuous infusion)
PROPHYLAXIS FOR RECURRENT ULCER	400 mg po, hs	150 mg po, hs	20 mg p.o., hs

*Oral dosage for nizatidine is identical to that for ranitidine; an intravenous preparation of nizatidine is not available.

Lifestyle Modification. A number of general therapeutic measures, including lifestyle modifications, dietary alterations, and psychotherapeutic interventions, are recommended in order to reduce the need for long-term maintenance therapy with H_2 blockers. Patients are encouraged to get adequate rest, relaxation, and sleep. The precise role that emotional factors such as anxiety, anger, frustration, and resentment play in the pathogenesis of peptic ulcer disease is hotly debated. In years past, they were widely thought to play a significant role, especially in duodenal ulcer disease, but in recent years their importance has been questioned. At any rate, anxiety and anger should probably be ameliorated as much as possible by simple means, such as by making patients aware of their feelings, encouraging them to vent their problems, manipulating their environments, encouraging participation in regular physical activity, and, when indicated, administering sedatives and tranquilizers. Ulcerogenic drugs, such as aspirin and NSAIDs, should be avoided or, if absolutely required, at least taken in smaller doses. Smoking and alcohol ingestion should also be minimized or completely eliminated if possible.

The role of diet in the treatment of peptic ulcer disease has been reevaluated in recent years. The traditional, restrictive bland diets, eaten in frequent, small meals, are unnecessary and may even be harmful. Patients should eat three regular meals a day while avoiding any foods noted to cause symptoms. Caffeine-containing beverages such as coffee, tea, and colas may also be restricted, although their effects are probably of little significance. Once recommended, frequent meals, and protein in particular, were meant to buffer the acid in the stomach. Unfortunately, these frequent meals also stimulated acid secretion for several hours, while providing satisfactory buffering of the gastric acid for only the first hour. Moreover, the traditional bedtime snack, which was recommended before the advent of H_2 blockers that could control nocturnal acid secretion, was especially harmful because it stimulated acid secretion for several hours, while the patient was asleep, and was unable to take antacids. The traditional bland diets are not only distasteful to patients, but also contain a lot of the milk sugar lactose, which causes abdominal cramps, gas, and even diarrhea in many patients with some degree of lactose intolerance. Bland diets also tend to be high in calories, and because of their high fat content, are possibly atherogenic.

Maintenance Therapy. Therapy of uncomplicated duodenal ulcer disease requires treatment with H_2 blockers or proton pump blockers. High-dose therapy for a period of 6 to 8 weeks usually results in ulcer healing. The indications for maintaining suppression of ulcer recurrence with chronic therapy using H_2 blockers remains controversial.[43,55,119] However, the preponderance of clinical trials strongly suggests that continued use of an H_2 receptor blocker (or any other ulcer-healing drug) at approximately *half* of the ulcer-healing dose is usually effective for prevention of ulcer recurrence. The mean recurrence rate for duodenal ulcer during maintenance therapy and placebo therapy is dramatically different. Only about 25% of patients taking continuous H_2 receptor blocker therapy experience ulcer recurrence, in contrast to approximately 75% of those patients receiving placebo. Thus, the overwhelming evidence shows that fewer duodenal ulcers recur during sustained maintenance therapy with an H_2 receptor blocker or with sucralfate than with placebo therapy. All of the H_2 receptor blockers appear equally effective in this regard.

Exactly how *long* maintenance therapy should be continued is uncertain.[55] The results of most studies show a consistently high relapse rate if maintenance drug treatment is withdrawn during the first year. Accordingly, maintenance therapy is approved and recommended for 12 months. However, it is also clear that once such maintenance treatment is discontinued, the same high rate of ulcer relapse is observed. This does *not* mean that therapy with H_2 blockers should be continued indefinitely. However, continuation of treatment beyond 1 year is effective in preventing both ulcer relapse and the development of ulcer complications such as hemorrhage and perforation. Accordingly, there is justification for continuing drug therapy, but only in patients who remain at high risk for ulcer recurrence, and in those with a medical condition that might be compromised by ulcer recurrence or complications. Certainly, patients who experience significant bleeding as a complication of their previous ulcers are at high risk for recurrent bleeding in the future, and, therefore, are reasonable candidates for indefinite maintenance therapy. Emerging evidence suggests that this specific patient group should be considered for prolonged maintenance therapy, even if other risk factors can be corrected.[43,55,119]

Exactly which schedule for maintenance therapy with H_2 blockers is best also remains uncertain. Physicians and pharmacists recognize that after ulcers heal, many patients follow a self-guided approach to care, even without our prescribing it. Many experts conclude that symptomatic self-care is an appropriate ulcer maintenance regimen for patients with healed, uncomplicated duodenal ulcer. However, self-care is not recommended for the following groups: elderly patients in whom ulcer relapse might present great risk; patients with serious concomitant illnesses; those with previous ulcer bleeding, with previous perforation, or frequent ulcer relapses (more than twice yearly); and those with ulcers that take a prolonged time to heal. Clearly, the approach to self-care with H_2 blocker maintenance therapy requires additional evaluation.

Cost Effectiveness. Although drug treatment trials adequately document the effectiveness of maintenance therapy in reducing ulcer recurrence and preventing complications, an important question is whether such treatment is also cost effective, especially in view of the high cost for many of these drugs. In making these determinations, it is important to remember that the overall costs related to ulcer disease include a number of different components. The direct costs that get early attention include medication acquisition costs, charges for physician visits, medical testing, expenses incurred by hospitalization, and treatment of complications associated with ulcer disease. However, in addition, there are also important indirect costs that must be considered. While not a complete list, these would include loss of work productivity, absenteeism from work, and overall quality-of-life issues.

A number of investigations in the last few years have specifically addressed the cost-benefit aspects of maintenance ulcer therapy. One such trial, evaluating short-term treatment with famotidine (6 months) concluded that the estimated direct cost for the care of the average ulcer patient prescribed maintenance therapy with famotidine was approximately 30% less than the cost would be if the patient received no maintenance H_2 antagonist therapy. In this study, most of the cost savings resulted from a reduction in risks for hospitalization and surgery. A number of other trials also support the cost-efficacy of maintenance therapy with H_2 blockers to prevent ulcer recurrence and emphasize that the added cost of the drug itself is more than offset by a reduction in other direct cost items such as repeated laboratory and endoscopic testing, and hospitalizations to treat complications of recurrent ulcer disease. In addition, the more difficult to measure quality-of-life issues are significantly improved with maintenance therapy. Therefore, it is reasonable to provide maintenance therapy for at least 6 to 12 months in all patients with documented peptic ulcer disease.

Guidelines. The goals for treating patients with ulcer disease are to relieve symptoms, heal the acute ulcer, reduce the risk of ulcer recurrence and complications, and decrease the economic impact of this chronic disease while maintaining the patient's quality of life. Assuming that a diagnosis of peptic ulcer is firmly established, an adequate period of drug treatment with H_2 blockers is indicated. If the patient is young and generally healthy, with an uncomplicated ulcer and few risk factors favoring relapse, the patient can be given a prescription for 3 to 6 months of medication, told to take full therapy for any recurrent symptoms, and to continue the treatment until symptoms are relieved. Failure of this treatment to relieve symptoms after 2 to 3 weeks, the onset of alarming symptoms such as intense pain, vomiting, or melena—or possibly, the exhaustion of the 6 month supply of medication with continued symptoms—should lead to reevaluation.

On the other hand, if the patient has had a complicated course of ulcer disease, such as bleeding, or has a significant number of risk factors—smoking, aspirin or NSAID use, etc.—that would make early ulcer relapse highly likely, it is most prudent to institute *continuous* maintenance therapy while working to reduce or eliminate the adverse risk factors. Any relapse of symptomatic ulcer disease during noncontinuous maintenance therapy should indicate the need for a return to a continuous-dosing regimen.

For ulcer disease that relapses during full-dose maintenance therapy, the clinician should consider permanent reduction of acid secretion by surgery or, more appropriately, search for gastric mucosal infection by *Helicobacter pylori*. In light of recent studies that show dramatic reductions in ulcer recurrence following successful eradication of *H. pylori*, it is clinically safe to consider treatment for this organism prior to more invasive procedures.[71] Early empiric treatment directed at *H. pylori* is also appropriate in patients with ulcer disease. While most of these recommendations are applicable primarily to duodenal ulcer disease, management of recurrent gastric ulcer is similar, once malignancy is excluded, in that risk factors for recurrence should be considered and corrected when possible. For gastric ulcer, these factors are use of NSAID and heavy cigarette smoking. Recurrent ulcerations should be treated by full-dose therapy, and then maintenance therapy instituted with continuous full-dose treatment. Duration of maintenance therapy is less well defined for gastric ulcer, but can be effective for years.

Recommendations for chronic maintenance therapy with H_2 blockers apply only to patients who have ulcer disease documented radiographically or endoscopically. Those patients who are taking long-term H_2 blocker therapy for symptomatic relief of gastrointestinal complaints, but who do not have documentation of peptic ulcer disease, can probably have H_2 blockers discontinued from their drug regimen. Unfortunately, encouraging patients to discontinue therapy with H_2 blockers may be difficult because many of these patients depend on this drug for symptomatic relief, either real or perceived. This is especially true when underlying symptoms are caused by gastroesophageal reflux (GERD).

Helicobacter Pylori

Helicobacter pylori is a curved gram-negative bacteria which was isolated and identified approximately a decade ago. It is uniquely adapted to survive in the hostile environment of the human stomach (or any area where gastric epithelium is found including metaplastic tissue in the esophagus, duodenum or Meckel's diverticulum) by invading the mucous layer and neutralizing the surrounding acid with a powerful urease enzyme. The organism was originally called *Campylobacter pylori* but was renamed in 1989 as part of the new genus *Helicobacter.* In retrospect, the organism was detected in animals during the 1800s and in humans in the early part of this century but because of misconceptions and faulty reasoning, it was ignored until interest was resurrected in the early 1980s by an Australian medical resident named Marshall. He proved that *H. pylori* can cause acute gastritis when he deliberately ingested an inoculum and subsequently subjected himself to repeated gastric endoscopies. There now is little dispute over *H. pylori's* role as the cause of chronic active gastritis. It is also integral to the pathogenesis of peptic ulcer disease and is epidemiologically linked to gastric cancer and lymphoma.

Transmission of *H. pylori* appears to occur via human-to-human spread since no environmental reservoir has been identified. Isolation of the organism in the stool implies that fecal-oral transmission is the likely route of infection. The exact mechanisms by which *H. pylori* produces the inflammatory and cellular destructive changes that accompany its infection remain unclear. The prevalence of infection in the United States is linked to lower socioeconomic class. An increased prevalence rate (up to 80%) is also found in family members of an affected patient. It appears that *H. pylori* is the predominant cause of type B antral, or environmental (as opposed to type A, or autoimmune) gastritis. This is based on several lines of evidence including a prevalence of the organism that approaches 100% in patients with type B antral gastritis and a decreased prevalence in those individuals with a specific gastritis precipitated by alcohol or nonsteroidal anti-inflammatory drugs (NSAIDs). Furthermore, the development of active gastritis in patients in volunteer ingestion studies as well as an epidemic of gastritis from accidental inoculation during the course of a study of acid secretory disorders, provide additional evidence. Finally, healing of gastritis upon treatment that eradicates *H. pylori* is the last parameter to fulfill Koch's postulates.

Disease Spectrum. Chronic active gastritis and associated infection with *H. pylori* are common, although infection is not necessarily associated with symptoms. There is conflicting evidence on whether nonulcer dyspepsia is associated with gastritis or *H. pylori* infection, but the balance of information does not support a relationship between the organism and dyspeptic symptoms. However, there has been tremendous interest in the link between *H. pylori* infection and duodenal ulcer. In the past it has been felt that the development of duodenal ulcer results from an imbalance between mucosal defensive factors and aggressive factors that insult the mucosa (acid and pepsin). It is now clear that *H. pylori* should also be considered an aggressive factor based upon several lines of evidence. There is the nearly uniform (>90%) finding of the organism, along with antral gastritis, in patients with duodenal ulcer. There are markedly reduced relapse rates of ulcer in patients in whom the organism is eradicated (0-25% relapse) compared to patients treated with conventional anti-secretory therapy alone (relapse of 70 to 90%).

One trial involved patients presenting at a Veterans Affairs Medical Center with dyspepsia or gastrointestinal hemorrhage who were endoscopically proven to have duodenal ulcers and were invited to participate in a randomized controlled trial to determine whether antibiotic therapy accelerates ulcer healing. All 105 patients who entered the study received ranitidine (Zantac) 300 mg each evening, with or without 2 weeks of "triple therapy" (a regimen with known activity against *H. pylori*). Healing was more rapid in patients receiving triple therapy and only two patients receiving triple therapy suffered persistent infection, whereas all patients treated with ranitidine alone remained positive for *H. pylori.* Although not as well studied as duodenal ulcer, there also is strong evidence for a causative role for *H. pylori* in gastric ulcer. Nearly 100% of patients with ulcers unrelated to NSAIDs have evidence of infection, and there are lower relapse rates in individuals in whom the organism is eradicated. An association between the organism and gastric malignancies is being actively studied.

Diagnosis. The diagnosis of *H. pylori* infection can be made by a variety of noninvasive and invasive tests some of which make use of the organism possessing a potent urease enzyme. Examples include the carbon 13 and carbon 14 urea breath tests which are simple, inexpensive and have sensitivity and specificity between 90 to 95% but will not be commercially available until sometime in the future. Other means to detect the organism include assaying a specimen obtained by biopsy at endoscopy for urease activity (e.g., Clo® test) or histological examination or culture of a mucosal biopsy specimen. Serologic tests are available but do not differentiate between active versus remote infection.

It is now appropriate to detect and eradicate *H. pylori* in patients with peptic ulcer since the natural history of the disease is then markedly improved. The goal of treatment of *H. pylori* infection should be the eradication of the organism since this has been associated with very low rates of recurrence of ulcer (<10% per year). Similar low recurrences are likely with eradication of the organism in patients with gastric ulcer. Patients who undergo upper gastrointestinal endoscopy can be tested for *H. pylori* by submitting a biopsy for culture or for an assay of bacterial urease activity (e.g., the CLO® test). Simple non-invasive tests for *H. pylori* are now widely available, allowing clinicians to definitively diagnose *H. pylori* infection and initiate antibiotic therapy. In patients in whom endoscopy is not performed, empiric antibiotic therapy directed at *H. pylori* is not unreasonable, although to date this has been reserved primarily for patients with recurrent disease. There is no indication to treat patients who have *H. pylori* and nonulcer dyspepsia or gastritis because eradication does not reliably affect their symptoms.

Drug Therapy. Many regimens for treatment of *H. pylori* have been evaluated, but the most sensible, compliance-sensitive approach involves short-term (i.e., 1 to 2 weeks) therapy with clarithromycin, omeprazole, and metronidazole.

Proton-Blockers

Omeprazole and Lansoprazole. Omeprazole and lansoprazole inhibit the gastrin/proton pump, which regulates the final pathway for acid secretion. These drugs are especially effective for patients with gastroesophageal reflux disease, who have not responded to traditional high-dose therapy with H_2 receptor antagonists and antacids.[120,121] They also provide more rapid symptom relief than H_2-blockers in patients with peptic ulcer disease, and are widely used as part of the drug regimen for *H. pylori* infection. Proton pump blockers are considerably more expensive than H_2 blockers; therefore, indications for their appropriate use in patients with gastroesophageal reflux disease need to be clarified. Candidates for omeprazole or lanasoprazole therapy include patients who have severe daytime symptoms, recurrent strictures requiring frequent dilations, or large esophageal ulcerations despite full-dose H_2 blocker therapy. As might be expected, omeprazole yields excellent results; after 4 weeks of treatment, 80% of patients with severe disease heal, and over 90% of patients are free of disease at 8 to 12 weeks. Cessation of the drug prompts recurrences in over 80% of patients by 6 months, and even 40% of patients relapse after switching to full-dose H_2 antagonist therapy for maintenance.[121]

An acceptable treatment strategy might be to cycle proton-blocker treatment for 4 to 8 weeks, followed by an H_2 blocker every 2 to 4 months, while monitoring the serum gastrin level. Recent studies suggest that maintenance therapy with these agents does not predispose patients to adverse side effects or to the development of tumors. Further investigations are required to confirm long-term safety of this class of medication.[121] In general, it is not appropriate to initiate therapy with proton-blockers until more conservative therapy with full-dose H_2 blockers is attempted. However, patients with documented severe, erosive gastroesophageal reflux disease (GERD) should be treated with proton-blockers initially, since superior healing rates and more rapid symptom relief are reported. Many patients cannot tolerate "stepdown" therapy to H_2-blockers, and will require long-term maintenance therapy with a proton pump blocker. Patients who are presently taking omeprazole and have never been treated with H_2 blocker maintenance therapy are appropriate candidates for discontinuation of omeprazole and substitution with H_2 blockers. It should be stressed that the relapse rate after healing is high when medication is stopped or if a lower dose of H_2 blocker is tried as maintenance therapy.

When discontinuing omeprazole or lansoprazole treatment, a *full dose* of an H_2 blocker (cimetidine, 800 mg/day; ranitidine, 300 mg/day; famotidine, 40 mg/day) is usually necessary on a continuous basis to control symptoms in most patients with gastroesophageal reflux disease.[122] Medication for primarily nocturnal symptoms can be initiated using the full dose administered only at night, preferably with the evening meal. Those with daytime reflux should have their medication divided into 12-hour portions. Ranitidine and famotidine are claimed by some to be marginally more effective than cimetidine. A higher dose of ranitidine, 300 mg every 12 hours, inhibits acid production almost to the same level as omeprazole, but a comparable healing rate is not proven. In general, the decision to maintain patients on H_2 blockers versus continuation of long-term therapy with proton-blockers is based on the patient's clinical response, ability to comply with a more expensive medication, and future studies demonstrating clinical superiority of omeprazole or lansoprazole therapy.[122-124]

Nonsteroidal Anti-inflammatory Drugs (NSAIDs)

Nonsteroidal anti-inflammatory drugs (NSAIDs) (see Tables 4-5 and 4-6) can precipitate gastrointestinal side effects. These adverse effects can range from minor gastric irritation to frank peptic ulceration and bleeding. The most serious of these effects result from NSAID-mediated inhibition of gastric prostaglandin synthesis, which is necessary for maintenance of gastric mucosal integrity. A new class of anti-inflammatory agents is currently in late phase clinical trials. This class does *not* inhibit gastric prostaglandin synthesis, and therefore, has the potential of providing pain relief without the adverse GI effects associated with NSAIDs. Although NSAIDs clearly can provide symptomatic relief for patients with chronic, inflammatory osteoarthritic disorders, there is also evidence to suggest that these drugs are over-used,[63] especially in light of their potentially serious, and sometimes life-threatening side effects.

There are many opportunities to discontinue NSAID therapy, and patient selection is of paramount importance.[12,118,125] Each year, more than 60 million prescriptions are written for NSAIDs, and more than 15 million patients are presently receiving long-term therapy. It is estimated that approximately 20% of patients receiving long-term NSAID therapy have some degree of gastric ulceration, with nearly one-half of these individuals having erosions verified by endoscopy. However, most of these upper gastrointestinal lesions remain clinically silent. The Food and Drug Administration estimates that each year, 2% to 4% of patients receiving long-term NSAID therapy are at risk of developing serious gastrointestinal complications.[126,127] These data translate into at least 300,000 to 600,000 cases of complicated ulcer disease annually in the United States occurring secondary to the use of NSAIDs.[128]

Reducing Toxicity. However, there are accepted guidelines for reducing the gastrointestinal toxicity associated with NSAIDs.[12,125] First, the risk of having a gastrointestinal hemorrhage is greatest during the first *6 months* of therapy. Consequently, physicians and pharmacists following patients on NSAID therapy should be especially vigilant during the early stages of therapy. Second, the risk of having gastrointestinal complications from NSAIDs is related to the *dose* of the medication. Consequently, it is prudent to begin NSAID therapy at a dose less than that recommended by the package insert, and to titrate the medication according to symptomatic response in the patient. In general, the initial dose should be approximately 50% of the average recommended dose in the package insert especially in the elderly patient. The dose should be increased only if symptomatic improvement is not reported by the patient.

Some experts recommend that NSAIDs be discontinued once gastrointestinal symptoms occur. Unfortunately, many older patients with NSAID-induced ulceration do not have symptoms of ulcer disease prior to a catastrophic gastrointestinal event. In many cases, the first evidence of ulceration is manifested by bleeding or perforation. Therefore, waiting for symptoms to occur and then intervening with drug discontinuation will probably not have a significant impact on either complication rates or morbidity. A more vigilant approach is to monitor the stool for occult bleeding and minimize the dose of NSAIDs to the lowest required to maintain symptom relief and adequate functional status of the patient.

Table 4-5

Potential Side Effects of Nonsteroidal Anti-inflammatory Drugs*	
System	**Symptoms or Findings**
Gastrointestinal	
	Anorexia, nausea, vomiting, dyspepsia, erosive gastritis, peptic ulcer Constipation Diarrhea† Hepatotoxicity
Hematologic	
	Impaired platelet aggregation and prolonged bleeding time Bleeding, especially in association with anticoagulants or clotting-factor deficiencies
Renal	
	Aggravation of renal failure during circulatory stress (e.g., congestive heart failure, nephrotic syndrome) Precipitation of renal failure in volume depleted, high risk patients Fluid retention and aggravation of congestive heart failure Hyperkalemia
Central nervous system	
	Headaches, dizziness, tinnitus, deafness, drowsiness, confusion, nervousness, profuse sweating Toxic amblyopia
Pulmonary	
	Aggravation of asthma and rhinosinusitis in patients with aspirin hypersensitivity
Obstetric	
	Delayed parturition Postpartum and neonatal bleeding Premature closure of the ductus arteriosus
Dermatologic	
	Allergic skin rashes

*Bone marrow toxicity as well as granulocytosis and aplastic anemia occur rarely. The best established example of bone marrow toxicity is that which occurs with phenylbutazone and oxyphenbutazone. Salicylates other than aspirin lack the gastric and antiplatelet side effects seen with aspirin and other nonsteroidal antiinflammatory drugs.

†Diarrhea is most frequently seen with meclofenamate (approximately 15% of patients).

Table 4-6

Generic Name	Trade Name	Usual Dosage*
Aspirin (plain, buffered, or enteric coated) **Salicylates** (eg, sodium, choline, or salicyl-salicylate)	(many)	2.4 to 6.0 g daily in four divided doses†
Diclofenac	Voltaren, Cefaflan	50 mg bid or tid or 75 mg bid
Diflunisal	Dolobid	500 mg bid
Etodolac	Lodine	600-1200 mg in divided doses
Fenoprofen	Nalfon	300-600 mg qid
Flurbiprofen	Ansaid	200-300 mg in divided doses bid, tid, or qid
Ibuprofen	Advil, Motrin, Nuprin, Rufen, others	200-800 mg qid
Indomethacin	Indocin	25 mg tid or qid 75 mg bid (slow-release preparation)
Ketoprofen	Orudis, Oruvail	50 mg qid or 75 mg tid
Meclofenamate	Meclomen	50-100 mg qid
Mefenamic acid	Ponstell	250 mg qid
Naproxen	Naprosyn, Anaprox, Aleve	250-500 mg bid
Nabumetone	Relafen	1000-2000 mg once or twice a day
Oxaprozin	Daypro	1200 mg once a day or 1800 mg in divided doses
Piroxicam	Feldene	10 or 20 mg once daily
Sulindac	Clinoril	150-200 mg bid
Tolmetin	Tolectin	200-400 mg qid

*Dosages recommended are for long-term therapy (longer than one week). Higher dosages of some of these drugs may be used for short-term therapy (e.g., in acute gouty arthritis). Lower dosages should be used in elderly patients or patients with impairment of kidney or liver function.

†Blood salicylate levels of 20-30 mg/dl should be reached for optimal effect.

One of the most important questions that should be addressed is, should geriatric patients who have a chronic, painful disease be treated with anti-inflammatory drugs known to have significant gastrointestinal toxicity? In fact, many experts now recommend that such patients be managed initially with analgesics such as acetaminophen that do not cause gastrointestinal side effects. Attempts to discontinue nonsteroidal therapy should be given high priority as part of a drug discontinuation program.[129-130] As a first step, whenever possible, NSAIDs should be used at the lowest dose possible to achieve relief of symptoms. In addition, patients should be closely monitored. In patients with non-inflammatory conditions, a trial with acetaminophen may be warranted. Drugs such as misoprostol or proton pump-blockers may be worth considering in high-risk patients (i.e., those with previous peptic ulceration).[131-134]

Oral Anticoagulants

Hemorrhage is the most serious complication of oral anticoagulant drugs (see Table 4-7), occurring in up to 30% of patients who receive these agents. Hemorrhagic complications associated with warfarin use range in severity from minor to life-threatening. Although bleeding can occur at virtually any body site, the gastrointestinal system is most often affected.[135,136]

Despite the risks associated with oral anticoagulants, these agents are indicated in several forms of arterial and venous embolic diseases common in the elderly population. Furthermore, recent studies demonstrate the efficacy of oral anticoagulants in reducing the risk of embolic stroke in patients with chronic atrial fibrillation, which occurs in 2% to 9% of patients over 60 years of age.[98] Despite the effectiveness of oral anticoagulants in reducing morbidity and mortality, some physicians are reluctant to use these agents in older patients because the perceived risk of bleeding complications outweighs the perceived benefits these drugs offer. This concern is supported by trials suggesting that even though older persons take lower doses of anticoagulants, age may increase the risk of hemorrhagic complications.[136,137]

Oral anticoagulants produce therapeutic results at much lower doses than previously suspected. At the present time, an International Normalized Ratio (INR) of 2 to 3 is sufficient to provide adequate thromboembolic prophylaxis in most patients.[138] Some studies suggest an INR of 2.0 to 2.5 is optimal for atrial fibrillation. Unfortunately, the opportunities for discontinuing anticoagulant therapy are few. For example, patients who take anticoagulants for prevention of embolic disease associated with chronic atrial fibrillation require lifelong therapy.[139] In addition, patients who are taking these agents for prophylaxis of embolic disease after mechanical cardiac valve replacement or tissue valve in the neutral position also require long-term maintenance therapy, and the opportunities for discontinuation are virtually nil. On the other hand, patients who take oral anticoagulation therapy for the treatment of venous embolic disease or nonlife-threatening pulmonary embolism can frequently have the medication withdrawn after 3 months, assuming risk factors that originally caused venous embolism are corrected. (See section, Indications and Guidelines for Antithrombotic Therapy.)

Of the factors that influence the risk of serious bleeding from oral anticoagulation, drug interactions play an important role (see Table 4-7). Many agents, including some NSAIDs, alter warfarin metabolism or protein binding and may theoretically increase the risk of bleeding. But of the many potential interactions, NSAIDs are of special interest because they are widely used by the elderly and substantially increase the risk of gastric erosions and ulceration.

Although it is frequently difficult to discontinue anticoagulant use, it is sometimes possible to eliminate medications from the drug regimen that are known to potentiate the risk of gastrointestinal hemorrhage. Combined use of NSAIDs and oral anticoagulants theoretically increases the risk of gastrointestinal hemorrhage in the elderly. Until recently, few studies supported the validity of this association. However, it is now clear that the concurrent use of NSAIDs and oral anticoagulants places elderly persons at risk for hemorrhagic peptic ulcer disease. Specifically, there is a nearly thirteen-fold increase in the risk of developing hemorrhagic peptic ulcer disease. This suggests that NSAIDs should be prescribed with extreme caution in patients undergoing anticoagulation therapy. Moreover, whenever it is possible to use medications other than NSAIDs to provide symptomatic relief, these agents are preferable to long-term NSAID therapy.[140]

Table 4-7

Warfarin antagonists and potentiators	
Antagonists	**Potentiators**
Barbiturates Carbamazepine Cholestyramine (when administered with warfarin) Glutethimide Griseofulvin Rifampin Vitamin K	Amiodarone Anabolic steroids Aspirin Chloramphenicol Cimetidine Ciprofloxacin Clofibrate Dextrothyroxine Disulfiram Erythromycin Fluconazole Hepatotoxins Metronidazole Miconazole Nalidixic Acid Norfloxacin Quinine Sulfinpyrazone Sulfonamides Tamoxifen Third-generation cephalosporins

Inhaled Beta Agonists

Numerous reports over the past several years suggested that regular use, and especially overuse, of inhaled beta agonists may lead to increased morbidity and mortality in patients with asthma. In particular, chronic use of inhaled beta agonists was implicated in the rising mortality associated with asthma; several mechanisms were proposed to explain why long-term use of these agents may lead to more severe complications. First, paradoxical bronchoconstriction from beta agonist use is reported, although this is more likely due to the propellant used in the metered dose inhaler than to the medication itself. Beta agonists also stimulate airway secretions, which may cause further narrowing of the airways. By using beta agonists regularly, patients may unwittingly cause greater exposure to asthma precipitants, which can exacerbate the disease. Whatever the mechanism, several well-publicized studies show that patients who use inhaled beta agonists regularly have accelerated decline in ventilatory function and higher asthma-related mortality than those who use the medication only *as needed* for exacerbations. Clearly, cautious use is warranted.

Although the opportunities for complete cessation of beta agonist therapy may be limited, patients should be instructed to use their inhalers primarily for acute symptomatic relief associated with exacerbations of asthma or prophylaxis of exercise-induced asthma. It is important to emphasize that asthma is fundamentally an inflammatory disease of the airways that can be triggered by numerous stimuli, including inhaled allergens, respiratory infections, exercise, cold, and other physical factors. Beta agonists can help alleviate the bronchospasm that results from airway inflammation, but they do little else. Corticosteroid therapy, preferably via inhalation, is more effective and appropriate as the mainstay of preventive and maintenance therapy in asthma and may help wean patients from chronic beta agonist therapy. Patient education also is important. Many asthmatics overuse beta agonists because of the relatively quick short-term relief they provide, but they fail to consider the long-term sequelae that are associated with chronic use of this medication.

Corticosteroids

Chronic corticosteroid therapy has a number of well-recognized side effects, including glucose intolerance, mental status changes, cataracts, osteoporosis, suppression of the immune system, and myopathy. Suppression of the hypothalamic-pituitary-adrenal (HPA) axis and inadequate intrinsic corticosteroid output by the adrenal gland is another widely known complication of chronic steroid treatment. This was initially recognized about 40 years ago when the first episodes of postoperative cardiovascular collapse and death were noted in association with steroid therapy withdrawal. Patients with insufficient adrenal function and a suppressed HPA axis are unable to increase corticosteroid output in the perioperative and postoperative settings and in response to other forms of stress. HPA axis suppression is related to a number of factors, including the duration of steroid therapy, the cumulative steroid dose, maximum steroid dose, and the current steroid dose just prior to discontinuation. Which of these factors is most important in producing suppression of the HPA axis is controversial. However, attempts should be made to reduce the dose or discontinue steroid therapy in patients who are being managed with this agent for long-term inflammatory conditions.

Naturally, discontinuation of steroid therapy or reduction of drug dosage will be dictated by symptomatic improvement of the patient, clinical stability, and monitoring of other laboratory parameters indicating the severity of the chronic inflammatory condition. When dose tapering is implemented, it is important to consider suppression of the HPA axis. Duration of therapy, dose interval, dose level, cumulative dose, and highest steroid dose are all thought to be contributing factors in HPA suppression. However, uncertainty about their significance has led to prolonged tapering courses of steroids, and frequent, empiric short-term increases in steroid dose to cover the stress of surgery and other medical illnesses. A recent study demonstrated that no patients receiving < 5 mg/day of prednisone had suppressed HPA axis function and that the dose of steroid to which the patient is tapered is more important than the rate of tapering.[103]

Accordingly, it is recommended that patients be weaned from steroid therapy by a stepwise reduction in daily dose as quickly as feasible, based on severity of illness and steroid withdrawal symptoms. Duration of chronic therapy, total cumulative dose, and highest steroid dose are not significant. An alternate-day steroid regimen is also unnecessary. With < 10 mg per day of prednisone, partial recovery of the HPA axis takes place. Provocative stress testing can serve to confirm adequacy of the adrenal gland. Alternatively, patients can receive supplemental stress steroid therapy. Below 7.5 mg of prednisone per day, full recovery is possible but variable, and patients should either have rapid intravenous adrenocorticotropic testing or empiric steroid stress therapy. Below 5 mg/day of prednisone, however, full recovery of the HPA axis is expected, and while provocative testing is probably unnecessary, a broader recommendation not to perform this requires larger confirmatory trials.

Steroid Tapering. Recommendations regarding tapering of short-term steroid courses are well established. The short-term side effects of corticosteroids include hyperglycemia, weight gain, fluid retention, peptic ulcer disease, hypertension, aseptic necrosis of the femoral head, and mood alterations. The corticosteroids of choice for use in the acute-care setting are prednisone or its active form, prednisolone, which is also available in an intravenous form, (methylprednisolone). Prednisone and prednisolone are five and six times more potent than endogenous hydrocortisone, respectively. Clinically significant improvement with these drugs is measurable 3 hours after administration, and peak effectiveness is reached at 6 to 12 hours. There is no question that steroids reduce the rate of relapse following acute treatment of asthma. More recently, there has been mounting evidence that early administration of steroids reduces admission rates for asthma in both adults and children.

In general, intravenous administration of steroids is indicated in patients with asthma who also require hospitalization. Despite routine use of intravenous steroids, there is no evidence that this route is any more effective than oral forms of steroids. In fact, recent studies show that there were no significant differences in peak expiratory flow, and ratio of forced expiratory flows at 25% and 75% of vital capacity between oral and intravenous steroid administration. The incidence of minor side effects was the same in both groups, and no patient had difficulty swallowing the large number of pills required for steroid therapy. Moreover, the number of days of hospitalization was similar in intravenous and oral steroid groups, and further analysis of subgroups revealed no differences between patients receiving 160 mg/day orally and those receiving the intravenous regimen. Based on this investigation, many experts conclude that oral methylprednisolone is safe and effective in the treatment of acute asthma.[141]

Inhaled steroids, while invaluable in the chronic management of outpatient asthma, do not have a role in acute exacerbations, and patients already receiving such therapy should be given oral steroids during acute exacerbations of their disease. A fear of corticosteroid-induced adrenal suppression has led many physicians to discharge patients with complicated steroid-tapering schedules. It now appears that this is unnecessary. Adrenal suppression is not usually seen until after at least 2 weeks of corticosteroid therapy, and most asthmatics require much shorter courses of therapy for control of their acute exacerbations. Tapering of steroid therapy is clearly indicated for asthmatic patients who are already taking oral steroids prior to their exacerbation and for those in whom a prolonged course of steroid therapy is anticipated. The majority of asthmatic patients, however, who are discharged on a 3 to 7 day course of steroids will benefit from high-dose "burst" therapy without the need to taper the drug. Such therapy results in clinical improvement that is comparable to longer tapering courses and does not increase the risk of asthma relapse or adrenal insufficiency. In conclusion, when administering oral steroids for a short-term course, short tapering courses over a 3 to 7 day period are sufficient.[141] Finally, it should be stressed that leukotriene inhibitors (Singulair, Accolate) have been shown to reduce oral steroid requirements in patients with asthma.

SUMMARY

This chapter has reviewed a number of commonly used medications that are amenable to discontinuation under appropriate clinical circumstances. The decision to discontinue a medication, or to reduce its dose, depends on specific clinical parameters, which take into account the patient's symptoms and severity of disease. Clearly, however, there are windows of opportunity available for discontinuing medications, thereby reducing toxicity and quality-of-life impairment. For example, in the nursing home setting, studies show that given the availability of alternative behavioral management techniques, antipsychotic medications such as amitriptyline, haloperidol, and benzodiazepines can be discontinued successfully in some geriatric patients. Of special note is the fact that this discontinuation can be accomplished without an increase in behavioral disturbances. It is encouraging to note that up to two thirds of elderly patients placed on an antipsychotic drug withdrawal program successfully completed it. In addition, cardiovascular, gastrointestinal, and central nervous system medications also can be discontinued successfully in a significant percentage of elderly patients, especially those lacking clinical indications for initiation of drug therapy. Although almost half of drug discontinuations were followed by an ADWE, these events were generally not serious and rarely required hospitalization. In fact, drugs that were discontinued were not reinstituted in 60% of patients, a finding that lends credence to the idea that drug reduction programs for such medications as digoxin, furosemide, H_2 blockers, and many other medications may be successful and have acceptable risk/benefit profiles. It should be stressed that careful clinical protocols should be followed when withdrawing medications, especially such drugs as benzodiazepines, H_2-blockers, or beta-adrenergic blockers, inasmuch as cessation of these drugs can cause serious withdrawal symptoms or exacerbation of underlying conditions.

In the case of hypertension, a strong case can be made for nonpharmacologic therapy with lifestyle modifications in a large percentage of patients with early, mild hypertension. Dose requirements for beta blockers and thiazide diuretics often times can be reduced in patients who are obese and who follow a successful weight loss program. Moreover, there are also opportunities for step-down therapy in patients who have adequate blood pressure control for at least one year and who are taking only a single antihypertensive agent. The best candidates are those on multiple drug therapy for hypertension; one or more agents can frequently be discontinued in this subgroup. In other cases, it may be preferable to *replace* a poorly performing anti-hypertensive drug with another *single* agent, rather than *adding* a drug, and thereby committing a patient to unnecessary multiple drug therapy. In the case of cardiovascular disease, additional opportunities for drug cessation exist in patients who are on digoxin therapy *and* have normal sinus rhythm but do *not* have left ventricular systolic dysfunction. Studies show that patients who have normal cardiac function and do not require digoxin for rate control usually can be discontinued from the medication without adverse clinical consequences. Furthermore, the use of type I antiarrhythmic agents does not seem to improve mortality outcomes in patients who are taking them for suppression of non life-threatening ventricular ectopy. Although long-term therapy with aspirin is necessary for the secondary prevention of myocardial infarction, dosages as low as 80 mg of aspirin per day appear to be sufficient to provide cardioprotective effects.

Opportunities exist for discontinuing medications used to treat neuropsychiatric conditions, although these cases require careful scrutiny. Patients who have a history of several depressive episodes frequently require lifelong therapy with antidepressant medications. However, those patients who have only a single episode of depression at a young age may be suitable candidates for gradual withdrawal of antidepressants. Individuals who are being treated with SSRIs for anxiety-related conditions associated with panic disorder may be considered for drug discontinuation after 12 months of treatment and clinical stabilization. Many patients, it should be emphasized, will require long-term treatment, however. Patients who are being treated with benzodiazepines such as alprazolam for long-term management of panic attacks can frequently be discontinued from this drug and managed with an SSRI. Patient selection must be careful; patients who have *not* had panic episodes for 6 to 12 months are considered most suitable for drug tapering and cessation of therapy. Studies show that benzodiazepines should be tapered gradually over a several-month period to improve clinical outcomes and reduce the incidence of undesirable side effects associated with benzodiazepine withdrawal.

In the case of gastrointestinal disorders, there is still considerable controversy concerning the wisdom of maintaining patients on long-term H_2 blocker or proton blocker therapy. However, the general consensus is that many patients are maintained on these agents unnecessarily. Patients with mild ulcer disease, as well as those taking H_2 blockers for dyspeptic symptoms, can be considered for withdrawal of H_2 blockers. On the other hand, those patients at high risk for recurrent complications associated with ulcer disease may require life-long maintenance therapy. Patients with suspected *H. pylori* infection should receive definitive therapy to eradicate the organism. Opportunities for discontinuation of corticosteroids, NSAIDs, and dipyridamole ought to be investigated for all patients on long-term therapy with these medications.

Ultimately, the decision to discontinue a medication depends on a combination of factors that includes patient compliance, severity of the underlying disease, and the response of the individual patient to the therapeutic agent being considered for discontinuation. Careful monitoring during the discontinuation process is always advised, and patients should be encouraged to report exacerbations of symptoms or clinical deterioration to their physician or pharmacist.

[1]Beers MH, Ouslander JG, Fingold SF, Morgenstern H, Reuben DB, Rogers W, Zeffren MJ, Beck JC. Inappropriate medication prescribing in skilled-nursing facilities [see comments]. Ann Intern Med 1992 Oct 15;117(8):684-9.

[2]Closser MH. Benzodiazepines and the elderly. A review of potential problems [Review]. J Subst Abuse Treat 1991;8(1-2):35-41.

[3]Beers MH, Ouslander JG, Rollingeer I, Reuben DB, Brooks J, Beck JC. Explicit criteria for determining inappropriate medication use in nursing home residents [Review]. Arch Intern Med 1991 Sep;151(9):1825-32.

[4]Gurwitz JH, Goldberg RJ, Chen Z, Gore JM, Alpert JS. Beta-blocker therapy in acute myocardial infarction: evidence for underutilization in the elderly. Am J Med 1992 Dec;93(6):605-10.

[5]Heston LL, Garrard J, Makris L, Kane RL, Cooper S, Dunham T, Zelterman D. Inadequate treatment of depressed nursing home elderly. J Am Geriatr Soc 1992 Nov;40(11):1117-22.

[6]Anonymous. Why do GPs overprescribe antibiotics? [news]. Br J Hosp Med 1991 Jul;46(1):59.

[7]Beers MH, Fingold SF, Ouslander JG, Reuben DB, Morgenstern H, Beck JC. Characteristics and quality of prescribing by doctors practicing in nursing homes. J Am Geriatr Soc 1993 Aug;41(8):802-7.

[8]Gilley J. Toward rational prescribing [editorial]. BMJ 1994 Mar 19;308(6931):731-2.

[9]Parrish RH. Understanding physician prescribing behavior [letter]. Am J Hosp Pharm 1991 Mar; 48(3):463.

[10]Rovner BW, Edelman BA, Cox MP, Shmuely Y. The impact of antipsychotic drug regulations on psychotropic prescribing practices in nursing homes. Am J Psychiatry 1992 Oct;149(10):1390-2.

[11]Willcox SM, Himmelstein DU, Woolhander S. Inappropriate drug prescribing for the community-dwelling elderly. JAMA 1994 Jul 27;272(4):292-6.

[12]Jordan LK 3d, Jordan LO. Prudent prescribing. Prescribing suggestions for physicians. N C Med J 1992 Nov;53(11):585-8.

[13]Kroenke K, Pinholt EM. Reducing polypharmacy in the elderly. A controlled trial of physician feedback [see comments]. J Am Geriatr Soc 1990;38(1):31-6.

[14]Colley CA, Lucas LM. Polypharmacy: the cure becomes the disease [Review]. J Gen Intern Med 1993 May;8(5):278-83.

[15]Soumerai SB, McLaughlin TJ, Avorn J. Quality assurance for drug prescribing [Review]. Qual Assur Health Care 1990;2(1):37-58.

[16]Col N, Fanale JE, Kronholm P. The role of medication noncompliance and adverse drug reactions in hospitalizations of the elderly. Arch Intern Med 1990 April;150(4):841-5.

[17]Deyo RA, Inui TS, Sullivan B. Noncompliance with arthritis drugs: magnitude, correlates, and clinical implications. J Rheumatol 1981;8:931-6.

[18]Halpern MT, Irwin DE, Brown RE, Clouse J, Hatziandreu EJ. Patient adherence to prescribed potassium supplement therapy. Clin Ther 1993 Nov-Dec;15(6):1133-45; discussion 1120.

[19]Hood JC, Murphy JE. Patient noncompliance can lead to hospital readmissions. Hospitals 1978; 52:79-82, 84.

[20]Weintraub M. Compliance in the elderly. Clin Geriatr Med 1990;6:445-52.

[21]DuBard MB, Goldenberg RL, Copper RL, Hauth JC. Are pill counts valid measures of compliance in clinical obstetric trials? Am J Obst Gynecol 1993 Nov;169(5):1181-2.

[22]Larson EB, et al. Adverse drug reactions associated with global cognitive impairment in elderly persons. Ann Intern Med 1987;107:169-73.

[23]Colley CA, Lucas LM. Polypharmacy: the cure becomes the disease. J Gen Intern Med 1993 May;8(5):278-83.

[24]Arstall MA, Beltrame JF, Mohan P, Wuttke RD, Esterman AJ, Horowitz JD. Incidence of adverse events during treatment with verapamil for suspected acute myocardial infarction. Am J Cardiol 1992 Dec 15;70(20):1611-2.

[25]Holden MD. Over-the-counter medications: Do you know what your patients are taking? Post-grad Med 1992 June;91(8):191-4, 199-200.

[26]Egstrup K. Transient myocardial ischemia after abrupt withdrawal of antianginal therapy in chronic stable angina. Am J Cardiol 1988;61:1219.

[27]File SE, Andrews N. Benzodiazepine withdrawal: behavioural pharmacology and neurochemical changes [Review]. Biochem Soc Symp 1993;59:97-106.

[28]Garner EM, Kelly MW, Thompson DF. Tricyclic antidepressant withdrawal syndrome [Review]. Ann Pharmacother 1993 Sep;27(9):1068-72.

[29]Ballenger JC, Pecknold J, Rickles K, Sellers EM. Medication discontinuation in panic disorder [Review]. J Clin Psychiatry 1993 Oct;54 Suppl:15-21; discussion 22-4.

[30]Burrows GD, Norman TR, Judd FK, Marriott PF. Short-acting versus long-acting benzodiazepines: discontinuation effects in panic disorders [Review]. J Psychiatr Res 1990;24 Suppl 2:65-72.

[31]Dilsaver SC. Withdrawal phenomena associated with antidepressant and antipsychotic agents [Review]. Drug Saf 1994 Feb;10(2):103-14.

[32]Gerety MB, Cornell JE, Plichta DT, Eimer M. Adverse events related to drugs and drug withdrawal in nursing home residents. J Am Geriatr Soc 1993 Dec;41(12):1326-32.

[33]Greenblatt RM, Hollander H, McMaster JR, Henke CJ. Polypharmacy among patients attending an AIDS clinic: utilization of prescribed, unorthodox, and investigational treatments. J Acquir Immune Defic Syndr 1991;4(2):136-43.

[34]Sadler C. A pill for every ill? Nurs Times 1991 Feb 27-Mar;87(9):21.

[35]Beers MH, Ouslander JG, Fingold SF, Morgenstern H, Ruben DB, Rogers W, Zeffren MJ, Beck JC. Inappropriate medication prescribing in skilled-nursing facilities.

[36]Bowler SD, Mitchell CA, Armstrong JG. Corticosteroids in acute severe asthma: effectiveness of low doses [see comments]. Thorax 1992 Aug;47(8):584-7.

[37]Rothschild AJ. Disinhibition, amnestic reactions, and other adverse reactions secondary to triazolam: a review of the literature [Review]. J Clin Psychiatry 1992 Dec;53 Suppl:69-79.

[38]Fries JF, Williams CA, Ramey DR, Bloch DA. The relative toxicity of alternative therapies for rheumatoid arthritis: implications for the therapeutic progression. Semin Arthritis Rheum 1993 Oct;23(2 Suppl 1):68-73.

[39]Alegro S, Fenster PE, Marcus FI. Digitalis therapy in the elderly. Geriatrics 1983; 38:98.

[40]Anonymous. Misoprostol for co-prescription with NSAID [Review]. Drug Ther Bull 1990 Apr 2; 28(7):25-6.

[41]DeSantis G, Harvey KJ, Howard D, Mashford ML, Moulds RF. Improving the quality of antibiotic prescription patterns in general practice. The role of educational intervention. Med J Aust 1994 Apr 18;160(8):502-5.

[42]Forman DE, Coletta D, Kenny D, Kosowsky BD, Stoukides J, Rohrer M, Pastore JO. Clinical issues related to discontinuing digoxin therapy in elderly nursing home patients. Arch Intern Med 1991 Nov;151(11):2194-8.

[43]Gurwitz JH, Noonan JP, Soumerai SB. Reducing the use of H_2-receptor antagonists in the long-term-care setting [see comments]. J Am Geriatr Soc 1992 Apr;40(4):359-64.

[44]Lamy PP. Renal effects of nonsteroidal anti-inflammatory drugs. Heightened risk to the elderly? J Am Geriatr Soc 1986;34:361-7.

[45]Green LW, Purrell CO, Koop CE, et al. Programs to reduce drug errors in the elderly: direct and indirect evidence from patient education. In: Improving Medication Compliance. Reston, Va: National Pharm Council, 1985.

[46]Lamy PP. Compliance in long-term care. Geriatrika 1985;1(8):32.

[47]Botelho RJ, Dudrak R 2d. Home assessment of adherence to long-term medication in the elderly. J Fam Prac 1992 July;35(1):61-5.

[48]Hamilton RA, Briceland LL. Use of prescription-refill records to assess patient compliance. Am J Hosp Pharm 1992 July;49(7):1691-6.

[49]Eisen SA, Miller DK, Woodward RS, Spitznagel E, Przybeck TR.The effect of prescribed daily dose frequency on patient medication compliance. Arch Intern Med 1990 Sept;150(9):1881-4.

[50]Keen PJ. What is the best dosage schedule for patients? J R Soc Med 1991 Nov;84(11):640-1.

[51]Litchman HM. Medication noncompliance: a significant problem and possible strategies. R I Med 1993 Dec;76(12):608-10.

[52]Kruse W, Weber E. Dynamics of drug regiment compliance—its assessment by microprocessor-based monitoring. Eur J Clin Pharmacol 1990;38:561-5.

[53]Rudd P, Marshall G. Resolving problems of measuring compliance with medication monitors. J Compliance Health Care 1987;2:23-35.

[54]Kirsten DK, Wegner RE, Jorres RA, Magnussen H. Effects of theophylline withdrawal in severe chronic obstructive pulmonary disease [see comments]. Chest 1993 Oct;104(4):1101-7.

[55]McCarthy DM. Maintenance therapy for peptic ulcer—who needs it? [Review]. Gastroenterol Jpn 1993 May;28 Suppl 5:172-7.

[56]Applegate WB, Miller ST, Elam JT, Cushman WC, el Derwi D, Brewer A, Graney MJ. Nonpharmacologic intervention to reduce blood pressure in older patients with mild hypertension. Arch Intern Med 1992 Jun;152(6):1162-6.

[57]Galimberti CA, Manni R, Parietti L, Marchioni E, Tartara A. Drug withdrawal in patients with epilepsy: prognostic value of the EEG. Seizure 1992 Sep;2(3):213-22.

[58]Jenck MA, Reynolds MS. Anticonvulsant drug withdrawal in seizure-free patients [Review]. Clin Pharm 1990 Oct;9(10):781-7.

[59]Semla TP, Palla K, Poddig B, Brauner DJ. Effect of the Omnibus Reconciliation Act 1987 on antipsychotic prescribing in nursing home residents. J Am Geriatr Soc 1994 Jun;42(6):648-52.

[60]Shorr RI, Fought RL, Ray WA. Changes in antipsychotic drug use in nursing homes during implementation of the OBRA-87 regulations [see comments]. JAMA 1994 Feb 2;271(5):358-62.

[61]Suck JA. Psychotropic drug practice in nursing homes. J Am Geriatr Soc 1988;36:409-18.

[62]Daly MP, Lamy PP, Richardson JP. Avoiding polypharmacy and iatrogenesis in the nursing home. Md Med J 1994 Feb;43(2):139-44.

[63]Edouard L, Rawson NS. Cutting costs by targeting prescribing practices [letter]. Can Med Assoc J 1994 July 1;151(1):14-5.

[64]Gilbert A, Owen N, Innes JM, Sansom L. Trial of an intervention to reduce chronic benzodiazepine use among residents of aged-care accommodation. Aust N Z J Med 1993 Aug;23(4):343-7.

[65]Lader M. Long-term anxiolytic therapy: the use of drug withdrawal. J Clin Psychiatry 1987; 48:12-6.

[66]Kaplan NM. Long-term effectiveness of nonpharmacological treatment of hypertension [Review]. Hypertension 1991 Sep;18(3 Suppl):I153-60.

[67]Kaplan NM. The potential benefits of nonpharmacological therapy. Am J Hypertens 1990 May; 3(5 Pt 1):425-7.

[68]Fuchs Z, Viskoper JR, Drexler I, Nitzan H, Lubin F, Berlin S, Almagor M, Zulty L, Chetrit A, Mishal J, et al. Comprehensive individualised nonpharmacological treatment programme for hypertension in physician-nurse clinics: two year follow-up. J Hum Hyptertens 1993 Dec;7(6):585-91.

[69]So N, Gotman J. Changes in seizure activity following anticonvulsant drug withdrawal. Neurology 1990 Mar;40(3 Pt1):407-13.

[70]Stults BM. Digoxin use in the elderly. J Am Geriatr Soc 1985;30(3):158.

[71]Hering R, Steiner TJ. Abrupt outpatient withdrawal of medication in analgesic-abusing migraineurs. Lancet 1991 Jun 15;337(8755):1442-3.

[72]Anonymous. The effects of nonpharmacologic interventions on blood pressure of persons with high normal levels. Results of the Trials of Hypertension Prevention, Phase I [published erratum appears in JAMA 1992 May 6;267(17):2330] [see comments]. JAMA 1992 Mar 4; 267(9):1213-20.

[73]Griffin JP, Griffin TD. The economic implications of therapeutic conservatism [see comments]. J R Coll Physicians Lond 1993 Apr;27(2):121-6.

[74]Tjoa HI, Kaplan NM. Nonpharmacological treatment of hypertension in diabetes mellitus [Review]. Diabetes Care 1991 Jun;14(6):449-60.

[75]Pickering TG. Predicting the response to nonpharmacologic treatment in mild hypertension [editorial; comment]. JAMA 1992 Mar 4;267(9):1256-7.

[76]Strasser T. Nonpharmacological treatment [Review]. J Hum Hypertens 1990 Feb;Suppl 1:39-42.

[77]Moriguchi Y, Consoni PR, Hekman PR. Systemic arterial hypertension: results of the change from pharmacological to nonpharmacological treatment. J Cardiovasc Pharmacol 1990;16 Suppl 8:S72-4.

[78]Dall JLC. Maintenance digoxin in elderly patients. Br Med J 1970;2:702.

[79]Packer M, Gheorghiade M, Young JB, et al. Withdrawal of digoxin from patients with chronic congestive heart failure treated with angiotensin-converting-enzyme inhibitors. N Engl J Med 1993;329:1-7.

[80]Akhtar M, Breithardt G, Camm AJ, Coumel P, Janse MJ, Lazzara R, Myerberg RJ, Schwartz PJ, Waldo AL, Wellens HJ, et al. CAST and beyond. Implications of the Cardiac Arrhythmia Suppression Trial. Task Force of the Working Group on Arrhythmias of the European Society of Cardiology [Review]. Circulation 1990 Mar;81(3):1123-7.

[81]Akiyama T, Pawitan Y, Greenberg H, Kuo CS, Reynolds-Haertle RA. Increased risk of death and cardiac arrest from encainide and flecainide in patients after non-Q-wave acute myocardial infarction in the Cardiac Arrhythmia Suppression Trial. CAST investigators. Am J Cardiol 1991 Dec 15;68(17):1551-5.

[82]Anonymous. Randomized antiarrhythmic drug therapy in survivors of cardiac arrest (the CASCADE Study). The CASCADE investigators. Am J Cardiol 1993 Aug 1;72(3):280-7.

[83]Mindardo JD, et al. Clinical characteristics of patients with ventricular fibrillation during antiarrhythmic drug therapy. N Engl J Med 1988;319:257.

[84]Peters RW, Mitchell LB, Brooks MM, Echt DS, Barker AH, Capone R, Liebson PR, Greene HL. Circadian pattern of arrhythmic death in patients receiving encainide, flecainide or moricizine in the Cardiac Arrhythmia Suppression Trial (CAST). J Am Coll Cardiol 1994 Feb;23(2):283-9.

[85]Prystowsky EN, Waldo AL, Fisher JD. Use of disopyramide by arrhythmia specialists after Cardiac Arrhythmia Suppression Trial: patient selection and initial outcome. Am Heart J 1991 May; 121(5):1571-82.

[86]Maynard C. Rehospitalization in surviving patients of out-of-hospital ventricular fibrillation (the CASCADE study). Cardiac Arrest in Seattle: Conventional Amiodarone Drug Evaluation. Am J Cardiol 1993 Dec 1;72(17):1295-300.

[87]Morganroth J, Bigger JT Jr, Anderson JL. Treatment of ventricular arrhythmias by United States cardiologists: a survey before the Cardiac Arrhythmia Suppression Trial results were available. Am J Cardiol 1990 Jan 1;65(1):40-8.

[88]Willund I, Gorkin L, Pawitan Y, Schron E, Schoenberger J, Jared LL, Shumaker S. Methods for assessing quality of life in the cardiac arrhythmia suppression trial (CAST). Qual Life Res 1992 Jun;1(3):187-201.

[89]Puech P. Practical aspects of the use of amiodarone [Review]. Drugs 1991;41 Suppl 2:67-73.

[90]Hine LK, Laird NM, et al. Meta-analysis of empirical long-term antiarrhythmic therapy after myocardial infarction. JAMA 1989;262:3037-40.

[91]Malik R, Ellenbogen KA, Stambler BS, Wood MA. Flecainide: its value and danger [Review]. Heart Dis Stroke 1994 Mar-Apr;3(2):85-9.

[92]Reiffel JA, Cook JR. Physician attitudes toward the use of type IC antiarrhythmics after the Cardiac Arrhythmia Suppression Trial (CAST). Am J Cardiol 1990 Nov 15;66(17):1262-4.

[93]Hirsh J. Oral anticoagulant drugs [see comments] [Review]. N Engl J Med 1991 Jun 27;324(26):1865-75.

[94]Hirsh J, Dalen JE, Fuster V, Harker LB, Slazman EW. Aspirin and other platelet-active drugs. The relationship between dose, effectiveness, and side effects [Review]. Chest 1992 Oct;102(4Suppl):327S-36S.

[95]Samuelsson K, Svensson J. Aspirin: optimal dose in stroke prevention [letter; comment]. Stroke 1993 Aug;24(8)1259-61.

[96]vanGijn J. Aspirin: dose and indications in modern stroke prevention. Neurologic Clin 1992 Feb; 10(1):193-207; discussion 208.

[97]Harker LA, Bernstein EF, et al. Failure of aspirin plus dipyridamole to prevent restenosis after carotid endarterectomy. Ann Intern Med 1992;116:731.

[98]Stroke Prevention in Atrial Fibrillation Study Group. Preliminary report of the stroke prevention in atrial fibrillation study. N Engl J Med 1990;322:863-8.

[99]Anonymous. Drugs for treatment of peptic ulcers. Med Lett Drugs Ther 1991 Nov 29; 33(858):111-4.

[100]Sessler CN. Theophylline toxicity: clinical features of 116 cases. Am J Med 1990;88:567-76.

[101]Hamilton RA, Gordon T. Incidence and cost of hospital admissions secondary to drug interactions involving theophylline. Ann Pharmacother 1992 Dec;26(12):1507-11.

[102]Richardson JP. Theophylline toxicity associated with the administration of ciprofloxacin in a nursing home patient. J Am Geriatr Soc 1990 Mar;38(3):236-8.

[103]LaRochelle GE, et al. Recovery of hypothalamic-pituitary-adrenal (HPA) axis in patients with rheumatic diseases receiving low-dose prednisone. Am J Med;95:258-64.

[104]Laan RF, et al. Low-dose prednisone induces rapid reversible axial bone loss in patients with rheumatoid arthritis. Ann Intern Med 1993;119:963-8.

[105]Broadhead WE, Larson DB, Yarnall KS, Blazer DG, Tse CK. Tricyclic antidepressant prescribing for nonpsychiatric disorders. An analysis based on data from the 1985 National Ambulatory Medical Care Survey [see comments]. J Fam Prac 1991 July;33(1):24-32.

[106]Huszonek JJ, Dewan MJ, Koss M, Hardoby WJ, Isphani A. Antidepressant side effects and physician prescribing patterns [Review]. Ann Clin Psychiatry 1993 Mar;5(1):7-11.

[107]Levin GM, DeVane CL. Prescribing attitudes of different physician groups regarding fluoxetine. Ann Pharmacother 1993 Dec;27(12):1443-7.

[108]Katon W, von Korff M, Lin E, Bush T, Ormel J. Adequacy and duration of antidepressant treatment in primary care. Med Care 1992 Jan;30(1):67-76.

[109]Keller MB, et al. Treatment received by depressed patients. JAMA 1982;248(15):1848.

[110]Greenblatt DJ, Miller LG, Shader RI. Benzodiazepine discontinuation syndromes [Review]. J Psychiatr Res 1990;24 Suppl 2:73-9.

[111]Pecknold JC. Discontinuation reactions to alprazolam in panic disorder. J Psychiat Res 1993;27 Suppl 1:155-70.

[112]Rosenbaum JF. Switching patients from alprazolam to clonazepam. Hosp Comm Psychiatry 1990 Dec;41(12):1302, 1305.

[113]Udelman HD, Udelman DL. Concurrent use of buspirone in anxious patients during withdrawal from alprazolam therapy. J Clin Psychiatry 1990 Sep;51 Suppl:46-50.

[114]Swantek SS, Grossberg GT, Neppe VM, Doubek WG, Martin T, Bender JE. The use of carbamazepine to treat benzodiazepine withdrawal in a geriatric population. J Geriatr Psychiatry Neurol 1991 Apr-Jun;4(2):106-9.

[115]Rickels, Schweizer, et al. Long-term therapeutic use of benzodiazepines: Part I, effects of abrupt discontinuation; Part II, effects of gradual taper. Arch Gen Psychiatry 1990;47:899-915.

[116]Anonymous. Anti-anxiety drug usage in the United States, 1989. Statistical Bulletin-Metropolitan Insurance Companies 1991 Jan-Mar;72(1):18-27.

[117]Bolten W, Gomes JA, Stead H, Geis GS. The gastroduodenal safety and efficacy of the fixed combination of diclofenac and misoprostol in the treatment of osteoarthritis. Br J Rheumatol 1992 Nov;31(11):753-8.

[118]MacWalter RS, Lindsay GH. A policy for minimising NSAID induced peptic ulcer. Scott Med J 1992 Feb;37(1):3-4.

[119]Penston JG, Dixon JS, Boyd EJ, Wormsley KG. A placebo-controlled investigation of duodenal ulcer recurrence after withdrawal of long-term treatment with ranitidine. Aliment Pharmacol Ther 1993 Jun;7(3):259-65.

[120]Creutzfeldt W. Risk-benefit assessment of omeprazole in the treatment of gastrointestinal disorders [Review]. Drug Saf 1994 Jan;10(1):66-82.

[121]Falk GW. Omeprazole: a new drug for the treatment of acid-peptic diseases [Review]. Cleve Clin J Med 1991 Sep-Oct;58(5):418-27.

[122]Hetzel DJ. Controlled clinical trials of omeprazole in the long-term management of reflux disease [Review]. Digestion 1992;51 Suppl 1:35-42.

[123]Holt S, Howden CW. Omeprazole. Overview and opinion [Review]. Dig Dis Sci 1991 Apr; 36(4):385-93.

[124]Maton PN. Omeprazole [Review]. N Engl J Med 1991 Apr 4;324(14):965-75.

[125]Ispano M, Fontana A, Scibilia J, Ortolani C. Oral challenge with alternative nonsteroidal anti-inflammatory drugs (NSAIDs) and paracetamol in patients intolerant to these agents. Drugs 1993; 46 Suppl 1:253-6.

[126]Lamy P. Adverse drug effects [Review]. Clin Geriatr Med 1990 May;6(2):293-307.

[127]Sager DS, Bennett RM. Individualizing the risk/benefit ratio of NSAIDs in older patients [Review]. Geriatrics 1992 Aug;47(8):24-31.

[128]World Health Organization. Health care in the elderly: report of the technical group on the use of medications in the elderly. Drugs 1981;22:279.

[129]Prichard P. The management of upper gastrointestinal problems in patients taking NSAIDs. Aust Fam Physician 1991 Dec;20(12):1739-41.

[130]Stalnikowicz R, Rachmilewitz D. NSAID-induced gastroduodenal damage: is prevention needed? A review and metaanalysis. J Clin Gastroenterol 1993 Oct;17(3):238-43.

[131]Gabriel SE, Campion ME, O'Fallon WM. A cost-utility analysis of misoprostol prophylaxis for rheumatoid arthritis patients receiving nonsteroidal anti-inflammatory drugs. Arthritis Rheum 1994 Mar;37(3):333-41.

[132]Walt RP. Misoprostol for the treatment of peptic ulcer and antiinflammatory-drug-induced gastroduodenal ulceration. N Engl J Med 1992;327:1575.

[133]Graham DY, White RH, Moreland LW, et al. Duodenal and gastric ulcer prevention with misoprostol in arthritis patients taking NSAIDs. Ann Intern Med 1993;119:257.

[134]Graham DY, White RH, Moreland LW, Schubert TT, Katz R, Jaszewski R, Tindall E, Triadafilopoulos G, Stromatt SC, Teoh LS. Duodenal and gastric ulcer prevention with misoprostol in arthritis patients taking NSAIDs. Misoprostol Study Group [see comments]. Ann Intern Med 1993 Aug 15;119(4):257-62.

[135]Bussey HI, Force RW, Bianco TM, et al. Reliance on prothrombin time ratios causes significant errors in anticoagulation therapy. Arch Intern Med 1992;152:278-82. See also the editorial by Hirsh J. Substandard monitoring of warfarin in North America. Arch Intern Med 1992; 152:257-8.

[136]Landefeld CS, Goldman, L. Major bleeding in outpatients treated with warfarin: incidence and prediction by factors known at the start of outpatient therapy. Am J Med 1989;87:144-52; Landefeld CS, Rosenblatt MW, Goldman L. Bleeding in outpatients treated with warfarin: relation to prothrombin time and important remediable lesions. Am J Med 1989;87:153-9.

[137]Jahnigens D, Cooper D, La Force M. Adverse events among hospitalized elderly patients. J Am Geriatr Soc 1988;36:65-72.

[138]Brigden ML. Oral anticoagulant therapy. Newer indications and an improved method of monitoring [Review]. Postgrad Med 1992 Feb 1;91(2):285-8, 293-6.

[139]Hirsh J, Dalen JE, Deykin D, Poller L. Oral anticoagulants. Mechanism of action, clinical effectiveness, and optimal therapeutic range [see comments] [Review]. Chest 1992 Oct;102(4 Suppl):312S-26S.

[140]Ansell JE. Oral anticoagulant therapy—50 years later [Review]. Arch Intern Med 1993 Mar 8; 153(5):586-96.

[141]Chapman KR, et al. Effect of a short course of prednisone in the prevention of early relapse after the emergency room treatment of acute asthma. N Engl J Med 1991;324:788.

[142]Aronow WS. Treatment of Ventricular Arrhythmias In Older Adults. JAGS 1995;43:688-95.

[143]Becker RC, Ansell J. Antithrombotic Therapy. An Abbreviated Reference for Clinicians. Arch Intern Med 1995;155:149.

[144]Bussey HI, Force RW, Bianco TM, et al. Reliance on prothrombin time ratios causes significant errors in anticoagulation therapy. Arch Intern Med 1992;152:278-82.

[145]Hirsh J. Substandard monitoring of warfarin in North America. Arch Intern Med 1992;152:257-8.

[146]A. Pini M. Prophylaxis of venous thromboembolism: the old and the new. Haematologica. 1995; 80(suppl 2):66-77.

[147]de Valk H, Banga J, Wester W, et al. Comparing subcutaneous danaparoid with intravenous unfractionated heparin for the treatment of venous thromboembolism. Ann Intern Med 1995;123-1-9.

[148]Meuleman D. Orgaran (Org 10172): its pharmacological profile in experimental models. Haemostasis 1992;22:58-65.

[149]Lindmarker P, Holmstrom M, Granqvist S, et al. Comparison of once daily subcutaneous Fragmin with continuous intravenous unfractionated heparin in the treatment of deep venous thrombosis. Thromb Haemostat 1994;72:186-190.

[150]Leizorovicz A, Simonneau G, Decousus H, et al. Comparison of efficacy and safety of low molecular weight heparins and unfractionated heparin in the initial treatment of deep venous thrombosis: a meta-analysis. Br Med J 1994;309-304.

[151]Lensing A, Prins M, Davidson B, et al. Treatment of deep venous thrombosis with low molecular weight heparins; a meta-analysis. Arch Intern Medical 1995;155:601-607.

[152]Koopman M, Prandoni P, Piovella F, et al. Treatment of venous thrombosis with intravenous unfractionated heparin administered in the hospital as compared with subcutaneous low-molecular-weight heparin administered at home. N Engl J Med 1996;334:628-687.

[153]Carter C, Kelton J, Hirsh J, et al. The relationship between the hemorrhagic and antithrombotic properties of low molecular weight heparins and heparin. Blood 1982;59:1239.

[154]Hirsh J, Levine M. Low molecular weight heparin. Blood 1992;79:1-17.

[155]Levine M, Gent M, Hirsh J, et al. A comparison of low molecular weight heparin administered primarily at home with fractionated heparin administered in the hospital for proximal deep vein thrombosis. N Engl J Med 1996;334:677-681.

[156]Wittkowsky AK. In Young LY, Koda-Kimble MA, eds. Applied therapeutics: the clinical use of drugs. Applied Therapeutics 6th ed Vancouver, WA 1995;12.1-12.25.

[157]Creager MA, Dzau VJ. Vascular diseases of the extremities. In Isselbacher KJ, Braunwald E, Wilson JD, eds. Principles of Internal Medicine. 13th ed. New York: McGraw-Hill; 1994:1135-43.

[158]Schafer AI. Low molecular weight heparin—an opportunity for home treatment of venous thrombosis. N Engl J Med. 1996;334:724-5. Editorial.

[159]Cziraky MJ, Spinler SA. Low molecular weight heparins for the treatment of deep-vein thrombosis. Clin Pharm. 1993;12:892-9.

[160]Gibaldi M, Wittkowsky AK. Contemporary use of and future roles for heparin in antithrombotic therapy. J Clin Pharmacol. 1995;35:1031-45.

[161]Leizorovicz A, Simonneau G, Decousus H, et al. Comparison of efficacy and safety of low molecular weight heparins and unfractionated heparin in initial treatment of deep venous thrombosis: a meta-analysis. BMJ. 1994;309:299-304.

[162]Lensing AWA, Prins MH, Davidson BL, et al. Treatment of deep venous thrombosis with low-molecular-weight heparins. Arch Intern Med. 1995;155:601-7.

[163]Siragusa S, Cosmi B, Piovella F, et al. Low-molecular weight heparins and unfractionated heparin in the treatment of patients with acute venous thromboembolism: results of a meta-analysis. Am J Med. 1996;100:269-77.

[164]Simonneau G, Charbonnier B, Decousus H, et al. Subcutaneous low-molecular-weight heparin compared with continuous intravenous unfractionated heparin in the treatment of proximal deep vein thrombosis. Arch Intern Med. 1993;153:1541-6.

[165]Levine M, Gent M, Hirsh J, et al. A comparison of low-molecular-weight heparin administered primarily at home with unfractionated heparin administered in the hospital for proximal deep-vein thrombosis. N Engl J Med. 1996;334:677-81.

[166]Lindmarker P, Homstrom M, Granqvist S, et al. Comparison of once-daily subcutaneous Fragmin with continuous intravenous unfractionated heparin in the treatment of deep vein thrombosis. Thromb Haemost. 1994;72:186-90.

[167]Koopman MMW, Prandoni P, Piovella F, et al. Treatment of venous thrombosis with intravenous unfractionated heparin administered in the hospital as compared with subcutaneous low-molecular-weight heparin administered at home. N Engl J Med. 1996;334:682-7.

[168]Garrett HM, ed. Red book. Montvale, NJ: Medical Economics; 1996.

[169]Sanchez LA. Pharmacoeconomic principles and methods: an introduction for hospital pharmacists. Hosp Pharm. 1994;29:774-9.

5

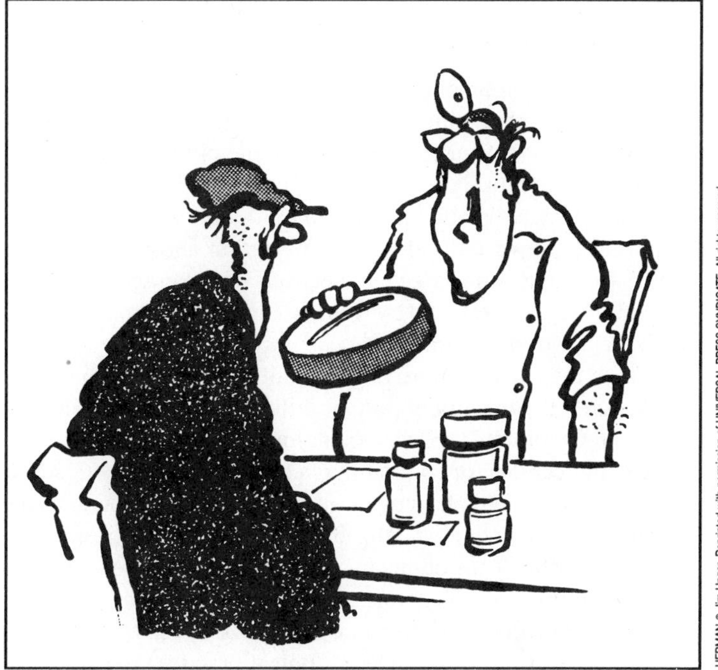

"I want you to take one of these with water every four years."

Pharmatectural Strategies for Antimicrobial Selection

The PPD® (Prescription Resistance, Patient Resistance, and Drug Resistance) System

Perhaps, in no single arena of drug prescribing, can pharmatectural principles make a greater impact on outcome-effectiveness than in the world of antibiotic use. Selecting antibiotics and managing an antibiotic formulary can be confusing, critical, and controversial exercises with formidable financial and clinical implications. With the introduction of so many new antimicrobial agents, the noise level in the "antibiotic of choice" arena has become almost deafening. There are claims and counter-claims for the superiority of one drug over another or of one class over another, with many of these opinions being rendered on the basis of personal anecdotal experience and selective interpretation of clinical trials. Since precise delineation of an etiologic agent is often impractical or unnecessary in the outpatient environment, antibiotic selection is almost always empiric and rarely benefits, at least initially, from microbiologic identification or susceptibility results.

There are other pitfalls as well. Many patients may not require antibiotic therapy, although distinguishing among patients who do and do not require antimicrobial intervention can be a formidable clinical challenge. Even if an antibiotic with an appropriate spectrum of coverage is identified, the issue of medication compliance remains, which can be woefully inadequate in the case of agents requiring multiple daily dose administration and prolonged courses of therapy. Aside from ensuring targeted spectrum of coverage, the issues of palatability, tolerance, side effects, and convenience are fundamental to maximizing cure rates in the real-world environment.

With the recent explosive growth of the antibiotic pharmacopoeia, appreciating subtle but clinically important differences among antimicrobials has become increasingly difficult. Newer quinolones have become available that have expanded indications for community-acquired pneumonia (CAP) and intra-abdominal infections, and one advanced generation macrolide is now indicated for parenteral therapy in hospitalized patients with lower respiratory tract infections. It may be difficult for clinicians to keep abreast of new indications, new agents, and their clinical implications.

Unfortunately, the selection process is never easy, even for well-educated practitioners at the front lines of clinical practice. Experienced clinicians, especially those who work in a managed care environment, are particularly aware of the debate: To choose a new, more conveniently dosed and, usually, more costly, antimicrobial with documented patient-friendliness and more predictable coverage or to choose a less expensive, vintage, warhorse drug with undesirable side effects—one that is "report card" and formulary-friendly—and that requires a 30-dose course of therapy. That is the question.

The fact remains that no matter how the issue is framed, nothing seems to produce more debate among health care practitioners than selection strategies for outpatient antibiotic therapy. In addition, it should be stressed that in clinical environments that are patient volume-driven and that are dominated by capitated reimbursement arrangements, there are powerful incentives to cure infections the first time around (i.e., within the framework of the first prescription generated in the initial visit).

Although optimizing cure rates with so-called convenient, dose- and duration-friendly branded agents that provide appropriate coverage may be perceived as costly on a course of therapy basis, it is important to stress that antimicrobials with these properties also can help avoid the unnecessary costs of patient re-evaluations, return visits, treatment failures, patient dissatisfaction, and the pharmacological reservicing cost associated with initiating a second course of antibiotics. In this sense, antibiotics that lower barriers to clinical cure can be seen as "productivity" tools that improve efficiency of clinical care and potentially reduce the overall costs associated with outpatient management of infections.

Clearly, coverage of implicated pathogens is critical for cost-effective care. Making matters worse is the difficulty of identifying an appropriate, cost-effective antibiotic that is "smart" enough to provide coverage against the most likely offending organisms in a particular patient. For example, in children with otitis media, a so-called "high-performing" antibiotic must be "smart" enough to cover appropriate species of *Streptococcus pneumoniae, Haemophilus influenzae,* and *Moraxella catarrhalis.* In adults with CAP, the corral of coverage must be expanded to include atypical organisms—*Mycoplasma pneumoniae, Legionella pneumophila,* and *Chlamydia pneumoniae*—which are now implicated in about 22% of cases of CAP.

The road from the clinician's prescription pad to clinical cure depends on many factors (i.e., beyond spectrum of coverage) including prescription, patient, drug, (PPD) and in the case of suspensions, parent-resistance. The PPD approach to antimicrobial selection in the emergency and primary care setting attempts to account for all the factors—and potential barriers—that go into the equation for clinical cure. These include cost of the medication, compliance profile, palatability issues, duration of therapy, GI side-effect profile, convenience of dosing, and spectrum of coverage.

Overcoming these barriers to clinical cure is essential for enhancing clinical outcomes and reducing the costs of therapy and complications of the disease. The goal, of course, is to identify an antibiotic that will simultaneously manage cost, manage coverage, and manage compliance, so that the clinician can manage care of the patient in an outcome-effective manner.

The Antimicrobial Armamentarium: Uses and Abuses

In addition to the older, so-called "standard" antibiotics—including the penicillins and sulfonamides—there are many newer oral agents, particularly cephalosporins, quinolones, and macrolides, that play a role in treating bacterial infections commonly encountered in the Emergency Department (ED) and primary care setting. Antibiotics typically have been evaluated by comparing spectrum of activity, clinical efficacy, toxicity (adverse drug reactions and interactions), pharmacokinetics (convenience and compliance with dosing), and cost. In addition to these parameters, there are at least two additional factors that must be taken into account when comparing antibiotics: 1) the selective pressure for the emergence of resistant organisms; and 2) the overall cost-effectiveness or outcome cost.

The newer antibiotics, although possessing variable increases in the spectrum of activity over older agents, have uniformly been shown in clinical trials to be equally, but rarely more efficacious, than standard therapy. It should be stressed, however, that within the context of clinical trials, patients are frequently given incentives through counseling and pill counts to comply with their regimens. Notably, outcomes in these studies may deviate from those seen in the "real world," where noncompliance with antibiotics is a major barrier to clinical cure. It may be difficult to extrapolate from cure rates published in idealized clinical trials to the front lines of clinical practice.

Generally speaking, most advantages associated with newer drugs are typically found in parameters rather than spectrum of coverage. For example, some of the newer agents have an improved toxicity or drug interaction profile compared with conventional therapy. One drawback of newer agents, even those that belong to familiar classes of antibiotics, is limited information regarding specific toxicity issues. In this regard, temafloxacin, a fluoroquinolone antibiotic, was withdrawn from the worldwide market just 4 months after approval in the United States because of subsequent reports of serious hemolysis, with or without other organ system dysfunction. This adverse reaction (temafloxacin syndrome) was not recognized in patients participating in the clinical trials, but became evident when nearly 200,000 prescriptions were written after approval.[1,2]

Outcome Considerations in Antibiotic Selection

In the best and most cost-effective of all worlds, the antibiotic selection process for common infections such as pneumonia, acute otitis media, cystitis, and pelvic inflammatory disease would be based on an outcome-oriented assessment of the total cost of cure associated with managing these conditions. This guide will underscore the importance of identifying therapeutic agents that, because of favorable cost, compliance, safety, and pathogen coverage features, are able to reduce barriers to clinical cure. In general, antimicrobial agents that satisfy these criteria will improve "first time around" cure rates and thereby reduce overall outcome costs.

Among the factors that could be included in a pharmatectural-based outcome analysis (i.e., the total costs associated with diagnosis, management, and cure of outpatient infection) are the following: cost of the initial physician visit; cost of the medication(s) used for the initial course of antibiotic therapy; human resource time (telephone time, revisits, etc.) required to service queries regarding the drug and/or its side effects; the cost of practitioner re-evaluations for treatment failures; hospitalization costs due to treatment failure; the cost of additional courses of therapy to achieve therapeutic endpoints (clinical improvement or bacterial eradication); the economic opportunity cost sustained by patients (or parents) because of time lost from work to care for themselves or their child; the cost of medications or other devices (diapers, etc.) to service the GI side effects (diarrhea) of the medications; and the short- and long-term sequelae of treatment failures or repeated episodes of infection.

Although comprehensive, outcome-directed studies addressing all of these variables for most outpatient infections are not currently available, other outcome-sensitive drug therapy assessment tools can be pressed into service for the purpose of drug selection. Using these parameters is fundamental to the pharmatectural approach to antibiotic selection. The prescription, patient, and drug resistance (PPD) approach to drug selection permits pharmacists and physicians to evaluate and compare the clinical success profiles of one antibiotic versus another. These comparisons are based on a synthetic approach constructed according to established specifications and parameters such as price, daily dose frequency, duration of therapy, palatability, side-effect profile, and spectrum of coverage.[3-15]

From the perspective of prescribing antibiotics in the outpatient setting, it must be emphasized that each of the PPD resistance barriers is important, and that if one or more of these barriers (cost, side-effect profile, lack of convenience, inadequate coverage of pathogens) is of sufficient magnitude, it may influence the overall real-world cure rate.[9,11,14,16] These barriers are discussed in the following sections.

Prescription Resistance, Patient Resistance, and Drug Resistance (PPD System)

The prescription, patient, and drug (PPD) resistance approach to drug selection permits primary care and emergency physicians to evaluate and compare the clinical success profiles of one antibiotic vs. another according to established specifications and parameters, such as price, daily dose frequency, duration of therapy, side-effect profile, and spectrum of coverage.[3-5]

Having a patient achieve a favorable outcome requires negotiating several real-world PPD resistance barriers. Using this outcome-based, cost-effectiveness-oriented, "real-world" approach, some antibiotics will fare better than others. It must be stressed that each of the three resistance barriers is equally important in determining whether clinical cure is likely. These barriers are discussed in the following sections.

Prescription Resistance

Prescription resistance refers to the likelihood that patients will actually fill their prescription. Studies show that up to 25% of patients given a prescription for an antibiotic never even fill their prescription, and the risk of non-filling increases with the cost of the medication.[3,5] Accordingly, the primary determinant of prescription resistance is the cost of the medication. In addition to the cost of the antibiotic, other factors affecting the patient's propensity for filling the prescription include: 1) The clinical provider's persuasiveness in convincing the patient he or she needs the antibiotic as part of their therapeutic program; 2) "word of mouth" about the drug (i.e., is it perceived by the community as a tolerable, or poorly tolerated, medication?); 3) previous experiences with the medication; and 4) the patient's perception of the seriousness of his or her condition.

Patient Resistance

Patient resistance refers to the likelihood that the patient will actually take the medication for the entire course of therapy, assuming that the prescription-resistance barrier was low enough to induce the patient to actually fill the prescription. Once filled there are a number of factors that determine whether patient resistance will be high or low—or, stated differently, how likely the patient is to be compliant with his or her medication.

The principal factors determining patient resistance are the daily dose frequency of the medication, the duration of therapy, the side-effect profile, and the discontinuation rate of the drug. Not surprisingly, the antibiotic with the lowest patient resistance profile would be characterized by a well-tolerated, single-dose therapy administered under supervision. Examples of low patient resistance regimens include a single 2 g dose of metronidazole for trichomoniasis, single-dose therapy for gonorrhea, a single 1 g dose of azithromycin for uncomplicated chlamydial cervicitis, or a single 150 mg dose of fluconazole for the treatment of candida vaginitis.

These approaches satisfy the criteria for Universal Compliance Precautions (UCP) because, in general, administration of single-dose therapy especially when given under supervision prevents noncompliance-mediated therapeutic failures from undermining the success of a drug regimen. Generally speaking, patient resistance is acceptable, but still less than perfect, for therapeutic courses based on antibiotics dosed on a once-daily basis and given for 5 or fewer days, and that have a low incidence of side effects (usually GI in origin). Patient resistance becomes an important barrier to clinical cure for medications given on a twice-daily or greater daily dose frequency, those given for 7 days or more, and for agents that have GI side effects that are severe enough to produce drug discontinuation.[4,5]

Special considerations apply to antibiotic suspensions for the pediatric age group. Since children do not self-administer medications, compliance in the pediatric age group depends greatly upon the parent's willingness and motivation to give the antibiotic. Similarly, medications that require refrigeration, must be administered by day care or school personnel or require special timing requirements with respect to food intake increase parent resistance and, therefore, may compromise proper, timely administration.[16,17] In particular, drugs with GI side effects, especially diarrhea, create a "clean-up" factor that may discourage parents from completing the entire course of therapy as prescribed. This can be called "parent" resistance. At least one study has shown that poor medication compliance is the most common cause of antibiotic treatment failures.[17]

The effect of patient resistance barriers (i.e., compliance profile) on clinical outcomes in outpatient infections should never be underestimated. Even when the cost of the medication is sufficiently low to encourage prescription fulfillment, if patient resistance factors are sufficiently imposing, clinical cure rates will be compromised.

Drug Resistance

Drug resistance refers to the spectrum of coverage (i.e., antimicrobial activity) provided by the antibiotic against the most likely organisms encountered in the specific infection against which the drug is directed. For example, organisms targeted for empiric therapy in community-acquired respiratory infections include *Streptococcus pneumoniae, Haemophilus influenzae, Mycoplasma pneumoniae,* and *Moraxella catarrhalis. Chlamydia pneumoniae* is also cited as an increasingly common etiologic agent.

An antibiotic with proven activity against all these organisms would provide optimal coverage and, therefore, would be associated with a low drug-resistance barrier. On the other hand, an antibiotic with activity against only three (or fewer) of these organisms might produce therapeutic failures in a significant percentage of cases and would be associated with a drug-resistance barrier obstructing the outcome highway. The risk of infection caused by specific organisms is often related to patient characteristics. *H. influenzae* is unusual in nonsmoking patients without COPD, and *M. pneumoniae* is less frequent outside the youngest adult age group.

Drug resistance must always be considered when selecting an antibiotic. Even when the medication is inexpensive and well-tolerated (i.e., prescription- and patient-resistance barriers are low), if the drug fails to provide optimal activity at the "business end" (it has poor spectrum of coverage against anticipated organisms at the site of infection), cure rates will be compromised.

Optimal PPD Profiles

Optimal PPD profiles are characterized by antibiotics with low prescription, patient, and drug resistance. The most desirable agent should be inexpensive enough to encourage the patient to have the prescription filled; well-tolerated by the patient to promote compliance; and active against all the anticipated pathogens, so as to prevent the necessity of retreatment due to resistant organisms.

Recent Advances in Antibiotic Therapy: New Agents, Formulations, Treatment Indications, and Antimicrobial Combinations

Among the most important advantages of the newer antibiotics is improved pharmacokinetics, which permits less frequent dosing, increased convenience, shorter duration of therapy, and increased compliance. Azithromycin is one important example of a newer agent with these features. In general, compliance is thought to be enhanced by once- or twice-daily dosing compared to more frequent administration.[3,4] Although this has been confirmed by "science of compliance" studies, other factors such as a good doctor-patient relationship reinforcing the importance of taking medications as prescribed also may be important in generating improved compliance.[5]

As a rule, the advantage of less-frequent dosing must always be weighed against the generally higher cost of newer antibiotics as well as the antibiotic's spectrum of activity. In this regard, although newer antibiotics are generally more expensive compared to established agents, there is considerable variability among the newer agents. (See Table 5-1)

Furthermore, the appropriateness of broad-spectrum antibiotic therapy in a setting in which narrower-spectrum therapy would suffice must be questioned, because of the selective pressure for resistance exerted. There are currently numerous examples of resistant organisms in both the community and hospital settings, including methicillin-resistant staphylococci, VISA, VRE, penicillin- and cephalosporin-resistant pneumococci, penicillin- and tetracycline-resistant gonococci, beta-lactamase-producing *H. influenzae* associated with amoxicillin resistance, and multiple antibiotic-resistant gram-negative bacilli.[6,7,18]

It appears that the increasing incidence of antibiotic resistance is in large part due to antibiotic prescribing and misuse.[19] Despite increased worry over antibiotic resistance, physicians are prescribing more expensive, broad-spectrum antibiotics (especially cephalosporins and quinolones) in the United States.[20] Because of uncertain benefits, there recently has been a plea to decrease inappro-

Table 5-1

Commonly Used Outpatient Antibiotics			
Antibiotic	**Brand Name**	**Usual Adult Dose***	**Cost†**
CEPHALOSPORINS			
First Generation:			
Cephalexin		250, 500 mg qid	$20, $39
Cefadroxil	Duricef	500, 1000 mg bid	$62, $116
Second Generation:			
Cefuroxime axetil	Ceftin	250, 500 mg bid	$63, $122
Cefprozil	Cefzil	250, 500 mg bid	$55, $107
Cefaclor	Ceclor	250, 500 mg tid	$56, $110
Loracarbef	Lorabid	200, 400 mg bid	$60, $76
Third Generation:			
Cefixime	Suprax	200, 400 mg qd	$31, $61
Cefpodoxime proxetil	Vantin	200, 400 mg bid	$63, $126
PENICILLINS			
Benzathine penicillin G		1.2 MU IM	$11
Penicillin V		250, 500 mg qid	$2, $4
Amoxicillin	Amoxil	250, 500 mg tid	$5, $10
Dicloxacillin		250, 500 mg qid	$15, $26
Amoxicillin-clavulanate	Augmentin	250, 875 mg bid	$57, $80

Table 5-1

Commonly Used Outpatient Antibiotics — cont'd.			
Antibiotic	**Brand Name**	**Usual Adult Dose***	**Cost†**
FLUOROQUINOLONES			
Ciprofloxacin	Cipro	250, 500, 750 mg bid	$54, $62, $110
Ofloxacin	Floxin	200, 300, 400 mg bid	$59, $70, $73
Norfloxacin	Noroxin	400 mg bid	$51
Lomefloxacin	Maxaquin	400 mg qd	$64
Enoxacin	Penetrex	200, 400 mg bid	$63, $63
Levofloxacin	Levaquin	500 mg qd x 7-14 days	$78
Sparfloxacin	Zagam	400 mg day 1, 200 mg days 2-10	$76
Trovafloxacin	Trovan	100 mg or 200 mg qd	$38-68
MACROLIDES			
Erythromycin		250, 500 mg qid	$6, $10
Clarithromycin	Biaxin	250, 500 mg bid	$63, $63
Azithromycin	Zithromax	500 mg day 1, 250 mg days 2-5	$36¥
MISCELLANEOUS			
Trimethoprim-sulfamethoxazole	Septa, Bactrim	1 double-strength bid	$4
Doxycycline	Vibramycin	100 mg bid	$4
Clindamycin	Cleocin	150, 300 mg qid	$36, $88
Metronidazole	Flagyl	500 mg tid	$7
Fosfomycin	Monurol	3 g (one dose)	$22

* Oral unless otherwise stated
† Average whole price (AWP) for 10 days of therapy unless otherwise stated (*1997 Red Book.* Montvale, JH: Medical Economics Data Production Co; 1997). The cost represents the average cost of generic formulations when brand name is not listed.
‡ A carbacephem antibiotic (see text)
¥ Five days of therapy constitutes an entire course of therapy

priate antibiotic use, especially in patients with acute bronchitis who do not have associated chronic obstructive pulmonary disease (COPD).[21] Patients with acute bronchitis unrelated to COPD probably do not benefit from antibiotic therapy. It should be stressed, however, that in patients with COPD, antibiotics do appear to have a role in the treatment of exacerbations caused by bacterial bronchitis.[22]

Although the newer antibiotics have a wide variety of approved indications (see Table 5-2), these agents should be used judiciously. Although studies generally stated that 5% to 16% of penicillin-allergic patients will have a reaction to cephalosporins, the true incidence may be much less (about 3% to 7%).[23] Consequently, cephalosporins may be cautiously administered to the majority of patients with a history of penicillin allergy; however, avoid such therapy in the case of a potential IgE-mediated allergy (anaphylaxis, urticaria).[24]

Cephalosporins. The extended-spectrum cephalosporins include the designated "second-generation" agents cefuroxime axetil and cefprozil.[25,26] The carbacephem antibiotic, loracarbef, has a spectrum of activity similar to these agents.[27] A minor modification of the cephalosporin ring of cefaclor results in the carbacephem designation. These antibiotics have good activity against common gram-positive organisms except for methicillin-resistant staphylococci and enterococci. They are reliably active against *H. influenzae, M. catarrhalis,* and many strains of *Escherichia coli, Proteus mirabilis,* and *Klebsiella pneumoniae.* (See Table 5-2)

In general, but not in all cases, these agents offer no significant advantage over trimethoprim-sulfamethoxazole (TMP/SMZ) for upper or lower respiratory tract pathogens, with the exception of *Streptococcus pyogenes,* which can cause pharyngitis or tonsillitis. Penicillin remains the drug of choice for pharyngitis, except in cases in which a high risk of noncompliance can be anticipated, in which case a macrolide with shorter duration of therapy should be considered. Skin and skin structure infections generally respond well to a first-generation cephalosporin or a penicillinase-resistant penicillin such as dicloxacillin. Cefuroxime axetil has been shown to be as effective as doxycycline in early Lyme disease.[28]

The "third-generation" cephalosporins include cefixime and cefpodoxime proxetil.[29,30] These antibiotics are characterized by an extended spectrum against gram-negative organisms such as *E. coli* and *Klebsiella*; nosocomial bacteria such as *Pseudomonas aeruginosa, Enterobacter, Serratia,* and others are generally resistant to these agents. Cefpodoxime proxetil has moderate gram-positive activity, while that of cefixime is poor. These antibiotics have a variety of approved indications but are generally not superior to established agents for the same indications. (See Table 5-2) Cefpodoxime proxetil has a lower cure rate for uncomplicated urinary tract infections than comparable agents.[31] Both of these agents are effective as one dose-therapy for uncomplicated gonorrhea.[32,33]

Penicillins. Although no dramatic advances have been reported in the penicillin-related antibiotics, the most important recent "modifications" among antimicrobials in this category has been the the new dosing schedule approved for amoxicillin-clavulanate in the treatment of otitis media. Recent approval for twice-daily administration of this antibiotic should be noted, although this agent

Table 5-2

Approved Indications for Newer Oral Antibiotics

ANTIBIOTIC	UPPER RESPIRATORY			LOWER RESPIRATORY TRACT		GENITOURINARY TRACT/SEXUALLY TRANSMITTED DISEASES					MISCELLANEOUS		
	Pharyngitis/ Tonsillitis	Otitis Media	Sinusitis	ABECB	CAP	Uncomp UTI	Comp UTI	Prostatitis	Uncomp GC	Uncomp NGU/C	USSSI	B&J	Infectious Diarrhea
Cefuroxime Axetil	X	X	X	X	X	X			X		X		
Cefprozil	X	X	X	X							X		
Cefaclor	X	X		X	X	X	X				X		
Loracarbef	X	X	X	X	X	X	X				X		
Cefixime	X	X		X		X			X				
Cefpodoxime Proxetil	X	X		X	X	X			X		X		
Amoxicillin/clavulanate		X	X	X	X	X	X						
Ciprofloxacin			X	X	X	X	X				X	X	X
Ofloxacin				X	X	X	X	X	X	X	X		
Norfloxacin						X	X		X				
Lomefloxacin				X†		X	X						
Enoxacin						X	X		X				
Levafloxacin			X	X	X	X	X				X		
Sparfloxacin				X	X								
Fosfomycin						X							
Clarithromycin	X	X	X	X	X						X		
Azithromycin	X	X		X	X				X	X	X		
Dirithromycin	X			X	X						X		
Trovafloxacin			X	X	X	X		X	X	X	X		

† Not *S. pneumoniae*
ABECB = Acute bacterial exacerbation of chronic bronchitis; CAP = Community-acquired pneumonia; Uncomp UTI = Uncomplicated urinary tract infection; Comp UTI = Complicated urinary tract infection; Uncomp GC = Uncomplicated gonorrhea; Uncomp NGU/C = Uncomplicated nongonococcal urethritis/cervicitis; USSSI = Uncomplicated skin and skin structure infection; B&J = Bone and joint infection

does not share the full compliance-promoting benefits of once-daily administration seen with other agents such as azithromycin, cefixime, and cefpodoxime. Although palatability of the amoxicillin is quite acceptable, the incidence of diarrhea is reported in large studies to be about 16%.[30] In vitro coverage of most bacterial offenders causing acute otitis media is favorable.

Amoxicillin-clavulanate. From a practical perspective, amoxicillin-clavulanate is now made in a 200 mg/5 mL and 400 mg/5 mL suspension, which can be administered on a twice daily basis, thus enhancing its compliance profile. This new suspension has a lower concentration of clavulanate and thus has fewer GI side effects (especially diarrhea). Furthermore, dosing differs for these two new suspensions. Otitis media should be treated with 45 mg/kg twice daily, a more convenient dosing pattern than the previous three times daily recommendations, if these suspensions are used. Finally, the new suspensions contain aspartame and should not be used by phenylketonurics.

Extended Spectrum Quinolones

The currently available quinolones include trovafloxacin, grepafloxacin, levofloxacin, sparfloxacin, ciprofloxacin, ofloxacin, norfloxacin, lomefloxacin, and enoxacin.[34-37] (See Table 5-2) Prior to the recent introduction of the extended spectrum fluoroquinolones (trovafloxacin, grepafloxacin, levofloxacin, and sparfloxacin) these antibiotics were characterized by extensive activity against gram-negative organisms including *H. influenzae, M. catarrhalis,* and most enteric bacilli. In addition, ciprofloxacin has good activity against *P. aeruginosa.*

Although most of the quinolones have no useful anaerobic activity except for trovafloxacin, they have moderate gram-positive activity, but resistance has emerged quickly in *S. aureus* and streptococcal activity is borderline, except in the case of the newer quinolones levofloxacin, trovafloxacin, and sparfloxacin (see below). There have been breakthrough bacteremias caused by *S. pneumoniae* reported with ciprofloxacin.[38,39] The older quinolones such as have excellent activity against bacteria commonly causing diarrheal illnesses, including *E. coli, Salmonella, Shigella, Campylobacter,* and *Yersinia.* This class of drugs is contraindicated in pregnancy and in children less than 18 years of age.

Levofloxacin. One of the most important developments in outpatient antibiotic therapy has been the introduction of the extended spectrum quinolones. In this regard, levofloxacin (Levaquin®), the S-enantiomer of ofloxacin, is a new fluoroquinolone antibiotic recently approved by the FDA. It is an extended spectrum quinolone that, compared with older quinolones, has improved activity against gram-positive organisms including *S. pneumoniae.* This has important drug selection implications for management of patients with community-acquired pneumonia and exacerbations of COPD. Levofloxacin, the active stereoisomer of ofloxacin, is available in a parenteral preparation or as a once daily oral preparation that is given for 7 to 14 days.

Levofloxacin is indicated for the treatment of adults (>18 years of age) with mild, moderate, and severe infections including acute maxillary sinusitis, acute bacterial exacerbation of chronic bronchitis, community-acquired pneumonia, uncomplicated skin and skin structure infections, and complicated urinary tract infections including acute pyelonephritis.[40] This antimicrobial is active against many gram-positive organisms including *S. pneumoniae, Enterococcus faecalis, S. aureus,* and *S. pyogenes,* and it also covers atypical pathogens including *Chlamydia pneumoniae, Legionella pneumophila,* and *M. pneumoniae.* It is also active against gram-negative organisms including *Enterobacter cloacae, E. coli, H. influenza, H. parainfluenzae, Klebsiella pneumoniae, M. catarrhalis, Proteus mirabilis,* and *P. aeruginosa.*

When given orally, levofloxacin is dosed once daily, is well absorbed orally, and penetrates well into lung tissue.[40] It is active against a wide range of respiratory pathogens including atypical pathogens and *S. pneumoniae* resistant to penicillin.[37,38] In general, levofloxacin has similar activity against gram-positive organisms such as ofloxacin and ciprofloxacin, and it is more active than ofloxacin and slightly less active than ciprofloxacin against gram-negative organisms.[41,42] In particular, it should be noted that levofloxacin is slightly less active against *P. aeruginosa* than ciprofloxacin.[41,42] Reflecting this sensitivity data, levofloxacin is FDA-approved for treating pseudomonal in the urinary tract only. In contrast, it has been reported to be more active than the older quinolones against *S. pneumoniae* resistant to penicillin.[43]

The drug is available as both an oral and parenteral form, and the oral and IV routes are interchangeable (i.e., same dose). Levofloxacin is generally well tolerated (incidence of adverse reactions <7%) with the most common side effects including nausea, diarrhea, headache, and constipation.[40] Levofloxacin is supplied in a parenteral form for IV use and in 250 mg and 500 mg tablets. The recommended dose is 500 mg IV or orally once daily for 7 to 14 days for upper or lower respiratory tract infections and uncomplicated skin and skin structure infections, and 250 mg once daily for 10 days for complicated UTI or acute pyelonephritis. Food does not affect the absorption of the drug, but it should be taken at least 2 hours before or two hours after antacids containing magnesium or aluminum, as well as sucralfate, metal cations such as iron, and multivitamin preparation with zinc. Dosage adjustment is recommended in patients with impaired renal function (clearance <50 mL/min).[40] All fluoroquinolones have been associated with cartilage damage in animal studies, and therefore, they are not recommended for use in children, adolescents, pregnant and nursing women.

Comparative trials (generally available in abstract form) suggest that levofloxacin is as effective as cefuroxime axetil, cefaclor, and amoxicillin/clavulanate in upper or lower respiratory infections.[44-46] In patients with community-acquired pneumonia, IV levofloxacin with step-down to oral therapy was superior to ceftriaxone with step-down therapy to cefuroxime axetil.[47] About 22% of patients in the cephalosporin arm required the addition of erythromycin or doxycycline due to the presence of atypical respiratory pathogens. The clinical response rates (cure plus improvement) were 88% to 97% for levofloxacin. Microbiological eradication was reported to be 94% to 98%; however, a large number of patients (32% to 43%) were not evaluated for this end point.[44,46,47]

Levofloxacin, ofloxacin, trovafloxacin, sparfloxacin, and grepafloxacin are the quinolones that currently are approved for respiratory tract infections, in particular, for empiric therapy for community acquired pneumonia. Currently, such macrolides as azithromycin or clarithromycin also are recommended for pneumonia in ambulatory, otherwise healthy adults. For older patients, an oral cephalosporin such as cefuroxime axetil, with or without the addition of a macrolide to provide coverage of atypical pathogens, may be considered.[43] In this patient subgroup, levofloxacin and trovafloxacin provide an effective, safe, and cost-attractive outpatient alternative to two-drug combinations, especially in the elderly patient who is deemed well enough to be treated as an outpatient and in whom coverage of gram-negative organisms in addition to coverage of *S. pneumoniae* and atypical pathogens are desirable. (Please refer to "Community-Acquired Pneumonia" section below for a more detailed analysis of drug options in CAP).

Sparfloxacin. Sparfloxacin (Zagan), another extended-spectrum fluoroquinolone antibacterial agent recently approved by the FDA, is a chemically unique fluoroquinolone, with an amino substituent in the five-position and a fluorine substituent in the eight-position of the quinolone nucleus. The amino substituent enhances gram-positive activity,[48] while the fluorine substituent increases plasma half-life[49] but also appears to increase the risk of phototoxicity (e.g., such as lomefloxacin).

Like levofloxacin, sparfloxacin is dosed once a day and provides a wide range of coverage including activity against common gram-positive and gram-negative respiratory pathogens, as well as against the atypical pathogens *Chlamydia pneumonia* and *Mycoplasma pneumonia.* Importantly, sparfloxacin shows excellent activity against penicillin-resistant pneumococcus and multidrug-resistant *H. influenzae* and *M. catarrhalis.*

Sparfloxacin is indicated for the treatment of adults (>18 years old) with the following infections caused by susceptible strains of the designated microorganisms: Community-acquired pneumonia (CAP) caused by *C. pneumoniae, H. influenzae, H. parainfluenzae, M. catarrhalis, M. pneumoniae,* or *S. pneumoniae,* and acute bacterial exacerbation of chronic bronchitis caused by *C. pneumoniae, E. cloacae, H. influenzae, H. parainfluenzae, K. pneumoniae, M. catarrhalis, S. aureus,* or *S. pneumoniae.*[49] In comparative trials, sparfloxacin was as effective as amoxicillin/clavulanate, cefaclor, erythromycin, amoxicillin, ofloxacin, or amoxicillin plus ofloxacin for clearing community-acquired pneumonia.[48,49,50-52] Sparfloxacin is more active than ciprofloxacin against *Mycobacterium tuberculosis,* but is less active against *P. aeruginosa* than ciprofloxacin with a median MIC90 two- to four-fold higher.[48]

Given this drug's excellent and appropriate spectrum of coverage for CAP and bacterial exacerbations of COPD, one issue that will clearly play a determining role in the acceptance of sparfloxacin among emergency medicine and primary care practitioners is the reported incidence of photosensitivity reactions (7.9%), which, in selected individuals (i.e., active, young, outdoor-oriented individuals who are not ill enough from their CAP to require bedrest indoors), can affect patient satisfaction, and potentially, be problematic.

To gain an accurate, balanced assessment of the photosensitivity dimension of this new antimicrobial, it is important to look at the rate of photosensitivity reactions in detail and their frequency in specific patient subgroups. First, it should be stressed that photosensitivity reactions were the most common adverse reaction observed, with an overall rate of 7.9% reported among patients enrolled in all clinical trials (126 of 1585) for the drug. Moderate to severe phototoxic reactions occurred in 3.9% of patients. It should be stressed, however, that these adverse event rates were generated from initial trial data that included a wide variety of active, minimally ill, younger individuals with infections such as UTI and sinusitis (two indications for which the drug is not FDA-approved or being marketed), that were not severe enough to prevent participation in normal daily activities, including outdoor exposure to sun or ultraviolet (UV) light. However, in patients with community-acquired pneumonia, a subgroup which, because of the morbidity and debilitation associated with this condition, is less likely to encounter sun or UV light exposure during their treatment course, the incidence of photosensitivity reaction diminished by almost 50%, to 4.1%. There were no severe (i.e., blister-forming) reactions in CAP group, and the discontinuation rate from photosensitivity problems was only about 1%.[49]

It appears as if patient selection can play a pivotal role in identifying clinical situations that will maximize the benefits of sparfloxacin, while reducing the potential side effects. Homebound patients and individuals who are not active in outdoor activities, are the most suitable candidates for this treatment. All patients must be instructed to avoid exposure to the sun, bright natural light, and UV rays throughout the duration of treatment and for 5 days after treatment is stopped. Phototoxic reactions have occurred even with the use of sun screens and can occur following a single dose.[49]

A moderate prolongation of the QTc interval (approximate 2% incidence) occurs with sparfloxacin. The mean prolongation is about 10 msec. A small percent of patients (0.7%) had a clinically significant QTc interval prolongation of more than 500 msec. Torsades de pointes has been reported in patients receiving sparfloxacin with disopyramide and amiodarone. Consequently, the drug is contraindicated in patients who are taking agents (e.g., astemizole, disopyramide, amiodarone, and others) known to prolong the QTc interval, and in individuals with a known QTc prolongation.[49] Other side effects include diarrhea (4.6%), nausea (4.3%), and headache (4.2%).[49]

Sparfloxacin is supplied in 200 mg tablets. The initial dose is 400 mg on the first day as a loading dose, then 200 mg every 24 hours for a total of 10 days. In patients with renal impairment (creatinine clearance < 50 mL/min), the 400 mg loading dose is used, but the maintenance dose should be reduced to 200 mg every 48 hours for a total of 10 days.[49] Sparfloxacin can be taken with food, but not with sucralfate or antacids because absorption may be decreased.

Sparfloxacin, trovafloxacin, and levofloxacin may be considered for the treatment of respiratory infections caused by penicillin-resistant *S. pneumoniae*.[53] Sparfloxacin has greater in vitro activity against this organism as well as more favorable pharmacodynamics (i.e., plasma levels relative to minimum inhibitory concentrations) than levofloxacin,[54] but the potential for phototoxicity and prolongation of QTc must be weighed against the potential advantages in selected patient subgroups. Prudent use of these new agents are essential. With the emergence of drug-resistant *S. pneumoniae,* the rational use of antibiotics is paramount in limiting the spread of this organism. These new fluoroquinolones, if used appropriately, can provide a useful alternative to older agents against this organism. Sparfloxacin is priced in the same range as levofloxacin, clarithromycin, and cefuroxime axetil and somewhat more than azithromycin.

Trovafloxacin. A recently introduced fluoroquinolone antibiotic, trovafloxacin (Trovan) has been approved by the FDA for several indications. An IV form of trovafloxacin is marketed as alatrofloxacin, an L-alanine form of trovafloxacin, and is similar pharmacokinetically to oral administration of similar doses.[55] As a rule, no adjustment is needed when switching from IV or oral for comparable dosages.[56]

Although similar in many respects to the extended spectrum quinolones (levofloxacin, sparfloxacin, and grepafloxacin), trovafloxacin is different among this group for its clinical effectiveness in selected infections involving anaerobic organisms, including *Bacteroides fragilis, Peptostreptococcus* sp., and *Prevotella* sp. This expanded spectrum accounts not only for its use in respiratory tract infections, but also for its usefulness as treatment for and/or prophylaxis of intra-abdominal, post-surgical, gynecologic, and pelvic infections. Because many polymicrobial infections, especially in the elderly, are treated on an empiric basis, and because etiologic confirmation is frequently not possible, especially in transient or poorly compliant patients, the antibiotic trovafloxacin may offer special therapeutic advantages in selected patients with compliance-compromising clinical profiles.

With respect to antibacterial activity, trovafloxacin is a broad spectrum naphthyridone fluoroquinolone with activity against such aerobic gram-positive organisms as *S. pneumoniae* and *S. aureus,* as well as atypical organisms, among them, *C. pneumoniae, C. trachomatis, M. pneumoniae,* and *L. pneumophila.* Trovafloxacin also is active against anaerobic organisms, including *Bacteroides* species, *Prevotella* species, *Peptostreptococcus* species, and *Clostridium perfringens* and difficile.[57-59] Some strains of *Enterococcus faecalis* are susceptible to trovafloxacin. About 30% of vancomycin-resistant enterococci were susceptible to the drug.[60,61] The activity of trovafloxacin against gram-negative organisms is similar to that of ciprofloxacin, although it exhibits poorer coverage of *Pseudomonas aeruginosa;* specifically, trovafloxacin is about two-fold less active than ciprofloxacin against *Pseudomonas aeruginosa.*[60,61]

From a practical, clinical perspective, trovafloxacin may be of special interest to the physicians and pharmacists: First, because the oral formulation of trovafloxacin is indicated for a wide range of infections, including those that involve the respiratory tract, skin and soft tissue structures, and genitourinary tract, which are commonly encountered in the outpatient setting. Second, because an IV formulation (alatrofloxacin mesylate) is available that can be initiated for patients with more severe infections requiring hospital admission. Dosages, routes of administration, and duration of therapy vary according to the specific condition and severity of illness. Trovafloxacin is supplied in 100 and 200 mg tablets. Parenteral: equivalent to 5 mg/mL (200 mg, 300 mg).

When prescribing trovafloxacin, physicians should note that some infections—depending upon their severity and anatomic location—can be treated with oral tablets only (e.g., uncomplicated urinary tract infection, cervicitis, acute bacterial exacerbation of chronic bronchitis). Other infections or prophylactic indications require either oral tablets or IV administration (e.g., community-acquired pneumonia, complicated skin and skin structure infections, etc.), whereas some infections should be treated initially with the IV formulation, followed by oral therapy (nosocomial pneumonia and complicated intra-abdominal infections). The daily cost of trovafloxacin is about $5.00 per day for the oral 100 mg tablet, and about $6.00 for the 200 mg oral tablet.

Trovafloxacin has been approved for the following respiratory tract infections: 1) Nosocomial pneumonia caused by *E. coli, P. aeruginosa, H. influenzae,* or *S. aureus;* 2) community-acquired pneumonia caused by *S. pneumoniae, H. influenzae, K. pneumoniae, S. aureus, M. pneumoniae, M. catarrhalis, L. pneumophila,* or *C. pneumoniae;* 3) acute bacterial exacerbation of chronic bronchitis caused by *Haemophilus influenzae, Moraxella catarrhalis, Streptococcus pneumoniae, Staphylococcus aureus,* or *Haemophilus parainfluenzae;* and 4) acute sinusitis caused by *H. influenzae, M. catarrhalis,* or *S. pneumoniae.*

As emphasized in previous sections, with development of increasing intermediate- and, even, complete-resistance of *S. pneumoniae* species to penicillins, macrolides, and other antimicrobial classes, the potential usefulness of such fluoroquinolones as trovafloxacin and levofloxacin for management of community-acquired pneumonia should be noted. In this regard, trovafloxacin has shown excellent in vitro activity against *S. pneumoniae,* including multiple-resistant strains.[60-63] In some studies, resistance to other antibiotics did not appear to affect the susceptibility to trovafloxacin.[57,60]

Skin and soft tissue infections, both uncomplicated and complicated—including those encountered in diabetic patients—can also be managed with this quinolone antibiotic. Trovafloxacin is indicated for uncomplicated skin and skin structure infections caused by *S. aureus, S. pyogenes,* or *S. agalactiae.* It also can be used to manage complicated skin and skin structure infections, including diabetic foot infections, caused by *S. aureus, S. agalactiae, P. aeruginosa, E. faecalis, E. coli,* or *P. mirabilis.* It should be stressed that trovafloxacin has not been studied in the treatment of osteomyelitis, nor has the safety or efficacy of this antibiotic when given for a period of greater than 4 weeks.

The drug also is indicated for a number of common GU conditions managed in the outpatient setting, in particular, uncomplicated urinary tract infection (cystitis) caused by *E. coli,* for which trovafloxacin is approved as a 100 mg PO daily regimen for a total of three days. Patients with chronic bacterial prostatitis caused by *E. coli, E. faecalis,* or *S. epidermidis* are treated with 200 mg PO once daily for 28 days. It is not indicated for pyelonephritis.

With respect to sexually transmitted diseases (STDs), trovafloxacin is effective in: 1) uncomplicated urethral gonorrhea in males, and endocervical and rectal gonorrhea in females caused by *N. gonorrheae,* and cervicitis caused by *C. trachomatis;* and 2) pelvic inflammatory disease (mild-to-moderate) caused by *N. gonorrheae* or *C. trachomatis.* In male patients with nongonococcal urethritis, trovafloxacin was somewhat less effective than doxycycline.[55] Because younger patients are becoming increasingly afflicted with STDs, it should be noted that the safety and efficacy of trovafloxacin in pediatric populations less than 18 years of age, pregnant women, and nursing women have not been established. It has a pregnancy category C rating.

The drug is indicated for gynecological and pelvic infections, including endomyometritis, parametritis, septic abortion, and post-partum infections caused by *E. coli, Bacteroides fragilis,* viridans group streptococci, *E. faecalis, S. agalactiae, Peptostreptococcus* sp., *Prevotella* sp., or *Gardinella vaginalis.* It is also approved for complicated intra- abdominal infections, including post-surgical infections caused by *E. coli, B. fragilis,* viridan group streptococci, *P. aeruginosa, K. pneumoniae, Peptostreptococcus* sp., or *Prevotella* sp. As with other antimicrobials, when *Pseudomonas* is a suspected or documented pathogen, combination therapy with either an aminoglycoside or aztreonam may be clinically indicated.

Trovafloxacin has been approved for prophylaxis of infections associated with elective colorectal surgery and vaginal or abdominal hysterectomy. In patients in whom surgical prophylaxis with oral trovafloxacin is indicated, Bicitra® should not be given within two hours, since absorption of the drug is reduced.

In worldwide, multidose clinical efficacy trials, the majority of adverse reactions were characterized as mild in nature, with more than 90% being described as mild or moderate. Trovafloxacin was discontinued for adverse events thought to be related to the drug in 5% of patients these included: dizziness (2.4%), nausea (1.9%), headache (1.1%), and vomiting (1%).

The most common side effect of trovafloxacin is lightheadedness (1% to 4%) and/or dizziness (reported in 2% to 11% of patients depending on dose and route of administration). The incidence of dizziness was reported more frequently in females under the age of 45 and may be reduced substantially if trovafloxacin is taken at bedtime or with food.[55] Nausea is reported with a frequency of 4% to 8%. Other drug-related adverse reactions with a frequency ≥1% include headache, vomiting, diarrhea, abdominal pain, insertion site reaction, and vaginitis.[55] Patients should know how they react to the drug before operating an automobile or machinery, and they should be advised to avoid excessive sunlight or artificial ultraviolet light and discontinue therapy if a sunburn-like reaction or skin eruption occurs (phototoxicity observed in less than 0.03% of patients).

Concomitant administration of IV morphine and oral trovafloxacin resulted in a reduction in bioavailability of trovafloxacin. Morphine should be administered at least two hours after oral trovafloxacin is taken on an empty stomach or at least four hours after oral trovafloxacin is taken with food.[55] Trovafloxacin can cause elevation of liver enzymes during or soon after prolonged therapy (21 days or more), and therefore, periodic assessment is advised.[55]

Trovafloxacin may be taken without regard to meals. However, because of impaired absorption, vitamins or minerals containing iron, aluminum, or magnesium-based antacids, antacids containing citric acid buffered with sodium citrate, or sucralfate should be taken at least 2 hours before or after trovafloxacin.[55] No adjustment is required in patients with impaired renal function, as the drug is eliminated primarily in the feces. Dosage adjustment, however, is recommended in patients with chronic hepatic disease.[55]

Comparative clinical trials have been reported in the package insert for trovafloxacin by the manufacturer. These trials suggest that trovafloxacin (100 mg/day) is at least comparable to clarithromycin (500 mg twice daily) for the treatment of acute bacterial exacerbation of chronic bronchitis. Sequential therapy (i.e., IV followed by oral administration) with IV alatrofloxacin and oral trovafloxacin appear comparable to sequential IV ciprofloxacin/ampicillin and oral ciprofloxacin/amoxicillin or IV ceftriaxone and oral cefpodoxime (with or without erythromycin) in hospitalized community-acquired pneumonia. Sequential therapy with alatrofloxacin and trovafloxacin also appeared comparable to sequential IV imipenem and amoxicillin/clavulanate in complicated intra-abdominal infections.[55]

Trovafloxacin's combination of approval for multiple indications, its broad spectrum of coverage, and high levels of activity against organisms that are becoming increasingly resistant to multiple antibiotics, suggest that it, as well as other extended spectrum quinolones, should be considered as an important alternatives to broad spectrum antibiotics such as ceftriaxone, which has been widely used in the emergency department and in-hospital setting.

Non-Extended Spectrum Quinolones

The so called, older non-extended spectrum quinolones still constitute the primary treatment modality for complicated bacterial infections of the urinary tract. Ciprofloxacin is still the mainstay of therapy for complicated infections of the urinary tract. In fact, the non-extended spectrum quinolones such as ciprofloxacin still play a very important role in and can be considered reasonable first-line agents for the following conditions: prostatitis in older men, invasive bacterial diarrheas with prolonged duration of symptoms, complicated urinary tract infections, otitis external, diabetic vasculopathic ulcers, one-dose therapy for gonorrhea, and selected cases of osteomyelitis.

Ciprofloxacin and ofloxacin have a wide variety of indications, while norfloxacin, lomefloxacin, and enoxacin are generally used only for infections of the urinary tract. More frequent use of quinolones has resulted in increasing resistance, which has been observed predominantly in methicillin-resistant staphylococci and *P. aeruginosa.*[64]

The quinolones are not presently recommended for use in patients younger than 18 years old or in pregnant or lactating women due to concerns over cartilage toxicity.[65] However, the quinolones may enjoy increased use in children if European safety data are further substantiated.[66] Because divalent and trivalent cations decrease quinolone absorption, concomitant antacids, calcium, sucralfate, iron, and zinc need to be avoided. The quinolones may decrease theophylline and caffeine metabolism by inhibiting the hepatic cytochrome P-4P-450 system, with enoxacin, ciprofloxacin, and norfloxacin being most often implicated.[64] Phototoxicity may occur most frequently with lomefloxacin and sparfloxacin.

Phosphonic Acids

Fosfomycin (Monurol®), a new single-dose antibiotic, has been approved by the FDA for the treatment of uncomplicated urinary tract infections in women, but not in men. This new synthetic antibiotic inhibits cell synthesis by inactivating the enzyme enolpyruvyl transferase, which catalyzes one of the early steps in cell wall synthesis. Extensively used in Europe since 1988, fosfomycin tromethamine represents the first in a new class of antibiotics that are derivatives of phosphonic acid. The drug is bactericidal against a wide range of common urinary tract pathogens and is well absorbed orally. A single dose results in high serum levels, which provides concentrations above the MIC for common urinary pathogens for up to 3.5 days. Supplied as a package of soluble granules that is mixed with water, fosfomycin is indicated for the treatment of uncomplicated UTIs (acute cystitis) in women, due to susceptible strains of *Escherichia coli* and *Enterococcus faecalis,* and there is generally little cross resistance between fosfomycin and other antibiotics.[68] It should be stressed, however, that in vitro data suggests that *Staphylococcus saprophyticus,* a common urinary pathogen, is resistant to fosfomycin.[59]

Fosfomycin carries a Pregnancy Category B rating (i.e., no documented evidence of risk in humans), the same as amoxicillin and nitrofurantoin, while TMP/SMZ and quinolones are in category C (i.e., risk cannot be ruled out and use in pregnancy not recommended). The most common side effect of fosfomycin is diarrhea (9%) which, on average, lasts for about two days.[70] Although the bacteriologic eradication rate with a single dose of fosfomycin (82%) is inferior to that of a seven-day course of ciprofloxacin (98%) or a 10-day course of TMP/SMZ (98%), it is comparable to eradication rates seen with 3-day courses of commonly used antimicrobials.[68] Because metoclopramide lowers the serum concentration and urinary excretion of fosfomycin, coadministration of these drugs is not recommended.

From a practical standpoint, fosfomycin is supplied in orange-flavored granules which are dissolved in 3 to 4 ounces of water taken as a single 3 g dose. The medication should not be mixed with hot water, and repeated daily doses do not appear to improve clinical success, but they do increase the incidence of adverse events. Fosfomycin may be taken without regard to food.[68]

The bacteriological cure rate for fosfomycin generally ranges between 69% to 96% as assessed 5 to 11 days post-treatment. In comparative clinical trials, fosfomycin was found to be less effective than 7 days of ciprofloxacin (250 mg twice daily) and 10 days of TMP/SMZ (960 mg daily), but was comparable to a seven-day course of nitrofurantoin (Macrodantin 100 mg twice daily).[68,69] A small, nonblinded study (n = 36) suggests that fosfomycin may be more effective than low-dose TMP/SMZ (960 mg) given for 3 days.[71] In a large, single-blind study (n = 308), however, fosfomcyin was comparable to a single dose of TMP/SMZ (1.92 g) and a single dose of ofloxacin (200 mg) in terms of bacteriologic rates.[72]

Although fosfomycin is the only FDA-approved, *single*-dose regimen for UTIs, current clinical data indicates that it may be no more effective than a single dose of two double strength TMP/SMZ tablets. In current practice, most physicians opt for the improved cure rates associated with a 3 day treatment of TMP/SMZ, one double strength tablet twice daily for 3 days, which is often considered to be optimal treatment due to effectiveness and reduced relapse rates.[73,74] Unfortunately, comparative studies between this regimen and fosfomycin have not been reported. Fosfomycin costs about $21 per treatment and, considering the other available, short-course alternatives, this drug should be reserved primarily for patients in whom TMP/SMZ is not appropriate (e.g., sulfa allergy, bacterial resistance, and third trimester of pregnancy).

Clearly, fosfomycin offers an alternative to standard therapy for UTIs in women. But because its cure rates are no better than standard therapy, even standard single-dose therapy, it is best reserved for women with multiple drug allergies or patients who are compliance risks.

Macrolides

The newer macrolide antibiotics include the erythromycin analogs, azithromycin, clarithromycin and dirithromycin.[75,76] Compared to erythromycin, the major advantages of these antibiotics are significantly decreased GI side effects, which produce enhanced tolerance, improved bioavailability, higher tissue levels, pharmacokinetic features that permit less frequent dosing and better compliance, as well as enhanced activity against *H. influenzae*.[77,78] In particular, the long tissue half-life of azithromycin allows this antibiotic to be prescribed for a shorter duration (5 days) than comparable antibiotics given for the same indications. (See Table 5-1)

Approved indications for the newer macrolides are listed in Table 5-2. A single 1 g dose of azithromycin has been shown to be as effective as 7 days of doxycycline in the treatment of uncomplicated chlamydial cervicitis and urethritis.[79] The availability of one-dose, "cure here now" therapy offers substantial compliance advantages in the Emergency Department setting. With the recent introduction of a 1 g sachet pack of azithromycin, which is priced at about $10 to $15 at many institutions and clinics, the Centers for Disease Control and Prevention (CDC) has advocated azithromycin as a drug of choice for uncomplicated chlamydia cervicitis.[80] A one-time 2 g oral dose has also been approved for the treatment of urethritis and cervicitis caused by *N. gonorrhoeae*.

In contrast, azithromycin, clarithromycin, and erythromycin should not be given with astemizole because of the risk of ventricular tachycardia. Both erythromycin and clarithromycin may increase theophylline levels. Clarithromycin, which has a pregnancy category C rating, is contraindicated in pregnancy because of fetal cardiovascular abnormalities discovered in animal toxicologic studies. Azithromycin, which has a category B rating, is appropriate for use in pregnant patients, but only when clinical findings indicate that antimicrobial treatment is warranted.

Because macrolides are one of the fastest-growing class of outpatient antimicrobials, comparing the advantages and disadvantages of these antibiotics is an important issue for the physician and pharmacist. Given the cost differences between azithromycin and clarithromycin, as well as the improved compliance patterns associated with short-duration therapy, any rational approach to distinguishing between these agents must consider prescription, patient, and drug resistance barriers.

From the outset, it is fair to say that these newer macrolides, to a great degree, have supplanted the use of erythromycin in community-acquired infections of the lower respiratory tract. Although erythromycin, in particular, has been considered by some to be the antibiotic of choice for community-acquired pneumonia, its lack of efficacy against *H. influenzae,* as well as its adverse GI side effects, potential for drug-drug interactions, and poor compliance profile are now recognized as clinically important liabilities in emergency practice. It is, however, effective against pneumococcal pneumonia, mycoplasma pneumonia, and many atypical infections, including *Legionella.* Food decreases the absorption of erythromycin, which interferes with drug metabolism. The drug should be used with caution in patients on theophylline or warfarin.

From the pharmactectural perspective of providing definitive, cost-effective, compliance-promoting, and drug-drug-interaction-minimizing therapy, the newer macrolide antibiotics, which include both azithromycin, clarithromycin, and dirithromycin have recently emerged as some of the drugs of choice for outpatient management of community-acquired pneumonia, as well as otitis media.[81] When used as oral agents, they play a central role in management of pneumonia in otherwise healthy individuals who do not require hospitalization. Recently, however, the IV formulation of azithromycin has been approved for hospitalized patients (see below). Unlike penicillins, cephalosporins, and sulfa-based agents, these drugs have the advantage of showing in vitro activity against both atypical and bacterial offenders implicated in community-acquired pneumonia. The most common side effects include GI upset and a metallic taste in the mouth which are more common in clarithromycin.

These agents also have the advantage of a simplified dosing schedule, especially azithromycin, which is given once daily for only five days (500 mg PO on day 1 and 250 mg PO once daily on days 2 to 5). Clarithromycin requires a longer course of therapy and is more expensive. In general, the decision to use a macrolide such as azithromycin rather than erythromycin is based on weighing the increased cost of a course of therapy with azithromycin against its real-world advantages, which include a more convenient dosing schedule, its broader spectrum of coverage, its favorable drug interaction profile, and its decreased incidence of GI side effects, which occur in 3% to 5% of patients taking a 5-day, multiple-dose regimen.[82] The recent introduction of a new oral tablet formulation permits consumption of the antibiotic without regard to food ingestion.

Azithromycin also has been approved in a palatable suspension formulation for the treatment of acute otitis media and pneumonia in children. The once-daily, 5-day course introduces compliance-enhancing features that, to a great degree, permit parental, day care, and grade school drug administration problems to be circumvented.[83] A well-accepted palatability profile, combined with an overall discontinuation rate of about 0.9%, are favorable as far as patient resistance is concerned.[84-86] When the 5-day course of the suspension is used for treatment of otitis media, the reported incidences of side effects includes diarrhea/loose stools (2%), abdominal pain (2%), vomiting (1%), and nausea (1%).

From the perspective of drug resistance, the oral suspension of azithromycin is characterized by excellent in vitro coverage of beta-lactamase-producing *H. influenzae* and *M. catarrhalis,* as well as in vitro coverage of *S. pneumoniae,* for which the overall resistance rate is estimated to be about 5% to 7%.[84-86] Some geographical areas or institutions may report higher rates. This second-generation macrolide has been used widely in the adult population, and more recently, azithromycin oral suspension for children recently has become available for use by pediatric specialists.

The clinical role of azithromycin in the Emergency Department, pediatric, and primary care setting is supported by rigorous clinical studies that have been published comparing the safety and efficacy of azithromycin to amoxicillin-clavulanate for the treatment of acute otitis media in children.[84,87,88] In these large trials, clinical cure rates of up to 87.5% are reported, and azithromycin was as effective as, but better tolerated than, amoxicillin-clavulanate for the treatment of acute otitis media in the pediatric age group.[83,87-89] Although azithromycin does not affect a single IV dose of theophylline, caution is advised if multiple doses of theophylline are used. Accordingly, prudent clinical monitoring of theophylline levels is recommended in these patients. Monitoring of the prothrombin time is also urged in patients taking warfarin.

Like azithromycin, clarithromycin suspension also has been shown to produce comparable cure rates to amoxicillin-clavulanate.[7] Finally, the potential for drug-drug interactions between clarithromycin and theophylline, or astemizole requires caution. From a prescription resistance perspective, the cost for a course of therapy for clarithromycin is more than it is for amoxicillin, TMP/SMZ, or azithromycin. Finally, with respect to medication compliance, twice daily dosing is less desirable than once-daily administration,[15] and unpleasant taste and palatability problems have been described for clarithromycin.[10,90,91]

From a practical clinical, and cost-effectiveness, perspective, the newest and, perhaps most important, advance in the area of macrolide therapy is the availability of IV azithromycin for the management of hospitalized patients with community-acquired pneumonia (CAP) as well as pelvic inflammatory disease (PID).[92,93] Currently, azithromycin is the only advanced generation macrolide indicated for parenteral therapy in hospitalized patients with CAP due to *C. pneumoniae, H. influenzae, Legionella pneumophila, M. catarrhalis, M. pneumoniae, S. pneumoniae,* or *S. aureus.*

The comparative trials demonstrating clinical success (patients who were cured or improved at 10 to 14 days post-therapy) rates of about 77%—with concomitant bacteriologic response rates of about 96% for frequently isolated pathogens—with azithromycin in CAP were conducted in a wide variety of patients. These included a significant percentage who were 65 years of age or older, had an abnormal respiratory rate (> 30 breaths per minute), a PaO_2 less than 60 mm Hg and/or BUN greater than 20 mg/dL. Many of these patients had concurrent diseases or syndromes, including emphysema, chronic obstructive airway obstruction, asthma, diabetes, and/or were cigarette smokers.[94] The efficacy of this macrolide was compared to clinical outcomes with a cephalosporin used with or without erythromycin. In a randomized comparative investigation, therapy with IV azithromycin alone plus oral azithromycin was as effective as IV treatment with the designated "second-generation" cephalosporin, cefuroxime followed by oral cefuroxime axetil, with or without the addition of oral or IV erythromycin.[94]

Azithromycin dosing and administration schedules for hospitalized patients are different than for the 5 day course used exclusively for outpatient management, and these differences should be noted. When this advanced generation macrolide is used for hospitalized patients with CAP, 2 to 5 days of therapy with azithromycin IV (500 mg once daily) followed by oral azithromycin (500 mg once daily to complete a total of 7 to 10 days of therapy) is clinically and bacteriologically effective. For patients requiring hospitalization, the initial 500 mg IV dose of azithromycin may be given in the Emergency Department.

Among all intent-to-treat patients with CAP receiving azithromycin evaluated in two studies, 24 were found to have *S. pneumoniae* bacteremia at baseline. Of these 24 patients, 19 (79%) achieved clinical cure, which was accompanied by eradication of the pathogen from the blood. Among the five patients considered to be clinical failures, three of the five had documented eradication of *S. pneumoniae* from the blood, and the remaining two did not have post-baseline cultures reported. All five patients had comorbid conditions that are predictive of poor outcomes, but none of the failures resulted in mortality.[94]

Like the oral formulation, IV azithromycin appears to be well-tolerated, with a low incidence of GI adverse events (4.3% diarrhea, 3.9% nausea, 2.7% abdominal pain, 1.4% vomiting), minimal injection-site reactions (>12% combined injection-site pain and/or inflammation or infection), and a low incidence of discontinuation (1.2% discontinuation of IV therapy) due to drug-related adverse patient events or laboratory abnormalities.[94]

Dirithromycin (Dynabac). Dirithromycin is a once-daily, expanded spectrum macrolide that, like azithromycin, offers the compliance and convenience advantages of short duration (5-day) therapy for acute bacterial exacerbations of chronic bronchitis due to *H. influenzae, M. catarrhalis,* or *S. pneumoniae.* The AWP price for a 5-day course of dirithromycin is about $21, compared to $38 for azithromycin and $45.64 for a 7-day course of clarithromycin, which makes this agent the most cost-attractive non-generic antibiotic indicated from management of acute bacterial exacerbations of COPD.

First-line use of dirithromycin is supported by one multicenter efficacy trial evaluating 212 patients, in which a 5-day, once daily course of dirithromycin demonstrated comparable efficacy-combined clinical cure or improvement rates—to a 7-day course of clarithromycin. In another trial, the dirithromycin 5-day course showed comparable efficacy to amoxicillin-clavulanate 500 mg 3 times/day for 7 to 10 days.

This cost-attractive drug is well-tolerated with a favorable discontinuation rate of only 3.8% in clinical trials evaluating the 5-day therapeutic course. The primary side effects and their frequency for the 5-day course include headache (7.7%), abdominal pain (7.1%), and diarrhea, which are seen in 7.7% to 9.7% of individuals requiring the 7 to 14 day course for treatment of secondary bacterial infection of acute bronchitis and community-aquired pneumonia (CAP), respectively. When used to treat CAP due to *S. Pneumoniae, Legionella,* and *M. pneumonia,* dirithromycin requires a 14-day therapeutic course. This antibiotic should be administered with food, or within one hour after having eaten.

Matching Drugs with Bugs: Outcome-Effective Antibiotic Selection

Recommendations for the empiric antibiotic therapy of bacterial infections commonly encountered in the ED, hospital, or primary care clinic are listed in Table 5-3. In addition, selected comments on some of the common indications for antibiotic therapy follow.

Community-Acquired Pneumonia

A variety of antibiotics are available for outpatient management of pneumonia. Although the selection process can be daunting, a sensible approach to antibiotic selection for patients pneumonia is provided by treatment categories for pneumonia generated by the Medical Section of the American Lung Association, and published under the auspices of the American Thoracic Society.[95] This classification scheme will not only help make clinical assessments useful for guiding therapy, but it is also predictive of ultimate prognosis and mortality outcome. (See Table 5-4) New, more recently devised consensus panel recommendations also are available, and will be discussed.

The most common pathogens responsible for causing community-acquired pneumonia include the typical bacteria: *S. pneumoniae, H. influenzae,* and *M. catarrhalis,* as well as the atypical pathogens: *Mycoplasma, Legionella,* and *Chlamydia pneumoniae.*[96] *H. influenzae* and *M. catarrhalis* are both found more commonly in patients with COPD. Clinically and radiologically, it is difficult to differentiate between the typical and atypical pathogens; therefore, coverage against all these organisms may be necessary. In patients producing sputum-containing polymorphonuclear leukocytes, the sputum Gram's stain may contain a predominant organism to aid in the choice of empiric therapy. For most patients, therapy must be entirely empiric and is based on the expected pathogens.[97,98]

It must be understood that outpatient therapy for pneumonia in emergency practice is almost always empiric in nature. For the vast majority of otherwise healthy patients who have community-acquired pneumonia, but who do not have comorbid conditions and who are deemed well enough to be managed as outpatients, therapy directed at *S. pneumoniae, H. influenzae, M. pneumoniae,* and *M. catarrhalis* is appropriate. In these cases, one of the newer macrolides, such as azithromycin, clarithromycin, or dirithromycin should be considered one of the initial agents of choice. The extended spectrum quinolones, such as trovafloxacin and levofloxacin provide similar coverage and are also approved as initial therapy in this patient subgroup. Because of their excellent in vitro activity against

Table 5-3

Empiric Antibiotic Therapy for Bacterial Infections Commonly Encountered in the Emergency Department

Clinical Indication	Usual Pathogens	Primary Treatment	Alternative Treatment	Comments
ABDOMINAL				
Biliary tract	Gram-negative aerobes *Peptostreptococcus* species, anaerobes	Antipseudomonal penicillin + metronidazole ± aminoglycoside *or* Imipenem or beta-lactam/ beta-lactamase inhibitor ± aminoglycoside	Third-generation cephalosporin + metronidazole ***or*** Aztreonam + clindamycin	Many acceptable regimens with requisite aerobic, anaerobic activity.
Abdominal infection, Peritonitis, appendicitis, diverticulitis, bowel perforation	Gram-negative aerobes, *E. coli*, anaerobes (occasionally *P. aeruginosa*)	Beta-lactam/ beta-lactamase inhibitor ***or*** Imipenem ± aminoglycoside; ***or*** IV alatrofloxacin ± aminoglycoside ***or*** ± aztreonam	Third-generation cephalosporin + metronidazole ***or*** Aztreonam + clindamycin	Many acceptable regimens with requisite aerobic, anaerobic activity. Usually combination therapy with severe disease.
Complicated post-surgical infections	Gram-negative aerobes, including *E. coli;* anaerobes including bacteroides; (occasionally *P. aeruginosa*)	IV alatrofloxacin ± aminoglycoside ***or*** ± aztreonam; ***or*** Imipenem ± aminoglycoside ***or*** ± aztreonam	See above	Many acceptable regimens
CENTRAL NERVOUS SYSTEM				
Meningitis	*S. pneumoniae*, meningococci, *L. monocytogenes*	Vancomycin + ceftriaxone ***or*** Cefotaxime + ampicillin	Penicillin allergy; vancomycin + chloramphenicol + TMP-SMX	Need for vancomycin dictated by incidence of penicillin-resistant pneumococci.

Table 5-3

Empiric Antibiotic Therapy for Bacterial Infections Commonly Encountered in the Emergency Department — cont'd.				
Clinical Indication	**Usual Pathogens**	**Primary Treatment**	**Alternative Treatment**	**Comments**
COMMUNITY-ACQUIRED PNEUMONIA				
Outpatient, < 60, no co-morbid conditions	*S. Pneumoniae, H. influenzae, M. pneumoniae, Legionella, Chlamydia*	A macrolide: azithromycin, clarithromycin, erythromycin (non-smokers and no COPD-see text)	Trovafloxacin ***or*** levofloxacin	
Outpatient, > 60 and/or co-morbid conditions	*S. aureus*, gram-negative, *S. pneumoniae*, Legionella	Trovafloxacin; *or* Amoxicillin/clavulanate *or* Extended-spectrum cephalosporin + *macrolide*	Levofloxacin	
Hospitalized	As per both above	Azithromycin IV; *or* Extended-spectrum cephalosporin IV + azithromycin IV; ***or*** alatrofloxacin IV; ***or*** levofloxacin IV	Substitute beta-lactam/beta-lactamase inhibitor ***or*** imipenem ***or*** others for cephalosporin	
Hospitalized (serious infection)	As per above	Alatrofloxacin IV ***or*** extended spectrum cephalosporin IV + azithromycin IV ***or*** levofloxacin IV		In selected cases (MRSA), vancomycin or adjunctive anti-pseudomonas antibiotics (aminoglycosides or aztreonam) may be required
GASTROINTESTINAL				
Infectious diarrhea	*Shigella, Salmonella, Campylobacter, E. coli*	Ciprofloxacin	TMP-SMX	

Table 5-3

Empiric Antibiotic Therapy for Bacterial Infections Commonly Encountered in the Emergency Department — cont'd.				
Clinical Indication	**Usual Pathogens**	**Primary Treatment**	**Alternative Treatment**	**Comments**
RESPIRATORY TRACT (UPPER)				
Acute otitis media	*Pneumococcus, Haemophilus, Moraxella,* Occasionally group A strep	Amoxicillin* ***or*** Azithromycin ***or*** Amoxicillin-clavulanate Extended-spectrum cephalosporin	TMP/SMZ *or* Clarithromycin	*Amoxicillin failure = 10-15%
Pharyngitis/tonsillitis	Beta-hemolytic strep (Group A, C, G) *A. haemolyticum,* Nonbacterial	Benzathine penicillin G ***or*** Penicillin V ***or*** Erythromycin	Extended-spectrum cephalosporin *or* Clarithromycin, *or* azithromycin	
Acute sinusitis	As per otitis media	Trovafloxacin ***or*** TMP-SMX ***or*** Amoxicillin-clavulanate	Extended-spectrum cephalosporin *or* clarithromycin	
RESPIRATORY TRACT (LOWER)				
Acute bacterial exacerbation of chronic bronchitis (ABECB)	*Pneumococcus, Haemophilus, Moraxella*	TMP-SMX ***or*** Azithromycin ***or*** Trovafloxacin	Extended-spectrum cephalosporin *or* Clarithromycin *or* Amoxicillin-clavulanate *or* Levofloxacin	
SEXUALLY TRANSMITTED DISEASES				
Uncomplicated gonorrhea	*N. gonorrhoeae*	Any single-dose regimen as per Table 7		
Uncomplicated nongonococcal urethritis, cervicitis	*C. trachomatis, Mycoplasma, Ureaplasma*	Azithromycin Doxycycline	Erythromycin *or* Ofloxacin	

Table 5-3

Empiric Antibiotic Therapy for Bacterial Infections Commonly Encountered in the Emergency Department — cont'd.				
Clinical Indication	**Usual Pathogens**	**Primary Treatment**	**Alternative Treatment**	**Comments**
PELVIC INFLAMMATORY DISEASE				
Outpatient (mild to moderate)	*Gonococcus, Chlamydia,* anaerobes	Trovafloxacin; ***or*** Ceftriaxone + doxycycline; *or* azithromycin IV + oral therapy for total of 7 days; ***or*** Ofloxacin ± clindamycin ***or*** metronidazole which may be added to any of the above regimens as required	Cefoxitin + probenecid + doxycycline	
Inpatient	As above	Cefoxitin/cefotetan + doxycycline ***or*** azithromycin IV ± metronidazole	Gentamicin + clindamycin	
SKIN AND SKIN STRUCTURE INFECTIONS				
Uncomplicated	*S. aureus, Streptococcal* species	Cephalexin ***or*** Azithromycin ***or*** Trovafloxacin	A macrolide Dicloxacillin	
Complicated	Polymicrobic	Amoxicillin-clavulanate *or* Trovafloxacin	Quinolone + clindamycin; TMP-SMX + clindamycin	
Diabetic foot	Polymicrobic; aerobic gram-positive, gram-negative, and anaerobes	Outpatient: Trovafloxacin; *or* ciprofloxacin + clindamycin	Hospitalized: alatrofloxacin, beta-lactam/beta-lactamase inhibitor, imipenem, or other with equivalent activity	

Table 5-3

Empiric Antibiotic Therapy for Bacterial Infections Commonly Encountered in the Emergency Department — cont'd.

Clinical Indication	Usual Pathogens	Primary Treatment	Alternative Treatment	Comments
URINARY TRACT INFECTIONS				
Uncomplicated	*E. coli*, occasionally other	TMP-SMX *or* Trovafloxacin	Extended spectrum cephalosporin Amoxicillin-clavulanate Fosfomycin (cystitis) Ciprofloxacin	
Chronic prostatitis		Trovafloxacin	TMP-SMX ***or*** Ofloxacin	
Complicated UTI	Gram-negative aerobes	Ciprofloxacin *or* amoxicillin clavulanate *or* other quinolones	Levofloxacin	

S. pneumoniae, the use of levofloxacin or trovafloxacin should be strongly considered as initial therapy in urban areas where surveillance studies demonstrate a high incidence of macrolide-resistant *S. pneumoniae* species.[86-89]

For the older patient with CAP who is considered stable enough to be managed as an outpatient, but in whom the bacterial pathogen list may also include gram-negative aerobic organisms, the combined use of a second-generation cephalosporin or amoxicillin-clavulanate plus a macrolide, or an advanced quinolone such as trovafloxacin or levofloxacin, is recommended. The advanced quinolones may be used as monotherapy, and, therefore, provide convenience and cost advantages in this high-risk subgroup. In those unusual cases in which a definitive, specific, etiologic diagnosis can be made (e.g., *Mycoplasma, C. pneumoniae, Legionella* sp.), agents with known activity against these organisms can be employed.[87-92]

Some experts emphasize that in non-smoking adults without COPD (i.e., patients at a low risk for having *H. influenzae*), therapy with erythromycin should be strongly considered.[98] This is a matter of clinical judgment, but in any event, the newer macrolides, azithromycin, clarithromycin, and dirithromycin are recommended in cases of erythromycin intolerance. In patients with COPD, TMP/SMZ or doxycycline usually provides adequate coverage against *S. pneumoniae* and *H. influenzae,* but TMP/SMZ will not cover atypical pathogens. Except for the newer quinolones such as levofloxacin or trovafloxacin, empiric use of the older quinolones is not recommended for treatment of community-acquired respiratory infections, primarily because of their variable activity against *S. pneumoniae* and overly broad gram-negative coverage. Although the older quinolones should generally not be used for the empiric treatment of community-acquired pneumonia, they may provide an alternative therapy for treatment of bronchiectasis, particularly when gram-negative organisms such as *Pseudomonas* are cultured from respiratory secretions.[99]

The use of trovafloxacin or levofloxacin as first-line drugs—in particular, as a substitute for the advanced generation macrolides—to treat uncomplicated community-acquired pneumonia or acute bacterial exacerbations of COPD in patients less than 60 years of age is more questionable and has become a matter of intense debate. Determining which of these antibiotics—macrolides vs. quinolones—should be considered "workhorse" drugs in the ED or primary care setting for treating bacterial "bugs and crud" above the belly button requires a thoughtful analysis that includes cost, convenience, spectrum, and potential for inducing resistance as part of the drug selection equation.

With its once-daily, minimum duration 7-day course, levofloxacin and trovafloxacin have dosing and duration advantages as compared to the macrolide clarithromycin, which requires 20 doses over 10 days. Moreover, the 7-day course of the extended spectrum quinolones is comparatively priced with clarithromycin. Based on this analysis, but excluding the potential pitfalls associated with "broad" or, so-called, "over-extended" (i.e., not absolutely necessary gram-negative) spectrum of coverage, these quinolones appear to provide a very reasonable alternative and, perhaps, even a slight advantage, to clarithromycin in managing patients with CAP.

Table 5-4

Empiric Antimicrobial Therapy of Choice for Outpatient and In-Hospital Management of Community-Acquired Pneumonia (CAP)*		
PATIENT PROFILE/ ETIOLOGIC AGENTS	**FIRST-LINE ANTIBIOTIC THERAPY∂**	**ALTERNATIVE FIRST-LINE ANTIBIOTIC THERAPY**
Otherwise healthy < 60 years of age	Azithromycin ***or*** Trovafloxacin ***or*** Levofloxacin	Clarithromycin ***or*** Erythromycin (in patient with no history of COPD and who has a low probability of *H. influenzae* infection)
Otherwise healthy > 60 years of age (patients deemed to be suitable, i.e., no systemic toxicity, high likelihood of compliance, and supportive home environment)	Trovafloxacin ***or*** Levofloxacin	Cefuroxime plus azithromycin ***or*** Amoxicillin-clavulanate plus azithromycin
> 60 years of age underlying risk factors or comorbid conditions: in-hospital management (malignancy, COPD, previous history of pneumonia, diabetes, etc.)	Trovafloxacin (alatrofloxacin) IV ***or*** Azithromycin IV ***or*** Ceftriaxone IV plus azithromycin IV	Levofloxacin IV ***or*** Ceftriaxone plus erythromycin IV ***or*** Imipenem IV plus azithromycin IV
CAP acquired in the nursing home environment (increased likelihood of gram negative, *E. coli, Klebsiella pneumoniae)*	Trovafloxacin (alatrofloxacin) IV ***or*** Ceftriaxone IV plus azithromycin IV	Levofloxacin IV ***or*** Ceftriaxone plus erythromycin IV ***or*** Imipenem IV plus azithromycin IV
CAP in the individual with chronic alcoholism (increased likelihood of *Klebsiella pneumoniae* infection)	Trovafloxacin (alatrofloxacin) IV ***or*** Ceftriaxone IV plus azithromycin IV ***or*** Levofloxacin IV	Ceftriaxone plus erythromycin IV ***or*** Cefepime IV plus azithromycin IV
Severe CAP acquired in an area or institution with significant prevalence (<20%) of *S. pneumoniae* species showing intermediate-to-complete resistance to macrolides, cephalosporins, and/or penicillin, but maintaining high sensitivity to extended spectrum quinolones)	Trovafloxacin (alatrofloxacin) IV ***or*** Vancomycin¶ plus azithromycin	Levofloxacin IV ***or*** Vancomycin¶ plus erythromycin

Table 5-4

Empiric Antimicrobial Therapy of Choice for Outpatient Management of Community-Acquired Pneumonia (CAP)* — cont'd.		
PATIENT PROFILE/ ETIOLOGIC AGENTS	**FIRST-LINE ANTIBIOTIC THERAPY∂**	**ALTERNATIVE FIRST-LINE ANTIBIOTIC THERAPY**
Severe CAP complicated by structural disease of the lung (bronchiectasis): increased likelihood of *Pseudomonas* and polymicrobial infection	Cefepime IV plus trovafloxacin IV plus aminoglycoside	Ciprofloxacin IV plus aminoglycoside IV plus azithromycin IV ***or*** Carbapenem IV plus azithromycin IV plus aminoglycoside
CAP in a patient with suspected aspiration (increases the likelihood of gram-negative and anaerobic infection**)	Trovafloxacin (alatrofloxacin) IV *plus* Clindamycin IV ***or*** *plus* ticarcillin/clavulanate IV	Trovafloxacin (alatrofloxacin) IV *plus* ampicillin-sulbactam IV
Severe CAP in a compromised host with a previous hospitalization for, or who resides in a community or facility with a high reported incidence of methicillin-resistant *S. aureus* (MRSA)***	Trovafloxacin (alatrofloxacin) IV plus vancomycin IV ***or*** Ceftriaxone IV plus azithromycin IV plus vancomycin IV	Levofloxacin IV plus vancomycin IV
CAP patient with severe pneumonia requiring ICU hospitalization***	Cefepime IV plus trovafloxacin IV plus aminoglycoside (*Pseudomonas* strongly suspected) ***or*** Trovafloxacin (alatrofloxacin) IV *plus* ceftriaxone IV ***or*** *plus* beta-lactam/beta-lactamase inhibitor	Ciprofloxacin IV plus aminoglycoside IV plus azithromycin IV ***or*** Ceftriaxone IV plus azithromycin IV plus aminoglycoside ***or*** Levofloxacin IV plus carbapenem IV

* Oral therapy/outpatient treatment recommendations are appropriate only for those otherwise healthy patients with community-acquired pneumonia of mild enough severity that they are judged to be suitable candidates for outpatient management with oral antibiotics.

¶ If *S. pneumoniae* demonstrates complete resistance to extended spectrum quinolones (rare), third-generation cephalosporin, and macrolides, vancomycin may be required as part of initial therapy.

∂ First line therapy recommendations take into consideration cost of the drug (which may vary from one institution to another), convenience of dosing, daily dose frequency, spectrum of coverage, and side effects, and risk of drug-drug interactions.

** When anerobic organisms are suspected as one of the possible etiologic pathogens in a patient with CAP, trovafloxacin in combination with clindamycin or a B-lactam/B-lactamase inhibitor (ampicillin/sulbactam, tricarcillin/clavulanate, or ticarcillin/tazobactam) is recommended.

*** High community prevalence of, previous history of hospitalization, or increasing local incidence of methicillin-resistant *Staphylococcal aureus* (MRSA) in a patient with a clinical presentation consistent with *S. aureus* pneumonia, vancomycin should be considered as component for initial therapy.

In the case of azithromycin, its 5-day duration of therapy, lower cost, and targeted coverage of *S. pneumoniae, H. influenzae, M. catarrhalis,* and *M. pneumoniae,* must be weighed against the longer duration and slightly greater cost per treatment course for the quinolones, and the fact that their spectrum of coverage includes not only the appropriately targeted, aforementioned organisms commonly implicated in CAP, but extensive activity against gram-negative organisms, to which resistance may develop with indiscriminate use.

From a pharmatectural and cost-effectiveness perspective, it appears that when gram-negative coverage of *Klebsiella* and other species is not required, the advanced generation macrolide azithromycin may still represent a more prudent, less costly choice as initial therapy, especially in individuals less than 60 years of age. However, in the older, sicker patient, in whom gram-negative infection is more of a concern, as well, as in areas in which there is a high prevalence of *S. pneumoniae* resistance, the newer quinolones are an important alternative to two-drug combinations, especially in the elderly patient where spectrum of coverage of polymicrobial infections may be especially important.

Finally, there is an increasing problem in the United States concerning the emergence of *S. pneumoniae* that is relatively resistant to penicillin and, less commonly, to extended-spectrum cephalosporins (see below). These isolates are often also resistant to macrolides, sulfonamides, and tetracyclines.[100-102] Except for vancomycin, the most favorable in vitro response rates to *S. pneumoniae* have been observed with the advanced macrolides and, more recently, with extended spectrum quinolones, especially trovafloxacin. Thus far, the majority of lower respiratory tract infections respond to standard therapy, though there have been profound implications for the empiric treatment of meningitis. Therapy for upper respiratory tract infections, such as sinusitis and otitis media, as well as for lower respiratory tract infections may be dramatically affected in the future if these mechanisms of resistance become more common.

Guidelines From the Infectious Diseases Society of America (IDSA) For Community-Acquired Pneumonia in Adults

The Infectious Disease Society of America (IDSA) through its Practice Guidelines Committee provides assistance to clinicians in the diagnosis and treatment of community-acquired pneumonia. The targeted providers are internists and family practitioners, and the targeted patient groups are immunocompetent adult patients. Criteria are specified for determining whether the inpatient or outpatient setting is appropriate for treatment. Differences from other guidelines written on this topic include use of laboratory criteria for diagnosis and approach to antimicrobial therapy. Panel members and consultants were experts in adult infectious diseases.

The guidelines are evidence-based where possible. A standard ranking system is used for the strength of recommendations and the quality of the evidence cited in the literature reviewed. The document has been subjected to external review by peer reviewers as well as by the Practice Guidelines Committee and was approved by the IDSA Council in September, 1998.

Role of Specific Pathogens in Community-Acquired Pneumonia

Prospective studies for evaluating the causes of CAP in adults have failed to identify the cause of 40% to 60% of cases of CAP, and two or more etiologies have been identified in 2% to 5% of cases. The most common etiologic agent identified in virtually all studies of CAP is *Streptococcus pneumoniae,* and this agent accounts for approximately two-thirds of all cases of cateremic pneumonia.

Other pathogens implicated less frequently include *Haemophilus influenzae* (most isolates of which are other than type B), *Mycoplasma pneumoniae, Chlamydia pneumoniae, S. aureus, Streptococcus pyogenes, Neisseria meningitidis, Moraxella catarrhalis, Klebsiella pneumoniae* and other gram-negative rods, *Legionella* sp., influenza virus (depending on the time of year), respiratory syncytial virus, adenovirus, parainfluenza virus, and other microbes. The frequency of other etiologies, e.g., *Chlamydia psittaci* (psittacosis), *Coxiella burnetii* (Q fever), *Francisella tularensis* (tularemia), and endemic fungi (histoplasmosis, blastomycosis, and coccidioidomycosis), is dependent on specific epidemiological factors.

The selection of antibiotics in the absence of an etiologic diagnosis (gram stains and culture results are not diagnostic) is based on multiple variables including severity of the illness, patient age, antimicrobial intolerance or side effects, clinical features, comorbidities, concomitant medications, exposures, and the epidemiological setting.

Preferred antimicrobials for most patients (in no specific order):

Macrolide*, fluoroquinolones**, or doxycycline

Alternative options: Amoxicillin/clavulanate and some second-generation cephalosporins (cefuroxime, cefpodoxime, or cefprozil)
Note: These will not be active versus atypical agents.

*Macrolide: erythromycin, clarithromycin, or azithromycin; clarithromycin, dirithromycin, or azithromycin are preferred if *H. influenzae* infection is suspected

**Fluoroquinolone: Levofloxacin, sparfloxacin, grepafloxacin, trovafloxacin, or another fluoroquinolone with enhanced activity against *S. pneumoniae*.

Preferred antimicrobials for most patients (in no specific order):

General medical ward

Preferred: a B-lactam (a) with or without a macrolide; (b) or a fluoroquinolone

Alternative: cefuroxime with or without a macrolide; (b) or azithromycin (alone)

Hospitalized in intensive care unit

Preferred: erythromycin, azithromycin, or a fluoroquinolone plus cefotaxime, ceftriaxone, or a B-lactam-\B-lactamase inhibitor

Modifying factors:

Structural disease of lung (bronchiectasis): antipseudomonal penicillin, carbapenem, or cefepime *plus* (a) macrolide (b) or fluoroquinolone (c) *plus* an aminoglycoside

Penicillin allergy: fluoroquinolone (c) with or without clindamycin

Suspected aspiration: fluoroquinolone (c) plus clindamycin or a B-lactam-\B-lactamase inhibitor (d)

(a) B-lactam: cefotaxime or ceftriaxone
(b) Macrolide: azithromycin, clarithromycin, dirithromycin, or erythromycin
(c) Fluoroquinolone: levofloxacin, sparfloxacin, grepafloxacin, trovafloxacin, or another fluoroquinolone with enhanced activity against *S. pneumoniae*
(d) B-lactam-\B-lactamase inhibitor: ampicillin/sulbactam, ticarcillin/clavulanate, or piperacillin/tazobactam; for structural disease of the lung; ticarcillin/clavulanate or piperacillin/clavulanate.

Bacterial Exacerbations of Chronic Obstructive Pulmonary Disease (COPD)

Chronic obstructive pulmonary disease (COPD) affects approximately 20% of all adults and is the fourth leading cause of death in the United States.[103] Exacerbations of COPD are usually manifested by an increase in cough, change in quantity or color of sputum, or worsening dyspnea and may lead to hospitalization. There are numerous possible causes of exacerbations of COPD but infection is one of the most common identifiable etiologies. As a result, antibiotics have become a mainstay in the treatment of patients with this disorder. Despite the widespread use of antibiotics in this setting, their efficacy remains somewhat uncertain.

In a landmark report, academic investigators performed a widespread literature search in order to conduct a meta-analysis to answer the question, "Are antibiotics beneficial in patients with COPD exacerbations?"[103] English language studies published in the last 40 years were included in the analysis if they were randomized trials comparing antibiotic to placebo in patients thought to be having an exacerbation of COPD and had follow-up for at least 5 days. Nine studies were included (230 studies were excluded for a variety of reasons) but there were no uniform outcome measures for all the trials.

These trials were conducted in both the outpatient and inpatient settings. The earliest trial included was from 1957 and the most recent was from 1992. Seven of the nine trials showed a benefit of antibiotics over placebo with the overall effect size indicating a small benefit in the antibiotic treated group. Patients who were hospitalized showed the greatest benefit. In 6 trials in which peak expiratory flow rates (PEFR) were one of the outcome measures, the summary effect size was also small, with a summary change in PEFR of 10.75 L/min in favor of the antibiotic treated group, which is small, but can be clinically significant, particularly in COPD patients with low baseline PEFR.

Exacerbations of COPD are commonly seen in the outpatient/ED setting and, not infrequently, lead to hospitalizations. Infection is believed to be a common cause of exacerbations, although they are often difficult to document definitively. Based on the evidence in this meta-analysis study, antibiotics should be used in this setting, although the benefit appears to be relatively small. Nevertheless, agents that cover common respiratory pathogens such as *Streptococcus pneumoniae, Hemophilus influenzae, Moraxella catarrhalis,* and perhaps, atypical organisms (*Chlamydiae, Legionella*) are reasonable for this problem. (See Table 5-5)

The shortest and most convenient regimens include azithromycin, trovafloxacin, or levofloxacin, whereas the least expensive regimens include TMP/SMZ or doxycycline. In addition to antibiotics, avoidance of airway irritants (tobacco, allergens), use of bronchodilators and systemic or inhaled corticosteroids are mainstays in the treatment of patients with exacerbations of COPD.

Stratification of Patients According to Risk Factors

Therapeutic failure might be expected to lead to more hospitalizations, increased costs due to extra physician visits, prolonged absences from work, further diagnostic tests, and repeated courses of antibiotics in high-risk individuals. Routine chemotherapy fails in 13% to 25% or more exacerbations. Stratification of patients into risk categories can identify high-risk patients and allow targeted antimicrobial therapy, particularly at resistant organisms. Treatment failure is particularly costly in these patients, since hospitalization and multiple courses of therapy are likely. All of the classification schemes are similar and define separate groups with increasing risk of significant impairment of health and possible adverse consequences of an acute exacerbation.

In patients with acute bronchitis with no underlying lung disease, the etiology is usually viral. No antibiotic is necessary for most patients. In the face of persistent symptoms, treatment with a macrolide or doxycycline is rational to eradicate potential infection with *Mycoplasma pneumoniae* or *Chlamydia pneumoniae.*

Table 5-5

Antibiotics for Acute Exacerbations of COPD

Antibiotic	Recommended Dose	Frequency	Duration
FIRST-LINE			
GENERICS			
Trimethoprim-sulfamethoxazole (Bactrim, Septra)	1 ds tab po	bid	7-14 d
Amoxicillin (Amoxil, Wymox)	500 mg	tid	7-14 d
Tetracycline	500 mg	qid	7-14 d
Doxycycline (Doryx, Vibramycin)	100 mg	bid	7-14 d
MACROLIDES/AZALIDES			
Azithromycin (Zithromax)	500 mg on 1st day, 250 mg qd x 4 days		5 d
Clarithromycin (Biaxin)	250 mg bid (for *S. pneumoniae/ M. catarrhalis*) 500 mg bid (for *H. influenzae*)		7-14 d
QUINOLONES			
Trovafloxacin (Trovan)	100 mg po qd		7-10 d
Levofloxacin (Levaquin)	500 mg qd		7-14 d

Table 5-5

Antibiotics for Acute Exacerbations of COPD — cont'd.

Antibiotic	Recommended Dose	Frequency	Duration
SECOND-LINE			
QUINOLONES			
Ofloxacin (Floxin)	400 mg	bid	10 d
Ciprofloxacin (Cipro)	500 mg	bid	10 d
Lomefloxacin (Maxaquin)	400 mg	qd	10 d
Sparfloxacin (Zagam)	400 mg qd day 1; 200 mg qd days 2-10		10 d
CEPHALOSPORINS			
Cefixime (Suprax)	400 mg	qd	
	200 mg	bid	10 d
Cefprozil (Cefzil)	500 mg	bid	10 d
Cefaclor (Ceclor)	250 mg	tid	10 d
PENICILLINS			
Amoxicillin/clavulanate (Augmentin)	875 mg	bid	10 d

The second category of patients are usually young (< 60 years), have only mild-to-moderate impairment of lung function (FEV1 < 50% predicted), and have less than four exacerbations per year. Common organisms found are *H. influenzae, S. pneumoniae,* and *M. catarrhalis,* although viral infections often precede bacterial superinfection. Treatment with a beta-lactam is usually successful, and the prognosis is excellent. Since most of these patients respond to therapy and the consequences of treatment failure are slight, virtually any antimicrobial could be used.

Patients in the third category are older, with poor underlying lung function (FEV1 > 50% predicted) or only moderate impairment of lung function (FEV1 between 50% and 65% predicted) but with concurrent significant medical illnesses (e.g., diabetes mellitus, congestive heart failure, chronic renal disease, chronic liver disease, etc.), and/or experience four or more exacerbations per year. *H. influenzae, S. pneumoniae,* and *M. catarrhalis* continue to be the predominant organisms. In this group of patients, initial treatment failure has major implications for the patient and health care system, including increased time lost from work and/or hospitalization. Treatment with medications directed toward resistant organisms, such as quinolone, amoxicillin-clavulanic acid, second- or third-generation cephalosporin, or second-generation macrolide, would be expected to demonstrate cost-effectiveness since the cost of therapeutic failure in this group of patients is high.

The last group is comprised of patients who have chronic bronchial suppuration with frequent exacerbations characterized by increased sputum production, increased sputum purulence, cough, and worsening dyspnea. These individuals tend to have a chronic progressive course, and an aggressive therapeutic approach should be offered. Beside the usual respiratory organisms, other Gram-negative organisms, including *Enterobacteriaceae* and *Pseudomonas* sp., are frequently isolated. The use of sputum cultures in this group of patients to identify potential multiresistant organisms and target specific therapy would be useful. Frequently, a quinolone is used for this group.

Upper Respiratory Tract Infection

Although penicillin remains the drug of choice in the treatment of pharyngitis caused by *S. pyogenes,* it appears that the newer cephalosporins and macrolides may yield a superior bacteriologic eradication rate and, possibly, a decreased relapse rate.[104,105] Since the prevention of rheumatic fever requires eradication of the infecting *Streptococcus,* the newer cephalosporins and the macrolides are assumed to be at least as effective as penicillin in achieving this goal. The more convenient dosing schedule of these newer agents may enhance compliance.

The most common etiologies of acute sinusitis include: *S. pneumoniae, H. influenzae, M. catarrhalis,* and a variety of less common organisms. Many antibiotic regimens have been shown to yield the expected bacteriologic cure rate of greater than 90%.[106] Interestingly, a recent trial using TMP/SMZ in the treatment of acute sinusitis indicates that a shorter treatment duration of 3 days

Figure 5-1

Management of Uncomplicated Sinusitis

History Physical Examination ± Plain Film Radiography

Treatment

Antibiotic, orally 10-14 days, repeat course with broader spectrum agent if no improvement after initial 7 days.
Antihistamine, orally, 4 weeks (if allergic symptoms present).
Decongestant, orally, 4 weeks.

Decongestant, intranasal topical, 3-5 days.
Consider adjunctive measures:
- Nasal saline irrigations
- Analgesics orally
- Mucolytics (e.g. guaifenesin orally)

3-4 week interval re-evaluation ± plain film radiography

Resolution

Treat any predisposing conditions (i.e., allergic, metabolic, or immunologic)

No Resolution

Antibiotic,† orally 3-6 weeks
Decongestant, orally, 6 weeks
Steroid, topical intranasal, 6 weeks
Antihistamine, orally, 6 weeks (if allergic symptoms present)
CT scan (axial and coronal views)
Continue adjunctive measures
Otolaryngology referral for surgical consideration

Antimicorobials

* First-line antibiotic recommendations:
- trovafloxacin 200 mg po qd x 10 days
- amoxicillin-clavulanate 500 mg po q8h
- clarithromycin 500 mg po bid x 10 days
- trimethoprim (160)/sulfamethoxazole (600 mg) po bid x 10 days
- levofloxacin 500 mg po 7-14 days

† Second-line antibiotic recommendations:
- cefuroxime axetil 500 mg po q12h
- cefprozil 500 mg po q12h
- cefpodoxime 200 mg po q12h
- loracarbef 400 mg po q12h
- or newer macrolides

may be as effective as a traditional 10 day course for selected patients with mild infections.[107] (See Figure 5-1)

Otitis Media In Children

The most commonly isolated bacterial pathogens in both acute and recurrent otitis media are *S. pneumoniae, H. influenzae* (nontypable), and *M. catarrhalis.*[85,86] Although there are studies that show high spontaneous cure rates in mild to moderate cases of acute otitis media, treatment with antibiotics is still the standard of care in the United States. Unfortunately, drug resistance among bacteria involved in otitis media is rapidly emerging.[85,86] In this regard, beta-lactamase production is common among isolates of *H. influenzae* and *M. catarrhalis,* rendering about 30% to 50% of *H. influenzae* and up to 80% of *M. catarrhalis* isolates resistant to ampicillin.[108]

Although variable from patient to patient and region to region, these emerging resistance patterns may explain the failure rates associated with such traditional therapeutic measures as amoxicillin.[84,86] Accordingly, the evolution of antibiotic-resistant bacterial strains implicated in otitis media has fueled interest in alternatives to amoxicillin, which, primarily because of its cost, has been the traditional first-line agent for this infection, despite showing increasing resistance. This problem can be circumvented by adding a beta-lactamase inhibitor such as clavulanic acid to amoxicillin (i.e., amoxicillin/clavulanate) or by choosing alternative antibiotics, among them, azithromycin, loracarbef, and second-generation cephalosporins.

Without question, as previously emphasized in the case of CAP for adults, a most disturbing trend is the emergence of penicillin-resistant *S. pneumoniae.* Although the incidence of resistant strains demonstrates regional variations, the continued prevalence of *S. pneumoniae* as the principal etiologic agent in otitis media has important therapeutic implications, especially in light of the trend toward emergence of penicillin- and cephalosporin-resistant strains of this organism. From a clinical perspective, it should be emphasized that the development of penicillin-resistant strains has been associated with increased resistance to other beta-lactam antibiotics, including amoxicillin, cefaclor, cefuroxime, and cefixime, as well as the non-beta-lactam antibiotics TMP/SMZ and erythromycin.[109,110]

Based on currently available studies, about 25% of *S. pneumoniae* isolates obtained by tympanocentesis from patients with otitis media in various regions of the United States demonstrated intermediate or complete resistance to penicillin. Currently, intermediate or complete resistance to the advanced macrolides, azithromycin, dirithromycin, and clarithromycin, has been identified in about 5% to 8% of *S. pneumoniae* isolates, as compared to 10% to 25% of isolates shown to be resistant to such antibiotics as penicillin, amoxicillin, cefixime, TMP/SMZ, and other cephalosporins.[84-86]

These findings suggest that in vitro resistance patterns to *S. pneumoniae* are one factor that should be considered in the selection process of an antibiotic for

Table 5-6

PPPD Approach to Selection of Oral Antibiotic Suspensions for Treatment of Acute Otitis Media in Children[3, 23, 26, 54, 66, 67]

ORAL ANTIBIOTIC SUSPENSION (Generic name)	**PRESCRIPTION RESISTANCE** (Cost for course of therapy < $40)	**PARENTAL RESISTANCE** (Once-daily dosing)	**PATIENT RESISTANCE** (Palatability and GI effect profile considered extremely favorable)	**DRUG RESISTANCE** (Less than 20% of *S. pneumoniae* isolates from middle ear show in vitro resistance and drug shows adequate coverage of beta-lactamase-producing *H. influenzae* and *M. catarrhalis*)
Amoxicillin	+ + ($6.02)	− (TID)	+	−
Amoxicillin-clavulanate	+ ($38.10)	±(BID)	− (diarrhea)	+
Azithromycin	+ ($28.40)	+	+	+
Cefaclor	+ ($38.20)	− (TID/BID)	+	±
Cefixime	− ($45.68)	+	+	±
Cefpodoxime	− ($54.00)	+	− (poor taste)	+
Cefprozil	− ($45.59)	±(BID)	− (poor taste)	+
Cefuroxime	− ($62.84)	±(BID)	+	+
Clarithromycin	− ($42.40)	±(BID)	− (poor taste)	+
Erythromycin-sulfisoxazole	+ ($22.77)	− (TID or QID)	− (poor taste, GI intolerance)	±
Loracarbef	− ($54.40)	±(BID)	+	+
Trimethoprim-sulfamethoxazole	+ + ($4.36)	±(BID)	− (allergic reactions)	±

(+) Satisfies specific PPPD category criterion
(−) Does not usually satisfy specific PPPD category criterion
(±) Possibly satisfies PPPD category criterion

treatment of otitis media. (See Table 5-6) The only antibiotic to which drug resistance has not been found is vancomycin.

Urinary Tract Infection

Cystitis, urethritis and pyelonephritis, and prostatitis are common infections managed in the primary care setting. An estimated 10% to 20% of women are afflicted at some point with a urinary tract infection (UTI) and the incidence in older men approaches that of women.[111] The development of new antibiotic agents, streamlining of the standard of care for young females with suspected UTI and the recognition that a wide array of clinical and microbiologic entities can present with dysuria, have led to a change in the approach to patients with UTI.

Acute cystitis and subclinical pyelonephritis are common in young females and are often impossible to distinguish clinically. Up to 25% of women presenting with the classic symptoms of lower UTIs actually suffer from "subclinical" pyelonephritis. Enterobacteriaceae (predominantly *E. coli*) account for 80% and *Staphylococcus saprophyticus* account for 10% to 15% of UTIs in young women when sexually transmitted pathogens are excluded. The precise etiology of UTIs in an individual patient may be difficult to determine. In one study, only 66% of young women presenting to a family practice setting with urinary tract symptoms could be assigned a specific microbiologic diagnosis despite an extensive work-up.[111]

In young women, acute cystitis and urethritis occur in the absence of classical criteria for bacteriuria (105 bacteria per mL of urine) in as many as 50% of cases.[111-113] The constellation of dysuria, frequency and pyuria in the absence of "significant" bacteriuria, has been termed the acute urethral syndrome. In many cases, this syndrome is caused by low level infections with *E. coli* (102 to 104 organisms per mL) or with a sexually transmitted pathogen such as *Chlamydia trachomatis.* The modern standard for a positive urine culture in a patient with dysuria is now widely accepted to be 102 rather than 105 organisms per mL.

Sexually transmitted pathogens can cause urethritis, vaginitis, and prostatitis, conditions that can clinically mimic the infections of classic uropathogens such as *E. coli.* Microorganisms including *Trichomonas vaginalis, Neisseria gonorrhoeae, C. trachomatis,* and *Ureaplasma urealyticum* are common offenders. Urethritis and epididymitis caused by sexually transmitted pathogens are increasingly common among promiscuous males, and UTI may be associated with HIV or herpes virus infection. With advancing age, the rate of UTI in males approaches that seen in females, and is often associated with prostate disease. Some unusual pathogens of iatrogenic origin are also found in the elderly. *Pseudomonas* and *Staphylococcus* sp. are associated with urinary tract manipulation, and enterococcus is found in patients who had previously received cephalosporin antibiotics.

Asymptomatic bacteriuria is diagnosed when more than 105 colonies of a single bacterial species are recovered on two consecutive urine cultures in patients without symptoms. In most of these patients, antibiotic therapy does not yield any lasting benefit. During pregnancy however, asymptomatic bacteriuria occurs in as many as 30% of women and commonly leads to full blown pyelonephritis if left untreated. Often, these infections are caused by *Streptococcus agalactiae,* a common flora of the female genitourinary tract that has been associated with premature delivery, neonatal sepsis, and postpartum endometritis. Asymptomatic bacteriuria can also be found in as many as 33% of residents of skilled nursing facilities, and may be a nidus for sepsis in some.[102]Antibiotic treatment in these patients is usually followed by relapse of bacteriuria and it is therefore not routinely recommended.

The majority of uncomplicated urinary tract infections, the diagnosis of which will usually not require cultures, are caused by *E. coli.*[103-105] However, insomuch as up to one-third of *E. coli* are resistant to amoxicillin, this antibiotic can no longer be recommended for treatment. In contrast, TMP/SMZ is reliably active and is considered one treatment of choice. A recent trial concluded that a 3 day regimen of TMP/SMZ was more effective and less expensive than 3 days of nitrofurantoin, amoxicillin, or cefadroxil in the treatment of uncomplicated cystitis in women.[114] Another approved 3 day regimen for uncomplicated UTI caused by *E. coli* is trovafloxacin. A new oral antibiotic, fosfomycin, is approved for single dose therapy, costs about $22, and has a success rate of about 70%.

In general, broader-spectrum agents offer no distinct advantage and are considerably more expensive than such agents as TMP/SMZ. Nevertheless, it should be stressed that the quinolones play a major role in the treatment of urinary tract infection, especially when allergy or intolerance, bacterial resistance, or complicated infection is present. The optimum duration of therapy for uncomplicated cystitis appears to be 3 days; however, a 7 day course is indicated in patients with diabetes, in individuals with more than 7 days of symptoms, a history of recent urinary tract infection, diaphragm use, age > 65 years, and in pregnant women.

As emphasized, for pyelonephritis, 14 days of therapy with TMP/SMZ, a fluoroquinolone, or a third-generation cephalosporin is indicated.[121,123] Treatment of asymptomatic bacteriuria is unnecessary except during pregnancy. Pregnant women should have a urinalysis and culture at their first prenatal visit and urine dipsticks during the course of pregnancy. Asymptomatic bacteriuria should be treated with 10 days of antibiotics and followed closely to assure that relapse does not occur. Antibiotics that are considered non-teratogenic include any of the beta-lactams, nitrofurantoin and sulfasoxazole. Trimethoprim and quinolone antibiotics should not be used in pregnant patients.

In sexually active patients, dysuria and pyuria may represent urethritis secondary to *N. gonorrhoeae* or chlamydia. A history of similar symptoms in a sexual partner or the presence of vaginal discharge may provide additional clues and prompt the appropriate genitourinary cultures. Some cases of acute urethral syndrome in females and most cases of epididymitis in young males are caused by chlamydia, which can be effectively treated with a 7 day course of doxycycline (100 mg twice daily). Trimethoprim and the fluoroquinolones have excellent penetration into inflamed prostatic tissue, making them excellent choices in elderly males where recurrent UTI is often associated with prostatitis. Nevertheless, relapses are common even after a month of antibiotic therapy.

Recurrent episodes of UTI may require a urologic evaluation for underlying problems such as urinary tract obstruction or stone disease. If no precipitating factors are discovered, prophylactic therapy should be considered. A nightly dose of 50 mg nitrofurantoin or 1 DS TMP/SMZ every other night will prevent recurrence in 90% of such patients. In a randomized, double-blind, placebo-controlled trial over eight months involving 93 postmenopausal women, investigators demonstrated that topical, intravaginal estrogen cream (0.5 mg estriol cream once each night for 2 weeks followed by 2 times per week for 8 months) led to a profound reduction in the rate of recurrent UTI and overall antibiotic use.[111,112,113,115] The mechanism appeared to be related to favorable alterations in vaginal pH and vaginal bacterial flora with increased presence of lactobacilli and reduced presence of Enterobacteriaceae.

Sexually Transmitted Diseases

Uncomplicated gonorrhea is treated with single-dose therapy. There are a variety of effective regimens based on quinolones, cephalosporins, and the macrolide azithromycin that vary considerably in cost. Chlamydia must always be empirically treated along with gonorrhea. The importance of effective communication in enhancing compliance with medication regimens cannot be overemphasized.[116] Current standards of care for the sexually transmitted diseases have been recommended by the CDC.[80] Because significant noncompliance has been reported with doxycycline, one-dose therapeutic modalities—azithromycin 1 g orally once for uncomplicated chlamydial infection and a choice of several agents for uncomplicated GC—are preferred. (See Table 5-7)

The chlamydia problem deserves special attention. From an emergency therapeutics perspective, what is instructive about the chlamydial epidemic is the fact that it has grown significantly, in large part because of poor compliance with the traditional, 7 day twice daily doxycycline regimen, which has been the weak link between the prescription pad and optimal clinical outcome.[117] In one "real world" study, only 65% of all patients prescribed a 7 day course of doxycycline therapy reported sufficient intake of the antimicrobial to achieve clinical cure of their chlamydial infection.[117-119] When this occurs, a sizable percentage of patients will return for retreatment because of noncompliance-mediated therapeutic failures. In addition, these patients are at risk for infecting other partners who must also access the health care system for treatment. The end result is "turnstyle STDs," a phenomenon in which pharmacologic reservicing for STDs and pelvic inflammatory disease (PID) is required because of therapeutic failures associated with inadequate adherence to medication regimens. These observations strongly support the use of single dose therapy given under supervision, on site, in the Emergency Department or clinic, for treatment of uncomplicated chlamydial infections.

Table 5-7

Treatment of Uncomplicated Chlamydia*	
FIRST-LINE THERAPY	**ALTERNATIVE THERAPY**
Azithromycin 1 g po once (This is the only single-dose therapy for chlamydia approved by the CDC.)	Erythromycin base 500 mg po qid x 7 days
or Doxycycline 100 mg po bid x 7-10 days (contraindicated in pregnancy)	**or** Erythromycin ethylsuccinate 800 mg po qid x 7 days
	or Tetracycline 500 mg po qid x 10-14 days (Although effective, compliance is less than adequate, and the drug is contraindicated in pregnancy.)
	or Ofloxacin 300 mg po bid x 7-10 days (contraindicated in pregnancy and in patients < 18 years)

Adapted from: McCormack WM. Pelvic inflammatory disease. *N Engl J Med* 1994;330:115-119; Therapy for sexually transmitted diseases. *Med Lett* 1994;36:1-4; Centers for Disease Control and Prevention. Sexually transmitted disease treatment guidelines.

MMWR Morb Mortal Wkly Rep 1993;42(number RR-14):i-102; Sweet RL, et al. Evaluation of new anti-infective agents for the treatment of acute pelvic inflammatory disease. *Clin Infect dis* 1992;15(supple): S33-42.

* A thorough discussion of the diagnosis and management of gonorrhea, chlamydia, and pelvic inflammatory disease appears in a previous issue of *Emergency Medicine Reports (Emerg Med Rep* 1994;15:251-260).

Pelvic Inflammatory Disease

Pelvic inflammatory disease (PID) is a term that is most commonly used to describe infection of the uterus, fallopian tubes, and adjacent pelvic structures that is not associated with surgery or pregnancy. An estimated 1 million women per year are diagnosed with PID, a condition that is particularly common and problematic among lower socioeconomic groups in urban areas.[119-122]

In addition to the acute manifestations of the infection, long-term sequelae such as ectopic pregnancy and infertility occur in 25% of cases.[118-120] In 1994, the direct and indirect costs of the disease and its complications were estimated to be greater than $4 billion. In view of the impact of this infection, a systematic approach to diagnosis and therapy is mandatory for all practitioners who encounter patients with this condition and its related complications.

In virtually all cases, PID results from ascending spread of organisms from the cervix and vagina to the upper genital tract. Sexual transmission of *Neisseria gonorrhoeae* and/or *Chlamydia trachomatis* account for more than half of all cases of PID, but *H. hominis* and other organisms have also been implicated.[119-121] *N. gonorrhoeae* is the major cause of PID in urban areas, where gonococcal infection is prevalent, whereas *C. trachomatis* is responsible for a greater proportion of cases among college students, in whom gonococcal infection is less common. Organisms such as *E. coli* and other enteric pathogens, as well as pathogens from the vaginal flora, also may cause PID, particularly when the normal vaginal flora (*lactobacilli*) are supplanted with other organisms. However, infection in the upper genital tract does not always result in clinically recognizable disease; indeed, many women with adverse sequelae associated with PID, such as infertility, have no known history of the disease.[110-112]

In one prospective study, infertility due to tubal occlusion occurred in 8% of women after one episode of PID, in 19.5% after two episodes, and in 40% after three or more episodes.[115] Furthermore, as previously mentioned, many cases of PID are clinically silent, but as many as 70% of women who are infertile due to tubal obstruction have serum antibodies against chlamydia vs. only about 25% of women who are infertile for other reasons.[118,120,122]

A high index of suspicion and a low threshold for initiating treatment are important for facilitating detection and appropriate management. This approach should be applied to all women of child-bearing age with pelvic pain. Although laparoscopic visualization of inflamed fallopian tubes and pelvic structures is possible and, according to some experts, serves as a "gold standard" for the diagnosis, it is seldom practical. As a rule, the emergency physician must initiate antibiotic therapy on clinical grounds, despite its limitations. In addition to the clinical symptoms, lower abdominal tenderness, adnexal tenderness, and pain on manipulation of the cervix are present in physical examination in up to 90% of women.[119,121,122] Other manifestations, such as elevated erythrocyte sedimentation rate or C-reactive protein and abnormal vaginal discharge vary widely in frequency. At present, there are no effective ways to detect clinically silent disease.

Because new and highly effective treatment regimens have been introduced for PID, pharmacists and physicians now have a number of therapeutic options available for managing these problematic—and, frequently, poorly compliant—patients with STDs and PID.[123-125] In this regard, the CDC recommend a number of possible regimens, most of which mandate the use of a broad-spectrum cephalosporin administered parenterally (initially) along with an oral agent effective against chlamydia such as doxycycline. Commonly used regimens for inpatient treatment of PID include the combination of cefoxitin, ceftriaxone, or cefotetan plus doxycycline; plus IV metronidazole followed by oral therapy with metronidazole plus doxycycline; gentamicin plus clindamycin; and IV ampicillin-sulbactam plus doxycycline.

As previously described, the oral formulation of azithromycin has been indicated for uncomplicated urethral and endocervical chlamydial infections and offers the unique advantage of efficacy with a single dose of 1 g orally. Recently, however, efficacy and safety, as well as FDA approval, have been established for IV azithromycin therapy followed by oral azithromycin for the treatment of PID.

One study evaluated results in a total of 221 women with PID treated with the following regimens: 1) azithromycin monotherapy (administered as 500 mg IV as the initial dose on day 1, followed by 250 mg/day for 6 additional days); 2) azithromycin in combination with metronidazole; and 3) metronidazole (either IV metronidazole 500 mg twice daily on day 1 followed by oral administration of 500 mg twice daily for 11 days or oral administration of 500 mg twice daily for 12 days), plus doxycycline (100 mg orally twice daily for 14 days), plus cefoxitin (2 g IV or IM) with probenecid 1 g on the first day of treatment.[92,94]

In an intent-to-treat analysis conducted 15 days after therapy with these regimens, 93% of the patients receiving azithromycin alone, 94% of patients receiving azithromycin plus metronidazole, and 93% of those receiving the triad of cefoxitin, doxycycline, and metronidazole were either cured or improved.[94] The bacteriologic eradication rates for all three regimens were in the 93% to 95% range. Azithromycin was well-tolerated in patients with PID. The most common side effects were diarrhea (8.5%) and nausea (6.6%). The addition of metronidazole to azithromycin increased slightly the incidence of GI side effects, with 10.3% reporting nausea, 3.7% abdominal pain, and 2.8% vomiting.[94]

Based on this data, azithromycin IV (500 mg once daily for 1 or 2 days) followed by oral azithromycin 250 mg PO once daily to complete a total of 7 days of therapy should be considered a primary treatment modality for managing patients who require initial IV therapy for PID caused by *C. trachomatis, N. gonorrhoeae,* or *M. hominis.* The timing of the switch from IV to oral therapy should be made by the physician, who should make this decision based on clinical parameters. Moreover, it should be stressed that when anaerobic infection is strongly suspected to play an etiologic role in any individual patient with PID, the physician should combine an antimicrobial agent such as metronidazole that provides anaerobic coverage along with azithromycin.

Although many patients with PID will require hospitalization, (especially those who appear to be systemically toxic, have abdominal rebound tenderness, have WBC counts greater than 15,000, have a unilateral mass suggestive of tubo-ovarian abscess, have a history or profile indicating risk for poor medication compliance, are in the adolescent age group, and those in whom preservation of fertility is a high priority) a significant percentage can be treated with initial IV or IM therapy in the ED, followed by oral therapy out of the hospital to complete the antimicrobial course.

Current options for out-of-hospital management of mild PID include trovafloxacin or other approved quinolones and the well-established regimen of ceftriaxone 500 mg IM, followed by doxycycline 100 mg PO twice daily for 14 days with or without metronidazole 500 mg PO three times daily for 10 to 14 days. With approval of the azithromycin IV/oral sequenced combination regimen outlined above, it is now possible to streamline therapy for PID into a 7 day course, and substantially reduce the number of oral doses required to complete the treatment course. The practical implications are as follows: If, on the basis of the clinical findings, the physician deems that a patient with mild PID can be managed out of the hospital, and that a single IV dose of azithromycin is sufficient prior to oral therapy, then azithromycin should be administered as an infusion at a rate of 2 mg/mL over one hour, or 1 mg/mL over three hours. Azithromycin IV should always be infused over a period of not less than one hour, and should never be administered by bolus or IM injection. If patients with PID have signs and symptoms that suggest the need for more than one intravenous dose, hospitalization will usually be necessary.

The 1-hour minimum infusion time required for this antibiotic is not as convenient as the IM route of administration required for the ceftriaxone (plus oral doxycycline) regimen. However, the post-parenteral therapy phase of the azithromycin treatment regimen (which requires only an additional 6 days of oral therapy following the IV dose) is considerably more convenient and compliance-enhancing, both with respect to daily dose frequency and duration of therapy, than the ceftriaxone regimen, which requires consolidation with 28 oral doses of doxycycline over a 14-day period. In a patient population at high risk for noncompliance, the azithromycin regimen offers a potential window of opportunity that should be considered in this difficult patient population.

An alternative for outpatient management is the quinolone antibiotic, trovafloxacin, which requires only once-daily administration for a 14-day course. For mild to moderate cases of PID, trovafloxacin can be dosed orally, without requiring IM or IV doses initially, as is the case for the doxycycline/ceftriaxone and IV/oral azithromycin regimens, respectively.

All women with suspected or confirmed PID require a pregnancy test to determine appropriate management. If present, intrauterine devices should be removed once antibiotic therapy is initiated. Close follow-up of outpatients within 24 to 48 hours after treatment is started is important. Failure to improve indicates the need for reassessment of the diagnosis (using laparoscopy, ultrasonography, or hospitalization) rather than a change in antibiotic therapy.

Male sexual partners of patients with PID need to be evaluated; this should include examination for sexually transmitted infections other than chlamydial and gonococcal disease, although, as a minimum, they must be treated for these two infections. Women who have had PID should be advised against the use of intrauterine devices and to protect themselves as much as possible against subsequent sexually transmitted infection to reduce their likelihood of infertility and other long-term sequelae. In women with concomitant HIV infection, hospitalization and IV therapy are indicated.

Skin and Skin Structure Infections

The majority of uncomplicated skin and skin structure infections are caused by *staphylococci* and *streptococci*. Conventional treatment with cephalexin or dicloxacillin is highly effective; the newer agents should be reserved for resistant organisms.[126] Diabetic foot infections are more frequently polymicrobial, and common offending agents include anaerobes, gram-positive organisms, and gram-negative bacteria. Consequently, treatment is often empiric. In the outpatient setting, an oral quinolone such as ciprofloxacin (plus clindamycin when anaerobic and enhanced gram-positive activity is required) is an appropriate first-line agent.[127] The availability of trovafloxacin, with its broad spectrum of coverage, offers the advantage of both monotherapy and once-daily dosing in the management of diabetic foot infections.

Pharmatectural Conclusions

The newer oral cephalosporins, quinolones, and macrolides often have an extended in vitro spectrum of activity, more desirable side-effect profiles, and improved pharmacokinetic patterns compared to older, conventional antibiotics. Frequently, there is a price to pay for such advances and advantages, including higher acquisition cost and increasing selective pressure for the emergence of resistant organisms. Although many common bacterial infections can usually be treated successfully with standard agents at a reduced cost, there are many circumstances when total outcome costs will be reduced by employing antibiotics with a shorter duration of therapy, less frequent daily dosing, and a more targeted spectrum of coverage that encompasses the most likely etiologic agents in specific patient subgroups. In particular, patient compliance with medications must always be considered when prescribing antibiotics in the outpatient setting.

[1]Temafloxacin withdrawn. FDA Med Bull 1992;22:4.

[2]Blum MD, Graham DJ, McCloskey CA. Temafloxacin syndrome: Review of 95 cases. Clin Infect Dis 1994;18:946-950.

[3]Cockburn J, Gibberd RW, Reid AL, et al. Determinants of non-compliance with short term antibiotic regimens. BMJ 1987;295:814-818.

[4]Eisen SA, Miller DK, Woodward RS, et al. The effect of prescribed daily dose frequency on patient medication compliance. Arch Intern Med 1990;150:1881-1884.

[5]Sanson-Fisher R, Bowman J, Armstrong, S. Factors affecting nonadherence with antibiotics. Diagn Microbiol Infect Dis 1992;15:103S-109S.

[6]Neu HC. The crisis in antibiotic resistance. Science 1992;257: 1064-1073.

[7]Murray BE. New aspects of antimicrobial resistance and the resulting therapeutic dilemmas. J Infect Dis 1991;163:1185-1194.

[8]Chater RW. Dosing tips for tots. Am Pharm 1993;NS33:55-56.

[9]Finney JW, Friman PC, Rapoff MA, et al. Improving compliance with antibiotic regimens for otitis media: Randomized clinical trial in a pediatric clinic. Am J Dis Child 1985;139:89-95.

[10]Demers DM, Scotik Chan D, Bass JW. Antimicrobial drug suspensions: a blinded comparison of taste of twelve pediatric drugs including cefixime, cefpodoxime, cefprozil, and loracarbef. Pediatr Infect Dis J 1994:13:87-89.

[11]Chinburapa V, Larson LN. The importance of side effects and outcomes in differentiating between prescription drug products. J Clin Pharm Ther 1992;17:333-342.

[12]Anonymous. Writing prescription instructions. Can Med Assoc J 1991;44:647-648.

[13]Coleman TJ. Non-redemption of prescriptions. BMJ 1994;308:135.

[14]Roth HP, Caron HS. Accuracy of doctor's estimates and patients' statements on adherence to a drug regimen. Clin Pharm Ther 1978;23:361-370.

[15]Eisen SA, Miller DK, Woodward RS, et al. The effect of prescribed daily dose frequency on patient medication compliance. Arch Intern Med 1990;150:1881-1884.

[16]Greenbery RN. Overview of patient compliance with medication dosing: A literature review. Clin Ther 1984;6:592-599.

[17]Bluestone CD, Klein JO. Management. In: Otitis Media in Infants and Children. Philadelphia: WB Saunders; 1988:121-201.

[18]Jacoby GA, Archer GL. New mechanisms of bacterial resistance to antimicrobial agents. N Engl J Med 1991;324:601-612.

[19]PÈchËre JC. Antibiotic resistance is selected primarily in our patients. Infect Control Hosp Epidemiol 1994;15:472-477.

[20]McCaig LF, Hughes JM. Trends in antimicrobial prescribing among office-based physicians in the United States. JAMA 1995;272:214-219.

[21]Gonzales R, Sande M. What will it take to stop physicians from prescribing antibiotics in acute bronchitis? Lancet 1995;345:665-666.

[22]Saint S, Bent S, Vittinghoff E, et al. Antibiotics in chronic obstructive pulmonary disease exacerbations. JAMA 1995;273:957-960.

[23]Hebel, S. Drug Facts and Comparisons. St. Louis. Facts and Comparisons;1998

[24]Anne S, Reisman RE. Risk of administering cephalosporin antibiotics to patients with histories of penicillin allergy. Ann Allergy Asthma Immunol 1995;74:167-170.

[25]Cefuroxime-axetil. Med Lett Drugs Ther 1988;30:57-60.

[26]Cefprozil. Med Lett Drugs Ther 1992;34:63-64.

[27]Loracarbef. Med Lett Drugs Ther 1992;34:87-88.

[28]Nadelman RB, Luger SW, Frank E, et al. A comparison of cefuroxime axetil and doxycycline in the treatment of early Lyme disease. Ann Intern Med 1992;117:273-280.

[29]Cefixime. Med Lett Drugs Ther 1989;31:73-75.

[30]Cefpodoxime proxetil. Med Lett Drugs Ther 1992;34:107-108.

[31]Vantin (Cefpodoxime proxetil) Prescribing Information. Kalamazoo, MI: Upjohn Co; 1992.

[32]Handsfield HH, McCormack WM, Hook EW, et al. A comparison of single-dose cefixime with ceftriaxone as treatment for uncomplicated gonorrhea. N Engl J Med 1991;325:1337-1341.

[33]Novak E, Paxton LM, Tubbs HJ, et al. Orally administered cefpodoxime proxetil for treatment of uncomplicated gonococcal urethritis in males: A dose-response study. Antimicrob Agents Chemother 1992;36:1764-1765.

[34]Ciprofloxacin. Med Lett Drugs Ther 1988;30:11-13.

[35]Ofloxacin. Med Lett Drugs Ther 1991;33:71-73.

[36]Mayer KH, Ellal JA. Lomefloxacin: Microbiologic assessment and unique properties. Am J Med 1992;92:58S-62S.

[37]Enoxacin. Med Lett Drugs Ther 1992;34:103-105.

[38]Cooper B, Lawer M. Pneumococcal bacteremia during ciprofloxacin therapy for pneumococcal pneumonia. Am J Med 1989;87:475.

[39]Gordon JJ, Kaufman CA. Superinfections with *Streptococcus pneumoniae* during therapy with ciprofloxacin. Am J Med 1990;89:383-384.

[40]Levaquin Product Information. Ortho-McNeil Pharmaceuticals. January 1997.

[41]Flynn CM, et al. J Chemother 1996;8:411-415.

[42]Dholakia N, et al. Antimicrob Agents Chemother 1994;38:848-852.

[43]Med Lett 1996;38:25-34.(d) references

[44]DeAbate LA, et al. Safety and Efficacy of Oral Levofloxacin versus Cefuroxime Axetil in Acute Bacterial Exacerbation of Chronic Bronchitis. Respir Care 1997;42:206-213.

[45]Adelglass J, et al. Abstr Infect Dis Soc Am 1996;34. 34th Annual Meeting Infectious Disease Society of America, New Orleans, Louisiana. September 18-20, 1996.

[46]Habib MP, et al. Abstr Intersci Conf Antimicrob Agents Chemother 1996;36. Abstract L002. 36th Interscience Conference on Antimicrobial Agents and Chemotherapy. New Orleans, Louisiana. September 15-18, 1996.

[47]File TM, et al. Abstr Intersci Conf Antimicrob Agents Chemother 1996;36. Abstract L001 (LM1). 36th Interscience Conference on Antimicrobial Agents and Chemotherapy. New Orleans, Louisiana. September 15-18, 1996.

[48]Goa KL, et al. Sparfloxacin: A Review of its Antibacterial Activity, Pharmacokinetic Properties, Clinical Efficacy and Tolerability in Lower Respiratory Tract Infections. Drugs 1997;53:700-725.

[49]Zagam Product Information. Rhone-Poulenc Rorer. January 1997.

[50]Portier H, et al. J Antimicrob Chemother 1996;37(Suppl. A):83-91.

[51]Lode H, et al. Eur Respir J 1995;8:1999-2007.

[52]Allegra L, et al. J Antimicrob Chemother 1996;37(Suppl. A):93-104.

[53]Med Lett Drugs Ther 1997;39:41-43.

[54]Stein GE. CID 1996;23(Suppl. 1):19-24.

[55]Trovan Product Information. Pfizer. December 1997.

[56]Vincent J, et al. Pharmacokinetics and safety of trovafloxacin in healthy male volunteers following administration of single intravenous doses of the prodrug, alatrofloxacin. J Antimicrob Chemother 1997;39(Suppl. B):75-80.

[57]Spangler SK, et al. Activity of CP 99,219 Compared with Those of Ciprofloxacin, Grepafloxacin, Metronidazole, Cefoxitin, Piperacillin, and Piperacillin-Tazobactam against 489 Anaerobes. Antimicrob Agents Chemother 1994;38:2471-2476.

[58]Child J, et al. J Antimicrob Chemother 1995;35:869-876.

[59]Brighty KE, et al. The chemistry and biological profile of trovafloxacin. J Antimicrob Chemother 1997;39(Suppl B):1-14.

[60]Hoogkamp-Korstanje JAA. In-vitro activities of ciprofloxacin, levofloxacin, lomefloxacin, ofloxacin, pefloxacin, sparfloxacin and trovafloxacin against Gram-positive and Gram-negative pathogens from respiratory tract infections. J Antimicrob Chemother 1997;40:427-431.

[61]Haria M, et al. Drugs 1997;54:435-445.

[62]Barry AL, et al. In Vitro Activities of Five Fluoroquinolone Compounds against Strains of *Streptococcus pneumoniae* with Resistance to Other Antimicrobial Agents. Antimicrob Agents Chemother 1996;40:2431-2433.

[63]Visalli MA, et al. Activity of CP 99,219 (trovafloxacin) compared with ciprofloxacin, sparfloxacin, clinafloxacin, lomefloxacin and cefuroxime against ten penicillin-susceptible and penicillin-resistant pneumococci by time-kill methodology. J Antimicrob Chemother 1996;37:77-84.

[64]Jones R. Fluoroquinolone resistance: An evolving national problem or just a problem for some physicians? Diagn Microbiol Infect Dis 1992;15:177-179.

[65]Gough AW, Kasali OB, Sigler RE, et al. Quinolone arthropathy—acute toxicity to immature articular cartilage. Toxicol Pathol 1992;20:436-450.

[66]Schaad UB, Wedgewood J. Lack of quinolone-induced arthropathy in children. J Antimicrob Chemother 1992;30:414-416.

[67]Rodvold KA, Piscitelli SC. New oral macrolide and fluoroquinolone antibiotics: An overview of pharmacokinetics, interactions, and safety. Clin Infect Dis 1993;17:S192-S199.

[68]Monurol Product Information. Forest Pharmaceuticals, Inc. January 1997.

[69]Patel SS, et al. Fosfomycin Tromethamine: A Review of its Antibacterial Activity, Pharmacokinetic Properties and Therapeutic Efficacy as a Single-Dose Oral Treatment for Acute Uncomplicated Lower Urinary Tract Infections. Drugs 1997;53(4):637-656.

[70]FDC Reports. The Pink Sheet. December 23, 1996.

[71]Crocchiolo P, et al. Chemotherapy 1990;36 Suppl 1:37-40.

[72]Naber KG, et al. Fosfomycin Trometamol versus Ofloxacin/Co-trimoxazole as Single Dose Therapy of Acute Uncomplicated Urinary Tract Infection in Females: A Multicentre Study. Infection 1990;18 Suppl 2:S70-76.

[73]Stamm WE, et al. Management of Urinary Tract Infections in Adults. N Engl J Med 1993;329:1328-1334.

[74]Med Lett Drugs Ther 1996;38:25-34.

[75]Clarithromycin and azithromycin. Med Lett Drugs Ther 1992;34:45-47.

[76]Whitman MS, Tunkel AR. Azithromycin and clarithromycin: Overview and comparison with erythromycin. Infect Control Hosp Epidemiol 1992;12:357-368.

[77]Periti P, Mazzei T, Mini E, et al. Adverse effects of macrolide antibiotics. Drug Safety 1993;9:346-364.

[78]Piscitelli SC, Danziger LH, Rodwold KA. Clarithromycin and azithromycin: New macrolide antibiotics. Clin Pharm 1992;11:137-152.

[79]Martin DH, Mroczkowski TF, Dalu ZA. A controlled trial of a single dose of azithromycin for the treatment of chlamydial urethritis and cervicitis. N Engl J Med 1992;327:921-925.

[80]Centers for Disease Control and Prevention: 1993 Sexually Transmitted Diseases Treatment Guidelines. MMWR Morb Mortal Wkly Rep 1998;42(RR-14):1-102.

[81]Watt B, Collee JG. Bacterial challenges and evolving antibacterial drug strategy. Postgrad Med J 1992;68:6-21.

[82]Pfizer, Inc. Azithromycin package insert.

[83]Khurana CM. Issues concerning antibiotic use in child care settings. Pediatr Infect Dis J 1995;14:S34-38.

[84]Neu HC. Otitis media: Antibiotic resistance of causative pathogens and treatment alternatives. Pediatr Infect Dis J 1995;14:S51-56.

[85]Data on file. New York. Pfizer, Inc.

[86]Barry AL, et al. In vitro activity of 12 orally administered antibiotics against four species of respiratory pathogens from US medical centers in 1992 and 1993. Antimicrob Agents Chemother 1994;38:2419-2425.

[87]Hopkins SJ, Williams D. Clinical tolerability and safety of azithromycin in children. Pediatr Infect Dis J 1995;14:S87-91.

[88]Khurana C, McLinn S, Block S, et al. Trial of Azithromycin (AZ) vs Augmentin (AUG) for treatment of acute otitis media (AOM) [Abstract M61-64 Presented at the 34th Interscience Conference on Antimicrobial Agents and Chemotherapy, Orlando, FL, October 4-7, 1994.

[89]McLinn S. Double blind and open label studies of azithromycin in the management of acute otitis media in children: A clinical review. Pediatr Infect Dis J 1995;14:S62-66.

[90]Nelson, JD. Clinical importance of compliance and patient intolerance. Infect Dis Clin Pract 1994;3:158-160.

[91]Schentag JJ. Antibiotic treatment of acute otitis media in children: Dosing consideration. Pediatr Infect Dis J 1995;14:S30-33.

[92]Pfizer product mongraph. Azithromycin for IV injection.

[93]Zimmerman T, Reidel K-D, Laufen H, et al. Intravenous toleration of azithromycin in comparison to clarithromycin and erythromycin. In Abstracts of the 36th Interscience Conference on Antimicrobial Agents and Chemotherapy. Washington, DC: American Society Microbiology; 1996:16 Abstract A82.

[94]Data on file, Pfizer, Inc. New York, NY

[95]American Thoracic Society, Medical Section of the American Lung Association. Am Rev Respir Dis 1993;148:1418-1426.

[96]Fang G-D, Fine M, Orloff J, et al. New and emerging etiologies for community-acquired pneumonia with implications for therapy. Medicine 1990;69:307-316.

[97]LaForce FM. Antibacterial therapy for lower respiratory tract infections in adults: A review. Clin Infect Dis 1992;14:S233-S237.

[98]American Thoracic Society. Guidelines for the initial management of adults with community-acquired pneumonia: Diagnosis, assessment of severity, and initial antimicrobial therapy. Am Rev Respir Dis 1993;148:1418-1426.

[99]Thys JP, Jacobs F, Byl B. Role of quinolones in the treatment of bronchopulmonary infections, particularly pneumococcal and community-acquired pneumonia. Eur J Clin Microbiol Infect Dis 1991;10:304-315.

[100]Jacoby GA. Prevalence and resistance mechanisms of common bacterial respiratory pathogens. Clin Infect Dis 1994;951-957.

[101]Friedland IR. Therapy of penicillin and cephalosporin-resistant pneumococcal infections. Ann Intern Med 1993;25:451-455.

[102]Steele RW. Drug-resistant pneumococci: What to expect, what to do. J Resp Dis 1995;16:624-633.

[103]Saint S, et al. Antibiotics in chronic obstructive pulmonary disease exacerbations. JAMA 1995;273:957-960.

[104]Pichichero ME. Group A streptococcal tonsillopharyngitis: Cost-effective diagnosis and treatment. Ann Emerg Med 1995;25:390-403.

[105]Vukmir RB. Adult and pediatric pharyngitis: A review. J Emerg Med 1992;10:607-616.

[106]Gwaltney JM Jr, Scheld WM, Sande MA et al. The microbial etiology and antimicrobial therapy of adults with acute community-acquired sinusitis: a 15-year experience at the University of Virginia and review of other selected studies. J Allergy Clin Immunol 1992;90:457-462.

[107]Williams JW, Holleman DR, Samsa GP, et al. Randomized controlled trial of 3 vs. 10 days of trimethoprim/sulfamethoxazole for acute maxillary sinusitis. JAMA 1995;273:1015-1021.

[108]Jacoby GA. Prevalence and resistance mechanisms of common bacterial respiratory pathogens. Clin Infect Dis 1994;18:951-957.

[109]Caputo GM, Singer M, White S, et al. Infections due to antibiotic-resistant gram-positive cocci. J Gen Intern Med 1993;8:626-634s.

[110]Friedland IR, McCracken GH. Management of infections caused by antibiotic-resistant *Streptococcus pneumoniae*. N Engl J Med

[111]Faro S. New considerations in treatment of urinary tract infections in adults. Urology 1992;39:1-11.

[112]Raz R, Stamm WE. A controlled trial of intravaginal estriol in postmenopausal women with recurrent urinary tract infections. N Engl J Med 1993; 329:753-756

[113]Arav-Boger R, et al. Urinary tract infections with low and high colony counts in young women. Spontaneous remission and single-dose vs multiple-day treatment. Arch Int Med 1994;154:300-304.

[114]Hooton TM, Winter C, Tiu F, et al. Randomized comparative trial and cost analysis of three-day antimicrobial regimens for treatment of acute cystitis in women. JAMA 1995;273:41-45.

[115]Hooton TM, et al. Randomized comparative trial and cost analysis of three-day antimicrobial regimens for treatment of acute cystitis in women. JAMA 1995;273:41-45.

[116]Dimateo MR. Patient adherence to pharmacotherapy: The importance of effective communication. Formulary 1995;30:596-605.

[117]Katz BP, Zwickl BW. Compliance with antibiotic therapy for *Chlamydia trachomatis* and *Neisseria gonorrheae*. Sex Trans Dis 1992;6:351-354.

[118]McCormack WM: Pelvic inflammatory disease. N Eng J Med 1994;330:115-119.

[119]Therapy for Sexually Transmitted Diseases. Med Lett 1994;913:1-4.

[120]Ambulatory PID Research Group. Multicenter randomized trial of ofloxacin versus cefoxitin and doxycycline in outpatient treatment of pelvic inflammatory disease. South Med J 1993;6:604-610.

[121]Soper DE, Brockwell NJ, Dalton HP. Microbial etiology of urban emergency department acute salpingitis: Treatment with ofloxacin. Am J Obstet Gynecol 1992;3:653-660.

[122]Sweet RL. Pelvic inflammatory disease. Hosp Pract 1993;28(Suppl 2):25-30.

[123]Rolle C. (Tuscon Medical Center, personal communication)

[124]Evaluation of new anti-infective agents for the treatment of acute pelvic inflammatory disease. Clin Infect Dis 1992;15(Suppl):S33-42.

[125]Witkin SS, Ledger WJ. New directions in diagnosis and treatment of pelvic inflammatory disease. J Antimicrob Chemother 1994;2:197-199.

6

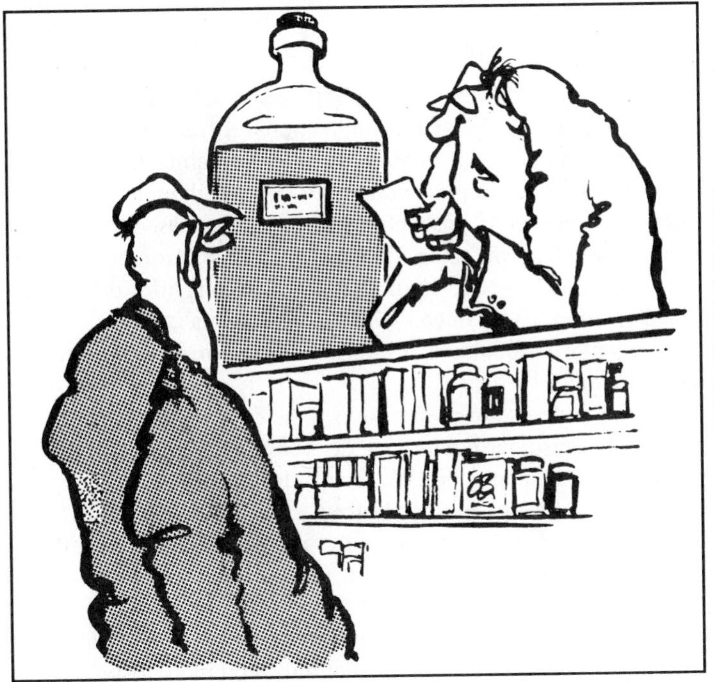

"That's what it says: 'one tablespoonful, 300 times a day.'"

Cocktails For Cardioprotection

A Systematic Approach for Improving Morbidity, Mortality, and Functional Status with Prevention-Based Pharmacotherapy in Heart Disease

Despite dramatic reductions in death from heart disease over the past three decades, our pharmacotherapeutic tools of defense remain underutilized against death and disability associated with cardiovascular disease.[1-4] The fact is, the declining incidence rate associated with heart disease is one of the formidable and quantifiable drug-based prevention—and life extension—success stories of modern medicine. It is now clear that better (and longer) living through chemistry is a claim amply supported by large evidentiary trials showing that prevention-oriented, pharmacological building blocks can play a pivotal role in reducing morbidity and mortality associated with heart disease.[1,5,6-8]

The pharmacoeconomic consequences are far-reaching. Constructing patient-specific, customized, medication-based "cocktails for cardioprotection" that can delay onset of myocardial infarction, reduce progression of left ventricular dysfunction, and prevent complications of CHD has the potential to reduce the frequency and costs of hospitalizations, to minimize the need for costly drug interventions (i.e., thrombolysis), and to maintain patients at higher levels of functional status and productivity.[1,2,24] Although pharmacological interventions—in particular, prevention-oriented drug-based therapies directed at specific cardiovascular risk factors such as hypercholesterolemia, hypertension, and platelet aggregation—have been shown to prolong life, delay onset of target organ deterioration, and reduce morbidity in patients at risk for ischemic heart disease, many reports document a consistent pattern of undertreatment in this patient population.[25,34,42,49]

The underuse of medications to achieve cardioprotective endpoints is unfortunate because cardiovascular disease is still the leading cause of death in the United States and most Western industrialized nations.[1,3,12] In fact, there are compelling incentives for ensuring adequate prophylaxis against coronary heart disease and its associated target organ complications. In 1997, there were more than 1.5 million cases of acute myocardial infarction (AMI) in the U.S., and almost 500,000 associated deaths.[1-3]

The most significant complication of ischemic cardiovascular disease, congestive heart failure (CHF), is the most common hospital discharge diagnosis in patients over the age of 65, and the fourth most common discharge diagnosis overall. In the United States alone, more than 400,000 new cases of heart failure are diagnosed annually, and CHF is the only major cardiovascular disease for which the incidence is increasing. As might be expected, the prognosis for patients with CHF is poor. Data from large clinical trials indicate that patients with CHF have a five-year mortality rate of approximately 50% and that patients with the most severe symptoms (Stages Class III-IV NYHA) have approximately a 50% one-year mortality.[52,53,57-59]

The economic impact of CHF, the majority of which is a clinical consequence of ischemic heart disease, also is significant. In the United States annual expenditures for the diagnosis and treatment of CHF exceed $10 billion. Of this amount, approximately $230 million is spent on drug therapy and $7.5 billion on hospitalizations.[54-57] The remainder is spent on nursing home days ($1.9 billion) and physician office visits ($690 million). The average length of hospitalization for CHF is approximately nine days, at an average cost of more than $12,000.[1-3,57] These patients frequently require recurrent hospitalizations, they require multiple drug therapy to maintain their functional status, and of course they require ongoing assessments and evaluations, which are oftentimes costly and invasive.

The Failure To Prevent Syndrome. Although costs, morbidity, and mortality associated with heart-related conditions can be minimized with vigilant pharmacotherapeutic measures directed at cardioprotection, it is remarkable how often patients do not receive adequate therapy directed at preventing death, acute MI, and heart failure associated with cardiovascular disease. Despite evidentiary studies conferring the role of such drugs as statins, beta-blockers, aspirin, ACE inhibitors, and antihypertensive agents, millions of Americans are underserved, underprotected, and undertreated. [6,17,18,28,29,34]

From a pharmatectural perspective, the objective is to identify outcome-effective, prevention-oriented medications that should be included in regimens designed to maximize protection against death and complications associated with heart disease.[13] An essential dimension of this "cocktail" approach is tailoring and customizing drug regimens for specific clinical needs of the *individual* patient. This comprehensive, "hit early, hit hard" strategy to cardioprotection not only stresses use of medications that treat and ameliorate *symptoms* of heart disease, it emphasizes use of drugs that can prolong life, improve functional status, and delay onset of adverse CAD-related end points in patients at risk for, or who already have heart disease.

In this analysis, cardioprotection is defined as reducing morbidity, mortality, exacerbations, and/or hospitalizations for either ischemia-related events (acute MI sudden death, angina, etc.) or left ventricular (LV) dysfunction associated with heart disease. For example, beta blockers are underused in patients following acute MI. Studies evaluating beta-blocker prescribing in managed care organizations reveal that only 35% to 65% of patients who are eligible for beta-blockers receive them following acute MI. Approximately 12,000 cases of MI could be prevented each year with adequate beta-blocker prophylaxis.[1-3,8,9]

Although aspirin is a relatively safe drug, especially when prescribed in the low-dose, cardioprotective formulation of 81 mg/day, it also is underused.[27,28] In particular, it is underused in men over the age of 45, in patients following acute MI, and in individuals at risk for coronary heart disease, such as diabetics and those with elevated LDL cholesterol levels. Over the next five years, about 500,000 MIs could be prevented if eligible patients received aspirin prophylaxis.[27,28] ACE inhibitors (ACEIs) also are underused (and underdosed) even though many evidentiary trials confirm their efficacy for reducing blood pressure, prolonging survival in patients with congestive heart failure (CHF), preventing progression of renal deterioration in Type 1 and Type 2 diabetes, and perhaps, preventing recurrent MI in selected high risk patient subgroups.[41,56,62,69,77] One study evaluating Medicare patients in California indicated that 40% of patients discharged from hospital, who had an echocardiographically confirmed diagnosis of CHF, did not have an ACE inhibitor included in their drug regimen.[1]

When it comes to cardioprotection, certain groups—especially women and the elderly—have become, to a significant and disturbing degree, "pharmacologic outcasts."[28,40,48] A recent study at the University of Iowa concluded that women were less likely to have their National Cholesterol Education Project (NCEP) Low Density Lipoprotein (LDL) cholesterol target goals met than were men. In fact, among all women who had clinically documented heart disease only 11% were meeting the NCEP target goals for LDL-cholesterol (LDL-C < 100 mg/dL). This means that about 90% of women were occupying a high risk category for recurrent coronary events, in large part because they were not extended the full benefits of drug-based cardioprotection.[45,50,51]

Eligible women are also undertreated with hormone (estrogen) replacement therapy.[13,51] This, despite the fact that estrogen replacement started at the time of menopause reduces coronary artery disease (CAD) related end points by about 50% over a ten year period.[1,13,51] Not all women benefit equally from estrogen replacement, and the risk for acquiring breast cancer must be considered in the decision to initiate therapy. As a general rule, however, the more CAD risk factors a woman has, the greater the potential benefits of estrogen replacement therapy.

The role of estrogen for secondary prevention of MI is more problematic. Recent studies have called into question the timing of estrogen use in women who already have had a heart attack and have not been on estrogen therapy. These preliminary studies (HERS) suggest that estrogen may not be useful—and may, in fact, be harmful—if initiated in women who have had a recent MI.[42] However, these results should not dissuade clinicians from initiating estrogen replacement in appropriate candidates at the time of menopause.[25,39,40,50] Other medications that are potentially underused in men and women include warfarin, vitamin E, folic acid, as well as antihypertensive drugs.

Compliance With Cardioprotective Cocktails. Achieving medication compliance can be difficult for cardioprotection, because: (a) multiple medication regimens are frequently required, and (b) drugs may have side effects that are problematic compared to the relatively asymptomatic nature of CAD risk factors. The fact is, if people feel better when they are *off* their medications than when they are *on* their medications, they will be noncompliant.[9,10] The cost-benefit equation as perceived by patients is frequently stacked against drug therapy because the individual must weigh the abstract benefit of consuming medications for the purpose of disease prevention—frequently, in the absence of any perceptible symptomatic or quality-of-life advantages—against the distress of ongoing medication-related side effects and the cost of therapy.

Cardioprotection presents a difficult challenge because most CAD risk factors for heart disease are relatively silent, that is, they produce minimal symptoms or have "low noise levels." People do not wake up in the morning and say, "Oh my, I have a backache. My blood pressure must be out of control today." Blood pressure, LDL-cholesterol elevations, increased glycosylated hemoglobin levels, obesity, and platelet adhesiveness are relatively silent risk factors. In order for patients to comply with prevention-oriented regimens, the noise levels of medications must be as low as possible, i.e., side effects must be minimal, daily dose frequency should be once daily, monitoring therapy should be as simple as possible, and the cost of therapy should be kept within the financial means of the patient.[11,12,13,20,21]

Selecting Cardioprotective Medications

Selecting specific agents that are uniquely targeted for specific patient CAD risk profiles is important, first, because some cardioprotective medications offer advantages over similar drugs in the same class; and second, because there frequently is a divergence between a drug that has worked well in a closely supervised clinical trial, and its outcome-effectiveness in the "real world." The reason for this discrepancy is that noncompliance with medications is oftentimes the weak link between the prescription pad and the desired clinical result.[10,11,12,19-22]

Accordingly, physicians must not only inquire about how much a medication will affect measurable parameters, but also how well does it achieve the target goals in typical patients who have to take the medication over the *long term*? Is this the kind of medication patients are motivated to take over the long haul? Or will side effects undetermine the stability of the regimen?[23,24,38,51]

Medication noncompliance is especially important for older individuals because multiple CAD risk factors frequently coexist in the same patient. But the challenge of building a cardioprotective regimen is even more complex—and the consequences of managing multiple risk factors with medications is potentially more harmful than it might appear on the surface because the greater the number of medications in a drug regimen, the greater the risk of incurring a drug-related adverse patient event (DRAPE).[22,23] This observation presents clinicians with a difficult-to-resolve therapeutic dilemma: On the one hand, multiple medication use is associated with an increased risk of drug-related problems; but, on the other, because many patients have multiple, coexisting CAD risk factors, polydrug therapy is virtually a *requirement* for maximizing life prolongation in the majority of patients.

Because individuals may require many different drugs for cardioprotection, the pharmatectural approach to streamlining drug regimens—a strategy that stresses consolidating, simplifying, and replacing ineffective, low productivity, or suboptimal medications—plays a critical role in constructing cardioprotective regimens.[13] This approach advocates the use of as few prescription ingredients as possible to manage risk factors and to achieve the desired cardiovascular clinical end points. In this scheme, if a patient has multiple CAD risk factors, it is preferable to find a *single* agent that can service each risk factor within the context of a single prescription ingredient, minimizing the need for multiple medications.

Pharmatectural Criteria for Optimizing Drug Choices. There are approximately 14,000 prescription drugs in America and often there are a number of different drugs available in each therapeutic class. As convenient as it might be to "lump" the currently approved 800 cardiovascular medications into distinct drug classes, and to consider the agents within each group as therapeutically equivalent, more often than not, there usually exist clinically significant distinctions among drugs that belong to the same class. These differences may help distinguish between safer, outcome-effective medications from those that are less outcome-effective. These distinctions are clinically important. For example, even though the clinician may recognize that a patient has an indication for a statin, a calcium blocker, a beta-blocker, or an ACEI, it is important to drill one layer deeper, and determine which medications—based on their potency profile, toleration, multiple indication advantages, convenience, and safety parameters—are more likely to yield better outcomes than similar drugs belonging to the same class.

To this end, the pharmatectural approach to drug selection takes into account multiple parameters of medications. It employs an *aggregate* analysis—one that considers many different dimensions and qualities of a pharmacotherapeutic agent—to determine which drugs, based on outcome-sensitive criteria, may have a tendency to perform better than others.[13] The parameters considered in this drug selection strategy for heart disease include the following:

Side Effects. Side effects may affect medication compliance, and therefore, may have an impact on clinical outcomes. For example, lipophilic beta blockers may cause decreased libido, depression, and sleep disorders, any of which may deter patients from long-term compliance. Statins may produce gastrointestinal side effects, estrogen replacement therapy can be associated with breakthrough bleeding, ACEIs may cause cough, and calcium blockers may be associated with peripheral edema. Irritating side effects may influence medication compliance.[10,11,51]

Compliance Profile. Because cocktails for cardioprotection usually require multiple medications, simplicity of drug intake may have advantages. Once-daily therapy is preferred, as are medications that can be taken without concern for food intake.[19]

Risk Management Issues (Drug-Drug and Drug-Disease Interactions). Drug-related adverse patient events (DRAPEs) are more common with cardiovascular medications than with any other group of drugs. For example, the combination of statins plus gemfibrozil increases the risk of rhabdomyolysis; high-dose beta blockers in combination with non-dihydropyridine calcium blockers may cause bradycardia; and potassium-sparing diuretics plus ACEIs can lead to hyperkalemia. Therefore, one fundamental, risk management-related question is: What is the risk of drug-drug interactions? And secondly, what is the risk of drug-disease interactions?[14] If two drugs are therapeutically equivalent, but one of them has a better risk management profile in terms of drug-drug or drug-disease interactions, from a risk management upgrade point of view, it is preferable—i.e., safer—to use the drug that has a "cleaner" drug-drug and/or drug-disease interaction profile.[12,13,21,23,24]

Productivity Level ("Smartness") of Medication. The "smartness" of a cardiovascular medication, also known as its clinical *productivity level* should also be factored into the drug selection scheme. For example, is this a medication that treats just *one* risk factor associated with heart disease, or does it address *multiple* risk factors, target organ needs, clinical objectives, and/or functional status end points. To minimize polypharmacy and its attendant risks, optimal drugs for cardioprotective are those agents that can carry the burden of a risk factor on their own "shoulders," i.e. within the framework of a single drug that provides "full service" management of a risk factor using monotherapy if possible.

In a patient with both elevated triglycerides and LDL-C levels, atorvastatin would be viewed as a high productivity statin because it is indicated for lowering both lipid fractions. In the patient with CHF, hypertension, and proteinuria associated with diabetes, an ACE inhibitor would be considered a high productivity intervention. Some calcium channel blockers have the advantage of treating high blood pressure and treating angina. Beta-blockers can be considered high-productivity drugs in patients who have had a MI and require treatment for high blood pressure.[70,77,88,89]

Regimen Durability (Effectiveness as Monotherapeutic Agent). One important and proven strategy for minimizing the risks of poly-drug toxicity is to identify medications that can be used as *monotherapeutic* agents to manage specific CAD risk factors. It is important to evaluate the "regimen durability" of the medication: How long can this individual ingredient be used without the need for add-on medications? In general, it is advantageous to identify medications that studies show can be used as monotherapy over an extended period, rather than agents that require add-on medications as pharmacological reinforcements. This is the regimen durability aspect of a medication, and the question it poses for any drug is "Is monotherapy a reasonable option with this medication over the long term?"[71]

Dose Stability. Dose stability reflects the capacity of a drug to produce desired target goals at the original starting dose. Can endpoints be achieved without raising the dose of the drug? Raising drug dose usually is associated with greater risk of drug-related side effects.

Cost. The cost of a medication should be entered into the equation for drug selection. If two drugs are equivalent in potency, indications, side effects, and drug-drug interactions, the less expensive medication usually is preferable.

Risk Management Profile (RMP). Consideration of the aforementioned pharmactectural selection factors will generate a risk management profile (RMP) for a specific drug or therapeutic class. From a practical, clinical perspective, when medications for cardioprotection are being considered, three questions should be asked: (1) What is the risk of *drug-drug interactions*? (2) What is the risk that the medication will cause *drug-disease interactions*? And (3) What is the risk that the drug might *not* be effective, i.e, what is the risk of *therapeutic failure*? In other words, what is the risk that a particular statin, in fact, will *not* bring a patient to NCEP LDL-C target goal? What is the risk that a blood pressure drug will not lower systolic or diastolic blood pressure in a particular patient population?[15] The risk of therapeutic failure depends on a drug's potency, its performance parameters, its compliance profile, and its pharmacologic productivity status.

Therapeutic-Efficacy Index (TE Index). How likely a drug is to perform over time is called the *T-E index*, or the Therapeutic-Efficacy Index. There are two major reasons a drug does not maintain its clinical efficacy over time: poor toleration or poor efficacy. (1) If a drug is not well tolerated, patients are at risk for compromised compliance; it follows that therapeutic efficacy will be compromised; (2) If the drug is not effective, even if it *is* well-tolerated and the patient complies with the regimen, it may be difficult to achieve desired end points.

Risk Management Upgrades (RMU). These principles can be used to implement *risk management upgrades* (RMUs) in the arena of cardiovascular drug selection. These RMUs are generated from the aforementioned pharmatectural criteria (see Table 6-1). From an historical, pharmacotherapeutic standpoint, RMUs in the world of cardiac medications explain the evolution from resins to statins for cholesterol management, from digoxin to ACEIs for treatment of CHF, and from myocardium-suppressing calcium blockers to dihydropyridines for blood pressure management. For example, physicians currently rely less on theophylline than in the past, and most patients requiring bronchodilation have been "upgraded" to inhaled beta agonists. Why is the pharmacotherapeutic transition from theophylline to inhaled beta agonists a legitimate risk-management upgrade? Because compared to theophylline, there is less risk of GI toxicity, a lower risk of drug interactions, less nausea and other drug-related side effects with inhaled beta-agonists, yet equal efficacy when used on a rescue basis to treat bronchoconstriction.

Table 6-1

Risk Management Upgrades (RMU) For Medications Commonly Used In Cardiovascular Disease and Associated Conditions

Original Medication/Therapeutic Class	Possible Risk Management Upgrade (RMU) Medication/Therapeutic Class
Theophylline	Inhaled beta-agonist
Systemic Corticosteroids	Inhaled corticosteroids
Beta-blockers	Alpha-beta blockers
Cholestyramine	Statins
Low potency statins	High potency statins
Hydralazine plus Nitrates	ACE Inhibitors
Cardiosuppressive calcium blockers	Long-acting dihydropyridines
H_2 Blockers	Proton pump blockers
Tricyclic antidepressants	SSRIs
Nonselective alpha blockers	Selective alpha blockers
Short-acting nitrates	Long-acting nitrates

In recent years, patients with post-MI depression have received an important risk management upgrade, from tricyclic antidepressants (TCAs) to selective serotonin reuptake inhibitors (SSRIs). Why is this a RMU? Because there is less anticholinergic toxicity, less risk of dry mouth, blurred vision, and orthostatic hypotension; there may also be less cardiotoxicity with SSRIs than with TCAs in patients with heart disease.

When considering RMUs for calcium channel blocker class, there has been an evolution from medications such as verapamil or diltiazem with potential myocardial-suppressing effects—properties that are more likely to be significant in older, vulnerable populations with CHF, brady-tachy syndrome, or conduction disturbances—to the dihydropyridines such as amlodipine and felodipine. The risk management upgrade (RMU) to these dihydropyridines is supported by the following: (1) Support for safe use of the dihydropyridine amlodipine in patients with all stages of CHF is documented in the PRAISE Trial and additional data evaluating therapeutic effectiveness in non-ischemic cardiomyopathy is under investigation in PRAISE-2; (2) The risk of peripheral edema, an irritative but important side effect, is slightly lower at the 5 mg dose of amlodipine (3% to 5%) than it is with some other calcium blockers; and (3) With respect to drug-drug and drug-disease interaction profiles, amlodipine usually will be compatible with other medications included in a cardioprotective cocktail and that may be required to manage or prevent heart disease. The role of calcium channel blockers in the treatment of high blood pressure has recently been elevated to first-line consideration by the JNC VI report, which cites the usefulness of using long-acting dihydropyridines in elderly patients with systolic hypertension.[68,87]

Risk management upgrades have also been implemented among cholesterol lowering medications.[34,35,36,82,83] Evaluated in the Lipid Research Clinical Trials, initial approaches to lowering serum cholesterol relied upon resins such as cholestyramine. Although these medications lowered LDL levels by about 12% to 14%, noncompliance rates with these agents were high and compromised their clinical efficacy.[34,35] Moreover, LDL-C reductions observed with cholestyramine was oftentimes insufficient to achieve desired cholesterol target goals. Accordingly, when HMG CoA Reductase Inhibitors (statins) became available, patients requiring significant cholesterol lowering were upgraded, initially, to the first HMG CoA-reductase available to market, lovastatin, and more recently, to other, even more potent statins.

Achieving 24% to 28% reductions in LDL-C levels, lovastatin recently has been shown in the TEX/CAPS AFACPS study to be effective in preventing first heart attacks.[32,37] Pravastatin is approved for prevention of first heart attacks. This suggests that primary prevention of heart disease, at least in part, is likely to be a "statin" class effect linked to LDL levels. To attain even greater LDL-C reductions, patients with CAD risk factors have been upgraded, over time, from lovastatin to pravastatin or simvastatin, which at their highest dose range are able to achieve greater LDL reductions than lovastatin.[33,70,80,83,84] At the 40 mg dose range, for example, simvastatin produces about a 40% reduction in LDL-C level, and at the newly available 80 mg dose, an average of 47% reduction in LDL-C level is achieved. On average, daily simvastatin doses of 5 mg, 10 mg, and 20 mg can be expected to produce LDL-C reductions of about 24%, 33%, and 34% respectively.

Extrapolating from studies evaluating the degree of LDL-C reduction at approved statin doses, the most potent drug in this class appears to be atorvastatin which, at the 10 mg dose (the lowest dose formulation), produces LDL-C reductions in the 39% to 41% range. The average monthly maintenance cost ($58 to $62/month) required to achieve a 39% to 41% LDL-C reduction using 10 mg of atorvastatin is significantly less than that required to achieve this degree of LDL-C reduction using the 40 mg dose of simvastatin ($87 to $102/month). Similarly, the average monthly maintenance cost ($78 to $84/month) required to achieve an approximately 50% LDL-C reduction using 20 mg of atorvastatin is significantly less than that required to achieve this degree of LDL-C reduction (47%) using the 80 mg dose of simvastatin ($92 to $105/month). Moreover, at this 10 mg dose, atorvastatin will lower the LDL-C level to the NCEP LDL-C target goal in about 75% of patients with the initial 10 mg starting dose.[82,85] At higher doses (20 to 80 mg/day), atorvastatin produces additional lowering of LDL-C levels; an average LDL-C reduction of 43%, 50%, and 60% is observed at the 20 mg, 40 mg, and 80 mg doses of atorvastatin, respectively. Atorvastatin is not only indicated for lowering LDL cholesterol but also for lowering triglycerides. Average serum triglyceride reductions of approximately 19%, 26%, 29%, and 37% are observed with daily atorvastatin doses of 10 mg, 20 mg, 40 mg, and 80 mg respectively.

Cocktails For Prolonging Life and Reducing Morbidity in Heart Disease

Cocktails for cardioprotection must account for "real world" clinical issues as part of the strategy for maximizing protection, while minimizing the risks of polypharmacy in patients at risk for heart disease.

What exactly is a cocktail for cardioprotection? And how do physicians go about constructing these cocktails for cardioprotection in patients at risk for heart disease? The concept of "cocktail" is relevant because it implies several ingredients; a mixture of medications that is customized for the patient's unique CAD risk factors, lifestyle patterns, functional needs, quality of life objectives, and financial status. It is a comprehensive approach to prevention of heart disease that includes lifestyle modification as well as medication-based interventions.[40]

One of the objectives of the cocktail philosophy is to customize the drug regimen for specific risk factors that coexist in the individual patient (See Table 6-2). There is no single cocktail "recipe" that fits all subjects. The concept focuses on the importance of tailoring the cardioprotective cocktail to the cardiac risk factors, past medical history, lifestyle, and functional needs of a specific patient. Streamlining and risk factor management also are given a high priority.

Table 6-2

COCKTAIL FOR CARDIOPROTECTION*
PATIENT SELECTION, INDICATIONS AND RISK STRATIFICATIONS

MEDICATIONS FOR POSSIBLE INCLUSION IN CARDIOPROTECTIVE COCKTAIL	CLINICAL INDICATIONS FOR INCLUSION IN PREVENTIVE REGIMEN	COMMENTS, WARNINGS AND SPECIAL CONSIDERATIONS
LOW-DOSE ASPIRIN (81MG/DAY)	Secondary prevention of MI in men and women well-established.	Slightly increases risk of hemorrhagic strokes in women with hypertension.
	Primary prevention in men with significant coronary artery disease risk factors and/or diabetes.	Booster doses of full-dose (325 mg) aspirin on weekends may augment cardioprotective effects.
	Primary prevention in men > 45 years of age with no risk factors is advocated by some consensus panels, but data is conflicting.	50% decrease in reinfarction at 30 days. Two year mortality decreased by 24%.
FULL-DOSE ASPIRIN (325 MG/DAY) **ANTI-PLATELET AGENTS:** **CLOPIDOGREL** **TICLOPIDINE**	Prevention of thromboembolic cerebrovascular complications associated with chronic atrial fibrillation (AF) in low-risk patients (i.e, no evidence of CHF, hypertension, CAD, stroke, valvular disease, LV dysfunction, and age < 65 years).	Risk reduction with aspirin in low-risk AF patients is about 35%. Patients should be followed closely since about 6% of low-risk patients enter high-risk category each year, requiring re-evaluation for possible Warfarin prophylaxis (See Warfarin).
	Alternative (second-line) therapy for patients with chronic AF who are intolerant of or ineligible for Warfarin (INR 2.0 - 3.0) prophylaxis, and who are at intermediate to high risk (i.e., > 2 risk factors cited above) for thromboembolic cerebrovascular complications of AF.	Aspirin is not as effective in reducing thromboembolic complications as Warfarin in high risk AF patients. Full-dose aspirin is associated with a higher risk of bleeding complications than low-dose aspirin.

Table 6-2

COCKTAIL FOR CARDIOPROTECTION*
PATIENT SELECTION, INDICATIONS AND RISK STRATIFICATIONS — cont'd.

MEDICATIONS FOR POSSIBLE INCLUSION IN CARDIOPROTECTIVE COCKTAIL	CLINICAL INDICATIONS FOR INCLUSION IN PREVENTIVE REGIMEN	COMMENTS, WARNINGS AND SPECIAL CONSIDERATIONS
WARFARIN (INR 2.0 - 3.0)	For prevention of thromboembolic complications in intermediate to high-risk patients with chronic AF. Effective for mortality reduction in patients with recent MI accompanied by heart failure and left ventricular ejection fraction < 35% greatest benefits seen in patients with anterior MI and stage III - IV NYHA functional class impairment.	Monitor INR closely and evaluate for bleeding complications if indicated. May occasionally need to add anti-platelet agent if thromboembolic complications are present while on Warfarin prophylaxis. Not to be used routinely for non- selective post-MI prophylaxis. Benefits-to-risk ratio most favorable in patients with poor ejection fractions. Two-year mortality reductions up to 30% reported in high risk groups.
(INR 3.0 - 4.0)	For reduction of thromboembolic complications in patients with prosthetic heart valves.	
BETA BLOCKERS **ATENOLOL** **CARVEDILOL** **METOPROLOL** **PROPRANOLOL**	Reduces morbidity and mortality following myocardial infarction. Recurrent MI reduced by 27% over 2-year period. Benefits of beta blockers extended to all MI sub groups including those with diabetes, heart failure, COPD, and the elderly. Primary prevention data with beta-blockers is contradictory. Some advocate beta-blockers for primary prevention in high-risk patients with hypertension, angina, and/or ventricular arrhythmias. Carvedilol may offer advantages in patients with MI complicated by CHF.	Beta-blockers should be used routinely in all patients post-MI, providing there are no contraindications for its use (i.e., asthma, brady-tachy syndrome). Greatest mortality and adverse event reductions are observed in the elderly, in diabetics, and in patients with large anterior MI. Overall mortality reduction of 12% in short-term post-MI, and 19% over long-term. Effective for reducing post-operative mortality in patients with CAD undergoing non-cardiac surgery. Avoid in asthma, AV-block.

Table 6-2

COCKTAIL FOR CARDIOPROTECTION*
PATIENT SELECTION, INDICATIONS AND RISK STRATIFICATIONS — cont'd.

MEDICATIONS FOR POSSIBLE INCLUSION IN CARDIOPROTECTIVE COCKTAIL	CLINICAL INDICATIONS FOR INCLUSION IN PREVENTIVE REGIMEN	COMMENTS, WARNINGS AND SPECIAL CONSIDERATIONS
STATINS (HMG CoA-REDUCTASE INHIBITORS) **ATORVASTATIN** **CERIVASTATIN** **FLUVASTATIN** **LOVASTATIN** **PRAVASTATIN** **SIMVASTATIN**	Effective for primary prevention of MI (up to 35% reductions in first MI) in individuals with and without risk factors for heart disease. NCEP guidelines recommend lowering LDL cholesterol levels to < 130 mg/dl in individuals with two or more CAD risk factors. Other studies demonstrate primary MI risk reduction in healthy individuals (TEXCAPS/AFCAPS) if LDL-C level lowered to less than 110 mg/dl. Effective for prevention of recurrent MI and/or adverse CAD-associated outcomes in wide range of high risk patients including: patients with MI, severe coronary artery disease, angina, coronary artery bypass, graft (CABG), or open-infarct procedure (angioplasty, stent, etc.). NCEP guidelines recommend lowering LDL-C levels to less than 100 mg/dl in this subgroup. Some authorities advocate more aggressive LDL-C reduction to 70-80 mg/dl based in sub-group re-analysis of 4S trial. Appears to be effective for lowering risk of first stroke, with meta-analysis trials showing 20% to 35% risk reductions in fatal and non-fatal stroke.	Some studies (WOSCOPS subgroup analysis) suggest maximal reduction observed with 24% lowering of LDL-C level, whereas other studies suggest a curvilinear (4S, AFCAPS/TEXCAPS) relationship between LDL-C lowering and risk reduction. Many authorities have expanded high-risk group (i.e., those individuals requiring LDL-C levels < 100 mg/dl) to include diabetics, individuals with family history of MI or stroke occurring at age < 50 years, individuals with greater than or equal to 3 coronary risk factors including smoking, obesity, and individuals with vascular disease. Statins vary with respect to potency and capacity for LDL-C reduction. Liver function tests should be monitored as indicated, and symptoms suggestive of myopathy of rhabdomyolysis require urgent evaluation. Possible drug interactions with cyclosporine, gemfibrozil, erythromycin, niacin, and digoxin.

Table 6-2

COCKTAIL FOR CARDIOPROTECTION*
PATIENT SELECTION, INDICATIONS AND RISK STRATIFICATIONS — cont'd.

MEDICATIONS FOR POSSIBLE INCLUSION IN CARDIOPROTECTIVE COCKTAIL	CLINICAL INDICATIONS FOR INCLUSION IN PREVENTIVE REGIMEN	COMMENTS, WARNINGS AND SPECIAL CONSIDERATIONS
STATINS—cont'd	New studies suggest triglyceride elevations may be a CAD risk factor in men as well as women. Statins effective in triglyceride lowering (atorvastatin) may play a role.	
ACE INHIBITORS (ACEIs) **CAPTOPRIL** **ENALAPRIL** **FOSINOPRIL** **LISINOPRIL** **QUINAPRIL** **RAMIPRIL** **TRANDOLAPRIL**	Effective for decreasing morbidity, reducing hospitalization, and prolonging survival in patients with heart failure. An essential component of cardioprotective cocktails designed to prolong life in patients with CHF. Effective for post-MI mortality reduction in patients with asymptomatic or symptomatic LV dysfunction (GISSI-3, AIRE). Selective use of ACEIs in diabetic patients post-MI decreases 6 week mortality by up to 30% (GISSI-3). Non-selective use of ACEIs in all patients post-MI is controversial. Overall 12-month mortality rate decreased by 5.4% (ISIS-4). Slightly better mortality reduction observed when ACEIs used in conjunction with nitrates post-MI.	In general, ACEI therapy for CHF or for post-MI cardioprotection should be continued indefinitely so long as drug is well tolerated and side effects do not require discontinuation. Avoid in renal artery stenosis and hypotension. Monitor for renal failure, hyperkalemia, azotemia and cough. Ensure sufficiently high doses are used for heart failure management.

Table 6-2

COCKTAIL FOR CARDIOPROTECTION*
PATIENT SELECTION, INDICATIONS AND RISK STRATIFICATIONS — cont'd.

MEDICATIONS FOR POSSIBLE INCLUSION IN CARDIOPROTECTIVE COCKTAIL	CLINICAL INDICATIONS FOR INCLUSION IN PREVENTIVE REGIMEN	COMMENTS, WARNINGS AND SPECIAL CONSIDERATIONS
ESTROGEN	Effective for primary prevention of MI when started at time of menopause women with no prior history of acute MI. Women with > 2 CAD risk factors benefit most from estrogen replacement therapy (ERT). Long-term reduction in coronary events of up to 47% reported. Currently *not* recommended for *secondary* prevention of MI. HERS study showed increased risk of recurrent MI in postmenopausal women started on estrogen. Estrogen therapy if started at time of menopause, appears to be effective (20% reduction) for stroke prevention.	Estrogen replacement therapy should be individualized according to patient's risk for family history of breast cancer which are "relative" contradictions to ERT. Raloxifene, an estrogen agonist/antagonist has positive effect on serum lipids, but its effect on cardiovascular mortality reduction in women at risk for heart disease is unproven. Studies are currently in progress. In addition to cardioprotection, ERT plays a role in prevention of osteoporosis, improves well-being, and may delay onset of Alzheimer's disease.

Table 6-2

COCKTAIL FOR CARDIOPROTECTION*
PATIENT SELECTION, INDICATIONS AND RISK STRATIFICATIONS — cont'd.

MEDICATIONS FOR POSSIBLE INCLUSION IN CARDIOPROTECTIVE COCKTAIL	CLINICAL INDICATIONS FOR INCLUSION IN PREVENTIVE REGIMEN	COMMENTS, WARNINGS AND SPECIAL CONSIDERATIONS
NITRATES	No convincing data that nitrates *alone* are cardioprotective, i.e. that they reduce first or recurrent MI or prolong survival in patients with CHF. When used *in combination* with ACE inhibitors post-MI, nitrates appear to provide additional cardioprotection in the form of decreasing recurrent adverse (fatal and non-fatal) coronary events (ISIS-4). When used *in combination* with hydralazine, nitrates appear effective for improving outcomes in patients with CHF.	Nitrates use primarily for symptomatic management of cardial ischemia and coronary hypoperfusion. Never use in combination with Viagra, under any circumstances. The hydralazine/nitrate cocktail for CHF management has been supplanted for the most part by ACE inhibitors.
DIGOXIN	No evidence that digoxin affects *overall* mortality in patients, but "DIG" study concluded that digoxin therapy in patients with CHF is associated with a reduction in the number of hospitalizations and combined outcome of death and hospitalization attributed to worsening heart failure.	In sicker patients with heart failure who have an ejection fraction < 30%, especially those who remain symptomatic on ACEIs, digoxin is an appropriate addition to the cardioprotective cocktail. In individuals with mild heart failure adequately managed with ACEIs, little justification for routine inclusion of digoxin in cardioprotective regimen.

Table 6-2

COCKTAIL FOR CARDIOPROTECTION* PATIENT SELECTION, INDICATIONS AND RISK STRATIFICATIONS — cont'd.		
MEDICATIONS FOR POSSIBLE INCLUSION IN CARDIOPROTECTIVE COCKTAIL	**CLINICAL INDICATIONS FOR INCLUSION IN PREVENTIVE REGIMEN**	**COMMENTS, WARNINGS AND SPECIAL CONSIDERATIONS**
ANTIHYPERTENSIVE MEDICATIONS **ACEIs** **CALCIUM BLOCKERS** **DIURETICS** **BETA-BLOCKERS** **PERIPHERAL ALPHA-BLOCKERS**	Systolic and diastolic hypertension are risk factors for both cardiovascular disease and stroke. Beta-blockers and thiazide diuretics have been shown to provide cerebrovascular protection (i.e., reduce incidence of stroke in treated hypertensives) but have demonstrated negligible or marginal prevention of CAD endpoints such as fatal and non-fatal MI. (Framingham). Inclusion of long-acting calcium blockers (dihydropyridines) and/or ACEIs for *cardioprotection* in patients with high blood pressure is supported by hypertension optimal treatment (HOT) trial, which shows cardioprotective benefits if diastolic blood pressure is reduced to 83-87 mm Hg using these drug classes.	Hypertension management is essential; choice of therapy is dictated by patient's cardiovascular risk profile, comorbid conditions, age, and other factors. Therapy should always be customized for the patient's clinical profile. ALLHAT study currently in progress, is designed to evaluate multiple endpoints in outcome-oriented trial comparing several antihypertensive drug classes. JNC recommends use of long-acting dihydropyridines for management of elderly patients with systolic hypertension; ACE inhibitors for diabetic hypertensives, as well as other strategies for targeting special therapeutic classes with patient subgroups.
VITAMIN E	Evidence is not definitive but supportive of antioxidant cardioprotection with vitamin E (400 IV) in patients at risk for MI and for post-MI secondary prevention.	Clinicians should follow continuing studies on role of vitamin E for primary and secondary cardioprotection. Insufficient evidence for inclusion of vitamin C or beta-carotene in cardioprotective regimen.

Table 6-2

COCKTAIL FOR CARDIOPROTECTION*
PATIENT SELECTION, INDICATIONS AND RISK STRATIFICATIONS — cont'd.

MEDICATIONS FOR POSSIBLE INCLUSION IN CARDIOPROTECTIVE COCKTAIL	CLINICAL INDICATIONS FOR INCLUSION IN PREVENTIVE REGIMEN	COMMENTS, WARNINGS AND SPECIAL CONSIDERATIONS
FOLATE AND B_6	Compelling evidence that *women* whose *diet* contains high levels of folate and B_6 had 50% reduction of non-fatal and fatal MIs over 14-year period (nurses' health study). This high folate/B_6 diet offered primary prevention benefits, presumably because these vitamins are important cofactors for homocysteine metabolism.	The value of multivitamin plus folate and B_6 supplementation is not known, but given potential benefits in women, a multivitamin containing folate, B_6 and B_{12} is a reasonable low-risk/possible benefit ingredient for cardioprotective cocktails in women. Women with mild-to-moderate (< 2 drinks/day) alcohol intake had much lower levels of cardiovascular disease, and these effects were additive to benefits delivered from high folate/B_6 intake.
ALCOHOL	Mild-to-moderate consumption of alcohol (< 2 oz. Eoh/day) is associated with significant reduction in coronary heart disease and overall mortality. This potential ingredient in the cardioprotective "cocktail" may take the form of either red wine, or etoh-containing mixed drinks.	Moderate consumption of alcohol may make blood pressure control more difficult. Alcohol consumption in greater than moderate quantities is associated with increased cardiovascular morbidity and increased total mortality from all causes.

Table 6-2

COCKTAIL FOR CARDIOPROTECTION*
PATIENT SELECTION, INDICATIONS AND RISK STRATIFICATIONS — cont'd.

MEDICATIONS FOR POSSIBLE INCLUSION IN CARDIOPROTECTIVE COCKTAIL	CLINICAL INDICATIONS FOR INCLUSION IN PREVENTIVE REGIMEN	COMMENTS, WARNINGS AND SPECIAL CONSIDERATIONS
CALCIUM CHANNEL BLOCKERS **AMLODIPINE** **FELODIPINE** **ISRADIPINE** **NICARDIPINE** **NISOLDIPINE**	No consistent body of evidence demonstrating reduction of ischemia-related coronary events (fatal and non-fatal MIs) in patients treated with calcium blockers. PRAISE trial demonstrated no overall benefit of amlodipine in patients with severe congestive heart failure. However, subgroup analysis indicated subjects with *non-ischemic* cardiomyopathy appeared to benefit, whereas CAD patients with ischemic class III-IV cardiomyopathy did *not* show a survival advantage. The PRAISE-2 trial will provide evidence of whether amlodipine is beneficial in patients with cardiomyopathy. Felodipine, evaluated in patients with stable class II-III heart failure, demonstrated no significant survival advantage, but appears to be safe in stage II-III heart failure if used for another indication.	Some calcium blockers may be detrimental in patients with acute MI associated with CHF or LV dysfunction. Amlodipine appears as if it can be used safely in all stages (I-IV) of heart failure in patients who require calcium blockers for clinical reasons. Possible benefit of amlodipine in heart failure in patients already on triple therapy (ACEI, digoxin, diuretic) awaits results of PRAISE-2 trial.

* Oral medications shown to be of possible or documented value for primary or secondary "cardioprotection," defined as reducing morbidity, mortality, exacerbations, and/or hospitalization for either ischemia-related events or LV dysfunction (heart failure) associated with heart disease or *cad* risk factors.

In addition, this approach stresses the importance of identifying those medications within a drug class that can modify each risk factor with monotherapy, if possible. It is generally more desirable to use a single agent to provide "full service management" of the patient's lipid profile, to use a single antihypertensive agent to manage the patient's blood pressure, and to employ a single drug to control diabetes and achieve target levels of glycosylated hemoglobin and blood glucose. Minimizing the number of medications required to manage risk factors and identifying high productivity agents that can shoulder the burden of a risk factor with monotherapy will reduce the risks of polypharmacy through streamlining.[13,20,21] It should be stressed that cocktails for cardioprevention are part of a comprehensive risk management program that also stressed lifestyle changes. It is a "medicate and modify" approach that also includes behavioral modifications—exercise, diet, smoking cessation, stress reduction—as well as pharmacology-based interventions. Over time, a number of medications have vied for entry into the cocktail for cardioprevention (See Table 6-3). These agents are discussed in the following sections according to therapeutic class.

Table 6-3

Possible Ingredients In The Cardioprotective Cocktail	
Aspirin	Fibric Acids (Gemfibrozil)
Warfarin	Vitamin E
Antiplatelet agents	Folic Acid
Statin Drugs	Vitamin B_6
ACE Inhibitors	Vitamin B_{12}
Digoxin	Coenzyme Q
Cholestyramine	Antihypertensive medications
Estrogen replacement therapy	Beta-blockers
Nitrates	Alcohol

Cholesterol Reducing Agents. The HMG CoA-reductase inhibitors (statins) are potentially revolutionary in the impact they can make on coronary heart disease. Despite evidence supporting their use in a wide range of risk groups, clinicians undertreat and underserve individuals with elevated LDL-cholesterol levels. Prevention-oriented medications—the HMG CoA reductase inhibitors or "statins"—are available for this large subgroup of people and clinicians should make them part of a cocktail for cardioprotection when indicated. Perhaps the most important thing is to recognize that it is possible to prolong life in patients who have—or are at risk for—heart disease by following NCEP guidelines.[33,34,36] Women in particular are underprotected in this category. A recent study investigating 2842 women demonstrated that only 9% of women with known heart disease met the life-prolonging, heart attack-preventing goals (i.e., an LDL blood cholesterol level of less than 100 mg/dL) of the NCEP Guidelines.[33,34,36] Although the undermanagement of cholesterol elevations in men is not as dramatic, it is estimated that up to 40% of men are not at NCEP target goals.[49,82,85]

There is ample evidence supporting use of LDL cholesterol-lowering medication in the patients with CAD, as well as in normal subjects with mild or in other words, a clear and graded relationship between absolute LDL nd adverse cardiac events. These studies conclude that the LDL levels at ear after treatment carry most of the prognostic information available from rotein analysis. They suggest, that in most high risk patients, lower is better, hat even for primary prevention, it is preferable to lower LDL levels to less 125 mg/dL, which is lower than the 130 mg/dL target goal established by the EP. The AFCAPS/TexCAPS target goal of 110 mg/dL would suggest an even wer threshold than that advocated by NCEP Guidelines for managing selected dividuals at risk for a first heart attack.[32-36]

For individuals with established vascular disease (i.e., those at extremely igh risk for a first heart attack as well as those with an established history of MI), he issue is more clear. It is advisable in these patients to lower LDL to less than 100 mg/dL, and in some cases to lower LDL even more. Pushing LDL levels o less than 100 mg/dL can be recommended in the following patient subgroups: (1) individuals with several CAD risk factors; (2) those with a history of MI, CABG, angioplasty, or stenting procedures; (3) individuals with diabetes; (4) patients whose parents died of a stroke or MI at less than 55 years of age; and (5) patients with a history of peripheral vascular disease, thromboembolic disease, or stroke. Evidence proving that maximal benefits are achieved when lowering LDL levels to the *lowest* range within NCEP target zones is not conclusive, however, and further studies under way are designed to provide definitive answers to this important question. It should be stressed that meta-analysis trials combining results from 16 cholesterol-lowering studies show that statin therapy also is effective in reducing the total stroke rate by as much as 29%, suggesting these agents also provide a basis for cerebrovascular protection as well as for reducing the rate of adverse CAD-related events.[45,46]

The need for aggressive lowering of triglyceride levels also has come under closer scrutiny. Choosing a specific cholesterol-lowering statin may be affected by the relationship between triglycerides and heart disease, since one statin, atorvastatin is approved for lowering LDL levels as well as serum triglycerides. The classic teaching has been that mild to moderate elevations in triglyceride level is not an independent risk factor for CAD in men, but it is a risk factor in women. A study by Jeppensen clearly indicates that the serum triglyceride level is an independent risk factor for men.[91] These investigators followed a group of 2906 men between the ages of 53 and 74. By stratifying the baseline triglyceride levels into the lowest, middle, and highest thirds and then comparing them to the known 229 fatal and non-fatal ischemic heart disease events, they generated a crude incidence rate for adverse cardiac events based on triglyceride level. It was 4.6% in the lowest third, 7.7% in the middle third, and 11.5% for the highest third of triglyceride levels.[91]

Although additional confirmation is necessary, this study indicates that triglyceride elevation is an independent risk factor for men as well as for women. This has implications for the clinician interested in designing cocktails for cardioprotection. Specifically, it suggests that individuals with both elevated LDL-C and triglyceride levels be started on a "high productivity" statin that is moderate dyslipidemia—with or without other C available data, the statins induce substantial reduc recurrent MI, unstable angina, and the need for Reductions in CHD presumably reflect improvement decreased propensity for plaque rupture and in situ thro are now also sufficient data in women (4S, CARE, LIP and the elderly to confirm that lipid lowering is at least as e in men and is beneficial in older individuals.[50,82,83,84] A recen confirms that LDL cholesterol-lowering also reduces cerebro populations free of overt cerebrovascular disease prior to entry.[4] the highest number of risk factors benefit most from statin therap

There is some debate about whether or not prolonging life in pa for heart disease because of elevated LDL-cholesterol levels is lin *relative* reduction of LDL levels, or to a predetermined target LDL-C go retrospective analyses of large studies, called subgroup analysis, suggest LDL cholesterol is lowered by 24%, it does not matter what the LDL-C measurement is on an absolute basis. In contrast, other studies sho curvilinear relationship between LDL-C and cardiac events, suggesting that wi greater reductions of LDL cholesterol, one observes a progressively lower risk of having a first or recurrent MI.[80,82] Confirmation of the curvilinear hypothesis has important treatment implications, because if, indeed, there is a curvilinear relationship between LDL levels and CHD risk reduction, it is sensible to argue that clinicians should strive to lower LDL-C levels to the lowest ranges of currently accepted NCEP guidelines.

For example, the patient with two CAD risk factors for heart disease, but no overt disease, and who, therefore, according to NCEP goals should have his or her LDL lowered to less than 130 mg/dL, might be even *better protected* if his or her LDL "NCEP Guideline-consistent" level of 128 mg/dL was lowered even *more* to 110 mg/dL. And similarly, the patient who has had an MI and has been maintained at an NCEP guideline-consistent LDL-C of 97 mg/dL might be *optimally* protected if his LDL-C level was decreased even lower to 75 mg/dL. Although there is data to suggest that "lower is better" and which supports the concept of bringing patients to "better goal" vs "worse goal," additional, prospective trials are needed to confirm what absolute levels of LDL-C confer the greatest degree of cardioprotection.[33,34,37,79,80,82]

It may be impossible to settle this debate given the current contradictory data, but, nevertheless, a number of studies, including West of Scotland Coronar Prevention Study (WOSCOPS), CARE, 4S (Simvastatin) Study, and mo recently, the AFCAPS/TexCAPS (Air Force/Texas Coronary Atheroscler Prevention Study) data, reinforce the powerful effect that statin drugs h on coronary artery disease, morbidity, and mortality.

In general, the greater the absolute risk for heart disease in any indiv the more aggressive therapy should be, leaving clinician judgment as an i tant factor in determining precisely how far one should lower LDL chol However, in both the TexCAPS study as well as the reanalysis of the there is a curvilinear relationship between LDL-C and risk for effective for lowering both LDL-C cholesterol and triglycerides. Atorvastatin may satisfy these requirements.[86]

Antihypertensive Medications. Hypertension is another cardiovascular risk factor the management of which is essential for disease prevention. Despite confirmed benefits of lowering blood pressure on stroke risk, many individuals with both diastolic and systolic hypertension are not adequately controlled. Unfortunately, observations from many trials showing that cardiovascular morbidity and mortality was still more frequent in treated hypertensives than normotensive individuals have raised concerns about the effectiveness of blood pressure-lowering drugs, and about the optimum level of blood pressure required to prevent adverse cardiac events.[71-73,81] Data is now available supporting the potential prevention-oriented benefits of antihypertensives in reducing cardiovascular morbidity and mortality. The results of the Hypertension Optimal Treatment (HOT) trial are of special interest because this investigation: (a) examines the role of newer agents (calcium channel blockers and ACEIs) for hypertensive management; (b) attempts to identify diastolic blood pressure target goals associated with maximal reduction of cardiovascular morbidity and mortality; and (c) attempts to clarify the risks and benefits of low-dose aspirin therapy in reducing adverse cardiac and neurovascular events.[81]

In this study of 18,790 patients, hypertension control was accomplished according to a sequence of therapy, beginning first with a calcium channel antagonist, then either an ACEI or beta-blocker, with the option of adding a diuretic if the first two drugs did not achieve blood pressure control. The results indicate that major cardiovascular events (MI, stroke, or cardiovascular death) were lowest at a diastolic blood pressure of 83 mm Hg and that cardiovascular mortality was lowest at a BP of 87 mm Hg. For stroke reduction, diastolic BP below 80 mm Hg showed the greatest benefit with no lower limit. Myocardial infarction was not affected by diastolic BP, but the incidence of MI was lowest with a systolic BP less than 142 mm Hg; diabetic patients showed the greatest reduction in cardiovascular events at diastolic BP less than 80 mm Hg.[81]

The HOT study provides new, important data demonstrating that more aggressive lowering of BP may be required to diminish the risk of cardiovascular events. Many have speculated that since older trials used beta-blockers and diuretics, the adverse effects of these agents on glucose metabolism and cholesterol levels may have abrogated any potentially beneficial effects associated with blood pressure reduction.[2,71,72,81] In that regard, the HOT study is important because it demonstrates that with use of newer agents such as calcium channel blockers and ACEIs—recently elevated to "first line" status by the JNC VI Report on Detection and Management of Hypertension—as primary therapeutic modalities for specific patients, it may be possible to positively affect both coronary as well as cerebrovascular endpoints.[74,87] Another difference that may explain the relatively beneficial effects of medications used in this study as opposed to agents employed in older trials is the fact that the newer agents (i.e., calcium blockers and ACEIs) achieved marked blood pressure reductions of up to 20 mm Hg, as opposed to 5 to 6 mm Hg decreased in previous trials. With respect to choice of antihypertensives, long acting dihydropyridines were used in 78% of patients, ACEIs in 41%, beta-blockers in 38%, and diuretics in 22%. Especially important is the finding in the HOT trial that calcium channel blockers were not associated with a higher mortality rate. And finally, although low-dose aspirin decreased major events by 15% and MI by 36%, it had no effect on stroke rates and almost doubled major bleeding episodes, suggesting therapy may have to be individualized.

One of the important parameters when selecting an antihypertensive agent is regimen durability; can it be used as monotherapy to achieve target blood pressure end points for several years without dose escalation or pharmacologic add-on drugs. The Treatment of Mild Hypertension Study (TOMHS) provides some direction. TOMHS was a double-blind, placebo-controlled randomized trial that compared six interventions—five antihypertensive agents (chlorthalidone, acebutolol, doxazosin, enalapril, and amlodipine) plus diet and exercise alone—for the long term treatment of patients with mild (stage 1) hypertensions. Four clinical centers enrolled 902 individuals (62% men, 38% women) who had a mean age of 54.8 years. The mean treatment pressure was 140/91 and patients were followed up for an average of 4.4 years.[71]

All treatment groups in TOMHS achieved substantial reductions in blood pressure, and except for enalapril, all interventions were significantly more effective ($p < .01$) than nonpharmacologic therapy in lowering blood pressure. Amlodipine had the highest percentage of patients—83%—remaining on monotherapy throughout the entire study period ($p < .01$ vs placebo).[71]

Estrogen Replacement Therapy. There is controversy about the precise timing of estrogen therapy. A recent study (HERS) questions the appropriateness of initiating estrogen replacement therapy in older women with preexisting heart disease who are not already on estrogen. In this study, women who had had an MI and were started on estrogen therapy were more likely to have a recurrent MI within the first year than those women not treated with estrogen. In a study of 2763 women who had not undergone hysterectomy and had CHD, subjects were entered into a randomized, blinded, placebo-controlled study, in which the treatment group received an estrogen/progestin combination. After an average of four years of follow-up, there was a slight improvement in LDL and HDL cholesterol levels in the treatment group, but there was no difference in the rate of MI or CHD death. Moreover, more women in the treatment group experienced venous thromboembolic events and gallbladder disease. Because there was no overall difference in mortality between treatment and placebo groups, the authors felt they could not recommend estrogen therapy for secondary prevention of MI.[42]

The use of estrogen for primary prevention, i.e., hormone replacement that is initiated at the onset of menopause, is much less controversial. In women at low risk for breast cancer, and without other contraindications who are eligible to receive estrogen, hormone replacement therapy should be included in the cocktail for cardioprotection in women.[1,2,13,25,47]

Aspirin/Antithrombotic Agents. An important ingredient in many cocktails for cardioprevention, aspirin is still under-utilized for prevention against recurrent MI.[1,2,26-28,78] The use of aspirin for primary prevention is still somewhat controversial, although most experts recommend its inclusion in cardioprotective regimens in high risk subgroups.[30] The 1988 American Physicians Health Study was stopped prematurely because of a 40% reduction in first, nonfatal MIs. The British Male Doctors study, however, did not show a reduction in first MIs.

The Thrombosis Prevention Trial (TPT) does not support the widespread use of aspirin for *primary* prevention, because even in high risk men the overall reduction in ischemic heart disease (IHD) events was a modest 20%, and aspirin had no effect on total mortality. Moreover, there is little data in women.

Low-intensity warfarin was also evaluated, and its cardioprotective effects for primary prevention was similar to aspirin. However, because warfarin was associated with an excess of dissecting and ruptured aortas, it cannot be recommended for *primary* prevention, especially in combination with aspirin. However, the case for using aspirin to prevent *recurrent* MI and coronary events in men at high risk is very strong. The appropriate dose is 81 mg of aspirin per day, with some experts recommending 162 mg/day. Moreover, there are now studies that indicate that booster doses of aspirin, i.e., a 325 mg dose of aspirin on weekends can increase cyclooxygenase inhibition and, may produce slightly better outcomes than just low-dose strategy of 81 mg per day. So who is eligible for aspirin therapy? Probably, most individuals over the age of 50 with no contraindications, diabetics, those with a history of coronary heart disease, stable or unstable angina, history of myocardial infarction, coronary angioplasty or coronary bypass graft. The use of aspirin for primary prevention in women at low risk for CAD is not settled because the risk of causing hypertensive hemorrhage is slightly greater in patients on than off aspirin.[43,90]

Atrial Fibrillation. The Stroke Prevention in Atrial Fibrillation (AF) (SPAF) III study has shown that aspirin is effective for preventing cerebrovascular events in *low* risk AF patients. On the other hand, patients with AF who are at *high* risk for embolic events—i.e., those with two or more risk factors from among the following: hypertension, valvular heart disease, elderly, women > 75 years, hypertension, prior stroke, and CHF or LV dysfunction—should be treated with warfarin to achieve an INR in the range of 2.0 to 3.0. Those at low risk (i.e., they do not have any of the risk factors cited above) can be treated with aspirin alone.

The value of antithrombotic therapy in patients with LV dysfunction was evaluated in the Studies of Left Ventricular Dysfunction (SOLVD) trial. The purpose of this investigation was to analyze the SOLVD database to assess the effects of antithrombotic therapy on risk for sudden cardiac death. A multivariate analysis revealed that antiplatelet therapy (primarily aspirin) was associated with a 24% reduction in sudden cardiac death risk, and anticoagulant (warfarin) therapy was associated with a 32% reduction in risk. Eligible candidates who have sustained an MI accompanied by an ejection fraction less than 35% will benefit most from warfarin-based anticoagulant therapy.[58]

New antiplatelet drugs are showing promise, although their use may be limited by cost or side effects. Ticlopidine (Ticlid) should be used cautiously based on recent reports that individuals taking this drug are at risk for acquiring thrombotic thrombocytopenic purpura (TTP) as well as neutropenia and agranulocytosis. The new antiplatelet agent clopidogrel (Plavix) is similar to ticlopidine, provides protection against recurrent MI that is similar or slightly better than aspirin, but is not associated with the hematological risks seen with ticlopidine.

Beta-Blockers. The benefits of beta-blockers to prevent recurrent MI has been well established.[1-3,16-18,29] Despite their effectiveness as cardioprotective agents, this medication class is underused in post-MI patients, with one study indicating that only 35% to 65% of eligible patients currently enrolled in managed care plans are currently receiving beta-blockers following their MI. This is unfortunate, because unlike calcium blockers and nitrates, for which there are no consistent data that cardiovascular morbidity or mortality can be influenced, post-MI studies in the pre-thrombolytic era, as well as recent studies in the setting of thrombolysis, continue to show a benefit for beta-blockers. Overall, studies with atenolol and propranolol show a 27% reduction in recurrent MI over a 2-year period, if beta-blockers are started at the time of acute MI and continued on an oral basis thereafter. Beta-blockers are useful for suppressing silent myocardial ischemia, they have a modest anti-arrhythmic effect, and when used carefully—especially, in low doses with incremental titration—also appear to be beneficial in heart failure and may prevent adverse remodeling of the left ventricle as well as improve survival. Beta-blockers improve survival post-MI especially in patients with large MIs and LV dysfunction, but the mechanism for these salutory effects has not been established.

It is possible that the beta blocker carvedilol, a non-selective beta-blocker with alpha-one mediated vasodilator properties as well as antioxidant activity, may play an important role not only for its approved indications—hypertension and mild congestive heart failure—but as a post-MI cardioprotective agent. A British study evaluated the role of carvedilol in acute MI, in which the drug was administered to patients intravenously and then after which subjects were converted to oral therapy. The 6-month end points consisted of all major cardiovascular events. Results of the study demonstrated a significant (42%) reduction in serious cardiac events in the carvedilol group. Adverse cardiac events—including reinfarction, unstable angina, and need for urgent revascularization—were also reduced in this group, confirming that post-MI patients with CHF on carvedilol not only did not suffer adverse events from the drug, but achieved a significant remodeling benefit.[70]

Of special note is the fact that about two-thirds of these MI patients received thrombolytic therapy, suggesting that improved survival benefits with beta-blockers such as carvedilol extend to patients who undergo clot lysis. Further studies are likely to be forthcoming. However, it appears as if carvedilol is safe to use after acute MI with or without associated heart failure. But whether this agent is different than other beta-blockers with established track records in long-term cardioprotection cannot be answered from this small trial. Moreover, whether the remodeling benefits demonstrated in this study can be extended to other beta-blockers cannot be answered at the present time. Carvedilol appears to be an appropriate addition to the cardioprotective cocktail of patients with MI and associated heart failure.[70]

ACE Inhibitors (ACEIs). Characterized by fatigue, exercise intolerance, shortness of breath, peripheral edema, and pulmonary congestion, congestive heart failure (CHF) is one of the most important cardiovascular diseases amenable to treatment with drug therapy. It affects approximately 1.5% of the U.S. adult population, causing a dramatic decline in quality of life and a shortened life expectancy among those who suffer from this condition.

It is estimated that approximately 3 million people in the United States are afflicted with CHF. The incidence of CHF is approximately 3 per 1000/year between the ages of 35 to 64 years, and increases with advancing age to about 10 per 1000 per year after 65 years of age. Accordingly, the prevalence of CHF approximately doubles for each decade of life. Because of the high morbidity, mortality, and cost associated with the disease, CHF is likely to remain a significant public health concern.[1-3,52,53] Innovations in the medical management of CHF should be evaluated for their ability to ameliorate symptoms, prevent hospitalizations, reduce medical costs, and increase life span. Recent trials with various angiotensin-converting-enzyme inhibitors (ACEIs) have documented progress toward these goals, and suggest drugs belonging to this class merit inclusion in cocktails for cardioprotection in a wide range of patients with ischemic, pump-related, and diabetes-mediated cardiovascular conditions.[58-60,61,63]

Approximately 35% of all patients diagnosed with CHF require at least one hospitalization for exacerbation of symptoms over the ensuing 12 months. Hospitalizations for CHF exacerbations are frequently due to progression of the disease, but noncompliance with diet or medications also is a major factor.[76]

Data from the SOLVD treatment trial indicate that ACEI therapy reduces the number of hospitalizations for exacerbations of CHF in patients with mild to moderate HF by approximately 30%.[58] The reduction in hospitalization frequency is greatest after one year of therapy (approximately 40%) and gradually declines to 27% after four years of therapy. The relative risk for first hospitalization for CHF was reduced by 36% in the SOLVD prevention trial with enalapril and by 22% in the SAVE trial with captopril. Other studies show that certain ACEIs (quinapril), and perhaps others, produce significant regression, and even, normalization of left ventricular hypertrophy (LVH) in patients with hypertension. The clinician should make every effort to include an ACEI in the therapy of every CHF patient.[1-3]

Despite the well-documented benefits of ACEIs therapy for patients with CHF, certain clinical situations represent either absolute or relative contraindications to ACEI therapy.[2,3,65-67] Absolute contraindications to ACEI therapy include pregnancy, history of angioedema or other documented hypersensitivity to an ACEI, bilateral renal artery stenosis, and history of well-documented intolerance due to hypotension, decline in renal function, hyperkalemia, or cough. Relative contraindications include hypotension (systolic blood pressure < 90 mm Hg), renal dysfunction, hyperkalemia (serum potassium > 5.5 meq/L), and cough documented as due to an ACEI.

Unfortunately, only 20% to 50% of patients with a diagnosis of CHF receive an ACEI as part of their cardioprotective cocktail, primarily because of concerns about hypotension, renal dysfunction, hyperkalemia, and cough. Therefore, awareness of the frequency and management of these conditions will allow patients to achieve optimal therapeutic outcomes with ACEIs.

Effect of ACEI Therapy on Mortality in CHF. ACEI therapy has been shown to reduce mortality from either symptomatic or asymptomatic left ventricular dysfunction. The defining criterion for left ventricular dysfunction is an ejection fraction of less than 40% (a normal ejection fraction is at least 50% to 55%). Although 10 ACEIs have received FDA approval for use in hypertension, only 7 agents bear FDA-approved labeling for CHF: captopril, enalapril, fosinopril, lisinopril, quinapril, trandolapril, and ramipril. Captopril, enalapril, lisinopril and ramipril have been studied for their effects on mortality in heart failure. Even when ACEIs are incorporated into regimens, they are frequently used at less than optimal doses. (See Table 6-4 for appropriate dosing of ACEIs in patients with heart failure.)

While the role of ACEIs in CHF patients is well-established—with ample trial justifying inclusion of this class in many cocktails for cardioprotection—the ELITE study suggested that angiotensin II receptor blockers (ARBs) may also eventually play a role in patients with left ventricular dysfunction. In this head-to-head comparison of 700 patients taking either captopril (50 mg tid) or losartan (titrated to a dose of 50 mg daily), there was a trend in favor of the combined endpoint of death and/or heart failure admission, with a 32% reduction for losartan vs. captopril. This study, while small and not definitive, suggests ARBs may one day play an important cardioprotective role (improving outcomes in CHF) in selected patient populations.[44,69] The precise role of ARBs in cardioprotection is likely to be elucidated in future studies.

Table 6-4

Dosing of Angiotensin-Converting-Enzyme Inhibitors (ACEIs) in Heart Failure

Drug	Initial Dose (mg)	Targeted Dosage (mg)	Maximum Dosage (mg)	Time (hr) to Peak Effect on Blood Pressure
Captopril	6.25-12.5	50 t.i.d.	100 t.i.d.	1-2
Enalapril maleate	2.5	10 b.i.d.	20 b.i.d.	4-6
Fosinopril sodium	5-10	20 daily	40 daily	2-6
Lisinopril	2.5-5 daily	10-20 daily	40 daily	4-6
Quinapril hydrochloride	5-10 b.i.d.	20 b.i.d.	20 b.i.d.	2-4
Ramipril	1.25-2.5 b.i.d	5 b.i.d.	10 b.i.d.	4-6
Trandolapril	1 daily	4 daily	4 daily	1-4

ACEIs Post-Myocardial Infarction. The primary value of ACE inhibitors is prolonging survival in patients who have left ventricular systolic dysfunction. However, studies also show that using ACE inhibitors in the post-MI period can reduce the risk of reinfarction. Apparently, this benefit extends not only to patients who have symptomatic or asymptomatic left ventricular (LV) dysfunction, but to other patients—in particular, *diabetics*—for post-MI reinfarction prevention.

The case for nonselective inclusion of ACE inhibitors in a cocktail for cardioprotection in all diabetic patients following MI has grown stronger in light of a recent reanalysis of the GISSI-3 trial. The European approach of treating all post-MI patients with ACEIs has not been widely followed in this country for a number of reasons. First, the large European studies supporting this practice (GISSI, ISIS-4) did not provide LV function measures on most of their patients, making it difficult to distinguish which groups might have benefited most from post-MI ACEI therapy. In contrast, the U.S. studies (SOLVD, SAVE) did analyze survival in post-MI patients treated with ACEIs, and concluded that cardioprotective benefits were seen almost exclusively in those with low ejection fractions. Given also that U.S. physicians have been more concerned about ACEI-related side effects such as hypotension, azotemia, and hyperkalemia, it is not surprising that ACEIs are currently being used selectively, and in very *specific* target groups, for cardioprotection in the post-MI period.[1-5,7,59]

Reanalysis of the GISSI-3 data, focusing especially on patients with a history of diabetes and insulin use, suggests that, perhaps, ACEIs should be used nonselectively in this patient population following MI. In the GISSI-3 trial, patients with suspected acute MI were randomized to receive lisinopril with or without nitrates, begun with 24 hours and continued for six weeks, or no therapy. The primary endpoint was 6-week mortality, and the secondary endpoint was combined mortality and severe LV dysfunction (EF < 35% or heart failure). Of the 2790 diabetic patients evaluated, ACEI treatment decreased mortality at 6 weeks from 12% in the no therapy group to 9% in the ACEI-treated patients, which translates into a relative risk reduction of about 25%.[4,57]

Based on these results, the investigators concluded that early treatment with ACEIs in diabetic patients with acute MI reduces morbidity and mortality at 6 weeks after the event. This reanalysis makes a compelling case that ACEIs might be used on a non-selective basis in diabetics with acute MI, even in those individuals who do not demonstrate LV dysfunction in the peri-infarction period. It can be argued that since LV dysfunction frequently evolves over time post-MI, initial hospital measures of ejection fraction may provide an unreliable trigger for ACEI use in this setting. One prudent approach for avoiding undertreatment of patients who might eventually develop LV dysfunction is to begin all post-MI patients on ACEIs, and then measure EF in 4 to 8 weeks. Those who have normal EFs may be discontinued from ACEIs, whereas those patients showing deterioration in LV function would be maintained on the medication indefinitely. In any event, it appears as if diabetics represent a special risk group which will benefit from ACEI therapy, regardless of LV function. Based on this data, ACEIs should be included as part of a cardioprotective cocktail in this subgroup of post-MI patients.

One of the issues regarding ACEI use post-MI is how long therapy should be continued. Recent studies suggest that once an ACEI is pressed into service post-MI, it should remain in the cardioprotective cocktail indefinitely. The Acute Infarction Ramipril Efficacy Study (AIRE) was a landmark randomized trial establishing a substantial mortality benefit (about a 33% reduction) using the ACEI ramipril in patients with acute MI who developed heart failure. In this study, patients were given ramipril for a period of 12 to 13 months. The extension analysis results indicate that the continuing survival benefit in the ACEI cohort at five years. Based on this data, the authors recommend that once an ACEI is introduced into a post-MI cocktail for cardioprotection, that treatment should be continued indefinitely.[59] Although the addition of nitrates to the cocktail was not examined in AIRE, the ISIS-4 trial showed that the cardioprotective effect of an ACE inhibitor following acute myocardial infarction is augmented if used in combination with nitrates.[8]

Calcium Channel Blockers. As far as cardioprotection with calcium blockers, there is no consistent body of evidence demonstrating reduction of ischemia-related coronary events (fatal and nonfatal MI) or overall improvements in mortality with this drug class. Early trials, in fact, with non-dihydropyridine calcium blockers (diltiazem), demonstrated an increased mortality risk post-MI when this agent was given to patients with acute MI associated with pulmonary congestion and an ejection fraction < 35%. Since this early study, subsequent data evaluating the efficacy of calcium blockers in patients with congestive heart failure is somewhat conflicting, but evolving. The PRAISE Trial demonstrated no *overall* benefit from the calcium blocker, amlodipine, in patients with severe (stage III-IV) congestive heart failure. However, a subgroup analysis indicated that subjects with *non-ischemic* cardiomyopathy appeared to benefit, whereas those individuals with severe CHF resulting from an ischemic etiology did not show a survival advantage. The possible benefits of amlodipine in patients with *non-ischemic* congestive heart failure currently is being evaluated in the PRAISE-2 Trial, which should shed more conclusive evidence on the value of adding amlodipine to triple drug therapy (ACEIs, digoxin, and diuretics) in patients whose LV dysfunction is non-ischemic in nature. Currently, however, amlodipine appears as if it can be used safely in patients with all stages of CHF, if they require calcium blocker therapy for clinical reasons.[68,75]

Felodipine, another dihydropyridine, has been evaluated in patients with stable Class II-III heart failure, but not Class IV. This calcium blocker showed no significant survival advantage, but it appears to be safe for use in patients with Class II-III heart failure if used for another indication.

Digoxin. The role of digoxin as a possible cardioprotective medication in the setting of heart failure has recently been clarified with publication of the results from the Digoxin (DIG) Trial.[52,53] This large clinical trial enrolled 6800 subjects with a clinical diagnosis of heart failure from 302 centers in the United States and Canada. The goals of the study were to assess whether digoxin has an impact on mortality and morbidity—as well as frequency of hospitalization—in patients with a wide variety of heart disease and a broad range of left ventricular

(LV) dysfunction. The main inclusion criteria were an established diagnosis of heart failure and an LV ejection fraction less than 45%.

The study concluded that digoxin had no effect on overall mortality, but it did reduce the number of hospitalizations and combined outcome of death or hospitalization attributed to worsening heart failure. In practical, clinical terms, the implication is that digoxin is likely to affect the frequency of hospitalization, but not survival. In sicker patients with heart failure who have an ejection fraction < 30%, especially those that remain symptomatic despite ACEI therapy, digoxin should be strongly considered for inclusion in the cardioprotective cocktail. There seems to be little justification for using digoxin for preventive purposes in patients who have only mild CHF and only moderate depression of LV function.[52,53]

Nutritional Supplementation. Finally, the use of nutritional supplements, among them antioxidants and vitamins—especially vitamin E—is now supported by a number of trials conducted in patients at high risk for coronary artery disease. In one large study, a group of investigators from the University of Pittsburgh and University of Miami reported in the *New England Journal of Medicine* (334:1156-62, 1996) that diets rich in vitamin E reduce fatal and nonfatal heart attacks by 35%. In addition to trials supporting inclusion of vitamin E, folate, and vitamin B_6, an interesting survey of cardiologists listed in the American College of Cardiology Directory suggests these specialty group practices primary prevention with antioxidants much more often than suspected.[48] Of 450 cardiologists asked about their own personal cocktails for cardioprotection, including intake of antioxidants, 181 responded (average age 46). Overall, 44% admitted to taking antioxidants, with vitamin E being the most commonly used antioxidant (39%), followed by vitamin C (33%) and beta carotene (19%). Interestingly, in those cardiologists who used aspirin as part of their cardioprotective cocktail, the most common dose was 325 mg/day, rather than 81 mg/day. As many of the respondents took antioxidants as took aspirin.

Alcohol. Finally, when it comes to "cocktails," it should be pointed out that low to moderate alcohol intake (< 2 oz/day) is associated with reduced risk of death from heart disease.[31] Greater than moderate intake of alcohol has been associated with an increase risk of cardiac and total mortality.

SUMMARY

A systematic patient evaluation is a prerequisite to drug therapy for patients with heart disease. Constructing a cocktail for cardioprotection requires a comprehensive patient and family history, laboratory evaluation of cardiac risk factors, ECG analysis, and other clinical data. Certain risk factors and clinical conditions will trigger consideration of preventive pharmacotherapy. These clinical triggers may include age, risk profile, lipid elevation, evidence of heart failure, rhythm disturbances, cardiac history, blood pressure, functional status, and many other factors. Unfortunately, although many single agents, as independent variables, have been shown to decrease morbidity and mortality associated with heart disease, the benefits or adverse effects of combining various cardioprotective agents has not been fully elucidated. Nevertheless, once the CAD risk profile and target goals are established for an individual patient, cocktails for cardioprotection can be customized using pharmatectural principles that minimize medications to maximize results. (See Table 6-5).

Table 6-5

Eligibility for Cardioprotective Cocktails: Patient Evaluation Checklist and Medication Options	
Patient Profile, Risk Factors, or Abnormal Measured Clinical Parameters	**Medications That Should Be Considered for Cardioprotection**
Men or women with CAD risk factors and LDL-C levels that exceed NCEP recommendations (> 130 mg/dL); Primary prevention	Statins (to lower LDL < 130 mg/dL) Aspirin (men > 45 years) Vitamin E (400 IU/day) Folate, B_6,B_{12} (women) Estrogen Replacement Therapy (in eligible women candidates) Exercise program
Men or women with no CAD risk factors; Primary Prevention of MI—AFCAPS/ TexCAPS study suggests lowering of LDL < 110 mg/dL may be of benefit	Same as above, except LDL target goal as low as < 110 mg/dl suggested for optimal primary prevention
Men or women with two or more CAD risk factor, strong history of family heart disease, or evidence of CAD with low HDL-C levels.	Niaspan® to elevate HDL levels; and/or statins in conjunction with niacin in order to increase the HDL/LDL ratio.
Men or women with Coronary Artery Disease (CAD): Secondary Prevention in the following risk groups: MI, documented CAD, angina, vascular disease, stroke, family history of death in parent from MI or stroke at age < 55 years, CABG surgery, angioplasty, stent, open-infarct procedure, diabetics.	Statins (to lower LDL < 100 mg/dl: NCEP Guidelines; to lower LDL to 75 mg/dl in selected high-risk patients with MI: 4S reanalysis) Aspirin 81 mg/day (booster dose of 325 mg on weekend days supported by some studies) Vitamin E (400 IU/day) Folate, B_6,B_{12} (women) Estrogen (currently not recommended for secondary prevention in women with MI not previously on estrogen therapy) ETOH: mild-to-moderate consumption is cardioprotective ACE Inhibitors (add to patients with Acute MI plus evidence of associated heart failure or diminished ejection fraction)

Table 6-5

Eligibility for Cardioprotective Cocktails: Patient Evaluation Checklist and Medication Options — cont'd.	
Patient Profile, Risk Factors, or Abnormal Measured Clinical Parameters	**Medications That Should Be Considered for Cardioprotection**
Men or Women Diabetic Patients with Acute MI	Same as above plus ACE Inhibitors for post-MI cardioprotection (GISSI-3), even if there is no associated heart failure
Men or Women with Acute MI (anterior wall) and evidence of heart failure with ejection fraction < 35%)	Same as above plus Warfarin to achieve INR 2.0-3.0 (aspirin may be discontinued if there are bleeding risks)
Hypertensive patients	Recommendations in abovementioned subgroups as applicable plus vigilant control of diastolic and systolic blood pressure: JNC VI Guidelines for management are available
	Hypertension Optimal Treatment (HOT) Trial suggests long-acting dihydropyridines and ACEIs are associated with reduced cardiovascular morbidity and mortality; recommends lowering of diastolic BP < 85 mm Hg.
Hypertriglyceridemia	Atorvastatin Fibric acids
Diabetics	Recommendations in abovementioned subgroups as applicable plus vigilant control of blood sugar and glycosylated hemoglobin A_1C levels.

[1]Califf R, Mark D, Wagner, S. Acute Coronary Care. St. Louis, Mo: Mosby, 1995.

[2]Ryan TJ, et al. ACA/AHA. Guidelines for management of patients with acute myocardial infarction. Task Force on Practice Guidelines. Am J Cardiol 1996;28:1328.

[3]Julian DG, Braunwald E, eds. Management of Acute Myocardial Infarction. London, England: WB Saunders Company, 1994.

[4]Gruppo Italiano per lo Studio della Sopravivenza nell' Infracto Miocardico. GISSI-3. Effects of lisinopril and transdermal nitroglycerin singly and together on six week mortality and LV function after acute myocardial infarction. Lancet 1994:343(8906):1115.

[5]Cutler, JA, MacMahon SW et al. Controlled clinical trials of drug treatment for hypertension. A Review. Hypertension 1998;13(suppl I): I:1989.

[6]Kaplan NM. Clinical Hypertension, ed 6. Baltimore, MD: Williams and Wilkins 1997.

[7]The MIAMI Trial Research Group. Metoprolol in acute myocardial infarction (MIAMI). A randomized placebo-controlled international trial. Eur Heart Journal 1985;6:199.

[8]ISIS-4 Collaborative Group. A randomized factorial trial assessing early captopril, oral mononitrate, and intravenous magnesium sulfate in 58,050 patients with suspected acute myocardial infarction. Lancet 1995;345:669.

[9]Berg JS, et al. Medication compliance: a health care problem. Ann Pharmacother 1993;27:(9 Suppl) S1-S24.

[10]Beardon PH, McGilchrist MM et al. Primary noncompliance with prescribed medication in primary care. BMJ 1993;307(6908):846.

[11]Conn VS, Taylor SG et al. Medication regimen complexity and adherence among adults. Image J Nurs Sch 1991;23(4):231.

[12]Lamy, PP. A risk approach to adverse drug reaction J Am Ger Soc 1988;36:79.

[13]Bosker, G. Pharmatecture: Minimizing Medications to Maximize Results. St. Louis, MO: Facts and Comparisons 1996.

[14]Estacio RO, et al. ABCD Trial Nisoldipine vs Enalapril on Cardiovascular outcomes in NIDDM and Hypertension. N Engl J Med 1998;338:645.

[15]Messerli FH, et al. Beta blockers for hypertension in the elderly. JAMA 1998;279:1903.

[16]Held P. Effects of beta-blockers on ventricular dysfunction after myocardial infarction: tolerability and survival effects. Am J Cardiol 25;71(9)39C.

[17]Hennekens, C, Jonas MA, et al. The benefits of aspirin in acute myocardial infarction: Still a well-kept secret in the United States. Arch Intern Med 1994;154(1):37-39.

[18]Frishman WH. Beta-adrenergic blockers as cardioprotective agents. Am J Cardiol 70(21):21.

[19]Eisen S, et al. The effect of prescribed daily dose frequency on patient medication compliance. Arch Intern Med 1990;150(9):1881.

[20]Keen PJ. What is the best dosing schedule for patients? J R Soc Med 1991;84(11):640.

[21]Ferguson, RP, Wetle T, et al. Relative importance to elderly patients of effectiveness, adverse side effects, convenience, and cost of antihypertensive medications. Drugs Aging 1994;4(1):56.

[22]Jahnigen D, Cooper D et al. Adverse events among elderly patients. J Am Ger Soc 1988;36:65.

[23]Black AJ, Somers K. Drug-related illness resulting in hospital admission. J R Coll Physicians 1989;18:40-44.

[24]Testa MA, Anderson RB et al. Quality of life and antihypertensive therapy in men. A comparison of captopril with enalapril. N Eng J Med 1993;328:907.

[25]Stampfer MJ, et al. Postmenopausal hormone replacement therapy and cardiovascular disease. N Eng J Med 1991;325:11.

[26]Steering Committee of the Physician's Health Study Research Group. Final report of the aspirin component of the ongoing Physicians' Health Study. N Eng J Med 1989;321:129.

[27]Peto R, Gray R, et al: Randomized trial of prophylactic aspirin in British male doctors. Br Med J 1988;296:313.

[28]McNally LE, Corn CR et al, Aspirin for prevention of vascular death in women. Ann Pharmacother 1992;26(12):1530.

[29]Gurwitz JH, Goldberg RJ, et al. Beta-blocker therapy in acute myocardial infarction: evidence for underutilization in the elderly. Am J Med 1992;93(6):605.

[30]Guazzi MD, et al. ACEIs and aspirin in attenuation of hypertension control. Clin Pharm Ther 1998;63:79.

[31]Vruzx O, et al. Alcohol consumption and mild hypertension. Am J Hypertens 1998;11:230.

[32]Downs JR, et al. The Air Force/Texas Coronary Atherosclerosis Prevention Study (AF/TEXCAPS). JAMA 1998;279:1615.

[33]Scandinavian simvastatin survival study group. Lancet 1994;344:1383.

[34]National Cholesterol Education Program Expert Panel. JAMA 1993;269:3015.

[35]Abramowicz M: Choice of cholesterol-lowering drugs. Med Lett Drugs Ther 1991;33:1.

[36]Brown WW. Review of clinical trials: proving the lipid hypothesis. Eur H Jour 1990;11(suppl H):15.

[37]Pearson TA. Editorial. TEXCAPS. JAMA 1998;279:1659.

[38]Avorn J, et al. Persistence of use of lipid-lowering medications: A Cross-national study. JAMA 1998;279:1458.

[39]Walsh BW, et al. Raloxifene, serum lipids, and coagulation factors. JAMA 1998;279:1445.

[40]Stefanick ML, et al. Diet, exercise, and cholesterol levels in men and women. N Eng J Med 1998;339:12.

[41]Roman MJ et al. Effects of ACE Inhibition and Diuretic Therapy on LVH. Am J Hypertens 1998;11:387.

[42]HERS. Estrogen for secondary prevention of heart disease. JAMA 1998;280.

[43]SPAF Investigators. Aspirin for Atrial Fibrillation Stroke Prevention. JAMA 1998;279:1273-1277

[44]Pitt B, et al. Benefit of Losartan in Congestive Heart Failure. Lancet 1997;349:747.

[45]Herbert PR, et al. Statins in on Stroke Prevention and Mortality Reduction. JAMA 1997;278:313;

[46]Bucher HC, et al. Statins for stroke prevention. Ann Intern Med 1998;128:89.

[47]Darling GM, et al. Postmenopausal HRT, Simvastatin and hyperlipidemia. NEJM 1997;337:595.

[48]Rimm EB, et al. Decreased CAD in Women with increased folate and Vitamin B6 intake. JAMA 1998;279:359-364.

[49]Kreisberg RA. Editorial of cholesterol reduction with statins. Am J Med 1996;101:445-457.

[50]Statins in women with elevated cholesterol levels. N Engl J Med 1995;333:1301.

[51]Ettinger B, et al. Continuation rates with hormone replacement therapy. Menopause 1996;3:1895.

[52]The Digitalis Investigation Group. N Engl J Med 1997;336:525.

[53]Packer, M. The Digitalis Investigation Group. N Engl J Med 1997;336:575.

[54]Australia/New Zealand Heart Failure Research Group. Carvedilol in heart failure. Lancet 1997;349:375.

[55]Cohn JN, et al. V-HeFT-III/Felodipine. Circulation. 96:856-863.

[56]Zuanetti G, et al. ACE Inhibitors Post-MI in Diabetics. Circulation 1997;96:4239-4245.

[57]Hall AS, et al. ACE inhibitor following acute myocardial infarction. AIRE Study follow-up. Lancet 1997;349:1493.

[58]SOLVD Investigators. Effect of enalapril on mortality and the development of heart failure in asymptomatic patients with reduced LV ejection fraction. N Eng J Med 1992;327:685.

[59]The Acute Infarction Ramipril Efficacy (AIRE) Study Investigators. Effect of ramipril on mortality and morbidity of survivors of acute myocardial infarction with clinical evidence of heart failure. Lancet 1993;342:821.

[60]Packer M, et al. Withdrawal of digoxin from patients with chronic heart failure treated with angiotensin-converting-enzyme inhibitors. N Engl J Med 1993;329:1.

[61]Kulick DL, Rahimtoola SH. Vasodilators have not been shown to be of value in all patients with chronic congestive heart failure due to left ventricular systolic dysfunction. Am J Cardiol 1990;66:435-8.

[62]Loeb HS, Johnson G, et al. Effect of enalapril, hydralazine plus isosorbide dinitrate, and prazosin on hospitalization in patients with chronic congestive heart failure. Circulation 1993;87(suppl 6):78.

[63]Schofield PM, Brooks NH, et al. Which vasodilator drug in patients with chronic heart failure? A randomised comparison of captopril and hydralazine. Br J Clin Pharmacol. 1991;31:25.

[64]Fonarow GC, Chelimsky-Fallick C, et al. Effect of direct vasodilation with hydralazine versus angiotensin-converting enzyme inhibition with captopril on mortality in advanced heart failure: the Hy-C Trial. Am J Cardiol. 1992;19:842.

[65]Van Vliet AA, Donker AJM, et al. Spironolactone in congestive heart failure refractory to high-dose loop diuretic and low-dose angiotensin-converting enzyme inhibitor. Am J Cardiol 1993;71:21A.

[66]Dahlstrom U, Karlsson E. Captopril and spironolactone therapy for refractory congestive heart failure. Am J Cardiol 1993;71:29A-33A.

[67]Dunselman PHJM, van der Mark TW, et al. Different results in cardiopulmonary exercise tests after long-term treatment with felodipine and enalapril in patients with congestive heart failure due to ischemic heart disease. Eur Heart J 1990;11:200.

[68]Packer M, O'Connor CM, et al. for the Prospective Randomized Amlodipine Survival Evaluation Study Group. PRAISE. Effect of amlodipine on morbidity and mortality in severe chronic heart failure. N Engl J Med 1996;335:1107-14.

[69]Crozier I, Ikram H, et al. Losartan in heart failure; hemodynamic effects and tolerability. Circulation 1995;91:691.

[70]Olsen SL, Gilbert EM, et al. Carvedilol improves left ventricular function and symptoms in chronic heart failure: a double-blind randomized study. Am J Cardiol 1995;25:1225.

[71]Grimm RH Jr, Flack JM et. al. Treatment of Mild Hypertension Study: final results. JAMA 1993;270:713.

[72]Collins R, Peto R et al. Blood pressure, stroke and coronary disease. Lancet 1990;335:827.

[73]Hansson L. Shortcomings of current antihypertensive therapy. Am J Hypertension. 1991;4:84S.

[74]Elliot, WJ. ALLHAT: the largest and most important clinical trial in hypertension ever done in the USA. Am J Hypertension 1996;9:409.

[75]Chen L, Haught, WH et al. Preservation of endogenous antioxidant activity and inhibition of lipid peroxidation as common mechanism of antioxidant effects of vitamin E, lovastatin, and amlodipine.

[76]Lee, J et al. Appointment attendance, pill counts, and achievement of blood pressure goals in the African American Study of Kidney Disease and Hypertension Pilot Study. Am J Kidney Dis 1997;29:720.

[77]Ravid M, et al. Long term renoprotective effects of ACEIs in non-insulin dependent diabetes mellitus: a 7-year follow-up study. Arch Intern Med 1996;156:286.

[78]Verhengt. L. Aspirin, the poor man's statin. Lancet 1998;352:227. Loh E, et al. Stroke following myocardial infarction. N Engl J Med 1997;336:251.

[79]Sacks FM, et al. Subgroup Renalaysis West of Scotland Coronary Prevention Study. Circulation 1998;97:1446.

[80]Pederson TR, et al. 4S Reanalysis Data. Circulation 1998;97:1453.

[81]Hansson L. Hypertension Optimal Treatment (HOT) Trial. Lancet 1998;351:1755.

[82]Grundy S. Statin Editorial. Circulation 1998;1436.

[83]Grundy, SM et al. Summary of the second report of the NCEP expert panel on detection, evaluation, and treatment of high blood cholesterol in adults. JAMA 1993;269(23):3015.

[84]Shepard J, et al. West of Scotland Coronary Prevention Study (WOSCOPS). N Eng J Med 1995;333:1301.

[85]Sacks et al. CARE Study. N Eng J Med 1998;335:1001.

[86]Bakker-Arkema RG, et al. Atorvastatin and triglycerides. JAMA 1996;275(2):128.

[87]JNC-VI Commission Report on Detection, Evaluation, and Treatment of Hypertension. JAMA 1998.

[88]The Medical Research Council's General Practice Research Framework. Lancet 1998;351:223.

[89]Mangano DT, et al. Beta-blockers for acute MI. N Engl Med 1996;335:1713.

[90]SPAF. Stroke prevention in atrial fibrillation investigators warfarin and aspirin. Lancet 1996;348:633.

[91]Jeppesen J, et al. Triglyceride levels as risk factor for heart disease in men and women. Circulation 1998;97:1029.

7

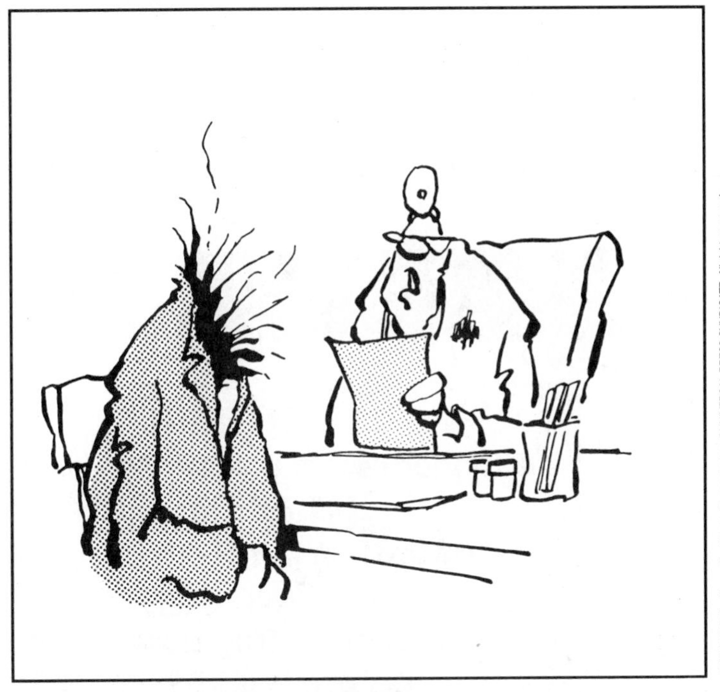

"I'm going to take you off the nitroglycerine pills."

The DRESC™ Program: Streamlining Drug Regimens Through Drug Reduction, Elimination, Simplification, and Consolidation

Minimizing medications to maximize results requires implementing a program of drug reduction, elimination, simplification, and consolidation (DRESC™ program). This represents a logical, systematic, and practical approach to streamlining therapeutic regimens and reducing polypharmacy. Based on these guiding principles, the DRESC program is designed for physicians or pharmacists as they deconstruct and reconstruct drug houses. The principle objective of the DRESC program is to *minimize* medications in order to *maximize* clinical results. Initially, the DRESC program requires a meticulous review of the patient's current drug regimen, including a careful reevaluation of the original indications for medication use (see Figure 7-1). Although this drug streamlining program usually requires several consultations, the elimination of unnecessary medications and dosage reductions, as well as a decrease in drug-related adverse patient events, (DRAPES)[1] will produce long-term cost savings for the patient and institution.[2,3]

Figure 7-1

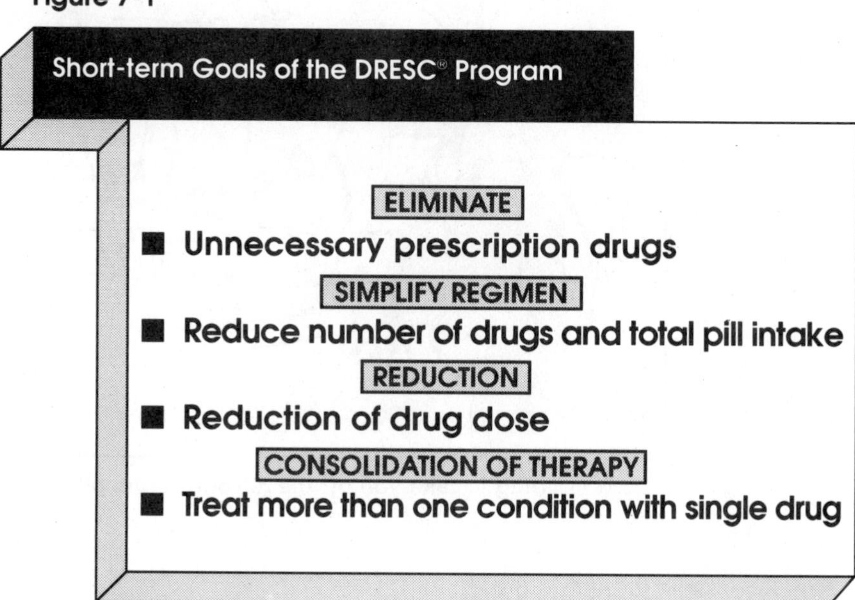

The *short*-term goals of the DRESC program include: (1) elimination of unnecessary prescription drugs; (2) reduction in the number of different medications; (3) decreasing the total number of pills taken daily; (4) decreasing the dose of one or more drugs; and (5) consolidation of drug therapy. *Long*-term goals of the DRESC program include: (1) improvement in quality of life;[4-8] (2) enhancing functional status[9,10] of the patient; (3) minimizing the potential for adverse drug reactions and interactions;[11-13] (4) improving patient education;[14-16] and (5) encouraging lifestyle modifications that permit nonpharmacologic management of chronic diseases. Generally speaking, patients who are taking four or more different prescription medications are excellent candidates for drug simplification, elimination, and consolidation. Nevertheless, individuals who take fewer than four drugs are still likely to benefit from dose reduction.

Potential benefits of the DRESC program are listed in Table 7-1. It should be stressed that the DRESC program plays a central role in total pharmacotherapeutic quality management (TPQM™) (see Table 7-2). Specifically, the DRESC program provides a practical, hands-on approach to the simplification and consolidation of complicated, polypharmacy drug regimens. Because the process of drug reduction, simplification, and consolidation requires frequent contact between patients and health care providers, this program promotes patient-physician and patient-pharmacist communication regarding medication-related issues.[14,16,19,20] Moreover, quality assurance objectives are fostered, because the three phases of drug regimen deconstruction and reconstruction—assessment, implementation, and evaluation—require regular reviews of the appropriateness of medication orders. It specifically encourages periodic reassessments of

Figure 7-2

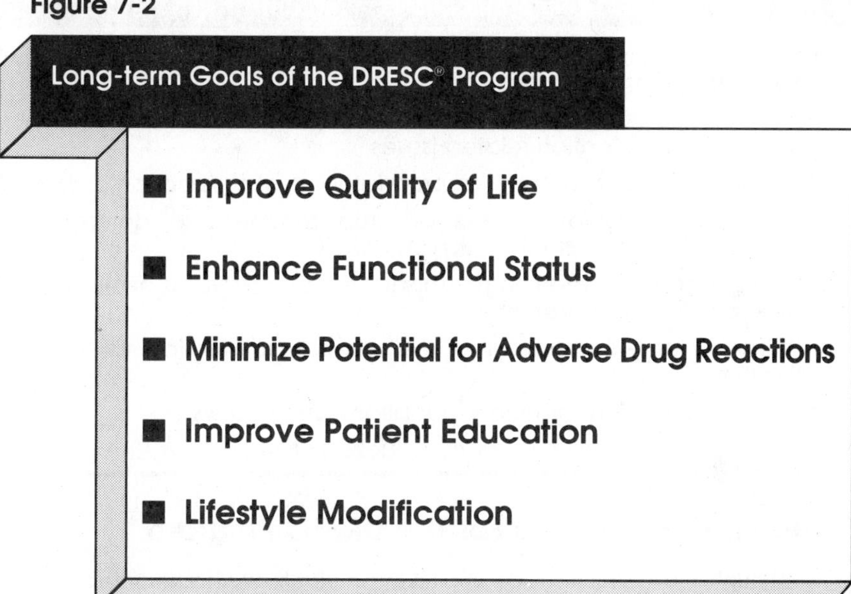

the drug regimen to determine whether stepdown therapy is possible. For these reasons, the DRESC program can easily be incorporated into risk management programs designed to evaluate drug safety and utilization. When successful, the DRESC program will promote long-term patient satisfaction with drug therapy, and can also be used as a centerpiece program for drug reduction clinics.

Table 7-1

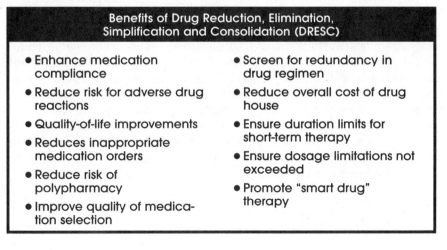

Benefits of Drug Reduction, Elimination, Simplification and Consolidation (DRESC)	
• Enhance medication compliance	• Screen for redundancy in drug regimen
• Reduce risk for adverse drug reactions	• Reduce overall cost of drug house
• Quality-of-life improvements	• Ensure duration limits for short-term therapy
• Reduces inappropriate medication orders	• Ensure dosage limitations not exceeded
• Reduce risk of polypharmacy	• Promote "smart drug" therapy
• Improve quality of medication selection	

Table 7-2

Total Pharmacotherapeutic Quality Management (TPQM): Role of The DRESC® Program
• Provides practical, hands-on approach to simplification and consolidation of drug regimens
• Promotes patient-physician and patient-pharmacist communication about medication-related issues
• Requires regular reviews of appropriateness of medication orders
• Encourages regular reviews of drug regimens to determine whether step-down therapy is possible
• Can be incorporated into risk-management programs evaluating drug safety and utilization
• Promotes long-term consumer (i.e., patient) satisfaction with drug therapy
• May influence P&T formulary adoptions and reviews
• Centerpiece program for drug reduction clinics

Screening Candidates For The DRESC Program

Although most patients who are taking multiple medications for chronic medical conditions will benefit from DRESC program strategies, not all individuals will benefit equally from attempts to streamline their medication intake. However, there are a number of risk factors, demographic characteristics, medication intake patterns, and clinical conditions that increase the likelihood that a patient will benefit from measures aimed at streamlining their medication intake (see Table 7-3). Programs oriented around TPQM should screen for these risk factors in order to identify patient candidates most likely to benefit from drug regimen redesign.

In particular, any patient who is taking *several* medications simultaneously is an excellent candidate for the DRESC program. In addition, four high-risk patient populations warrant special attention because of their increased risk of incurring drug-related toxicity. In this regard, DRESC strategies should be considered for patients who are critically ill,[21] for the elderly,[22-25] for persons with AIDS, and for individuals with cardiovascular or neuropsychiatric disease who are on multiple drug therapy. Generally speaking the risk of having a drug-related adverse patient event is linked to the number of *diseases* a person is burdened with, as well as the number of different *prescription ingredients* in the drug regimen. Inasmuch as little can be done to reduce disease burden, attention must be focused primarily on *reducing pharmacologic burden* to decrease the risk of drug-related toxicity and associated complications.

Table 7-3

Screening for and Identifying Candidates Appropriate For DRESC® Program
PATIENTS WITH THE FOLLOWING DRUG REGIMENS, RISK FACTORS, DEMOGRAPHIC CHARACTERISTICS, AND CLINICAL CONDITIONS SHOULD BE CONSIDERED FOR DRUG REDUCTION, ELIMINATION, SIMPLIFICATION, AND CONSOLIDATION.
• Patients taking three or more drugs
• 65 years of age and older
• A history of unexplained fatigue, sexual dysfunction, sleep disturbance, depression, mood disturbance, cough.
• Six or more physician visits within a 1-year period
• A history of adverse drug reactions or interactions
• Perception that drug regimen is too costly
• Regimen contains drugs dosed at multiple daily dose frequencies
• Medications with only one end-organ salvage function
• Medications considered inappropriate for age group (e.g., the elderly)
• Medications consumed at highest recommended dose
• Patients taking more than 9 doses per day
• Patients taking medications beyond normally accepted duration limits (H2 blockers, antibiotics, corticosteroids, etc.)
• Regimen consists of primarily generic medications
• Complaints of medication side effects

Patient Factors. Patients who complain of unexplained fatigue, sexual dysfunction, sleep disturbance, depression, mood disturbance, or cough, require meticulous screening of their drug intake to determine whether any of these symptoms are the result of pharmacologic toxicity.[10] Agents used to treat neuropsychiatric disorders, hypertension, and cardiovascular diseases require special scrutiny.[26-29] Studies show that individuals who make six or more physician visits within a one-year period also are at increased risk for having drug-related toxicity. In addition, when these physician encounters occur with more than one practitioner, the risk of pharmacologic mismanagement is even greater. Hence, patients taking multiple medications who have made more than six physician visits within a one-year period, and who acknowledge that they have multiple prescribing sources, will almost always benefit from streamlining programs aimed at reduction, simplification, and consolidation.

Individuals with a history of adverse drug reactions,[13,30] medication compliance problems,[20,31-33] or drug interactions also require careful evaluation. These patients may be extremely susceptible to pharmacologic intervention, and therefore, DRESC program strategies can help reduce the risk of drug-related problems. In addition, if patients perceive that their drug regimen is too costly, the practitioner should determine whether medication compliance has been affected by drug cost. In this patient subgroup, simple alterations that reduce drug acquisition costs for the patient can produce dramatic improvements in compliance, and, therefore, enhance therapeutic outcomes.

Drug Factors. Most drug regimens require careful screening and assessment to uncover suboptimal drugs, dosing patterns, combinations, or prescribing practices. For example, a regimen that contains many medications given at multiple daily dose frequencies will usually be less than satisfactory from a compliance perspective. In these cases, a streamlining program aimed at consolidating the regimen with primarily once-daily medications may improve drug compliance and, in the process, enhance therapeutic results. The regimen should also be screened to determine if medications that salvage only one target organ, treat only one symptom, or have only one function are being used. For example, if a patient with diabetes is taking one medication to treat high blood pressure, a different medication to treat congestive heart failure, and yet another drug to treat renal dysfunction, it may be more appropriate to consolidate this patient's drug regimen with a single agent, such as an ACE inhibitor, which is able to service several target organs simultaneously. Similarly, if a patient is consuming one drug to treat angina and another drug to treat high blood pressure, it may be therapeutically far more effective to identify a *single* agent, such as a calcium channel blocker, that can provide both symptomatic relief and treatment for hypertension using only one medication.

As a general rule, patients who have multiple clinical disorders and are being treated with many different medications—each of which is targeted at only *one* disease or clinical problem—are likely to benefit from DRESC program *consolidation* strategies; whenever possible, the objective is to treat multiple conditions with a single prescription drug (see Table 7-4). Drug regimens should also be screened for medications considered to be inappropriate or unsuitable for use in the elderly. In particular, drug houses that include sedative or hypnotic agents, tricyclic antidepressants, nonsteroidal anti-inflammatory drugs (NSAIDs), unproven dementia therapies, muscle relaxants, and bronchodilators will almost always benefit from DRESC program modifications.

The need for drug house deconstruction and reconstruction is also suggested when treatment regimens contain medications prescribed at levels that approach their highest recommended daily dose. Although not always the case, when medications are used at their maximal dosage strength, it is possible that the patient may be more responsive to an agent belonging to a different drug class. For example, a non-diabetic African American patient whose blood pressure is marginally controlled on a maximum dose of an ACE inhibitor may respond favorably by switching to a calcium blocker. In these cases, DRESC program strategies aimed at selecting drugs that are dosed at lower levels will oftentimes improve side effect profiles and medication compliance. DRESC program strategies also deserve application in patients who are taking more than 10 pills per day, in individuals who are taking medications that are frequently prescribed beyond their normally accepted duration limits (eg, H_2 blockers, antibiotics, corticosteroids), and in persons whose drug regimens consist primarily of *generic medications.* Finally, any patient complaining of side effects or quality-of-life impairments that may be attributable to their medication intake requires a careful review to see whether DRESC program strategies are indicated.

Table 7-4

CONSOLIDATION OF REGIMENS WITH SMART DRUGS	
SMART DRUG	**CONDITIONS/SYMPTOMS**
AMLODIPINE	
	Hypertension Angina
DILTIAZEM	
	Angina Hypertension Supraventricular tachycardia
PROPRANOLOL	
	Arrhythmia prophylaxis Post-MI cardioprotection Hypertension Migraine prophylaxis Angina
ATENOLOL	
	Arrhythmia prophylaxis Angina Hypertension Secondary prevention of myocardial infarction
ACE INHIBITORS	
	Hypertension Congestive heart failure Prevention of renal disease in diabetes Prevention of CHF, post-MI
DOXAZOSIN	
	Symptoms of benign prostatic hypertrophy Hypertension
DIGOXIN	
	Chronic atrial fibrillation Congestive heart failure
ASPIRIN	
	Secondary prevention of MI Stroke prevention

Table 7-4

CONSOLIDATION OF REGIMENS WITH SMART DRUGS — cont'd.	
SMART DRUG	**CONDITIONS/SYMPTOMS**
ATORVASTATIN	
	Elevated cholesterol levels Elevated triglycerides
CETIRIZINE	
	Seasonal allergic rhinitis Perennial allergic rhinitis Chronic urticaria
ESTROGEN REPLACEMENT THERAPY (WITH PROGESTERONE IF NECESSARY)	
	Delay onset of Alzheimer's disease? Cardioprevention Osteoporosis prevention Amelioration of postmenopausal symptoms
SEROTONIN SELECTIVE REUPTAKE INHIBITORS (eg, SERTRALINE)	
	Obsessive-Compulsive Disorder (OCD) Depression Panic disorder
TRICYCLIC ANTIDEPRESSANT	
	Diabetic neuropathy pain Depression
SHORT-ACTING BENZODIAZEPINE	
	Insomnia Panic disorder

Establishing Patient Confidence and Cooperation

Experienced clinicians and pharmacists understand that streamlining a patient's drug house is much easier said than done. No matter how logical, practical, or pharmacologically justified a program of drug reduction, simplification, and consolidation may be, it always requires the patient's cooperation to put such a program into practice; and while many drugs in a regimen may be problematic for one reason or another, patients don't always perceive it that way. In fact, patients often depend heavily on their medications for reasons that may not be logical or scientific. Consequently, implementation of the DRESC program requires patient confidence and cooperation, two barriers that can be difficult to overcome. For example, older patients who have been taking multiple medications for many years often believe that drugs help them feel secure and can control symptoms that otherwise might be incomprehensible, painful, or frightening. Consequently, these individuals may resist attempts at pharmacologic weaning.

On occasion, a practitioner may be too busy to review medication-related information from the patient's chart. Insufficient time spent taking a case history is also a risk factor for polypharmacy. For example, a physician may fail to associate the onset of a new symptom with the introduction of a new medication into the therapeutic regimen. Patients who suffer from anxiety, somatization disorder, depression, and multiple medical conditions also are prone to the pitfalls of polypharmacy. These individuals often consult various physicians about vague and numerous complaints. Consequently, they may have a tendency to accumulate drugs.

Successful implementation of the DRESC program requires planning, education, and patience. As a preliminary step to drug regimen simplification, the patient's current medications should be grouped into three categories: (1) drugs that are clearly not needed and can be toxic in normal doses or lethal in overdose, thus giving them the greatest potential for harm; (2) drugs that are probably unnecessary but in normal doses are not harmful; (3) those drugs that are reasonably safe and for which there is some medical indication.

Physician Factors. Preparing a patient to comply with the DRESC program is often a delicate process. Too often, physicians or pharmacists may simply tell their patients what to do, rather than explain why they want them to do it. In general, a patient is more likely to comply with a streamlining program if a credible reason is offered for discontinuing or substituting certain drugs. For example, the practitioner may point out that not only are some of the medications in the drug regimen potentially harmful, but they also may not have worked as well as expected, and a different pharmacologic approach should be tried. If the patient has more than one physician, it is imperative that all participate in the DRESC program. Usually however, the primary care practitioner or consulting pharmacist will be the liaison person for all individuals involved in writing prescriptions for the patient. Ideally, only one physician should write prescriptions. If this is not possible, all participating physicians should write prescriptions only in their specialty fields, and each should notify the others when medications are added, changed, or deleted. In addition, all medications should be filled at one pharmacy. This will reduce the likelihood that multiple or duplicate medications are prescribed for the same symptom or clinical disorder. In general, patient cooperation will be facilitated if physicians and other prescibers collaborate on a drug reduction program.

Patient Factors. Despite initial patient reluctance to consider modifications in the drug regimen, a number of strategies are useful for informing, reassuring, and guiding patients through the DRESC program. As a prelude to drug house redesign, the patient should be educated about the risks associated with inappropriate drug prescribing and the necessity for constant reevaluation of drug house building blocks. Specifically the patient should be taught that many medications once considered state-of-the-art therapy for a particular condition have been replaced by better drugs that are dosed less frequently and produce fewer side effects.

Interestingly, many patients feel insecure about reducing daily dose frequency of a medication because they think that drugs taken more frequently are better equipped to treat their condition. Physicians and pharmacists should reassure patients that medications with a long half-life, when indicated, can produce around-the-clock coverage with simpler dosing regimens. In this regard, many patients need special reassurance that *once-daily* medications used to manage high blood pressure, inflammatory osteoarthritic conditions, pain-producing syndromes, and depression are proven to be just as effective as medications previously dosed on a more frequent basis (see Table 7-5). Reassurance and education are especially necessary for patients who suffer from symptomatic clinical disorders because these individuals may tend to associate pain relief with consumption of many pills throughout the day. Informing the patient that medications dosed less frequently are able to achieve constant blood levels throughout the day—therefore, providing adequate protection against pain—may be all that is necessary to induce patient acceptance of and compliance with once-daily medications.

Reluctance to permit streamlining of drug therapy is also observed in patients who are accustomed to taking a 10- to 14-day course of antibiotic therapy to treat common infectious diseases such as pneumonia, sinusitis, cellulitis, and sexually transmitted diseases. In such cases, it may be helpful for the clinician to point out that "less is sometimes more," and that one-dose or short-duration therapeutic courses can treat infections just as effectively as older regimens requiring a longer duration of therapy (see Table 7-6).

Program Factors. As previously mentioned, patients should be reassured that the DRESC program is a *collaborative* process between physician, pharmacist, and patient (see Table 7-7). It is especially helpful to stress the importance of

Table 7-5

DRESC® Strategies: Once-A-Day Drug Therapy
Selected Medications With Clinical Effectiveness

ONCE-DAILY DRUG	COMMENTS AND ANALYSIS
SULFONYLUREAS	
Glipizide GITS Glyburide	Diabetes
H_2 BLOCKERS	
Famotidine Ranitidine Nizatidine Cimetidine	Ulcer disease

Table 7-5

DRESC® Strategies: Once-A-Day Drug Therapy Selected Medications With Clinical Effectiveness — cont'd.	
ONCE-DAILY DRUG	**COMMENTS AND ANALYSIS**
BETA-BLOCKERS	
Metoprolol Atenolol Acebutolol	Hypertension
PERIPHERAL ALPHA-BLOCKER	
Doxazosin	Hypertension BPH symptoms
CALCIUM CHANNEL BLOCKERS	
Amlodipine Felodipine Diltiazem Verapamil	Hypertension
ACE INHIBITORS	
Enalapril Lisinopril	Hypertension CHF
LIPID LOWERING DRUGS	
Atorvastatin Pravastatin Simvastatin Lovastatin Fluvastatin	Cholesterol reduction
ANTIDEPRESSANTS	
Sertraline Paroxetine Fluoxetine	Depression

maintaining both patient-physician and patient-pharmacist communication regarding drug-induced side effects and concerns about drug costs. Cooperation is more likely if the patient is informed that only drugs deemed to be unnecessary, redundant, outdated, prescribed for excessive duration, or prescribed at inappropriately high doses will be considered for deletion or modification. Once again, education and reassurance are essential for establishing patient confidence and cooperation. It is also useful to stress that the patient's overall clinical status, as well as such parameters as blood pressure, symptom level, and pain patterns will be carefully monitored during the DRESC program.

Sometimes, patient cooperation is facilitated if individuals are presented with opportunities for lifestyle modification that will enable nonpharmacologic management of their chronic conditions. Patients frequently welcome the opportunity to be a coparticipant in a drug streamlining program, especially if they can be convinced that drug reduction and elimination will be facilitated by lifestyle modifications that include weight loss, regular physical activity, and cessation of cigarette smoking.

In general, individuals do not respond well to *precipitous* changes in their therapeutic regimen. Consequently, it is often helpful to reassure the patient that the DRESC program will be a *gradual* process, usually involving no more than one to two drug substitutions per 12-week cycle (see Chapter 8). Initial patient enthusiasm for a drug streamlining program frequently can be generated by stressing that significant cost savings may result from drug elimination or substitution. In those cases in which *increased* drug expenditures are required, the patient should be reassured that benefits such as quality-of-life improvements, simplified dosing, enhanced compliance, and reduced risk of drug interactions are well worth the price. Finally, it should be stressed that gaining patient confidence and cooperation for participation in a drug simplification program can be a time-consuming process. In the long run, however, laying the groundwork that will make the patient a full-fledged collaborator in the DRESC program is essential for maximizing pharmacotherapeutic results.

Cost Considerations and Potential Risks

One of the principal objectives of the DRESC program is to *reduce* overall medical expenditures associated with a long-term therapeutic regimen (see Table 7-8). To achieve this objective, however, increased *short-term* costs associated with multiple consultations may be required. It is important to remember, however, that the purpose of these visits is to identify medications that are unnecessary and/or that can be eliminated, thereby producing *long-term cost savings* to the patient. In general, when generic medications are replaced by brand-name products, increases in drug costs can be expected. However, the newer, more expensive medications may be associated with better compliance, dose stability, regimen durability, and fewer side effects. Often these advantages will justify the increased costs. There are many opportunities for offsetting the costs associated with introducing more expensive and better-tolerated agents into the drug house.

Table 7-6

DRESC PROGRAM: ONE DOSE/SHORT DURATION THERAPEUTIC OPTIONS FOR INFECTIONS

Condition/Disease	One Dose/Short Course Option
Nonspecific bacterial vaginosis	Metronidazole, 2 g PO
Trichomoniasis	Metronidazole, 2 g PO (contraindicated during first trimester of pregnancy)
Candida vaginitis	Fluconazole, 150 mg PO or tioconazole 6.5% vaginal ointment

Table 7-6

DRESC PROGRAM: ONE DOSE/SHORT DURATION THERAPEUTIC OPTIONS FOR INFECTIONS — cont'd.	
Condition/Disease	**One Dose/Short Course Option**
Gonorrhea	Ceftriaxone, 125 mg IM or cefixime, 400 mg PO or ciprofloxacin, 500 mg PO or ofloxacin, 400 mg PO or azithromycin 2 g PO once
Chlamydia (uncomplicated) (cervicitis, urethritis)	Azithromycin 1 g PO
Cellulitis *(Staphylococcus aureus, Streptococcus)*	Azithromycin, 500 mg PO day 1, 250 mg PO x 4 days
Otitis media (children)	Ceftriaxone, 50 mg/kg IM once or Azithromycin oral suspension x 5 days
Urinary tract infection (uncomplicated)	TMP/SMZ 1 tab PO bid × 3 days
Whipworm Infection *(Truchuris trichiuria)*	Albendazole, 400 mg PO
Pinworm Infection *(Enterobius vermicularis)*	Mebendazole, 100 mg PO and repeat after 2 weeks
Hookworm *(Necator Americanus)*	Albendazole, 400 mg PO or mebendazole, 100 mg PO
Scabies/Mites *(Sarcoptes scabei)*	Permethrin (5%) massage from head to soles; wash off after 8-14 hours
Body Lice *(Pediculus huanus coporis)*	Pyrethrin with piperonyl butoxide; apply lotion for 10 minutes, then bathe

Table 7-7

The DRESC® Program: Establishing Patient Confidence and Cooperation
THE FOLLOWING STRATEGIES WILL HELP INFORM, REASSURE, AND GUIDE PATIENTS THROUGH REGIMEN STREAMLINING:
• Educate patient about risks associated with inappropriate drug prescribing and necessity of evaluation of drug house building blocks

Table 7-7

The DRESC® Program: Establishing Patient Confidence and Cooperation — cont'd.
• Emphasize that DRESC® program is a collaborative process between physician, pharmacist, and patient
• Stress that significant cost savings may be accomplished with DRESC® changes
• Inform patient that original indications for using certain drugs may have changed and that it is possible that medications can be deleted without adverse effects
• Reassure patient that clinical status and parameters (blood pressure, symptom level, pain patterns, etc.) will be carefully monitored during DRESC® program
• Reassure patient that only drugs deemed to be unnecessary, redundant, outdated, prescribed for excessive duration, or at inappropriately high doses will be considered for modification
• Inform patient of opportunities for nonpharmacologic management (weight loss, dietary modifications, etc.) for certain disorders
• Emphasize importance of medication compliance and its relation to daily dose frequency
• Stress advantages of simplified drug regimens
• Reassure patient that DRESC® program is a gradual process, involving no more than 1-2 drug substitutions per cycle
• Stress importance of patient-physician communication regarding drug-induced side effects and lifestyle changes noted during DRESC® process

Clearly, the most desirable approach is to selectively eliminate medications that are unnecessary from the therapeutic regimen, consolidate two or more drugs with the use of a single agent, and/or introduce better agents that are of similar cost. Nevertheless, it should be stressed that if the improved drug regimen is, indeed, more costly than the original regimen, this increase in drug cost may be justified.

Although the DRESC program is designed to produce more streamlined, better tolerated pharmacotherapeutic regimens, there are potential risks (see Table 7-9). For example, the practitioner may discontinue a medication that is needed by the patient. Naturally, precautions should be taken to avoid elimination of necessary medications. Discontinuation of medications such as digoxin, theophylline, antidepressants, or corticosteroids requires careful clinical monitoring and evaluation. Inappropriate elimination of medications can be prevented by establishing strict criteria for drug discontinuation. For example, digoxin should not be discontinued in patients who have documented congestive heart failure. However, it may be appropriate to attempt discontinuation of this agent in individuals who have normal sinus rhythm and who have echocardiographic confirmation of normal ventricular function.

Table 7-8

Cost Considerations Associated With DRESC® Program
• Increased short-term cost of multiple physician/pharmacist consultations will be more than offset by reduction in long-term cost savings associated with a streamlined drug regimen
• Potential increases in cost of some drug substitutions may be offset by reduction in total outcome costs produced by better medication compliance
• Post-DRESC® program (i.e., reconstructed) drug regimen may be less costly than original therapeutic regimen
• If post-DRESC® program drug regimen is more costly than original therapeutic regimen, these potential increases in drug cost may still be associated with reduced costs associated with return visits, drug monitoring costs, and therapeutic failures caused by poor compliance

Table 7-9

Potential Risks of the DRESC® Program
• Elimination of necessary medications
• Clinical deterioration caused by reduction of drug dosage
• Erosion of patient confidence in drug regimen
• Introduction of unexpected side effects
• Introduction of unexpected drug interactions
• Reduced clinical efficacy of reconstructed drug regimen
• Increased cost of reconstructed drug regimen

Discontinuation of antidepressants may precipitate episodes of severe clinical depression. Elimination of these agents is more likely to be successful in patients with limited, situational depression and in those persons who have had no more than one episode of serious depression in the last 5 years. Clinical deterioration can result not only from drug cessation but from reduction of drug dosage. Many of these problems can be avoided by careful screening and clinical monitoring of patients in whom drugs have been withdrawn, or have had dose reductions (see Tables 7-10 and 7-11).

Other potential risks of the DRESC program include introduction of unexpected side effects from the addition of new agents or the precipitation of unexpected drug interactions. As a rule, however, the purpose of DRESC program drug substitutions is to identify medications with fewer side effects and a lower risk of drug interactions. Nevertheless, sometimes the reconstructed drug regimen may produce undesirable side effects, in which case other therapeutic alternatives should be considered. Whenever drug deletions, substitutions, or additions are made, it is always possible that the reconstructed drug house will not be as clinically effective as the original regimen. For example, a patient who is taking a thiazide diuretic and beta-blocker for the management of hypertension may find that his blood pressure is not as well controlled with the ACE inhibitor that is substituted for the two original antihypertensive agents. In such cases, it may be worth considering the use of another antihypertensive agent, such as a calcium blocker, instead of the ACE inhibitor, before returning the patient to the original drug regimen. The point is, reduction of clinical efficacy is a potential liability of any reconstructed drug regimen, and therefore, careful clinical monitoring is mandatory whenever drug substitutions or consolidations are made.

ELIMINATION OF UNNECESSARY PRESCRIPTION DRUGS

Elimination of potentially unnecessary prescription drugs is one of the cornerstones of the DRESC program. The process of drug elimination begins with a careful review of the patient's current medication list. There are many opportunities and indications for cessation of prescription medications, all of which deserve careful consideration (see Table 7-12). For example, some commonly used medications can be discontinued simply because the *initial* indications for starting the drug were insufficient in the first place. In other cases, drugs can be eliminated because they are being used for a duration of time that extends beyond the window of therapeutic opportunity (see Table 7-11). For example, maintenance therapy with H_2 blockers beyond 12 months duration is usually not required for patients with mild peptic ulcer disease, especially those with no history of gastrointestinal hemorrhage. Patients with *H. pylori* infection who have had their infection eradicated may not require maintenance therapy with H_2-blockers at all. Similarly, short-acting benzodiazepines should initially be prescribed for brief duration courses only. The original indications for initiating drugs from this class should always be reviewed, and unless there are continuing indications for long-term maintenance therapy, drug discontinuation should be considered. Sometimes a drug can be eliminated because new clinical trials demonstrate that the agent is not useful in the condition for which it was thought to be effective. For example, dipyridamole is sometimes used in patients with cerebrovascular disease, despite the fact that a number of well-designed clinical trials confirm that it offers no advantages over aspirin in the prevention of transient ischemic attacks, stroke, or myocardial infarction. Similar justifications can be given for discontinuing cyclandelate and isoxsuprine, both of which have been shown to be ineffective for the treatment of chronic dementia. Antiarrhythmic agents represent some of the most important examples of medications that should be evaluated for clinical usefulness, based on recent clinical trials that show many agents in the Type I drug class do not prevent morbidity or mortality in patients who have nonlife-threatening ventricular ectopy.

Table 7-10

Medications That May Be Suitable For Elimination Because of Inappropriate or Questionable Indications For Clinical Use	
DRUG	**COMMENTS AND ANALYSIS**
DIGOXIN	
	Useful in patients with *documented* CHF and for rate control in chronic atrial fibrillation. Digoxin is sometimes overused in patients with normal sinus rhythm and a presumptive diagnosis of CHF, which should be confirmed with objective criteria such as echocardiography.
MISOPROSTOL	
	Cost-effectiveness is optimized in patients who require NSAIDs and who also have a documented history of peptic or gastric ulcer disease.
DIPYRIDAMOLE	
	Aspirin is more effective at lower cost for prevention of secondary MI, TIAs, and stroke. Persantine may have role as adjunct therapy in patients with prosthetic heart valves.
CHOLESTYRAMINE	
	Noncompliance is extremely common and frequently undermines clinical efficacy of the drug. Statins are generally preferrable, and more effective for cholesterol reduction.
THEOPHYLLINE	
	This drug is frequently overused in treatment of bronchospastic pulmonary disease, COPD, and asthma. Prior to inclusion of theophylline in a drug regimen, inhaled beta-agonists or inhaled corticosteroids (in asthmatic patients) should be tried, and compliance with metered-dose inhalers should be ensured by providing instructions to patients or using spacer.
PROPOXYPHENE	
	Equally effective analgesics available with less toxicity.

Table 7-10

Medications That May Be Suitable For Elimination Because of Inappropriate or Questionable Indications For Clinical Use — cont'd.	
DRUG	**COMMENTS AND ANALYSIS**
BENZODIAZEPINES	
Diazepam Chlordiazepoxide Clonazepam Flurazepam Oxazepam Lorazepam	Review original indications for drug. Many patients, especially those who have been clinically stable for at least 12 months, can have benzodiazepines slowly discontinued over several weeks.
OMEPRAZOLE	
	This agent is sometimes introduced into regimen for treatment of mild erosive esophagitis or peptic ulcer disease before attempting less costly therapy with H_2 blockers.
NSAIDS	
	In many cases, acetaminophen should be tried for analgesia before committing patients to long-term NSAID use.

Table 7-11

DRESC® Screening For Drugs With Established or Possible Duration Limits	
DRUG	**COMMENTS AND ANALYSIS**
HISTAMINE ANTAGONISTS	
Cimetidine Ranitidine Famotidine Nizatidine	Maintenance therapy for 12 months is indicated in most patients with documented peptic or gastric ulceration. Long-term maintenance therapy (ie, > 12 months) is generally not indicated, except in patients who continue to be at high risk for complications such as hemorrhage.

Table 7-11

DRESC® Screening For Drugs With Established or Possible Duration Limits — cont'd.	
DRUG	**COMMENTS AND ANALYSIS**
SHORT-ACTING BENZODIAZEPINES	
	Therapy for sleep disorders, anxiety, and panic attacks should initially be short-term. Patients with panic disorders who are symptom-free for at least 6 months may be appropriate candidates for gradual discontinuation of benzodiazepines.
ORAL ANTIBIOTICS	
	Long-term suppressive therapy is indicated in selected patients only, especially in those with HIV infection.
PHENYTOIN	
	Selected patients who have an idiopathic seizure disorder, normal sleep deprivation ECG, and are seizure-free for 3 years or longer may be considered for discontinuation, but with careful clinical monitoring only.
ANTIHYPERTENSIVE AGENTS	
	Step-down therapy may be attempted in selected patients with mild hypertension who have excellent control with monotherapy. Tapering dose and/or elimination of antihypertensive agents is also encouraged, especially in patients who have implemented lifestyle changes (ie, weight reduction, increased exercise, etc.) conducive to nonpharmacologic management of hypertension.

Table 7-11

DRESC[R] Screening For Drugs With Established or Possible Duration Limits — cont'd.	
DRUG	**COMMENTS AND ANALYSIS**
ANTIDEPRESSANTS	
	Step-down therapy may be advisable in some patients with self-limited, situational depression, and in those individuals with no more than one episode of serious depression in the last 3 years. Lifetime maintenance *usually* is required in patients who are 50 years old or more at the onset of their first major depressive episode, aged 40 or more at onset with two or more depressive episodes, or with more than three prior episodes at any age. Patients who are committed to a trial of antidepressants should generally be given a 9-12 month trial to achieve desired clinical effects and stabilization.
ORAL SULFONYLUREAS	
	Dose reduction or discontinuation may be possible in patients who pursue active lifestyle modifications (weight reduction, exercise, etc.) known to lower blood glucose.
CORTICOSTEROIDS	
	Short duration tapering course of 7-10 days are as effective as long tapering courses (ie, 2-3 weeks) in preventing exacerbations of asthma.

Table 7-12

Opportunities and Indications For Possible Elimination of Unnecessary Prescription Drugs
• Inadequate initial indications for beginning medication (example: digoxin, benzodiazepine, misoprostol etc.)
• Drug can be eliminated because it has been used for duration that extends beyond window of opportunity (example: H2 blocker)
• Drug can be eliminated because new clinical trials show it is not useful in condition for which it was thought to be effective (example: dipyridamole, isoxsuprine, hydergine)
• Drug can be eliminated because less toxic agents are available that produce equivalent clinical result (example: theophylline, indocin, indomethacin)
• Drug may be eliminated because patient is clinically stable for long periods without exacerbations of disease state (example: dilantin, corticosteroids)
• Drug can possibly be eliminated because condition has stabilized and pharmacologic therapy is no longer required for clinical maintenance (example: antihypertensive medications, antiulcer drugs, theophylline)
• Drug can be eliminated because less expensive, equally effective agents are available (ticlodipine, dipyridamole)
• Drug can be eliminated because it is associated with noncompliance (example: cholestyramine)

In some cases, medications can be eliminated because less toxic agents are available that produce equivalent clinical results. For example, a prescriber may eliminate theophylline in an asthmatic patient experiencing gastrointestinal side effects and replace it with an inhaled beta-agonist, producing equivalent relief with far less toxicity. *Oral* prednisone therapy—including frequency and dosage—can sometimes be eliminated in patients treated with potent, high dose *inhaled* steroids such as Flovent. Systemic steroid requirements may also be reduced in asthmatics who respond to leukotriene inhibitors such as Singulair or Accolate. Drug cessation may be especially successful in individuals who are clinically stable for long periods of time and have no exacerbations of their disease. For example, a patient with an idiopathic seizure disorder who is epilepsy-free for three or more years while taking dilantin may be a candidate for drug discontinuation. Similarly, patients who remain clinically stable for long periods while taking corticosteroids, NSAIDs, and benzodiazepines should be considered for drug discontinuation. Migraine sufferers may find intermittent use of sumatriptan (Imitrex) as effective as long term suppressive therapy. Naturally, drug substitution should be attempted when less expensive, equally effective agents are available. Finally, some drugs can be eliminated simply because they are associated with patient noncompliance.[33] Although cholestyramine, when taken as prescribed, will lower serum cholesterol levels, few patients are able to tolerate a drug with the consistency of liquid sand. There are many other drugs which, because they require a complicated dosing schedule, produce virtually intolerable side effects, or are associated with extraordinary financial expenditures, may require evaluation for drug cessation or substitution, simply because they are associated with poor compliance patterns that undermine therapeutic efficacy. In each case, the decision to discontinue or replace a medication should be made on a case-by-case basis.

Drug Discontinuation in the Elderly

The opportunities and indications for medication discontinuation in the *elderly* warrant special attention (see Table 7-13). Individuals aged 65 years or older account for about 25% of all prescription drug use in the United States and are at high risk for adverse drug effects. Polypharmacy, which is common in the geriatric population, sharply increases the risk of side effects.

A comprehensive set of explicit criteria has been published for inadequate drug-prescribing practices in the elderly based on the following three concepts: (1) prescription medications that should be entirely avoided in the elderly; (2) excessive dosage; and (3) excessive duration of treatment. Using these criteria, a recent report presented conservative estimates of the incidence of potentially inappropriate prescribing practices for community-dwelling elderly persons in the United States.[34]

The investigators reported an alarming incidence of prescriptions in the elderly for 20 potentially inappropriate drugs, using explicit criteria previously developed by Canadian and American geriatric experts. This landmark study demonstrated that a total of 23.5% of people aged 65 years or older living in the community, or about 6.64 million Americans, received *at least one* of the 20 contraindicated drugs. While 79.6% of the people receiving potentially inappropriate medications received only one such drug, about 20% received two or more of these contraindicated agents. Among the drugs considered inappropriate in this population, the most commonly prescribed medications were dipyridamole, propoxyphene, amitriptyline, chlorpropamide, diazepam, indomethacin, and chlordiazepoxide, each of which was taken by at least 600,000 individuals aged 65 years or older. If one includes three controversial cardiovascular agents (propranolol, methyldopa, and reserpine) in the list of contraindicated drugs, the incidence of inappropriate medication use rose to 32%, or 9 million people. The study concluded that physicians prescribed potentially inappropriate medications for nearly a quarter of all older people living in the community, placing them at risk for adverse drug effects such as cognitive impairment and sedation.[34-36]

Inappropriate Medications In The Elderly

Anxiolytics. Medications considered to be inappropriate in the geriatric age group include those that ought to be entirely avoided, those used in excessive dosages, and drugs used for an excessive duration. Among the sedative or hypnotic agents, diazepam, chlordiazepoxide, flurazepam, and meprobamate

Table 7-13

DRESC® Program Summary of Inappropriate Medication Use: Drugs To Be Avoided In The Elderly	
DRUG CLASS	**REASON FOR AVOIDANCE**
SEDATIVE OR HYPNOTIC AGENTS	
Diazepam Chlordiazepoxide Flurazepam	Prolonged half-life, increased daytime sedation, increased risk of falls and hip fractures. Shorter acting benzodiazepines such as lorazepam, temazepam, etc. considered safer.
Meprobamate	Considered to be less safe than short-acting benzodiazepines for treatment of anxiety and sleep disturbance.
SHORT-DURATION BARBITURATES	
Pentobarbital	Shorter-acting benzodiazepines safer for sedation in the elderly and phenobarbital preferable in epilepsy
TRICYCLIC ANTIDEPRESSANTS	
Amitriptyline Doxepin	Anticholinergic side effects, orthostatic hypotension, and sedation more pronounced than with serotonin selective reuptake inhibitors (ie, sertraline, etc.)
COMBINATION ANTIDEPRESSANTS/ANTIPSYCHOTICS	
	Geriatric doses are difficult to titrate in fixed-dose combinations
NONSTEROIDAL ANTIINFLAMMATORY DRUGS (NSAIDS)	
Indomethacin	Greater CNS, gastrointestinal, and renal toxicity, than other NSAIDs. Colchicine may be a better option for treatment of gout in the elderly.

Table 7-13

DRESC[R] Program Summary of Inappropriate Medication Use: Drugs To Be Avoided In The Elderly — cont'd.	
DRUG CLASS	**REASON FOR AVOIDANCE**
ANALGESICS	
Propoxyphene	Relatively ineffective (perhaps no better pain relief than acetaminophen) and low toxic-to-therapeutic ratio may cause CNS and cardiac toxicity from accumulation of toxic metabolites.
Pentazocine	Overdose is associated with seizures and cardiotoxicity.
PLATELET INHIBITORS	
Dipyridamole	Useful only as adjunct to warfarin therapy in patients with artificial heart valves. Use for prophylaxis in other conditions not substantiated. Can cause headache, dizziness, and CNS disturbances at higher doses.
MUSCLE RELAXANTS/ANTISPASMODICS	
Cyclobenzaprine Orphenadrine Methocarbamol Carisoprodol	Potential CNS side effects may outweigh benefits.
ANTIEMETIC AGENTS	
Trimethobenzamide	Less effective than other agents and may cause drowsiness, rash, diarrhea, and extrapyramidal reactions.
ANTIHYPERTENSIVES	
Propranolol Methyldopa Reserpine Verapamil	Agents of equal efficacy with fewer side effects are oftentimes available.
BRONCHODILATORS	
Theophylline Terbutaline	Toxicity increased in the elderly. Inhaled beta agonists and inhaled steroids should be the first tier of therapy.

Table 7-13

DRESC® Program Summary of Inappropriate Medication Use: Drugs To Be Avoided In The Elderly — cont'd.	
DRUG CLASS	**REASON FOR AVOIDANCE**
H_2 BLOCKERS	
Cimetidine	Inhibits P_{450} cytochrome oxidase system and, therefore, it has the potential to cause drug interactions with a wide range of commonly used therapeutic agents. Although not contraindicated in the elderly, H_2 blockers (eg, famotidine) that do not inhibit drug metabolism may be preferable, especially in patients on polypharmacy.

should generally be considered inappropriate for use in the elderly patient. Many of these benzodiazepines have a prolonged half-life, produce increased daytime sedation, and are associated with an increased risk of falls and hip fractures. When benzodiazepine use *is* indicated in an elderly patient, shorter-acting agents such as lorazepam, temazepam, or oxazepam are considered to be safer. Meprobamate is considered to be less safe than short-acting benzodiazepines for the treatment of anxiety and sleep disturbances. Short duration barbiturates such as pentobarbital and secobarbital are generally not advised for the geriatric patient, in whom shorter-acting benzodiazepines have proven safer for sedation. In general, patients should be converted from long-acting to short-acting benzodiazepine therapy. In many cases, benzodiazepine therapy may be eliminated altogether, and if gradual tapering programs are followed, withdrawal symptoms can be minimized.[17,26,40]

The decision to discontinue use of a benzodiazepine can be difficult. After all, patients frequently take these anxiolytic agents for many years and depend on them for behavioral and emotional stability. On the other hand, these drugs are frequently started for management of short-term, situational crises and then become permanent fixtures in the drug house. On occasion, the patient is unaware that physical or psychological dependence has occurred and may pressure the physician into long-term maintenance therapy.[26,43] These cases can be difficult to manage because the patient believes that the anxiolytic agent is still required for symptomatic relief. Also, the physician may be reluctant to withdraw a drug that has the potential for producing withdrawal symptoms.

Despite these obstacles to benzodiazepine cessation, physicians and pharmacists should carefully evaluate the original reasons for prescribing drugs in this class. Ideally, this review is conducted in collaboration with the patient, who may provide valuable information. Patients often express their own willingness to attempt a program of drug cessation under careful physician supervision. Benzodiazepines that should be targeted for elimination, when appropriate, include diazepam, chlordiazepoxide, flurazepam, oxazepam, lorazepam, and alprazolam. Success rates are improved when the tapering process is extremely gradual (over 3 to 6 months), if the patient is informed about the likely withdrawal symptoms and if supportive counseling is provided.

The elimination of amitriptyline and doxepin and substitution with an SSRI is usually justified in this age group because anticholinergic side effects such as orthostatic hypotension, sedation, and confusion are more pronounced with tricyclic antidepressants than with serotonin selective reuptake inhibitors (SSRI) (eg, sertraline, fluoxetine). Use of combination antidepressant/antipsychotic agents are discouraged because geriatric doses are difficult to titrate in fixed-dose combinations.[37,38] If behavioral disturbances, symptoms related to anxiety, aggressive behavior, and sleep patterns are well-controlled it is appropriate to consider incremental elimination or dosage reduction of psychotropic medications. (See Table 7-14)[39] This is especially true if excessive sedation or lethargy is a problem. In addition, it is reasonable to reduce antidepressant drug use to 50% of the recommended dose and evaluate the patient for clinical deterioration. If antidepressant medications *are* needed, it is usually preferable to convert patients from tricyclic antidepressants to SSRIs.

NSAIDs. The use of NSAIDs remains controversial, and all opportunities for eliminating this drug class from a patient's regimen should be pursued. In particular, indomethacin and phenylbutazone usually are inappropriate medications for the geriatric patient. Indomethacin is associated with greater central nervous system, gastrointestinal, and renal toxicity than other NSAIDs.

Table 7-14

DRESC® PROGRAM STRATEGIES FOR REDUCTION AND CONSOLIDATION OF PSYCHOTROPIC MEDICATIONS
• Review original indications for psychotropic drug use: if behavioral disturbance, symptoms
• In elderly, reduce antidepressant to 50% of recommended dose and evaluate for clinical deterioration
• Convert patient from long-acting to short-acting benzodiazepines (if benzodiazepine therapy is still required)
• Convert patient from tricyclic antidepressant to serotonin selective reuptake inhibitor, if there are no contraindications
• In elderly patient on multiple medications, consider converting from fluoxetine (P450 cytochrome oxidase inhibitor) to sertraline (minimal P450 cytochrome oxidase inhibition).
• Alprazolam: Patients with panic attacks who have been symptom-free for at least six months are appropriate candidates for gradual discontinuation of alprazolam.

Although this drug is indicated for the treatment of acute gout, colchicine may be a better, less toxic option. Phenylbutazone, which is no longer available in the U.S., is more likely than other NSAIDs to cause bone marrow toxicity and renal deterioration and should be eliminated from the drug houses of all older patients. Recent studies have shown that people taking NSAIDs have a 2.24 times higher risk of developing diverticular disease, while those taking acetominophen had a 1.81 times greater risk. In those with asymptomatic diverticular disease, the risk of bleeding is increased by both NSAIDs and acetominophen. The decision to eliminate an NSAID from the therapeutic regimen of an older patient requires consideration of multiple clinical factors. If an agent from this drug class is indicated, phenylbutazone and indomethacin should be avoided, and preference should be given to once-daily NSAIDs that cause less GI toxicity. Finally, some patients may achieve adequate symptomatic or pain relief with acetaminophen.

Analgesics. The appropriateness of analgesic drug use in the elderly requires evaluation on a case-by-case basis. It should be stressed that patients with chronic pain, terminal malignancy, and other disabling inflammatory disorders should not be deprived of narcotic pain medication. In fact, there are many studies that indicate that pain medications are *underused* in older patients. Nevertheless, there are better and worse choices when it comes to selecting analgesics in this patient population. Propoxyphene should be avoided because it is relatively ineffective. When taken in excessive quantities, propoxyphene can cause central nervous system, hepatic, and cardiac toxicity due to accumulation of toxic metabolites. Similarly, pentazocine should be avoided in the elderly because overdose is associated with seizures and cardiotoxicity. Consequently, when either propoxyphene or pentazocine appear in the drug regimen of an older individual, strong consideration should be given to their elimination. If pain relief is needed, therapy with either codeine or hydrocodone is preferable.

Neuromuscular Agents. Although there are strong pressures to use therapies aimed at improving cognitive and behavioral function in patients with chronic dementia, there is no justification for maintaining patients on medications that have no demonstrated efficacy in this condition. Therefore, cyclandelate and isoxsuprine can be eliminated from the drug houses of older patients. Although their toxicity may be minimal, ineffective treatments are difficult to justify. Dipyridamole, which is prescribed for many patients with cerebrovascular disease, does not improve clinical outcomes in patients with transient ischemic attacks, strokes, carotid stenosis, or cardiovascular disease. Its use for prophylaxis in these conditions cannot be substantiated, and, therefore, the drug should be eliminated from most drug regimens. It may, however, be useful as an adjunct to warfarin therapy in patients with artificial heart valves. Elimination of this drug is justified not only because it can cause headache, dizziness, and central nervous system disturbances at higher doses, but also because it is relatively expensive.

There are a number of reasons to discontinue use of muscle relaxants and antispasmodic drugs such as cyclobenzaprine, orphenadrine, methocarbamol, and carisoprodol. Several of these agents have anticholinergic side effects. In others, the potential central nervous system toxicity of the agent outweighs its potential benefits. Trimethobenzamide should be avoided in older patients because it is less effective than other antiemetic agents, and may cause drowsiness, rash, diarrhea, and extrapyramidal reactions.

Antihypertensive Agents. The elimination of specific antihypertensive agents from the drug houses of older individuals is a highly controversial topic. Most geriatric experts agree that propranolol, methyldopa, reserpine, and verapamil should be avoided in the majority of elderly patients. Propranolol is a lipophilic agent, and, therefore, is more likely to penetrate the central nervous system and cause such symptoms as lethargy, fatigue, and depression. Methyldopa and reserpine also can cause sedation, sexual dysfunction, and mood disturbances. Verapamil should be avoided because of its propensity to produce bradyarrhythmias, AV node conduction disturbances, and myocardial suppression that can sometimes lead to congestive heart failure, especially in the elderly with poor LV function or sinoatrial node disease. Naturally, caution is required when eliminating these medications from a drug regimen.[41,42] Precipitous withdrawal of a beta blocker such as propranolol can precipitate rebound angina; therefore, if discontinuation of one beta blocker is contemplated, substitution with another agent from the same therapeutic class is usually recommended. When antihypertensive medications are withdrawn, it should be gradual and the patient should be monitored closely; if blood pressure rises, new agents may be required.

As a rule, drugs used to treat hypertension are used for appropriate reasons.[44-46] However, because the decision to start antihypertensive therapy has long-term implications, it is prudent to review the original indications for beginning blood pressure-lowering medications. Patients who have normal or subnormal blood pressure recordings on *multiple* clinic visits while taking medication may be candidates for discontinuation of treatment, or reduction of drug dose. An examination of the medical records should attempt to establish that the diagnosis of hypertension was not made on the basis of a single measurement. Patients on monotherapy who are consistently normotensive over a one-year period should have their records reviewed to ensure that their initial elevated blood pressure measurements were confirmed on at least two subsequent visits over a period of several weeks. In addition, patients who were not given a 3- to 6-month trial of nonpharmacologic therapy (i.e., lifestyle changes and modifications known to reduce blood pressure) should: (1) be instructed in a weight reduction program if the patient is overweight; (2) be encouraged to engage in aerobic exercise regularly; and (3) be persuaded to limit alcohol intake. Although discontinuation of antihypertensive medications is oftentimes *not* possible, those patients who are taking a single drug, who are consistently normotensive, and whose records fail to confirm multiple elevated blood pressure measurements at the onset of therapy, constitute the best candidates for discontinuation of blood pressure lowering medications (see Table 7-15).

Bronchodilators. Bronchodilators such as theophylline and terbutaline should be eliminated from the drug regimens of older patients whenever possible. Side effects associated with these agents are increased in the elderly, in whom life-threatening toxicity is not uncommon. In general, inhaled beta agonists and inhaled corticosteroids are preferable to theophylline for the management of bronchospastic pulmonary disease. Finally, elimination of cimetidine and substitution with another H_2 blocker is recommended in all older patients who are taking three or more different prescription ingredients.

Gastrointestinal Agents. Among drugs used to treat gastrointestinal disorders, a careful evaluation of medications such as misoprostol, H_2 blockers, and omeprazole may reveal situations in which these agents were started or continued for inappropriate or questionable reasons. Therapy with misoprostol should be limited to patients who require NSAID therapy and who *also* have a documented history of peptic or gastric ulcer disease. And although omeprazole is a highly effective treatment for erosive esophagitis and peptic ulcer disease, as a rule, this agent should not be used until more conservative, less costly therapy with H_2 blockers is attempted. Finally, the use of H_2 blockers should be limited to short-term therapy for those individuals with suspected peptic ulcer disease. Long-term maintenance therapy is justified only in patients with recurrent disease, as well as those who are at high risk for incurring complications such as gastrointestinal hemorrhage.

Digoxin. Although cardiovascular drugs are important for the management of patients with congestive heart failure, hypertension, and cardiac arrhythmias, a number of medications used for these conditions can be eliminated. Unfortunately, there is still considerable confusion about the role of digoxin therapy in patients with congestive heart failure. Digoxin is a useful agent for patients with left ventricular dysfunction. In fact, numerous trials show that when digoxin is discontinued in patients with mild to moderate congestive heart failure, clinical deterioration is likely. Therefore, patients whose medical records contain diagnostic studies that confirm the presence of left ventricular systolic dysfunction

Table 7-15

DRESC® PROGRAM STRATEGIES FOR ANTIHYPERTENSIVE THERAPY: Indications for treatment, step-down therapy, discontinuation, and lifestyle modifications
Step 1: Ensure that blood pressure requires therapy before initiating pharmacotherapeutic intervention
• Hypertension should *not* be diagnosed on the basis of a single measurement • Blood pressure ≥ 140/90 justifies treatment • Initial elevated readings should be confirmed on at least two subsequent visits during one to several weeks (unless systolic BP > 210 mm Hg and/or diastolic BP > 120 mm Hg, in which case immediate therapy is justified) • When readings are obtained, two or more measurements separated by two minutes should be recorded and averaged. If the first two readings differ by more than 5 mm Hg, additional readings should be obtained.

Table 7-15

DRESC[R] PROGRAM STRATEGIES FOR ANTIHYPERTENSIVE THERAPY: Indications for treatment, step-down therapy, discontinuation, and lifestyle modifications — cont'd.
• Measurements should be taken after 5 minutes at rest, and it is important to ensure that patient has not ingested caffeine, a phenylpropanolamine-containing compound, or smoked cigarettes 30 minutes prior to recording. • Blood pressure characterized by systolic readings in the 130-139 mm Hg range and diastolic blood pressure in the 85-89 mm Hg range should be rechecked in 1 year; systolic readings in the 140-159 mm Hg range and diastolic blood pressure in the 90-99 mm Hg range should be confirmed within 2 months; systolic readings in the 160-179 mm Hg range and diastolic blood pressure in the 100-109 mm Hg range require evaluation and referral to definitive source of care within 1 month. • The presence of target organ disease is an indicate for evaluation, prompt referral, and treatment.
Step 2: Attempt a 3-6 month trial of nonpharmacologic therapy (i.e., in cases of mild to moderate hypertension, vigorously encourage the following lifestyle modifications known to reduce blood pressure)
• Instruct patient in weight reduction program if the patient is overweight • Limit alcohol intake to < 1 oz per day of ethanol (24 oz beer, 8 oz of wine, or 2 oz of 100 proof whiskey) • Aerobic exercise regularly • Reduce sodium intake to < 100 mmol/d (< 2.3 g of sodium or approximately < 6 g of sodium chloride) • Stop smoking • Reduce dietary intake of saturated fat and cholesterol for overall cardiovascular health.
Step 3: If measures outlined under Step 2 above produce inadequate blood pressure control, then lifestyle modifications should continue and pharmacologic therapy should be initiated.
• Initial choice of agent is controversial, but in general, therapy with a beta blocker, diuretic, calcium blocker, ACE inhibitor, or alpha-blocker is recommended (See Table 3-4). The agent should be started at the lowest recommended daily dose. • When cost is the principal barrier to drug acquisition and compliance, therapy with a thiazide diuretic or beta-blocker is appropriate. • If an inadequate response is observed, it is preferable to maintain a single agent at a higher dose level, but only if no side effects are observed at this dose. • If side effects are observed at any dose, substitute another agent or reduce dose of the drug and start additional agent at low dose.

Table 7-15

DRESC® PROGRAM STRATEGIES FOR ANTIHYPERTENSIVE THERAPY: Indications for treatment, step-down therapy, discontinuation, and lifestyle modifications — cont'd.
Step 4: Situations in which automated, noninvasive ambulatory blood pressure monitoring devices may be useful
• "Office" or "white-coat" hypertension (i.e. blood pressure is repeatedly elevated in office or clinic setting but is repeatedly normal in other environments). • Unexplained drug resistance • Unexplained nocturnal blood pressure changes • Episodic hypertension
Step 5: Is ongoing drug therapy still required for hypertension?
• "Step Down" approach is encouraged, which includes elimination of drug or dose reduction if blood pressure is controlled for more than 1 year.

should not have digoxin discontinued from their therapeutic regimen. In addition, patients who require digoxin for ventricular rate control are appropriate for long-term maintenance therapy with digoxin. Occasionally, however, congestive heart failure is overdiagnosed in the outpatient population. If physicians rely *solely* on physical examination and history to diagnose congestive heart failure in the ambulatory patient, approximately 25% of these individuals will be inappropriately treated with digoxin because subsequent echocardiography will reveal normal left ventricular function. It is this overdiagnosis of congestive heart failure that is primarily responsible for the excessive prescribing of digoxin. Therefore, if a careful review of the medical records of a patient who is taking digoxin therapy fails to turn up objective, confirmatory evidence for congestive heart failure, and the patient is in normal sinus rhythm, echocardiography is indicated to evaluate LV function. If LV is normal, discontinuation should be considered.

Antiarrhythmic Agents. Antiarrhythmic agents are generally not indicated for outpatient management of nonlife-threatening ventricular arrhythmias. Even the use of quinidine to maintain patients in normal sinus rhythm after being pharmacologically cardioverted from atrial fibrillation has been seriously questioned. There is now strong evidence to suggest that patients with coronary heart disease and congestive heart failure who once had atrial fibrillation but are now maintained in normal sinus rhythm with quinidine, have twice the mortality rate as patients who remain in atrial fibrillation and have their ventricular rates controlled with digoxin alone. Therefore, physicians and pharmacists should review the original reasons for initiating quinidine therapy. If medical records indicate that quinidine was started to maintain normal sinus rhythm after atrial fibrillation, careful consideration should be given to discontinuing the drug, observing the patient for recurrence of the arrhythmia, and, if ventricular rate problems emerge, treating them with AV node blocking agents such as digoxin.

Drugs with Duration Limits

One of the principal objectives of the DRESC program is to screen for drugs that can be eliminated because they are being used beyond their established *duration limits.* There are many reasons that drugs are not withdrawn from a drug regimen even though they no longer serve a useful purpose. Often, the patient will continue to fill the prescription because he or she is not aware that the medication has duration limits. In other cases, physicians maintain individuals on drugs as a preventive measure, even though continued therapy with the drug is not strictly indicated. Sometimes patients are lost to follow-up and continue filling the prescription, assuming that this is what their physician would have recommended. Those drug classes which require evaluation regarding duration of use include the following: H_2-blockers, proton pump blockers, antiseizure medications, anxiolytics, antidementia medications, antidepressants, and analgesics.

Antidementia Therapy. Constructing drug houses that are fit for individuals who suffer from chronic dementia is one of the most important challenges facing American physicians and pharmacists.[43,50] Alzheimer's disease is the most common cause of chronic dementia, affecting approximately 2.5 million people older than 65 years of age in the United States and Canada. Not surprisingly, the pressures to pharmacologically manage behavioral disturbances, cognitive dysfunction, and memory loss associated with this devastating illness are intense. Patients may require significant levels of care, and intensive pharmacotherapy for many years, resulting in a tremendous toll for patients, family, and society as a whole. Aggressive pharmacologic management with antipsychotic medications such as haloperidol and prochlorperazine, as well as anxiolytics, has been the mainstay of drug therapy for many years.[17,39]

HIV Infection. Decisions regarding discontinuation of medications in patients with HIV infection presents a particularly vexing and difficult clinical problem. Most of these patients require polypharmacy, both for the purpose of antiretroviral therapy, and as preventive therapy for a number of opportunistic infections. It is not uncommon for a patient with advanced HIV infection to tolerate a drug house consisting of trimethoprim/sulfamethoxazole, pentamidine isethionate, fluconazole, clarithromycin, and one of a number of antiretroviral agents, including protease inhibitors, zidovudine, didanosine, or zalcitabine. Discontinuation of medications used for prophylaxis and antiretroviral therapy is not recommended. Unfortunately, however, a large percentage of patients with AIDS develop toxicity from their medication regimens and discontinuation of drugs becomes absolutely necessary. The decision to discontinue a drug is always based on laboratory parameters, the patient's previous clinical course, and symptomatic complaints related to pharmacotherapy. (See Tables 7-16 through 7-18 for dosages and adverse effects requiring possible discontinuation for drugs used to treat HIV disease).

Table 7-16

Dosages and Adverse Effects of Medications Used For PCP Prophylaxis

Medication	Dosage Adult/Tanner stage IV and V Adolescents[3]	Dosage Infants/children/ Tanner stage I and II adolescents	Adverse Effects
Trimethoprim-Sulfamethoxazole (TMP-SMZ) Bactrim® Septra® Formulations: Single-strength tablet: 80 mg TMP 400 mg SMZ Double-strength tablet: 160 mg TMP 800 mg SMZ Pediatric suspension: (per 5 ml) 40 mg TMP 200 mg SMZ	Most commonly used regimens: one double-strength tablet taken orally three times per week on alternate days or daily 7 days per week.	150 mg/m² TMP 750 mg/m² SMZ Total oral daily dose given 3 times/week Can be divided into two doses or administered as a single daily dose and given on 3 consecutive days or 3 alternate days per week This same oral daily dose divided into 2 doses can be given 7 days per week	Drug allergy: Skin rash Stevens-Johnson syndrome Fever Arthralgia Toxic epidermal necrolysis Hematologic: Anemia Neutropenia Thrombocytopenia Gastrointestinal: Elevation of serum transaminase Nausea Vomiting Anorexia Fulminant hepatic necrosis (rare)

Table 7-16

Dosages and Adverse Effects of Medications Used For PCP Prophylaxis — cont'd.

Medication	Dosage Adult/Tanner stage IV and V Adolescents[3]	Dosage Infants/children/ Tanner stage I and II adolescents	Adverse Effects
Pentamidine Isethionate NebuPent® 300 mg The vial must be dissolved in 6 ml sterile water and used with Respirguard® nebulizer	Aerosolized pentamidine (AP) (NebuPent®) is given as single 300 mg (one vial) dose every 4 weeks. Nebulized dose given over 30-45 min at a flow rate of 5-9 liters/min from a 40-50 lb per square inch air or oxygen source Alternative: If a Fisons ultrasonic nebulizer is used, dose of pentamidine is 60 mg given every 2 weeks after a loading dose of five treatments given over 2 weeks	Children over 5 yr can receive same inhalation dose as adults	Pulmonary: Bronchospasm with cough Pneumothorax Other: Extrapulmonary *P. carinii* infection Increased risk of environmental transmission of *M. tuberculosis*

Table 7-16

Dosages and Adverse Effects of Medications Used For PCP Prophylaxis — cont'd.			
Medication	**Dosage Adult/Tanner stage IV and V Adolescents[3]**	**Dosage Infants/children/ Tanner stage I and II adolescents**	**Adverse Effects**
Dapsone Formulation: 25 and 100 mg tablets	50-100 mg total daily dose divided into two doses or administered as a single daily dose given 2-7 times per week daily dose given 7 days per week	1 mg/kg administered orally as a single daily dose given 7 days per week	Hematologic: Agranulocytosis Aplastic anemia Hemolytic anemia in G6PD deficiency Methemoglobinemia Cutaneous reactions: Bullous and exfoliative dermatitis Erythema nodosum Erythema multiform Peripheral neuropathy Gastrointestinal: Nausea Vomiting

Table 7-17

Dosages and Adverse Effects Requiring Possible Discontinuation of Antiretroviral Drugs Used in HIV Infection			
Medication	**Dosage Adult/Tanner Stage IV and V adolescents**	**Dosage Infants/children/Tanner stage I and II adolescents**	**Adverse effects**
Zidovudine (ZDV) formerly azidothymidine (AZT) Retrovir® Formulation: 100 mg capsules Pediatric syrup 50 mg/5 ml	100 mg/dose administered orally every 4 hours or 5 doses given 7 days/week	180 mg/m^2 dose administered orally every 6 hours given 7 days/week	Granulocytopenia Anemia Nausea Headache Confusion Myositis Anorexia Hepatitis Seizures Nail discoloration
Protease Inhibitors	As directed	As directed	Drug interactions GI complaints Nausea Fatigue Insomnia

Table 7-17

Dosages and Adverse Effects Requiring Possible Discontinuation of Antiretroviral Drugs Used in HIV Infection — cont'd.

Medication	Dosage Adult/Tanner Stage IV and V adolescents	Dosage Infants/children/Tanner stage I and II adolescents	Adverse effects
Didanosine (ddI) (dideoxyinosine) Videx® Formulation: 25, 50, 100, 150 mg tablets Pediatric powder for oral solution 10 mg/ml	Patients under 45 kg: 100 mg/dose orally given every 12 hours 7 days/week Patients over 45 kg: 200 mg/dose administered orally every 12 hours given 7 days/week (Tablet should be chewed and taken on an empty stomach)	200 $mg/m^2/day$ administered orally every 12 hours given 7 days per week	Pancreatitis, potentially fatal Peripheral neuropathy Peripheral retinal atrophy (in children only) Nausea Diarrhea Confusion Seizures
Zalcitabine (ddC) (dideoxycitidine) Formulation: 0.375 mg tablets 0.750 mg tablets Pediatric 0.1 mg/ml syrup	Patients under 45 kg: 0.375 mg/dose administered orally every 8 hours given 7 days/week Patients over 45 kg: 0.750 mg dose administered orally every 8 hours given 7 days/week	0.005-0.01 mg/kg/dose administered orally every 8 hours given 7 days/week	Aphthous ulcers Esophageal ulcers Peripheral neuropathy Stomatitis Cutaneous eruptions Thrombocytopenia Pancreatitis

Table 7-18

Dosages and Adverse Effects Requiring Possible Discontinuation For Antimycobacterial Drugs Used in HIV Infection

Medication	Dosage Adult/Tanner stage IV and V adolescents	Dosage Infants/children/Tanner stage I and II adolescents	Adverse Effects
Isoniazid INHR Nydrazid® Formulation: 50 mg, 100 mg, 300 mg tablets 1 gram vial Syrup 50 mg/5 ml	300 mg administered orally as a single daily dose given 7 days/wk for 12 mo or 900 mg administered orally as a single daily dose given 2 days/week for 12 mo	10-15 mg/kg/day (max 300 mg/day) administered orally as a single daily dose given 7 days/wk for 12 mo	Gastrointestinal: Hepatotoxicity (rare in children) Nausea, vomiting, anorexia Neurologic: Peripheral neuropathy Neuritis, fatigue Weakness

Table 7-18

Dosages and Adverse Effects Requiring Possible Discontinuation For Antimycobacterial Drugs Used in HIV Infection — cont'd.

Medication	Dosage Adult/Tanner stage IV and V adolescents	Dosage Infants/children/Tanner stage I and II adolescents	Adverse Effects
Isoniazid (cont'd)			Hematologic: Agranulocytosis Hemolytic and aplastic anemia Thrombocytopenia Eosinophilia Drug allergy: Skin rash Fever Lymphadenopathy and vasculitis (SLE-like syndrome)

REDUCTION OF DRUG DOSE

Screening drug houses for opportunities to lower drug dosage is one of the most important guiding principles of the DRESC program. It is staggering to think how many medications are used today at far lower doses than they were in the past, without any compromise in clinical efficacy. In fact, a number of medications are presently used at doses far lower than originally recommended and are more *effective* at these lower doses because they are associated with fewer side effects. For example, when the anxiolytic triazolam was introduced into the market, the manufacturer recommended using this medication at a dose of about 0.5 mg at night for sleep. After sufficient clinical experience with the drug, it became clear that doses of this magnitude, especially in the elderly, could produce a number of undesirable side effects, including memory loss, confusion, and disorientation. When dosage recommendations were lowered to 0.125 mg, the safety and side effect profile of the drug improved considerably, and the drug maintained its therapeutic efficacy for management of sleep disorders and anxiety-related conditions.

Anticoagulants. Unfortunately, despite rigorous FDA mandates governing clinical trials of new pharmaceuticals, some drugs are still introduced into the market at doses that exceed what is necessary to produce excellent clinical outcomes. For example, there was a time when physicians and pharmacists believed that to achieve adequate thromboembolic prophylaxis in patients with venous occlusive disease, stroke, and atrial fibrillation, that warfarin doses producing prothrombin times that were 2 to 2.5 times the control value were needed for clinical efficacy. Subsequently, we have learned that equally effective outcomes are obtained when warfarin is dosed to achieve prothrombin times that are 1.3 to 1.5 times the control value. In the process of reducing the drug's dose, therapeutic efficacy is maintained, but the risk of hemorrhagic complications is reduced.

H_2 Blockers. When cimetidine, the first H_2 blocker approved for use in the management of peptic ulcer disease, was introduced into the market, daily doses as high as 1,600 mg to 2,000 mg were advocated for routine clinical management of acute or recurrent peptic disease. These levels were associated with a significant incidence of central nervous system toxicity including confusion, that frequently necessitated discontinuation of the medication. Subsequent experience demonstrated that doses as low as 400 mg were sufficient for achieving desired therapeutic objectives, such as ulcer healing and symptomatic relief. Hence, it is important to ensure that the lowest acceptable doses are prescribed.

Cardiovascular Drugs. Some of the most dramatic effects of lowering medication dosage are observed with drugs used to treat hypertension. For example, when ACE inhibitors were first introduced, captopril doses as high as 25 mg to 50 mg three times daily were recommended for treatment of hypertension. A significant minority of patients developed acute renal dysfunction. Subsequent experience with this drug demonstrated that far lower doses (ie, 12.5 mg of captopril t.i.d.) could achieve the desired antihypertensive effects with a much lower risk of renal toxicity. Recent studies suggest that dose reduction is especially important for thiazide diuretics. As recently as 10 years ago, it was not uncommon for patients to be treated with hydrochlorothiazide doses in the range of 100 to 150 mg per day. Although these dosages were clearly effective in lowering blood pressure and treating symptoms of congestive heart failure, they were also associated with a number of side effects, ranging from hypokalemia and other electrolyte disturbances to hypercholesterolemia and, in some patient subgroups, sudden death.

In fact, recent trials using high dose thiazide diuretics in patients with coronary heart disease and hypertension have revealed an unexpected, dose-related increase in rates of cardiac sudden death. In the high-dose (100 mg thiazide/day) group the risk of sudden cardiac death negated more than 50% of the expected cardiovascular benefit from improved blood pressure control. The suspected thiazide-related precipitants of cardiac arrest have included reductions in serum potassium and magnesium. In particular, the study was designed to assess the relationship between thiazide treatment for hypertension and occurrence of primary cardiac arrest; a dose-response relationship between thiazide dose and risk of primary cardiac sudden death was confirmed. Compared to low-dose thiazide therapy (25 mg/day), high-dose therapy (100 mg/day) was associated with the greatest risk of sudden death. For intermediate-dose thiazide therapy (50 mg/day), the risk of sudden death compared to low dose therapy was still elevated, but less so. Patients prescribed a potassium-sparing diuretic in conjunction with thiazide treatment manifested a reduction in risk for cardiac death. Similarly, adding a potassium-sparing agent to preexisting thiazide therapy also reduced the risk of sudden death. Potassium supplementation, however, did little to reduce the risk.

This study demonstrates the importance of DRESC program strategies aimed at evaluating dosage levels of commonly prescribed medications such as thiazide diuretics. When appropriate, initial therapy for hypertension should begin with a low-dose thiazide diuretic, (ie, 12.5 to 25 mg per day). If higher thiazide doses are required (50 to 100 mg/day), consideration should be given to adding a potassium-sparing diuretic to the program or switching to another agent.

Other Drugs. The wisdom of using lower doses has been confirmed for a number of other medications, including heparin, beta agonists, misoprostol, antidepressants, levothyroxine, and NSAIDs (see Table 7-19).

Table 7-19

Reduction of Drug Dose: Medications That May Be Effective At Lower Doses Than Originally Prescribed	
• Aspirin	• Cimetidine
• Triazolam	• Misoprostol
• Warfarin	• Heterocyclic antidepressants
• Heparin	• H2 Blockers
• Hydrochlorothiazide	• NSAIDs
• Beta-agonists	• Synthroid
• Estrogen (ie, in birth control pills)	• Digoxin
	• AZT
• ACE Inhibitors	• SSRIs

As discussed earlier, the risk of producing gastrointestinal toxicity with aspirin and NSAIDs is dose-related, and therefore, it is imperative that regimens be reviewed to confirm that these medications are prescribed at the *lowest* effective maintenance dosage. Given the widespread use of antidepressants, ascertaining the appropriate dosage for this drug class presents a particularly difficult problem. Although many patients require maximal doses, it is reasonable to consider dosage reduction in patients who have stabilized clinically for a minimum of 12 months, and who report adverse side effects.

DRESC program strategies aimed at dosage reduction are designed not only to produce less expensive therapeutic regimens, but to improve the overall side effect profile of the drug regimen. In general, adverse side effects are a function of drug dose. Consequently, when a review of the regimen uncovers medications that are being used at the maximal dosage, the possibility that patient symptoms or complaints might reflect drug-induced side effects should be strongly considered. Because side effects tend to be dose related, it is frequently difficult to decide which is preferable: to maintain a patient on a high dose of a *single* agent, or to prescribe *two* medications, each of which is given at the lowest recommended dose. The latter approach has the benefit of producing excellent clinical results using medications that are dosed in a range that is unlikely to produce bothersome side effects. On the other hand, converting a patient from monotherapy to two-drug therapy may involve increasing the cost of the therapeutic regimen. Another option is to replace one drug class with another. In the end, the decision to use a single agent at a maximal dose versus two drugs, each of which is prescribed at a very low dose, depends on a number of factors including side effect profiles, cost issues, and medication compliance patterns. It should be emphasized that patients are just as likely to comply with a drug therapy program if they are taking two different medications once each day as they would on a regimen consisting of only one drug given once daily.

SIMPLIFICATION OF DRUG REGIMENS

Simplifying the drug regimen is a DRESC program strategy designed to prevent and treat noncompliance, as well as reduce the risks of drug interactions. To implement these changes, physicians and pharmacists should examine each regimen and make sure that it represents the safest, simplest and most effective therapy available. Every effort should be made to simplify scheduling. When appropriate, medications with a long half-life that can be given on a once daily basis will offer significant advantages over drugs dosed three or four times daily. When several once-daily medications can be taken simultaneously, at the same time of day, compliance will be enhanced. Medications that require special precautions (ie, food intake) should be avoided, if possible. In general, the total number of pills consumed on a daily basis should be kept to a minimum (see Table 7-20).

Universal Compliance Precautions. Measures aimed at simplifying the drug regimen are part of a DRESC program strategy called Universal Compliance Precautions (UCP™). UCPs are necessary because studies show that physicians and pharmacists are very poor at predicting which patients will take their medications as prescribed.[20,33] Consequently, the most prudent approach for ensuring medication compliance is simply to assume that all patients are noncompliant, and to implement UCP. The most important features of Universal Compliance Precautions include: (1) once-daily dosing; (2) short duration therapies; (3) one-dose therapy (if available); (4) patient education; (5) selecting medications with tolerable side effects; and (6) providing follow-up to ensure medications are taken as prescribed (see Table 7-21).

Table 7-20

Opportunities and Strategies For Simplifying Drug Regimens
• Reduce the total number of pills consumed on a daily basis
• Attempt to construct regimen using once-daily medications consumed simultaneously at the same time of day
• Decrease daily dose frequency of medication
• Avoid medications that require special precautions (ie, food intake considerations)
• Avoid medications with complex dosing schedules
• Avoid medications that are known to produce drug interactions

Table 7-21

Universal Compliance Precautions UCP®	
• Once daily dosing	• Patient education
• Short duration therapy	• Tolerable side effect profile
• One-dose therapy (if available)	• Follow-up

Once-Daily Therapy. As might be expected, identifying once-daily medications with proven clinical effectiveness is an important objective of the DRESC program. The DRESC program generally advocates once-daily medications, *except* when side effects produced by a long half-life are likely to cause complications that require prolonged management until drug levels return to normal limits. For example, the use of once-daily verapamil is not recommended in older patients with conduction disturbances caused by cardiovascular disease, because if the drug happens to produce symptomatic or life-threatening bradycardia, intensive monitoring and management may be required for up to 24 hours. On the other hand, there is no particular advantage to using a short-acting NSAID dosed four times a day, as opposed to a long half-life NSAID, which is dosed once daily, because if either drug results in a gastrointestinal hemorrhage, the treatment is the same and independent of the half-life of the medication.

Within each drug class, some once-daily preparations appear to offer more advantages than others (see Table 7-5). Among the sulfonylureas, chlorpropamide should be avoided because of its long half-life. Oral hypoglycemics such as glipizide and glyburide offer 24-hour effectiveness and fewer side effects than are seen with chlorpropamide. Metformin and Rezulin also offer 24-hour control. All H_2 blockers are equally effective, but famotidine and nizatidine may have a lower risk of drug interactions. Among the beta blockers, hydrophilic agents such as atenolol generally are preferable to drugs that penetrate the central nervous system, such as propranolol. Among the calcium channel blockers, amlodipine is useful for the management of both angina and hypertension. In patients who have underlying congestive heart failure, amlodipine may be preferable because it does not cause clinically significant suppression of myocardial pump function. Once-daily ACE inhibitors are useful for the management of hypertension, congestive heart failure, and for preventing progression of diabetic renal disease.

Selection of a once-daily antidepressant presents a unique clinical challenge. The primary care physician now has five distinct classes of antidepressant medications that may be used for treating depression, including tricyclic antidepressants (TCAs); monoamine oxidase inhibitor (MAOIs); SSRIs (e.g., fluoxetine, sertraline, and paroxetine); aminoketones (bupropion); and triazolopyridines (trazodone). Although all these medications are effective antidepressants, recent studies suggest that the SSRI drug class may be the best for treating elderly depressed patients and for those in whom maintenance of work and psychomotor function are important considerations. In particular, the SSRIs have a broad range of antidepressant activity, a wide therapeutic index, and are free of many of the adverse effects associated with other antidepressants, such as cardiovascular toxicity, orthostatic hypotension, and sedation.

In addition to once-daily medications, the DRESC program also encourages the use of one-dose/short-duration therapies as part of its simplification strategy. The rationale for using one-dose/short-duration therapies is supported by a large number of studies that show noncompliance-mediated therapeutic failures are not only a problem for long-term management of chronic conditions, but also short-term therapy. A number of one-dose therapies are now available for treating many common infections (see Table 7-6).

Simplification of drug regimens takes many forms, from once-daily dosing and reduction of daily pill consumption, to implementation of UCP and use of one-dose therapies. It should be stressed that simplification strategies are useful for both long-term and short-term drug regimens. Finally, identifying once-daily medications which are best suited to a particular patient is a process that takes into account a number of factors, including cost of the medication, side effect profile, and the risk for drug interactions (see Chapter 3).

CONSOLIDATION OF DRUG REGIMENS

From a pharmatectural perspective, consolidating therapeutic regimens is an essential strategy for minimizing medications in order to maximize results. Fortunately, there are many opportunities for treating multiple conditions, symptoms, and disease states with a single active prescription ingredient (see Table 7-4). In general, opportunities for implementing consolidation strategies are most easily recognized by listing all the patient's conditions, abnormal laboratory values, target goals, and symptoms on one side of the page, and then trying to match this list with the fewest number of drugs possible to treat these clinical abnormalities.

Consolidating therapeutic regimens will be facilitated by gaining familiarity with those drugs that have established indications for treating *more than one* clinical disorder. For example, the elderly patient who has systolic hypertension and angina is most appropriately treated with a calcium channel blocker such as amlodipine. On the other hand, for younger patients who have recurrent episodes of supraventricular tachycardia and hypertension, the calcium channel blocker verapamil has the advantage of both lowering blood pressure and being useful for the prevention of supraventricular tachyarrhythmia. When hypertension must be treated in a patient who also requires secondary prevention of myocardial infarction, a beta blocker such as atenolol is a reasonable choice. However, when hypertension is encountered along with congestive heart failure or diabetes with microalbuminuria, an ACE inhibitor such as captopril, enalapril, or lisinopril is most appropriate for consolidating the drug regimen.

A significant percentage of diabetic patients who have hypertension also have clinically important elevations in their serum cholesterol *and* triglyceride levels. In these situations, an HMG Co-A reductase inhibitor such as atorvastatin has the advantages of lowering both serum LDL cholesterol and triglyceride levels. Similarly, older patients who have high blood pressure *and* obstructive symptoms of benign prostatic hypertrophy can benefit from the use of a peripheral alpha blocker such as doxazosin. The postmenopausal woman who requires prophylaxis against cardiovascular disease, osteoporosis prevention, and amelioration of postmenopausal symptoms is best managed with estrogen replacement therapy. In the case of neuropsychiatric disorders, the combination symptom complex of anxiety associated with panic attacks and depression, is best managed with an SSRI such as sertraline, whereas treatment of diabetic mononeuropathy and depression can be consolidated by using a tricyclic antidepressant. Managing symptoms of CHF and rapid ventricular rate associated with atrial fibrillation is consolidated with digoxin therapy, whereas a thiazide diuretic may be helpful for ameliorating symptoms of CHF in a patient who is also hypertensive.

Although attempts at consolidating drug therapy are an important part of the DRESC program, it should be emphasized that streamlining drug regimens is not always successful. Some patients, especially those with severe or longstanding disease, may simply *require* two or three different prescription ingredients to manage their constellation of clinical disorders. However, in the majority of cases in which a drug has approved indications for managing more than one condition, consolidation strategies that match single drugs to multiple clinical abnormalities or symptoms will be successful. Consolidation strategies are most likely to succeed if withdrawal symptoms are prevented, if medications are tapered within accepted duration limits, and if the patient becomes an active participant in the streamlining process. Finally, when replacing two, three, or more medications with a single drug, it may be necessary to introduce the consolidating agent at its mid-dosage range. In other words, it is sometimes necessary to use monotherapeutic regimens at higher doses to achieve the same therapeutic goals that were previously maintained by two or more drugs. When this is the case, the physician or pharmacist will have to weigh the potential disadvantages of possible side effects that are incurred at higher dosage ranges against the potential advantages of a simplified and consolidated drug regimen. The final decision is best made through a collaborative process that includes patient, physician, and pharmacist.

DRESC PROGRAM DRUG SURVEILLANCE

Screening for and identifying patient candidates who are appropriate for the DRESC program requires a meticulous review of the safety of pharmacologic building blocks that constitute the patient's regimen. A number of risk factors, demographic characteristics, and clinical conditions have been highlighted that suggest drug streamlining will be of benefit. Patients on polypharmacy, the elderly, individuals who are receiving medications from more than three physicians, and drug regimens consisting primarily of generic medications are just some of the risk factors that should prompt physicians and pharmacists to evaluate the safety and effectiveness of the therapeutic regimen. Perhaps no risk factor is more important than the presence of medications that are known to cause drug interactions (see Tables 7-22 and 7-23).

Table 7-22

Drugs That May Cause Drug-Drug Interactions in Patients On Polypharmacy	
• Warfarin	• Propulsid
• Cimetidine	• Erythromycin
• Fluoxetine	• Verapamil
• Statins	• Ketoconazole

For example, drugs known to inhibit the P450 cytochrome oxidase system, among them cimetidine, fluoxetine, and erythromycin, should at least raise a red flag in patients who are on polypharmacy. When one or more anticholinergic agents are in a single regimen, careful evaluation should be made for anticholinergic signs and symptoms. Anticholinergic drugs that are frequently encountered in the *treatment plans* of older individuals include tricyclic antidepressants, scopolamine-containing anti-diarrheal agents, antihistamines such as diphenhydramine, muscle relaxants, antiparkinsonian drugs, and antipsychotic agents such as phenothiazines. Sedative hypnotics in the benzodiazepine class can produce sedation, drowsiness, memory disturbance, and confusion in both younger and older patients. If patients on long-term benzodiazepine therapy have agitation, diaphoresis, or dehydration, the physician or pharmacist should consider the possibility of withdrawal syndrome.

Among cardiovascular agents, the calcium channel blockers verapamil and diltiazem can, in susceptible individuals—those with CHF or brady-tachy syndrome—cause bradycardia, AV node conduction inhibition, myocardial suppression, constipation, and congestive heart failure. It should be stressed that some of the adverse effects of these calcium channel blockers may be potentiated by concurrent use of high doses of beta blockers. Special vigilance is required when using these agents, especially in older patients with underlying cardiovascular disease characterized by conduction disturbances or congestive heart failure. When beta blockers are in a therapeutic regimen, the history should focus on symptoms related to depression, fatigue, sexual dysfunction, or sleep disturbances. ACE inhibitors, which are frequently used in diabetic patients with hypertension, produce cough that is serious enough to prompt discontinuation of this drug in up to 15% of all patients. ACE inhibitor-induced cough is more likely to occur in elderly females with hypertension. Not infrequently, it may be difficult to distinguish between ACE inhibitor-induced cough, and coughing symptoms that reflect progression of underlying disease. Consequently, cigarette smokers, and patients with asthma, chronic obstructive pulmonary disease, or occupational lung disease may not be ideal candidates for ACE inhibitor therapy because it may be difficult to distinguish between drug-induced cough and disease-induced cough. Nevertheless, when there are strong indications for the use of ACE inhibitors, the drug should not be denied to those patients who need them, even if they have underlying conditions known to cause cough. The use of angiotensin receptor blockers (ARBs) such as losartan is advisable in hypertensive patients who are unable to tolerate ACE inhibitors because of cough. Although *long-term* survival studies confirming efficacy of ARBs for prolonging survival in patients with CHF are not yet available, short-term studies comparing losartan to captopril suggest this ARB reduces the number of exacerbations of CHF and need for hospitalization to the same degree as the ACE inhibitor.

The presence of NSAIDs, corticosteroids, and aspirin could cause gastrointestinal side effects. In addition to producing gastric erosions and ulceration, NSAIDs also can produce renal deterioration, hyperkalemia, and azotemia. These adverse effects are potentiated by concurrent thiazide use and by the presence of renal disease, coronary artery disease, or diabetes. When corticosteroids are added to a regimen consisting of nonsteroidal drugs, the risk of GI tract hemorrhage is increased by fourfold. As a result, NSAIDs and corticosteroids should not be used concurrently unless absolutely indicated.

The presence of any antihypertensive drug in a patient's drug house should prompt the physician or pharmacist to look for symptoms of sexual dysfunction.[53-56] Not surprisingly, many patients are reluctant to complain about sexual function, unless asked directly. Virtually all antihypertensive drugs are associated with sexual dysfunction (see Figure 7-6), and, therefore, when any of these agents are encountered in the patient's drug house, a careful sexual history is mandatory. Spironolactone, alpha methyldopa, clonidine, and propranolol are among those most likely to cause sexual problems. In general, the calcium channel blockers, ACE inhibitors, and peripheral alpha blockers are relatively preserving of sexual function.

Table 7-23

DRESC® PROGRAM DRUG SURVEILLANCE	
Drug or Drug Class	**Monitor Patient For Side Effects/Drug Interactions**
NSAIDS	
	Gastrointestinal hemorrhage, gastritis, renal deterioration, hyperkalemia, azotemia. Adverse effects potentiated by concurrent thiazide use and presence of renal disease, coronary artery disease, or diabetes.
CORTICOSTEROIDS	
	Psychosis, confusion, fluid retention, osteoporosis, hyperglycemia, GI hemorrhage (especially when used in combination with NSAIDs or aspirin)

Table 7-23

DRESC® PROGRAM DRUG SURVEILLANCE — cont'd.	
Drug or Drug Class	**Monitor Patient For Side Effects/Drug Interactions**
DIGOXIN	
	Nausea, visual disturbances, conduction disturbances, arrhythmias. Blood levels increased by quinidine and some calcium channel blockers.
CALCIUM CHANNEL BLOCKERS	
Verapamil Diltiazem	These calcium blockers can cause bradycardia, AV node conduction inhibition, myocardial suppression, constipation, and congestive heart failure in vulnerable individuals. Adverse effects are potentiated by concomitant use of high doses of beta-blockers, especially in older patients with underlying cardiovascular disease (ie, conduction disturbances, CHF).
BETA-BLOCKERS	
Propranolol Atenolol Metoprolol Acebutolol	May produce depression, fatigue, sexual dysfunction, and sleep disturbances. When used in high doses in combination with calcium blockers such as verapamil or diltiazem, beta-blockers may produce bradycardia, AV node blocker, myocardial suppression, or congestive heart failure, especially in susceptible elderly individuals.
ANTIDEPRESSANTS	
Tricyclics Heterocyclics	Anticholinergic side effects, including dry mouth, visual disturbance, orthostatic hypotension, urinary retention, low-grade fever, and disorientation can result from such agents as amitriptyline, doxepin, nortriptyline, etc. These effects can be potentiated by concomitant use of other drugs with anticholinergic properties, including diphenhydramine, muscle relaxants, antipsychotics (phenothiazines), and scopolamine-containing antidiarrheal agents.

Table 7-23

DRESC[R] PROGRAM DRUG SURVEILLANCE — cont'd.	
Drug or Drug Class	**Monitor Patient For Side Effects/Drug Interactions**
ANTIPSYCHOTICS	
	Phenothiazines are noted for their anticholinergic side effects, whereas haloperidol-like agents are more likely to cause tardive dyskinesia. Both classes can cause CNS sedation and other mental status changes.
ANTICHOLINERGIC MEDICATIONS	
Tricyclic antidepressants Scopolamine Diphenhydramine Muscle relaxants Phenothiazines	When one or more of these agents is in a single regimen, careful evaluation should be made for anticholinergic signs and symptoms (i.e., dry mouth, confusion, excessive sedation, orthostatic hypotension, urinary retention, etc.)
SEDATIVE HYPNOTICS	
	Sedation, drowsiness, memory disturbance, and confusion can be seen in both younger and older patients. Long-acting agents (diazepam, flurazepam, and chlordiazepoxide) are to be avoided in older patients, because there is an increased risk of falling, daytime sleepliness, and hip fractures associated with their use. If patient on long-term benzodiazepine therapy presents with agitation, diaphoresis, and dehydration, consider withdrawal syndrome.
CIMETIDINE	
	This drug is an inhibitor of the P450 cytochrome oxidase system and, therefore, can potentially elevate the blood levels of a number of commonly used medications including: theophylline, warfarin, narcotics, antidepressants, beta-blockers, verapamil, and many others.

Table 7-23

DRESC® PROGRAM DRUG SURVEILLANCE — cont'd.	
Drug or Drug Class	**Monitor Patient For Side Effects/Drug Interactions**
ERYTHROMYCIN/CLARITHROMYCIN	
	Theophylline levels can be elevated and, therefore, careful monitoring of drug levels during concurrent administration is advisable. Erythromycin and clarithromycin should not be used in conjunction with such nonsedating antihistamines as astemizole, because cardiac arrhythmias may result. Erythromycin can produce clinically important elevations in carbamazepine (*Tegretol®*) blood levels.
KETOCONAZOLE	
	Potentiates cyclosporine renal toxicity; can cause cardiac arrhythmias in combination with certain nonsedating antihistamines (astemizole), and potentiate quinidine toxicity.
QUINIDINE	
	May potentiate toxic effects of digoxin, amiodarone, beta-adrenergic blockers (including ophthalmic medications), procainamide, and others.
THEOPHYLLINES	
	Toxic levels of theophylline can produce gastrointestinal upset, seizures, cardiac arrhythmias, and mental status changes. Their action is potentiated by concurrent use with erythromycin, cimetidine, fluoroquinolones, neuromuscular blocking agents, thiabendazole, and other agents.

SUMMARY

The three main objectives of the DRESC program are to be simple, to be safe, and to be certain. In most patients taking multiple medications, a meticulous review of the drug regimen and a thorough history that includes the patient's social, cognitive, and sexual well-being will usually uncover opportunities for making alterations that will enhance medication compliance, reduce the risk of adverse drug interactions, improve quality of life, and in many circumstances, reduce the total cost of the therapeutic regimen.

[1]Ahronheim J. Practical pharmacology for older patients; avoiding adverse drug effects. Mt Sinai J Med 1993 Nov;60(6):497-501.

[2]Bailey RA, Ashcraft NA. Pharmacist-physician drug fair for educating physicians in cost-effective prescribing. Am J Hosp Pharm 1993 Oct;50(10):2088-9.

[3]Jolicoeur LM, Jones-Grizzle AJ, Boyer JG. Guidelines for performing a pharmacoeconomic analysis. Am J Hosp Pharm 1992 July;49(7):1741-7.

[4]Bulpitt CJ, Fletcher AE. Drug treatment and quality of life in the elderly [Review]. Clin Geriatr Med 1990 May;6(2):309-17.

[5]Coons SJ, Kaplan RM. Assessing health-related quality of life: application to drug therapy. Clin Ther 1992;14(6):850-8; discussion 849.

[6]Fletcher AE, Battersby C, Adnitt P, Underwood N, Jurgensen HJ, Bulpitt CJ. Quality of life on antihypertensive therapy: a double-blind trial comparing quality of life on pinacidil and nifedipine in combination with a thiazide diuretic. European Pinacidil Study Group. J Cardiovasc Pharmacol 1992 July;20(1):108-14.

[7]Limouzin-Lamothe MA, Mairon N, Joyce CR, Le Gal M. Quality of life after the menopause; influence of hormonal replacement therapy. Am J Obstet Gynecol 1994 Feb;170(2):618-24.

[8]Wiklund I, Karlberg J, Mattsson LA. Quality of life of postmenopausal women on a regimen of transdermal estradiol therapy; a double-blind placebo-controlled study. Am J Obstet Gynecol 1993 Mar;168(3 Pt 1):824-30.

[9]deBoer JB, van Dam FS, Sprangers MA, Frissen PH, Lange JM. Longitudinal study on the quality of life of symptomatic HIV-infected patients in a trial of zidovudine versus zidovudine and interferon-alpha. AIDS 1993 July;7(7):947-53.

[10]LeMay P. Quality of life—measuring outcomes of pharmaceutical management. Summary of workshop proceedings. Can J Public Health 1992 May-June;83(3):S5-16.

[11]Hallas J, Harvald B, Worm J, Beck-Nielsen J, Gram LF, Grodum E, Damsbo N, Schou J, Kromann-Andersen H, Frolund F. Drug related hospital admissions. Results from an intervention program. Eur J Clin Pharmacol 1993;45(3):199-203.

[12]Hallas J, Worm J, Beck-Nielsen J, Gram LF, Grodum E, Damsbo N, Brosen K. Drug related events and drug utilization in patients admitted to a geriatric hospital department. Dan Med Bull 1991 Oct;38(5):417-20.

[13]Lamy P. Adverse drug effects [Review]. Clin Geriatr Med 1990 May;6(2):293-307.

[14]De Geest S, Abraham I, Gemoets H, Evers G. Development of the long-term medication behavior self-efficacy scale: qualitative study for item development. J Adv Nurs 1994 Feb;19(2):233-8.

[15]Mawhinney H, Spector SL, Heitjan D, Kinsman RA, Dirks JF, Pines I. As-needed medication use in asthma usage patterns and patient characteristics. J Asthma 1993;30(1):61-71.

[16]Opdycke RA, Ascione FJ, Shimp LA, Rosen RI. A systematic approach to educating elderly patients about their medications. Pat Ed Coun 1992 Feb;19(1):43-60.

[17]Carlyle W, Ancill RJ, Sheldon L. Aggression in the demented patient: a double-blind study of loxapine versus haloperidol. Intern Clin Psychopharmacol 1993 Summer;8(2):103-8.

[18]Thomas DR. "The brown bag" and other approaches to decreasing polypharmacy in the elderly. N C Med J 1991 Nov;52(11):565-6.

[19]Barry K. Patient self-medication: an innovative approach to medication teaching [Review]. J Nurs Care Qual 1993 Oct;8(1):75-82.

[20]McNally DL, Wertheimer D. Strategies to reduce the high cost of patient noncompliance. Md Med J 1992 Mar;41(3):223-5.

[21]Nielson C. Pharmacologic considerations in critical care of the elderly [Review]. Clin Geriatr Med 1994 Feb;10(1):71-89.

[22]Anonymous. Medication use and the elderly. Can Med Assoc J 1993 Oct 15;149(8):1152A-D.

[23]Gainsborough N, Powell-Jackson P. Prescribing for the elderly. Practitioner 1990 Mar 8; 234(1484):246-8.

[24]Harris R. Pharmacological and nonpharmacological approaches to the treatment of cardiovascular disease in the geriatric patients. Geriatr Med Today 1982;1(3):47.

[25]Newton PF, Levinson W, Maslen D. The geriatric medication algorithm; a pilot study. J Gen Intern Med 1994 Mar;9(3):164-7.

[26]Busto UE, Sellers EM. Anxiolytics and sedative/hypnotics dependence. Br J Addict 1991 Dec; 86(12):1647-52.

[27]Morss SE, Lenert LA, Faustman WO. The side effects of antipsychotic drugs and patients' quality of life; patient education and preference assessment with computers and multimedia. Proceedings - the Annual Symposium on Computer Applications in Medical Care 1993; :17-21.

[28]Amir M, Cristal N, Bar-On D, Loidl A. Does the combination of ACE inhibitor and calcium antagonist control hypertension and improve quality of life? The LOMIR-MCT-IL study experience. Blood Pres 1994;Suppl 1:40-2.

[29]Palmer AJ, Fletcher AE, Rudge PJ, Andrews CD, Callaghan TS, Bulpitt CJ. Quality of life in hypertensives treated with atenolol or captopril: a double-blind crossover trial. J Hyptertens 1992 Nov;10(11):1409-16.

[30]Sager DS, Bennett RM. Individualizing the risk/benefit ratio of NSAIDs in older patients [Review]. Geriatrics 1992 Aug;47(8):24-31.

[31]Buchanan N. Noncompliance with medication amongst persons attending a tertiary referral epilepsy clinic: implications, management and outcome. Seizure 1993 Mar;2(1):79-82.

[32]Phillips SL, Carr-Lopez SM. Impact of a pharmacist on medication discontinuation in a hospital-based geriatric clinic. Am J Hosp Pharm 1990 May;47(5):1075-9.

[33]Weintrub M. Compliance in the elderly. Clin Geriatr Med 1990 May;6(2):445-52.

[34]Wilcox SM, Himmelstein DU, Woolhander S. Inappropriate drug prescribing for the community-dwelling elderly. JAMA 1994 July 27;272(4):292-6.

[35]Burris JF. Hypertension management in the elderly [Review]. Heart Dis Stroke 1994 Mar-Apr;3(2):77-83.

[36]Report of the Royal College of General Physicians: Medication for the elderly. J R Coll Physicians Lond 1984;18:7.

[37]Anonymous. Medication use and the elderly. Canadian Medical Association. Can Med Assoc J 1993 Oct 15;149(8):1152A-D.

[38]Cadieux RJ. Geriatric psychopharmacology. A primary care challenge [Review]. Postgrad Med 1993 Mar;93(4):281-2, 285-8, 294-301.

[39]Ancill RJ, Carlyle WW, Liang RA, Holliday SG. Agitation in the demented elderly: a role for the benzodiazepines? Int Clin Psychopharmacol 1991 Winter;6(3):141-6.

[40]Burrows GD, Norman TR, Judd FK, Marriott PF. Short-acting versus long-acting benzodiazepines: discontinuation effects in panic disorders. J Psychiatr Res 1990;24 Supp 2:65-72.

[41]Frank T. Tapering antihypertensives: avoiding the rebound. Senior Patient. 1990 16, June.

[42]Frishman WH. Beta-adrenergic blocker withdrawal. Am J Cardiol 1987;59:26F-32F.

[43]Coccaro EF, Kramer E, Zemishlany Z, Thorne A, Rice CM 3d, Giordani B, Duvvi K, Patel BM, Torres J, Nora R, et al. Pharmacologic treatment of noncognitive behavioral disturbances in elderly demented patients. [see comments]. Am J Psychiatry 1990 Dec;147(12):1640-5.

[44]Amery A, et al. Mortality and morbidity results from the European working party on high blood pressure in the elderly. Lancet 1985;1:1349-54.

[45]Applegate WB, Rutan GH. Advances in management of hypertension in older persons [see comments] [Review]. J Am Geriatr Soc 1992 Nov;40(11):1164-74.

[46]Avanzini F, Alli C, Bettelli G, Corso R, Colombo F, Mariotti G, Radice M, Torri V, Tognoni G. Antihypertensive efficacy and tolerability of different drug regimens in isolated systolic hypertension in the elderly. Eur Heart J 1994 Feb;15(2):206-12.

[47]Jenck MA, Reynolds MS. Anticonvulsant drug withdrawal in seizure-free patients [Review]. Clin Pharm 1990 Oct;9(10):781-7.

[48]Hetzel DJ. Controlled clinical trials of omeprazole in the long-term management of reflux disease [Review]. Digestion 1992;51 Suppl 1:35-42.

[49]Maton PN. Omeprazole [Review]. N Engl J Med 1991 Apr 4;324(14):965-75.

[50]Eagger SA, Levy R, Sahakian BJ. Tacrine in Alzheimer's disease [see comments]. Lancet 1991 Apr 27;337(8748):989-92.

[51]Levine M, Hirsh J, Gent M, et al. Double blind randomized trial of very-low-dose warfarin for prevention of thromboembolism in stage IV breast cancer. Lancet 1994;343:886-9.

[52]Aguglia E, Casacchi GB, et al. Double blinded study of the efficacy and safety of sertraline versus fluoxetine in major depression. Int Clin Psychopharmacol 1994;8:197-202.

[53]Avanzini F, Alli C, Bettelli G, Corso R, Colombo F, Mariotti G, Radice M, Torri V, Tognoni G. Antihypertensive efficacy and tolerability of different drug regimens in isolated systolic hypertension in the elderly. Eur Heart J 1994 Feb;15(2):206-12.

[54]Borland C, et al. Biochemical and clinical correlates of diuretics therapy in the elderly. Age Ageing 1986;15:357-63.

[55]Coope J, Warrender TS. Randomized trial of treatment of hypertension in elderly patients in primary care. BMJ 1986;293:1145,1148.

[56]Wassertheil-Smoller S, Blaufox DM, et al. Effect of antihypertensives on sexual function and quality of life: The TAIM study. Ann Intern Med 1991;114:613-20.

8

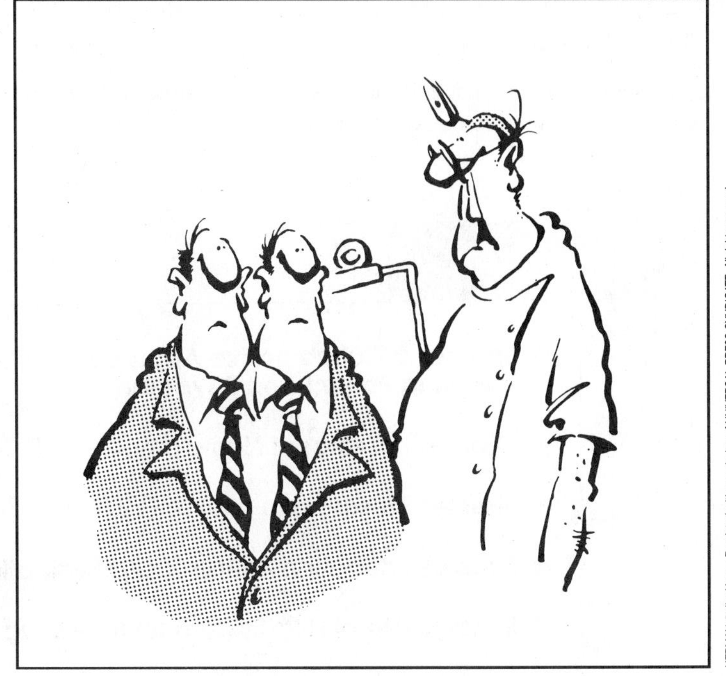

"Take four aspirin and call me in the morning."

Streamlining Drug Therapy in Clinical Practice: A Systematic Approach to Drug Regimen Design

It is now time to put the DRESC program into practice. This requires not only specific information regarding opportunities for applying drug reduction, elimination, simplification, and consolidation as outlined in previous chapters, but a practical step-by-step approach that can be implemented by physicians and pharmacists in an outpatient setting.

The most common questions asked by prescribing practitioners when implementing the DRESC program are the following: (1) which medications should be discontinued first; (2) how rapidly should medication additions, substitutions, or deletions should be made; (3) how many physician visits, pharmacist consultations, or telephone consultations are required to monitor the effects—and establish the effectiveness—of DRESC program strategies; (4) what instruments can be used to measure patient satisfaction and response to the reconstructed drug regimens; and (5) what endpoints should be monitored to ensure that the remodeled drug regimen is outcome-effective.[1]

Figure 8-1

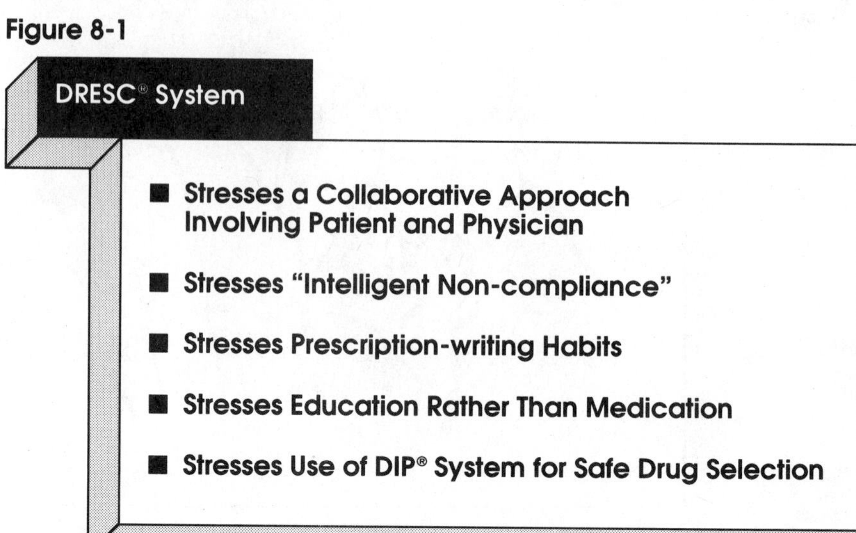

DRESC® System
Stresses a Collaborative Approach Involving Patient and Physician
Stresses "Intelligent Non-compliance"
Stresses Prescription-writing Habits
Stresses Education Rather Than Medication
Stresses Use of DIP® System for Safe Drug Selection

Because establishing patient confidence is a priority, physicians and pharmacists should *first* identify those medications that in all likelihood, can be discontinued *without* adversely affecting the patient's clinical condition. In other words, before discontinuing a medication that can produce significant exacerbations of the underlying disease if *inappropriately* discontinued, it is preferable to start with a medication that has a *low* probability of producing clinical deterioration if deleted from the regimen.

Time Framework. In general, up to a 12-week period may be required to implement, monitor, and fully assess the clinical effectiveness of any single-drug deletion, substitution, or addition. This 12-week period is divided into three phases: (1) assessment; (2) implementation; and (3) evaluation (see Figure 8-2). Following the initial encounter, a physician visit is required at week 4, week 8, and week 12. If, at that time, alterations in the drug regimen have produced the desired therapeutic effects, the physician can begin a second 12-week cycle for modifications that apply to a second drug, and so on. As a rule, only one drug deletion, alteration, or substitution is made per 12-week period. This incremental approach encourages patient monitoring for side effects, measurement of clinical goals, and opportunities to evaluate dosages. In some cases especially when adverse side effects are troubling for the patient, more rapid substitutions or deletions can be made. In addition, when switching from one drug to another drug in the *same* class (i.e., replacing pravastatin with atorvastatin) the substitution can be made quickly, but it may require several weeks to document the full therapeutic impact (i.e., changes in the LDL level) of the change. Because the step-by-step approach to drug house remodeling usually is gradual, it may take several weeks, or months to complete the entire process of deconstruction and reconstruction.[2-4] As a result, however, not only will the drug regimen be more durable, but physicians and pharmacists will be able to better assess patient attitudes and responses to changes in their medications.

Figure 8-2

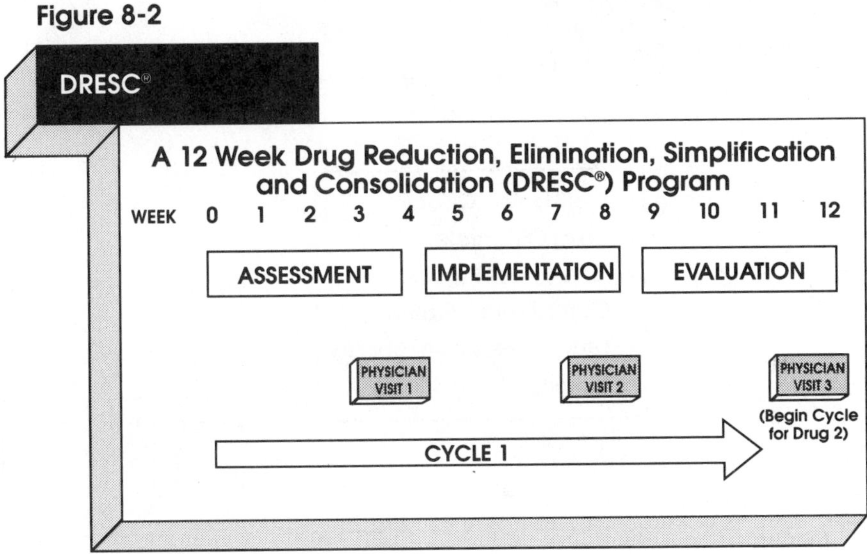

PHASE I: ASSESSMENT

The first phase of the DRESC program is a 4-week period of comprehensive assessment of the patient's drug house (see Figure 8-1).[3] During this 4-week period, the physician or pharmacist will explore a number of features related to the patient's drug regimen. Thorough questioning is necessary to assess the current regimen's side effects, compliance pattern, and quality-of-life impact. A careful history will reveal the patient's overall well-being, preferences regarding medication intake, and provide information that will help construct a drug chronicle.

The purpose of the assessment phase is to help the physician or pharmacist determine just how comfortable the patient is with the current medication regimen and how well the pharmacotherapeutic program is meeting its objectives. As part of the assessment, inquiries should be made about a wide range of symptoms and patient concerns (see Table 8-1). For example, the patient should be asked whether he or she has noticed any significant changes in energy levels while on the current drug regimen. Have there been problems sleeping through the entire night? Quality-of-life issues are important in making drug selections. Consequently, questioning regarding the patient's sex life is appropriate. The physician should ask whether the patient's desire for sex has decreased significantly since beginning the current regimen and whether there are specific impairments in the performance of sexual activities or other daily functions.

Figure 8-3

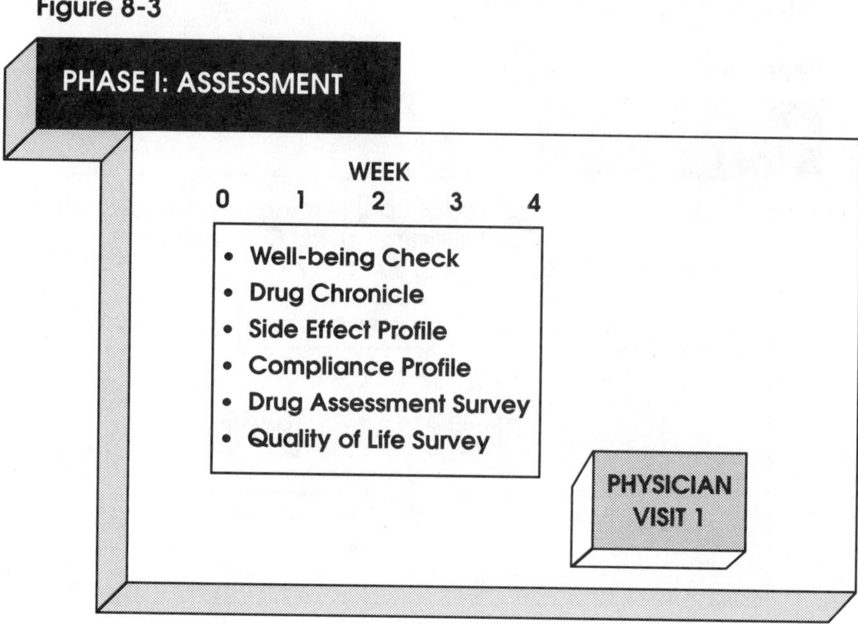

Because older patients may be on one or more anticholinergic medications, questions regarding the presence of dry mouth, visual disturbances, difficulty voiding, constipation, or excessive daytime sleepiness are appropriate. Does the patient have excessive fatigue, lethargy, or lack of energy, and is the patient still interested in participating in hobbies, work activities, or social functions while on the current medication? Finally, the patient should be asked to document any skin changes, peripheral edema, changes in appetite, or unexplained headaches.

Before DRESC program strategies are implemented, it is sometimes helpful to ask patients which specific drugs they might feel comfortable doing without and which medications they feel are particularly valuable. This assessment phase also requires the patient to document drug intake in the form of a chronicle. Table 8-1 suggests one scheme that is useful for documenting medication intake.[5] Finally, the drug chronicle should also include any over-the-counter drugs the patient is taking.

Table 8-1

DRESC[R] Program Drug Regimen/Assessment Questionnaire
Well-Being Check and Side-Effect Profile Assessment
1. Have you noticed significant changes in your energy level while on the current drug regimen?
2. Are you sleeping the entire night? Do you have problems going to sleep or awakening in the morning?
3. Has your desire for sex decreased significantly since beginning your current drug regimen?
4. Have you noted any of the following symptoms: dry mouth, visual disturbances, difficulty voiding, constipation, excessive daytime sleepiness, or light-headedness?
5. Have you noticed an unexplained cough since starting your medication?
6. Have you experienced shakiness, palpitations, anxiety, or rapid heart rate?
7. Have you experienced excessive fatigue, lethargy, or lack of energy?
8. Do you still have the desire and energy to engage in hobbies and social activities since beginning your current medications?
9. Have you experienced any unusual, undesirable, or unexplained tastes in your mouth?
10. Have you had any unexplained headaches or difficulty concentrating?
11. Have you noticed any burning in your stomach, nausea, constipation, diarrhea, or abdominal discomfort while on the current drug regimen?
12. Have you noticed any unusual swelling in your legs?
13. Are there any medications in the drug regimen that you feel might be responsible for producing undesirable side effects?
14. Are there any medications you are taking that do not agree with you?
15. Has your appetite either increased or decreased significantly?

Table 8-1

DRESC[R] Program Drug Regimen/Assessment Questionnaire — cont'd.

Drug Chronicle and Assessment Survey

1. Please list the medications you are currently taking, and the time of day you take them. (You may use your medication bottles or any other sources you require to provide this information.)

   Medication 1 ____________________

   Time of Day Taken ____________________

   Medication 2 ____________________

   Time of Day Taken ____________________

   Medication 3 ____________________

   Time of Day Taken ____________________

2. Do you regularly take any over-the-counter drugs? If so, which ones and when do you take them? What do you take for a headache? How often? When was last time?

   OTC Medication 1 ____________________

   Time of Day Taken ____________________

   OTC Medication 2 ____________________

   Time of Day Taken ____________________

   OTC Medication 3 ____________________

   Time of Day Taken ____________________

3. Are there any medications in your drug regimen that you would prefer not to take? If so, which one(s) and why?
4. Are you happy with your current drug regimen? If not, please explain why.
5. Are there any medications in your regimen that you feel are too expensive? If so, which ones?
6. Would you be interested in trying other medications that are just as effective for your medical problem, but are much less likely to cause side effects?
7. Would you be interested in being on medications that are less expensive than the ones you are currently taking?
8. Would you be willing to make regular visits to the physician over the next several weeks to make medication adjustments that would help streamline your drug regimen?
9. Is there any single medication you feel you absolutely must stay on because it has produced such dramatic improvements in your condition?
10. Is there any single medication you feel you should absolutely stop taking because it has produced such a dramatic worsening in your medical condition?

Table 8-1

DRESC[R] Program Drug Regimen/Assessment Questionnaire — cont'd.
Quality-of-Life Survey
1. In general, do you feel better or worse than you did before starting your current medication regimen?
2. Do you think you would feel better or worse if you were taken off all your medications?
3. Do you think the quality of your life would improve if you were taking smaller doses of the medications?
4. In general, what makes you feel worse—your medical condition or your medications?

Patient Perspective. Although drug substitutions, eliminations, additions, and deletions should be based on sound pharmacologic principles, important information can be gleaned, and a sense of collaboration is fostered, if patients are asked *their preferences* about how they want their drug regimen to be remodeled. For example, it is valuable to ask if there are any medications in the drug regimen that the patient would prefer *not* to take. If so, which medications and why? Financial considerations can be a deterrent to drug intake; therefore, patients should be asked to identify any medications that they perceive as being too expensive. Does the patient indicate an interest in trying medications that are much less expensive than the ones they are currently taking? Occasionally, patients perceive that some of their medications as extremely valuable and dislike others. Finally, a valuable index of the patient's willingness to cooperate with the DRESC program can be gleaned from the following question: "Would you be willing to visit your physician or pharmacist regularly over the next several weeks or months to make medication adjustments that would help streamline your drug regimen?" This important question reveals the prescriber's intentions and educates the patient as to the sacrifices and cooperation necessary to implement a program of drug house reconstruction.

Compliance Profile. Compliance is also necessary to set the stage for remodeling the therapeutic regimen. Patients should be asked whether or not they take their medications as prescribed. Those patients who acknowledge that their medication compliance is less than perfect should fill out a compliance profile assessment questionnaire (Table 8-2) that may reveal specific reasons for poor medication intake. The purpose of this questionnaire is to uncover both objective and subjective features of the current drug house that may deter a patient from taking their medications as prescribed. For example, the patient is asked if the medications are too expensive, whether they are taken too frequently, how the patient feels after taking the medication, and whether or not they think the medication is working. In addition, patients are encouraged to indicate whether or not they have received adequate instructions regarding medication intake, whether or not they believe better medications are available to treat their condition, and if they know of undesirable side effects and potential interactions. As part of the compliance profile assessment, patients should be asked directly whether or not they would be interested in trying other medications that might produce the same or better results with fewer side effects and a reduction in their total pill intake.

Table 8-2

DRESC® Program Drug Regimen/Assessment Questionnaire

Compliance Profile Assessment

1. For the most part, do you take your medications exactly as prescribed?

   (If your answer to Question 1 was "No," "Maybe," "Some of the time," or something similar, please complete Question 2)

2. In your view, the failure to take your pills as prescribed is best explained by the following factors (Please check all the answers that apply to your situation):
   ( ) The medications are too expensive
   ( ) I have to take them too often
   ( ) I don't like the way they make me feel
   ( ) They don't seem to be working
   ( ) The medication(s) seem to make me feel worse than I did before starting them
   ( ) I don't think I need as much medication as I once did
   ( ) The medication(s) seem(s) not to work as well as it once did
   ( ) I am a forgetful person
   ( ) It is too complicated to take them the way they are prescribed
   ( ) I haven't been told exactly how these medications should be taken
   ( ) I haven't been given written instructions on how to take my medications
   ( ) In general, I just don't like taking pills
   ( ) I believe there may be better medications available to treat my medical problem
   ( ) I have heard that this medication produces undesirable side effects

3. Would you be interested in having your medications adjusted so that you could take fewer pills less frequently?

4. Would you be interested in trying other medications that might produce fewer side effects?

The first follow-up visit occurs approximately 4 or 5 weeks after the patient has stabilized on an established drug regimen. Preferably, patient assessment should occur after the patient is stabilized on a regimen for at least 2 to 3 months.

Based on the information, perceptions, and impressions collected during this first phase, specific drug additions, deletions, or substitutions can be made. Implementation of DRESC program strategies can occur during either the first or second follow-up visit. If the physician or pharmacist feels there is enough information to initiate a single drug elimination, substitution, or addition, this modification to the drug house can be made after the first 4-week assessment phase.

PHASE II: IMPLEMENTATION

DRESC program strategies are implemented in a systematic fashion, but only after the assessment phase of the program is completed.[6,7] The assessment phase, if successful, provides the physician and pharmacist with valuable information about the patient's willingness to cooperate with a drug streamlining program, about medications thought to be troublesome, and about side effect issues that may be undermining medication compliance or patient well-being. During the implementation phase, which includes weeks 5 through 8, the physician or pharmacist should discuss the drug assessment survey, as well as opportunities for making specific changes in the therapeutic regimen that are tailored to the specific patient. The patient should be reassured that implementation of DRESC strategies will require ongoing collaboration between physician, patient, and pharmacist. Both oral and written instructions regarding drug changes must be provided during the implementation phase. The patient should be encouraged to immediately report any side effects from medication discontinuation, substitution, or additions.

If one medication is being tapered while another drug is gradually being introduced, explain to the patient the rationale of slow medication tapering. If tapering a medication is known to cause withdrawal symptoms, the patient should be alerted to expect these symptoms and reassured that reintroduction of the drug is always possible if withdrawal symptoms are intolerable. During the implementation phase, the physician or pharmacist has the option of either gradually decreasing the dose of a medication or stopping the drug immediately. This decision depends on specific pharmacologic and pharmacokinetic properties of the drug and how strongly the physician believes that the patient does not need the medication to maintain clinical stability.

If changes to the drug regimen are made during the first follow-up visit (i.e., after 4 weeks into the DRESC program cycle), the purpose of the next visit is to evaluate the clinical response to these changes and to make necessary changes. By the end of the second follow-up visit, a specific strategy for drug reduction, simplification, and consolidation should be formulated. It is preferable to begin with drug elimination or dose reduction. If there are no opportunities for drug elimination or dosage reduction, it is appropriate to proceed with consolidation of the drug regimen, (ie, identifying a single prescription ingredient that can be substituted for two different drugs currently in the regimen). After alterations are made as part of the implementation phase, the patient undergoes an evaluation phase lasting for an additional 4 weeks to determine if remodeling strategies have proved beneficial to the patient's clinical condition, target goals, and well-being.

Figure 8-4

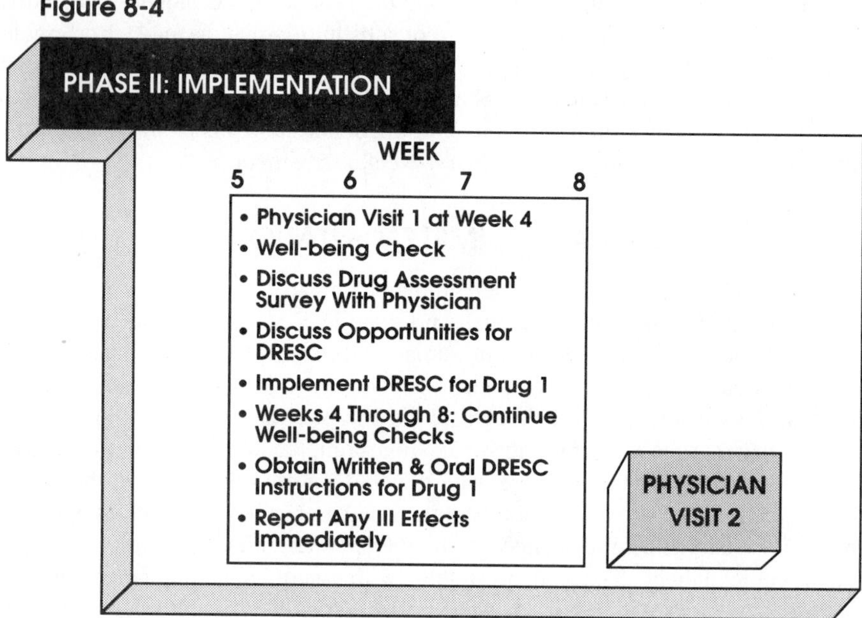

PHASE II: IMPLEMENTATION
WEEK
5
6
7
8
• Physician Visit 1 at Week 4
• Well-being Check
• Discuss Drug Assessment Survey With Physician
• Discuss Opportunities for DRESC
• Implement DRESC for Drug 1
• Weeks 4 Through 8: Continue Well-being Checks
• Obtain Written & Oral DRESC Instructions for Drug 1
• Report Any Ill Effects Immediately
PHYSICIAN VISIT 2

PHASE III: EVALUATION

The purpose of Phase III is to evaluate the patient's clinical, psychological, and symptomatic response to modifications in the drug regimen. During this phase, the patient is asked to report any subjective or objective changes that seem related to modifications made in the drug house. This is the time to assess the need for minor DRESC program changes, adjustments, and drug house repairs. For example, should the tapering of a medication occur over a longer duration than originally planned? By the tenth week, it should be apparent whether or not the patient is tolerating changes in the drug regimen.

Objective parameters such as blood pressure, lipid profile, liver function tests, electrocardiogram, drug levels, glycosylated hemoglobin, etc. are monitored as necessary. At this point in the DRESC Program, it is also useful to review the well-being profile and quality-of-life assessment questionnaire that was completed during phase I. During the third physician visit, the patient might be asked to complete the questionnaire again, and the results from each phase of the DRESC program cycle can be compared. The purpose of this comparison, which can be conducted either through a formal, written questionnaire or as a part of the patient's history, is to determine if the patient's attitudes about his or her reconstructed drug regimen have improved since the first visit. If changes to the drug house meet with patient approval, opportunities for additional medication changes should be presented at this time.

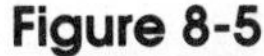
Figure 8-5

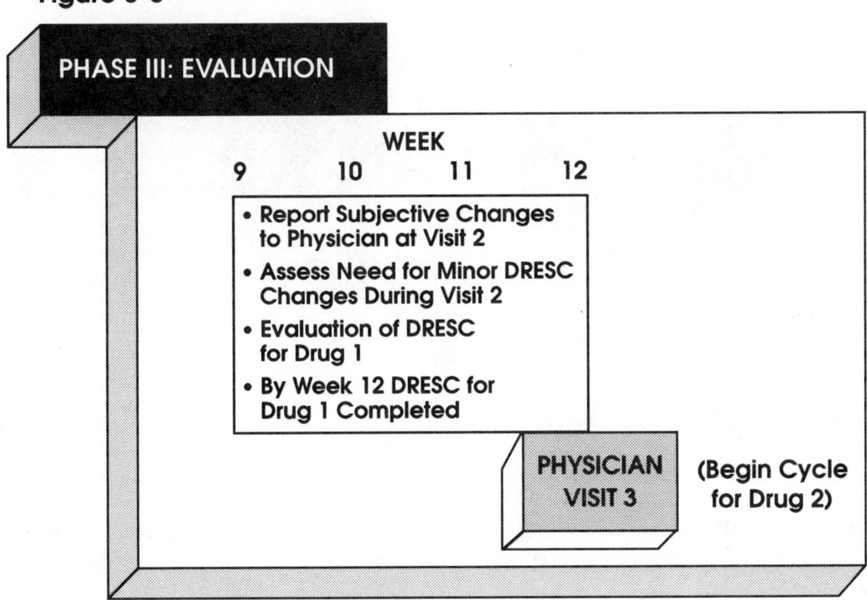

By the end of week 12, the physician and patient can assess whether or not symptoms, clinical condition, side effects, and the patient's overall sense of well-being have improved or deteriorated as a result of DRESC program strategies. If significant benefits are observed from the first DRESC program cycle, it is appropriate to start a new three-phase DRESC cycle for another drug. In general, one 12-week DRESC program cycle is required for each significant drug elimination, substitution, or consolidation, although in each case, there may be exceptions to this rule. Simplification of the drug regimen and reductions in dosage can occur at any time during the course of this cycle.

ADRESC: APPLYING DRUG REDUCTION, ELIMINATION, SIMPLIFICATION AND CONSOLIDATION

Not surprisingly, the opportunities for implementing DRESC program strategies are wide and varied. It is helpful, however, to evaluate some actual case studies to fully appreciate the benefits that can be derived from streamlining pharmacotherapeutic regimens.

DRESC PROGRAM CASE STUDY NUMBER 1

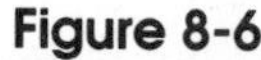

Figure 8-6

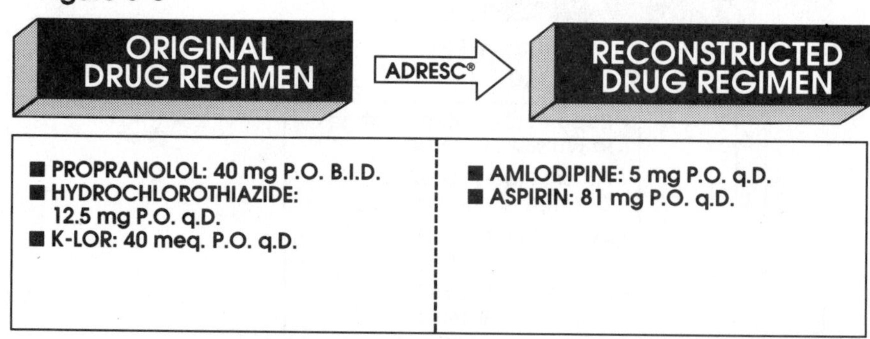

ORIGINAL DRUG REGIMEN
ADRESC®
RECONSTRUCTED DRUG REGIMEN
■ PROPRANOLOL: 40 mg P.O. B.I.D.
■ HYDROCHLOROTHIAZIDE: 12.5 mg P.O. q.D.
■ K-LOR: 40 meq. P.O. q.D.
■ AMLODIPINE: 5 mg P.O. q.D.
■ ASPIRIN: 81 mg P.O. q.D.

A 67-year-old man with a history of hypertension and a family history of heart disease had been maintained for three years on a three-drug regimen consisting of a beta-blocker (propranolol), diuretic (hydrochlorothiazide), and potassium supplementation (see Figure 8-6). There was no history of myocardial infarction. His blood pressure was reasonably well controlled at 130/90. His LDL-C cholesterol level had increased slightly over the treatment period from 120 mg/dl to 128 mg/dl, which his physician felt may have been due, in part, to the possible mild cholesterol-elevating effects associated with combination of beta-blocker and thiazide therapy. In addition, the patient reported decreased libido, late afternoon fatigue, and occasional noncompliance with the potassium supplement. On one occasion, the serum potassium was slightly below normal limits, at which time the man complained of muscle weakness.

It was felt that applying drug reduction, elimination, simplification, and consolidation would be useful in this gentleman. Over a period of 12 weeks, the propranolol was very gradually decreased and the antihypertensive agent, amlodipine (5 mg daily) was started. Over the next 12 week period, the patient's blood pressure had decreased to 118/82 and stabilized at that level. This reading was observed in the office on three occasions. Hence, it was felt that perhaps the patient could be discontinued from his low dose thiazide therapy and achieve BP control with amlodipine monotherapy. Over the next 12 week (ADRESC) cycle, the thiazide and potassium were discontinued, while blood pressure was closely monitored every two weeks. At week 12, of the next cycle, the patient's blood pressure had stabilized at 120/85 on a single agent (amlodipine).

In addition, the patient noted improved energy and vigor—as well as the perception that his libido had improved—and it was felt by his physician that some of the possible depressive effects associated with lipophilic beta-blockers such as propranolol may have been ameliorated by substitution therapy with a calcium blocker. Six months after monotherapy with amlodipine, the patient's LDL-C level decreased to its original level of 120 mg/dl. It was speculated that the neutral effect on serum lipids observed with calcium blockers may have partly explained the normalization of his LDL-C level. Finally, low dose aspirin therapy was started for cardioprotection.

DRESC PROGRAM CASE STUDY NUMBER 2

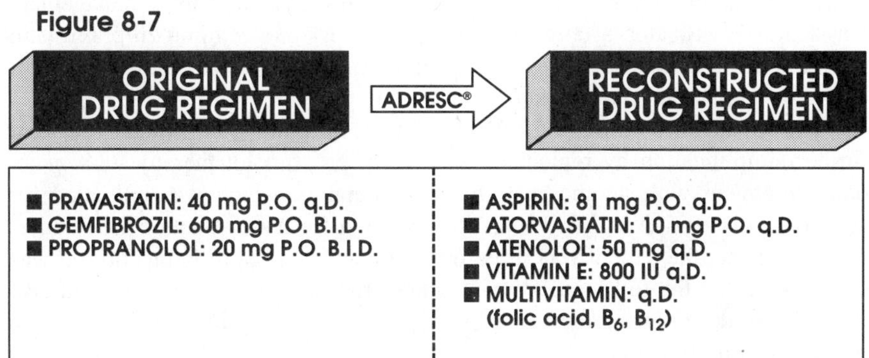

ORIGINAL DRUG REGIMEN
ADRESC®
RECONSTRUCTED DRUG REGIMEN
■ PRAVASTATIN: 40 mg P.O. q.D.
■ GEMFIBROZIL: 600 mg P.O. B.I.D.
■ PROPRANOLOL: 20 mg P.O. B.I.D.
■ ASPIRIN: 81 mg P.O. q.D.
■ ATORVASTATIN: 10 mg P.O. q.D.
■ ATENOLOL: 50 mg q.D.
■ VITAMIN E: 800 IU q.D.
■ MULTIVITAMIN: q.D.
(folic acid, B_6, B_{12})

Figure 8-7

This 58-year-old woman with a history of breast cancer, elevated LDL-C and triglyceride levels had a myocardial infarction one year prior to being evaluated for muscle cramps, fatigue, vague gastrointestinal complaints, and noncompliance with her drug regimen (see Figure 8-7). The patient had been on estrogen therapy at the time of her breast cancer, was found to be estrogen-receptor positive. She was discontinued from hormone replacement therapy (HRT) after in-depth discussions with her physician. Despite the cardioprotective benefits that have been observed with hormone replacement therapy, it was felt this individual was not an ideal candidate for HRT because of her past history of breast cancer.

When she was first seen the patient's LDL-C cholesterol level was 113 mg/dl and her triglyceride level was 425 mg/dl. Her CPK level was slightly elevated at 286 IU.

The patient was evaluated for opportunities to optimize management of her cardiovascular risk factors and reduce the risk of possible drug-drug interactions (gemfibrozil-statins). During the first ADRESC cycle, it was determined that the patient, who had a history of myocardial infarction, was not achieving NCEP (National Cholesterol Education Project) goals for LDL-C level. Given her history of MI, it was felt her LDL-C level should be less than 100 mg/dl. Moreover, it was felt her triglyceride level of 425 mg/dl was also in poor control, and reduction to a level less than 300 mg/dl was considered an appropriate target. It was noted that such cardioprotective measures as aspirin, vitamin E, and multivitamins (including folic acid) had been initiated as part of her pharmacological prevention program. Finally, the elevated CPK and muscle cramps were of concern, because of the known increased risk of rhabdomyolysis from the combination of statins and gemfibrozil.

During the first 12 weeks, a primary objective was to determine whether NCEP target goals for LDL-C and lowering of elevated triglyceride level could be achieved with monotherapy. To evaluate this possibility, the patient was discontinued from pravastatin and started on atorvastatin 10 mg P.O. q.D. By the second 12-week ADRESC® cycle the patient's LDL-C level had dropped to 91 mg/dl, thus achieving NCEP target goals for high-risk patients. In addition, the triglyceride level had fallen from 425 mg/dl to 318 mg/dl, and was within a more acceptable range for her clinical status. Once consolidation of lipid management was achieved with atorvastatin *monotherapy*, the risk of a gemfibrozil/pravastatin interaction was eliminated. The patient reported a reduction in GI symptomatology and the muscle cramps abated.

During the third 12-week ADRESC® cycle, the patient's regimen underwent further simplification by replacing twice daily propranolol therapy with once-daily treatment with another beta-blocker, atenolol, which was indicated for secondary prevention of MI. During this cycle a further evaluation was undertaken to ensure the patient was receiving full benefits of cardioprotection. It was determined that the full medication "cocktail for cardioprevention" should also include low-dose (81 mg/day) aspirin, vitamin E, and a multivitamin consisting of B_6, B_{12}, and folic acid.

The final regimen permitted once-daily consumption of five prescription ingredients and/or supplements directed at aggressive lipid, platelet, antioxidant, and homocysteine management for the purpose of lowering risk for recurrent cardiovascular disease and stroke.

DRESC PROGRAM CASE STUDY NUMBER 3

Figure 8-8

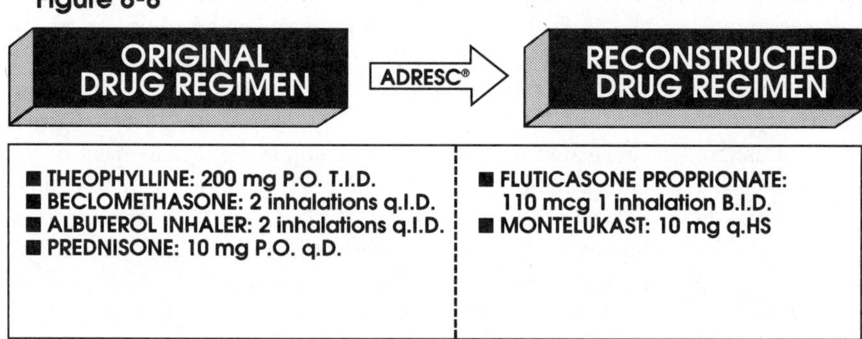

This 42-year-old obese woman with a long history of bronchial asthma had been maintained on a complex regimen consisting of theophylline, steroid inhaler, beta-agonist inhaler, and low-dose prednisone therapy. Over the past year she had made several emergency department visits, one of which required a two-day hospitalization. Complicating optimization of her drug regimen was the fact that she was being seen by three different physicians, none of which was identified by her as the primary physician. Moreover, she had reported difficulty complying with her regimen, which required up to 16 inhalations and 4 pills per day and complained of nausea, which she associated with the theophylline. Over the past six months, she had twice required high-dose, rapid taper steroid therapy, but found it difficult to maintain an adequate respiratory status without chronic prednisone therapy.

The goal of the first 12-week cycle was to assess opportunities for streamlining the drug regimen and identifying medications that would maximize anti-inflammatory effects through streamlined, high potency treatment. During this first cycle, it was determined that a prevention- and maintenance-oriented drug house build around NIH-endorsed recommendations for steroid-based anti-inflammatory therapy should be given high priority. During this cycle, the low-dose beclomethasone inhaler was replaced with a higher potency fluticasone preparation, initially at the 220 mcg dose per inhalation. During the second 12-week cycle, the theophylline was gradually discontinued without adverse effects on clinical status. During this period, the patient also noted decreasing reliance on the albuterol inhaler, and was well-maintained with PRN use of the beta-agonist.

The goal of the second 12-week ADRESC® cycle was to evaluate the possibility of eliminating dependence on chronic low-dose systemic steroid therapy, and in the process reduce risk of steroid-related adverse side effects. To achieve this objective, the patient's physician initiated treatment with a once-daily leukotriene antagonist, montelukast (Singulair®). During this cycle, the prednisone was gradually tapered and, by week 8 of the second cycle, was eliminated entirely.

By the end of the second 12-week cycle, the patient reported excellent respiratory functional status, elimination of theophylline-related nausea, dramatic improvements in medication compliance, and required no emergency department visits for exacerbations of her asthma.

DRESC PROGRAM CASE STUDY NUMBER 4

Figure 8-9

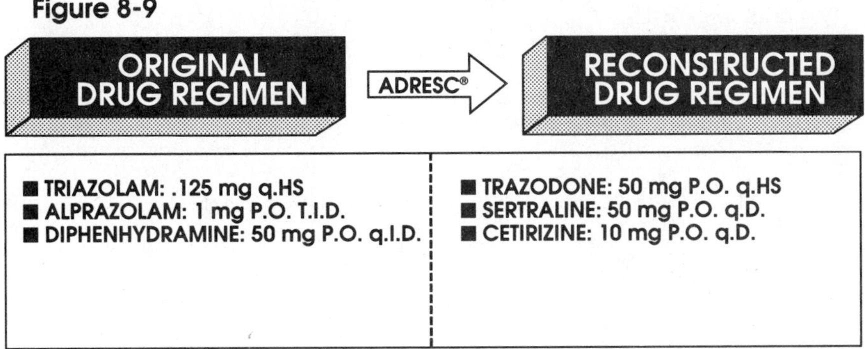

ORIGINAL DRUG REGIMEN
ADRESC®
RECONSTRUCTED DRUG REGIMEN
■ TRIAZOLAM: .125 mg q.HS
■ ALPRAZOLAM: 1 mg P.O. T.I.D.
■ DIPHENHYDRAMINE: 50 mg P.O. q.I.D.
■ TRAZODONE: 50 mg P.O. q.HS
■ SERTRALINE: 50 mg P.O. q.D.
■ CETIRIZINE: 10 mg P.O. q.D.

This 38-year-old woman has a history of anxiety symptoms associated with panic disorder, insomnia, and seasonal allergic rhinitis. She has a previous history of alcohol abuse. The patient has been adequately maintained for four months on three medications, including two benzodiazepines, but complains of dry mouth, occasional memory lapses, and feelings of drowsiness, especially during the spring and summer months, when her antihistamine therapy is continuous. She also expresses sincere concern about developing physiological dependency on the benzodiazepine medications, and consults with her physician about alternative treatment for her clinical disorders.

The principal goal of the first 12-week cycle is to determine whether or not the patient is able to undergo a very gradual tapering of her alprazolam (Xanax), while substitution with an SSRI, sertraline (Zoloft), is being initiated in order to manage anxiety symptoms associated with panic disorder. The sertraline is started on week 4 of the first ADRESC® cycle and is well tolerated. On week 12, very gradual tapering of alprazolam is undertaken, and with strong support from her physician and family, the patient tolerates the elimination of the benzodiazepine without rebound anxiety, and without significant withdrawal symptoms. By the end of the second 12-week ADRESC® cycle, the patient is free of panic-related symptoms, and is maintained on sertraline 50 mg P.O. q.D.

The goal of the third cycle is to evaluate the possibility of replacing triazolam, which may be responsible for her reports of occasional memory lapses, with another medication known to treat insomnia. The antidepressant trazodone is introduced into the regimen for qiHS dosing, and over the next several weeks, the woman reports she no longer requires triazolam for sleep induction.

Finally, to treat symptoms of seasonal allergic rhinitis, the antihistamine sertraline is used to replace diphenhydramine. This substitution is accompanied by improvement in allergy-related symptoms and a reduction in daytime sleepiness.

[1]Stander PE, Yates GR. Modifying physician prescribing patterns of H2 receptor antagonists in an ambulatory setting. QRB 1988 July;14(7):206-9.

[2]Phillips SL, Carr-Lopez SM. Impact of a pharmacist on medication discontinuation in a hospital-based geriatric clinic. Am J Hosp Pharm 1990 May;47(5):1075-9.

[3]Schainen JS. Screening for polypharmacy in a nursing home care unit. Journal of Gerontol Nurs 1994 Mar;20(3):41,44.

[4]Sherman D. Reducing unnecessary psychoactive drugs. Contem Longterm Care 1992 Oct;15(10):76,78.

[5]Steiner JF, Fihn SD, Blair B, Inut TS. Appropriate reductions in compliance among well-controlled hypertensive patients. J Clin Epidemiol 1991;44(12):1361-71.

[6]Laucka PV, Hoffman NB. Decreasing medication use in a nursing-home patient-care unit. Am J Hosp Pharm 1992 Jan;49(1):96-9.

[7]Lipowski EE, Becker M. Presentation of drug prescribing guidelines and physician response. QRB 1992 Dec;18(12):461-70.

9

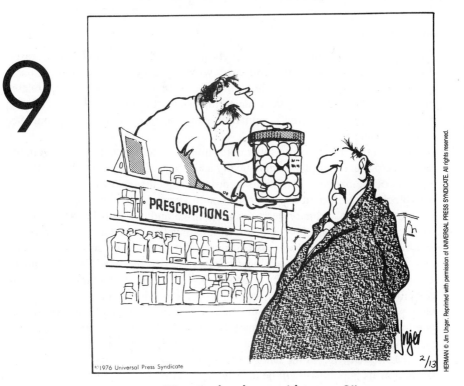

"Can I take them with water?"

Pharmatectural Strategies for Cardiovascular Drug Therapy and Disease Prevention in the Elderly

A rational, systematic approach to construction of drug regimens in the geriatric patient should be guided by several unique aspects of pharmacotherapy in this patient population. They include quality-of-life maintenance, the pitfalls of polypharmacy, prevention-oriented drug therapy, drug-drug interactions, and noncompliance-induced disease deterioration.[1-3] Even with meticulous attention to drug regimen design and vigilant monitoring of drug-related adverse patient events (DRAPEs), the older patient frequently requires pharmacologic maintenance with three or more medications, a therapeutic reality that places such individuals at high risk of incurring clinically important side effects and interactions.[4]

Oftentimes, side effects in the elderly are quietly festering, insidious, and ascribed by the patient or physician to nonpharmacologic factors, making drug regimen deconstruction and reconstruction especially difficult. In other cases, drug therapy may have been initiated without adequate indications. Consequently, pharmatectural strategies aimed at reducing the risk of drug-related problems in the geriatric patient must emphasize not only drug dose reduction but, when appropriate, drug elimination, simplification and consolidation. (See Chapters 7 and 8).

Put simply, the principal pharmatectural objective in treating the geriatric patient is to use as *few* pharmacologically active ingredients as possible to service as many of the patient's conditions as possible. Agents of low toxicity—aspirin, beta-blockers, ACE inhibitors, estrogen, antihypertensives, etc.—that have been shown to prevent coronary heart disease, stroke and/or renal deterioration, and which have significant potential for eliminating the need for more aggressive pharmacotherapy with more toxic drugs, offer special windows of opportunity.[2,5,6] By reducing pharmacologic burden, the risk of DRAPEs is minimized and quality-of-life maintenance is preserved.[7,8] The pharmatectural approach to constructing a therapeutically effective, prevention-oriented drug regimen in the older patient requires not only application of the general principles emphasized in previous chapters, but a careful analysis of clinical trials that identify specific pharmacotherapeutic options that are useful in the elderly.[9-11]

Background. As the United States enters the twenty-first century, a large fraction of its population will be elderly. Mean survival has increased more than 60% since the turn of the last century, and Americans 65 years and older will comprise 20% of the population by the year 2010.[12,13] Moreover, in the year 2000 there will be 15 million Americans over the age of 85, the fastest growing segment of the geriatric population.

With advancing age, individuals are susceptible to a number of clinical disorders. Current approaches to most geriatric disorders use drug therapy.[14] As a result, the elderly are burdened not only by diseases of old age, but with the consumption of an ever-increasing number of potent drugs, many of which can precipitate adverse side effects.[15-18]

No other risk factor compares with polypharmacy as a cause of adverse drug reactions and interactions in the geriatric population.[14,19] A number of British and American studies corroborate that persons over 65 years of age living independently take an average of 2.8 drugs per day. In skilled nursing facilities the number increases to an average of 3.4, while about 9 drugs per day are prescribed for the hospitalized elderly[20,21] (Table 9-1).

Table 9-1

Causes of Unintentional Drug Toxicity Among the Elderly	
• Duplications	• Omissions
• Self selection of drugs	• Pharmacy error
• Taking p.r.n. drugs too frequently	• Drug-induced confusion
	• Recreational misuse
• Automatic refills	• Multiple MDs

A study conducted by Larson at the University of Washington demonstrated that there is a ninefold increased risk of having an adverse drug reaction when four or more drugs are taken simultaneously.[22,23] Not surprisingly, 3% to 5% of all hospital admissions are related to adverse drug reactions, and of all hospital admissions for the elderly, 15% to 25% are complicated by an adverse drug reaction.[7,24,25] Some of these reactions are life threatening, and it is estimated that adverse drug reactions in the United States may account for up to 100,000 deaths each year.[19,26,27]

The potential toxicity of drugs in the elderly is exacerbated by a burgeoning and increasingly complex pharmaceutical landscape. At present, 14,000 prescription drugs are available in the United States, including at least 14 beta-blockers, 15 cephalosporins, 16 nonsteroidal anti-inflammatory drugs (NSAIDs), 8 oral sulfonylureas, 13 diuretic preparations, 10 ACE inhibitors, 15 penicillins, and 11 calcium channel blockers. A new entity is approved for human use every 2 to 3 weeks and two-thirds of all physician visits culminate in a prescription for a drug. In 1981, American physicians wrote 1.8 billion prescriptions, an average of 6.2 prescriptions for every person in the country. Over the past 8 years, it is estimated that the total number of prescriptions and "pills" have increased by 27% and 35%, respectively.[28]

Assessment of Drug Therapy. As the number of geriatric patients receiving pharmacologic treatment continues to rise, physicians are increasingly challenged with the diagnosis, identification, and management of adverse drug reactions among the elderly.[14,29] Inaccurate diagnoses of adverse drug reactions in these patients are common. Patients often experience multiple, nonspecific symptoms, a problem that is further complicated by the fact that many elderly patients suffer from dementia, depression, or other psychiatric disturbances. In addition, in this age group drug toxicity usually affects the central nervous system, and its symptoms are frequently attributed to other underlying causes, such as sepsis, neurologic disease, and metabolic derangements.[27,30,31]

Complicating assessment of drug-related toxicity is poor drug compliance,[32] which is frequent among the elderly (Table 9-2). In addition to not taking their medications, some elderly patients make unauthorized changes in their dosing intervals. Up to 70% of the geriatric population take OTC drugs that may interfere with, inhibit, or potentiate the effects of prescribed medications.[33,34]

Table 9-2

Risk Factors for Adverse Drug Reactions	
• Multiple drug regimens	• Changes in drug metabolism
• Incorrect diagnosis	• Changes in drug effect
• Lack of compliance	• Multiple physicians
• Poor OTC drug history	• Generic versus trade names

Complex drug regimens can confuse the geriatric patient, particularly if the patient has cognitive impairments. Physical limitations may also hinder drug compliance.

Pharmacologic therapy of the elderly, therefore, requires knowledge not only of appropriate drug dosages, potential side effects, and altered pharmacokinetics of drugs, but an increased awareness of potential drug interactions. Although it is generally assumed that the elderly inherently are more susceptible to adverse drug reactions, some investigators argue that no good evidence exists in the medical literature to support this contention.[7] Rather, these experts suggest that drug treatment of the elderly is complicated by the presence of coexisting diseases, multiple medications, self-selection of drugs, inappropriate dosing, multiple doctors, difficulty with compliance, and other factors common to the geriatric age group.[16,19,35]

Based on numerous reports and clinical reviews, it is clear that to reduce the risks of drug therapy in the elderly, it is useful to categorize precipitating factors into physician-, patient-, and drug-related groups.[26,36-38]

Physician-Related Risk Factors for Adverse Drug Reactions

The majority of adverse drug reactions in the elderly are difficult to detect because symptoms are vague and nonspecific and, not infrequently, mimic symptoms of *illnesses* common to the geriatric age group. As a result, manifestations of many drug reactions and side effects are often overlooked or ignored by the physician. Difficulty in obtaining a history in this age group, the lack of specific physical findings, and the inability to alter the progression of disease can lull the clinician into unsafe prescribing habits and poor case detection patterns.

For example, physicians who prescribe drugs primarily in response to symptoms may fail to detect adverse drug reactions and interactions which, in many cases, obscure the underlying medical condition that prompted initial drug therapy.

Table 9-3

Causes of Adverse Drug Reactions in the Elderly
PHYSICIAN FACTORS
• Physician prescribes a high-risk drug to vulnerable host (i.e., ASA for patient with peptic ulcer disease) • Physician prescribes highly interactive drug to "pharmacologically vulnerable" patient (i.e., captopril to patient on potassium-sparing agent, diphenhydramine to patient on anticholinergics, etc.) • Physician prescribes inappropriate compensatory drug for unrecognized drug effect (i.e., tricyclic antidepressant to treat beta-blocker depression, major tranquilizer to treat benzodiazepine agitation, etc.)

Table 9-3

Causes of Adverse Drug Reactions in the Elderly — cont'd.
• Automatic drug prescribing (i.e., standard orders for ICU, CCU, or chronic care facilities)
• Lack of follow-up on drug effects or poor longitudinal monitoring of drug interactions
• Failure to adjust dosage

without exception, pharmaceutical trials are short-term, and, oftentimes, do not exceed 6 months in duration. Consequently, it is safest for the clinician to wait until careful trials with older patients are available.

It is estimated that 75% of all geriatric patient-physician contacts result in the addition of a prescription drug to the patient's therapeutic program (Table 9-4). Part of the problem is a discrepancy between physician and patient expectations regarding the necessity for drug administration. One large study has shown that 80% to 90% of physicians are under the impression that their patients expect a prescription drug as part of their outpatient therapy.[39] However, patients primarily indicate the need for a thorough examination, consultation, and reassurance and expect a prescription in only 30% to 50% of physician contacts. It appears that the unfounded expectations of both physicians and patients contribute to excessive prescribing of medications.

Table 9-4

Physician Prescribing Behavior: Patterns and Pitfalls
• Two thirds of all physician visits lead to prescription for drug.
• American patients receive about four times more medication for a specific complaint than patients in Scotland.
• In one study, 60% of physicians prescribed antibiotics for common cold.
• Duke University study suggested 64% of antibiotic usage in hospitalized patients was either unnecessary or inappropriately dosed.

Until recently, physician prescribing knowledge in geriatric therapeutics was not examined in a systematic way. Early studies documented significant misuse of psychotropic drugs in nursing homes and suggested that the physician's knowledge base in geriatric clinical therapeutics may be inadequate. In one study, a questionnaire was devised to test the prescribing knowledge of primary care physicians in Pennsylvania. This investigation concluded that fewer than 30% of responding doctors "exhibited adequate knowledge of prescribing for the elderly." They also identified physician variables positively and negatively associated with an adequate knowledge of geriatric pharmacotherapy.[28] Positive associations included the importance of professional meetings, perception of the need for continuing medical education, board eligibility or certification, group (rather than solo) practice, and a practice which had at least 25% to 50% geriatric patients. Negative associations were the number of years since licensure and the belief that drug advertisements are an important source of drug information.[5,11,24]

Physician supervision of medications for the elderly, particularly in the nursing home environment, was judged inadequate by several authors in England who reviewed repeated prescriptions for psychotropic drugs without a physician visit.[41,42] These studies demonstrated a strong association between the number of times a prescription was refilled without seeing a physician and the age of the patient. In a large general practice in England, 70% of patients taking psychotropic or cardiovascular drugs had not contacted their physician in more than a month, and, of these, half had not been in contact with their physicians for a 6-month period.[43] Inasmuch as psychotropic drugs are capable of producing a variety of adverse reactions, their use demands constant vigilance. Ironically, those patients least able to monitor their own medications, (i.e., the oldest and most frail elderly) were most likely to be taking these drugs without supervision. Attitude surveys of these older patients found them very receptive to physician intervention aimed at withdrawing drugs judged detrimental or no longer useful.

Patient-Related Risk Factors for Adverse Drug Reactions

The two major patient-related risk factors associated with adverse drug reactions are compliance and age-associated changes in drug distribution and metabolism. Noncompliance with medications is an important therapeutic problem in patients taking multiple medications. Noncompliance with prescribed medications can lead to therapeutic failure and end-organ damage and, not infrequently, can induce the physician to prescribe additional—albeit unnecessary—medications to correct the clinical disorder.

Common noncompliance errors include: (1) deleting a prescribed drug; (2) continuing to take a dose of a drug that the physician has discontinued; (3) taking an incorrect dose; (4) taking the correct dose but at the wrong time interval. With respect to medication errors, polypharmacy drug regimens and daily dose frequency have been identified as important risk factors precipitating noncompliance.

If perfect compliance is defined as taking prescribed medications in a specified manner, then the elderly as a group are noncompliant at least 50% of the time in the community setting.[32] The complexity of a three-drug regimen, for example, is sufficiently great so that even patients under age 45 demonstrate noncompliance rates equal to those of the elderly. Patient noncompliance is a diverse category that includes errors of *omission* and *commission.* In a group of elderly diabetic patients with heart failure, analysis of noncompliance rates identified several factors that were associated with altered or inappropriate drug intake. These include age, number of associated diseases, functional impairment of the patient, and frequency of hospitalization. Only one factor clearly correlated with both errors of omission and commission: the *number* of drugs in the patient's regimen. Level of confusion and dementia were not assessed in this study, but other investigations suggest that compliance is threatened because of the forgetfulness so common in this age group.[7,21]

Compliance errors of commission include mixing of alcohol or over-the-counter drugs with prescribed drugs. It is estimated that alcoholism is present in up to 10% of the elderly population. Alcohol interacts adversely with sedative drugs, and such OTC drugs as antihistamines may add to the anticholinergic effects of prescribed antipsychotics, antidepressants, and antiparkinsonian medications. Laxative abuse is thought to increase with age, and this may result in fluid and electrolyte disorders.

Environmental limitations are a major obstacle to compliance and play an important role in inappropriate drug intake in the elderly. For example, the elderly patient with arthritis may be unable to open childproof bottles or to split pills to obtain a fractional dose. A patient with limited mobility may have difficulty getting to the bathroom, and, therefore, discontinue regular use of diuretics. Retinopathy and peripheral neuropathy may preclude use of insulin for the older patient who lives alone.

Changes in drug effect and metabolism vary widely among individuals in old age. Biologic functions decline at varying rates. Consequently, the appropriate dose will usually follow the maxim, "Start low, go slow" to accommodate patient variability in the elderly. A number of recent studies and position statements published in the medical literature suggest that we are in the midst of an epidemic characterized by excessive, inappropriate, and suboptimal drug prescribing in middle-aged and older Americans. Less-than-satisfactory patient compliance with prescription medications ranks among the most problematic aspects of outpatient therapy, with some clinical experts claiming that poor drug compliance is a bona fide public health problem.

Poor medication compliance is a multifaceted problem that has the potential for: (1) preventing effective treatment of a clinical condition; (2) compromising the natural history of a disease; (3) coaxing out additional, unnecessary prescription medications to compensate for subtherapeutic drug levels and inadequate clinical effects; (4) inducing patients to self-medicate with OTC drugs or make alterations in their drug regimens; and (5) causing drug-induced side effects.

PATHOPHYSIOLOGY AND PHARMACOKINETICS

A number of age-related changes in pharmacokinetics can affect drugs commonly prescribed for the elderly. In this regard, alterations in absorption, distribution, metabolism, and elimination can precipitate adverse reactions or potentiate drug toxicity. Because drugs are absorbed passively and are not transported in active forms, absorption generally does not change with increasing age. However, distribution may be altered because the fat to muscle ratio increases with age. The fat portion of body weight increases from mid-life averages of about 18% for men and 33% for women, to 36% and 48% respectively for individuals aged 65 or over. As a result, the volume of distribution for water-soluble drugs decreases with age, whereas that for fat-soluble drugs increases.

Relatively water-soluble drugs include acetaminophen and alcohol. Diazepam and lidocaine are examples of fat-soluble drugs. In the elderly, acetaminophen and other water-soluble drugs will attain higher plasma levels. On the other hand, diazepam and lidocaine will be distributed across a greater volume of fat, causing markedly delayed metabolism and a prolonged half-life elimination.

Serum albumin also decreases with age.[4] This alteration is important for highly protein-bound drugs, such as sulfonylureas, for which effective concentrations depend on the amount of unbound drug. Accordingly, drug interactions that decrease protein binding for such drugs as chlorpropamide (Diabinese®) and tolbutamide (Orinase®) may lead to toxicity in the elderly patient.

Renal and hepatic clearance of drugs may also be affected by the aging process.[4,6] Liver blood flow is decreased 40% to 50% in the elderly. But hepatic drug metabolism varies widely with individuals, and there are no predictable age-related alterations.

The glomerular filtration rate (GFR), however, is reduced by approximately 35% in the geriatric age group.[46] Unlike hepatic clearance, the GFR reduction leads to predictable, directly proportional decreases in the clearance of drugs dependent on the kidney for excretion. Examples of such drugs include lithium, digoxin, cimetidine, procainamide, most commonly used antimicrobials, and chlorpropamide.[4] Age-related changes in pharmacodynamics affect the use of a number of drugs. For example, the number of beta-adrenergic receptors is markedly reduced on lymphocytes of elderly patients. Therefore, plasma levels of propranolol and metoprolol are higher and can cause marked hypotension, bradycardia, or central nervous system depression.

CATEGORIES OF ADVERSE DRUG REACTIONS

When evaluating and identifying potential drug reactions in the elderly, it is helpful to classify them into four groups (Tables 9-5 and 9-6):

1. Primary drug reactions
2. Secondary drug interactions
3. Drug withdrawal syndromes
4. Tertiary extrapharmacologic drug effects

Primary drug reactions. These occur when a *single* medication is responsible for the patient's symptoms. Examples include cimetidine psychosis, NSAID gastritis, ACE inhibitor cough, theophylline-induced seizures, propranolol depression, and digitalis toxicity. Other primary reactions are narcotic-induced respiratory depression, chronic salicylism, and lidocaine psychosis.

Secondary drug reactions. These reactions result from the *interaction* between two medications, with one causing an increased plasma level of the other drug. Examples include the interaction between first-generation sulfonylurea agents and sulfonamide antibiotics. The sulfonamides impair hepatic metabolism of sulfonylureas, causing elevated plasma levels, which may lead to increased insulin release and hypoglycemia. Salicylates and NSAIDs also can displace first sulfonylureas from serum protein binding sites, causing hyperinsulinemia and hypoglycemia.

Because it is an inhibitor of the P450 cytochrome oxidase system in the liver, cimetidine has the potential for increasing the plasma concentration of several important drugs that undergo hepatic metabolism. These drugs include alcohol, lidocaine, phenytoin, aminophylline, benzodiazepines, propranolol, and warfarin. Thus, any elderly patient who is taking cimetidine in addition to one of these medications is at risk for developing a secondary drug interaction.

Erythromycin, clarithromycin, and ciprofloxacin inhibit hepatic breakdown of theophylline compounds, terfenadine, and carbamazepine and, therefore, can cause elevation in blood levels of these drugs.

Drug withdrawal syndromes. In the elderly, drug withdrawal syndromes caused by medications such as phenobarbital and benzodiazepines usually do not differ in their clinical presentations from those seen in younger patients. However, older patients carry an additional risk of drug withdrawal syndromes from such medications such as beta-blockers or other antihypertensives.

Sudden cessation of beta-blockers, for example, can produce angina and rebound hypertension in susceptible elderly patients. In fact, myocardial infarction is precipitated in 2% to 3% of patients when propranolol is abruptly withdrawn, especially in elderly patients at high cardiovascular risk. The proposed mechanism for rebound symptoms is an extended period of beta-receptor supersensitivity to endogenous catecholamine stimulation.

Extrapharmacologic effects. Finally, tertiary extrapharmacologic effects are a consideration for elderly patients taking many medications. One study reports that the elderly have a 50% to 150% increased risk of falling and sustaining a hip fracture when taking cyclic antidepressants, long-acting anxiolytics, or antipsychotic medications.[43]

Table 9-5

Evaluation of Drug Toxicity in the Elderly
TOXIC/THERAPEUTIC RATIO:
A time-honored concept that is valuable primarily when measuring dose-related adverse effects of a single drug in a patient with uncomplicated disease pattern.
INTERDRUG TOXICITY:
An important concept in the elderly, in whom there is a ninefold increase in adverse drug toxicity with consumption of four or more drugs.
EXTRAPHARMACOLOGIC TOXICITY:
Tertiary clinical pathology (falls, hip fractures) not included in classic categories of drug toxicity and measurable only through large-scale epidemiologic surveys; not included as "adverse" drug reaction in package insert (i.e., propensity to cause falling)

Table 9-6

Types of Adverse Drug Reactions in the Elderly
PRIMARY DRUG REACTIONS
(One drug—one side effect) • Cimetidine psychosis • Narcotic-induced respiratory depression • Lidocaine psychosis • Theophylline seizures • Insulin reaction • Chronic salicylism
SECONDARY DRUG INTERACTIONS
(Requires at least two drugs to cause interaction) • Sulfonylurea/sulfonamide • Cimetidine/lidocaine • Erythromycin/theophylline • Statin/gemfibrozil • Tricyclic antidepressant/alpha-sympatholytic
DRUG WITHDRAWAL SYNDROMES
(Addictive and nonaddictive withdrawal) • Beta-blocker withdrawal (angina) • Withdrawal syndromes (benzodiazepines, narcotics,etc.)
TERTIARY "EXTRAPHARMACOLOGIC" EFFECTS
(Measurable only by epidemiologic studies) • Falls caused by tricyclics, anxiolytics, and antipsychotics (short half-life versus long half-life agents) • Traumatic injuries caused by drug-induced orthostatic hypotension

GENERAL PRINCIPLES AND PATIENT EVALUATION

Clinical manifestations of drug toxicity may be particularly subtle in the elderly (Tables 9-7 and 9-8). In the case of digoxin or insulin toxicity, the nature of the drug reaction can frequently be diagnosed from the history, physical examination, and laboratory results alone. However, when a drug reaction produces a minimal alteration in mental status or mood, fatigue, focal neurologic lesion, coma, seizure disorder, cardiac arrest, myopathy, or nonspecific symptom complex, the diagnosis may be much more difficult. In such cases, if the clinician does not use a systematic approach to drug evaluation, the drug reaction may go undiagnosed and untreated.

A British study of nearly 2000 geriatric patients admitted to the hospital examined the drugs most often associated with adverse reactions.[44] Diuretics were responsible for the greatest absolute number of side effects, but they were also the most frequently used medications. Drug groups with the highest risk of adverse reactions were antihypertensives and antiparkinsonian drugs (13%), diuretics (11%), psychotropic drugs (12%), and digitalis (11.5%). Smaller studies in both the extended care and home settings have confirmed these findings.

Table 9-7

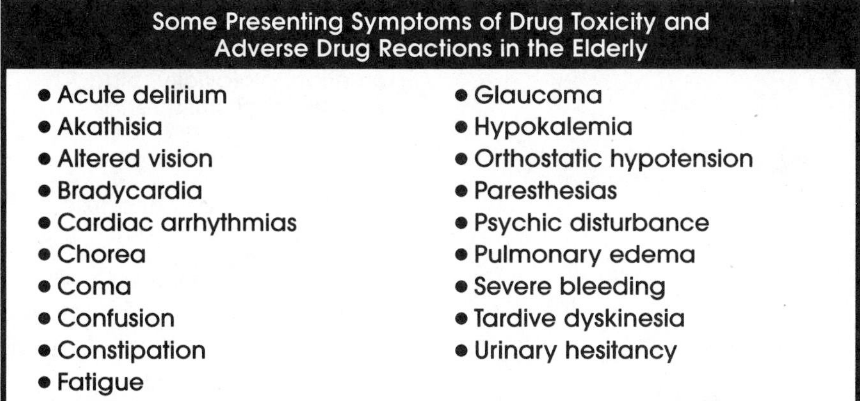

Some Presenting Symptoms of Drug Toxicity and Adverse Drug Reactions in the Elderly	
• Acute delirium	• Glaucoma
• Akathisia	• Hypokalemia
• Altered vision	• Orthostatic hypotension
• Bradycardia	• Paresthesias
• Cardiac arrhythmias	• Psychic disturbance
• Chorea	• Pulmonary edema
• Coma	• Severe bleeding
• Confusion	• Tardive dyskinesia
• Constipation	• Urinary hesitancy
• Fatigue	

To ensure rapid recognition of adverse drug reactions and the institution of appropriate therapy, familiarity with common medications and the ability to assess drug toxicity are essential. Aspirin-containing compounds can lead to chronic salicylism as well as gastritis. Moreover, antihistamines such as diphenhydramine can produce anticholinergic symptoms that may be potentiated by other commonly prescribed medications, such as cyclic antidepressants and antipsychotics. Finally, sympathomimetics such as pseudoephedrine and phenylpropanolamine-containing compounds can precipitate hypertension, angina, or even myocardial infarction.

Table 9-8

Indicators of Possible Toxicity	
Selected Drugs	**Reactions**
DIGITALIS	
	Anorexia, nausea, vomiting, arrhythmias, blurred vision, other visual disturbances (colored halos around objects).
FUROSEMIDE (LASIX)	
	Severe electrolyte imbalance, impaired hearing and/or balance (ototoxicity), hepatic changes, pancreatitis, leukopenia, thrombocytopenia.

Table 9-8

Indicators of Possible Toxicity — cont'd.	
Selected Drugs	**Reactions**
NSAIDS	
	Nephrotic syndrome, fluid retention, ototoxicity, blood dyscrasias, gastritis, renal toxicity.
LITHIUM	
	Diarrhea, drowsiness, anorexia, vomiting, slurred speech, tremors, blurred vision, unsteadiness, polyuria, seizures.
METHYLDOPA	
	Hepatic changes, mental depression, nightmares, dyspnea, fever, tachycardia, tremors.
PHENOTHIAZINE TRANQUILIZERS	
	Tachycardia, arrhythmias, dyspnea, hyperthermia, excessive anticholinergic effects.
PROCAINAMIDE	
	Arrhythmias, mental depression, leukopenia, agranulocytosis, thrombocytopenia, joint pain, fever, dyspnea, skin rash.
THEOPHYLLINE	
	Anorexia, nausea, vomiting, GI bleeding, tachycardia, arrhythmias, irritability, insomnia, muscle twitching, seizures.
TRICYCLIC ANTIDEPRESSANTS	
	Arrhythmias, congestive heart failure, seizures, hallucinations, jaundice, hyperthermia, excessive anticholinergic effects.

Alterations in body temperature such as hypothermia are associated with drug-induced hypoglycemia, whereas temperature elevations may be caused by anticholinergic drugs. Elevated blood pressure may reflect abrupt withdrawal from beta-blockers or clonidine. Increases in resting heart rate may indicate not only beta-blocker *withdrawal,* but occult toxicity due to cyclic antidepressants or aminophylline. Profound, symptomatic bradycardia may be the first manifestation of beta-blocker toxicity, which is potentiated by concomitant use of calcium channel blockers such as verapamil or diltiazem.

Hyperventilation, especially when associated with respiratory alkalosis, is a nonspecific finding but may be the first manifestation of chronic salicylism in the elderly patient. An irregular or rapid pulse may reflect digoxin, aminophylline, or cyclic antidepressant toxicity. Neurologic findings, such as nystagmus, may suggest sedative intoxication or phenytoin toxicity, while constricted pupils may reflect opiate intoxication. Wheezing may be the first sign of beta-blocker or salicylate toxicity.

The laboratory exam is invaluable and may reveal metabolic and electrolyte abnormalities associated with drug toxicity. Thiazide and loop diuretics may cause hyponatremia and hypokalemia, the former sometimes severe enough to induce coma and seizures. A decreased serum bicarbonate level may indicate chronic salicylism or anion gap acidosis. Azotemia may reflect not only excessive diuretic use, but also renal failure precipitated by NSAIDs, especially in patients with pre-existing renal disease.

CARDIOVASCULAR MEDICATIONS

Beta-Blockers

Toxicity from beta-blockers primarily affects the cardiovascular and central nervous systems. The most common cardiovascular side effects include hypotension, congestive heart failure, bradycardia, and heart block. The most common respiratory manifestation is bronchoconstriction. Central nervous system alterations include depression, altered mental status, and decreased libido. Hydrophilic agents, such as atenolol, are associated with less CNS toxicity.

A number of medications, including cimetidine, oral contraceptives, furosemide, and hydralazine, increase beta-blocker effects and may produce clinical symptoms. Concomitant use of *intravenous* verapamil and propranolol is contraindicated in patients with CHF because the combination may produce profound hypotension and profound bradycardia.

Cardiovascular Medications: Optimal Use

For a variety of reasons, patients with heart disease frequently require adjustments in their drug regimen. However, dramatic cardiac events, including unstable angina, rebound hypertension, and myocardial infarction, have been described following abrupt cessation of beta-blocking agents such as propranolol.[49] While such events are sufficient to argue persuasively against the abrupt withdrawal of antianginal agents in patients with chronic stable angina, the association and frequency of silent myocardial ischemia from withdrawal is less well studied. The results of one important investigation make it clear that abrupt withdrawal from beta-blocker therapy may result in transient myocardial ischemia *whether or not* patients have angina.[51,52] In fact, the finding of predominantly *silent* ischemia with beta-blocker cessation suggests that *all* patients should be considered at risk for potentially morbid cardiac events when such therapy is abruptly discontinued.

Adverse effects of drugs used to treat high blood pressure require special consideration. A significant percentage of elderly individuals treated with antihypertensive medications show symptoms of sadness, fatigue, apathy, agitation, or insomnia.[60] T Reserpine, propranolol, and methyldopa cause these symptoms most often, but clonidine, guanethidine, and hydralazine are also capable of producing symptoms of mental depression. Other nonantihypertensive agents that can produce similar effects include neuroleptics, tranquilizers, hypnotics, digoxin, antiparkinsonian drugs, anticancer agents, corticosteroids and NSAIDs. Drug interactions also are common (see Table 9-12).

Thiazide diuretics are associated with a number of adverse reactions.[62] They are also among the most commonly prescribed drugs for the elderly. Hypovolemia and postural hypotension, electrolyte imbalances (hyponatremia, hypercalcemia, and hypokalemia), glucose intolerance, and hyperuricemia are the most common adverse reactions (Table 9-9).

Table 9-9

Side Effects of Commonly Used Diuretics

Diuretic	Thiazide	Loop Diuretic	Potassium-sparing
Hypokalemia	+	+	–
Hyperkalemia	–	–	+
Acidosis	–	–	+
Alkalosis	+	+	–
Hyperuricema	+	+	–
Hypercalcemia	+	+	–
Hyperglycemia	+	+	–
Hypertriglyceridemia	+	+	–
Hyponatremia	+	+	–
Hypomagnesemia	+	+	+

Hypokalemia may induce or augment digoxin toxicity, while severe hyponatremia may produce stupor, seizures, and coma. Mild hyperuricemia is common but rarely induces an acute gout attack. Obtaining serum uric acid levels, however, can be helpful when the patient presents with a monarthric arthritis. Finally, loop diuretics can induce urinary retention and symptoms of prostatism in elderly men with gland enlargement. Spironolactone and triamterene may be associated with hyperkalemia in patients with reduced renal failure and in those taking ACE inhibitors.

Clonidine and methyldopa can cause postural hypotension, CNS depression, and sexual dysfunction (Table 9-10). The CNS depression associated with clonidine can decrease mental acuity, causing patients to seem senile or demented in addition to feeling tired or drowsy. Moreover, sudden discontinuation of clonidine can cause a withdrawal syndrome of headache, sweating, and rebound hypertension. Consequently, if a patient on clonidine therapy presents with symptoms of rebound hypertension, insomnia, headache, or arrhythmia, inquire if the patient has discontinued the drug abruptly.

Table 9-10

Potential Adverse Side Effects of Antihypertensive Drugs

	Impotence	Ejaculation difficulties	Decreased libido	Gyneco-mastia
Thiazides	?	–	+	–
Spironolactone	+	–	+	+
Methyldopa	+	+	+	+
Clonidine	+	+	–	+
Propranolol	+	–	+	–
Hydralazine	?	–	–	–
Prazosin	+	–	–	–

Elderly patients may experience sudden syncope after taking the first dose of prazosin or report some combination of dizziness, headache, or lethargy. Usually, these symptoms will subside after 2 or 3 days of therapy. A number of medications can cause orthostatic hypotension (Table 9-11).

Table 9-11

Drugs Causing Orthostatic Hypotension

Benzothiadiazides	Methotrimeprazine
Bretylium	Methyldopa
Captopril	Methysergide
Clonidine	Minoxidil
Cyclic antidepressants	Nifedipine
Furosemide	Nitroglycerin
Guanethidine	Pentolinium
Guanidine	Phenothiazines
Hexamethonium	Phenoxybenzamine
Hydralazine	Prazosin
Iopanoic acid	Procarbazine
Levodopa	Reserpine
Lidocaine	Thiothixene

Table 9-12

Drug Interactions in Antihypertensive Therapy
Diuretics
■ Diuretics can raise lithium blood levels by enhancing proximal tubular reabsorption of lithium ■ NSAIDs, including aspirin, may antagonize antihypertensive and natriuretic effectiveness of diuretics, and perhaps, ACE inhibitors ■ ACE inhibitors magnify potassium-sparing effects of triamterene, amiloride, or spironolactone ■ ACE inhibitors blunt hypokalemia induced by thiazide diuretics
Sympatholytic Agents
■ Guanethidine monosulfate and guanadrel sulfate. Ephedrine and amphetamine displace guanethidine and guanadrel from storage vesicles. Tricyclic antidepressants inhibit uptake of guanethidine and guanadrel into these vesicles. Cocaine may inhibit neuronal pump that actively transports guanethidine and guanadrel into nerve endings. These actions may reduce antihypertensive effects of guanethidine and guanadrel ■ Hypertension can occur with concomitant therapy with phenothiazines or sympathomimetic amines ■ Monoamine oxidase inhibitors may prevent degradation and metabolism of released norepinephrine produced by tyramine-containing foods and may thereby cause hypertension ■ Tricyclic antidepressant drugs may reduce effects of clonidine
Beta-blockers
■ Cimetidine may reduce bioavailability of beta-blockers metabolized primarily by the liver by inducing hepatic oxidative enzymes. Hydralazine, by reducing hepatic blood flow, may increase plasma concentration of beta-blockers ■ Cholesterol-binding resins, i.e., cholestyramine and colestipol, may reduce plasma levels of propranolol hydrochloride ■ Beta-blockers may reduce plasma clearance of drugs metabolized by the liver (e.g., lidocaine, chlorpromazine, warfarin) ■ Combinations of calcium channel blockers and beta-blockers may promote negative inotropic effects on the failing myocardium ■ Combinations of beta-blockers and reserpine may cause marked bradycardia and syncope ■ Nonsteroidal anti-inflammatory drugs, including aspirin, may magnify potassium-retaining effects of ACE inhibitors
Calcium Antagonists
■ Combinations of calcium antagonists with quinidine may induce hypotension, particularly in patients with idiopathic hypertrophic subaortic stenosis ■ Calcium antagonists may induce increase in plasma digoxin levels ■ Cimetidine may increase blood levels of nifedipine

Given the wide variety and proven efficacy of the many available agents, optimal antihypertensive therapy has become less a matter of selecting a drug that adequately controls diastolic and systolic blood pressure than of selecting an agent or regimen that is predictably associated with high patient compliance, a low incidence of adverse drug reactions, minimal interdrug toxicity (see Table 9-12), and preservation of quality of life, including cognitive and sexual function. As better-tolerated agents become available and long-term, large-scale studies on hypertension begin to yield statistically significant morbidity and mortality data, the focus has now shifted to the comparative ability of different antihypertensives to reduce total, cardiac, and stroke morbidity and mortality.

In general, the elderly respond to all available antihypertensive agents. Some trials suggest they may respond to a calcium channel blocker better than to a beta-blocker or an ACE inhibitor, although any one of these classes may be used as monotherapy in the elderly. Since concomitant diseases are prevalent in the elderly, tailoring therapy to these disorders and vigilant anticipation of side effects is the most important part of antihypertensive management. Hypertensive patients with angina may improve with a beta-blocker or a calcium channel blocker. When congestive heart failure accompanies hypertension, patients may benefit from diuretics and/or ACE inhibitors.[61]

Studies show that physicians may find it difficult to evaluate effects of hypertensive therapy on quality of life. Interestingly, patients were found to be only marginally better at assessing their general well-being in a British study of the effects of antihypertensive therapy. The spouse or house mate was the most sensitive indicator of adverse effects on well-being. Failure of the regimen to lower blood pressure must not necessarily be assumed to be a failure of the drug. Compliance must be verified before additional drugs are added to prevent hypotension.

As far as systolic hypertension, it should be noted that the SHEP study provides conclusive evidence, heretofore lacking, that treatment of isolated systolic hypertension (ISH; SBP > 160 mm Hg) can reduce the incidence of stroke in the elderly. The 36% reduction demonstrated in the trial may actually underestimate the true benefit because many subjects initially in the placebo group ultimately received active treatment. Treatment of systolic hypertension can also reduce other cardiovascular morbidity, although to a lesser degree. Some caution must be exercised in extrapolating these results to a less healthy population, since only 1% of all those initially screened for the trial were ultimately enrolled. Many were excluded because of co-existing cardiovascular disease or liver or renal dysfunction, which raises the possibility of significant selection bias.

This SHEP study further debunks numerous *myths* that are still somewhat prevalent regarding hypertension in the elderly: hypertension cannot be safely or effectively treated in the elderly, there are no benefits of therapy, and the elderly population does not tolerate treatment well. Based on this study, all persons older than 60 years of age (including those older than 75 years) with isolated systolic hypertension should be treated to reduce the risk of stroke and other cardiovascular diseases unless the presence of co-existent illness or poor overall functional status makes this unreasonable.[63]

Thromboembolic Prophylaxis

Overall, the stroke rate for patients with chronic atrial fibrillation is about 5% per year. However, this arrhythmia is a heterogeneous disorder, and in certain subgroups, (i.e., the elderly, those with recent myocardial infarction, and those with history of hypertension), the stroke rate is greater than 5% per year. At one time, rheumatic heart disease was the disorder most commonly associated with atrial fibrillation, but currently, nonvalvular heart disease accounts for more than 70% of the cases of atrial fibrillation. Despite the clear association between atrial fibrillation and stroke, the role of long-term anticoagulant therapy or long-term antiplatelet therapy for prevention of thromboembolic cerebral infarction remains unclear.

With its propensity for causing thromboembolic cerebrovascular infarction, atrial fibrillation is a common disease that has the potential for killing and disabling thousands of elderly Americans each year. It should be emphasized that atrial fibrillation has a prevalence of about 2% in the general population and is more common in the elderly, affecting about 5% of persons older than 60 years of age. Clinicians now recognize that chronic atrial fibrillation in older patients with coronary artery disease is a quietly festering but deadly condition. Previously, many physicians chose not to treat it because of the perception that the hemorrhagic risks of anticoagulant therapy would outweigh the benefits.

It now appears that most patients with nonvalvular atrial fibrillation, especially those at high risk for stroke and who are candidates for anticoagulation therapy, will benefit from chronic warfarin therapy. The elderly patient with chronic nonvalvular atrial fibrillation and underlying coronary heart disease is perhaps the most likely to benefit from chronic low-intensity warfarin therapy. If attempts at restoration of normal sinus rhythm have failed or are contraindicated, patients should be started on long-term warfarin therapy, although it should be stressed that the precise benefits and risks of long-term anticoagulation are simply not known.

Monitoring Anticoagulation Therapy. An important empirical observation is that a significant minority of patients who sustained a thromboembolus while taking warfarin had a subtherapeutic PT ratio at the time of their morbid event. This observation stresses the importance of vigilant monitoring of warfarin therapy to prevent morbidity.

Warfarin and Myocardial Infarction. Following a myocardial infarction (MI), reinfarction and stroke are major causes of subsequent morbidity and mortality. Arterial thrombosis (or embolism in the case of stroke) is the primary pathogenic event in each of these, implying that anticoagulant therapy after a MI might be a beneficial prophylactic measure. In the past, high dose warfarin was often used during the postinfarction period, but hemorrhagic complications were common, and studies evaluating this therapy reached conflicting conclusions regarding the risk to benefit ratio. Therefore, routine administration of anticoagulants in the post-infarction period fell out of favor.

At present, routine warfarin therapy cannot be recommended for patients: (l) who have had thrombolytic therapy, a revascularization procedure, or are taking aspirin for secondary prevention of MI; and 2) who have had an inferior, uncomplicated MI, inasmuch as the morbidity and mortality is already so favorable in these groups that the benefits of warfarin therapy may outweigh the risks.

Who then should receive warfarin therapy following MI? Patients who have had a large anterior MI, as well as those at high risk for subsequent complications and increased mortality but who have not been thrombolyzed, revascularized, and are not *already* on aspirin for secondary prevention, can be expected to benefit from warfarin therapy, if this therapy is started within 1 month following acute MI.

Finally, it should be emphasized that some kind of therapy directed at thrombus prevention is essential following MI. Whether aspirin or warfarin is preferable is still a matter of debate, inasmuch as at least one study has shown that 650 mg aspirin is just as effective as warfarin in preventing thrombus formation in high-risk patients.

Thromboembolism and Mechanical Heart Valves

There is general agreement that patients with mechanical heart valves require lifelong anticoagulation therapy with warfarin to reduce the risk of systemic embolization associated with the use of these prostheses. Controversy remains, however, regarding the optimal dosage. The major controversy concerns weighing the potential risk of increased thromboembolic events seen with inadequate anticoagulation against the increased bleeding complications seen with more intensive warfarin therapy. Recent randomized studies of anticoagulation for other medical conditions, such as venous thromboembolism, have shown that less intense anticoagulation therapy was just as effective as, but safer than, the usual recommended dose of warfarin therapy. It is important to determine the efficacy and safety of different anticoagulation regimens in patients with mechanical heart valves.

Long-term anticoagulation therapy is effective in limiting thromboembolic events in many clinical situations, including patients with mechanical heart valves. Such therapy is not benign, however, and can be complicated by potentially serious bleeding episodes. Several studies have demonstrated equal efficacy but greater safety with lower-intensity anticoagulation regimens than previously recommended. It appears prudent for clinicians to strive for an INR of 1.5 when treating patients with mechanical heart valves with oral warfarin. Lower prothrombin ratios (i.e., < 1.5) are likely to be associated with a greater risk of thromboembolic events, while higher ratios are known to cause more bleeding complications.

Aspirin and Transient Ischemic Attacks (TIAs)

Aspirin reduces the risks of vascular death, stroke, and nonfatal MI in patients with a prior stroke or TIA. Dosages ranging from 300 to 1500 mg/day have been used. Such doses diminish platelet adhesiveness by inhibiting thromboxane A2 production. Theoretically, a lower dose of aspirin sufficient to inhibit thromboxane, but not prostacyclin, may be even more effective in preventing vascular complications in high-risk patients. In patients with a history of TIA or ischemic stroke, the annual risk for a serious vascular event is almost 10%. Even a very small dose of aspirin (30 mg/day) effectively reduces the chances of a thrombotic event in high-risk patients, with fewer minor bleeding complications. However, the degree of thrombotic risk reduction equals, but does not exceed, that of a higher-dose regimen. Even at low doses, aspirin retains a potent antiplatelet effect that should be respected. The decision to implement low-dose antiplatelet therapy must still be made with the risk of a hemorrhagic complication in mind. In the future, a low-dose aspirin regimen will probably be the preferred program for prevention of a thrombotic event in high-risk patients because it is equally effective, better tolerated, and associated with a reduction in risk of minor bleeding episodes.

SALICYLATES

More than 200 OTC preparations contain aspirin, which can adversely affect the elderly. Presenting symptoms can include gastritis with gastrointestinal blood loss leading to iron deficiency anemia and peptic ulcer with or without serious hemorrhagic manifestations. The elderly are particularly prone to chronic salicylate intoxication, which presents as tinnitus, confusion, respiratory alkalosis, and noncardiogenic pulmonary edema. Even patients taking therapeutic analgesic doses of salicylates are prone to chronic salicylism. Consequently, any elderly patient who presents with confusion, respiratory alkalosis, and pulmonary edema of unknown etiology should have a salicylate blood level determined. The diagnosis depends on a thorough drug history and elevated blood salicylate level.

Treatment for primary prevention of stroke in high-risk patients has been rather disappointing. Endarterectomies, bypass procedures, and dipyridamole therapy are without proven efficacy. There is no evidence that anticoagulant therapy prevents strokes due to atheromatous cerebrovascular disease, although it is useful for prevention of systemic embolization. Aspirin lowers the risk of stroke in men, but the effect has not been demonstrated convincingly in women.

Ticlopidine is a new antiplatelet agent. Its mode of action is the irreversible inhibition of ADP-dependent platelet aggregation pathways. Unlike aspirin and NSAIDs, it does not impair prostaglandin synthesis and thromboxane production. Ticlopidine is capable of lowering the risk of fatal and nonfatal stroke in high-risk patients and is more effective than aspirin, the only other agent previously shown to have such an effect. However, the risk of severe neutropenia, although infrequent and fully reversible, means that ticlopidine should be used cautiously, with blood counts monitored frequently. Most episodes of neutropenia occurred within 1 to 3 months of onset of therapy. Moreover, diarrhea can be a troublesome side effect. Nonetheless, if prescribed carefully, this agent is a useful and important addition to the limited choices available for stroke prevention in patients unable to take aspirin.

MANAGEMENT OF HYPERCHOLESTEROLEMIA IN THE ELDERLY

Patients over 60 years of age have a higher prevalence of elevated serum cholesterol and coronary heart disease than any other segment of the population, yet no prospective trial has been performed solely to examine the benefits of treating hypercholesterolemia in the elderly. Consequently, the decision to initiate therapy in these patients is often difficult. Furthermore, concern has been raised over the value of the total serum cholesterol level for predicting coronary artery disease in the geriatric population.

Total cholesterol levels generally increase with age. In men, cholesterol rises continuously between the ages of 18 and 55, while in women a large increase in cholesterol occurs at menopause. By the age of 60, these levels reach a plateau, but by this time one third of men and one half of women have total cholesterol levels > 240 mg/dl, and low-density lipoprotein levels > 160 mg/dl. By consensus of the National Cholesterol Education Program, these individuals fall into the high-risk group. The number of elderly candidates for lipid-lowering therapy is, therefore, immense, and policy regarding management has an enormous impact on society.

Several studies have demonstrated diminution in the predictive value of total cholesterol levels with increasing age. In the Framingham Heart Study, the relative risk of developing coronary artery disease for patients younger than 50 years of age with severe hypercholesterolemia was 3.58%; but in similar patients older than 50 years, the risk ratio fell to 2.18%. This is due in part to the increased impact of competing risk factors such as diabetes and hypertension in the elderly, which tend to obscure the relationship between hypercholesterolemia and coronary artery disease. However, in the Multiple Risk Factor Intervention Trial (MRFIT), although the risk ratio declined with age, the attributable risk of coronary artery disease related to hypercholesterolemia actually increased between the ages of 35 and 60 years.

Although definitive, prospective data specific to the elderly are as yet unavailable, the potential benefits of lowering cholesterol may be greater in the elderly than in any other age group. Other studies also have suggested that lipid-lowering therapy in the elderly is effective.[64] For instance, the Lipid Research Clinics Primary Prevention Trial (LRC-PPT) enrolled male patients up to 59 years old and followed them for up to 10 years. It documented substantial reductions of LDL levels with combined dietary and pharmacologic intervention in elderly subjects; there were significant reductions in myocardial infarction, cerebrovascular accidents, and cardiovascular mortality. It is important to note that in this and most other trials, 2 to 3 years of follow-up were necessary before significant benefits became apparent. LDL and HDL levels retain strong relative risk values with advancing age. The inverse correlation between HDL and coronary disease is the most powerful of these relationships. HDL and LDL levels should, therefore, be determined in elderly patients, even in the absence of other risk factors.

Most experts agree that the following three questions emerge that should be answered before embarking on lipid lowering therapy in the elderly. First, does the patient have a reasonable remaining life expectancy? Advanced age alone should not exclude a patient from therapy, but an octogenarian should probably be treated only if the patient is physiologically young, has a history of cardiovascular disease, and is able to enjoy an active lifestyle. Second, does the patient have an acceptable quality of life that would be lost if cardiovascular disease became apparent? The authors suggest that patients with end stage diseases such as crippling rheumatoid arthritis or dementia are unlikely to benefit from aggressive treatment of hypercholesterolemia. Third, can the patient be reasonably expected to comply with therapy? It is often difficult for elderly patients to make major changes in dietary habits, to pay for expensive medications, or to tolerate side effects. The decision to treat hypercholesterolemia in the elderly must be viewed in perspective. Furthermore, since hypertension and diabetes increase morbidity and mortality in the elderly, treatment of these disorders should always accompany treatment of elevated cholesterol levels.

When the decision to institute treatment for hypercholesterolemia is made, dietary modification usually is the first step and should be carried out for at least 6 months before drug therapy is instituted. However, if the patient has had a recent MI or is at high risk for heart disease, medications should be initiated promptly, while lifestyle changes are being implemented. In general, drug treatment should be started with statins as first-line therapy.[65]

Until definitive, prospective data exist regarding the treatment of hypercholesterolemia in the elderly, decisions about such therapy will be difficult to make and are somewhat controversial. It seems reasonable at this point to base decisions about therapy primarily on the levels of LDL and HDL rather than on total serum cholesterol. Age alone should not be an exclusion for any particular treatment regimen in an otherwise healthy elderly individual. As with virtually all disorders in the geriatric population, the physiologic age and functional status of the patient are far more important determinants of the value of therapy than chronologic age.

Nitrate Therapy

The sublingual (nitroglycerin) and oral (isosorbide dinitrate) nitrate preparations are antianginal agents that promote vasodilation of both venous and, to a lesser extent, arterial vascular beds. In the coronary beds, nitrates redistribute blood flow along collateral routes to the underperfused myocardium.

Orthostatic hypotension can occur in the elderly. Tolerance and cross-tolerance between nitrates develops with prolonged usage. Headache occurs early after consumption and with excessive doses. Angina may develop or worsen with sudden withdrawal of nitrates. Sildenafil (Viagra®) should *never* be prescribed in patients who require either intermittent (PRN) or chronic nitrate therapy. The combination of nitrates and Viagra can produce life-threatening hypotension.

Patients inexperienced with nitrates should lie down for the first few doses in case of hypotension, which is usually due to dehydration or excessive preload reduction. The onset of action of nitroglycerin topical ointment takes 20 to 60 minutes, and the transdermal patch takes 40 to 60 minutes. These preparations are adequate for prophylaxis, but their onset of action is too slow for acute angina. Only sublingual nitroglycerin, nasal, or sublingual-chewable isosorbide, with an onset of action of 1 to 3 minutes, should be used for acute anginal attacks.

ESTROGEN AND CARDIOVASCULAR DISEASE IN POSTMENOPAUSAL WOMEN

All postmenopausal women should be considered candidates for ERT. The final decision as to whether estrogen is appropriate should be made by the patient and her physician after weighing all relevant factors. A history of breast cancer or other estrogen-sensitive malignancy is the only true absolute contraindication to estrogen use. Initiating estrogen therapy in women who already have a history of MI may require caution. A history of thromboembolic disease is a common relative contraindication but does not generally preclude therapy. In women who were treated with a hysterectomy, the benefits of ERT generally greatly outweigh the risks because there is obviously no risk of endometrial cancer or the annoying recurrence of menstrual bleeding. (Please see Chapter 2 for a complete discussion of ERT).

In women who still have a uterus, progestins should be added to the regimen to minimize the risk of endometrial cancer. There is no evidence that this combination blunts the beneficial lipid-lowering effects of estrogen. The standard cyclical estrogen/progestin regimen frequently results in withdrawal bleeding, which usually affects long-term compliance. The use of continuous low-dose progesterone along with daily estrogen use can greatly reduce the frequency of bleeding and thereby improve the tolerability of ERT. Unusually heavy or irregular bleeding should be investigated by endometrial biopsy or curettage. Doses greater than 1.25 mg of conjugated estrogen (or its equivalent) per day should be avoided.

Estrogen Replacement Therapy and Risk of Venous Thrombosis

Of special concern is the possible risk of venous or arterial thrombosis in patients receiving ERT. Although epidemiologic data fail to demonstrate an association between ERT and thrombosis, the well-known and documented association between contraceptive estrogens and thrombosis has deterred some practitioners from long-term ERT in women suspected to be at high risk for thrombotic complications.[67]

Characterizing the precise relationship between estrogen use and thrombosis in middle-aged and older women is problematic because idiopathic thrombosis and conditions that predispose to thrombosis are more commonly seen with increasing age, making it difficult to implicate estrogens as independent risk factors for thrombosis. Clearly, this issue must be clarified, and the safety of postmenopausal estrogen use should be well-established before women are encouraged to consider long-term ERT for cardioprotection. In addition, there is some debate as to the best medication for oral estrogen replacement. Although the use of synthetic oral estrogens is discouraged by most experts, these preparations are the most widely used. Additional data regarding their safety would be useful.

A study at the University of California,[67] was conducted to test the association of estrogen with thrombophlebitis in postmenopausal women. The investigators reviewed consecutive hospital admissions of women aged 45 years or older from 1980 through 1987. Cases were defined as all women with a diagnosis of thrombophlebitis, deep venous thromboembolism, or pulmonary embolism. Women were considered current hormone users if they were taking hormones at the time of admission. Two controls per case were identified through a computer search of women aged 45 years or older whose diagnoses did not include one of the thrombotic diagnoses listed above. There were 121 cases and 236 controls identified, with a mean age of 65.4 years (range, 48 to 87). Overall, the three most common nonthrombotic diagnoses were hypertension, diabetes, and coronary artery disease.

Current use of exogenous estrogens was reported by 5.1% of cases and 6.3% of controls. Hormone regimens varied considerably, so that determining an average dose for controls and cases was not possible. Although not statistically significant, several purported risk factors for thrombosis were more prevalent in estrogen users than nonusers. The presence of these factors would tend to increase the incidence of thrombosis, thus strengthening the probability that there was no association demonstrated between estrogen use and thrombosis.

The investigators conclude that although an estrogen-mediated shift toward hypercoagulability would be expected to increase the incidence of thrombosis, this study found no evidence that long-term estrogen therapy was a risk factor for clinically significant venous thrombosis. This study should be reassuring to physicians and patients who are considering the use of ERT but are concerned about the potential for venous or arterial thrombosis.[67]

Although the study finds no increased risk of thrombosis with estrogen use, unfortunately, the investigators were not able to determine the precise dose of estrogen, a central issue in risk-factor analysis. At present, ERT can be prescribed for women at low risk for endometrial carcinoma and for those without a prior risk of thrombotic episodes. In women with a history of thrombotic episodes, lower doses of non-oral estrogen are preferred. Generally, on the basis of current information, postmenopausal estrogen therapy is of proven value and should be prescribed routinely unless contraindicated.[68]

VITAMIN D AND OSTEOPOROTIC FRACTURES IN POSTMENOPAUSAL WOMEN

Osteoporosis is now widely recognized as a major public health problem in the United States that results in significant morbidity and mortality, particularly among postmenopausal women. Estrogen, calcium supplementation, weight-bearing exercise, calcitonin, and diphosphonates such as alendronate (Fosamax) are all effective to varying degrees in preventing or treating osteoporosis. Calcitriol, the physiologically active form of vitamin D, is also considered potentially useful therapy for osteoporosis because of its ability to enhance calcium absorption in the gastrointestinal tract and, at least in vitro, to stimulate bone mineralization.

Three previous studies of calcitriol for osteoporosis produced conflicting results. Two studies showed bone-mass stabilization in patients who received calcitriol, while the third showed no difference from placebo in slowing bone loss. No study showed that calcitriol improved bone formation, and all the trials were too small to evaluate fracture rates. The criteria for efficacy and the numbers of patients in these studies were all different, making it difficult to draw definite conclusions about the benefits of calcitriol.

Investigators at the University of Otago in New Zealand performed a prospective, randomized trial of the effects of calcitriol on the development of new vertebral fractures in 622 ambulatory postmenopausal women.[72] All subjects had osteoporosis but no other severe medical problems. None of the women was taking estrogen before or during the study. Subjects were randomized to receive either 0.25 pg calcitriol twice daily or 1 g calcium daily. The subjects and the physicians were aware of the treatment assignment after randomization.

Subjects were observed for 3 years and were assessed periodically regarding routine biochemical and renal function, calcium absorption, and urinary calcium excretion. The major outcome studied was the development of new vertebral fractures. Roentgenograms of the thoracic and lumbar spine were obtained each year. A fracture was defined as the decrease of 15% or more in any 1 year in the anterior or posterior height of the body of any vertebra from T4 through L4.

Treatment with calcitriol for 3 years resulted in a three-fold reduction in the rate of new vertebral fractures as compared with treatment with calcium alone. The effect of calcitriol was evident only during the second and third years of therapy (second-year fracture rate 9.3, versus 25 fractures per 100 patient years; third year, 9.9, versus 31.5 fractures per 100 patient years; $p < 0.001$). The benefit from calcitriol was clear *only* in women with *mild to moderate* osteoporosis, defined as those with five or fewer vertebral fractures at baseline entry into the study. Calcitriol treatment was effective in women with normal calcium absorption as well as those with calcium malabsorption and was not associated with hypercalcemia or other side effects.

Therapy for osteoporosis should be directed toward those at highest risk by taking steps to prevent falls, eliminate smoking and excessive alcohol intake, and to avoid medications known to increase bone loss, such as corticosteroids and high doses of thyroid hormone. Moderate degrees of weight-bearing exercise and calcium supplementation are prudent and helpful for most individuals. ERT is effective in reducing bone loss and fractures even in older women and exerts benefits on the cardiovascular system as well. Calcitonin is effective in preserving bone mass, but it must be given by injection and is expensive. Etidronate improves spinal bone mass and prevents spinal fractures.

Based on this trial, calcitriol should potentially be considered for treating patients with osteoporosis. Further studies are required to define its exact role. Until then, its use is most appropriate in high-risk individuals, without severe osteoporosis and multiple fractures. For instance, those with inadequate calcium intake, evidence of calcium malabsorption, or limited sun exposure may be particularly appropriate candidates for vitamin D supplementation. Close monitoring of serum and urine calcium levels and renal function is essential during therapy with calcitriol. Therapy should be prolonged because it appears that no benefit accrues until after at least several years of treatment.

Pharmacotherapy and Impotence: The Clinical Decision Tree

There has been debate, discussion, guidelines-generation, misinformation, and confusion about the safety of sildenafil (Viagra®) therapy for the treatment of male impotence in the elderly population. Concerns about the safety of this pharmacological agent have been generated largely by case reports submitted to the FDA by physicians and the manufacturer regarding patients who died while taking sildenafil and/or participating in sexual activity. Although a number of these cases seem to have been caused by the interaction between sildenafil and nitrates, which must *never* be used in combination under any circumstances, in other cases, they were not. Most of the deaths occurred in elderly individuals in their 60s, 70s, and 80s, and, because a number of these individuals had a history of heart disease, it is postulated that many of them may have suffered acute coronary or cerebrovascular ischemic events precipitated by excessive physical activity that frequently accompanies sexual activity.

After reviewing these cases (at the time of this book's printing, about 103 cases had been documented) the FDA panel monitoring sildenafil has continued to rule that this drug for male impotence is safe and effective if used appropriately in eligible patient populations. Prudent use includes individuals who: (1) are suitable candidates for the drug on the basis of demonstrating a clinical indication for its use; (2) are appropriately screened to ensure they are not at risk for incurring potential harmful drug-drug or drug-disease interactions; and (3) are evaluated for their suitability (i.e., exercise capacity and lack of contraindications) for participating in sex-related activity. This assessment requires a complete history and discussion that should document past, current, and anticipated levels of aerobic expenditure required to participate in sex-related exertion. It is less the safety of the impotence drug that requires consideration, than it is the safety of participating in the *activity* (i.e., sex) that the drug is facilitating in a group of potentially older individuals with limited cardiac reserve or neurovascular conditions that place them at risk for strenuous physical activity.

Moreover, it should be stressed that, on a statistical basis, it is very difficult, given the widespread use of sildenafil, to determine conclusively whether the reported deaths were related to the medication, or whether they reflected *expected* mortality patterns in older individuals with cardiac or neurovascular disease, who may have succumbed as a result of excessive aerobic demands triggered by "sexual exercise."

In any event, because of the sildenafil's proven effectiveness in the treatment of psychogenic and organic impotence, and because of its growing use within a potential target group of 30 million U.S. men who may have some degree of erectile dysfunction, it is important to develop guidelines for its use. These guidelines should be designed to minimize any possible risks associated with this and other effective pharmacological approaches to the treatment of male impotence. As simple as it may sound, the most important aspect of determining the appropriateness of sildenafil therapy is, "common sense." By this is meant the understanding that, perhaps, the most critical decision that must be made when clinicians are contemplating the use of sildenafil is whether or not engaging in *sex is safe for the patient.*

Generally speaking, the physician should determine if the patient can have safe sex (as predicted by the patient's exercise capacity, documentation of current or recent participation in sexual activity without adverse consequences). Sexual activity must be seen as a strenuous exercise program. As such, sex may not be suitable for all individuals; and when participation in *sex* is not deemed to be safe for the patient with erectile dysfunction, then the introduction of any medication or device—regardness of its pharmacological or mechanical properties—is not in the patient's best interest.

Sexual stress testing is not an established procedure for evaluating cardiovascular reserve, and therefore, medications or devices that facilitate unsupervised "sexual stress testing" should not be introduced into treatment regimen until it is considered safe for the patient to participate in these activities. A number of conditions may exclude a patient from being "fit enough" to participate in vigorous sexual activity. These conditions include, but are not limited to angina, severe coronary heart disease, cardiac arrhythmias, congestive heart failure, and neurovascular disease.

Accordingly, identifying patients who can have sex safely is a high priority, since those who *can* will generally be suitable candidates for drug treatment of erectile dysfunction. In order to accomplish this, the physician and/or the pharmacist should ask patients in whom sildenafil is being considered a few basic, but important, questions: "What is your general state of health?" "What is your pattern of recent sexual activity?" If the patient has not had sex for 10 years and he is 70 years old, then the individual has to be evaluated for his cardiovascular suitability for embarking upon a sexual exercise resumption program. On the other hand, if a 70-year old individual has been having sex without exercise-related complications, has demonstrated the aerobic capacity and the cardiac capacity to have sex at that age, and manifests erectile dysfunction (and there are no contraindications in terms of drug interaction issues), this patient may be a suitable candidate for pharmacotherapy aimed at treatment of erectile dysfunction.

If a patient with erectile dysfunction has *not* been sexually *or* physically active for many years, and he is in an age group at risk for coronary heart disease, the use of drug therapy to facilitate the patient's escalation to a new level of aerobic exercise capacity that is not part of their normal pattern is unwise. There are important questions that can be asked: Do you regularly exericse? Can you play 18 holes of golf? Can you walk up two flights of stairs? Can you carry the groceries up the steps? Do you run on a treadmill? Do you play tennis? Do you have sexual activity? If the physician can document that the patient is participating in aerobic/exercise activities that are equivalent in energy expenditure to those of having strenuous sex, then the patient is likely a very reasonable candidate for sildenafil therapy.

Once suitability for sexual activity is established and clinical indications for drug treatment of erectile dysfunction are satisfied, what other parameters require evaluation prior to initiation of sildenafil therapy? What are the absolute contraindications to sildenafil? The answer is, patients who are on nitrates or have a medical condition that has any reasonable chance of requiring nitrate therapy should be not treated with sildenafil. Put simply, nitrates and sildenafil do not belong in the "same medicine cabinet," and therefore, patients with conditions (angina) that currently or are likely to require nitrate-based intervention are not appropriate candidates for sildenafil treatment of erectile dysfunction.

What about intermittent, chronic stable angina? The answer is, "No." Although there are some patients who have angina that only rarely requires nitrate therapy, safety would say that because anyone with angina may encounter a time when they are going to need nitrate therapy—perhaps during the stress of sexual activity, or upon arrival in the emergency department with unstable angina or myocardial infarction—the more prudent approach is not to use sildenafil in patients who have angina. If they want to have sex, they can have sex. But not with sildenafil, since this drug and nitrates should be prevented from crossing the road at the same time.

If these guidelines are followed, and clinicians use common sense and take a comprehensive exercise, drug, coronary, and neurovascular history, drug-based approaches for treating male impotence will improve the quality of life for up to 30 million Americans.

PROSTATIC HYPERTROPHY

Benign prostatic hypertrophy (BPH) is an extremely common condition among elderly men. Accordingly, transurethral resection of the prostate (TURP), the mainstay of therapy for symptomatic BPH, is one of the most frequently performed surgeries in the elderly population. For years, medical alternatives for the treatment of BPH were sought but remained limited. Because of the rich alpha-adrenergic innervation of the smooth muscles in the prostate and the bladder neck, medical therapy directed at blockade of these receptors, resulting in smooth muscle relaxation, relieves symptoms of prostatism. This was the basis of the treatment of BPH with phenoxybenzamine, a pure alpha blocker, which although somewhat effective, had unacceptable side effects making clinical use impractical. Terazosin and doxazosin are approved as useful and safe options for medical therapy of BPH. Although transurethral resection remains the definitive treatment for this disorder, patients with mild to moderate prostatism and those who are poor surgical candidates or wish to avoid surgery should be considered for medical therapy to relieve symptoms.

Doxazosin and terazosin (and probably other $alpha_1$ blockers) provide symptomatic relief without significant side effects in approximately one half of these individuals. If improvement is to occur, it is generally present by 2 months after starting therapy; if no benefit is noted during this period, the medication should be stopped.

[1]Ahronheim J. Practical pharmacology for older patients: avoiding adverse drug effects. Mt Sinai J Med 1993 Nov;60(6):497-501.

[2]Canadian Medical Association. Medication use and the elderly. Can Med Assoc J 1993 Oct 15; 149(8):1152A-D.

[3]Hallas J, Worm J, Beck-Nielsen J, Gram LF, Grodum E, Damsbo N, Brosen K. Drug related events and drug utilization in patients admitted to a geriatric hospital department. Dan Med Bull 1991 Oct;38(5):417-20.

[4]Lamy PP. Comparative pharmacokinetic changes and drug therapy in an older population. J Am Geriatr Soc 1982;30:S11-9.

[5]Delafuente JC. Perspectives on geriatric pharmacotherapy. Pharmacotherapy 1991;11(3):222-4.

[6]Greenblatt DJ, Sellers EM, Shader RI. Drug therapy: drug disposition in old age. N Eng J Med 1982;306(18):1081.

[7]Hutchinson TA, et al. Frequency, severity, and risk factors for adverse drug reactions in adult outpatients: prospective study. J Chronic Diseases 1986;39(7):533.

[8]Kernan WN, Castellsague J, Perlman GD, Ostfeld A. Incidence of hospitalization for digitalis toxicity among elderly Americans. Am J Med 1994 May;96(5):426.

[9]Lamy PP. Drug therapy in the elderly. Pharmacy International 1986;7:46.

[10]Lamy PP. Geriatric pharmacology. Geriatrics 1986;36(12):41-49.

[11]Lamy PP. Medication management. Clin Geriatr Med 1984;4:623-638.

[12]U.S. Department of Health and Human Services Guidelines for the study of drugs likely to be used in the elderly. Rockville, Md: FDA, Center for Drug Evaluation and Research, 1989.

[13]World Health Organizations. Health care in the elderly: report of the technical group on the use of medications in the elderly. Drugs 22:279.

[14]Michocki RJ, Lamy PP, Hooper FJ, Richardson JP. Drug prescribing for the elderly [see comments] [Review]. Arch Fam Med 1993 Apr;2(4):441-4.

[15]Lamy PP. Prescribing for the Elderly. Littleton, Mass: PSG Publishing, Inc., 1980.

[16]Leach S, Roy SS. Adverse drug reactions: an investigation on an acute geriatric ward. Age Ageing 1986;15:241.

[17]Fletcher A, Bulpitt C. Quality of life and antihypertensive drugs in the elderly [Review]. Aging (Milano) 1992 Jun;4(2):115-23.

[18]Hall RCW, et al. Anticholinergic delirium: etiology, presentation, diagnosis, and management. J Psychedelic Drugs 1978;10:237.

[19]Pollow RL, Stoller EP, Forster LE, Duniho TS. Drug combinations and potential for risk of adverse drug reaction among community-dwelling elderly. Nurs Res 1994 Jan-Feb;43(1):44-9.

[20]Christopher CD. The role of the pharmacist in a geriatric nursing home: a literature review. Drug Intell Clin Pharm 1984;18:428-33.

[21]Darnell JC, et al. Medication used by ambulatory elderly: an inhome survey. J Am Geriatr Soc 1986;34:1.

[22]Larson EB, Kukull WA, Buchner D, et al. Adverse drug reactions associated with global cognitive impairment in elderly persons. Ann Intern Med 1987;107:169-73.

[23]Craft JC, Siepman N. Overview of the safety profile of clarithromycin suspension in pediatric patients. Pediatr Infect Dis J (12 Suppl 3):S142-7.

[24]Knapp DA, et al. Drug prescribing for ambulatory patients 85 years of age and older. J Am Geriatr Soc 1984;32(2):138.

[25]Wilcox SM, Himmelstein DU, Woolhander S. Inappropriate drug prescribing for the community-dwelling elderly. JAMA 1994 July 27;272(4):292-6.

[26]Shrimp LA, et al. Potential medication-related problems in noninstitionalized elderly. Drug Intell Clin Pharm 1985;19:766.

[27]Williamson J, Chopin JM. Adverse reactions to prescribed drugs in the elderly: a multicenter investigation. Age Ageing 1980;9:73.

[28]American College of Physicians. Improving medical education in therapeutics. Ann Intern Med 1988;108:145-147.

[29]Newton PF, Levinson W, Maslen D. The geriatric medication algorithm: a pilot study. J Gen Intern Med 1994 Mar;9(3):164-7.

[30]Symposium: managing medication in an aging population: physician, pharmacist, and patient perspectives. J Am Geriatr Soc 1985;Supp 30:11.

[31]Vestal R.E. Drug use in the elderly: a review of problems and special considerations. Drugs 1978; 16:358.

[32]Gryfe CI, Gryfe BM. Drug therapy for the aged: the problems of compliance and the roles of physicians and pharmacists. J Am Geriatr Soc 1984;32(4):301.

[33]Hale WE, May FE, Marks RG, Stewart RM. Drug use in an ambulatory elderly population: a five-year update. Drug Intell Clin Pharm 1987;21:530-5.

[34]Helling DK, Lemke LH, Semia TP, et al. Medication use characteristics in the elderly: the Iowa 65+ Rural Health Study. J Am Geriatr Soc 1987;35:4-12.

[35]Report of the Royal College of General Physicians: Medication for the elderly. J R Coll Physicians Lond 1984;18:7.

[36]Sloan RW. Principles of drug therapy in geriatric patients [Review]. Am Fam Phys 1992 June; 45(6):2709-18.

[37]Thomas DR. The brown bag and other approaches to decreasing polypharmacy in the elderly. N C Med J 1991 Nov;52(11):565-6.

[38]Thompson JF, et al. Clinical pharmacists prescribing drug therapy in a geriatric setting: outcome of a trial. J Am Geriatr Soc 1984;32(2):154.

[39]Furguson RP, Wetle T, Dubitzky D, Winsemius D. Relative importance to elderly patients of effectiveness, adverse effects, convenience and cost of antihypertensive medications. A pilot study. Drugs Aging 1994 Jan;4(1):56-62.

[40]Nathan A, Sutters CA. A comparison of community pharmacists' and general practitioners' opinions on rational prescribing, formularies and other prescribing-related issues. J R Soc Health 1993 Dec;113(6):302-7.

[41]Gosney M, Tallis RL. Prescription of contraindicated and interacting drugs in elderly patients admitted to hospital. Lancet 1984;2:564-567.

[42]Jue SG, Vestal RE. Adverse drug reactions in the elderly: a critical review. O'Malley K. Ed. Medicine in Old Age-Clinical Pharmacology and Drug Therapy London, 1985.

[43]Ray WA, Griffin MR, Schaffner W, et al. Psychotropic drug use and the risk of hip fracture. N Engl J Med 1987;316:363.

[44]Montamat SC, Cusak B. Overcoming problems with polypharmacy and drug misuse in the elderly. Clin Geriatr Med 1992 Feb:8(1):143-58.

[45]Hallas J, Worm J, Beck-Nielsen, Gram LF, Grodum E, Damsbo N, Brosen K. Drug related events and drug utilization in patients admitted to a geriatric hospital department. Dan Med Bull 1991 Oct; 38(5):417-20.

[46]Haves LP, Stewart CJ, et al. Timolol side effects and inadvertent overdosing. J Am Geriatr Soc 1989;37:261-2.

[47]Nelson WL, Fraunfelder FT, et al. Adverse respiratory and cardiovascular events attributed to timolol ophthalmic solution, 1978-1985. Am J Ophthalmol 1986;102:606-11.

[48]Diggory P, Heyworth P, Chau G, McKenzie S, Sharma A. Unsuspected bronchospasm in association with topical timolol—a common problem in elderly people: can we easily identify those affected and do cardioselective agents lead to improvement? Age Ageing 1994 Jan;23(1):17-21.

[49]Psaty BM, Koepsell TD, et al. The relative risk of incident coronary heart disease associated with recently stopping the use of B-blockers. JAMA 1990; 263.

[50]Vidt DG, Borazanian RA. Calcium channel blockers in geriatric hypertension [Review]. Geriatrics 1991 Jan;46(1):28-30, 33-4, 36-8.

[51]Schwartz JS, Abernethy DR. Cardiac drugs: adjusting their use in aging patients. Geriatrics 1987; 42(8):31.

[52]Held PH, Yusuf S, Furberg CD. Calcium channel blockers in acute myocardial infarction and unstable angina: an overivew. BMJ 1989;299:1187-1192.

[53]Tonkin A, Wing L. Aging and susceptibility to drug-induced orthostatic hypotension. Clin Pharmacol Ther 1992 Sept;52(3):277-85.

[54]O'Malley K, Cox JP, O'Brien E. Choice of drug treament for elderly hypertensive patients [Review]. Am J Med 1991 Mar;90(3A):27S-33S.

[55]Nestico PF, Morganroth J. Cardiac arrhythmias in the elderly: antiarrhythmic drug treatment. Cardiol Clin; 4(2):285-303. 199866

[56]Hine LK, Laird NM, et al. Meta-analysis of empirical long-term antiarrhythmic therapy after myocardial infarction. JAMA 1989;262:3037-40.

[57]Morganroth J. Bigger JT Jr, Anderson JL. Treatment of ventricular arrhythmias by United States cardiologists: a survey before the Cardiac Arrhythmia Suppression Trial results were available. Am J Cardiolog 1994 Feb;23(2):283-9.

[58]Peters RW, Mitchell LB, Brooks MM, Echt DS, Barker AH, Capone R, Liebson PR, Greene HL. Circadian pattern of arrhythmic death in patients receiving encainide, flecainide or moricizine in the Cardiac Arrhythmia Suppression Trial (CAST). J Am Coll Cardiol 1994 Feb;23(2):283-9.

[59]Willund I, Gorkin L, Pawitan Y, Schron E, Schoenberger J, Jared LL, Shumaker S. Methods for assessing quality of life in the cardiac arrhythmia suppression trial (CAST). Qual Life Res 1992 Jun;1(3):187-201.

[60]Burris JF. Hypertension management in the elderly [Review]. Heart Disease Stroke 1994 Mar-Apr; 3(2):77-83.

[61]Flack JM, Wolley A, Esunge P, Grimm RH. A rational approach to hypertension treatment in the older patient [Review]. Geriatrics 1992 Nov;47(11):24-8,33-8.

[62]Warram JH, Laffel LMB, et al. Excess mortality associated with diuretic therapy in diabetes mellitus. Arch Intern Med 1991;151:1350-6.

[63]SHEP Cooperative Research Group. Prevention of stroke by antihypertensive drug treatment in older persons with isolated systolic hypertension. JAMA 1991;265:3255-65.

[64]Lewis B, et al. On lowering lipids in the post-infarction patients. J Intern Med 1991;229:483-8.

[65]Denke MA, Grundy SM. Hypercholesterolemia in the elderly: resolving the treatment dilemma. Ann Intern Med 1990;112:780-92.

[66]Stampfer MJ, et al. Postmenopausal estrogen therapy and cardiovascular disease. N Engl J Med 1991;325:11.

[67]Devor M, Barrett-Connor E, et al. Estrogen replacement therapy and risk of venous thrombosis. Am J Med 1992;92:271-82.

[68]Falkeborn M, et al. Hormone replacement therapy and the risk of stroke. Arch Intern Med 1993;153:1201-9.

[69]Tilyard MW, et al. Treatment of postmenopausal osteoporosis with calcitriol or calcium. N Engl J Med 1992;326(6):33357-362.

[70]Prince RL, Smith M, Dick IM, et al. Prevention of postmenopausal osteoporosis: A comparative study of exercise, calcium supplementation, and hormone replacement therapy. N Engl J Med 1991;325:1189-95.

[71]Dawson-Hughes B, Dallal GE, Krall EA, et al. Effect of vitamin D supplementation on wintertime and overall bone loss in healthy postmenopausal women. Ann Intern Med 1991;115:505-12.

[72]Aloia JF, Vaswani A, Yeh JK, et al. Calcium supplementation with and without hormone replacement therapy to prevent postmenopausal bone loss. Ann Intern Med 1994;120:97.

10

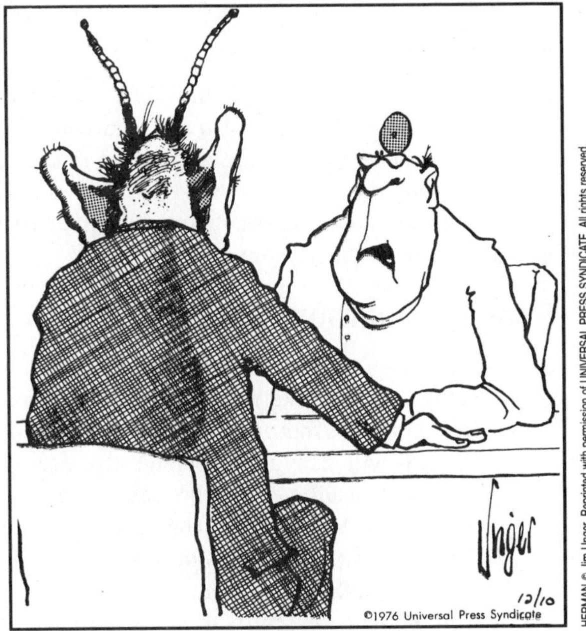

"If you remember, I did mention possible side-effects."

Pharmatectural Strategies for Psychiatric, Arthritic, Pulmonary, and Gastrointestinal Drug Therapy in the Elderly

Nonsteroidal anti-inflammatory drugs (NSAIDs) (See Table 10-1) including aspirin, are among the most important causes of drug-related morbidity and mortality in the elderly. Important forms of toxicity include gastritis, peptic ulceration, and renal insufficiency.[2,3,4,5] Aspirin has an *irreversible* effect on platelet function that lasts for the life of the platelet (4 to 7 days). NSAIDs also can cause allergic reactions, ranging from rash to anaphylaxis in patients allergic to aspirin.[6] Chronic consumption of aspirin, even in recommended amounts, may lead to chronic salicylism, which is characterized by deafness, marked fatigue, confused and withdrawn behavior, metabolic acidosis, and noncardiogenic pulmonary edema.[7] CNS effects include dizziness, anxiety, tinnitus, and confusion, which may occur in up to 10% to 20% of the elderly on chronic salicylate therapy.

Hepatic reactions are usually mild when they occur, but severe hepatitis has been reported. Aplastic anemia is also reported with NSAIDs.

Women older than 65 are at greatest risk of gastrointestinal bleeding and gastric perforation associated with NSAIDs.[8] A history of gastrointestinal bleeding and concomitant diuretic therapy are the two risk factors identified in this group of patients that predict poor outcome.

Renal Impairment Associated with NSAIDs

A review of elderly patients on Medicaid with diagnoses of nephritis, nephropathy, and hyperkalemia showed a strong correlation with NSAID use. Three distinct renal syndromes are now associated with NSAIDs.[9]

1. Patients with dehydration, congestive heart failure, nephrosis, or preexisting renal insufficiency who develop acute renal failure within days of starting NSAID therapy. The urine sediment is normal.
2. Acute interstitial nephritis may occur at any time but usually presents after months of NSAID exposure. There is no eosinophilia, eosinophiluria, or rash. Patients present with the nephrotic syndrome (usually edematous).
3. Chronic interstitial nephritis is associated with high-dose NSAID therapy and other analgesics. Papillary necrosis is frequently present.

Table 10-1

Current NSAIDs
Aspirin
Diclofenac
Diflunisal (Dolobid)
Etodolac
Fenoprofen (Nalfon)
Flurbiprofen
Ibuprofen
Indomethacin (Indocin)
Ketoprofen (Orudis)
Ketoralac
Meclofenamic acid (Ponstel)
Mefenamic Acid
Nabumetone
Naproxen (Naprosyn)
Oxaprozin
Piroxicam (Feldene)
Sulindac (Clinoril)
Tolmetin (Tolectin)

Numerous clinical studies have raised questions regarding the overall safety of ibuprofen and other NSAIDs with respect to renal toxicity.[9] Based on acute interventional studies, patients at unusually high risk for NSAID-associated renal impairment are those with clinical disorders and underlying conditions that depend on renal prostaglandin synthesis, such as renal disease, heart failure, cirrhosis, old age, volume depletion, ACE inhibitor therapy, and diuretic use. Despite the lack of well-designed, large-scale investigations, smaller trials have caused some experts to recommend that all elderly patients taking NSAIDs have their renal function closely monitored.

Some authorities, it should be pointed out, are less certain about the evidence linking ibuprofen to renal damage. They emphasize that, in contrast to experimental and interventional studies, previous epidemiologic investigations did not show a major degree of NSAID-associated renal impairment. Critics of these findings, however, note that such studies may have lacked the sensitivity to detect ibuprofen-associated renal impairment, since investigators used a diagnosis of renal disease as opposed to a deterioration in serum creatine or creatinine clearance as the primary criteria for renal impairment from NSAIDs. They also emphasize that other epidemiologic studies of ibuprofen-associated renal impairment may have excluded patients at high risk for adverse toxicity from these agents.

Not surprisingly, the seemingly contradictory findings between acute interventional studies and epidemiologic data have left many clinicians in a quandary as to precisely what the actual risks of adverse renal effects of NSAIDs are and, as a corollary, what the parameters for appropriate patient monitoring should be. Given the widespread use of NSAIDs, it is critical to clarify these issues for the primary care practitioner and pharmacist so that subgroups of patients who might be at increased risk can be identified.

To address the aforementioned issues, investigators from the Indiana University School of Medicine performed a controlled, retrospective cohort study using a computerized medical record system that contained complete patient laboratory and clinical data, diagnoses, and drug prescriptions for patients in a large internal medicine practice.[9] In particular, they studied the medical records of 1908 patients taking ibuprofen for about 15 months, and compared them to 3933 patients from the same practice who were taking acetaminophen for a similar duration of time. They attempted to: (1) determine the incidence of renal impairment in patients taking ibuprofen; (2) identify predictors for the development of renal impairment; (3) determine which univariate predictors are independently predictive of renal impairment and which ones are merely confounders of this event; and (4) determine whether the risk of renal impairment among patients taking ibuprofen differs from that of a control group of patients taking acetaminophen.

Only those patients who had at least one determination of serum creatinine (SCR) and blood urea nitrogen (BUN) within the year preceding the first ibuprofen or acetaminophen prescription date, and at least one SCR and BUN determination within the year following this date were included in the study. Renal impairment was defined according to either SCR or BUN criteria as follows: (1) In patients with a normal initial creatinine level, ibuprofen-associated renal impairment was defined by a post-prescription date determination documenting an increase in SCR >1.2 mg/dl. Serious impairment was defined as a two-fold increase in SCR, or any final SCR value >2.5 mg/dl; (2) patients with an elevated initial SCR (>1.2 mg/dl) were defined as having ibuprofen-associated renal impairment if the post-prescription SCR determination revealed a 10% increase over baseline, while serious impairment was defined as any two-fold increase in SCR; (3) in patients with a normal initial, pre-prescription BUN level, ibuprofen-associated renal impairment was defined as an increase >40 mg/dl; (4) in patients with elevated BUN levels, a 10% increase in BUN was considered indicative of ibuprofen-induced renal impairment, whereas any two-fold increase was defined as serious renal impairment.

Risk Factors. Of the 1,908 patients in the study group, investigators found that renal impairment occurred in 343 patients (18%). Of the 1,658 ibuprofen-treated patients with normal baseline SCR and BUN, 8.6% developed renal impairment, whereas, of the 250 patients with elevated initial renal function parameters, 25.2% developed renal impairment, 0.7% of which could be characterized as serious. Multivariate analyses indicated five independent predictors of renal impairment: age, prior renal insufficiency, coronary artery disease, elevated systolic blood pressure, and diuretic use. Interestingly, when these investigators tested the degree to which ibuprofen contributed to renal impairment by evaluating the control group of 3,933 acetaminophen recipients, they found that neither ibuprofen nor acetaminophen was among the independent predictors of risk when all the patients were considered. Rather, as these researchers carefully note, these risk factors reflect the likelihood of developing renal impairment by general internal medicine patients and are not specific to ibuprofen therapy.

However, multivariate analyses of patients in both study and control groups at high-risk for renal impairment revealed that compared to the acetaminophen recipients, ibuprofen was indeed a risk factor for renal impairment in patients more than 65 years of age (odds ratio, 1.34) and those with a diagnosis of coronary artery disease.

These investigators conclude that within the year following the receipt of a prescription for ibuprofen, patients over the age of 65 years and those with clinically documented coronary artery disease are at greater risk of renal impairment than patients receiving acetaminophen. Because ibuprofen does not appear to contribute to renal impairment in healthier, younger patients, the authors suggest that such individuals do not require special monitoring of renal function. In contrast, however, they note that in the elderly and in patients with known or suspected coronary heart disease, renal monitoring is warranted with long-term ibuprofen therapy.[5]

NSAIDS and Gastrointestinal Hemorrhage

Although NSAIDs are effective in the management of acute and chronic pain syndromes associated with osteoarthritis and other inflammatory musculoskeletal disorders, the propensity of these drugs to cause gastrointestinal side effects remains a significant deterrent to their use, especially in the elderly.[1,4] Fortunately, the incidence of consequential gastrointestinal hemorrhage, defined as the need for hospitalization, or death resulting from ulcer-induced bleeding, is reported to be 1.6% to 1.8% among long-term users of NSAIDs.[10] These data provide some comfort for practitioners who rely on NSAIDs to improve functional status in patients with chronic, debilitating disease. However, the risk of ulceration in the elderly may be higher, with many recent studies reporting a threefold risk or greater for peptic ulcer disease and upper gastrointestinal tract bleeding associated with NSAID use. The problem with most of these studies, however, is that they fail to generate conclusions and guidelines regarding the effect of NSAID drug dose, duration of use, and specific drug therapy on the development of gastrointestinal hemorrhage, ulceration, or both. Clearly, a need exists for a large-scale investigation that would help clinicians identify factors that increase or, conversely, decrease the risk of NSAID-induced toxicity.[2,3]

To address these issues, a group of investigators from Vanderbilt University School of Medicine conducted a case-control study of Tennessee Medicaid enrollees who were 65 years of age or older.[11] The study included 1,415 patients who were hospitalized for confirmed peptic ulcer disease or upper gastrointestinal tract hemorrhage sometime between 1984 and 1986. The 7,063 control persons represented a stratified random sample of other Medicaid enrollees. Subjects with confirmed peptic ulcer disease or hemorrhage were then categorized according to recency of NSAID use, filled prescriptions, dose, and duration of use. The investigators then defined four categories of exposure according to recency of use.

Current users were defined as patients who had filled a prescription before the index date with a supply of the drug that ended on or after the index date. Indeterminate users were defined as those persons whose prescribed supply of NSAIDs ended 1 to 60 days before the index date. Former users were defined as persons who had received a prescription for NSAIDs 365 days before the index date, but whose supply ended more than 60 days before the index date. Nonusers were classified as subjects with no prescription for NSAIDs for 365 days before the index date.

Overall, of those patients hospitalized with peptic ulcer disease, 34% were *current* users of NSAIDs, compared with 13% of control persons, for an estimated relative risk of 4.1 for development of peptic ulcer disease or upper gastrointestinal tract hemorrhage among NSAID users. Current NSAID use was associated with an elevated risk of development of peptic ulcer in each of three diagnostic categories. The risks were 5.5 for gastric ulcer, 4.3 for duodenal ulcer, and 2.4 for upper gastrointestinal tract hemorrhage. Moreover, the risk of developing peptic ulcer disease increased with increasing dose. It appears as if subjects with a short duration of exposure to the NSAID were at increased risk for developing peptic ulcer disease (i.e., that risk for NSAID-induced complications was greater during the first month of therapy).

Relative Risks. Although the design of this study did not permit investigators to monitor compliance associated with specific NSAIDs, they attempted to compare risks for peptic ulcer disease among current users of specific agents. The relative risks of current users of naproxen, piroxicam, tolmetin, and meclofenamate were significantly greater than those of current users of ibuprofen.

These investigators conclude that current elderly users of prescription nonaspirin NSAIDs are about four times more likely to be hospitalized for confirmed peptic ulcer disease or upper gastrointestinal tract hemorrhage than a control group not on NSAID therapy.

The authors note that the finding of reduced risk among ibuprofen users must be interpreted cautiously because: (l) the lower risk associated with this drug might have resulted from poorer compliance associated with agents given on a three or four times daily basis, as opposed to other NSAIDs (piroxicam, sulindac, etc.), which are given once or twice daily; (2) the 1200 mg standard daily dose of ibuprofen used in this study is, in fact, much lower than the dosage rate customarily used by most practitioners to achieve anti-inflammatory effects and substantial improvements in functional capacity (i.e., 1600 to 2400 mg of ibuprofen daily); and (3) the 1200 mg standard daily dose of ibuprofen used as a benchmark in this study probably does not have the same anti-inflammatory activity or therapeutic efficacy as do the other agents evaluated at their recommended daily dose. As a result of these clinically important dose- and compliance-dependent limitations and variations, interdrug comparisons, especially as they relate to the propensity of therapeutically equivalent doses of NSAIDs to cause peptic ulcer pathology, cannot be fully substantiated from the results reported in this study.

Prescribing Guidelines. This study provides further confirmatory evidence that non-aspirin prescription NSAID use is associated with an increased risk of developing peptic ulcer disease, upper gastrointestinal tract disease, or both, in patients 65 years of age or older. This is not new information. What this study reports, however, that *is* new and clinically useful is: (1) the significant association between increasing dose of NSAIDs and the risk of developing peptic ulcer disease and complications requiring hospitalization; and (2) the finding that the greatest risk for developing NSAID-induced complications is observed during the first 30 days of drug therapy. Based on these findings, prescribers are advised to use the lowest dose of NSAID possible to achieve acceptable functional status and pain control in patients with osteoarthritic disorders. It should be emphasized, however, that achieving an adequate clinical response at the standardized recommended dose of ibuprofen (1200 mg) cited in this study will not be possible in a significant percentage of cases, and that higher and, therefore, potentially more toxic doses of ibuprofen may be required. Moreover, given the increased risk observed early in the course of NSAID therapy, patients should be followed very carefully, especially during the first month of NSAID therapy. The presence of gastrointestinal complaints, weakness, melena, or other symptoms referable to the gastrointestinal or cardiovascular system necessitate immediate follow-up. Stool guaiac monitoring is strongly recommended in older patients using NSAIDs.

Elderly patients at risk of renal failure or GI bleeding need to be advised of these risks when taking ibuprofen. If at all possible, NSAID use should be reserved for acute inflammation associated with rheumatoid arthritis or osteoarthritis. GI blood loss is usually minimal even in predisposed patients during the first 7 to 10 days unless an active ulcer is present. After the acute flare, NSAIDs should be withdrawn in favor of acetaminophen for chronic pain control. Hypertensive patients should be advised that OTC ibuprofen and all NSAIDs may elevate blood pressure. Patients should be warned to stop NSAID use if they become weak or dizzy or develop diarrhea, vomiting, or loss of appetite.

Misoprostol for Preventing NSAID Gastropathy

Nonsteroidal anti-inflammatory drugs (NSAIDs) continue to be among the most widely prescribed medications in ambulatory populations for a variety of rheumatologic and pain disorders. The chronic use of NSAIDs is also associated with an increased frequency of peptic ulcers and ulcer complications, including bleeding and perforation. Although endoscopically confirmed upper gastointestinal ulcers have been estimated to occur in between 15-31% of chronic NSAID users, the incidence of clinically significant ulcers is certainly less than this although not exactly defined. The morbidity, mortality and overall costs of NSAID induced gastrointestinal problems are quite substantial and have led to efforts to use other agents to help prevent or lessen their severity. H_2 receptor antagonists such as ranitidine (Zantac®) have been shown to inhibit the development of duodenal ulcers in NSAID users but neither these agents nor sucralfate (Carafate®) are useful in reducing the incidence of NSAID induced gastric ulcers. Misoprostol (Cytotec®), a synthetic prostaglandin analog, affords significant protection against NSAID-induced gastropathy. This has been documented in terms of both reduced endoscopic lesions as well as fewer clinically significant ulcers and upper gastrointestinal bleeding episodes in *high risk individuals.*

Studies confirm that misoprostol reduces the risk of clinically serious UGI complications in patients taking NSAIDs.[62-64] *Routine use* of misoprostol in all patients taking NSAIDs cannot be recommended, however, because of its expense and frequent side effects. A more practical approach for misoprostol use, therefore, is to stop NSAIDs in high risk individuals, and whenever possible, target misoprostol mainly for individuals at high risk for serious UGI complications.

Table 10-2

Pharmacologic and Pharmacokinetic Activity of Sulfonylurea Agents

Generic name	Brand	Daily dose range (mg)	Duration of effect (hr)	Elimination of half-life (hr)
Tolbutamide	Orinase	500-3,000	6-12	4-5
Tolazamide	Tolinase	100-750	10-16	7
Acetohexamide	Dymelor	500-1,500	12-24	5
Chlorpropamide	Diabinese	100-500	24-60	35
Glyburide	Micronase	2.5-20	24	10
Glipizide	Glucotrol	2.4-50	24	2-4

Table 10-3

Sedative-Hypnotic and Anxiolytic Drugs in the Elderly

Drug	FDA approved	Half-life (hr)	Usual initial dose for the elderly	Brand
Flurazepam	Hypnotic	50-100 (major metabolite)	15 mg at bedtime	Datmane
Temazepam	Hypnotic	5-15	15 mg at bedtime	Restoril
Oxazepam	Anxiolytic	5-20	10 mg three times a day	Serax
Diazepam	Anxiolytic	20-100 (major metabolite)	2 mg per day or twice a day	Valium
Lorazepam	Anxiolytic	10-20	0.5-2 mg/day	Ativan
Triazolam	Hypnotic	2,3	0.125 mg or 0.0612 mg	Halcion
Alprazolam	Anxiolytic	12-15	0.25 mg-1.0 mg three times a day	Xanax

ANXIOLYTIC AND SEDATIVE-HYPNOTIC DRUGS

Although morbidity precipitated by psychoactive drug use in the elderly is well recognized, recent epidemiologic data suggest that the geriatric population,[15] especially the institutionalized elderly, is at continued risk for toxicity and functional impairment associated with polypharmacy. Given the potential morbidity associated with suboptimal drug administration in this vulnerable subgroup, a Harvard-based study[16] attempted to characterize patterns of psychoactive medication use for 850 residents of intermediate-care facilities (ICF) in Massachusetts. The investigators reported all prescriptions and patterns of actual drug use for patients during a 1-month period to arrive at a comprehensive profile of how such medications are being prescribed and consumed in these facilities.

On average, ICF residents were prescribed 8.1 medications during the study month and actually received 4.7 medications during this period. Nearly two-thirds (65%) of the residents were prescribed psychoactive medications. Of ICF inhabitants, 53% actually received psychoactive drugs on 5 or more days during the month, with 26% receiving antipsychotic medication; haloperidol (Haldol®) was given to 43% of those receiving antipsychotics and to 10% of the total sample. Twenty-eight percent of patients were receiving sedative/hypnotic drugs, primarily on a scheduled (82%) rather than on an as-needed basis. Of all patients receiving a sedative/hypnotic, about one-fourth (26%) were taking diphenhydramine hydrochloride (Benadryl®), a strongly anticholinergic agent used frequently for nighttime sedation. Of those residents receiving one or more of the benzodiazepines as a sedative/hypnotic, 30% were receiving such long-acting drugs as flurazepam (Dalmane®), diazepam (Valium®), and chlordiazepoxide (Librium®); 87% of benzodiazepine orders were prescribed as a standing order.

Of special note is the fact that 41% of patients with a diagnosis of Alzheimer's disease were receiving sedative/hypnotic drugs, although most experts agree that these agents have little therapeutic value in these patients and, in some studies, have been shown to induce agitation and increase the frequency of cognitive dysfunction. Amitriptyline hydrochloride, the most sedating and anticholinergic antidepressant presently available, was the most commonly prescribed agent in this therapeutic class. Overall, 14% of all patients studied were prescribed an antidepressant, although only 31% of this group had a *diagnosis* of depression noted in the record. Based on their findings, the investigators conclude that ICF patients were exposed to high levels of sedative/hypnotic and antipsychotic drug use. Suboptimal choice of medications within a drug class was common, and use of standing versus as-needed orders was often not in keeping with current concepts in geriatric psychopharmacology.

Prescribing Guidelines. Despite a barrage of carefully wrought admonitions regarding excessive prescribing and misuse in the geriatric age group,[17-18] practitioners frequently encounter geriatric patients for whom a sedative/hypnotic, antidepressant, or antipsychotic, either alone or in some combination, is indicated.[19-22] Although this study concentrated on psychoactive drug use in ICF residents, the conceptual points and suboptimal prescribing patterns flagged by this important investigation can easily be applied to the outpatient sphere, where psychoactive drugs are so often prescribed in geriatric patients.[23]

Anticholinergic toxicity in the elderly must be avoided.[24-26] Amitriptyline, for example, is a sedating drug with potent anticholinergic activity, two properties that make it especially undesirable for elderly patients.[27-29] SSRIs such as fluoxetine (Prozac®), sertraline (Zoloft®), and paroxetine (Paxil®), which possess less anticholinergic toxicity, may be preferable for the treatment of depression.[30] The use of diphenhydramine,[31-33] a strongly sedating agent whose use is also characterized by undesirable anticholinergic side effects, can be especially problematic when combined with other strongly anticholinergic agents in the antipsychotic and antidepressant class.[34,35] Practitioners, therefore, should recognize that diphenhydramine is not the sedative of choice for the elderly,[36,37] nor are such long-acting benzodiazepines as flurazepam hydrochloride, diazepam, or chlordiazepoxide, which also present an increased risk of toxicity for this vulnerable population. When benzodiazepines are required, low doses of shorter-acting agents are generally preferable.

Benzodiazepines. These agents are frequently used to relieve short-term anxiety in geriatric patients.[38] In general, agents with long half-lives should be avoided in the elderly population (See Table 10-3, page 438). Somnolence, confusion, and depression are the most common presenting symptoms of anxiolytic toxicity associated with long-acting benzodiazepines. Drugs with shorter half-lives are preferable anxiolytics for the elderly. Benzodiazepines are also effective sedative hypnotics. Flurazepam is the most common but has a long half-life. Thirty-nine percent of elderly patients receiving the usual 30 mg dose of flurazepam have significant CNS depression due to accumulation of the drug. A shorter-acting benzodiazepine, such as temazepam (Restoril®), may be a better choice.[38]

Triazolam is a widely prescribed hypnotic. Its relatively short serum half-life (approximately 6 hours) reduces the risks of daytime sedation and cumulative sedation compared with longer-acting hypnotics such as flurazepam. However, behavioral disturbances and impairment of memory have been reported,[39] with particular concern for the elderly who seem to be more sensitive to the medication. The mechanism(s) and severity of the adverse effects of triazolam remain incompletely defined and the subject of considerable research.[39]

The approximately 50% reduction in drug clearance and the absence of evidence for a specific drug sensitivity suggests the dosage of triazolam should be cut by 50% from that which would be appropriate for a young patient. A reasonable single dose might be 0.125 mg. One might even consider prescribing just half of a 0.125 mg tablet, as this is likely to have the same sedative effect 0.125 mg would have in a young person. It is important to note that the etiology of insomnia must be determined before it can be deemed safe to use any sedative. Nocturnal heart failure, sleep apnea, and depression are among the very important conditions that might cause insomnia but not be appropriate for sedative use. Even when it is deemed appropriate to use triazolam, only a small number of pills should be dispensed at any one time, and the patient and family should be carefully instructed against the routine or daily use of the medication.[40] The issue of an idiosyncratic behavioral disturbance triggered by triazolam remains a concern and the literature should be followed carefully for more details about its occurrence and identifying patients at risk.[41]

PHARMACOTHERAPY FOR ALZHEIMER'S DISEASE (AD): TREATMENT TRIGGER THRESHOLDS FOR DRUG THERAPY AND MEASURING CLINICAL OUTCOMES

Alzheimer's disease (AD), the most common cause of dementia in the elderly, affects approximately 4 million persons in the United States.[67] A prolonged course of deterioration in cognition, functioning, and behavior exacts a profound physical and emotional toll on family members and caregivers. The overall economic burden on society is enormous.[68]

Although there currently is no known cure for AD, recent investigations attribute at least some of the cognitive and memory manifestations of this disorder to a relative, disease-induced deficiency in the neurotransmitter acetylcholine. Accordingly, medications that increase the concentration of acetylcholine in neurosynapses have been shown to improve or stabilize, on a temporary basis, but for significantly long periods to improve quality of life and reduce the need for placement in skilled nursing facilities, these characteristic symptoms in patients with mild-to-moderate Alzheimer's dementia.[67-69]

The first drug approved for this purpose, tacrine (Cognex®), a cholinesterase inhibitor, showed a modest but statistically significant reduction in the rate of cognitive deterioration in patients with mild-to-moderate AD. Unfortunately, the drug required multiple daily administrations and monitoring of liver function tests, two features that prevented its widespread adoption for managing patients in the early stages of AD.[70-72]

Donepezil hydrochloride (Aricept®), a recently introduced reversible inhibitor of the enzyme acetylcholinesterase with more than 55 million estimated patient-days of exposure, appears to offer significant promise for patients who are in the early stages of their disease. One of the most important issues regarding the use of donepezil is timing of initiation of therapy, i.e. introducing the drug into the patient's regimen as early in the natural history of the disease as possible. Many physicians and pharmacists have come to recognize that donepezil, which is indicated for the treatment of mild-to-moderate AD, is time-sensitive, which means its benefits are maximized if the medication is given as early as possible after the diagnosis of AD has been established.

Donepezil doesn't produce dramatic clinical improvements or stabilization in *all* individuals to whom the drug is prescribed. The enhancements of cognitive function, delay of symptomatic deterioration, and the stabilization of mental decline are impressive enough in a significant percentage of people (up to 50% of those studied on the 5 mg/day donepezil dose, and up to 60% of those evaluated on the 10 mg/day dose report stabilization, delay of decline, or improvement in AD markers) to justify inclusion of this drug as part of a comprehensive (behavioral, psychosocial, and pharmacotherapeutic) AD treatment program.[67-71] Consequently, if the diagnosis of mild-to-moderate AD is strongly suspected, then donepezil should be started without delay. Other promising drug-based strategies, including vitamin E, NSAIDs, and estrogen must be considered investigational as their efficacy and optimal therapeutic dose has not been confirmed in prospective randomized, placebo-controlled trials.

Treatment Trigger Threshold (TTT). Despite the availability of FDA-approved medications to treat AD, drug-based therapy remains underutilized. There are many reasons for this "failure to treat" phenomenon, the most important of which are: (a) failure to diagnose the condition; (b) a lack of consensus among clinicians as to what the treatment trigger threshold should be for initiation of drug-based management; (c) an insufficiently formalized approach among physicians and pharmacists regarding the value of drug-based intervention for delaying disease deterioration of AD; and (4) failure to appreciate the potential benefits to total outcome costs that accompany pharmacologic intervention and delay of clinical deterioration in AD.

From a practical, real world perspective, many disease entities trigger drug therapy when objective measurements of organ dysfunction are present. When blood pressure, blood sugar, or cholesterol levels fall out of normal parameters, physicians and pharmacists feel justified in initiating drug therapy. Measured values can be normalized and target goals are concrete. In contrast, in AD, although mini-mental status examinations and other assessment tools are available to monitor patient status, progress, and deterioration, the end points are less well defined. In this regard, physicians and pharmacists should recognize that delay of disease progression and stabilization of patients with AD is a clinically important target goal that has important cost, family-related, and functional benefits. Moreover, in much the same way that clinicians initiate therapy with ACEIs to delay progression of renal disease or heart failure, in much the same way inhaled corticosteroids are used to prevent disease deterioration in asthma, drug-mediated disease progression and stabilization strategies for AD are also outcome-effective, even though stabilization of patients with mild-to-moderate AD is possible for only a limited time period.

Physicians may fail to recognize early signs of AD or to correctly diagnose the condition, perhaps as the result of insufficient attention to cognitive functioning on routine medical examinations.[68] Clinical suspicion for symptoms of AD should be increased if there is a family history of this disease, which is known to have a genetic basis. Although AD is considered nonreversible at present, accurate diagnosis in the early stages can be beneficial.[69] Primary therapeutic goals are to improve quality of life and maximize function by enhancing cognition, mood, and behavior.[68] Both pharmacologic and nonpharmacologic approaches are available. Evaluation by a neurologist or geriatric psychiatrist may be required, but much of the treatment can be managed in the primary-care setting. Recently published guidelines on diagnosis and assessment of dementia are among the resources helpful to primary-care physicians.[70]

Drug Therapy. Pharmacologic approaches to AD have attempted to stabilize or improve cognitive function or relieve worrisome behavioral symptoms; future strategies are to slow (or even reverse) neuronal damage or delay its onset.[71,72] Treatments to ameliorate cognitive impairment by improving cholinergic neurotransmission are emerging and physicians will face increasingly numerous choices for psychopharmacologic agents; attention to potential interactions with concomitant medications also will be particularly important.[68] As the population of older Americans increases, so will the challenge of diagnosing this condition for primary care physicians.

Currently, underdetection of and failure-to-treat patients during the early stages of AD constitutes a major public health awareness and intervention problem. In recent data from the ongoing Honolulu-Asia Aging study, it was clear that AD remains unreported and undiagnosed in large segments of the population.[9A] As characterized by this study, symptoms in over 50% of patients with *very mild* dementia went unnoticed significantly more often ($P < 0.001$) by *family* members—who are critical for detecting symptoms that may suggest early AD—than did mild or more severe dementia. In this study, both patients and caregivers often mistook these mild or early signs of dementia as a part of normal aging. (10A) As might be expected, patients with dementia are often unaware of a problem, since the illness may reduce both insight and judgment. On the other hand, family members may not recognize or report memory difficulties in an aging loved one for such reasons as: (1) diminished expectations relating to cognitive function in the elderly; (2) denial that symptoms represent a dementing illness; and (3) fear of embarrassment. To ensure that potentially valuable therapeutic agents are used early enough in the natural history of the disease to maximize their effectiveness, specific cognitive screening techniques by physicians are warranted.

As already mentioned, among the most promising, currently approved agents, cholinesterase inhibitors have attracted the greatest interest. Cholinesterase inhibitors actually represent one subtype of cholinergic agents. The rationale for cholinesterase inhibition is to delay degradation of the neurotransmitter acetylcholine, thereby prolonging its physiologic effect in the synapse. These agents have proved the most effective in clinical trials, and secondly, tacrine and donepezil are currently available.

Current theories on the pathogenesis of the cognitive signs and symptoms of AD attribute some of them to a deficiency of cholinergic neurotransmission. Donepezil is postulated to exert its therapeutic effect by enhancing cholinergic function. This is accomplished by increasing the concentration of acetylcholine through reversible inhibition of its hydrolysis by acetylcholinesterase. If this proposed mechanism of action is correct, donepezil's effect may lessen as the disease process advances and fewer cholinergic neurons remain functionally intact. There is no evidence that donepezil alters the course of the underlying dementing process.

Important pharmacologic issues in drug selection include linearity of pharmacokinetics, drug half-life and dosage schedules, complexity of dose titration, and potential for side effects or drug interactions. For example, tacrine has a 4-times/day dosage schedule, nonlinear kinetics, and a significant potential for drug-drug interactions. Moreover, slow dose titration and frequent monitoring or serum transaminase levels are recommended because of the possibility for hepatotoxic effects.

Donepezil has a relative oral bioavailability of 100% and linear pharmacokinetics over a dose range of 1 to 10 mg given once daily. Highly bound to plasma proteins, donepezil has a low rate of binding to drug-metabolizing enzymes. In laboratory studies, it demonstrated no significant effects on the pharmacokinetics of theophylline, cimetidine, warfarin, or digoxin.

Cholinesterase inhibitors have not been directly compared in head-to-head in formal trials, and it is unclear what role differences in selectivity for enzyme types or duration of inhibition will have at the clinical level. Therefore, emerging clinical experience will help to delineate any differences in side effects or other issues. From a side effect perspective, diarrhea, nausea, and vomiting are a predicable consequence of cholinesterase inhibition but have been generally mild and transient. These agents should be prescribed cautiously to patients with cardiac conduction abnormalities or a history of asthma or obstructive pulmonary disease.

Dosage schedule is important, because the easier an agent is to administer, the more likely it will be taken as directed—which improves the chances for a favorable response. Even for patients whose treatment is supervised by a caregiver, multiple daily doses are an increased burden. Drug interactions are always of concern in the elderly, who are more likely to use a variety of medications for concurrent conditions.[69]

Clinical Trials in Alzheimer's Disease. Although clinical trials are designed to show a difference between drug and placebo in cognitive function and a measure of global function, most trials last only 6 months. AD is progressive, however, and requires prolonged follow-up. As a class, cholinesterase inhibitors may exert a measurable and significant effect on the long-term course of AD. Two-year clinical trial extensions have demonstrated that cognitive and related functions are maintained *above* status at baseline with donepezil[71] and that placement in nursing homes was delayed in patients receiving tacrine.[72] Thus, we must be aware that positive effects at 6 months do not imply that therapy works only for that length of time. Moreover, patients who do not show immediate improvement should be monitored longer to determine whether they are declining or not.

Accurate diagnosis and establishment of baseline status are very important. The Mini-Mental State Examination (MMSE) and a measure of activities of daily living are helpful for these purposes. Noting in detail the patient's major functional, cognitive, and behavioral difficulties also clarifies later evaluations of response. Once therapy has begun, careful monitoring for adverse effects is prudent practice.

Some patients may show improvement during the first few months of treatment, but stabilization without evident improvement from baseline also constitutes a favorable response. Moreover, continued deterioration—although at a rate slower than expected—may designate therapeutic success. Quantitative instruments like the Mini-Mental State Examination can facilitate the assessment of change from baseline. In some instances, response may be accompanied by improvement in functional performance or behavior, or some combination of these manifestations. Behavioral symptoms, such as delusions, anxiety, and sleep disturbances, are usually considered secondary manifestations, but they have a major impact on quality of life, functional ability, and caregiver burden.[69]

The important thing for physicians and pharmacists to understand is that AD patients can be evaluated on a systematic basis to document effects of drug therapy. The effectiveness of donepezil as a treatment for this condition is demonstrated by the results of randomized, double-blind, placebo-controlled clinical investigations in patients with AD (diagnosed by NINCDS and DSM III-R criteria, Mini-Mental State Examination). The mean age of patients participating in trials was 73 years with a range of 50 to 94. Approximately 62% of patients were women and 38% were men. The racial distribution was white 95%, black 3% and other races 2%.

In most studies, the effectiveness of treatment with donepezil was evaluated using a dual outcome assessment strategy. The ability of donepezil to improve cognitive performance was assessed with the cognitive subscale of the *Alzheimer's Disease Assessment Scale* (ADAS-cog), a multi-item instrument that has been extensively validated in longitudinal cohorts of AD patients. The ADAS-cog examines selected aspects of cognitive performance including elements of memory, orientation, attention, reasoning, language and praxis. The ADAS-cog scoring range is from 0 to 70, with higher scores indicating greater cognitive impairment. Healthy elderly adults may score as low as 0 or 1, but it is not unusual for non-demented adults to score slightly higher.

The patients recruited as participants in each study had mean scores on the ADAS-cog of approximately 26 units, with a range from 4 to 61. Experience gained in longitudinal studies of ambulatory patients with mild-to-moderate AD suggest that they gain 6 to 12 units a year on the ADAS-cog. However, lesser degrees of change are seen in patients with very mild or very advanced disease because the ADAS-cog is not uniformly sensitive to change over the course of the disease. The annualized rate of decline in the placebo patients participating in trials was approximately 2 to 4 units per year. The ability of donepezil to produce an overall clinical effect also was assessed using a Clinician's Interview Based Impression of Change that required the use of caregiver information, the CIBIC plus. The CIBIC plus is not a single instrument and is not a standardized instrument like the ADAS-cog.

Clinical trials support the use of donepezil for use in patients with mild-to-moderate AD. In a 15-week, double-blind, placebo-controlled clinical trial, improvement in cognitive function vs placebo is seen as early as the third week in patients treated with both 5 and 10 mg/day. Improvement in ADAS-cog mean scores was significant for both donepezil-treated groups vs placebo at weeks 3, 6, 9, and endpoint. During the 12-week active-treatment phase, approximately 60% of patients treated with donepezil (10 mg/day) and approximately 50% of patients treated with 5 mg/day achieved a best-change score of 4 points or more on the ADAS-cog vs approximately 30% of placebo-treated patients.[67] The study also showed that treatment effects begin to abate after a 3-week discontinuation period.[67] A longer, 30-week, double-blind, placebo-controlled clinical trial further demonstrates enhanced cognitive function in both the 5 and 10 mg/day donepezil groups. ADAS-cog performance for treated groups remained above baseline at all assessment times.

The long-term use of donepezil have recently been evaluated in an interim analysis conducted in mild-to-moderate AD patients who were taking this agent for a period of 98 weeks.[68] A multicenter, non-randomized, open-label extension study enrolled 133 individuals (mean age 71, 61% female) with mild to moderate AD who had completed a previous 14-week (including a 2-week placebo washout), double-blind, placebo-controlled clinical trial of donepezil.

An analysis of the first 98 weeks of treatment (at week 98: donepezil-treated, n=43, ADAS-cog analysis, n=37), reveals that the majority of patients in the study were receiving the maximum dose of 10 mg/day by week 60 from the beginning of the open-label phase. Interim analysis from this clinical trial data suggests possible treatment effects for up to 98 weeks. Cognitive function scores were at or above baseline for 38 weeks, as measured by ADAS-cog. Overall, donepezil-treated patients' ADAS-cog scores were estimated to decline an average of 6.6 points per year.[68] In a degenerative disease, improvement or less than expected decline is considered a clinical success.[70]

Common adverse events in this study were consistent with results of placebo-controlled studies and included diarrhea (11%), nausea (9%), pain (8%), accident, abdominal disturbance, insomnia, agitation, and dizziness (6%). Clinical studies of donepezil have shown no increase, relative to placebo, in the incidence of either peptic ulcer disease or GI bleeding. Nevertheless, cholinesterase inhibitors may be expected to increase gastric acid secretion. Therefore, patients (especially those at increased risk for developing ulcers i.e., history of ulcer disease, receiving concurrent NSAIDs) should be monitored closely for GI bleeding. In clinical trials, syncopal episodes have been reported in association with the use of donepezil (2% vs 1% for placebo).

The dosages shown to be effective in controlled clinical trials are 5 and 10 mg administered once per day. The higher dose of 10 mg did not provide statistically significantly greater clinical benefit than 5 mg. There is a suggestion, however, based on order of group mean scores and dose tread analyses of data from these clinical trials, that a daily dose of 10 mg of donepezil might provide additional benefit for some patients. Accordingly, whether or not to employ a dose of 10 mg is a matter of prescriber and patient preference.

Evidence from the controlled trials indicates that the 10 mg dose, with a 1 week titration, is likely to be associated with a higher incidence of cholinergic adverse events than the 5 mg dose. In open label trials using a 6 week titration, the frequency of these same adverse events was similar between the 5 and 10 mg dose groups. Therefore, because steady state is not achieved for 15 days and because the incidence of untoward effects may be influenced by the rate of dose escalation, treatment with a dose of 10 mg should not be contemplated until patients have been on a daily dose of 5 mg for 4 to 6 weeks. Donepezil should be taken in the evening, just prior to retiring. It can be taken with or without food.

Safety Profile of Drug Therapy. The long-term clinical trial data confirm favorable safety and tolerability of donepezil. There was no evidence of hepatotoxicity and no clinically significant changes in renal function, metabolic function, or vital signs. Common adverse events in this open-label, long-term extension trial, including agitation, dizziness, nausea, diarrhea, and headache were often mild and transient.[68]

Whether donepezil has any potential for enzyme induction is not known. Ketoconazole and quinidine, inhibitors of CYP450, 3A4 and 2D6, respectively, inhibit donepezil metabolism in vitro. Whether there is a clinical effect of these inhibitors is not known. Inducers of CYP 2D6 and CYP 3A4 (e.g., phenytoin, carbamazepine, dexamethasone, rifampin, phenobarbital) could increase the rate of elimination of donepezil. Because of their mechanism of action, cholinesterase inhibitors have the potential to interfere with the activity of anticholinergic medications. A synergistic effect may be expected when cholinesterase inhibitors are given concurrently with succinylcholine, similar neuromuscular blocking agents or cholinergic agonists such as bethanechol. Therefore, caution with anesthesia is advised.

MANAGEMENT OF PAIN IN PATIENTS WITH CANCER

The prevalence of cancer in the United States continues to increase. Cancer is newly diagnosed in approximately one million individuals per year and one out of every five deaths in the US (about 1400 per day) is caused by cancer. One of the most debilitating and recalcitrant symptoms in patients with metastatic or recurrent cancer is severe pain, which often develops well before the terminal stages of disease. Even when pain is treated, relief is often inadequate and patients have persistent functional impairment in their activities of daily living. Despite guidelines for pain management in cancer patients, there remains significant variability in treatment regimens. This is unfortunate since in the majority of patients, pain can be controlled through a comprehensive, multidisciplinary approach that incorporates both pharmacologic and non-pharmacologic modalities. Many factors contribute to the inadequacy of pain management in cancer patients incuding inadequate knowledge amongst clinicians, negative attitudes of patients and clinicians toward medications and a variety of reimbursement problems.

In order to address the scope of pain management regimens employed and characteristics of cancer patients whose pain is well controlled versus those in whom it is not, investigators at multiple academic cancer centers around the United States evaluated 1,308 patients with metastatic or recurrent cancer.[61] Sixty-seven percent of the subjects admitted having pain beyond common everyday types (headache, sprains, etc.), reported that they took analgesic medications on an everyday basis, or were identified by their physicians as having pain. Of those with pain, 62% were considered to have substantial pain, defined as a score of at least 5 on a scale of zero to ten, that was sufficient to interfere with activities of daily living. At subsequent office visits, all patients completed a pain severity scale as well as rating how much the pain interfered with their enjoyment of life and their activities of daily living and the degree of pain relief (pain management index) they were receiving from treatment (a negative score represented inadequate treatment). Physicians caring for the subjects were asked to assess the same features in order to determine the degree of discrepancy between the two.

In 42% of those with pain, there were negative pain management scores indicating inadequate analgesia. Factors associated with increased likelihood of inadequate analgesia included discrepancy between patients and physician in judging the severity of pain, pain not attributed to cancer by the physician, better functional status, age greater than 70, female sex and being seen at a center that predominantly cared for minority groups. Patients with less adequate analgesia also reported greater pain-related impairment of function.

Prescribing Guidelines. Pain management is frequently inadequate for many patients with cancer. In order to minimize this, clinicians need to take a collaborative, interdisciplinary approach to pain management, develop an individualized plan for pain management with patients and their families, perform thorough ongoing assessments of the patient's pain and effects of treatment, and use both pharmacologic and non-pharmacologic interventions for pain relief. In assessing pain, patients should be the primary source of information, but they need to be questioned frequently since some may be reluctant to volunteer information. In addition to obvious sources of pain (eg, bone fractures), clinicians must be able to recognize other common conditions that can cause pain in cancer patients (eg, bone metastases, epidural metastases with spinal cord compression, peripheral neuropathies, mucositis).

Medications are the cornerstone of pain management in the cancer patient because they are relatively inexpensive, usually work fairly quickly and generally entail acceptable risks. Although the specific regimen needs to be tailored to the individual patient, a workable protocol has been developed by the World Health Organization. Initially, aspirin, acetaminophen or a non-steroidal anti-inflammatory drug is instituted followed by the addition of an opioid such as codeine or hydrocodone (often as a fixed combination pill because of synergistic effects). These more potent agents should be started initially for patients who present with moderate to severe pain. More potent opioids such as morphine, methadone and fentanyl should be instituted for patients with persistent severe pain and should be given on an around-the-clock basis with additional doses available on an as-needed basis.

Tolerance and dependence are predictable consequences of use of potent high dose opioid analgesics, but this should not preclude the use of adequate doses to achieve acceptable pain relief while balancing side effects (constipation, sedation, nausea, etc.). The sequential trial of more than one opioid is usually preferrable before switching to another method of administration of medication or more invasive procedures. Patient-controlled analgesia involving programmable pumps to deliver drugs intravenously, subcutaneously or epidurally are most useful to treat breakthrough pain. Physical modalities such as cold, heat, electrical stimulation, and acupuncture may reduce the need for medication but should not be used as a substitute for drugs. Furthermore, psychosocial support and antidepressant and other medications (eg, carbamazepine, phenytoin) may be useful adjuncts to opioid medications. For severe, refractory pain syndromes, radiation therapy, nerve blocks or invasive surgical procedures should be considered.

Aspirin, acetaminophen or non-steroidal anti-inflammatory drugs are the initial agents of choice followed by the addition of an opioid such as codeine or hydrocodone (often as a fixed combination pill because of synergistic effects). Morphine, methadone and fentanyl are appropriate for patients with persistent severe pain and should be given on an around-the-clock basis with additional doses available on an as-needed basis. Tolerance and dependence are predictable consequences of use of potent high dose opioid analgesics, but this should not preclude the use of adequate doses to achieve acceptable pain relief. Antidepressant and other medications (eg, carbamazepine, phenytoin) may be useful adjuncts to opioid medications.

ANTIDEPRESSANTS

The elderly are particularly sensitive to the adverse effects of tricyclic antidepressants (See Table 10-4).[42] As discussed previously, these agents are *not* recommended as drugs of choice for treatment of depression in the elderly. The most common presenting symptoms of toxicity include sedation, anticholinergic effects, adrenergic hyperactivity (tremulousness, sweating), and cardiovascular toxicity. Anticholinergic effects include dry mouth, constipation, blurred vision, urinary retention, decreased sweating, and hyperthermic reactions.

Researchers at the National Institutes of Health conducted a series of randomized, double-blind, crossover studies of patients with painful diabetic peripheral neuropathy, comparing amitriptyline, desipramine and fluoxetine. The study objectives were to assess relative efficacy and to better understand the mechanism(s) of action on diabetic neuropathic pain.

Two separate studies were conducted: one compared desipramine with amitriptyline; the other compared fluoxetine with a placebo. The outcome measures examined were daily pain score and end-of study global pain rating. Each treatment phase lasted 7 weeks, followed by a washout period and crossover for another 7 weeks of treatment. Recruitment was done by advertisement: 57 patients qualified and entered one or both studies.

Mean daily dose was 105 mg for amitriptyline, 111 mg for desipramine and 40 mg for fluoxetine. Seventy-four percent of patients reported moderate or greater pain relief during the blinded use of amitriptyline; 61% during the use of desipramine; and 41% during the use of the placebo. The differences between amitriptyline and desipramine were not significant, nor were those between fluoxetine and the placebo. Amitriptyline and desipramine were effective even in patients who were not depressed, whereas fluoxetine worked only when there was an underlying depression. Some of the study's findings include:

Amitriptyline and desipramine are equally effective for treatment of pain caused by diabetic peripheral neuropathy, regardless of the presence of depression. Fluoxetine appears to work *only in the context of depression,* suggesting it

Table 10-4

Adverse Effects and Toxicity of Tricyclic and Tetracyclic Antidepressants					
Structural class	**Trade name**	**Young adult daily dose**	**Elderly daily dose**	**Sedative properties**	**Anticholinergic properties**
Tricyclic					
Tertiary amine					
Amitriptyline	Elavil	100-300 mg	25-150 mg	+++	++++
Imipramine	Tofranil	100-300 mg	25-150 mg	++	+++
Doxepin	Sinequan	100-300 mg	25-150 mg	+++	++++
Trimipramine	Surmontil	100-300 mg	25-150 mg	+++	+++
Secondary amine					
Nortriptyline	Pamelor	50-100 mg	10-60 mg	+	+++
Desipramine	Norpramin	100-300 mg	25-150 mg	0	++
Protriptyline	Vivactil	20-60 mg	5-30 mg	0	+++
Dibenzoxazepine (amoxapine)	Asendin	150-300 mg	25-150 mg	++	+++
Triazolopyridine (trazodone)	Desyrel	150-400 mg	50-300 mg	+++	+
Tetracyclic maprotiline	Ludiomil	100-300 mg	25-150 mg	++	+++
Selective serotonin reuptake inhibitor (SSRI)					
Sertraline	Zoloft	50-200 mg	50-100 mg	0	0
Fluoxetine	Prozac	20-40 mg	10-20 mg	0	0
Paroxetine	Paxil	20-50 mg	10-40 mg	0	0
Venlafaxine	Effelor	75-150 mg	75-150 mg	0	0

has no direct effect on the mechanism of pain in diabetic peripheral neuropathy. Desipramine and other tricyclics with lesser anticholinergic activity (eg, nortriptyline), might be reasonable alternatives to amitriptyline, which many patients find difficult to tolerate.

Anticholinergic effects—which may cause delirium, agitation, visual hallucinations, and decreased thirst—precipitated by tricyclic antidepressants are frequently underdiagnosed. Lack of sweating and decreased thirst can produce dehydration and electrolyte imbalances that can be fatal in the elderly population. Orthostatic hypotension due to anticholinergic toxicity can cause falls, myocardial infarction, and cerebrovascular events.[43] Cardiovascular effects due to antidepressant toxicity in the elderly include an anticholinergic effect that can increase the heart rate and a quinidine-like effect that may increase PR, QRS, and QTC intervals.

Tricyclic antidepressant overdose has serious cardiotoxic effects that are not usually present at the therapeutic doses. Because of the cardiovascular effects associated with overdose, researchers anticipated an increased incidence of sudden death and arrhythmia among elderly patients using these antidepressants. The Boston Collaborative Drug Surveillance Program, however, demonstrated that neither occurs, even in the presence of organic heart disease, which is so common in the elderly.[39] The toxicity of TCAs in elderly patients with heart disease remains controversial.

Monoamine oxidase inhibitors should be avoided in the elderly because of the risks of serious drug interactions and the frequency of orthostatic hypotension.

ANTIPSYCHOTIC DRUGS

Several major psychiatric disorders in the elderly are treated with antipsychotic and neurologic drugs (See Table 10-5). Complications of this treatment include tardive dyskinesia (five times more common in the elderly), akathisias, dystonias, pseudoparkinsonism, and anticholinergic side effects.[46,47] A major adverse reaction to neuroleptics is neuroleptic malignant syndrome (NMS), which is frequently unrecognized in the elderly. NMS consists of fever, rigidity, autonomic instability, and mental status changes.

With the widespread use of both tricyclic antidepressants and antipsychotics, 12% of all elderly ambulatory patients and 25% of those hospitalized in nursing homes now receive two or more drugs with anticholinergic effects.[48] In general, studies show that clinicians do not choose drugs within a given class to minimize anticholinergic effects. Consequently, suspect an anticholinergic reaction in elderly patients with symptoms of urinary retention, acute glaucoma, delirium, hallucinations, seizures, dysarthria, hyperthermia, tachycardia, and even heart block—especially if the patient has taken drugs in one or more of the anticholinergic classes.[49,50] Newer antipsychotics such as Risperdol are less likely to produce movement disorders.

Table 10-5

Adverse Effects of Antipsychotic Medications in the Elderly					
Drug and dose for elderly	**Relative potency**	**Sedation**	**Extra-pyramidal**	**Anticholinergic**	**Orthostatic hypotension**
Chlorpromazine					
(Thorazine) 10-25 mg b.i.d. t.i.d.	100	+++	++	+++	++
Thioridazine					
(Mellaril) 10-25 mg b.i.d. t.i.d.	95-100	+++	+	+++	++
Thiothixene					
(Navane) 2-3 mg	5	+	+++	+	+
Haloperidol					
(Haldol) 0.5-2 mg	2	+	+++	+	+
Fluphenazine					
(Prolixin) 0.5-2 mg	2	+	+++	+	+

MANAGEMENT OF DEPRESSION FOLLOWING MYOCARDIAL INFARCTION

Depression is not uncommon following acute, life-threatening illnesses, but the majority of patients have resolution of depressive symptoms and return to normal function. It is estimated, however, that 15-20% of patients who suffer an acute myocardial infarction (MI) have a major depressive episode in the post-infarction period, and a substantial number of these individuals have persistent emotional difficulties which have been correlated with increased mortality. Surprisingly, the severity of the cardiac illness and the degree of emotional problems are unrelated in these patients. Although persistent depression has been linked to increased mortality following myocardial infarction, less is known about outcomes in *survivors* of MI who have persistent depression.

In one analysis,[65] 552 male myocardial infarction patients between the ages of 29 and 65 years were evaluated beginning 17 to 21 days following an acute myocardial infarction with follow-up six months later. Subjects underwent a comprehensive phychodiagnostic evaluation and were allocated into one of three groups: low, moderate or severe depression. At baseline, 15% patients were identified with severe depression, 22% with moderate depression, and 63% with a low degree of depression. Follow-up information on fatal and nonfatal cardiac events (reinfarction, syncope, severe angina, coronary bypass surgery, coronary angioplasty) and functional and emotional status after discharge were obtained for all 552 subjects for the six month study. Taking all of these assessments into account, the relative risks were significantly increased for those patients with high degrees of post-MI depression at baseline in terms of ongoing angina, emotional instability, and continued smoking, and the likelihood of return to work was significantly less in the high depression group.

Cardiac patients who develop significant post-MI depression fail to convalesce as well as those who are without significant symptoms of depression. Depressed individuals are in a psychological state of reduced vigor, with a lack of initiative and detachment from activities of daily living. They have a reduced ability to comply with risk factor modification efforts and may develop feelings of hopelessness. Ultimately, individuals with significant depression can lapse into a prolonged invalid state with a tendency to remain in the sick role for possible secondary benefits. Patients with depression have increased episodes of angina, an increased risk for recurrent infarction and a reduced quality of life. The exact reasons for this are not entirely clear. While the degree of myocardial damage and consequent left ventricular function are critical factors in determining post-MI morbidity and mortality, the degree of depression and emotional difficulties following MI, surprisingly, is not well correlated to the severity of the cardiac problem itself.

Clinicians need to be vigilant in identifying patients with depression following an MI and stratify the individual into a higher risk status. As with other cases of depression, it may be misdiagnosed or under-recognized in cardiac patients who may deny or downplay depressive symptoms. The exact role of antidepressant medication in this situation is not entirely defined but certainly should be considered for those individuals with persistent significant symptoms. Avoidance of agents with high anticholinergic potential that carry some added risk in the cardiac patient is advisable.

Post-MI depression is an independent and significant source of morbidity and reduced quality of life at least for the first six months (the highest risk period) following myocardial infarction. Depression appears to have the greatest impact on pain perception and illness behavior. The diagnosis of depression can be difficult in cardiac patients who may deny or downplay depressive symptoms. Patients with depression following an MI should be considered at high risk status. Antidepressants are generally indicated for those individuals with persistent significant symptoms.

Predicting Major Bleeding Complications in Patients on Long-Term Anticoagulants

It is estimated that two million Americans are treated with warfarin as outpatients each year. Although long-term anticoagulant therapy has been demonstrated to be effective in preventing thromboembolism, the key issue for these patients is whether the benefit of such therapy outweighs the risk of hemorrhagic complications in an individual patient. Predictors of major bleeding complications at the start of outpatient therapy in those treated with warfarin would be of great benefit to clinicians faced with the challenge of initiating and monitoring the effects of anticoagulation. In addition to knowing just how frequently bleeding complications occur and what subgroups are at greatest risk, practitioners would also benefit from knowing: (1) the relationship of bleeding to prothrombin time during outpatient therapy with warfarin; (2) the yield of diagnostic evaluation of bleeding in terms of previously unknown, remediable lesions; and (3) whether the yield of discovering a remediable lesion varies according to the prothrombin time at the time of hemorrhagic episode.

Two back-to-back, retrospective studies shed important light on these critical issues in outpatient drug therapy. The records of 565 patients starting outpatient therapy with warfarin upon discharge from a university hospital were reviewed. Bleeding was classified as *major* if it was fatal, life-threatening, led to severe blood loss, to surgical intervention, or to moderate blood loss that was acute or subacute and could not be explained by trauma or surgery. *Minor* bleeding included other internal bleeding (including overt or occult gastrointestinal bleeding, hemoptysis, and gross hematuria), symptomatic anemia ascribed to acute but occult blood loss, or chronic bleeding with moderate blood loss.

Based on these criteria, investigators found that major bleeding occurred in 65 patients (12%) and was fatal in 10 patients (2%). Minor bleeding also occurred in 65 patients (12%). The cumulative incidences of major bleeding at 1, 12, and 48 months were 3%, 11%, and 22% respectively. Five independent risk factors for major bleeding—age 65 years or greater, history of stroke, history of gastrointestinal bleeding, a serious comorbid condition (recent myocardial infarction, renal insufficiency, or severe anemia), atrial fibrillation—predicted bleeding in the test group. The cumulative incidence of major bleeding was 2% in 57 low-risk patients and 63% in 20 high-risk patients. As expected, the gastrointestinal tract was the most frequent location of bleeding but was fatal in only one case. Intracranial bleeding was the most common cause of fatal hemorrhage. It is important to note that the researchers observed a significant association between a history of hypertension and intracranial bleeding. This association was significant even if blood pressure was adequately controlled at the time of warfarin therapy. Interestingly, patients with a history of stroke had increased rates of gastrointestinal bleeding as well as intracranial hemorrhage.

Those 130 patients (24%) with either major or minor bleeding were then studied to determine the relation of bleeding to prothrombin times and important *remediable* lesions. Important remediable lesions were classified as those lesions or injuries for which specific therapy is routinely indicated (ie, esophageal, gastric, or duodenal ulcers; colonic diverticula, colon cancer; bladder cancer, etc.). Using these criteria, it was found that for each 1.0 increase in the prothrombin time-to-control ratio, the odds ratio for major bleeding during the week after a prothrombin time measurement increased 80%; the odds ratio for minor bleeding increased 50%. Bleeding complications are related to important remediable lesions in 49 of 130 cases (38%), although these lesions were unknown before bleeding in only 22 cases (17%). New, previously unknown lesions were discovered in 20 of 59 case subjects of (34%) with gastrointestinal bleeding or hematuria, but in only 2 of 71 case subjects (3%) with bleeding from other sites. Finally, of special clinical importance is the observation that prothrombin times rose precipitously at the time of bleeding in patients *without* important remediable lesions, whereas prothrombin times tended to be in the therapeutic range in those *with* significant remediable lesions.

The overall rates of major and fatal bleeding (12% and 2%, respectively) as well as for the rates of major and fatal bleeding *per year of outpatient anticoagulant therapy* (7% and 1%, respectively) are striking. Put simply, these investigations dramatize the potential risks of long-term warfarin therapy and convincingly demonstrate that this form of pharmacologic intervention is associated with significantly higher morbidity in individuals 65 years of age or older, in those with recent myocardial infarction or a comorbid condition, and in patients with atrial fibrillation. Clinicians should also note that a previous history of stroke or hypertension (even if blood pressure is normal at the time anticoagulant therapy is initiated) is associated with a significantly increased risk of intracranial hemorrhage.

With respect to the prothrombin time, it appears as if increases in the ratio of measured to controlled values are related to predictable increases in major and minor bleeding during the weeks following such measurements. Moreover, it appears that remediable lesions most often surface at a time when prothrombin times or INR are in the therapeutic range, whereas nonremediable lesions declare themselves following precipitous rises in prothrombin time. Given these observations, clinicians should aggressively pursue diagnostic evaluation in all patients who present with bleeding, especially when their prothrombin times or INR are in the therapeutic range and have been stable for quite some time prior to the hemorrhagic complication. For now, the decision to proceed with long-term anticoagulation continues to present a formidable dilemma in which the predictable risks must be weighted against not-so-predictable benefits in a vulnerable patient population. See Tables 10-6 through 10-8 for possible drug interactions that can effect bleeding times.

Table 10-6

Possible Drug Interactions with Anticoagulants			
Decrease vitamin K	**Displace anticoagulant**	**Inhibit metabolism**	**Other**
Antibiotics Cholestyramine Mineral oil	Salicylates Sulfonamides Sulfonylureas Ethacrynic acid Mefenamic acid Naldixic acid Diazoxide	Chloramphenicol Allopurinol Nortriptyline Disulfiram Metronidazole Alcohol (acute ingestion) Cimetidine Fluconazole	Thyroid drugs Anabolic steroids Quinidine Glucagon

Table 10-7

Drugs That Diminish Anticoagulant Drug Activity	
Induction of Enzymes	**Increased Procoagulant factors**
Barbiturates Glutethimide Ethchlorvynol Griseofulvin Phenytoin Carbamazepine Rifampin Chlorinated insecticides	Estrogens Oral contraceptives Vitamin K

Table 10-8

Drugs Potentiating Anticoagulant Drug Effects		
Inhibition of platelet aggregation	**Inhibition of procoagulant factors**	**Ulcerogenic drugs**
Salicylates Sulfinpyrazone Dipyridamole NSAIDs	Quinidine Antimetabolites Alkylating agents Salicylates	Sulfinpyrazone Salicylates Adrenal corticosteroids

H_2 ANTAGONISTS

A commonly prescribed drug among the elderly population, cimetidine (Tagamet®) can cause sedation and confusion, especially in doses above 1000 mg/day. Aside from this direct adverse reaction, side effects are very usually tolerable. However, because cimetidine is an inhibitor of the p-450 hepatic microsomal oxidation enzymes, it blocks metabolism of many other drugs that may be taken concurrently, increasing their effect on plasma levels. This leads to a number of potentially dangerous drug interactions. In patients taking warfarin, the prothrombin time can rise 20% to 200%. Both diazepam and chlordiazepoxide can cause increased sedation. Theophylline levels can increase from the therapeutic to the toxic range in patients who are on cimetidine therapy. Toxic effects, such as bradycardia, hypotension, and arrhythmias, may appear with beta-blockers. Elevated levels of anticonvulsants, especially in the elderly, can be seen within a period of several days in patients taking carbamazepine (Tegretol®) and phenytoin (Dilantin®). With lidocaine, an increase in serum levels of 60% to 90% can occur with maintenance infusions in patients on cimetidine therapy.

Table 10-9

Adverse Drug Interactions in Combination with Cimetidine (Tagamet)
• With warfarin, prothrombin time rises 20 to 200%.
• With benzodiazepines, increases sedation.
• With theophylline, increases in theophylline from therapeutic to toxic range (narrow therapeutic range).
• With beta-blockers, toxic effects may appear, such as bradycardia, hypotension, arrhythmias.
• With carbamazepine (Tegretol) and phenytoin (Dilantin), elevated levels of anticonvulsants, especially in the elderly, over several days.
• With lidocaine, 60 to 90% increase in serum levels occurred with maintenance infusion; study conducted in the elderly. Cimetidine therapy was new in these patients.

Selective H_2 antagonists, ranitidine (Zantac®) and famotidine (Pepcid®), have the advantage of producing less inhibition of the hepatic microsomal oxidation system.

BRONCHODILATORS

Aminophylline and theophylline once represented the cornerstone of oral bronchodilator therapy for the elderly asthmatic, bronchitic. These drugs are metabolized by the liver, and clearance is remarkably sensitive to hepatic dysfunction. Complications of aminophylline include seizures, which may even occur at therapeutic levels, increased angina, palpitations, and arrhythmias.

Nervousness and lack of sleep are also encountered in the geriatric population. Theophylline toxicity in the elderly may also mimic chronic organic brain syndrome, multiinfarct dementia, and psychosis. Draw blood levels on patients who have this constellation of symptoms and are taking a theophylline preparation.

Certain drug interactions may precipitate aminophylline toxicity. Cimetidine and other liver-metabolized antibiotics (erythromycin) decrease excretion of aminophylline. Ephedrine and other sympathomimetic agents in combination with aminophylline may cause excessive CNS stimulation, precipitating bizarre behavior and sleeplessness.

ANTIHISTAMINES

The early stages of diphenhydramine intoxication are characterized by acute psychosis, hallucinations, autism, loosened associations, affective blunting, and inappropriate behavior.[54] As time passes, the symptom complex may become more similar to an acute brain syndrome with confusion, disorientation, inability to concentrate, and loss of short-term memory.[34] These symptoms present an interesting differential diagnosis. However, based on the physical exam, drug overdose should always be suspected. Initial lab analysis should include serum electrolytes, prothrombin time, calcium, BUN, glucose, arterial gases, blood alcohol, and urine toxicologic screening. In addition, an ECG, chest and skull x-rays, and lumbar puncture may be necessary, depending on the clinical presentation.

A history of drug ingestion is frequently unreliable or unobtainable from the patient. Friends or relatives may be questioned concerning the drug intake. Autonomic signs or symptoms may be the key to diagnosis. Anticholinergic poisoning is associated with tachycardia, mydriasis, flushing, hyperpyrexia, urinary retention, decreased intestinal motility, hypertension, dry skin and decreased salivation.

A vast array of antihistamines, hypnotics, antidepressants, and tranquilizing agents pose significant anticholinergic activity (Table 10-10). An increasing number of these drugs are now available in OTC preparations and may, in acute poisoning, produce a picture typical of central anticholinergic toxicity. This syndrome refers to an acute psychosis of delirium resulting from a primary blockade of cerebral cholinergic inhibitory pathways accompanied by signs of peripheral muscarinic blockage.[55]The presentation may vary from confusion, hallucinations, and convulsions to deepening coma and respiratory arrest (Table 10-11). Toxic psychosis is a recognized complication of antihistamine poisoning.

Table 10-10

Anticholinergic Agents
Antihistamines
Antiparkinsonian drugs
Antipsychotics (phenothiazines and butyrophenones)
Antispasmodics
Belladonna alkaloids
Ophthalmic products (mydriatics)
Plants (jimsonweed)
Thioxanthenes
Tricyclic antidepressants

Table 10-11

Central Effects of Anticholinergic Toxicity	
Anxiety	Hyperactivity
Ataxia	Lethargy
Choreoathetoid movements	Loss of short-term memory
Coma	Myoclonus
Delirium	Paranoid ideation
Disorientation	Respiratory failure
Dizziness	Seizures
Dysarthria	Tinnitus
Expressive aphasia	Tremor
Frank psychosis	
Hallucinations (visual/auditory)	

Low sedating or non-sedating antihistamines are preferred in the elderly. Once-daily options include loratidine (Clariton®) which produces sedation or somnolence in about 1%-2% of patients and cetirizine, which produces these symptoms in about 14% of patients, as compared to about 7% in the placebo group.

VACCINES

Pneumococcal infection represents a substantial threat to the health of the elderly, the immunocompromised, and those with serious underlying illness. Polyvalent pneumococcal polysaccharide vaccine was developed to address this threat. There are two formulations of the vaccine: the original one contained the polysaccharides of 14 species, whereas the currently available vaccine contains the polysaccharides of 23 species of Streptococcus pneumoniae. Although the vaccine has been available for more than a decade, evidence of its efficacy is limited. One study demonstrated the vaccine to be effective, but the protection decreases with time (especially after 5 years), advancing age, and immunoincompetence.

A recent summary of recommendations from the Advisory Committee on Immunization Practices (ACIP) of the CDC updates previous recommendations concerning the use of pneumococcal polysaccharide vaccines. Indications include individuals > 65 years of age; functional or anatomic asplenia; immunocompromise or immunosuppression; HIV infection; malignancies; chronic renal failure, hemodialysis, nephrotic syndrome; chronic cardiovascular or pulmonary disease; and Alaskan and American Indians. Revaccination is recommended in individuals 65 years or older (every 5 years); those with immunosuppression (every 5 years); and asplenia (every 5 years in those > 10 years of age).

Despite being effective and safe, pneumococcal vaccine is underused. It should be administered to all patients with moderately high risk of serious pneumococcal infection, including the elderly.

Investigators designed a case-control study comparing pneumococcal vaccine status in 1,054 patients with documented pneumococcal infection and in 1,054 carefully matched controls (similar age, gender, underlying illnesses) who had not had pneumoccal infection. Thirteen percent of those with pneumococcal infection had received the vaccine versus 20% of the controls (P<0.001).

Aggregate protective efficacy of the 14-and 23-valent vaccines was 56% against serotypes represented by the vaccines. Efficacy was 65% in immunocompetent patients but fell to 21% in immuncompromised persons. In addition, efficacy declined with age and time from immunization, five-year protective efficacy was 85% in patients less than age 55, but declined to 32% in those aged 75 to 84. Efficacy declined by about 30% after five years from the time of vaccination. There was no difference among the vaccinated and the nonvaccinated in terms of mortality from pneumococcal infection.

SUMMARY

Although the elderly constitute only 12% of the U.S. population, they consume approximately 20% to 30% of all drugs.[56,57] Moreover, many of the elderly are simultaneously taking prescription drugs for more than one chronic condition over variable periods of time, and they may supplement their prescription drugs with OTC medications and alcohol. For these reasons, this age group is at high risk for sustaining drug toxicity and adverse drug interactions.[58]

One large study of hospitalized elderly patients with a mean age of 71 years found that each patient consumed an average of 3.1 prescription drugs and one OTC preparation. Initially, one sixth of the persons surveyed denied using OTC medications, but further questioning revealed that these patients did, in fact, take OTC drugs. Moreover, 50% of these elderly patients needed prompting to remember to take their medications, so noncompliance was a serious problem.[59]

Among the implications of that study for the diagnosis and identification of adverse drug reactions in the emergency setting is the importance of focused assessment and interview techniques to examine drug-taking behavior and compliance in the elderly, particularly for OTC drugs.

Finally, any elderly patient with nonspecific CNS, cardiac, or gastrointestinal signs and symptoms must provide a careful drug history, including OTC medications, antiulcer agents, cardiac medications, and antihypertensive drugs. Always consider adverse drug reactions, especially the anticholinergic syndrome, and secondary drug interactions, as a cause of illness.

[1]Albrich JM. Geriatric pharmacology. In: Schwartz GR, Bosker G, Grigsby JW, eds. Geriatric Emergencies. Bowie, Md.: Robert J. Brady Co., 1984.

[2]Walt RP. Misoprostol for the treatment of peptic ulcer and antiinflammatory-drug-induced gastroduodenal ulceration. N Engl J Med 1992;327:1575.

[3]Graham DY, White RH, Moreland LW, et al. Duodenal and gastric ulcer prevention with misoprostol in arthritis patients taking NSAIDs. Ann Intern Med 1993;119:257.

[4]Lamy PP. A consideration of NSAID use in the elderly. Geriatric Medicine Today 1988;7(4):30.

[5]Lamy PP. Renal effects of nonsteroidal anti-inflammatory drugs. Heightened risk to the elderly? J Am Geriatr Soc 1986;34:361-7.

[6]Hogan DB, Campbell NR, Crutcher R, Jennett P, MacLeod N. Prescription of nonsteroidal anti-inflammatory drug for elderly people in Alberta. Can Med Assoc J 1994 Aug 1;151(3):315-22.

[7]Durnas C, Cusak BJ. Salicylate intoxication in the elderly. Recognition and recommendations on how to prevent it [Review]. Drugs Aging 1992 Jan-Feb;2(1):20-34.

[8]Sager DS, Bennett RM. Individualizing the risk/benefit ration of NSAIDs in older patients [Review]. Geriatrics 1992 Aug;47(8):24-31.

[9]Whelton A, et al. Renal effects of ibuprofen, piroxican, and sulindac in patients with asymptomatic renal failure. Ann Intern Med 1990;112:568-76.

[10]Shorr RI, Ray WA, Daugherty JR, Griffin MR. Concurrent use of nonsteroidal antiinflammatory drugs and oral anticoagulants places elderly persons at high risk for hemorrhagic peptic ulcer disease. Arch Intern Med 1993 July 26;153(14):1665-70.

[11]Griffin MR, et al. NSAID use and death from peptic ulceration in the elderly. Ann Intern Med 1988;109:359-63.

[12]Melander A. Clinical pharmacology of sulfonylureas. Metabolism 1987;36(2)(supp 1).

[13]Leichter S. A prospective double-blind clinical trial of glipizide and glyburide in type II diabetes mellitus. Communication 1986.

[14]Asplund K, Wilholm BE, Lithner F. Glibenclamide-associated hypoglycemia: a report on 57 cases. Diabetologia 1984;26:412.

[15]Cadieux RJ. Geriatric psychopharmacology. A primary care challenge [Review]. Postgrad Med 1993 Mar;93(4):281-2, 285-8, 294-30.

[16]Mayer-Oakes SA, Kelman G, Beers MH, DeJong F, Matthias R, Atchison KA, Lubben JE, Schweitzer SO. Benzodiazepine use in older, community-dwelling southern Californians: prevalence and clinical correlates. Ann Pharmacother 1993 Apr;27(4):416-21.

[17]Stewart RM, Marks RG, Padgett PD, Hale WE. Benzodiazepine use in an ambulatory elderly population: a 14-year overview. Clin Ther 1994 Jan-Feb;16(1):118-24.

[18]Takami N, Okada A. Triazolam and nitrazepam use in elderly outpatients. Ann Pharmacother 1993 Apr;27(4):506-9.

[19]Cancellaro LA. Appropriate use of neuroleptics and antidepressants in the geriatric patient. South Med J 1991 May;84(5 Suppl):S53-6.

[20]Freeman C. Drug treatment of insomnia in the elderly. Conn Med 1992 Jan;56(1):35-7.

[21]Garrard J, Makris L, Dunham T, Heston LL, Cooper S, Ratner ER, Zelterman D, Kane RL. Evaluation of neuroleptic drug use by nursing home elderly under proposed Medicare and Medicaid regulations [see comments]. JAMA 1991 Jan 23-30;265(4):463-7.

[22]Katz IR. Drug treatment of depression in the frail elderly: discussion of the NIH Consensus Development Conference on the Diagnosis and Treatment of Depression in Late Life [Review]. Psychopharmacol Bull 1993;29(1):101-8.

[23]Monroe R, Jacobson G, Ervin F. Activation of psychosis by combination of scopolamine and alpha-chloralose. Arch Neurol 1957;76-536.

[24]Blazer DG, et al. The risk of anticholinergic toxicity in the elderly: a study of prescribing practices in two populations. J Gerontol 1983;38(1):31.

[25]Granacher RP, Baldessarini RJ. Physostigmine: its use in acute anticholinergic syndrome with antidepressant and antiparkinson drugs. Arch Gen Psychiatry 1975;32:375.
[26]Kulig K, Rumack BH. Anticholinergic poisoning. In Haddad LM, Winchester JF, eds. Clinical management of poisoning and drug overdose. Philadelphia: W.B. Saunders Co., 1983
[27]Bressler R, Katz MD. Drug therapy for geriatric depression [Review]. Drugs Aging 1993 May-Jun;3(3):195-219.
[28]Cassel CK, Walsh JR, eds. Medical, psychiatric, and pharmacological topics. Geriat Med 1984;1:554.
[29]Glassman AH, Roose SP. Risks of antidepressants in the elderly: tricyclic antidepressants and arrhythmia-revising risks [Review]. Gerontology 1994;40(Supp):15-20.
[30]Dunner DL. An overview of paroxetine in the elderly [Review]. Gerontology 1994;40(Supp):21-7.
[31]Sachs BA. The toxicity of benadryl: report of a case and review of the literature. Ann Intern Med 1948;29:135.
[32]Tune L, Carr S, Hoag E, Cooper T. Anticholinergic effects of drugs commonly prescribed for the elderly: potential means for assessing risk of delirium [see comments]. Am J Psychiatry 1992 Oct;149(10):1393-4.
[33]Wyngaarden JB, Severs MH. The toxic effects of antihistamine drugs. JAMA 1951;145:277.
[34]Hestand HE, Teske DW. Diphenhydramine hydrochloride intoxication. J Pediatr 1977; 90(6):1017.
[35]Iserson KV, Hackney KU. Antihistamines. In Haddad LM and Winchester JF. Clinical management of poisoning and drug overdose. Philadelphia: WB Saunders Co., 1983
[36]National Poison Center Network. Annual statistical report. Pittsburgh 1979.
[37]Nigro SA. Toxic psychosis due to diphenhydramine hydrochloride. JAMA 1968;203(4):139.
[38]Shorr RI, Robin DW. Rational use of benzodiazepines in the elderly [Review]. Drugs Aging 1994 Jan;4(1):9-20.
[39]Greenblatt DJ, Harmatz JS, et al. Sensitivity to triazolam in the elderly. N Engl J Med 1991;324:1691-8.
[40]Michocki RJ, Lamy PP, Hooper FJ, Richardson JP. Drug prescribing for the elderly [see comments] [Review]. Arch Fam Med 1993 Apr;2(4):441-4.
[41]Longe RL. Triazolam dose in older patients [letter]. J Am Geriatr Soc 1992 Jan;40(1):103-4.
[42]McCue RE. Using tricyclic antidepressants in the elderly [Review]. Clin Geriatric Med 1992 May; 8(2):323-34.
[43]Smith M, Buckwalter KC. Medication management, antidepressant drugs, and the elderly: an overview [Review]. J Psychosoc Nurs Ment Health Serv 1992 Oct;30(10):30-6.
[44]Thapa PB, Meador KG, Gideon P, Fought RL, Ray WA. Effects of antipsychotic withdrawal in elderly nursing home residents. J Am Geriatr Soc 1994 Mar;42(3):280-6.
[45]Todd B. Drugs and the elderly: identifying drug toxicity. Geriatr Nurs 1985;12:213.
[46]Lindley CM, Tully MP, Paramsothy V, Tallis RC. Inappropriate medication is a major cause of adverse drug reactions in elderly patients. Age Ageing 1992 July;21(4):294-30.
[47]Livingston J, Reeves RD. Undocumented potential drug interactions found in medical records of elderly patients in a long-term care facility. J Am Diet Assoc 1993 Oct;93(10):1168-70.
[48]Raskind MA. Geriatric psychopharmacology. Management of late-life depression and the noncognitive behavioral disturbances of Alzheimer's disease [Review]. Psychiatr Clin N Am 1993 Dec;16(4):815-27.
[49]Stewart RB. Advances in pharmacotherapy: depression in the elderly—issues and advances in treatment [Review]. J Clin Pharm Ther 1993 Aug;18(4):243-53.
[50]Swift CG. Prescribing in old age. BMJ 1988;296:913-15.
[51]Gurwitz JH, Avorn J, Ross-Degnan D, Choodnovskiy I, Ansell J. Aging and the anticoagulant response to warfarin therapy [see comments]. Ann Intern Med 1992 June 1;116(11):901-4.
[52]Stroke Prevention in Atrial Fibrillation Study Group. Preliminary report of the stroke prevention in atrial fibrillation study. N Engl J Med 1990;322:863-8.
[53]Becker RC, Ansell J. Antithrombotic therapy. An abbreviated reference for clinicians. Arch Intern Med 1995;155:149.
[54]Gibian T. Rational drug therapy in the elderly or how not to poison your elderly patients [Review]. Aust Fam Physician 1992 Dec;21(12):1755-60.
[55]Sternberg L. Unusual side reactions of hysteria from Benadryl. J Allergy 1947;18:417.

[56]Benson JW. Drug utilization patterns in geriatric drugs in the US-1986. J Geriatric Drug Ther In press.

[57]Bloom JA, Frank JW, Shafir MS, Martiquet P. Potentially undesirable prescribing and drug use among the elderly. Measurable and remediable [see comments]. Can Fam Physician 1993 Nov;39:2337-45.

[58]Eng HJ, Lee ES. The role of prescription drugs in health care for the elderly. Journal of Health and Human Resources Administration 1987;9:306-18.

[59]May FE, Stewart RM, Hale WE, et al. Prescribed and nonprescribe drug use in an ambulatory elderly population. South Med J 1982;75:522-8.

[60]Expert Panel on Detection, Evaluation, and Treatment of High Blood Cholesterol in Adults. Summary of the Second Report of the National Cholesterol Education Program. JAMA 1993;269:3015.

[61]Cleeland CS, et al. Pain and its treatment in outpatients with metastatic cancer. NEJM 1994 March 3;330:592-6.

[62]Graham DY, et al. Duodenal and gastric ulcer prevention with misoprostol in arthritis patients taking NSAIDs. Ann Int Med Aug 15, 1993;119:257-62.

[63]Silverstein FE, et al. Misoprostol reduces serious gastrointestinal complications in patients with rheumatoid arthritis receiving nonsteroidal anti-inflammatory drugs. Ann Int Med Aug 15, 1995;123:241-49.

[64]Raskin JB, et al. Misoprostol dosage in the prevention of nonsteroidal anti-inflammatory drug-induced gastric and duodenal ulcers: a comparison of three regimens. Ann Int Med Sept 1, 1995;123:344-50.

[65]Ladwig KH, et al. Post-infarction depression and incomplete recovery six months after acute myocardial infarction. Lancet 1994 Jan 1;343:20-3.

[66]Juniper EF, et al. Quality of life in asthma clinical trials: comparison of salmeterol and salbutamol. Am J Respir Crit Care Med 1995;151:66-70.

[67]Tariot PN, Schneider L, Porsteinsson AP, Treating Alzheimer's disease: pharmacologic options now and in the near future. Postgrad Med 1997; 101(6):73-90.

[68]Schneider LS, Tariot PN. Emerging drugs from Alzheimer's disease: mechanisms of action and prospects of cognitive enhancing medications. Med Clin North Am 1994;78:911.

[69]Knopman DS, Morris JC. An update on primary drug therapies for Alzheimer disease. Arch Neurol 1997;54:1406.

[70]Schneider LS. New therapeutic approaches to Alzheimer's disease. J Clin Psychiatry 1996; 57(suppl 14):30.

[71]Rogers SL, Perdomo C, Friedhoff LT. Clinical benefits are maintained during long-term treatment of Alzheimer's disease with the acetylcholinesterase inhibitor, E2020. Eur Neuropsychopharmacol (Abstract P-8-21) 1995;5:386.

[72]Tacrine Study Group. Long-term tacrine (Cognex) treatment: effects on nursing home placement and mortality. Neurology 1996;47:166.

POCKET VERSION

drug facts and comparisons®

Drug Facts and Comparisons® Pocket Version, Third Edition, 1999

Printed in the United States of America

Published by
Facts and Comparisons®
111 West Port Plaza, Suite 300
St. Louis, Missouri 63146-3098
314/216-2100

ANTICOAGULANTS

Blood coagulation resulting in the formation of a stable fibrin clot involves a cascade of proteolytic reactions involving the interaction of clotting factors, platelets and tissue materials. Clotting factors (see table) exist in the blood in inactive form and must be converted to an enzymatic or activated form before the next step in the clotting mechanism can be stimulated. Each factor is stimulated in turn until an insoluble fibrin clot is formed.

Two separate pathways, intrinsic and extrinsic, lead to the formation of a fibrin clot. Both pathways must function for hemostasis.

Intrinsic pathway: All the protein factors necessary for coagulation are present in circulating blood. Clot formation may take several minutes and is initiated by activation of factor XII.

Extrinsic pathway: Coagulation is activated by release of tissue thromboplastin, a factor not found in circulating blood. Clotting occurs in seconds because factor III bypasses the early reactions.

Refer to the next page for the complete coagulation pathway.

Anticoagulants used therapeutically include heparin, warfarin (a coumarin derivative) and anisindione (an indandione derivative).

Blood Clotting Factors

Factor	Synonym	Vitamin K-dependent
I	Fibrinogen	no
II	Prothrombin	yes
III	Tissue thromboplastin, tissue factor	no
IV	Calcium	no
V	Labile factor, proaccelerin	no
VII	Proconvertin	yes
VIII	Antihemophilic factor, AHF	no
IX	Christmas factor, plasma thromboplastin component, PTC	yes
X	Stuart factor, Stuart-Prower factor	yes
XI	Plasma thromboplastin antecedent, PTA	no
XII	Hageman factor	no
XIII	Fibrin stabilizing factor, FSF	no
HMW-K	High molecular weight Kininogen, Fitzgerald factor	no
PL	Platelets or phospholipids	no
PK	Prekallikrein, Fletcher factor	no
Protein C[1]		yes
Protein S[2]		yes

[1] Partially responsible for inhibition of the extrinsic pathway. Inactivates factors V and VIII and promotes fibrinolysis. Activity declines following warfarin administration.

[2] A cofactor to accelerate the anticoagulant activity of protein C. Decreased levels occur following warfarin administration.

COAGULATION PATHWAY

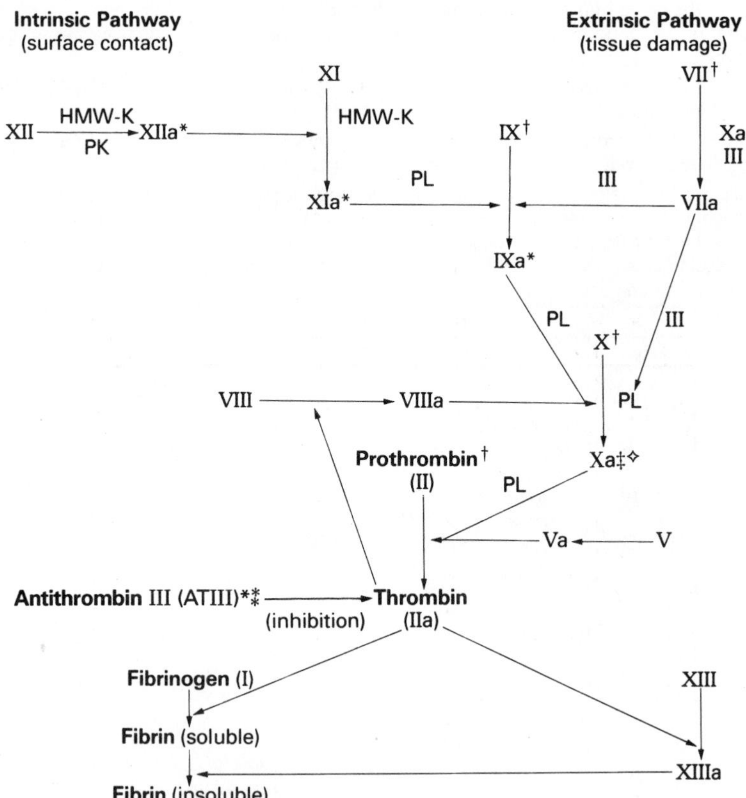

* Major site of activity for unfractionated heparin
† Site of activity for warfarin and anisindione
‡ Major site of activity for fractionated heparin
⁑ Minor site of activity for fractionated heparin
✧ Minor site of activity for unfractionated heparin

LOW MOLECULAR WEIGHT HEPARINS

ARDEPARIN SODIUM	
Injection: 5000 anti-Xa U in 0.5 ml and 10,000 anti-Xa U in 0.5 ml (*Rx*)	*Normiflo* (Wyeth)
DALTEPARIN SODIUM	
Solution: 16 mg/0.2 ml and 32 mg/0.2 ml (*Rx*)	*Fragmin* (Pharmacia)
ENOXAPARIN SODIUM	
Injection: 30 mg/0.3 ml and 40 mg/0.4 ml (*Rx*)	*Lovenox* (Rhone-Poulenc Rorer)

Actions:

Pharmacology: **Enoxaparin, ardeparin** and **dalteparin** are low molecular weight heparins (LMWHs) with antithrombotic properties. These agents enhance the inhibition of Factor Xa and thrombin by antithrombin III and potentiate preferentially the inhibition of coagulation factor Xa, while only slightly affecting thrombin and clotting time (eg, activated partial thromboplastin time [APTT] or prothrombin time [PT]).

Ardeparin binds to and accelarates the activity of antithrombin III, thereby inhibiting thrombosis by inactivating Factor Xa and thrombin and also inhibits thrombin by binding to heparin cofactor II.

Pharmacokinetics:

Pharmacokinetic Parameters of LMWHs Based on Anti-Xa Activity					
LMWH	Bioavailability (%)	T_{max} (hrs)	Vd (L)	Cl (ml/min)	Terminal t½ (hrs)
Ardeparin	76 to 108	2.1 to 3.3	4.3 to 9.5[1]	26.8 to 43.1[1,2]	NA
Dalteparin	81 to 93	4	2.8 to 4.2[1]	35 to 15.4[1]	3 to 5
Enoxaparin	92	3 to 5	6	25	4.5

[1] Based on a 70 kg patient.
[2] Following 30 and 120 IU/kg doses, respectively.
NA = Not available.

Indications:

Ardeparin: Prevention of deep-vein thrombosis, which may lead to pulmonary embolism, following knee replacement surgery.

Dalteparin: Prevention of deep-vein thrombosis, which may lead to pulmonary embolism in patients undergoing abdominal surgery who are at risk for thromboembolic complications.

Enoxaparin: Prevention of deep-vein thrombosis, which may lead to pulmonary embolism, following hip replacement surgery or abdominal surgery who are at risk for thromboembolic conplications.

Unlabeled uses: Systemic anticoagulation in venous and arterial thromboembolic complications (1 mg/kg **enoxaparin** SC twice daily); secondary prophylaxis for recurrent thromboembolic events (40 mg enoxaparin SC once daily, 35 to 50 U/kg **ardeparin** SC twice daily).

Contraindications:

Active major bleeding; thrombocytopenia associated with a positive in vitro test for antiplatelet antibody in the presence of an LMWH; hypersensitivity to LMWHs, heparin or pork products; methylparaben or propylparaben (**ardeparin**).

Warnings:

Interchangeability with heparin: LMWHs cannot be used interchangeably (unit for unit) with unfractionated heparin or other low molecular weight heparins.

Spinal/Epidural anesthesia: As with other anticoagulants, there have been rare cases of neuraxial hematomas reported with the concurrent use of **enoxaparin** and spinal/epidural anesthesia resulting in long-term or permanent paralysis.

Hemorrhage: Like other anticoagulants, use with extreme caution in conditions with increased risk of hemorrhage. Bleeding can occur at any site during therapy with enoxaparin.

Discontinue agents that might affect hemostatis (eg, oral anticoagulants, platelet inhibitors) prior to therapy with LMWHs. Concomitant use may increase the risk of hemorrhage.

Thrombocytopenia: Moderate thrombocytopenia occurred at a rate of about 2% in patients given **enoxaparin** and **ardeparin**, and < 1% with **dalteparin**. Closely monitor thrombocytopenia of any degree. If platelet count falls to < 100,000/mm^3, discontinue **enoxaparin**.

Heparin-induced thrombocytopenia: Use with extreme caution in patients with a history of this condition.

Renal function impairment: Delayed elimination of LMWHs may occur.

Elderly: Delayed elimination of **enoxaparin** may occur.

Pregnancy: Category B (**enoxaparin, dalteparin**), *Category* C (**ardeparin**).

Lactation: It is not known whether this drug is excreted in breast milk.

Children: Safety and efficacy in children have not been established.

Precautions:

Monitoring: Periodic complete blood counts, including platelet count, urinalysis and stool occult blood tests are recommended during the course of treatment.

Lipid effects: **Ardeparin** is known to increase lipoprotein lipase activity. Paradoxical elevations in serum triglyceride levels have occurred.

Special risk patients: Use with care in patients with a bleeding diathesis, uncontrolled arterial hypertension or a history of recent GI ulceration and hemorrhage and diabetic retinopathy.

Thromboembolic events: If thromboembolic events occur despite LMWH prophylaxis, discontinue and initiate appropriate therapy.

Sulfite sensitivity: **Ardeparin** contains metabisulfite, a sulfite that may cause allergic-type reactions including anaphylactic symptoms and life-threatening or less severe asthmatic episodes.

Drug Interactions:

Anticoagulants and platelet inhibitors: Use LMWHs with care.

Adverse Reactions:

Adverse reactions associated with LMWHs include hemorrhage, thrombocytopenia, local irritation following SC administration, fever, nausea, edema, peripheral edema and hyochromic anemia.

Lab test abnormalities:

Asymptomatic increases in transaminase levels (AST and ALT) > 3 times the upper limit of normal of the laboratory reference range have been reported in 1.7% to 5.5% and 4.3% to 8.7% of patients, respectively, during treatment with LMWHs. Such elevations are fully reversible and are rarely associated with increases in bilirubin. Since transaminase determinations are important in the differential diagnosis of myocardial infarction, liver disease and pulmonary emboli, interpret elevations that might be caused by drugs like LMWHs with caution.

Administration and Dosage:

ENOXAPARIN: In patients undergoing hip or knee replacement, the recommended dose is 30 mg twice daily administered by SC injection with the initial dose given as soon as possible after surgery, but not more than 24 hours postoperatively. Continue treatment throughout the period of postoperative care until the risk of deep-vein thrombosis has diminished. Up to 14 days administration has been well tolerated in controlled clinical trials. The average duration of administration is 7 to 10 days.

Screen all patients prior to prophylactic administration of enoxaparin to rule out a bleeding disorder. There is usually no need for daily monitoring of the effect of enoxaparin in patients with normal presurgical coagulation parameters.

Abdominal surgery – In adults undergoing abdominal surgery who are at risk for thromboembolic complications, the recommended dose of **enoxaparin** is 40 mg once/day administered SC with the initial dose given 2 hours prior to surgery. The usual duration of administration is 7 to 10 days; up to 12 days.

Administration – Administer by SC injection. Do not administer by IM injection.

SC injection technique – Patients should be lying down; administer by deep SC injection. Alternate administration between the left and right anterolateral and left and right posterolateral abdominal wall. Introduce the whole length of the needle into a skin fold held between the thumb and forefinger; hold the skin fold throughout the injection.

DALTEPARIN:

Administration – Administer by SC injection, not by IM injection.

Adults – In patients undergoing abdominal surgery with a risk of thromboembolic complications, administer 2500 IU each day, SC only, starting 1 to 2 hours prior to surgery and repeated once daily for 5 to 10 days postoperatively. Dosage adjustment and routine monitoring of coagulation parameters are not required if these dosage and administration recommendations are followed.

High risk patients – In patients at high risk for thromboembolic complications (eg, malignancy), administer 5000 IU, SC only, the evening before surgery and repeat once daily for 5 to 10 days postoperatively. Alternatively, in patients with malignancy, the first 5000 IU dose can be administered as 2500 IU SC 1 to 2 hours prior to surgery with an additional 2500 IU SC dose 12 hours later and then 5000 IU once daily for 5 to 10 days.

Systemic anticoagulation – 200 IU/kg SC daily or 100 IU/kg SC twice daily.

SC injection technique – Administer while patient is sitting or lying down by deep SC injection. Dalteparin may be injected in a U-shaped area around the navel, the upper outer side of the thigh or the upper outer quadrangle of the buttock. Vary the injection site daily. When the area around the navel or the thigh is used, use the thumb and forefinger to lift up a fold of skin while giving the injection. Insert the entire length of the needle at a 45 to 90 degree angle.

Admixture incompatibility – Do not mix with other injections or infusions unless specific compatibility data are available that support such mixing.

ARDEPARIN: Administer by deep SC injection. Do not give IM in order to avoid the possible occurrence of hematoma at the injection site.

The recommended SC injection is 50 anti-Xa U/kg every 12 hours. Begin treatment the evening of the day of surgery or the following morning and continue for ≤ 14 days or until the patient is fully ambulatory.

HEPARIN

HEPARIN SODIUM	
Injection: 1000, 5000, 10,000 and 20,000 units/ml (multiple dose vials) (*Rx*)	Various, *Liquaemin Sodium* (Organon)
Injection: 1000, 5000, 10,000 and 20,000 units/ml (single dose amps and vials) (*Rx*)	Various, *Liquaemin Sodium Preservative Free* (Organon)
Injection: 1000, 2500, 5000, 7500, 10,000 and 20,000 units/ml (unit dose vials) (*Rx*)	Various
HEPARIN SODIUM AND SODIUM CHLORIDE	
Injection: 1000 and 2000 units (*Rx*)	*Heparin Sodium and 0.9% Sodium Chloride-* (Clintec)
Injection: 12,500 and 25,000 units (*Rx*)	*Heparin Sodium and 0.45% Sodium Chloride* (Abbott)
HEPARIN SODIUM LOCK FLUSH	
Injection: 10 and 100 units/ml (*Rx*)	Various, *Hep-Lock* (Elkins-Sinn)

Actions:

Pharmacology: The major rate-limiting step in the coagulation cascade is the activation of factor X, which is involved in both intrinsic and extrinsic pathways. Small amounts of heparin in combination with antithrombin III (heparin cofactor) inhibit thrombosis by inactivating factor Xa and inhibiting the conversion of prothrombin to thrombin. Once active thrombosis has developed, larger amounts of heparin can inhibit further coagulation by inactivating thrombin and preventing the conversion of fibrinogen to fibrin. In combination with antithrombin III, heparin inactivates factors IX, X, Xa, XI, XII and thrombin, inhibiting conversion of fibrinogen to fibrin. The heparin-antithrombin III complex is 100 to 1000 times more potent as an anticoagulant than antithrombin III alone. Heparin also prevents the formation of a stable fibrin clot by inhibiting the activation of factor XIII (the fibrin stabilizing factor). Other effects include the inhibition of thrombin-induced activation of factors V and VIII.

Commercial products contain both low and high molecular weight heparin fractions. Low molecular weight heparin has a greater inhibitory effect on factor Xa, and less antithrombin activity than the high molecular weight fraction.

Heparin inhibits reactions that lead to clotting, but does not significantly alter the concentration of the normal clotting factors of blood. Although clotting time is prolonged by full therapeutic doses, in most cases it is not measurably affected by low doses of heparin. Bleeding time is usually unaffected.

Heparin also enhances lipoprotein lipase release, (which clears plasma of circulating lipids), increases circulating free fatty acids and reduces lipoprotein levels.

Pharmacokinetics:

Absorption/Distribution – Heparin is not adsorbed from the GI tract. An IV bolus results in immediate anticoagulant effects. The duration of action is dose-dependent. Peak plasma levels of heparin are achieved 2 to 4 hours following SC use. Once absorbed, heparin is distributed in plasma and is extensively protein bound.

Metabolism/Excretion – Following administration, heparin demonstrates a biphasic elimination curve. The lack of relationship between plasma and pharmacologic half-lives may reflect factors such as protein binding. Heparin is rapidly cleared from plasma with an average half-life of 30 to 180 minutes. Half-life is dose-dependent and may be significantly prolonged at higher doses. Heparin is partially metabolized by liver heparinase and the reticuloendothelial system. There may be a secondary site of metabolism in the kidneys. Apparent volume of distribution is 40 to 60 ml/kg. In patients with deep venous thrombosis, plasma clearance is more rapid and half-life is shorter than in patients with pulmonary embolism. Heparin is excreted in urine as unchanged drug (up to 50%) particularly after large doses. Some urinary degradation products have anticoagulant activity.

Indications:

Prophylaxis and treatment of venous thrombosis and its extension; pulmonary embolism; peripheral arterial embolism; atrial fibrillation with embolization.

Diagnosis and treatment of acute and chronic consumption coagulopathies (disseminated intravascular coagulation [DIC]).

Postoperative: Low dose regimen for prevention of postoperative deep venous thrombosis (DVT) and pulmonary embolism in patients undergoing major abdominothoracic surgery or patients who are at risk of developing thromboembolic disease.

According to National Institutes of Health Consensus Development Conference, low-dose heparin is treatment of choice as prophylaxis for DVT and pulmonary embolism in urology patients > 40 years old; pregnant patients with prior thromboembolism; stroke patients; those with heart failure, acute MI or pulmonary infection; also recommended as suggested prophylaxis in high-risk surgery patients, moderate and high-risk gynecologic patients without malignancy, neurology patients with extracranial problems and patients with severe musculoskeletal trauma.

Prevention of clotting in arterial and heart surgery, blood transfusions, extracorporeal circulation, dialysis procedures and blood samples for laboratory purposes.

Unlabeled uses: Prophylaxis of left ventricular thrombi and cerebrovascular accidents post-MI.

Continuous infusion for treatment of myocardial ischemia in unstable angina refractory to conventional treatment. Heparin decreases the number of anginal attacks and silent ischemic episodes and reduces the daily duration of ischemia. Intermittent heparin is not as effective.

Prevention of cerebral thrombosis in the evolving stroke.

As an adjunct in treatment of coronary occlusion with acute myocardial infarction (MI). Although there is some controversy regarding the efficacy of heparin therapy with concurrent antiplatelet therapy (eg, aspirin) in the prevention of rethrombosis/reocclusion after primary thrombolysis with thrombolytics during acute MI, it is recommended by the American College of Cardiology and the American Heart Association. Generally, administer heparin IV immediately after thrombolytic therapy, usually within 2 to 8 hours (depending on the thrombolytic used), and maintain the infusion for at least 24 hours. Begin aspirin therapy immediately as soon as the patient is admitted, and continue its administration.

Contraindications:

Hypersensitivity to heparin; severe thrombocytopenia; uncontrolled bleeding (except when it is due to DIC); any patient for whom suitable blood coagulation tests cannot be performed at the appropriate intervals (there is usually no need to monitor coagulation parameters in patients receiving low-dose heparin).

Warnings:

Hemorrhage can occur at virtually any site in patients receiving heparin. An unexplained fall in hematocrit, fall in blood pressure or any other unexplained symptom should lead to serious consideration of a hemorrhagic event. An overly prolonged coagulation test or bleeding can usually be controlled by withdrawing the drug. Signs and symptoms will vary according to the location and extent of bleeding and may present as paralysis, headache, chest, abdomen, joint or other pain, shortness of breath, difficulty breathing or swallowing, unexplained swelling or unexplained shock. GI or urinary tract bleeding may indicate an underlying occult lesion. Certain hemorrhagic complications may be difficult to detect.

Use heparin with extreme caution in disease states in which there is increased danger of hemorrhage. These include:

Cardiovascular – Subacute bacterial endocarditis; arterial sclerosis; dissecting aneurysm; increased capillary permeability; severe hypertension.

CNS – During and immediately following spinal tap, spinal anesthesia or major surgery, especially of the brain, spinal cord or eye.

Hematologic – Hemophilia; some vascular purpuras; thrombocytopenia.

GI – Ulcerative lesions, diverticulitis or ulcerative colitis; continuous tube drainage of the stomach or small intestine.

Obstetric – Threatened abortion; menstruation.

Other – Liver disease with impaired hemostasis; severe renal disease.

Hyperlipidemia: Heparin may increase free fatty acid serum levels by induction of lipoprotein lipase. The catabolism of serum lipoproteins by this enzyme produces lipid fragments which are rapidly processed by the liver. Patients with dysbetalipoproteinemia (type III) are unable to catabolize the lipid fragments, resulting in hyperlipidemia.

Resistance: Increased resistance to the drug is frequently encountered in fever, thrombosis, thrombophlebitis, infections with thrombosing tendencies, MI, cancer and postoperative states.

Thrombocytopenia has occurred in patients receiving heparin. The incidence of heparin-associated thrombocytopenia is higher with bovine than with porcine heparin. The severity also appears to be related to heparin dose.

Early thrombocytopenia (Type I) develops 2 to 3 days after starting heparin, tends to be mild and is due to a direct action of heparin on platelets.

Delayed thrombocytopenia (Type II) develops 7 to 12 days after either low-dose or full-dose heparin, can have serious consequences and may reflect the presence of an immunoglobulin that induces platelet aggregation.

Mild thrombocytopenia may remain stable or reverse even if heparin is continued. However, closely monitor thrombocytopenia of any degree. If a count falls below 100,000/mm^3 or if recurrent thrombosis develops, discontinue heparin. If continued heparin therapy is essential, administration of heparin from a different organ source can be reinstituted with caution.

White clot syndrome – Rarely, patients may develop new thrombus formation in association with thrombocytopenia resulting from irreversible aggregation of platelets induced by heparin, the so-called "white clot syndrome." The process may lead to severe thromboembolic complications. Monitor platelet counts before and during therapy. If significant thrombocytopenia occurs, immediately terminate heparin and institute other therapeutic measures.

Hypersensitivity: Heparin is derived from animal tissue; use with caution in patients with a history of allergy. Before a therapeutic dose is given, a trial dose may be advisable. Have epinephrine 1:1000 immediately available.

Vasospastic reactions may develop 6 to 10 days after starting therapy and last 4 to 6 hours. The affected limb is painful, ischemic and cyanotic. An artery to this limb may have been recently catheterized. After repeated injections, the reaction may gradually increase to generalized vasospasm with cyanosis, tachypnea, feeling of oppression and headache. Itching and burning, especially on the plantar side of the feet, is possibly based on a similar allergic vasospastic reaction. Chest pain, elevated blood pressure, arthralgias or headache have also been reported in the absence of definite peripheral vasospasm.

Hepatic function impairment: Heparin half-life may be prolonged in liver disease.

Elderly: A higher incidence of bleeding has occurred in women > 60 years of age.

Pregnancy: Category C. Safety for use during pregnancy has not been established. Heparin does not cross the placenta. However, its use during pregnancy has been associated with 13% to 22% unfavorable outcomes, including stillbirths and prematurity. This contrasts with a 31% incidence with coumarin derivatives. Heparin is probably the preferred anticoagulant during pregnancy, but it is not risk free.

Lactation: Heparin is not excreted in breast milk.

Children: Safety and efficacy have not been determined in newborns; germinal matrix intraventricular hemorrhage occurs more often in low-birth-weight infants receiving heparin.

Use heparin lock flush solution with caution in infants with disease states in which there is an increased danger of hemorrhage. The use of the 100 unit/ml concentration is not advised because of bleeding risk, especially in low-birth-weight infants.

Precautions:

Monitoring: The most common test used to monitor heparin's effect is APTT. Other tests used include Activated Coagulation Time (ACT) and Lee White-Whole Blood Clotting Time (WBCT). If the coagulation test is unduly prolonged or if hemorrhage occurs, discontinue the drug promptly. Perform periodic platelet counts, hematocrit and tests for occult blood in stool during the entire course of therapy, regardless of route of administration.

Hyperkalemia may develop, probably due to induced hypoaldosteronism. Use with caution in patients with diabetes or renal insufficiency. Monitor patient closely.

Drug Interactions:

Drugs that may interact include cephalosporins, nitroglycerin, penicillins and salicylates.

Drug/Lab test interactions: Significant elevations of **aminotransferase** (AST and ALT) levels have occurred in a high percentage of patients. Cautiously interpret aminotransferase increases that might be caused by heparin.

If heparin comprises ≥ 10% of the total volume of a sample for blood gas analysis, errors in measurements of **carbon dioxide pressure, bicarbonate concentration** and **base excess** may occur.

Adverse Reactions:

Adverse reactions associated with heparin include hemorrhage, chills, fever, urticaria and thrombocytopenia.

Administration and Dosage:

Give by intermittent IV injection, continuous IV infusion or deep SC (ie, above the iliac crest of abdominal fat layer) injection. Continuous IV infusion is generally preferable due to the higher incidence of bleeding complications with other routes. Avoid IM injection because of the danger of hematoma formation.

Adjust dosage according to coagulation test results prior to each injection. Dosage is adequate when WBCT is ≈ 2.5 to 3 times control value, or when APTT is 1.5 to 2 times normal.

When given by continuous IV infusion, perform coagulation tests every 4 hours in the early stages. When administered by intermittent IV infusion, perform coagulation tests before each dose during early stages and at appropriate intervals thereafter. After deep SC injection, perform tests 4 to 6 hours after the injections.

General heparin dosage guidelines: Although dosage must be individualized, the following may be used as guidelines:

Heparin Dosage Guidelines

Method of administration	Frequency	Recommended dose[1]
Subcutaneous[2]	Initial dose	10,000 – 20,000 units[3]
	Every 8 hours	8000 – 10,000 units
	Every 12 hours	15,000 – 20,000 units
Intermittent IV	Initial dose	10,000 units[4]
	Every 4 to 6 hours	5000 – 10,000 units[4]

Heparin Dosage Guidelines		
Method of administration	Frequency	Recommended dose[1]
IV Infusion	Continuous	20,000 – 40,000 units/day[3]

[1] Based on a 68 kg (150 lb) patient.
[2] Use a concentrated solution.
[3] Immediately preceded by IV loading dose of 5000 units.
[4] Administer undiluted or in 50 to 100 ml 0.9% NaCl.

Children: In general, the following dosage schedule may be used as a guideline:

Initial dose – 50 units/kg IV bolus.

Maintenance dose – 100 units/kg/dose IV drip every 4 hours, or 20,000 units/m^2/24 hours continuous IV infusion.

Low-dose prophylaxis of postoperative thromboembolism: Low-dose heparin prophylaxis, prior to and after surgery, will reduce the incidence of postoperative DVT in the legs and clinical pulmonary embolism. Give 5000 units SC 2 hours before surgery and 5000 units every 8 to 12 hours thereafter for 7 days or until the patient is fully ambulatory, whichever is longer. Administer by deep SC injection above the iliac crest or abdominal fat layer, arm or thigh using a concentrated solution. Use a fine gauge needle (25 to 26 gauge) to minimize tissue trauma. Reserve such prophylaxis for patients > 40 years of age undergoing major surgery. Exclude patients on oral anticoagulants or drugs that affect platelet function or in patients with bleeding disorders, brain or spinal cord injuries, spinal anesthesia, eye surgery or potentially sanguineous operations.

If bleeding occurs during or after surgery, discontinue heparin and neutralize with protamine sulfate. If clinical evidence of thromboembolism develops despite low-dose prophylaxis, give full therapeutic doses of anticoagulants until contraindicated. Prior to heparinization, rule out bleeding disorders; perform appropriate coagulation tests just prior to surgery. Coagulation test values should be normal or only slightly elevated at these times.

Surgery of the heart and blood vessels: Give an initial dose of not less than 150 units/kg to patients undergoing total body perfusion for open heart surgery. Often, 300 units/kg is used for procedures < 60 minutes and 400 units/kg is used for procedures > 60 minutes.

Extracorporeal dialysis: Follow equipment manufacturers' operating directions.

Laboratory samples: Add 70 to 150 units per 10 to 20 ml sample of whole blood to prevent coagulation of sample.

Clearing intermittent infusion (heparin lock) sets: To prevent clot formation in a heparin lock set, inject dilute heparin solution (Heparin Lock Flush Solution, USP; or a 10 to 100 units/ml heparin solution) via the injection hub in a quantity sufficient to fill the entire set to the needle tip. Replace this solution each time the heparin lock is used. If the administered drug is incompatible with heparin, flush the entire heparin lock set with sterile water or normal saline before and after the medication is administered; following the second flush, the dilute heparin solution may be reinstilled into the set. Consult the set manufacturer's instructions.

Converting to oral anticoagulant therapy: Perform baseline coagulation tests to determine prothrombin activity when heparin activity is too low to affect PT or INR. When the results of the initial prothrombin determinations are known, initiate the oral anticoagulant in the usual amount. Thereafter, perform coagulation tests and prothrombin activity at appropriate intervals. When the prothrombin activity reaches the desired therapeutic range, discontinue heparin and continue oral anticoagulants.

COUMARIN AND INDANDIONE DERIVATIVES

WARFARIN SODIUM
Tablets: 1, 2, 2.5, 4, 5, 7.5 and 10 mg (*Rx*) — *Coumadin* (DuPont)

ANISINDIONE
Tablets: 50 mg (*Rx*) — *Miradon* (Schering)

DICUMAROL
Tablets: 25 mg (*Rx*) — *Dicumarol* (Abbott)

Actions:

Pharmacology: Coumarins (dicumarol and warfarin) and indandiones (anisindione) interfere with the hepatic synthesis of vitamin K-dependent clotting factors which results in an in vivo depletion of clotting factors VII, IX, X and II (prothrombin). Anticoagulant effects are dependent on the half-lives of these clotting factors, which are 6, 24, 36 and 50 hours, respectively. Hence, the reduction in the rate of synthesis of the clotting factors determines the clinical response. Although factor VII is quickly depleted and an initial prolongation of the prothrombin time (PT) is seen in 8 to 12 hours, maximum anticoagulation (thus, antithrombotic effects) is not approached for 3 to 5 days as the other factors are depleted and the drug achieves steadystate.

Oral anticoagulants have no direct effect on an established thrombus, nor do they reverse ischemic tissue damage. However, once thrombosis has occurred, anticoagulant treatment may prevent further extension of the formed clot and prevent secondary thromboembolic complications which may result in serious and possibly fatal sequelae.

Warfarin is available as a racemic mixture containing the R(+) and S(–) enantiomers in equal proportions; however, the S-isomer is 3 to 6 times more potent as an anticoagulant than the R-isomer.

Pharmacokinetics:

Absorption – The oral anticoagulants are generally rapidly and completely absorbed.

Distribution – Oral anticoagulants are highly bound to plasma proteins (97% to > 99%), primarily albumin.

Metabolism/Excretion – These agents are metabolized by hepatic microsomal enzymes and are excreted primarily in the urine and feces as inactive metabolites.

Various Pharmacokinetic Parameters of Oral Anticoagulants

Oral anticoagulant	Half-life (days)	Peak activity (days)	Duration[1] (days)
Coumarin derivatives			
Dicumarol	1-2	1.5-2	5-6
Warfarin	1-2.5[2]	1.5-3	2-5
Indandione derivative			
Anisindione	3-5	2-3	1-3

[1] Following drug discontinuation
[2] S-isomer ≈ 2 days; R-isomer ≈ 1.33 days

Indications:

Warfarin/Anisindione/Dicumarol: Prophylaxis and treatment of venous thrombosis and its extension; treatment of atrial fibrillation with embolization; prophylaxis and treatment of pulmonary embolism.

Warfarin: Prophylaxis of atrial fibrillation with embolism. As an adjunct in the prophylaxis of systemic embolism after myocardial infarction (MI).

Anisindione/Dicumarol: As an adjunct in the treatment of coronary occlusion. Warfarin is generally the drug of choice.

Unlabeled uses: Oral anticoagulants have been used to prevent recurrent transient ischemic attacks and to reduce the risk of recurrent MI, but data conflict. Warfarin has shown potential benefit as an adjunct in the treatment of small cell carcinoma of the lung, given concomitantly with chemotherapy and radiation.

Contraindications:

Pregnancy (see Warnings); hemorrhagic tendencies; hemophilia; thrombocytopenic purpura; leukemia; recent or contemplated surgery of the eye or CNS, major regional lumbar block anesthesia, or surgery resulting in large, open surfaces; patients bleeding from the GI, respiratory or GU tract; threatened abortion; aneurysm (cerebral, dissecting aortic); ascorbic acid deficiency; history of bleeding diathesis; prostatectomy; continuous tube drainage of the small intestine; polyarthritis; diverticulitis; emaciation; malnutrition; cerebrovascular hemorrhage; eclampsia and preeclampsia; blood dyscrasias; severe uncontrolled or malignant hypertension; severe renal or hepatic disease; pericarditis and pericardial effusion; subacute bacterial endocarditis; visceral carcinoma; following spinal puncture and other diagnostic or therapeutic procedures (ie, IUD insertion) with potential for uncontrollable bleeding; unsupervised senility; alcoholism; psychosis; open wounds; history of warfarin-induced necrosis.

Warnings:

Monitoring:

PT – Treatment is highly individualized. Control dosage by periodic determination of PT or other suitable coagulation tests (eg, INR). Monitor PT daily during the initiation of therapy and whenever any other drug is added to or discontinued from therapy which may alter the patient's response. Concurrent heparin therapy will elevate the PT 10% to 20%; if target PT levels are not increased by the same percentage during concurrent therapy, the patient could be inadequately anticoagulated when the heparin therapy is discontinued. Once stabilized, monitor PT every 4 to 6 weeks.

INR is based on the determination of an International Normalized Ratio which provides a common basis for PT results and interpretations of therapeutic ranges. For a discussion of the relationship between PT and INR in clinical practice, refer to Administration and Dosage.

Hemorrhage/Necrosis: The most serious risks associated with anticoagulant therapy are hemorrhage in any tissue or organ and, less frequently, necrosis or gangrene of skin and other tissues; this has resulted in death or permanent disability. The risk of hemorrhage is related to the level of intensity and duration of therapy. Discontinue therapy when anticoagulants are the suspected cause of developing necrosis; consider heparin therapy.

Hemorrhagic tendency may be manifested by hematuria, skin petechiae, hemorrhage into or from a wound or ulcerating lesion or petechial and purpuric hemorrhages throughout the body.

Bleeding during anticoagulant therapy does not always correlate with prothrombin activity. Bleeding that occurs when the PT or INR is within the therapeutic range warrants investigation since it may unmask a previously unsuspected lesion (eg, tumor, ulcer).

Independent risk factors that may provide a basis for predicting major bleeding with anticoagulants include: ≥ 65 years of age; history of stroke; history of GI bleeding; serious comorbid condition (eg, recent MI, renal insufficiency, severe anemia); atrial fibrillation.

"Purple toe syndrome" – Anticoagulant therapy may enhance the release of atheromatous plaque emboli thereby increasing the risk of complications from systemic cholesterol microembolization including the "purple toe syndrome."

Excessive uterine bleeding may occur, but menstrual flow is usually normal. Women may be at risk of developing ovarian hemorrhage at the time of ovulation.

Oral anticoagulants should not be used in the treatment of acute completed strokes due to the risk of fatal cerebral hemorrhage.

Adrenal hemorrhage with resultant acute adrenal insufficiency has occurred.

Special risk patients: There is an increased risk with use of anticoagulants in the following conditions: Trauma; infection (concomitant antibiotic therapy may alter intestinal flora); renal insufficiency; prolonged dietary insufficiencies (eg, sprue, vitamin K deficiency); severe to moderate hypertension; polycythemia vera; vasculitis; severe allergic disorders; anaphylactic disorders; indwelling catheters; severe diabetes; surgery or trauma resulting in large exposed raw surfaces.

Use with caution in patients with active tuberculosis, severe diabetes, history of ulcerative disease of the GI tract and during menstruation and the postpartum period.

Protein C deficiency: Known or suspected hereditary, familial or clinical deficiency in protein C has been associated with necrosis following warfarin therapy.

Agranulocytosis and hepatitis have been associated with anisindione use.

Rebound hypercoagulability was thought to occur upon sudden anticoagulant withdrawal, but has not been reproducible. Also there is no evidence that thrombosis will recur following abrupt withdrawal. Therefore, tapering the dose to discontinuation appears unnecessary, although tapering the dose gradually over 3 to 4 weeks is recommended if possible.

CHF: Patients with CHF may become more sensitive to dicumarol.

Hypersensitivity: Delayed reactions are rare and occur within 1 to 3 months following the start of anisindione; 10% of cases are fatal. Discontinue the medication at the first sign of hypersensitivity reactions.

Renal/Hepatic function impairment: Use with caution.

Elderly: Older patients may be more sensitive to these agents.

Pregnancy: *Category* X.

If oral anticoagulants are used in pregnant women, do not administer during the first trimester, and discontinue prior to labor and delivery.

Some clinicians suggest the replacement of oral anticoagulants with heparin therapy before term. After 5 to 7 days, therapy with oral anticoagulants may be resumed if indicated.

Lactation: Warfarin appears in breast milk in an inactive form. Infants nursed by warfarin-treated mothers had no change in PT.

Anisindione and dicumarol or their metabolites may be excreted in breast milk in amounts sufficient to cause a prothrombopenic state and bleeding in the newborn.

Children: Safety and efficacy in children < 18 years old have not been established. Oral anticoagulants may be beneficial in children with rare thromboembolic disorder secondary to other disease states such as the nephrotic syndrome or congenital heart lesions. Heparin is probably the initial anticoagulant of choice because of its immediate onset of action.

Precautions:

Enhanced anticoagulant effects: Several endogenous factors that may result in an increased response to the oral anticoagulants or an increased PT or INR include: Carcinoma; hepatic disorders including hepatitis or obstructive jaundice; biliary fistula; febrile states; preparatory bowel sterilization; recent surgery; x-ray therapy; vitamin K deficiency; steatorrhea; CHF; diarrhea; poor nutritional state or collagen disease; renal insufficiency; hyperthyroidism; elevated temperature. Also, female and elderly patients are more sensitive to these agents.

Decreased anticoagulant effects: Endogenous factors that may reduce the response to the oral anticoagulants or decrease the PT or INR include: Edema; hyperlipidemia; diabetes mellitus; hypothyroidism; hereditary resistance to oral anticoagulants.

Drug Interactions:

Oral anticoagulants have a great potential for clinically significant drug interactions. Warn all patients about potential hazards and instruct against taking **any** drug, including nonprescription products, without the advice of a physician or pharmacist.

Careful monitoring and appropriate dosage adjustments usually will permit safe administration of combined therapy. Critical times during therapy occur when an interacting drug is added to or discontinued from a patient stabilized on anticoagulants.

Coumarin and indandione derivatives are affected by many drugs. Those that may significantly affect coumarin and indandione derivatives include amiodarone, 17–alkyl androgens, barbiturates, clofibrate, dextrothyroxine, erythromycin, histamine H_2 antagonists, metronidazole, miconazole, phenylbutazones, quinine derivatives, salicylates, sulfinpyrazone, sulfonamides, thioamines, thyroid hormones and vitamin E.

Drug/Lab test interactions: Oral anticoagulants may cause red-orange discoloration of alkaline urine; this may interfere with some lab tests.

Adverse Reactions:

Hemorrhage is the principal adverse effect of oral anticoagulants.

Other adverse reactions include nausea; diarrhea; pyrexia; dermatitis; exfoliative dermatitis; urticaria; alopecia; sore mouth; mouth ulcers; fever; abdominal cramping; leukopenia; red-orange urine; priapism (causal relationship not established); paralytic ileus and intestinal obstruction from submucosal or intramural hemorrhage.

Administration and Dosage:

Dosage: Individualize dosage.

Available clinical evidence indicates that prolongation of the PT to 1.2 to 1.5 times control, when measuring with the less sensitive thromboplastin reagents, is sufficient for prophylaxis and treatment of venous thromboembolism and minimizes the risk of hemorrhage associated with more prolonged PT values. In cases where the risk of thromboembolism is great, such as in patients with recurrent systemic embolism, maintain a PT of 1.5 to 2 times control. A ratio of > 2 appears to provide no additional therapeutic benefit in most patients and is associated with a higher risk of bleeding.

For the three commercial rabbit brain thromboplastins currently used in North America, a PT ratio of 1.3 to 2 is equivalent to an INR of 2 to 4. For other thromboplastins, the INR can be calculated as:

$$\text{INR} = (\text{observed PT ratio})^{\text{ISI}}$$

where the ISI (International Sensitivity Index) is the calibration factor and is available from the manufacturers of the thromboplastin reagent and observed PT ratio is:

$$\frac{\text{PT observed}}{\text{PT control}}$$

Following are the recommended therapeutic ranges for oral anticoagulant therapy from the American College of Chest Physicians (ACCP) and the National Heart, Lung and Blood Institute (NHLBI):

ACCP/NHLBI Recommended Therapeutic Range for Oral Anticogulant Therapy

Condition	PT Ratio[1]	INR
Acute MI[2]	1.3 to 1.5	2 to 3
Atrial fibrillation[2]	1.3 to 1.5	2 to 3
Mechanical prosthetic valves	1.5 to 2	3 to 4.5
Pulmonary embolism, treatment	1.3 to 1.5	2 to 3
Systemic embolism		
Prevention	1.3 to 1.5	2 to 3
Recurrent	1.5 to 2	3 to 4.5
Tissue heart valves[2]	1.3 to 1.5	2 to 3
Valvular heart disease[2]	1.3 to 1.5	2 to 3
Venous thrombosis		
Prophylaxis (high-risk surgery)	1.3 to 1.5	2 to 3
Treatment	1.3 to 1.5	2 to 3

[1] ISI of 2.4
[2] To prevent systemic embolism

Transfer from heparin therapy: To provide continuous adequate anticoagulation in a patient on heparin, switch to oral anticoagulation. Since there is a delayed onset of oral anticoagulant effects, give heparin and warfarin simultaneously from the first day, or alternatively, start warfarin on the third to sixth day of heparin therapy. Use concurrent therapy until a therapeutic PT or INR is achieved.

Elderly: Lower dosages are recommended.

Duration of therapy: In the determination of the duration of long-term anticoagulant therapy, consider history of recurrent thromboembolism, underlying diseases, reason for anticoagulant therapy (eg, atrial fibrillation) and risks of adverse effects.

WARFARIN:

Induction – Initiate with 10 mg/day for 2 to 4 days; adjust daily dosage according to PT or INR determinations. Use of a large loading dose (eg, 30 mg) may increase the incidence of hemorrhagic and other complications, does not offer more rapid protection against thrombi formation and is not recommended.

Maintenance – 2 to 10 mg daily, based on PT or INR.

Bioequivalence problems have been documented for warfarin sodium products marketed by different manufacturers. Brand interchange is not recommended.

Treatment during dentistry and surgery – In patients who must be anticoagulated prior to, during or immediately following dental or surgical procedures, adjusting the dosage to maintain the PT at the low end of the therapeutic range (or maintain the corresponding INR value) may safely allow for continued anticoagulation. Limit the operative site to permit effective use of local measures for hemostasis. Under these conditions, dental and surgical procedures may be performed without undue risk of hemorrhage.

Minidose warfarin may be beneficial as prophylaxis against venous thrombosis after major surgery. In one study, 1 mg daily given before surgery (mean 20 days) significantly lowered the incidence of DVT compared to controls; there was no difference between the 1 mg/day and the full-dose anticoagulation group. APTT and PT were not prolonged beyond normal on the day of surgery using the minidose therapy.

ANISINDIONE: 300 mg the first day, 200 mg the second day, 100 mg the third day and 25 to 250 mg daily for maintenance.

DICUMAROL: 200 to 300 mg the first day, 25 to 200 mg on subsequent days.

Treatment during dentistry and surgery – If it is elected to administer anticoagulants prior to, during or immediately following dental or surgical procedures, it is recommended that the dosage of dicumarol be adjusted to maintain the prothrombin time at
≈ 1½ to 2½ times the control level.

ESTROGENS

ESTRONE AQUEOUS	
Injection: 2 and 5 mg per ml (*Rx*)	Various, *Aquest* (Dunhall), *Estrone 5* (Keene), *Kestrone 5* (Hyrex)
ESTROGENIC SUBSTANCE OR ESTROGENS (MAINLY ESTRONE) AQUEOUS SUSPENSION	
Injection: 2 mg per ml estrogenic substance or estrogens (mainly estrone) (*Rx*)	Various
ESTRADIOL TRANSDERMAL SYSTEM	
Transdermal Patch: 0.0375 mg, 0.05 mg, 0.075 mg and 0.1 mg per 24 hours (*Rx*)	*Estraderm* (Ciba), *Climara* (Berlex), *Vivelle* (Ciba)
ESTRADIOL, ORAL	
Tablets: 0.5, 1 and 2 mg micronized estradiol (*Rx*)	*Estrace* (Bristol-Myers Squibb)
ESTRADIOL VALERATE IN OIL	
Injection: 10, 20 and 40 mg per ml (*Rx*)	Various, *Delestrogen* (Mead Johnson), *Dioval* (Keene), *Estra-L* (Pasadena), *Gynogen L.A.* (Forest), *Valergen* (Hyrex)
CONJUGATED ESTROGENS, ORAL	
Tablets: 0.3, 0.625, 0.9, 1.25 and 2.5 mg (*Rx*)	*Premarin* (Wyeth-Ayerst)
CONJUGATED ESTROGENS, PARENTERAL	
Injection: 25 mg conjugated estrogens (*Rx*)	*Premarin Intravenous* (Wyeth-Ayerst)
ESTERIFIED ESTROGENS	
Tablets: 0.3, 0.625, 1.25 and 2.5 mg (*Rx*)	*Estratab* (Solvay Pharm.), *Menest* (SK-Beecham)
ESTROPIPATE	
Tablets: 0.75, 1.5 and 3 mg estropipate (*Rx*)	Various, *Ogen* (Abbott), *Ortho-Est* (Ortho)
QUINESTROL	
Tablets: 100 mcg (*Rx*)	*Estrovis* (Parke-Davis)
ETHINYL ESTRADIOL	
Tablets: 0.02, 0.05, 0.5 mg (*Rx*)	*Estinyl* (Schering)
DIETHYLSTILBESTROL (DES)	
Tablets: 1 and 5 mg (*Rx*)	Various
CHLOROTRIANISENE	
Capsules: 12 and 25 mg (*Rx*)	*Tace* (Marion Merrell Dow)
ESTRADIOL CYPIONATE IN OIL	
Injection: 5 mg per ml (*Rx*)	Various, *depGynogen* (Forest), *Depo-Estradiol, Cypionate* (Upjohn), *Depogen* (Hyrex), *Estro-Cyp* (Keene)

Warning:

Estrogens have been reported to increase the risk of endometrial carcinoma.

When estrogens are used for the treatment of menopausal symptoms, use the lowest dose and discontinue medication as soon as possible. When prolonged treatment is indicated, reassess the patient at least semiannually to determine the need for continued therapy. Cyclic administration of low doses of estrogen may carry less risk than continuous administration.

Do not use estrogens during pregnancy.

The use of female sex hormones (both estrogens and progestins) during early pregnancy may seriously damage the offspring.

If estrogens are used during pregnancy, or if the patient becomes pregnant while taking estrogens, inform her of the potential risks to the fetus.

Actions:

Pharmacology: Although six different natural estrogens have been isolated from the human female, only three are present in significant quantities: Estradiol, estrone and estriol. The most potent and major secretory product of the ovary, estradiol, is rapidly oxidized to estrone. Hydration of estrone produces the much weaker estriol. The estrogenic potency of estradiol is 12 times estrone's and 80 times estriol's.

Estrogens, important in developing and maintaining female reproductive system and secondary sex characteristics, promote growth and development of vagina, uterus, fallopian tubes and breasts. They affect release of pituitary gonadotropins; cause capillary dilatation, fluid retention, protein anabolism and thin cervical mucus; inhibit or facilitate ovulation; prevent postpartum breast discomfort. Indirectly, they contribute to: Shaping the skeleton (conserving calcium and phosphorus and encouraging bone formation); maintenance of tone and elasticity of urogenital structures; changes in epiphyses of long bones that allow for pubertal growth spurt and its termination; growth of axillary and pubic hair; pigmentation of nipples and genitals.

Menstruation – Decline of estrogenic activity at the end of the menstrual cycle can induce menstruation, although cessation of progesterone secretion does the same to an estrogen-primed endometrium. However, in the preovulatory or nonovulatory cycle, estrogen withdrawal is the primary determinant of the onset of menstruation.

Menopause – The beginning of menopause is marked by hot flushes, decreasing frequency and quality of ovulation, associated with skips and delays of menses or variable periods of amenorrhea and later by decreasing estrogen secretion. Estrogen production, first to appear at menarche, is last to decline at menopause. The declining estrogen secretion is accompanied by signs and symptoms of hormone deficits in the estrogen-dependent organs, including pituitary, uterus, cervix, vagina and breasts. Pituitary gonadotropin secretion rises, reflected by increased quantities of gonadotropin in blood and urine. The endometrium becomes atrophic, myometrial mass decreases and the vaginal epithelium becomes thin as, deficient in glycogen, it fails to become keratinized. The ovarian stroma producing androgens persist at variable amounts of time.

Pharmacokinetics:

Absorption/Distribution – Absorption of most natural estrogens and their derivatives from the GI tract is complete. The limited oral effectiveness of natural estrogens and their esters is due to their metabolism. About 80% of estradiol is bound to sex hormone binding globulin; most of the rest is loosely bound to albumin and about 2% is unbound. Estrone is highly bound to protein as it circulates in the blood, primarily as a conjugate with sulfate.

Transdermal system: In contrast to oral estradiol, the skin metabolizes estradiol via the transdermal system only to a small extent. Therefore, transdermal use produces therapeutic serum levels of estradiol with lower circulating levels of estrone and estrone conjugates, and requires smaller total doses. Transdermal use produces mean serum estradiol concentrations comparable to those produced by daily oral administration at about 20 times the daily transdermal dose.

Metabolism/Excretion – Metabolism and inactivation occur primarily in the liver. During cyclic passage through the liver, estrogens are degraded to less active estrogenic compounds conjugated with sulfuric and glucuronic acids.

Indications:

Moderate to severe vasomotor symptoms associated with menopause: The primary indication is to treat hot flushes. Sleep deprivation associated with this can aggravate depression. Estrogens are not the drug of choice for treating depression.

Atrophic vaginitis; kraurosis vulvae.

Female hypogonadism; female castration; primary ovarian failure.

Breast cancer: Palliation only in selected women and men or those with metastatic disease.

Prostatic carcinoma: Palliative therapy of advanced disease.

Osteoporosis: **Conjugated estrogens** are indicated in postmenopausal women, with evidence of loss or deficiency of bone mass, to retard further bone loss and estrogen-deficiency-induced osteoporosis. Use with other important measures such as diet, calcium and physiotherapy. A more favorable benefit/risk ratio exists if women have had a hysterectomy; there is no risk of endometrial carcinoma.

The FDA has also approved the use of the other oral short-acting estrogens (DES, esterified estrogens, estradiol, ethinyl estradiol and estropipate) in the treatment of osteoporosis.

Abnormal uterine bleeding due to hormonal imbalance in the absence of organic pathology **(conjugated estrogens, parenteral)**.

Unlabeled uses: Oral DES is an effective postcoital contraceptive when given in doses of 25 mg twice daily for 5 days if therapy is started no later than 72 hours after intercourse. Ethinyl estradiol, conjugated estrogens and other estrogens have also been evaluated for postcoital contraception.

Ethinyl estradiol – A 5 mcg tablet is being investigated for use in the treatment of Turner's syndrome.

Contraindications:

Breast cancer, except in appropriately selected patients being treated for metastatic disease; estrogen-dependent neoplasia; undiagnosed abnormal genital bleeding; active thrombophlebitis or thromboembolic disorders; history of thrombophlebitis, thrombosis or thromboembolic disorders associated with previous estrogen use (except when used in treatment of breast or prostatic malignancy); known or suspected pregnancy.

Warnings:

Induction of malignant neoplasms: Estrogens may increase the risk of endometrial carcinoma.

Gallbladder disease: There is a 2– to 3–fold increase in risk of gallbladder disease in women receiving postmenopausal estrogens. This may be related to large doses.

Effects similar to those caused by estrogen-progestin oral contraceptives (OCs): Consider the following effects noted in OC users as potential risks of estrogen use:

Elevated blood pressure is common, but is less frequent with estrogen replacement therapy than with OC use.

Thromboembolic disease – OC users have an increased risk of thromboembolic and thrombotic vascular diseases, including thrombophlebitis, pulmonary embolism, stroke and myocardial infarction. Cases of retinal thrombosis, mesenteric thrombosis and optic neuritis have been reported. The risk of several of these adverse reactions is dose-related. An increased risk of postsurgical thromboembolic complications has also been reported.

Do not use in persons with active thrombophlebitis or thromboembolic disorders or in persons with a history of such disorders associated with estrogen use (except in treatment of malignancy).

Large doses (conjugated estrogens 5 mg/day), comparable to those used to treat prostate and breast cancer, have increased risk of nonfatal MI, pulmonary embolism and thrombophlebitis in men. When such estrogen doses are used, the thromboembolic and thrombotic adverse effects associated with OC use are a clear risk.

Hypercalcemia: Estrogens may lead to severe hypercalcemia in patients with breast cancer and bone metastases. If this occurs, discontinue the drug and take appropriate measures to reduce the serum calcium level.

Glucose tolerance: Usual replacement doses of estrogen improve insulin sensitivity.

Hepatic function impairment: Patients with a history of jaundice during pregnancy have an increased risk of recurrence while on estrogen-containing OCs. If jaundice develops in any patient on estrogen, discontinue medication and investigate the cause. Estrogens may be poorly metabolized in impaired liver function; use with caution.

Pregnancy: *Category* X (See Warning Box).

Lactation: Estrogens have been shown to decrease the quantity and quality of breast milk and may be excreted in breast milk. Administer only when clearly needed.

Children: Safety and efficacy are not established. Because of effects on epiphyseal closure, use judiciously in young patients in whom bone growth is incomplete.

Precautions:

History/Physical exam: Before initiating estrogens, take complete medical and family history. Pretreatment and periodic history and physical exams every 6 to 12 months should include blood pressure, breasts, abdomen, pelvic organs and a Papanicolaou smear. Generally, do not prescribe for > 1 year between physical examinations.

Excessive estrogenic stimulation: Certain patients may develop undesirable manifestations of excessive estrogenic stimulation (eg, abnormal or excessive uterine bleeding, mastodynia). Advise the pathologist of estrogen therapy when relevant specimens are submitted.

Fluid retention: Estrogens may cause some degree of fluid retention; conditions which might be influenced by this factor (eg, asthma, epilepsy, migraine and cardiac or renal dysfunction) require careful observation.

Calcium and phosphorus metabolism is influenced by estrogens; use caution in patients with metabolic bone diseases associated with hypercalcemia or in renal insufficiency.

Prolonged unopposed estrogen therapy may increase risk of endometrial hyperplasia.

Acute intermittent porphyria may be precipitated by estrogens.

Benzyl alcohol, contained in some of these products as a preservative, has been associated with a fatal "gasping syndrome" in premature infants.

Photosensitivity: Photosensitization may occur; therefore, caution patients to take protective measures (ie, sunscreens, protective clothing) against exposure to ultraviolet light or sunlight until tolerance is determined.

Tartrazine sensitivity: Some of these products contain tartrazine which may cause allergic-type reactions (including bronchial asthma) in susceptible individuals. Although the incidence of sensitivity is low, it is frequently seen in patients who also have aspirin hypersensitivity.

Drug Interactions:

Drugs that may be affected by estrogens include oral anticoagulants, tricyclic antidepressants, dantrolene, hydantoins and corticosteroids.

Drugs that may affect estrogens include barbiturates, rifampin and hydantoins.

Drug/Lab test interactions: Certain endocrine and liver function tests may be affected by estrogen-containing OCs. Expect these similar changes with larger doses:

Increased **sulfobromophthalein retention.**

Increased **prothrombin** and **factors** VII, VIII, IX and X; decreased **antithrombin III**; increased norepinephrine-induced **platelet aggregability.**

Increased **thyroid binding globulin (TBG)** leading to increased circulating total thyroid hormone, as measured by **PBI,** T_4 by column or T_4 by radioimmunoassay. **Free T_3 resin uptake** is decreased, reflecting the elevated TBG; **free T_4** concentration is unaltered.

Impaired **glucose tolerance**; decreased **pregnanediol excretion**; reduced response to **metyrapone test**; reduced **serum folate** concentration; increased **serum triglyceride** and **phospholipid** concentration.

Adverse Reactions:

Significant adverse reactions include breakthrough bleeding; spotting; change in menstrual flow; dysmenorrhea; premenstrual-like syndrome; amenorrhea during and after treatment; nausea; vomiting; abdominal cramps; bloating; cholestatic jaundice; chloasma or melasma (may persist when drug is discontinued); erythema nodosum/multiforme; hemorrhagic eruption; urticaria; dermatitis; steepening of corneal curvature; intolerance to contact lenses; headache; migraine; dizziness; mental depression; convulsions; pain at injection site; sterile abscess; postinjection flare; redness and irritation at application site with the estradiol transdermal system (17%); aggravation of porphyria; edema; changes in libido; breast tenderness, enlargement or secretion.

Administration and Dosage:

Concomitant progestin therapy: Addition of a progestin for 7 or more days of a cycle of estrogen has lowered the incidence of endometrial hyperplasia. Morphological and biochemical studies of endometrium suggest that 10 to 13 days of progestin are needed to provide maximal maturation of the endometrium and to eliminate any hyperplastic changes.

ESTRONE: Administer IM only. Shake vial and syringe well prior to withdrawal and injection (using a 21 to 23 gauge needle) to properly suspend medication.

Cyclically –

Replacement therapy of estrogen deficiency associated conditions (eg, hypogonadism, female castration, primary ovarian failure): Initial relief of symptoms may be achieved through the administration of 0.1 to 1 mg of estrone weekly in single or divided doses. Some patients may require 0.5 to 2 mg weekly.

Senile vaginitis and kraurosis vulvae: Generally, 0.1 to 0.5 mg 2 or 3 times/week.

Abnormal uterine bleeding due to hormone imbalance: May respond to brief courses of intensive therapy. Usual dose range is 2 to 5 mg daily for several days.

Chronically –

Inoperable progressing prostatic cancer: For palliation in prostatic cancer, use estrone at 2 to 4 mg, 2 or 3 times/week. If a response to therapy is going to occur, it should be apparent within 3 months of beginning therapy. If a response does occur, continue the hormone until the disease is again progressive.

Inoperable progressing breast cancer in appropriately selected men and postmenopausal women: 5 mg ≥ 3 times/week according to severity of pain.

ESTRADIOL TRANSDERMAL SYSTEM:

Initiation of therapy –

Treatment of menopausal symptoms: Start with the 0.05 mg system applied to the skin twice weekly. Adjust dose as necessary to control symptoms. Use the lowest dosage necessary to control symptoms, especially in women with an intact uterus. Make attempts to taper or discontinue the drug at 3 to 6 month intervals.

Prophylaxis to prevent postmenopausal bone loss: Initiate with 0.05 mg/day as soon as possible after menopause. Adjust dosage if necessary to control concurrent menopausal symptoms. Discontinuation may reestablish natural rate of bone loss.

In women who are not taking oral estrogens, start treatment immediately. In women who are currently taking oral estrogens, start treatment 1 week after withdrawal of oral therapy or sooner if symptoms reappear in < 1 week.

Therapeutic regimen – Therapy may be given continuously in patients who do not have an intact uterus. In patients with an intact uterus, therapy may be given on a cyclic schedule (eg, 3 weeks therapy followed by 1 week off).

Estraderm and *Vivelle* are applied twice a week; the *Climara* patch lasts for 7 days.

Application of system – Place adhesive side of the system on a clean, dry area on the trunk of the body (including the buttocks and abdomen). Do not apply to breasts. Rotate application site with an interval of at least 1 week between applications to a particular site. The area should not be oily, damaged or irritated. Avoid the waistline, since tight clothing may rub the system off. Apply the system immediately after opening pouch and removing protective liner. Press firmly in place with the palm for ≈ 10 seconds. Make sure there is good contact, especially around the edges. In the unlikely event that a system should fall off, the same system may be reapplied. If necessary, apply a new system. In either case, continue the original treatment schedule.

ESTRADIOL, ORAL:

Moderate to severe vasomotor symptoms, vulva/vaginal atrophy associated with menopause, female hypogonadism, female castration, primary ovarian failure – Initiate treatment with 1 or 2 mg/day; adjust to control presenting symptoms. Titrate to determine the minimal effective dose for maintenance therapy.

Prostatic cancer (androgen-dependent, inoperable, progressing) – Administer 1 to 2 mg 3 times daily. Judge the effectiveness of therapy by phosphatase determinations and by symptomatic improvement of the patient.

Breast cancer (inoperable, progressing) – Given chronically in appropriately selected men and women, the usual dose is 10 mg 3 times daily for at least 3 months.

Osteoporosis prevention – Administer cyclically (eg, 23 weeks on, 5 days off) 0.5 mg/day as soon as possible after menopause. Adjust dosage if necessary to control concurrent menopause symptoms. Discontinuation may reestablish natural rate of bone loss.

ESTRADIOL VALERATE IN OIL: Provides 2 to 3 weeks of estrogenic effect from a single IM injection. For IM injection only.

Moderate to severe vasomotor symptoms, atrophic vaginitis or kraurosis vulvae associated with menopause, female hypogonadism, female castration or primary ovarian failure – 10 to 20 mg every 4 weeks.

Prostatic carcinoma – 30 mg or more every 1 or 2 weeks.

CONJUGATED ESTROGENS, ORAL: Administer cyclically (3 weeks of daily estrogen and 1 week off) for all indications except selected cases of carcinoma.

Moderate to severe vasomotor symptoms associated with menopause – 1.25 mg/day. If the patient has not menstruated in 2 months or more, administration is started arbitrarily. If the patient is menstruating, begin administration on day 5 of bleeding.

Atrophic vaginitis and kraurosis vulvae associated with menopause – 0.3 to 1.25 mg or more daily, depending on tissue response of the patient.

Female hypogonadism – 2.5 to 7.5 mg daily, in divided doses for 20 days, followed by a rest period of 10 days. If bleeding does not occur by the end of this period, repeat dosage schedule. The number of courses of estrogen therapy necessary to produce bleeding may vary, depending on the responsiveness of the endometrium.

If bleeding occurs before the end of the 10 day period, begin a 20 day estrogen-progestin cyclic regimen with estrogen, 2.5 to 7.5 mg daily in divided doses. During the last 5 days of estrogen therapy, give an oral progestin. If bleeding occurs before this regimen is concluded, discontinue therapy and resume on the fifth day of bleeding.

Female castration and primary ovarian failure – 1.25 mg/day. Adjust according to severity of symptoms and patient response. For maintenance, adjust to lowest effective level.

Osteoporosis – 0.625 mg/day, cyclically.

Mammary carcinoma (for palliation) – 10 mg 3 times daily for at least 3 months.

Prostatic carcinoma (for palliation) – 1.25 to 2.5 mg 3 times daily. Effectiveness can be judged by phosphatase determinations as well as by symptomatic improvement.

CONJUGATED ESTROGENS, PARENTERAL: Treatment of abnormal uterine bleeding due to hormonal imbalance in the absence of organic pathology. Administration IV produces a more rapid response and is preferred. Usual dose is one 25 mg injection IV or IM. Repeat in 6 to 12 hours if necessary. Inject slowly to obviate the occurrence of flushes.

Compatibility – Infusion of conjugated estrogens with other agents is not recommended. In emergencies, however, when an infusion has already been started, make the injection into the tubing just distal to the infusion needle. Solution is compatible with normal saline, dextrose and invert sugar solutions. It is not compatible with protein hydrolysate, ascorbic acid or any solution with an acid pH.

ESTERIFIED ESTROGENS:

Moderate to severe vasomotor symptoms, atrophic vaginitis or kraurosis vulvae associated with menopause – Cyclic therapy for short-term use. Average dose is 0.3 to 1.25 mg daily. Adjust dosage to the lowest effective level and discontinue as soon as possible.

Female hypogonadism – Administer 2.5 to 7.5 mg daily in divided doses for 20 days followed by a 10 day rest period. If bleeding does not occur by the end of this period, repeat the same dosage schedule. The number of courses of estrogen therapy necessary to produce bleeding varies, depending on endometrial responsiveness.

If bleeding occurs before the end of the 10 day period, begin a 20 day estrogen-progestin cyclic regimen of 2.5 to 7.5 mg daily in divided doses for 20 days. During the last 5 days of estrogen therapy, give an oral progestin. If bleeding occurs before this regimen is concluded, discontinue therapy; resume on the fifth day of bleeding.

Female castration and primary ovarian failure – Give 1.25 mg daily, cyclically.

Prostatic carcinoma (inoperable, progressing) – 1.25 to 2.5 mg 3 times a day. Judge the effectiveness of therapy by symptomatic response and phosphatase determinations.

Breast cancer (inoperable, progressing) – In appropriately selected men and postmenopausal women, give 10 mg 3 times a day for at least 3 months.

QUINESTROL:

Moderate to severe vasomotor symptoms associated with menopause, atrophic vaginitis, kraurosis vulvae, female hypogonadism, female castration and primary ovarian failure – Initially, 100 mcg daily for 7 days; follow with 100 mcg once weekly for maintenance starting 2 weeks after treatment begins. Increase dosage to 200 mcg per week if the therapeutic response is not desirable or optimal.

ESTROPIPATE (Piperazine Estrone Sulfate):

Moderate to severe vasomotor symptoms, atrophic vaginitis or kraurosis vulvae associated with menopause – Give cyclically for short-term use. The lowest dose and regimen that will control symptoms should be chosen. Usual dosage range is 0.625 to 5 mg/day.

Female hypogonadism, female castration or primary ovarian failure – Administer cyclically, 1.25 to 7.5 mg/day for the first 3 weeks, followed by a rest period of 8 to 10 days. Repeat if bleeding does not occur by the end of the rest period. The duration of therapy necessary to produce withdrawal bleeding will vary according to the responsiveness of the endometrium. If satisfactory withdrawal bleeding does not occur, give an oral progestin in addition to estrogen during the third week of the cycle.

Osteoporosis prevention – 0.625 mg daily for 25 days of a 31 day cycle per month.

ETHINYL ESTRADIOL:

Moderate to severe vasomotor symptoms associated with menopause – Usual dosage range is 0.02 to 0.5 mg/day. The effective dose may be as low as 0.02 mg every other day. Dosage schedule for early menopause, while spontaneous menstruation continues, is 0.05 mg once/day for 21 days followed by a 7-day rest period. May add a progestational agent during the latter part of the cycle.

For initial treatment of late menopause, the same regimen is indicated with 0.02 mg for the first few cycles, after which the 0.05 mg dosage may be substituted. In more severe cases, such as those due to surgical and roentgenologic castration, give 0.05 mg 3 times daily at the start of treatment. With adequate clinical improvement, usually obtainable in a few weeks, dosage may be reduced to 0.05 mg/day. A progestational agent may be added during the latter part of a planned cycle.

Female hypogonadism – 0.05 mg 1 to 3 times daily during the first 2 weeks of a theoretical menstrual cycle. Follow with a progestin during the last half of the arbitrary cycle. Continue for 3 to 6 months. The patient is then untreated for 2 months. Prescribe additional therapy if the cycle cannot be maintained without hormonal therapy.

Cancer of the female breast (inoperable, progressing) – In appropriately selected postmenopausal women, 1 mg 3 times daily given chronically for palliation.

Prostatic carcinoma (inoperable, progressing) – 0.15 to 2 mg/day given chronically for palliation.

DIETHYLSTILBESTROL (DES):

Prostatic carcinoma (inoperable, progressing) – Given chronically, the usual dosage is 1 to 3 mg/day initially, increased in advanced cases; dosage may later be reduced to an average of 1 mg/day.

Breast cancer (inoperable, progressing) – Given chronically in appropriately selected men and postmenopausal women, the usual dosage is 15 mg/day.

CHLOROTRIANISENE:

Moderate to severe vasomotor symptoms associated with menopause – 12 to 25 mg/day given cyclically for 30 days; one or more courses may be prescribed.

Atrophic vaginitis and kraurosis vulvae – 12 to 25 mg/day cyclically for 30 to 60 days.

Female hypogonadism – 12 to 25 mg/day given cyclically for 21 days. May be followed immediately by 100 mg progesterone IM or by an oral progestin during the last 5 days of therapy. Next course may begin on the fifth day of induced uterine bleeding.

Prostatic carcinoma (inoperable, progressing) – Given chronically, the usual dose is 12 to 25 mg/day.

ESTRADIOL CYPIONATE IN OIL:

Moderate to severe vasomotor symptoms associated with menopause – Usual dosage range is 1 to 5 mg IM, every 3 to 4 weeks.

Female hypogonadism – 1.5 to 2 mg IM at monthly intervals.

SULFONYLUREAS

ACETOHEXAMIDE	
Tablets: 250 and 500 mg (*Rx*)	Various, *Dymelor* (Lilly)
CHLORPROPAMIDE	
Tablets: 100 and 250 mg (*Rx*)	Various, *Diabinese* (Pfizer)
GLIMEPIRIDE	
Tablets: 1, 2 and 4 mg (*Rx*)	*Amaryl* (Hoechst-Roussel)
GLIPIZIDE	
Tablets: 5 and 10 mg (*Rx*)	Various, *Glucotrol* (Roerig)
Tablets, extended release: 5 and 10 mg (*Rx*)	*Glucotrol XL* (Pfizer)
GLYBURIDE	
Tablets: 1.25, 2.5 and 5 mg (*Rx*)	Various, *DiaBeta* (Hoechst-Roussel), *Micronase* (Upjohn)
Tablets, micronized: 1.5, 3 and 6 mg (*Rx*)	*Glynase PresTab* (Upjohn)
TOLAZAMIDE	
Tablets: 100, 250 and 500 mg (*Rx*)	Various, *Tolinase* (Upjohn)
TOLBUTAMIDE	
Tablets: 500 mg (*Rx*)	Various, *Orinase* (Upjohn)

Actions:

Pharmacology: The sulfonylurea hypoglycemic agents are sulfonamide derivatives, but are devoid of antibacterial activity. They are used as adjuncts to diet and exercise in the treatment of non-insulin-dependent diabetes mellitus (NIDDM). NIDDM is characterized by insulin resistance and defects in insulin secretion. The sulfonylurea hypoglycemic agents appear to lower blood glucose by stimulating insulin release from beta cells in the pancreatic islets possibly due to increased intracellular cAMP. These agents are only effective in patients with some capacity for endogenous insulin production. They may improve the binding between insulin and insulin receptors or increase the number of insulin receptors.

Guidelines for oral hypoglycemic therapy in NIDDM patients may include:

- Onset of diabetes at ≥ 40 years of age
- Obese or normal body weight
- Duration of diabetes < 5 years
- Absence of ketoacidosis
- Fasting serum glucose ≤ 200 mg/dl
- Insulin requirement < 40 units/day
- Absence of renal or hepatic dysfunction

Pharmacokinetics: All sulfonylureas are strongly bound to plasma proteins, primarily albumin.

Major Pharmacokinetic Parameters of the Sulfonylureas

Sulfonylureas	Equivalent doses (mg)	Doses/day	Serum t½ (hrs)	Onset (hrs)	Duration (hrs)	Metabolism
First generation						
Acetohexamide	500	1-2	6-8 (parent drug = metabolite)	1	12-24	Reduced in liver to potent active metabolite
Chlorpropamide	250	1	36	1	Up to 60	80% metabolized in liver; metabolite activity unknown
Tolazamide	250	1	7	4-6	12-24	Several mildly active metabolites
Tolbutamide	1000	2-3	4.5-6.5	1	6-12	Oxidized in liver to inactive metabolites
Second generation						
Glipizide	10	1-2	2-4	1-1.5	10-16	Liver metabolism to inactive metabolites
Glyburide Nonmicronized	5	1-2	10	2-4	24	Liver metabolism to weakly active metabolites
Micronized	3	1-2	≈ 4	1	24	

Indications:

As an adjunct to diet to lower the blood glucose in patients with non-insulin-dependent diabetes mellitus (Type II) whose hyperglycemia cannot be controlled by diet alone.

Unlabeled uses: Chlorpropamide has been used in the treatment of neurogenic diabetes insipidus.

Sulfonylureas have been used as temporary adjuncts to insulin therapy in selected NIDDM patients to improve diabetic control.

Contraindications:

Hypersensitivity to sulfonylureas; diabetes complicated by ketoacidosis, with or without coma; sole therapy of insulin-dependent (Type I) diabetes mellitus; diabetes when complicated by pregnancy.

Warnings:

The administration of oral hypoglycemic drugs has been associated with increased cardiovascular mortality as compared to treatment with diet alone or diet plus insulin.

Patients treated for 5 to 8 years with diet plus tolbutamide (1.5 g/day) had a rate of cardiovascular mortality approximately 2.5 times that of patients treated with diet alone. A significant increase in total mortality was not observed. Consider this for other sulfonylureas as well.

Bioavailability: Micronized glyburide 3 mg tablets provide serum concentrations that are *not* bioequivalent to those from the conventional formulation (nonmicronized) 5 mg tablets.

Renal/Hepatic function impairment: Hepatic impairment may result in inadequate release of glucose in response to hypoglycemia. Renal impairment may cause decreased elimination of sulfonylureas leading to accumulation producing hypoglycemia.

Elderly: Elderly and debilitated patients are particularly susceptible to the hypoglycemic action of the sulfonylureas. Hypoglycemia may be difficult to recognize in the elderly.

Pregnancy: Category C; Category B (glyburide).

Because abnormal blood glucose levels during pregnancy may be associated with a higher incidence of congenital abnormalities, insulin is recommended to maintain blood glucose levels as close to normal as possible. If used during pregnancy, discontinue at least 2 days to 4 weeks before expected delivery date.

Lactation: Chlorpropamide and tolbutamide are excreted in breast milk. It is not known if other sulfonylureas are excreted in breast milk.

Children: Safety and efficacy in children have not been established.

Precautions:

Monitoring: During the transitional period, test the urine for glucose and acetone at least 3 times daily and have the results reviewed by a physician frequently. Measurement of glycosylated hemoglobin is also useful. It is important that patients be taught to correctly and frequently self-monitor blood glucose.

Hypoglycemia: All sulfonylureas may produce severe hypoglycemia. Proper patient selection, dosage and instructions are important to avoid hypoglycemic episodes.

Asymptomatic patients: Controlling blood glucose in NIDDM with sulfonylureas has not been definitely established to be effective in preventing the long-term cardiovascular or neural complications of diabetes.

Loss of blood glucose control: When a patient stabilized on any diabetic regimen is exposed to stress such as fever, trauma, infection or surgery, a loss of control may occur. At such times, it may be necessary to discontinue drug and give insulin.

The effectiveness of any oral hypoglycemic in lowering blood glucose to a desired level decreases in many patients over time (secondary failure). Primary failure occurs when the drug is ineffective in a patient when first given. Certain patients who demonstrate an inadequate response or true primary or secondary failure to one sulfonylurea may benefit from a transfer to another sulfonylurea.

Disulfiram-like syndrome: A sulfonylurea-induced facial flushing or breathlessness reaction may occur when some sulfonylureas are administered with alcohol.

Syndrome of inappropriate secretion of antidiuretic hormone (SIADH): Water retention and dilutional hyponatremia have occurred after administration of sulfonylureas to NIDDM patients, especially those with congestive heart failure or hepatic cirrhosis.

Drug Interactions:

Drugs that may affect sulfonylureas include androgens, anticoagulants, beta blockers, charcoal, chloramphenicol, cholestyramine, clofibrate, diazoxide, ethanol, fenfluramine, fluconazole, gemfibrozil, histamine H_2 antagonists, hydantoins, magnesium salts, methyldopa, MAO inhibitors, probenecid, rifampin, salicylates, sulfinpyrazone, sulfonamides, thiazide diuretics, tricyclic antidepressants, urinary acidifiers and urinary alkalinizers. Drugs that may be affected by sulfonylureas include digitalis glycosides.

Drug/Lab test interactions: A metabolite of tolbutamide in the urine may give a false-positive reaction for **albumin** if measured by the acidification-after-boiling test, which causes the metabolite to precipitate. There is no interference with the sulfosalicylic acid test.

Drug/Food interactions: Absorption of glipizide is delayed by about 40 minutes when taken with food; the drug is more effective when given approximately 30 minutes before a meal. The other sulfonylureas may be taken with food.

Adverse Reactions:

GI disturbances (eg, nausea, epigastric fullness, heartburn) are the most common reactions. Other adverse reactions may include hypoglycemia, disulfiram-like reactions; allergic skin reactions; eczema; pruritus; erythema; urticaria; photosensitivity reactions; leukopenia; thrombocytopenia; aplastic anemia; agranulocytosis; hemolytic anemia; pancytopenia; weakness; paresthesia; tinnitus; fatigue; dizziness; vertigo; malaise; elevated liver function tests.

Administration and Dosage:

Short-term administration of sulfonylureas may be sufficient during periods of transient loss of control in patients usually well controlled on diet.

Transfer from other hypoglycemic agents:

Sulfonylureas – When transferring patients from one oral hypoglycemic agent to another, no transitional period and no initial or priming dose is necessary. However, when transferring patients from chlorpropamide, exercise particular care during the first 2 weeks because the prolonged retention of chlorpropamide in the body and subsequent overlapping drug effects may provoke hypoglycemia.

Insulin – During insulin withdrawal period, test blood for glucose and urine for ketones 3 times daily and report results to physician daily.

Insulin Requirement When Instituting Sulfonylurea Therapy	
Insulin dose	Insulin requirement
< 20 units	Start directly on oral agent and discontinue insulin abruptly.
20-40 units	Initiate oral therapy with concurrent 25% to 50% reduction in insulin dose. Further reduce insulin as response is observed. With glyburide, insulin may be discontinued immediately.
> 40 units	Initiate oral therapy with concurrent 20% to 50% reduction in insulin dose. Further reduce insulin as response is observed.

Elderly patients may be particularly sensitive to these agents; therefore, start with a lower initial dose before breakfast, and check blood and urine glucose during the first 24 hours of therapy.

Acute complications: During the course of intercurrent complications (eg, ketoacidosis, severe trauma, major surgery, infections, severe diarrhea, nausea, vomiting), supportive therapy with insulin may be necessary.

Combination insulin therapy: Concurrent administration of insulin and an oral sulfonylurea (generally glipizide or glyburide) has been used with some success in Type II diabetic patients who are difficult to control with diet and sulfonylurea therapy alone.

ACETOHEXAMIDE:

Initial dose – 250 mg to 1.5 g/day. Patients on ≤ 1 g daily can be controlled with once daily dosage. Those receiving 1.5 g/day usually benefit from twice daily dosage before morning and evening meals. Doses > 1.5 g/day are not recommended.

CHLORPROPAMIDE:

Initial dose – 250 mg/day in the mild to moderately severe, middle-aged, stable diabetic patient; use 100 to 125 mg/day in older patients.

Maintenance therapy – ≤ 100 to 250 mg/day. Severe diabetics may require 500 mg/day. Avoid doses > 750 mg/day.

GLIMEPIRIDE:

Initial dose – 1 to 2 mg once daily, given with breakfast or the first main meal. Patients sensitive to hypoglycemic drugs should begin at 1 mg once daily; titrate carefully.

Maximum starting dose is ≤ 2 mg.

Maintenance dose – 1 to 4 mg once daily. The maximum recommended dose is 8 mg once daily. After a dose of 2 mg is reached, increase dose at increments of ≤ 2 mg at 1 to 2 week intervals based on the patient's blood glucose response.

Combination insulin therapy – The recommended dose is 8 mg once daily with the first main meal with low-dose insulin.

Transfer from other hypoglycemic agents –

Sulfonylureas: When transferring patients to glimepiride, no transition period is necessary.

GLIPIZIDE: Give approximately 30 minutes before a meal to achieve the greatest reduction in postprandial hyperglycemia.

Initial dose – 5 mg, given ≈ 30 minutes before breakfast. Geriatric patients or those with liver disease may be started on 2.5 mg.

Adjust dosage in 2.5 to 5 mg increments, as determined by blood glucose response. Several days should elapse between titration steps. If response to a single dose is not satisfactory, dividing that dose may prove effective. The maximum recommended once daily dose is 15 mg. The maximum recommended total daily dose is 40 mg.

Maintenance dose – Some patients may be controlled on a once-a-day regimen, while others show better response with divided dosing. Divide total daily doses > 15 mg and give before meals of adequate caloric content. Total daily doses > 30 mg have been safely given on a twice daily basis to long-term patients.

GLYBURIDE (Glibenclamide):

DiaBeta/Micronase –

Initial dose: 2.5 to 5 mg daily, administered with breakfast or the first main meal. For patients who may be more sensitive to hypoglycemic drugs, start at 1.25 mg daily.

Maintenance dose: 1.25 to 20 mg daily. Give as a single dose or in divided doses. Increase in increments of no more than 2.5 mg at weekly intervals based on the patient's blood glucose response. Daily doses > 20 mg are not recommended.

Glynase –

Initial dose: 1.5 to 3 mg/day, administered with breakfast or the first main meal. For patients who may be more sensitive to hypoglycemic drugs, start at 0.75 mg/day.

Maintenance dose: 0.75 to 12 mg/day. Give as a single dose or in divided doses; some patients, particularly those receiving > 6 mg/day, may have a more satisfactory response with twice-daily dosing. Increase in increments of no more than 1.5 mg at weekly intervals based on the patient's blood glucose response. Daily doses > 12 mg are not recommended.

TOLAZAMIDE:

Initial dose – 100 to 250 mg/day with breakfast or the first main meal. If fasting blood sugar (FBS) is < 200 mg/dl, use 100 mg/day, or 250 mg/day if FBS is > 200 mg/dl. If patients are malnourished, underweight, elderly or not eating properly, use 100 mg once a day. Adjust dose to response. If > 500 mg/day is required, give in divided doses twice daily. Doses > 1 g/day are not likely to improve control.

TOLBUTAMIDE:

Initial dose – 1 to 2 g/day (range, 0.25 to 3 g). A maintenance dose > 2 g/day is seldom required. Total dose may be taken in the morning, but divided doses may allow increased GI tolerance.

TROGLITAZONE

Tablets: 200, 300 and 400 mg (*Rx*)	*Rezulin* (Parke-Davis)

Actions:

Pharmacology: Troglitazone is a thiazolidinedione antidiabetic agent that lowers blood glucose by improving target cell response to insulin, without increasing pancreatic insulin secretion. It decreases insulin resistance. It has a unique mechanism of action that is dependent on the presence of insulin for activity. Troglitazone decreases hepatic glucose output and increases insulin-dependent glucose disposal in skeletal muscle and possibly liver and adipose tissue.

Pharmacokinetics:

Absorption – Following daily drug administration, steady-state plasma concentrations of troglitazone are reached within 3 to 5 days.

Troglitazone is absorbed rapidly following oral administration; the time for maximum plasma concentration (T_{max}) occurs within 2 to 3 hours.

Distribution – Mean apparent volume of distribution of troglitazone following multiple-dose administration ranges from 10.5 to 26.5 L/kg. Troglitazone is extensively bound (> 99%) to serum albumin.

Metabolism – After 14 days of treatment with 400 mg troglitazone, the major metabolites found in the plasma were the sulfate conjugate, followed by the quinone metabolite. Only 3.1% of the dose was detected in the urine; this was primarily in the form of the glucuronide conjugate, which is present in negligible amounts in the plasma.

Excretion – Following oral administration of troglitazone, ≈ 85% is recovered in feces and 3% in urine. Unchanged troglitazone is not recovered in urine following oral administration. Mean plasma elimination half-life ranges from 16 to 34 hours.

Indications:

Type 2 diabetes: Concomitantly with a sulfonylurea or insulin to improve glycemic control.

Monotherapy as an adjunct to diet and exercise to lower blood glucose.

Unlabeled uses: A study showed troglitazone may be beneficial in the productive and metabolic consequences of polycystic ovary syndrome and less essential hypertension with NIDDM.

Contraindications:

Known hypersensitivity or allergy to troglitazone or any of its components.

Warnings:

Hepatotoxicity: Rare cases of severe idiosyncratic hepatocellular injury have occurred. The hepatic injury is usually reversible, but very rare cases of hepatic failure, including death, have occurred. Injury has occurred after both short- and long-term troglitazone treatment.

Hepatic function impairment: Troglitazone and its metabolites plasma concentrations in patients with chronic liver disease were increased compared with those in healthy subjects without hepatic dysfunction. Use troglitazone with caution in patients with hepatic disease.

Pregnancy: Category B.

Lactation: It is not known whether troglitazone is secreted in breast milk. Do not administer to breastfeeding women.

Children: Safety and efficacy in pediatric patients have not been established.

Precautions:

Monitoring: It is recommended that serum transaminase levels be checked within the first 1 to 2 months and then every 3 months during the first year of troglitazone therapy, and periodically thereafter. Obtain liver function tests for patients at the first symptoms suggestive of hepatic dysfunction (eg, nausea, vomiting, abdominal pain, fatigue, anorexia, dark urine). Discontinue if the patient has jaundice or if laboratory measurements suggest liver injury (eg, ALT > 3 times the upper limit of normal).

Type 1 diabetes: Because of its mechanism of action, troglitazone is active only in the presence of insulin. Therefore, do not use in type 1 diabetes or for the treatment of diabetic ketoacidosis.

Hypoglycemia: Patients receiving troglitazone in combination with insulin may be at risk for hypoglycemia, and a reduction in the dose of insulin may be necessary. Hypoglycemia has not been observed during the administration of troglitazone as monotherapy and would not be expected based on the mechanism of action.

Drug Interactions:

Troglitazone may induce drug metabolism by CYP3A4. Consider this when prescribing other CYP3A4 substrates such as astemizole, calcium channel blockers, cisapride, corticosteroids, cyclosporine, tacrolimus, triazolam, trimetrexate and some HMG-CoA reductase inhibitors.

Drugs that may affect troglitazone include cholestyramine.

Drugs that may be affected by troglitazone include oral contraceptives and terfenadine.

Drug/Lab test interactions:

Hematologic – Small decreases in hemoglobin, hematocrit, and neutrophil counts (within the normal range) may be related to increased plasma volume observed with troglitazone treatment.

Lipids – Small changes in serum lipids have been observed.

Serum transaminase levels – 2.2% of troglitazone-treated patients had reversible elevations in AST or ALT > 3 times the upper limit of normal.

Drug/Food interactions: Food increases the extent of troglitazone absorption by 30% to 85%; therefore, take with food.

Adverse Reactions:

Adverse reactions that were reported in ≥ 3% of patients include infection; headache; pain; accidental injury; asthenia; dizziness; back pain; nausea; rhinitis; diarrhea; urinary tract infection; peripheral edema; pharyngitis.

Other adverse reactions include: Jaundice, hepatitis, liver transplant and death (see Warnings).

Administration and Dosage:

Continue the current insulin or sulfonylurea dose upon initiation of troglitazone therapy. Initiate therapy at 200 mg once daily in patients on insulin therapy. Do not use troglitazone as monotherapy in patients previously well controlled with a sulfonylurea alone. It should be added to, not substituted for, a sulfonylurea. Take troglitazone with a meal. For patients not responding adequately, increase the dose after ≈ 2 to 4 weeks. The usual dose is 400 mg/day. The maximum recommended dose is 600 mg/day. It is recommended that the insulin dose be decreased by 10% to 25% when fasing plasma glucose concentrations decrease to < 120 mg/dl in patients receiving concomitant insulin and troglitazone.

Monotherapy: Initiate at 400 or 600 mg once daily for patients not adequately controlled with diet alone. For patients not responding to 400 mg once daily, increase the dose to 600 mg after 6 to 8 weeks. For patients not responding adequately to 600 mg after 6 to 8 weeks, consider alternative therapeutic options.

Use with caution in patients with hepatic disease.

BISPHOSPHONATES

ALENDRONATE **Tablets:** 10 and 40 mg (*Rx*)	*Fosamax* (Merck)
ETIDRONATE DISODIUM (ORAL) **Tablets:** 200 and 400 mg (*Rx*)	*Didronel* (Procter & Gamble Pharm.)
ETIDRONATE DISODIUM (PARENTERAL) **Injection:** 300 mg per amp (*Rx*)	*Didronel IV* (MGI Pharma)
PAMIDRONATE DISODIUM **Powder for injection, lyophilized:** 30, 60 and 90 mg (*Rx*)	*Aredia* (Ciba)
TILUDRONATE SODIUM **Tablets:** 240 mg (*Rx*)	*Skelid* (Sanofi Winthrop)

Actions:

Pharmacology: Bisphosphonates act primarily on bone. Their major pharmacologic action is the inhibition of normal and abnormal bone resorption.

Pharmacokinetics:

Alendronate – There is no evidence that the bisphosphonates are metabolized. Mean steady-state volume of distribution (exclusive of bone) is ≥ 28 L. Protein binding in plasma is ≈ 78%.

Etidronate – Most absorbed drug is cleared from blood in 6 hours. Within 24 hours, about half the absorbed dose is excreted in urine. The remainder is chemically adsorbed to bone and is slowly eliminated. Unabsorbed drug is excreted intact in feces.

Pamidronate – A mean of 51% (32% to 80%) was excreted unchanged in urine within 72 hours. Urinary excretion rate profile after 60 mg over 4 hours exhibited biphasic disposition characteristics with an alpha half-life of 1.6 hours and a beta half-life of 27.2 hours.

Tiludronate – After administration of a single dose equivalent to 400 mg tiludronic acid to healthy male subjects, tiludronic acid was rapidly absorbed with peak plasma concentrations of ≈ 3 mg/L occurring within 2 hours.

Indications:

Alendronate: Osteoporosis in postmenopausal women.

Paget's disease of the bone.

Etidronate:

Paget's disease of bone, symptomatic (oral) –

Heterotopic ossification (oral) – Prevention and treatment following total hip replacement or due to spinal injury.

Hypercalcemia of malignancy inadequately managed by dietary modification or oral hydration (parenteral).

Hypercalcemia of malignancy which persists after adequate hydration has been restored (parenteral).

Pamidronate: Paget's disease of bone.

Hypercalcemia of malignancy.

Breast cancer/multiple myeloma

Tiludronate: Paget's disease of bone.

Unlabeled uses:

Etidronate has been used to treat postmenopausal osteoporosis.

Pamidronate may be useful in treating the following conditions: Postmenopausal osteoporosis; hyperparathyroidism; to prevent glucocorticoid-induced osteoporosis; to reduce bone pain in patients with prostatic carcinoma; immobilization-related hypercalcemia.

Contraindications:

Hypersensitivity to bisphosphonates or any component of the products; hypocalcemia (alendronate); Class Dc and higher renal impairment (serum creatinine > 5 mg/dl; etidronate only).

Warnings:

Osteoporosis (alendronate): Consider causes other than estrogen deficiency and aging.

Paget's disease (etidronate): Response may be slow and may continue for months after treatment discontinuation. Do not increase dosage prematurely or resume treatment before there is evidence of reactivation of disease process.

Renal function impairment: It is likely that **alendronate** elimination via the kidney will be reduced in impaired renal function. Therefore, somewhat greater accumulation of alendronate in bone might be expected in impaired renal function. No dosage adjustment is necessary in mild-to-moderate renal insufficiency; alendronate use is not recommended in more severe renal insufficiency. Occasional mild-to-moderate renal function abnormalities (elevated BUN or serum creatinine) have occurred when **etidronate** was given to patients with hypercalcemia of malignancy. Reduction of the etidronate dose, if used at all, may be advisable in Class Cc renal functional impairment. In patients with Class Dc and higher renal functional impairment, withhold etidronate. Patients with hypercalcemia who receive an IV infusion of **pamidronate** should have periodic lab and clinical evaluations of renal function.

Tiludronate is not recommended for patients with severe renal failure (creatinine clearance < 30 ml/min). The plasma elimination half-life is longer.

Pregnancy: *Category B (oral etidronate); Category C (alendronate, parenteral etidronate, pamidronate and tiludronate).*

Lactation: It is not known whether these drugs are excreted in breast milk. Do not give alendronate to a nursing mother.

Children: Safety and efficacy for use in children have not been established. Children have been treated with **etidronate** at doses recommended for adults, to prevent heterotopic ossifications or soft tissue calcifications.

Precautions:

Monitoring: Carefully monitor standard hypercalcemia-related metabolic parameters, such as serum levels of calcium, phosphate, magnesium and potassium following pamidronate initiation. Asymptomatic hypophosphatemia (16%), hypokalemia (7% to 9%), hypomagnesemia (11% to 12%) and hypocalcemia (5% to 12%) have occurred. Also, closely monitor electrolytes, creatinine as well as CBC, differential and hematocrit/hemoglobin. Carefully monitor patients who have preexisting anemia, leukopenia or thrombocytopenia in the first 2 weeks following treatment.

Nutrition: Patients should maintain adequate nutrition, particularly an adequate intake of calcium and vitamin D.

GI disorders: Use caution when using bisphosphonates in patients with active upper GI problems. Etidronate therapy has been withheld from patients with enterocolitis because diarrhea is seen in some patients, particularly at higher doses.

Osteoid: **Etidronate** suppresses bone turnover and may retard mineralization of osteoid laid down during the bone accretion process.

Fracture: In Paget's patients, treatment regimens of **etidronate** exceeding the recommended daily maximum dose of 20 mg/kg or continuous administration for periods > 6 months may be associated with an increased risk of fracture.

Hormone replacement therapy: Concomitant use with **alendronate** for osteoporosis in post-menopausal women is not recommended.

Hypocalcemia: Hypocalcemia has occurred with **etidronate** and **pamidronate**.

Hypocalcemia must be corrected before therapy initiation with **alendronate**.

Drug Interactions:

Drugs that may interact with **alendronate** include ranitidine and aspirin. Drugs that may interact with **tiludronate** include aspirin and indomethacin. Calcium supplements and antacids may interact with **alendronate, etidronate** or **tiludronate**. The patient should wait ≥ 30 minutes after taking alendronate before taking any other drug.

Drug/Food interactions: Absorption of **etidronate,** complete in 2 hours, may be reduced by foods or other preparations containing divalent cations. The bioavailability of **tiludronate** is reduced by food. Do not take within 2 hours of food.

Adverse Reactions:

Alendronate: Musculoskeletal pain; asymptomatic, mild and transient decreases in serum calcium and phosphate.

Etidronate: GI complaints. Increased or recurrent bone pain at pagetic sites, occasional mild-to-moderate abnormalities in renal function, metallic, altered or loss of taste.

Pamidronate: Transient mild temperature elevation occurred in some, also redness, swelling or induration and pain on palpation. Adverse reactions in at least 15% of patients include fluid overload; generalized pain; hypertension; abdominal pain; anorexia; constipation; nausea; vomiting; urinary tract infection; bone pain; anemia; hypokalemia; hypomagnesemia; hypophosphatemia. Other adverse reactions include hypertension; arthrosis; bone pain; headache; fever; nausea; back pain.

Bisphosphonate Adverse Reactions (%)[1]

	Pamidronate			Etidronate (n = 35)	Alendronate (n = 196)[2]	Tiludronate (n = 75)
Adverse reaction	60 mg over 4 hr (n = 23)	60 mg over 24 hr (n = 17)	90 mg over 24 hr (n = 17)	7.5 mg/kg x 3 days	10 mg/day	400 mg/day
General						
Fever	26	19	18	9	0	0
Infusion site reaction	0	4	18	0	0	0
Fatigue	0	0	12	0	0	≥ 1
Moniliasis	0	0	6	0	0	0
Fluid overload	0	0	0	6	0	0

Bisphosphonate Adverse Reactions (%)[1]						
	Pamidronate			Etidronate (n = 35)	Alendronate (n = 196)[2]	Tiludronate (n = 75)
Adverse reaction	60 mg over 4 hr (n = 23)	60 mg over 24 hr (n = 17)	90 mg over 24 hr (n = 17)	7.5 mg/kg x 3 days	10 mg/day	400 mg/day
Respiratory						
Rales/Rhinitis	0	0	6	0	0	5.3
URI	0	3	0	0	0	5.3
Sinusitis	0	0	0	0	0	5.3
Dyspnea	0	0	0	3	0	0
Cardiovascular						
Atrial fibrillation	0	0	6	0	0	0
Hypertension	0	0	6	0	0	≥ 1
Syncope	0	0	6	0	0	≥ 1
Tachycardia	0	0	6	0	0	0
GI						
Nausea	4	0	18	6	3.6	9.3
Anorexia	4	1	12	0	0	≥ 1
Constipation	4	0	6	3	3.1	≥ 1
GI hemorrhage	0	0	6	0	0	0
Abdominal pain	0	1	0	0	6.6	≥ 1
Stomatitis	0	1	0	3	0	0
Diarrhea	0	1	0	0	3.1	9.3
Dyspepsia	4	0	0	0	3.6	5.3
Vomiting	4	0	0	0	1	4
CNS						
Headache	0	0	0	0	0	6.7
Somnolence	0	1	6	0	0	≥ 1
Psychosis	4	0	0	0	0	0
Dizziness	0	0	0	0	0	4
Paresthesia	0	0	0	0	0	4
Convulsions	0	0	0	3	0	0
Hemic/Lymphatic						
Anemia	0	0	6	0	0	0
Leukopenia	4	0	0	0	0	0
Lab abnormalities						
Hypophosphatemia	0	9	18	3	0	0
Hypokalemia	4	4	18	0	0	0
Hypomagnesemia	4	10	12	3	0	0
Hypocalcemia	0	1	12	0	0	0
Abnormal hepatic function	0	0	0	3	0	0
Other						
Hypothyroidism	0	0	6	0	0	0
Uremia	4	0	0	0	0	0
Taste perversion	0	0	0	3	0.5	0

[1] Data are pooled from separate studies and are not necessarily comparable.
[2] Alendronate was used for osteoporosis in postmenopausal women in this study.

Administration and Dosage:

ETIDRONATE DISODIUM (ORAL): Administer as a single dose. However, if GI discomfort occurs, divide the dose.

Paget's disease –

Initial treatment: 5 to 10 mg/kg/day (not to exceed 6 months) or 11 to 20 mg/kg/day (not to exceed 3 months). Reserve doses > 10 mg/kg/day for use when lower doses are ineffective, when there is an overriding requirement for suppression of increased bone turnover or when prompt reduction of elevated cardiac output is required. Doses > 20 mg/kg/day are not recommended.

Retreatment: Initiate only after an etidronate-free period of at least 90 days and if there is biochemical, symptomatic or other evidence of active disease process. Retreatment regimens are the same as for initial treatment.

Heterotopic ossification –

Due to spinal cord injury: 20 mg/kg/day for 2 weeks, followed by 10 mg/kg/day for 10 weeks; total treatment period is 12 weeks. Institute as soon as feasible following the injury, preferably prior to evidence of heterotopic ossification.

Complicating total hip replacement: 20 mg/kg/day for 1 month preoperatively, then 20 mg/kg/day for 3 months postoperatively; total treatment period is 4 months.

ETIDRONATE DISODIUM (PARENTERAL):

Recommended dose is 7.5 mg/kg/day for 3 successive days.

Infusion time – Administer the diluted dose IV over a period of at least 2 hours. Slow infusion is important. The usual course of treatment is one infusion of 7.5 mg/kg/day on each of 3 consecutive days, but some patients have been treated for up to 7 days.

Retreatment may be appropriate if hypercalcemia recurs. There should be at least a 7-day interval between courses of treatment. With renal impairment, dose reduction may be advisable.

Oral etidronate may be started on the day after the last infusion. The recommended oral dose for patients who have had hypercalcemia is 20 mg/kg/day for 30 days. If serum calcium levels remain normal or clinically acceptable, treatment may be extended. Use for > 90 days is not adequately studied and is not recommended.

PAMIDRONATE DISODIUM:

Hypercalcemia of malignancy –

Moderate hypercalcemia: The recommended dose in moderate hypercalcemia is 60 to 90 mg. The 60 mg dose is given as an initial, *single-dose*, IV infusion over at least 4 hours. The 90 mg dose must be given by an initial, *single-dose*, IV infusion over 24 hours.

Severe hypercalcemia: Recommended dose (corrected serum calcium > 13.5 mg/dl) is 90 mg, which must be given by initial *single-dose*, IV infusion over 24 hrs.

Retreatment: Retreatment, in patients who show complete or partial response initially, may be carried out if serum calcium does not return to normal or remain normal after initial treatment. Allow a minimum of 7 days to elapse before retreatment to allow for full response to the initial dose. The dose and manner of retreatment are identical to that of the initial therapy.

Paget's disease – The recommended dose in patients with moderate-to-severe Paget's disease of bone is 30 mg daily, given as a 4 hour infusion on 3 consecutive days for a total dose of 90 mg.

Retreatment: When clinically indicated, retreat at the dose of initial therapy.

ALENDRONATE: Alendronate must be taken at least 30 minutes before the first food, beverage or medication of the day with plain water only. Other beverages (including mineral water), food and some medications are likely to reduce the absorption of alendronate. Waiting > 30 minutes or taking the drug with food, beverages (other than plain water) or other medications will lessen the effect of the drug by decreasing its absoprtion. To facilitate delivery to the stomach, take with a full glass of water (6 to 8 oz) and avoid lying down for at least 30 minutes thereafter.

Osteoporosis in postmenopausal women – 10 mg once a day. Safety of treatment for > 4 years has not been studied (extension studies are ongoing).

Paget's disease of bone – 40 mg once a day for 6 months.

Retreatment: Relapses during the 12 months following therapy occurred in 9% of patients who responded to treatment. Retreatment with alendronate may be considered, following a 6-month post-treatment evaluation period, in patients who have relapsed based on increases in serum alkaline phosphatase.

TILUDRONATE: Administer a single 400 mg daily oral dose, taken with 6 to 8 ounces of plain water only for a period of 3 months. Beverages other than plain water (including mineral water), food and some medications are likely to reduce the absorption of tiludronate. Do not take within 2 hours of food. Take calcium or mineral supplements at least 2 hours before or after tiludronate. Take aluminum- or magnesium-containing antacids at least 2 hours after taking tiludronate. Do not take within 2 hours of indomethacin.

Retreatment – Following therapy, allow an interval of 3 months to assess response.

THIAZIDES AND RELATED DIURETICS

BENDROFLUMETHIAZIDE
Tablets: 5 and 10 mg (*Rx*) — *Naturetin* (Princeton)

BENZTHIAZIDE
Tablets: 50 mg (*Rx*) — *Exna* (Robins)

CHLOROTHIAZIDE
Tablets: 250 and 500 mg (*Rx*) — Various, *Diuril* (Merck), *Diurigen* (Goldline)
Suspension: 250 mg/5 ml (*Rx*) — *Diuril* (Merck)
Powder for injection, lyophilized: 500 mg (as sodium) (*Rx*) — *Sodium Diuril* (Merck)

CHLORTHALIDONE
Tablets: 15, 25, 50 and 100 mg (*Rx*) — Various, *Hygroton* (Rhone-Poulenc Rorer), *Thalitone* (Horus Therapeutics)

HYDROCHLOROTHIAZIDE
Tablets: 25, 50 and 100 mg (*Rx*) — Various, *Esidrix* (Ciba), *Ezide* (Econo Med), *HydroDIURIL* (Merck), *Hydro-Par* (Parmed), *Oretic* (Abbott)
Solution: 50 mg per 5 ml (*Rx*) — *Hydrochlorothiazide* (Roxane)

HYDROFLUMETHIAZIDE
Tablets: 50 mg (*Rx*) — Various, *Diucardin* (Wyeth-Ayerst), *Saluron* (Apothecon)

INDAPAMIDE
Tablets: 1.25 and 2.5 mg (*Rx*) — Various, *Lozol* (Rhone-Poulenc Rorer)

METHYCLOTHIAZIDE
Tablets: 2.5 and 5 mg (*Rx*) — Various, *Aquatensen* (Wallace), *Enduron* (Abbott)

METOLAZONE
Tablets: 2.5, 5 and 10 mg (*Rx*) — *Zaroxolyn* (Fisons)
Tablets: 0.5 mg (*Rx*) — *Mykrox* (Fisons)

POLYTHIAZIDE
Tablets: 1, 2 and 3 mg (*Rx*) — *Renese* (Pfizer)

QUINETHAZONE
Tablets: 50 mg (*Rx*) — *Hydromox* (Lederle)

TRICHLORMETHIAZIDE
Tablets: 2 and 4 mg — Various, *Diurese* (American Urologicals), *Metahydrin* (Marion Merrell Dow), *Naqua* (Schering)

Actions:

Pharmacology: Thiazide diuretics increase the urinary excretion of sodium and chloride in approximately equivalent amounts. They inhibit reabsorption of sodium and chloride in the cortical thick ascending limb of the loop of Henle and the early distal tubules. Other common actions include: Increased potassium and bicarbonate excretion, decreased calcium excretion and uric acid retention. At maximal therapeutic dosages all thiazides are approximately equal in diuretic efficacy.

The antihypertensive action requires several days to produce effects. Administration for up to 2 to 4 weeks is usually required for optimal therapeutic effect. The duration of the antihypertensive effect of the thiazides is sufficiently long to adequately control blood pressure with a single daily dose.

Pharmacokinetics:

Pharmacokinetics of Thiazides and Related Diuretics

Diuretic	Onset (hours)	Peak (hours)	Duration (hours)	Equivalent dose (mg)	Percent absorbed	Half-life (hours)
Bendroflumethiazide	2	4	16 to 12	5	≈ 100	3 to 3.9
Benzthiazide	2	4 to 6	16 to 18	50	nd[1]	nd[1]
Chlorothiazide	2[2]	4[2]	16 to 12	500	10 to 21[3]	0.75 to 2
Chlorthalidone	2 to 3	2 to 6	24 to 72	50	64[3]	40
Hydrochlorothiazide	2	4 to 6	16 to 12	50	65 to 75	5.6 to 14.8
Hydroflumethiazide	2	4	16 to 12	50	50	≈ 17
Indapamide	1 to 2	within 2	up to 36	2.5	93	≈ 14
Methyclothiazide	2	6	24	5	nd[1]	nd[1]
Metolazone[4]	1	2	12 to 24	5	65	nd[1]

Pharmacokinetics of Thiazides and Related Diuretics						
Diuretic	Onset (hours)	Peak (hours)	Duration (hours)	Equivalent dose (mg)	Percent absorbed	Half-life (hours)
Polythiazide	2	6	24 to 48	2	nd[1]	25.7
Quinethazone	2	6	18 to 24	50	nd[1]	nd[1]
Trichlormethiazide	2	6	24	2	nd[1]	2.3 to 7.3

[1] nd = No data.
[2] Following IV use, onset of action is 15 minutes; peak occurs in 30 minutes.
[3] Bioavailability may be dose-dependent.
[4] *Mykrox only:* Peak plasma concentrations reached in 2 to 4 hrs, t½ ≈ 14 hrs.

Indications:

Edema: Adjunctive therapy in edema associated with congestive heart failure (CHF), hepatic cirrhosis and corticosteroid and estrogen therapy. Useful in edema due to renal dysfunction (ie, nephrotic syndrome, acute glomerulonephritis, chronic renal failure).

Indapamide alone is indicated for edema associated with CHF.

Metolazone, rapidly acting (Mykrox) has not been evaluated for the treatment of CHF or fluid retention due to renal or hepatic disease, and the correct dosage for these conditions and other edematous states has not been established.

Hypertension: As the sole therapeutic agent or to enhance other antihypertensive drugs in more severe forms of hypertension.

Unlabeled uses:

Calcium nephrolithiasis – Thiazide diuretics have been used alone and in combination with amiloride or allopurinol to prevent formation and recurrence of calcium nephrolithiasis in hypercalciuric and normal calciuric patients.

Osteoporosis – Thiazide diuretics may be useful in reducing the incidence of osteoporosis in postmenopausal women, either alone or in combination with calcium or estrogen.

Diabetes insipidus – Thiazide diuretics reduce urine volume by 30% to 50%. They constitute the mainstay of therapy for nephrogenic diabetes insipidus.

Contraindications:

Anuria; renal decompensation; hypersensitivity to thiazides or related diuretics or sulfonamide-derived drugs; hepatic coma or precoma (metolazone).

Warnings:

Parenteral use: Use IV **chlorothiazide** only when patients are unable to take oral medication or in an emergency. In infants and children, IV use is not recommended.

Lupus erythematosus exacerbation or activation has occurred.

Hypersensitivity: Hypersensitivity reactions may occur in patients with or without a history of allergy or bronchial asthma; cross-sensitivity with sulfonamides may also occur. Refer to Management of Acute Hypersensitivity Reactions.

Renal function impairment: Use with caution in severe renal disease since these agents may precipitate azotemia. Cumulative effects of the drug may develop in patients with impaired renal function. Monitor renal function periodically. **Metolazone** is the only thiazide-like diuretic that may produce diuresis in patients with GFR < 20 ml/min. Indapamide may also be useful in patients with impaired renal function.

Pregnancy: *Category* B (chlorothiazide, chlorthalidone, hydrochlorothiazide, indapamide, metolazone); *Category* C (bendroflumethiazide, benzthiazide, hydroflumethiazide, methyclothiazide, trichlormethiazide). Routine use during normal pregnancy is inappropriate.

Lactation: Thiazides may appear in breast milk. Discontinue nursing or the drug.

Children: Bendroflumethiazide, benzthiazide, chlorthalidone, hydrochlorothiazide, methyclothiazide, metolazone, hydroflumethiazide, trichlormethiazide – Safety and efficacy have not been established. Metolazone is not recommended for use in children. In infants and children, IV use of chlorothiazide has been limited and is generally not recommended.

Precautions:

Fluid/Electrolyte balance: Perform initial and periodic determinations of serum electrolytes, BUN, uric acid and glucose. Observe patients for clinical signs of fluid or electrolyte imbalance (eg, hyponatremia, hypochloremic alkalosis, hypokalemia, changes in serum and urinary calcium).

Hypokalemia may develop during concomitant corticosteroids, ACTH and especially with brisk diuresis, with severe liver disease or cirrhosis, vomiting or diarrhea, or after prolonged therapy.

Hyponatremia/Hypochloremia – A chloride deficit is generally mild and usually does not require specific treatment, except in extraordinary circumstances (as in liver or renal disease). Thiazide-induced hyponatremia has been associated with death and neurologic damage in elderly patients.

Hypomagnesemia – Thiazide diuretics have been shown to increase urinary excretion of magnesium, resulting in hypomagnesemia.

Hypercalcemia – Calcium excretion may be decreased by thiazide diuretics.

Hyperuricemia may occur or acute gout may be precipitated in certain patients receiving thiazides, even in those patients without a history of gouty attacks.

Glucose tolerance – Hyperglycemia may occur with thiazide diuretics.

Lipids: Thiazides may cause increased concentrations of total serum cholesterol, total triglycerides and LDL (but not HDL) in some patients, although these appear to return to pretreatment levels with long-term therapy.

Photosensitivity: Photosensitization may occur.

Drug Interactions:

Drugs that may be affected by thiazides include: Allopurinol; anesthetics; anticoagulants; antigout agents; antineoplastics; calcium salts; diazoxide; digitalis glycosides; insulin; lithium; loop diuretics; methyldopa; nondepolarizing muscle relaxants; sulfonylureas; vitamin D. Drugs that may affect thiazides include: Amphotericin B; anticholinergics; bile acid sequestrants; corticosteroids; methenamines; NSAIDs.

Drug/Lab test interactions: Thiazides may decrease serum PBI levels without signs of thyroid disturbance. Thiazides may also cause diagnostic interference of serum electrolyte levels, blood and urine glucose levels (usually only in patients with a predisposition to glucose intolerance), serum bilirubin levels and serum uric acid levels. In uremic patients, serum magnesium levels may be increased. **Bendroflumethiazide** and **trichlormethiazide** may interfere with the **phenolsulfonphthalein test** due to decreased excretion. In the **phentolamine** and **tyramine tests,** bendroflumethiazide may produce false-negative and trichlormethiazide may produce false-positive results.

Adverse Reactions:

Adverse Reactions of Thiazides and Related Diuretics

Adverse reaction	Bendroflumethiazide	Benzthiazide	Chlorothiazide	Chlorthalidone	Hydrochlorothiazide	Hydroflumethiazide	Indapamide	Methyclothiazide	Metolazone	Polythiazide	Quinethazone	Trichlormethiazide
Cardiovascular												
Orthostatic hypotension	✓	✓	✓		✓	✓	<5%	✓	<2%[1]	✓	✓	✓
Palpitations							<5%		<2%[2]			✓
CNS												
Dizziness/Lightheadedness	✓	✓	✓	✓	✓	✓	≥5%	✓	10%[2]	✓	✓	✓
Vertigo	✓		✓	✓	✓	✓	<5%	✓	✓[3]	✓	✓	✓
Headache	✓	✓	✓	✓	✓	✓	≥5%	✓	9%[2]	✓	✓	✓
Paresthesias	✓	✓	✓	✓	✓	✓		✓	✓[3]	✓	✓	✓
Xanthopsia	✓	✓	✓	✓	✓	✓		✓		✓	✓	✓
Weakness	✓	✓	✓	✓	✓	✓	≥5%	✓	<2%[4]	✓	✓	✓
Restlessness/Insomnia	✓	✓	✓	✓	✓	✓	<5%	✓	✓[3]	✓	✓	✓
Drowsiness							<5%		✓[3]			✓
Fatigue/Lethargy/Malaise/Lassitude							≥5%		4%[2]			✓
Anxiety							≥5%		<2%[3]			
Depression							<5%		<2%[2]			✓
Nervousness							≥5%		<2%[3]			
Blurred vision (may be transient)	✓		✓		✓	✓	<5%		✓[3]			
GI												
Anorexia	✓	✓	✓	✓	✓	✓	<5%	✓	✓[3]	✓	✓	✓
Gastric irritation/epigastric distress	✓	✓	✓	✓	✓	✓	<5%	✓		✓	✓	✓
Nausea	✓	✓	✓	✓	✓	✓	<5%	✓	<2%[2]	✓	✓	✓
Vomiting	✓	✓	✓	✓	✓	✓	<5%	✓	<2%[4]	✓	✓	✓
Abdominal pain/cramping/bloating	✓	✓	✓	✓	✓	✓	<5%	✓	<2%[2]	✓	✓	✓
Diarrhea	✓	✓	✓	✓	✓	✓	<5%	✓	<2%[2]	✓	✓	✓
Constipation	✓	✓	✓	✓	✓	✓	<5%	✓	<2%[2]	✓	✓	✓
Jaundice (intrahepatic/cholestatic)	✓	✓	✓	✓	✓	✓		✓	✓[3]	✓	✓	✓
Pancreatitis	✓	✓	✓	✓	✓	✓		✓	✓[3]	✓	✓	✓
Dry mouth							<5%		<2%[1]			✓
GU												
Nocturia							<5%		<2%[1]			
Impotence/Reduced libido	✓	✓	✓	✓	✓	✓	<5%	✓	<2%[2]	✓	✓	✓
Hematologic:												
Leukopenia	✓	✓	✓	✓	✓	✓		✓	✓[3]	✓	✓	✓
Thrombocytopenia	✓	✓	✓	✓	✓	✓		✓		✓	✓	✓
Agranulocytosis	✓	✓	✓	✓	✓	✓		✓	✓[3]	✓	✓	✓
Aplastic/Hypoplastic anemia	✓	✓	✓	✓	✓	✓		✓	✓[3]	✓	✓	✓
Dermatologic												
Purpura	✓	✓	✓	✓	✓	✓		✓	✓[3]	✓	✓	✓
Photosensitivity/Photosensitivity dermatitis	✓	✓	✓	✓	✓	✓		✓	✓[3]	✓	✓	✓
Rash	✓	✓	✓	✓	✓	✓	<5%	✓	<2%[2]	✓	✓	✓

Adverse Reactions of Thiazides and Related Diuretics												
Adverse reaction	Bendroflumethiazide	Benzthiazide	Chlorothiazide	Chlorthalidone	Hydrochlorothiazide	Hydroflumethiazide	Indapamide	Methyclothiazide	Metolazone	Polythiazide	Quinethazone	Trichlormethiazide
Urticaria	✓	✓	✓	✓	✓	✓			✓[3]	✓	✓	✓
Necrotizing angiitis, vasculitis, cutaneous vasculitis	✓	✓	✓	✓	✓	✓	<5%	✓	✓[2]	✓	✓	✓
Pruritus	✓						<5%		<2%[1]			
Metabolic												
Hyperglycemia	✓	✓	✓	✓	✓	✓	<5%	✓	✓[3]	✓	✓	✓
Glycosuria	✓	✓	✓	✓	✓	✓	<5%	✓	✓[3]	✓	✓	✓
Hyperuricemia	✓	✓	✓	✓	✓	✓	<5%	✓		✓[3]		✓
Miscellaneous												
Muscle cramp/spasm	✓	✓	✓	✓	✓	✓	≥5%	✓	6%[2]	✓	✓	✓

[1] Percentage of occurrence refers to rapidly acting doseform; however this adverse reaction also occurred with the slow acting doseform.
[2] IV doseform.
[3] Possibly with life-threatening anaphylactic shock.
[4] Slow acting doseform only.
[5] Rapidly acting doseform only.

Administration and Dosage:

BENDROFLUMETHIAZIDE:

Edema – 5 mg once daily, preferably in the morning.

Initial: Up to 20 mg once daily or divided into 2 doses.

Maintenance: 2.5 to 5 mg daily.

Hypertension –

Initial: 5 to 20 mg daily.

Maintenance: 2.5 to 15 mg/day.

BENZTHIAZIDE:

Edema –

Initial: 50 to 200 mg daily for several days, or until dry weight is attained. If dosages exceed 100 mg/day, give in 2 doses, following morning and evening meal.

Maintenance: 50 to 150 mg daily.

Hypertension –

Initial: 50 to 100 mg daily. Give in 2 doses of 25 or 50 mg each, after breakfast and after lunch.

Maintenance: Maximal effective dose is 200 mg daily.

CHLOROTHIAZIDE:

Adults –

Edema: 0.5 to 1 g once or twice a day, orally or IV. Reserve IV route for patients unable to take oral medication or for emergency situations.

Hypertension (oral forms only): Starting dose is 0.5 to 1 g/day as a single or divided dose. Rarely, some patients may require up to 2 g/day in divided doses.

Infants and children –

Oral: 22 mg/kg/day (10 mg/lb/day) in 2 doses. Infants < 6 months may require up to 33 mg/kg/day (15 mg/lb/day) in 2 doses.

On this basis, infants up to 2 years of age may be given 125 to 375 mg daily in 2 doses. Children from 2 to 12 years of age may be given 375 mg to 1 g daily in 2 doses.

IV use is not generally recommended.

CHLORTHALIDONE: Give as a single dose with food in the morning. Maintenance doses may be lower than initial doses.

Edema – Initiate therapy with 50 to 100 mg (*Thalitone*, 30 to 60 mg) daily, or 100 mg (*Thalitone*, 60 mg) on alternate days. Some patients may require 150 or 200 mg (*Thalitone*, 90 to 120 mg) at these intervals, or 120 mg *Thalitone* daily. Dosages above this level, however, do not usually create a greater response.

Hypertension – Initiate therapy with a single dose of 25 mg/day (*Thalitone*, 15 mg). If response is insufficient after a suitable trial, increase to 50 mg (*Thalitone*, increase from 30 to 50 mg). For additional control, increase dosage to 100 mg once daily (except *Thalitone*), or add a second antihypertensive.

Note: Doses > 25 mg/day are likely to potentiate potassium excretion but provide no further benefit in sodium excretion or blood pressure reduction.

HYDROCHLOROTHIAZIDE:

Adults –

Edema:

Initial – 25 to 200 mg daily for several days, or until dry weight is attained.

Maintenance – 25 to 100 mg daily or intermittently. Refractory patients may require up to 200 mg daily.

Hypertension –

Initial: 50 mg daily as a single or two divided doses. Doses > 50 mg are often associated with marked reductions in serum potassium. Patients usually do not require doses > 50 mg daily when combined with other antihypertensives.

Infants and children: Usual dosage is 2.2 mg/kg (1 mg/lb) daily in two doses. Pediatric patients with hypertension only rarely will benefit from doses > 50 mg daily.

Infants (< 6 months) – Up to 3.3 mg/kg (1.5 mg/lb) daily in two doses.

Infants (6 months to 2 years of age) – 12.5 to 37.5 mg daily in two doses. Base dosage on body weight.

Children (2 to 12 years of age) – 37.5 to 100 mg daily in two doses. Base dosage on body weight.

HYDROFLUMETHIAZIDE:

Edema –

Initial: 50 mg once or twice a day.

Maintenance: 25 mg to 200 mg daily. Administer in divided doses when dosage exceeds 100 mg daily.

Hypertension –

Initial: 50 mg twice daily.

Maintenance: 50 to 100 mg/day. Do not exceed 200 mg/day.

INDAPAMIDE:

Edema of congestive heart failure –

Adults: 2.5 mg as a single daily dose in the morning. If response is not satisfactory after 1 week, increase to 5 mg once daily.

Hypertension –

Adults: 1.25 mg as a single daily dose taken in the morning. If the response to 1.25 mg is not satisfactory after 4 weeks, increase the daily dose to 2.5 mg taken once daily. If the response to 2.5 mg is not satisfactory after 4 weeks, the daily dose may be increased to 5 mg taken once daily, but consider adding another antihypertensive.

METHYCLOTHIAZIDE:

Edema –

Adults: 2.5 to 10 mg once daily. Maximum effective single dose is 10 mg.

Hypertension –

Adults: 2.5 to 5 mg once daily. If blood pressure control is not satisfactory after 8 to 12 weeks with 5 mg once daily, add another antihypertensive.

METOLAZONE: Individualize dosage.

Zaroxolyn –

Mild to moderate essential hypertension: 2.5 to 5 mg once daily.

Edema of renal disease/cardiac failure: 5 to 20 mg once daily.

Mykrox –

Mild to moderate hypertension: 0.5 mg as a single daily dose taken in the morning. If response is inadequate, increase the dose to 1 mg daily. Do not increase dosage if blood pressure is not controlled with 1 mg. Rather, add another antihypertensive agent with a different mechanism of action.

Brand interchange – The metolazone formulations are not bioequivalent or therapeutically equivalent at the same doses. Mykrox is more rapidly and completely bioavailable. Do not interchange brands.

POLYTHIAZIDE:

Edema – 1 to 4 mg daily.

Hypertension – 2 to 4 mg daily.

QUINETHAZONE:

Adults – 50 to 100 mg once daily. Occasionally, 50 mg twice daily; 150 to 200 mg daily may be necessary infrequently.

TRICHLORMETHIAZIDE:

Edema – 2 to 4 mg once daily.

Hypertension – 2 to 4 mg once daily. In initiating therapy, doses may be given twice daily.

LOOP DIURETICS

BUMETANIDE	
Tablets: 0.5, 1 and 2 mg (*Rx*)	Various, *Bumex* (Roche)
Injection: 0.25 mg per ml (*Rx*)	
ETHACRYNIC ACID	
Tablets: 25, 50 mg (*Rx*)	*Edecrin* (Merck)
Powder for Injection: 50 mg (as ethacrynate sodium) per vial (*Rx*)	*Edecrin Sodium* (Merck)
FUROSEMIDE	
Tablets: 20, 40 and 80 mg (*Rx*)	Various, *Lasix* (Hoechst-Roussel)
Oral Solution: 10 mg/ml (*Rx*)	
Injection: 10 mg/ml (*Rx*)	
TORSEMIDE	
Tablets: 5, 10, 20 and 100 mg (*Rx*)	*Demadex* (Boehringer Mannheim)
Injection: 10 mg/ml (*Rx*)	

Warning:

These agents are potent diuretics; excess amounts can lead to a profound diuresis with water and electrolyte depletion.

Actions:

Pharmacology: Furosemide and ethacrynic acid inhibit primarily reabsorption of sodium and chloride, not only in proximal and distal tubules, but also the loop of Henle. In contrast, bumetanide is more chloruretic than natriuretic and may have an additional action in the proximal tubule; it does not appear to act on the distal tubule. Torsemide acts from within the lumen of the thick ascending portion of the loop of Henle, where it inhibits the $Na^+/K^+/2Cl^-$-carrier system.

Pharmacokinetics: These agents are metabolized and excreted primarily through the urine. Protein binding of these agents exceeds 90%. Furosemide is metabolized approximately 30% to 40%, and its urinary excretion is 60% to 70%. Oral administration of bumetanide revealed that 81% was excreted in urine, 45% of it as unchanged drug. Torsemide is cleared from the circulation by both hepatic metabolism (≈ 80% of total clearance) and excretion into the urine (≈ 20% of total clearance).

Pharmacokinetic Parameters of the Loop Diuretics

Diuretic	Bioavailability (%)	Half-life (min)	Onset of action (min)	Peak (min)	Duration (hr)	Dosage (mg)	Relative potency	Doses/ day
Furosemide								
Oral	60-64[1]	≈ 120[2]	within 60	60-120[3]	6-8	20-80	1	1-2
IV or IM			within 5[4]	30	2	20-40	1	
Ethacrynic acid								
Oral	≈100	60	within 30	120	6-8	50-100	0.6-0.8	1-2
IV			within 5	15-30	2	50	0.6-0.8	1-2
Bumetanide								
Oral	72-96	60-90[5]	30-60	60-120	4-6	0.5-2	≈ 40	1
IV			within minutes	15-30	0.5-1	0.5-1	≈ 40	1-3
Torsemide								
Oral	≈ 80	210	within 60	60-120	6-8	5-20	2-4	1
IV			within 10	within 60	6-8	5-20	2-4	1

[1] Decreased in uremia and nephrosis.
[2] Prolonged in renal failure, uremia and in neonates.
[3] Decreased in CHF.
[4] Somewhat delayed after IM administration.
[5] Prolonged in renal disease.

Indications:

Edema associated with CHF, hepatic cirrhosis and renal disease, including the nephrotic syndrome. Particularly useful when greater diuretic potential is desired.

Parenteral administration is indicated when a rapid onset of diuresis is desired (eg, acute pulmonary edema), when GI absorption is impaired or when oral use is not practical for any reason. As soon as it is practical, replace with oral therapy.

Hypertension (furosemide, oral; torsemide, oral): Alone or in combination with other antihypertensive drugs.

Ethacrynic acid:

Ascites – Short-term management of ascites due to malignancy, idiopathic edema and lymphedema.

Congenital heart disease, nephrotic syndrome – Short-term management of hospitalized pediatric patients, other than infants.

Pulmonary edema, acute – Adjunctive therapy.

Unlabeled uses: Ethacrynic acid is being investigated for the treatment of glaucoma; a single injection into the eye may reduce intraocular pressure for a week or more.

Bumetanide may be beneficial in the treatment of adult nocturia; it is not effective in males with prostatic hypertrophy.

Contraindications:

Anuria; hypersensitivity to these compounds or to sulfonylureas; infants (ethacrynic acid); patients with hepatic coma or in states of severe electrolyte depletion until the condition is improved or corrected (bumetanide).

Warnings:

Dehydration: Excessive diuresis may result in dehydration and reduction in blood volume with circulatory collapse and the possibility of vascular thrombosis and embolism, particularly in elderly patients.

Hepatic cirrhosis and ascites: In these patients, sudden alterations of electrolyte balance may precipitate hepatic encephalopathy and coma. Do not institute therapy until the basic condition is improved.

Ototoxicity: Tinnitus, reversible and irreversible hearing impairment, deafness and vertigo with a sense of fullness in the ears have been reported. Deafness is usually reversible and of short duration (1 to 24 hours); however, irreversible hearing impairment has occurred. Usually, ototoxicity is associated with rapid injection, with severe renal impairment, with doses several times the usual dose and with concurrent use with other ototoxic drugs.

Systemic lupus erythematosus may be exacerbated or activated.

Thrombocytopenia: Since there have been rare spontaneous reports of thrombocytopenia with **bumetanide,** observe regularly for possible occurrence.

Hypersensitivity: Patients with known sulfonamide sensitivity may show allergic reactions to **furosemide, torsemide** or **bumetanide**. Bumetanide use following instances of allergic reactions to furosemide suggests a lack of cross-sensitivity. Refer to Management of Acute Hypersensitivity Reactions.

Renal function impairment: If increasing azotemia, oliguria or reversible increases in BUN or creatinine occur during treatment of severe progressive renal disease, discontinue therapy.

Pregnancy: Category B (ethacrynic acid, torsemide); *Category* C (furosemide, bumetanide). Since furosemide may increase the incidence of patent ductus arteriosus in preterm infants with respiratory-distress syndrome, use caution when administering before delivery.

Lactation: **Furosemide** appears in breast milk; such transfer of **ethacrynic acid, torsemide** and **bumetanide** is unknown.

Children: Safety and efficacy for use of **torsemide** in children, **bumetanide** in children < 18 years old, and **ethacrynic acid** in infants (oral) and children (IV) have not been established.

Furosemide stimulates renal synthesis of prostaglandin E_2 and may increase the incidence of patent ductus arteriosus when given in the first few weeks of life, to premature infants with respiratory-distress syndrome.

Precautions:

Monitoring: Observe for blood dyscrasias, liver or kidney damage or idiosyncratic reactions. Perform frequent serum electrolyte, calcium, glucose, uric acid, CO_2, creatinine and BUN determinations during the first few months of therapy and periodically thereafter.

Cardiovascular effects: Too vigorous a diuresis, as evidenced by rapid and excessive weight loss, may induce an acute hypotensive episode. In elderly cardiac patients, avoid rapid contraction of plasma volume and the resultant hemoconcentration to prevent thromboembolic episodes, such as cerebral vascular thromboses and pulmonary emboli.

Electrolyte imbalance may occur, especially in patients receiving high doses with restricted salt intake. Perform periodic determinations of serum electrolytes.

Hypokalemia prevention requires particular attention to the following: Patients receiving digitalis and diuretics for CHF, hepatic cirrhosis and ascites; in aldosterone excess with normal renal function; potassium-losing nephropathy; certain diarrheal states; or where hypokalemia is an added risk to the patient (eg, history of ventricular arrhythmias).

Hypomagnesemia – Loop diuretics increase the urinary excretion of magnesium.

Hypocalcemia – Serum calcium levels may be lowered (rare cases of tetany have occurred).

Hyperuricemia: Asymptomatic hyperuricemia can occur, and rarely, gout may be precipitated.

Glucose: Increases in blood glucose and alterations in glucose tolerance tests (fasting and 2 hour postprandial sugar) have been observed.

Lipids: Increases in LDL and total cholesterol and triglycerides with minor decreases in HDL cholesterol may occur.

Photosensitivity: Photosensitization (photoallergy or phototoxicity) may occur.

Drug Interactions:

Loop diuretics may affect the following drugs: Aminoglycosides; anticoagulants; chloral hydrate; digitalis glycosides; lithium; nondepolarizing neuromuscular blockers; propranolol; sulfonylureas; theophyllines. Loop diuretics may be affected by the following drugs: Charcoal; cisplatin; clofibrate; hydantoins; NSAIDs; probenecid; salicylates; thiazide diuretics.

Drug/Food interactions: The bioavailability of **furosemide** is decreased and its degree of diuresis reduced when administered with food. Simultaneous food intake with **torsemide** delays the time to C_{max} by about 30 minutes, but overall bioavailability and diuretic activity are unchanged.

Adverse Reactions:

Adverse reactions associated with loop diuretics include nausea; vomiting; diarrhea; gastric irritation; headache; fatigue; dizziness; thrombocytopenia; rash; orthostatic hypotension; hyperuricemia; hyperglycemia; electrolyte imbalance (decreased chloride, potassium and sodium); dehydration.

Furosemide: Adverse reactions may include anorexia, cramping, constipation, blurred vision, hearing loss, restlessness, fever, anemia, purpura, thrombocytopenia, agranulocytosis, photosensitivity, urticaria, pruritus, thrombophlebitis, muscle spasm, weakness.

Ethacrynic acid: Adverse reactions may include anorexia, pain, GI bleeding, severe neutropenia, agranulocytosis, fever, chills, confusion, fatigue, malaise, sense of fullness in the ears, blurred vision, tinnitus, hearing loss (irreversible), rash.

Bumetanide: Adverse reactions may include impaired hearing, ear discomfort, dry mouth, pain, renal failure, weakness, arthritic pain, muscle cramps, ECG changes, chest pain, hives, pruritus, itching, sweating, hyperventilation.

Torsemide: Adverse reactions may include excessive urination.

Administration and Dosage:

BUMETANIDE:

Oral – 0.5 to 2 mg/day, given as a single dose. If diuretic response is not adequate, give a second or third dose at 4 to 5 hour intervals, up to a maximum daily dose of 10 mg. An intermittent dose schedule, given on alternate days or for 3 to 4 days with rest periods of 1 to 2 days in between, is the safest and most effective method for the continued control of edema. In patients with hepatic failure, keep the dose to a minimum, and if necessary, increase the dose carefully.

Parenteral – Initially, 0.5 to 1 mg IV or IM. Administer IV over a period of 1 to 2 minutes. If the initial response is insufficient, give a second or third dose at intervals of 2 to 3 hours; do not exceed a daily dosage of 10 mg. End parenteral treatment and start oral treatment as soon as possible.

Renal function impairment – In patients with severe chronic renal insufficiency, a continuous infusion of bumetanide (12 mg over 12 hours) may be more effective and less toxic than intermittent bolus therapy.

ETHACRYNIC ACID:

Oral –

Initial therapy: Give minimally effective dose (usually, 50 to 200 mg daily) on a continuous or intermittent dosage schedule to produce gradual weight loss of 2.2 to 4.4 kg/day (1 to 2 lb/day). Adjust dose in 25 to 50 mg increments. Higher doses, up to 200 mg twice daily, achieved gradually, are most often required in patients with severe, refractory edema.

Children: Initial dose is 25 mg. Make careful increments of 25 mg to achieve maintenance. Dosage for infants has not been established.

Maintenance therapy: Administer intermittently after an effective diuresis is obtained using an alternate daily schedule or more prolonged periods of diuretic therapy interspersed with rest periods.

Parenteral – Do not give SC or IM because of local pain and irritation. The usual IV dose for the average adult is 50 mg, or 0.5 to 1 mg/kg. Give slowly through the tubing of a running infusion or by direct IV injection over several minutes. Usually, only one dose is necessary; occasionally, a second dose may be required; use a new injection site to avoid thrombophlebitis. A single IV dose, not exceeding 100 mg, has been used. Insufficient pediatric experience precludes recommendation for this age group.

FUROSEMIDE:

Oral –

Edema: 20 to 80 mg/day as a single dose. Depending on response, administer a second dose 6 to 8 hours later. If response is not satisfactory, increase by increments of 20 or 40 mg, no sooner than 6 to 8 hours after previous dose, until desired diuresis occurs. This dose should then be given once or twice daily (eg, at 8 am and 2 pm). Dosage may be titrated up to 600 mg/day in patients with severe edema.

Mobilization of edema may be most efficiently and safely accomplished with an intermittent dosage schedule; the drug is given 2 to 4 consecutive days each week. With doses > 80 mg/day, clinical and laboratory observations are advisable.

Hypertension: 40 mg twice a day; adjust according to response. If the patient does not respond, add other antihypertensive agents. Reduce dosage of other agents by at least 50% as soon as furosemide is added to prevent excessive drop in blood pressure.

Infants and children: 2 mg/kg. If diuresis is unsatisfactory, increase by 1 or 2 mg/kg, no sooner than 6 to 8 hours after previous dose. Doses > 6 mg/kg are not recommended. For maintenance therapy, adjust dose to the minimum effective level. A dose range of 0.5 to 2 mg/kg twice daily has also been recommended.

CHF and chronic renal failure: It has been suggested that doses as high as 2 to 2.5 g/day or more are well tolerated and effective in these patients.

Parenteral –

Edema: Initial dose: 20 to 40 mg IM or IV. Give the IV injection slowly (1 to 2 minutes). If needed, another dose may be given in the same manner 2 hours later. The dose may be raised by 20 mg and given no sooner than 2 hours after previous dose, until desired diuretic effect is obtained. This dose should then be given once or twice daily. Administer high-dose parenteral therapy as a controlled infusion at a rate ≤ 4 mg/min.

Acute pulmonary edema: The usual initial dose is 40 mg IV (over 1 to 2 minutes). If response is not satisfactory within 1 hour, increase to 80 mg IV (over 1 to 2 minutes).

Infants and children: 1 mg/kg IV or IM given slowly under close supervision. If diuretic response after the initial dose is not satisfactory, increase the dosage by 1 mg/kg, no sooner than 2 hours after previous dose, until desired effect is obtained. Doses > 6 mg/kg are not recommended.

CHF and chronic renal failure: It has been suggested that doses as high as 2 to 2.5 g/day or more are well tolerated and effective in these patients. For IV bolus injections, the maximum should not exceed 1 g/day given over 30 minutes.

TORSEMIDE: Torsemide may be given at any time in relation to a meal.

Because of high bioavailability, oral and IV doses are therapeutically equivalent, so patients may be switched to and from the IV form with no change in dose. Administer the IV injection slowly over a period of 2 minutes.

Congestive heart failure/chronic renal failure – The usual initial dose is 10 or 20 mg once daily oral or IV. If the diuretic response is inadequate, titrate the dose upward by approximately doubling until the desired diuretic response is obtained. Single doses > 200 mg have not been adequately studied.

Hepatic cirrhosis – The usual initial dose is 5 or 10 mg once daily oral or IV, administered together with an aldosterone antagonist or a potassium-sparing diuretic. If the diuretic response is inadequate, titrate the dose upward by approximately doubling until the desired diuretic response is obtained. Single doses > 40 mg have not been adequately studied.

Hypertension – The usual initial dose is 5 mg once daily. If the 5 mg dose does not provide adequate reduction in blood pressure within 4 to 6 weeks, the dose may be increased to 10 mg once daily.

POTASSIUM-SPARING DIURETICS

Actions:

Pharmacology: In the kidney, potassium is filtered at the glomerulus and then absorbed parallel to sodium throughout the proximal tubule and thick ascending limb of the loop of Henle, so that only minor amounts reach the distal convoluted tubule. As a result, potassium appearing in urine is secreted at the distal tubule and collecting duct. The potassium-sparing diuretics interfere with sodium reabsorption at the distal tubule, thus decreasing potassium secretion. They exert a weak diuretic and antihypertensive effect when used alone. Their major use is to enhance the action and counteract the kaliuretic effect of thiazide and loop diuretics.

Spironolactone, a competitive inhibitor of aldosterone, binds to aldosterone receptors of the distal tubule and prevents the formation of a protein important in sodium transport. It is effective in both primary and secondary hyperaldosteronism. Spironolactone is effective in lowering systolic and diastolic blood pressure in both primary hyperaldosteronism and essential hypertension, although aldosterone secretion may be normal in benign essential hypertension.

Amiloride and *triamterene* not only inhibit sodium reabsorption induced by aldosterone, but they also inhibit basal sodium reabsorption. They are not aldosterone antagonists, but act directly on the renal distal tubule, cortical collecting tubule and collecting duct. They induce a reversal of polarity of the transtubular electrical-potential difference and inhibit active transport of sodium and potassium. Amiloride may inhibit sodium, potassium-ATPase.

Potassium-Sparing Diuretics: Pharmacological and Pharmacokinetic Properties

Parameters	Amiloride	Spironolactone	Triamterene
Pharmacology			
Tubular site of action	Proximal = distal	Distal	Distal
Mechanism of action	Na^+, K^+–ATPase inhibition; Na^+/H^+ exchange mechanism inhibition (proximal tubule)	Aldosterone antagonism	Membrane effect
Action:			
Onset (hours)	2	24 to 48	2 to 4
Peak (hours)	6 to 10	48 to 72	6 to 8
Duration (hours)	24	48 to 72	12 to 16
Pharmacokinetics			
Bioavailability	15% to 25%	> 90%	30% to 70%
Protein binding	23%	≥ 98%[1]	50% to 67%
Half-life (hours)	6 to 9	20[2]	3
Active metabolites	none	canrenone	hydroxytriamterene sulfate
Peak plasma levels (hours)	3 to 4	canrenone: 2 to 4	3
Excreted unchanged in urine	≈ 50%[3]	†[4]	≈ 21%
Dosage			
Daily dose (mg)	5 to 20	25 to 400	200 to 300

[1] Canrenone > 98%.
[2] 10 to 35 hours for canrenone.
[3] 40% excreted in stool within 72 hours.
[4] Metabolites primarily excreted in urine, but also in bile.

NITRATES

ISOSORBIDE MONONITRATE (ORAL)
Tablets: 10 and 20 mg (*Rx*) — *Monoket* (Schwarz Pharma), *ISMO* (Wyeth-Ayerst)
Tablets, extended release: 60 and 120 mg (*Rx*) — *Imdur* (Key)

NITROGLYCERIN (IV)
Injection: 0.5 and 5 mg/ml (*Rx*) — Various, *Tridil* (Faulding)
Injection solution: 25, 50, 100 and 200 mg in 5% Dextrose (*Rx*) — Various

NITROGLYCERIN (TRANSMUCOSAL)
Tablets, buccal, controlled release: 1, 2 and 3 mg (*Rx*) — *Nitrogard* (Forest)

AMYL NITRITE
Inhalant: 0.3 ml (*Rx*) — *Amyl Nitrite Vaporole* (Glaxo Wellcome)

NITROGLYCERIN (SUBLINGUAL)
Tablets, sublingual: 0.3, 0.4 and 0.6 mg (*Rx*) — *Nitrostat* (Parke-Davis)

NITROGLYCERIN (TRANSLINGUAL)
Spray: 0.4 mg/dose (*Rx*) — *Nitrolingual* (Rhone-Poulenc Rorer)

NITROGLYCERIN (SUSTAINED RELEASE)
Tablets, sustained release: 2.6, 6.5 and 9 mg (*Rx*) — *Nitrong* (Rhone-Poulence Rorer)
Capsules, sustained release: 2.5, 6.5, 9 and 13 mg (*Rx*) — Various, *Nitroglyn* (Kenwood), *Nitro-Time* (Time-Cap Labs)

NITROGLYCERIN TRANSDERMAL SYSTEMS
Patch: 0.1, 0.2, 0.3, 0.4, 0.6 and 0.8 mg/hr (*Rx*) — *Nitro-Dur* (Key)

NITROGLYCERIN (TOPICAL)
Ointment: 2% in a lanolin-petroleum base (*Rx*) — Various, *Nitrol* (Adria)

ISOSORBIDE DINITRATE (SUBLINGUAL AND CHEWABLE)
Tablets, sublingual: 2.5, 5 and 10 mg (*Rx*) — Various, *Isordil* (Wyeth-Ayerst)
Tablets, chewable: 5 and 10 mg (*Rx*) — *Sorbitrate* (ICI Pharma)

ISOSORBIDE DINITRATE (ORAL)
Tablets: 5, 10, 20, 30 and 40 mg (*Rx*) — Various, *Isordil Titradose* (Wyeth-Ayerst)
Tablets, sustained release: 40 mg (*Rx*) — Various, *Isordil Tembids* (Wyeth-Ayerst)
Capsules, sustained release: 40 mg (*Rx*) — Various, *Isordil Tembids* (Wyeth-Ayerst), *Dilatrate-SR* (Schwarz Pharma)

Actions:

Pharmacology: Relaxation of vascular smooth muscle via stimulation of intracellular cyclic guanosine monophosphate production is the principal pharmacologic action of nitrates. Although venous effects predominate, nitroglycerin produces a dose-dependent dilation of both arterial and venous beds. Dilation of the postcapillary vessels, including large veins, promotes peripheral pooling of blood and decreases venous return to the heart, reducing left ventricular end-diastolic pressure (preload). Arteriolar relaxation reduces systemic vascular resistance and arterial pressure (afterload).

Pharmacokinetics:

Doseform, Onset and Duration of Available Nitrates

Nitrates	Dosage form	Onset (minutes)	Duration
Amyl nitrate	Inhalant	0.5	3 to 5 min
Nitroglycerin	IV	1 to 2	3 to 5 min
	Sublingual	1 to 3	30 to 60 min
	Translingual spray	2	30 to 60 min
	Transmucosal tablet	1 to 2	3 to 5 hours[1]
	Oral, sustained release	20 to 45	3 to 8 hours
	Topical ointment	30 to 60	2 to 12 hours[2]
	Transdermal	30 to 60	up to 24 hours[3]
Isosorbide dinitrate	Sublingual	2 to 5	1 to 3 hours
	Oral	20 to 40	4 to 6 hours
	Oral, sustained release	up to 4 hours	6 to 8 hours
Isosorbide mononitrate	Oral	30 to 60	nd

Doseform, Onset and Duration of Available Nitrates			
Nitrates	Dosage form	Onset (minutes)	Duration
Erythrityl tetranitrate	Sublingual & chewable	5	3 hours
	Oral	15 to 30	6 hours
Pentaerythritol tetranitrate	Oral	20 to 60	≈ 5 hours
	Oral, sustained release	30	up to 12 hours

[1] A significant antianginal effect can persist for 5 hours if the tablet has not completely dissolved.
[2] Depends on total amount used per unit of surface area.
[3] Tolerance may develop after 12 hours.
nd = No data.

Indications:

Acute angina (nitroglycerin sublingual, transmucosal or translingual spray; isosorbide dinitrate sublingual; amyl nitrite): For relief of acute anginal episodes; prophylaxis prior to events likely to provoke an attack.

Angina prophylaxis (nitroglycerin topical, transdermal, translingual spray, transmucosal and oral sustained release; isosorbide dinitrate; isosorbide mononitrate; erythrityl tetranitrate; pentaerythritol tetranitrate): Prophylaxis and long-term management of recurrent angina.

Nitroglycerin IV: Control of blood pressure in perioperative hypertension associated with surgical procedures, especially cardiovascular procedures, such as endotracheal intubation, anesthesia, skin incision, sternotomy, cardiac bypass and in the immediate postsurgical period.

CHF associated with acute myocardial infarction (MI); treatment of angina pectoris unresponsive to organic nitrates or β-blockers; production of controlled hypotension during surgical procedures.

Unlabeled uses: Sublingual and topical nitroglycerin and oral nitrates have been used to reduce cardiac workload in patients with acute MI and in CHF.

Nitroglycerin ointment has been used as adjunctive treatment of Raynaud's disease and other peripheral vascular diseases.

IV nitroglycerin may be used in the treatment of hypertensive crisis, specifically in patients who have hypertension with angina or MI.

Contraindications:

Hypersensitivity or idiosyncrasy to nitrates; severe anemia; closed-angle glaucoma; postural hypotension; early MI (sublingual nitroglycerin); head trauma or cerebral hemorrhage; allergy to adhesives (transdermal).

Amyl nitrate: Pregnancy.

Nitroglycerin IV: Hypotension or uncorrected hypovolemia; inadequate cerebral circulation; increased intracranial pressure; constrictive pericarditis; pericardial tamponade.

Warnings:

MI: In acute MI, use nitrates only under close clinical observation and with hemodynamic monitoring. In general, do not use a long-acting form because its effects are difficult to terminate rapidly if excessive hypotension or tachycardia develop.

Arcing: A cardioverter/defibrillator should not be discharged through a paddle electrode that overlies a transdermal nitroglycerin system.

Postural hypotension may occur, even with small doses.

Angina: Nitrates may aggravate angina caused by hypertrophic cardiomyopathy.

Nitroglycerin IV:

Hepatic or renal disease, severe – Use with caution.

Hypotension – Avoid excessive prolonged hypotension, because of possible deleterious effects on the brain, heart, liver and kidney from poor perfusion and the attendant risk of ischemia, thrombosis and altered organ function. Paradoxical bradycardia and increased angina pectoris may accompany nitroglycerin-induced hypotension.

Alcohol intoxication has developed in patients on high-dose IV nitroglycerin.

Sublingual nitroglycerin: Absorption is dependent on salivary secretion. Dry mough decreases absorption.

Transdermal nitroglycerin is not for immediate relief of anginal attacks.

Pregnancy: *Category C; Category X (amyl nitrite).*

Lactation: It is not know whether nitrates are excreted in breast milk.

Children: Safety and efficacy for use in children have not been established.

Precautions:

Tolerance to vascular and antianginal effects of nitrates may develop. The use of a low-nitrate or nitrate-free period should be part of the therapeutic strategy.

Nitrates that appear least likely to associated with tolerance are the short-acting formulations (eg, sublingual, translingual spray), with the exception of the IV form. The transmucosal formulation also appears to be associated with minimal tolerance.

Glaucoma: Intraocular pressure may be increased; therefore, caution is required in administering to patients with glaucoma.

Excessive dosage may produce severe headache.

Volume depletion/hypotension: Severe hypotension (particularly with upright posture) may occur with even small doses of isosorbide mononitrate.

Withdrawal: In terminating treatment of angina, gradually reduce the dosage to prevent withdrawal reactions.

Drug Interactions:

Drugs that may interact with nitrates include alcohol, aspirin, calcium channel blockers, dihydroergotamine and heparin.

Drug/Lab test interactions: Nitrates may interfere with the *Zlatkis-Zak* color reaction causing a false report of decreased serum cholesterol.

Adverse Reactions:

GI: Nausea; vomiting; diarrhea; dyspepsia; involuntary passing of urine and feces; abdominal pain.

CNS: Headache which may be severe and persistent (up to 50%); apprehension; restlessness; weakness; vertigo; dizziness; agitation; anxiety; confusion; insomnia; nervousness.

Cardiovascular: Tachycardia; palpitations; hypotension (sometimes with paradoxical bradycardia and increased angina pectoris); postural hypotension.

Dermatologic: Drug rash or exfoliative dermatitis; cutaneous vasodilation with flushing; crusty skin lesions; pruritus; rash.

Sublingual nitroglycerin tablets may cause a local burning or tingling sensation in the oral cavity at the point of dissolution. Absence of this effect does not indicate loss of potency; some older patients may not experience this effect. The stabilized tablets may be less likely to product these sensations.

GU: Dysuria; impotence; urinary frequency.

Miscellaneous: Arthralgia; bronchitis; muscle twitching; pallor; perspiration; cold sweat; asthenia; blurred vision; diplopia; edema; malaise; neck stiffness; increased appetite.

Administration and Dosage:

ISOSORBIDE MONONITRATE:

Tablets – 20 mg twice daily, with the two doses given 7 hours apart. A starting dose of 5 mg might be appropriate for persons of particularly small stature, but should be increased to at least 10 mg by the second or third day of therapy. Suggested regimen is to give first dose on awakening and second dose 7 hours later.

Tablets, extended release – Initially, 30 or 60 mg once daily. After several days, the dosage may be increased to 120 mg once daily. Rarely 240 mg may be required. Suggested regimen is to give in the morning on arising. Do not crush or chew extended release tablets, and swallow them with a half glassful of liquid.

AMYL NITRITE: Usual adult dose is 0.3 ml by inhalation, as required.

Crush the capsule and wave under the nose; 1 to 6 inhalations from one capsule are usually sufficient to produce the desired effect. May repeat in 3 to 5 minutes.

NITROGLYCERIN, INTRAVENOUS:

Dosage requirements – Initially, 5 mcg/min delivered through an infusion pump. Titrate to the clinical situation, initially in 5 mcg/min increments with increases every 3 to 5 minutes until some response is noted. If no response occurs at 20 mcg/min, use increments of 10 to 20 mcg/min. Once a partial blood pressure response is observed, reduce the dose and lengthen the interval between increments.

NITROGLYCERIN, TRANSMUCOSAL: 1 mg every 3 to 5 hours during waking hours. Place tablet between lip and gum above incisors, or between cheek and gum.

NITROGLYCERIN, SUBLINGUAL: Dissolve 1 tablet under tongue or in buccal pouch (between cheek and gum) at first sign of an acute anginal attack. Repeat approximately every 5 minutes until relief is obtained. Take no more than 3 tablets in 15 minutes. May be used prophylactically 5 to 10 minutes prior to activities which might precipitate an acute attack.

NITROGLYCERIN, TRANSLINGUAL: At the onset of attack, spray 1 or 2 metered doses onto or under the tongue. No more than 3 metered doses are recommended within 15 minutes. May use prophylactically 5 to 10 minutes prior to activities which might precipitate an acute attack. Do not inhale spray.

NITROGLYCERIN SUSTAINED RELEASE: The usual starting dose is 2.5 or 2.6 mg, 3 or 4 times daily. The dose generally may be increased by 2.5 or 2.6 mg increments 2 to 4 times daily over a period of days or weeks. Doses as high as 26 mg given 4 times daily have been reported effective.

Give the smallest effective dose 2 to 4 times daily.

Capsules must be swallowed; not for chewing or sublingual use.

NITROGLYCERIN TRANSDERMAL SYSTEMS: Patient instructions for application are provided with products.

Apply once daily to a skin site free of hair and not subject to excessive movement. Do not apply to distal parts of extremities. Avoid areas with cuts/irritations.

Starting dose – 0.2 to 0.4 mg/hr. Doses between 0.4 and 0.8 mg/hr have shown continued effectiveness for 10 to 12 hours daily for at least 1 month of intermittent administration. Although the minimum nitrate-free interval has not been defined, data show that a nitrate-free interval of 10 to 12 hours is sufficient. Thus, an appropriate dosing schedule would include a daily "patch-on" period of 12 to 14 hours and a "patch-off" period of 10 to 12 hours. Tolerance is a major factor limiting efficacy when the system is used continuously for > 12 hours each day.

NITROGLYCERIN, TOPICAL:

Usual therapeutic dose – 1 to 2 inches (25 to 50 mm) every 8 hours, up to 4 to 5 inches (100 to 125 mm) every 4 hours. Start with ½ inch (12.5 mm) every 8 hours; increase by ½ inch with each application to achieve desired effects.

One inch (25 mm) of ointment contains ≈ 15 mg nitroglycerin.

ISOSORBIDE DINITRATE, SUBLINGUAL AND CHEWABLE:

Angina pectoris – Usual starting dose is 2.5 to 5 mg for sublingual tablets and 5 mg for chewable tablets.

Acute prophylaxis – 5 to 10 mg sublingual or chewable tablets every 2 to 3 hours. Limit use of sublingual or chewable isosorbide dinitrate for aborting an acute anginal attack in patients intolerant of or unresponsive to sublingual nitroglycerin.

Do not crush or chew sublingual tablets; do not crush chewable tablets before administering.

ISOSORBIDE DINITRATE, ORAL:

Tablets – Initial dose is 5 to 20 mg; maintenance dose is 10 to 40 mg every 6 hours.

Sustained release – The initial dose is 40 mg; maintenance controlled release dose is 40 to 80 mg every 8 to 12 hours. Do not crush or chew these preparations.

Tolerance to these agents may develop. Consider administering the short-acting preparations 2 or 3 times daily (last dose no later than 7 pm) and the sustained release preparations once daily or twice daily at 8 am and 2 pm.

CALCIUM CHANNEL BLOCKING AGENTS

AMLODIPINE	
Tablets: 2.5, 5, 10 mg (*Rx*)	*Norvasc* (Pfizer)
BEPRIDIL HCl	
Tablets: 200, 300, 400 mg (*Rx*)	*Vascor* (McNeil)
DILTIAZEM HCl	
Tablets: 30, 60, 90, 120 mg (*Rx*)	Various, *Cardizem* (Marion Merrell Dow)
Capsules, sustained release: 60, 90, 120, 180, 240, 300, 360 mg (*Rx*)	Various, *Cardizem SR* (Marion Merrell Dow), *Cardizem CD* (Marion Merrell Dow), *Dilacor XR* (Rhone-Poulenc Rorer), *Tiazac* (Forest)
Injection: 25 mg (5 mg/ml), 50 mg (5 mg/ml) (*Rx*)	*Cardizem* (Marion Merrell Dow)
FELODIPINE	
Tablets, extended release: 2.5, 5, 10 mg (*Rx*)	*Plendil* (Merck)
ISRADIPINE	
Capsules: 2.5, 5 mg (*Rx*)	*DynaCirc* (Sandoz)
NICARDIPINE HCl	
Capsules: 20, 30 mg (*Rx*)	*Cardene* (Syntex)
Capsules, sustained release: 30, 45, 60 mg (*Rx*)	*Cardene SR* (Syntex)
Injection: 2.5 mg/ml (*Rx*)	*Cardene I.V.* (Wyeth)
NIFEDIPIINE	
Capsules: 10, 20 mg (*Rx*)	Various, *Procardia* (Pfizer), *Adalat* (Bayer)
Tablets, sustained release: 30, 60, 90 mg (*Rx*)	*Procardia XL* (Pfizer), *Adalat CC* (Bayer)
NIMODIPINE	
Capsules, liquid: 30 mg (*Rx*)	*Nimotop* (Bayer)
NISOLDIPINE	
Tablets, extended release: 10, 20, 30, 40 mg (*Rx*)	*Sular* (Zeneca)
VERAPAMIL HCl	
Tablets: 40, 80, 120 mg (*Rx*)	Various, *Calan* (Searle), *Isoptin* (Knoll)
Tablets, sustained release: 120, 180, 240 mg (*Rx*)	Various, *Calan SR* (Searle), *Isoptin SR* (Knoll), *Covera-HS* (Searle)
Capsules, sustained release: 120, 180, 240 mg (*Rx*)	*Verelan* (Lederle)
Injection: 5 mg/2 ml (*Rx*)	Various, *Isoptin* (Knoll)
MIBEFRADIL	
Tablets: 50, 100 mg (*Rx*)	*Posicor* (Roche)

Actions:

Pharmacology: The calcium channel blockers share the ability to inhibit movement of calcium ions across the cell membrane. The effects on the cardiovascular system include depression of mechanical contraction of myocardial and smooth muscle and depression of both impulse formation (automaticity) and conduction velocity. **Bepridil** also inhibits fast sodium inward channels. Calcium channel blockers are classified by structure as follows: Diphenylalkylamines – verapamil; benzothiazepines – diltiazem; dihydropyridines – amlodipine, felodipine, isradipine, nicardipine, nifedipine, nimodipine, nisoldipine.

Although these agents are similar in that they all act on the slow (calcium) channel, they have different degrees of selectivity in their effects on vascular smooth muscle, myocardium or specialized conduction and pacemaker tissues. The resulting clinical effects depend on the direct activity of the drug, reflex physiological responses (primarily β-adrenergic response to vasodilation) and the patient's cardiovascular status. This heterogeneity of the calcium blockers, in part, determines their clinical application and the different side effects produced by each agent.

Pharmacokinetics:

	Parameters	Nifedipine/SR	Verapamil	Diltiazem/SR	Nicardipine	Nisoldipine
Calcium Channel Blocking Agents: Pharmacology/Pharmacokinetics						
Pharmacokinetics	Extent of absorption (%)[1]	90	90	80-90	≈ 100	nd
	Absolute bioavailability (%)[1]	45-70/86	20-35	40-67	35	5
	Onset of action - oral (min)	20	30[2]	30-60	20	nd
	Time of peak plasma levels (hrs)	0.5/6	1-2.2	2-3/6-11	0.5-2	6-12
	Protein binding (%)	92-98	83-92	70-80	> 95	> 99
	Therapeutic serum levels (ng/ml)	25-100	80-300	50-200	28-50	nd
	Metabolite	Acid or lactone[3]	Norverapamil[4]	Desacetyl-diltiazem[5]	Glucuronide conjugates	5 major urinary metabolites
	Excreted unchanged in urine (%)	1-2	3-4	2-4	< 1	trace
	Half-life, elimination (hrs)	2-5	3-7[7]	3.5-6/5-7	2-4	7-12
Electrophysiology	Effective refractory period (ERP)					
	Atrium	0	0	0	0	0
	AV node	±	↑↑*	↑*	↑↓*	0
	His-Purkinje	0	0	0	↓*	0
	Ventricle	0	0	0	0	0
	Accessory pathway	0	±	na	0	0
	SA node automaticity[8]	0	↓↓*	↓*	0	0
	AV node conduction[8]	±	↓↓↓*	↓↓*	0-↑*	0
	Sinus node recovery time	0	0[9]	0[9]	0	0
ECG Changes	Heart rate	↑*	↑↓*	↓*-0	↑*	±
	QRS complex	0	0	0	0	0
	PR interval	0	↑*	↑*	nd	0
	QT interval	nd	nd	nd	↑*	0
Hemodynamics	Myocardial contractility[8]	↓*	↓↓*	↓*	0	0
	Cardiac output	↑↑*	↑↓*	0-↑*	↑↑*	0
	Peripheral vascular resistance	↓↓↓*	↓↓*	↓*	↓↓↓*	↓↓↓

* ↑↑↑ or ↓↓↓ = pronounced effect; ↑↑ or ↓↓ = moderate effect; ↑ or ↓ = slight effect; ± = negligible effect; nd = no data; na = not applicable

[1] Although these agents are well absorbed (80% to 90%) following oral administration, they are subject to extensive first-pass effects, resulting in an absolute bioavailability that is considerably less.

[2] Peak therapeutic effects occur within 3 to 5 minutes after IV administration.

[3] Inactive.

[4] Pharmacologic activity 20% of verapamil.

[5] Pharmacologic activity 25% to 50% of diltiazem; plasma levels 10% to 20% of parent drug.

[6] Of 6 metabolites identified, account for > 75%.

[7] 4.5 to 12 hours with multiple dosing; may be prolonged in elderly.

[8] Direct effects may be counteracted by reflex activity.

[9] Prolonged in sick sinus syndrome.

[10] Dose-related.

Calcium Channel Blocking Agents: Pharmacology/Pharmacokinetics						
	Parameters	Nimodipine	Isradipine	Bepridil	Felodipine	Amlodipine
Pharmacokinetics	Extent of absorption (%)[1]	nd	90-95	≈ 100	≈ 100	nd
	Absolute a vailability (%)[1]	13	15-24	59	20	64-90
	Onset of action - oral (min)	nd	120	60	120-300	nd
	Time of peak plasma levels (hrs)	≤ 1	1.5	2-3	2.5-5	6-12
	Protein binding (%)	> 95	95	> 99	> 99	93
	Therapeutic serum levels (ng/ml)	nd	nd	1-2	nd	nd
	Metabolite	Unknown[3]	Monoacids and cyclic lactone[6]	4-OH-N-phenyl-bepridil	Six inactive[2]	90% converted to inactive
	Excreted unchanged in urine (%)	< 1	0	±	< 0.5	10
	Half-life, elimination (hrs)	1-2	8	24	11-16	30-50
Electrophysiology	Effective refractory period					
	Atrium	na	0	↑*	0	0
	AV node		0	↑*	0	0
	His-Purkinje		0	↑*	0	0
	Ventricle		0	↑*	0	0
	Accessory pathway		nd	↑*	0	0
	SA node automaticity		0	↓*	0	0
	AV node conduction		0	↓*	0	0
	Sinus node recovery time		±	nd	0	0
ECG Changes	Heart rate		±	↓*	±	±
	QRS complex		0	0	0	0
	PR interval		0	↑*	0	0
	QT interval		↑*	↑↑[10]	0	0
Hemodynamics	Myocardial contractility		0	↓*	↑*	↑*
	Cardiac output		↑*	0	↑*	↑*
	Peripheral vascular resistance		↓↓↓*	↓*	↓↓↓*	↓↓↓*

* ↑↑↑ or ↓↓↓ = pronounced effect; ↑↑ or ↓↓ = moderate effect; ↑ or ↓ = slight effect; ± = negligible effect; nd = no data; na = not applicable

[1] Although these agents are well absorbed (80% to 90%) following oral administration, they are subject to extensive first-pass effects, resulting in an absolute bioavailability that is considerably less.

[2] Peak therapeutic effects occur within 3 to 5 minutes after IV administration.

[3] Inactive.

[4] Pharmacologic activity 20% of verapamil.

[5] Pharmacologic activity 25% to 50% of diltiazem; plasma levels 10% to 20% of parent drug.

[6] Of 6 metabolites identified, account for > 75%.

[7] 4.5 to 12 hours with multiple dosing; may be prolonged in elderly.

[8] Direct effects may be counteracted by reflex activity.

[9] Prolonged in sick sinus syndrome.

[10] Dose-related.

Indications:

Calcium Channel Blocking Agents – Summary of Indications

Indications	Amlodipine	Bepridil	Diltiazem	Diltiazem SR	Diltiazem IV	Felodipine	Isradipine	Mibefradil	Nicardipine	Nicardipine SR	Nicardipine IV	Nifedipine	Nifedipine SR	Nimodipine	Nisoldipine	Verapamil	Verapamil SR	Verapamil IV
Angina pectoris																		
Vasospastic	✓			✓								✓	✓			✓		
Chronic stable	✓	✓	✓	✓				✓	✓							✓		
Unstable																✓		
Hypertension, essential	✓			✓		✓	✓	✓	✓	✓	✓		✓		✓	✓	✓	
Arrhythmias					✓											✓		
Supraventricular tachyarrhythmias																		✓
Subarachnoid hemorrhage														✓				

Unlabeled uses:

Nifedipine – Preliminary studies suggest nifedipine may be useful for hypertensive emergencies, prophylaxis in migraine headache and in the treatment of primary pulmonary hypertension, asthma, preterm labor, severe pregnancy-associated hypertension, esophageal disorders, biliary and renal colic, cardiomyopathy, to reduce progression of coronary artery disease, CHF and Raynaud's syndrome.

Verapamil (oral), has been used for PSVT. It has also been studied for the prophylaxis of migraine headache, cluster headache and exercise-induced asthma, for treatment of hypertrophic cardiomyopathy, as alternate therapy in manic depression and for recumbent nocturnal leg cramps.

Diltiazem has been investigated in the prevention of reinfarction of non-Q-wave myocardial infarction, tardive dyskinesia and Raynaud's syndrome.

Nimodipine appears to be beneficial in patients with common and classic migraine and chronic cluster headache.

Nicardipine may be useful in the treatment of congestive heart failure and in combination with aminocaproic acid for SAH.

Isradipine may be beneficial in the treatment of chronic stable angina.

Contraindications:

Hypersensitivity to the drug; sick sinus syndrome or second- or third-degree AV block except with a functioning pacemaker, hypotension < 90 mm Hg systolic (bepridil, diltiazem and verapamil).

Diltiazem: Acute MI and pulmonary congestion.

Verapamil: Severe left ventricular dysfunction; cardiogenic shock and severe CHF, unless secondary to a supraventricular tachycardia amenable to verapamil therapy and in patients with atrial flutter or atrial fibrillation and an accessory bypass tract.

Verapamil IV – Do not administer concomitantly with IV β-adrenergic blocking agents (within a few hours), since both may depress myocardial contractility and AV conduction; ventricular tachycardia, since use in patients with wide-complex ventricular tachycardia (QRS ≥ 0.12 sec) can result in marked hemodynamic deterioration and ventricular fibrillation.

Nicardipine: Advanced aortic stenosis.

Bepridil: History of serious ventricular arrhythmias; uncompensated cardiac insufficiency; congenital QT interval prolongation; use with other drugs that prolong QT interval.

Warnings:

Induction of new serious arrhythmias (bepridil): Bepridil has Class I antiarrhythmic properties and, like other such drugs, can induce new arrhythmias, including VT/VF. In addition, because of its ability to prolong the QT interval, bepridil can cause torsades de pointes-type ventricular tachycardia (VT). Because of these properties, reserve for patients in whom other antianginal agents do not offer a satisfactory effect.

While the safe upper limit of QT is not defined, it is suggested that the interval not be permitted to exceed 0.52 seconds during treatment. If dose reduction does not eliminate the excessive prolongation, stop the drug. If concomitant diuretics are needed, consider low doses and the addition or primary use of a potassium-sparing diuretic and monitor serum potassium.

Hypotension, usually modest and well tolerated, may occasionally occur during initial therapy or with dosage increases, and may be more likely in patients taking concomitant β–blockers.

CHF has developed rarely, usually in patients receiving a β-blocker, after beginning **nifedipine.**

Oral verapamil, 1.8% developed CHF or pulmonary edema.

Use **diltiazem, nicardipine, isradipine, felodipine, amlodipine** and **bepridil** with caution in CHF patients.

Cardiac conduction: **IV verapamil** slows AV nodal conduction and SA nodes; it rarely produces second- or third-degree AV block, bradycardia, and in extreme cases, asystole. This is more likely to occur in patients with sick sinus syndrome.

Oral verapamil may lead to first-degree AV block and transient bradycardia, sometimes accompanied by nodal escape rhythms.

Premature ventricular contractions (PVCs): During conversion or marked reduction in ventricular rate, benign complexes of unusual appearance (sometimes resembling PVCs) may occur after **IV verapamil.** Verapamil IV may produce potentially fatal ventricular fibrillation in patients with atrial fibrillation (AF) and WPW syndrome.

Hypertrophic cardiomyopathy (IHSS): Serious adverse effects were seen in 120 patients with IHSS (most refractory or intolerant to propranolol) who received oral **verapamil** at doses up to 720 mg/day. Sinus bradycardia occurred in 11%, second-degree AV block in 4% and sinus arrest in 2%.

β-blocker withdrawal/nifedipine: Patients recently withdrawn from β-blockers may develop a withdrawal syndrome with increased angina, probably related to increased sensitivity to catecholamines. Initiation of nifedipine will not prevent this occurrence and might exacerbate it by provoking reflex catecholamine release. Taper β-blockers rather than stopping them abruptly before beginning nifedipine.

Hepatic function impairment: The pharmacokinetics, bioavailability and patient response to **verapamil** and **nifedipine** may be significantly affected by hepatic cirrhosis.

Since **amlodipine, diltiazem, nicardipine, bepridil, felodipine** and **nimodipine** are extensively metabolized by liver, use with caution in impaired hepatic function or reduced hepatic blood flow.

Renal function impairment: The pharmacokinetics of **diltiazem** and **verapamil** in patients with impaired renal function are similar to the pharmacokinetic profile of patients with normal renal function. However, caution is still advised. **Nifedipine's** plasma concentration is slightly increased in patients with renal impairment. **Nicardipine's** mean plasma concentrations, AUC and maximum concentration were ≈ 2–fold higher in patients with mild renal impairment. Use **bepridil** with caution in patients with serious renal disorders since the metabolites of bepridil are excreted primarily in the urine.

Increased angina: Occasional patients have increased frequency, duration or severity of angina on starting **nifedipine** or **nicardipine** or at the time of dosage increases.

Duchenne's muscular dystrophy: **Verapamil** may decrease neuromuscular transmission in patients with Duchenne's muscular dystrophy, and prolong recovery from the neuromuscular blocking agent vecuronium.

Elderly: **Verapamil, nifedipine** and **felodipine** may cause a greater hypotensive effect than that seen in younger patients, probably due to age-related changes in drug disposition.

Pregnancy: *Category* C.

Lactation: **Verapamil, diltiazem** and **bepridil** are excreted in breast milk. One report suggests that diltiazem concentrations in breast milk may approximate serum levels. Bepridil is estimated to reach about one third the concentration in serum. Significant concentrations of **nicardipine** and **nimodipine** appear in maternal milk of rats. An insignificant amount of **nifedipine** is transferred into breast milk (over 24 hours, < 5% of a dose). It is not known if **isradipine, amlodipine** or **felodipine** are excreted in breast milk.

Children: Safety and efficacy of **diltiazem, bepridil, felodipine, amlodipine** and **isradipine** have not been established.

Controlled studies of **IV verapamil** have not been conducted in pediatric patients, but uncontrolled experience indicates that results of treatment are similar to those in adults. Patients < 6 months of age may not respond to IV verapamil; this resistance may be related to a developmental difference of AV node responsiveness.

Precautions:

Acute hepatic injury: In rare instances, symptoms consistent with acute hepatic injury, as well as significant elevations in enzymes such as alkaline phosphatase, CPK, LDH, AST and ALT have occurred with **diltiazem** and **nifedipine**.

Elevations of transaminases with and without concomitant elevations in alkaline phosphatase and bilirubin have occurred with **verapamil**.

Isolated cases of elevated LDH, alkaline phosphatase and ALT levels have occurred rarely with **nimodipine.**

Clinically significant transaminase elevations have occurred in approximately 1% of patients receiving **bepridil;** however, no patient became clinically symptomatic or jaundiced, and values returned to normal when the drug was stopped.

Edema, mild to moderate, typically associated with arterial vasodilation and not due to left ventricular dysfunction, occurs in 10% of patients receiving **nifedipine**. It occurs primarily in the lower extremities and usually responds to diuretics. In patients with CHF, differentiate this peripheral edema from the effects of decreasing left ventricular function.

Peripheral edema, generally mild and not associated with generalized fluid retention, may occur with **felodipine** within 2 to 3 weeks of therapy initiation. The incidence is both age- and dose-dependent, with frequency ranging from 10% in patients < 50 years of age taking 5 mg/day to 30% in patients > 60 years of age taking 20 mg/day.

Drug Interactions:

Drugs that may affect calcium blockers include barbiturates, calcium salts, dantrolene, erythromycin, histamine H_2 antagonists, hydantoins, quinidine, rifampin, sulfinpyrazone, vitamin D and carbamazepine. Drugs that may be affected by calcium blockers include quinidine, anticoagulants, beta blockers, carbamazepine, cyclosporine, digitalis glycosides, encainide, etomidate, fentanyl, lithium, magnesium sulfate (parenteral), nondepolarizing muscle relaxants, prazosin and theophyllines.

Drug/Food interactions: **Nifedipine, amlodipine** and **verapamil** may be administered without regard to meals.

Bioavailability of **felodipine** is not affected by food, but increased > 2–fold when taken with doubly concentrated grapefruit juice vs water or orange juice.

High-fat meals and grapefruit juice with **nisolodipine** should be avoided.

Adverse Reactions:

Generally not serious; rarely requires discontinuation or dosage adjustment.

Adverse Reactions of Calcium Channel Blockers (%)

	Adverse Reactions	Nifedipine[1]	Nisoldipine	Verapamil (IV)	Diltiazem[1]	Nicardipine	Nimodipine	Bepridil	Isradipine	Felodipine	Amlodipine
Central Nervous System	Dizziness/Lightheadedness	4.1-27	5	3.5 (1.2)	1.5-7	4-6.9	< 1	11.6-27	7.3	5.8	1.1-3.4[2]
	Drowsiness							≥ 7	≤ 1		
	Nervousness	≤ 7			< 1	0.6		7.4-11.6	≤ 1	≤ 1.5	≤ 1
	Headache	10-23	22	2.2 (1.2)	2.1-12	6.4-8.2	1.4-4.1	7-13.6	13.7	18.6	7.3
	Weakness/Shakiness/Jitteriness	≤ 12		< 1	1.2	0.6			1.2		
	Asthenia	< 3		1.7	2.8-5	4.2-5.8		6.5-14		4.7	1-2
	Fatigue/Lethargy								3.9		4.5[2]
	Tremor/Hand tremor		≤ 1		< 1			≤ 9.3			≤ 1
Gastrointestinal	Nausea	3.3-11	2	2.7 (0.9)	1.6-1.9	1.9-2.2	0.6-1.4	7-26	1.8	1.9	2.9[2]
	Diarrhea	< 3	≤ 1	< 1	< 1		1.7-4.2	0-10.9	1.1	1.6	≤ 1
	Constipation	≤ 3.3		7.3	1.6	0.6		2.8	≤ 1	1.6	≤ 1
	Dry mouth/Thirst	< 3	≤ 1	< 1	< 1	0.4-1.4		3.4	≤ 1	≤ 1.5	≤ 1
	Flatulence	≤ 3	≤ 1					≤ 2		≤ 1.5	≤ 1

Adverse Reactions of Calcium Channel Blockers (%)											
	Adverse Reactions	Nifedipine[1]	Nisoldipine	Verapamil (IV)	Diltiazem[1]	Nicardipine	Nimodipine	Bepridil	Isradipine	Felodipine	Amlodipine
Cardiovascular	Pharyngitis		5								
	Peripheral edema	10-30	22	2.1	2.4-9	7.1-8	0.4-1.2	≤ 2	7.2	22.3	1.8-14.6[2]
	Hypotension	≤ 5		2.5 (1.5)	1	< 0.4	1.2-8.1		≤ 1	≤ 1.5	≤ 1
	Palpitations	≤ 7	3	< 1	< 1	3.3-4.1	< 1	≤ 6.5	42[2]	1.8	0.7-4.5[2]
	AV block (1°, 2° or 3°)		≤ 1	0.8-1.2	0.6-7.6	< 0.4				≤ 1.5	
	Bradycardia			1.4 (1.2)	1.5-6		0.6-1	≤ 2			≤ 1
	Congestive heart failure	2-6.7	≤ 1	1.8	< 1		< 1		≤ 1		
	Myocardial infarction	4-6.7	≤ 1	< 1		< 0.4			≤ 1	≤ 1.5	
	Pulmonary edema	7		1.8							
	Angina	≤ 1	2		< 1	5.6			2.4	≤ 1.5	
	Tachycardia	≤ 1		(1)	< 1	0.8-3.4	1	≤ 2	1.5	≤ 1.5	≤ 1
	Abnormal ECG				4.1	0.6	0.6-1.4				
	Vasodilation		4								
Dermatologic	Dermatitis/Rash	≤ 3	2	1.2	1-1.5	0.4-1.2	0.6-2.4	≤ 2	1.5	1.5	1-2
	Pruritus/Urticaria	≤ 3	≤ 1	< 1 (†)	< 1		< 1		≤ 1	≤ 1.5	1-2
Other	Flushing	< 3-25	4	< 1	1.7-3	5.6-9.7	1-2.1		2.6	6.4	0.7-4.5[2]
	Nasal or chest congestion/ sinusitis/rhinitis	≤ 6	≤ 3	†	< 1	†		≤ 2		≤ 1.5	≤ 0.1
	Sexual difficulties	≤ 3		< 1	< 1	†		≤ 2	≤ 1	≤ 1.5	1-2
	Shortness of breath/ dyspnea/ wheezing	≤ 8		1.4	< 1	0.6	1.2	≤ 8.7	1.8	≤ 1.5	1-2
	Muscle cramps/ pain/inflammation	≤ 8		< 1			0.2-1.4			≤ 1.9	1-2
	Joint stiffness/ pain/ arthritis	≤ 3			< 1	†					≤ 1
	Cough	6						≤ 2	≤ 1	2.9	≤ 0.1
	Anorexia				< 1			≤ 7			≤ 1
	Respiratory infection	≤ 1						2.8		≤ 5.5	

[1] Includes data for sustained release form.
[2] Appears to be dose-related.
†Occurs, no incidence reported.

Administration and Dosage:

NISOLDIPINE: Administer nisoldipine orally once daily. Administration with a high fat meal can lead to excessive peak drug concentration and should be avoided. Avoid grapefruit products before and after dosing. Nisoldipine is an extended release dosage form; swallow whole, do not bite or divide.

Initiate therapy with 20 mg orally once daily, then increase by 10 mg per week, or longer intervals, to attain adequate control of blood pressure. The usual maintenance dosage is 20 to 40 mg once daily. Blood pressure (BP) response increases over the 10 to 60 mg daily dose range, but adverse event rates also increase. Doses > 60 mg once daily are not recommended.

Elderly/Hepatic function impairment – Patients over age 65 or patients with impaired liver function are expected to develop higher plasma concentrations of nisoldipine. Monitor blood pressure closely during any dosage adjustment. A starting dose not exceeding 10 mg daily is recommended in these patient groups.

NIFEDIPINE: Individualize dosage. Excessive doses can result in hypotension.

Initial dosage (capsule) – 10 mg 3 times/day. Usual range is 10 to 20 mg 3 times/day. Some patients, especially those with coronary artery spasm, respond only to higher doses, more frequent administration or both. In such patients, 20 to 30 mg 3 or 4 times/day may be effective. Doses > 120 mg/day are rarely necessary. More than 180 mg/day is not recommended.

Titrate throughout 7 to 14 days to assess response to each dose level; monitor blood pressure before proceeding to higher doses.

Sustained release –

Procardia XL: 30 or 60 mg once daily. Do not chew or divide tablet. Titrate over a 7 to 14 day period. Titration may proceed more rapidly if the patient is frequently assessed. Titration to doses > 120 mg is not recommended.

Angina patients maintained on the nifedipine capsule formulation may be switched to the sustained release tablet at the nearest equivalent total daily dose. Experience with doses > 90 mg in angina is limited; therefore, use with caution and only when clinically warranted.

Adalat CC: Adjust dosage according to the patient's needs. Administer once daily on an empty stomach. Swallow tablets whole; do not bite, chew or divide. In general, titrate over a 7 to 14 day period starting with 30 mg once daily. Base upward titration on therapeutic efficacy and safety. Usual maintenance dose is 30 to 60 mg once daily. Titration to doses > 90 mg daily is not recommended.

Concomitant drug therapy with β-blockers may be beneficial in chronic stable angina; however, the effects of concurrent treatment cannot be predicted, especially in patients with compromised left ventricular function or cardiac conduction abnormalities.

NICARDIPINE HCl:

Oral –

Angina (immediate release only): Usual initial dose is 20 mg 3 times/day (range, 20 to 40 mg 3 times/day). Allow at least 3 days before increasing dose to ensure achievement of steady-state plasma drug concentrations.

Hypertension:

Immediate release – Initial dose is 20 mg 3 times daily (range 20 to 40 mg 3 times daily). The maximum BP lowering effect occurs ≈ 1 to 2 hours after dosing. Allow at least 3 days before increasing dose to ensure achievement of steady-state plasma drug concentrations.

Sustained release – Initial dose is 30 mg twice daily. Effective doses have ranged from 30 to 60 mg twice daily. The maximum BP lowering effect at steady-state is sustained from 2 to 6 hours after dosing.

The total daily dose of immediate release nicardipine may not be a useful guide in judging the effective dose of the sustained release form. Titrate patients currently receiving the immediate release form with the sustained release form starting at their current daily dose of immediate release, then re-examine to assess adequacy of BP control.

Renal impairment: Titrate dose beginning with 20 mg 3 times a day (immediate release) or 30 mg twice daily (sustained release).

Hepatic impairment: Starting dose is 20 mg twice a day (immediate release) with individual titration.

Parenteral –

Dosage:

Substitute for oral nicardipine – The IV infusion rate required to produce an average plasma concentration equivalent to a given oral dose at steady state is shown in the following table:

Equivalent Nicardipine Doses: Oral vs IV Infusion	
Oral dose	Equivalent IV infusion rate
20 mg q 8 hr	0.5 mg/hr
30 mg q 8 hr	1.2 mg/hr
40 mg q 8 hr	2.2 mg/hr

Initiation in a drug free patient – The time course of blood pressure decrease is dependent on the initial rate of infusion and the frequency of dosage adjustment. Administer by slow continuous infusion at a concentration of 0.1 mg/ml. With constant infusion, blood pressure begins to fall within minutes. It reaches about 50% of its ultimate decrease in about 45 minutes and does not reach final steady state for about 50 hours.

When treating acute hypertensive episodes in patients with chronic hypertension, discontinuation of infusion is followed by a 50% offset of action in 30 minutes but plasma levels of drug and gradually decreasing antihypertensive effects exist for ≈ 50 hours.

Titration – For gradual reduction in blood pressure, initiate therapy at 50 mg/hr (5 mg/hr). If desired reduction is not achieved at this dose, the infusion rate may be increased by 25 ml/hr (2.5 mg/hr) every 15 minutes up to a maximum of 150 ml/hr (15 mg/hr) until desired reduction of blood pressure is achieved. For more rapid reduction of blood pressure, initiate at 50 ml/hr. If desired reduction is not achieved at this dose, the infusion rate may be increased by 25 ml/hr every 5 minutes up to a maximum of 150 ml/hr until desired reduction of blood pressure is achieved. Following achievement of the blood pressure goal, decrease the infusion rate to 30 ml/hr.

Maintenance – Adjust the rate of infusion as needed to maintain desired response.

Conditions requiring infusion adjustment –

Hypotension or tachycardia: If there is concern of impending hypotension or tachycardia, discontinue the infusion. When blood pressure has stabilized, infusion may be restarted at low doses (eg, 30 to 50 ml/hr) and adjusted to maintain desired blood pressure.

Infusion site changes: Continue IV use as long as bp control is needed. Change the infusion site every 12 hours if administered via peripheral vein.

Cardiac/Renal/Hepatic function impairment: Use caution when titrating in patients with CHF or renal or hepatic function impairment

Transfer to oral antihypertensives – If treatment includes transfer to an oral antihypertensive other than nicardipine, generally initiate therapy upon discontinuation of the infusion. If oral nicardipine is to be used, administer the first dose of a 3-times-daily regimen 1 hour prior to discontinuation of the infusion.

BEPRIDIL HCl: Usual initial dose is 200 mg/day. After 10 days, dosage may be adjusted upward depending on response. Most patients are maintained at 300 mg. Maximum daily dose is 400 mg; minimum effective dose is 200 mg.

Elderly – Starting dose does not differ from that for younger patients; however, after therapeutic response is demonstrated, the elderly may require more frequent monitoring.

ISRADIPINE: Recommended initial dose is 2.5 mg twice daily. An antihypertensive response usually occurs within 2 to 3 hours; maximal response may require 2 to 4 weeks. If a satisfactory response does not occur after this period, the dose may be adjusted in increments of 5 mg/day at 2 to 4 week intervals up to a maximum of 20 mg/day. However, most patients show no additional response to doses > 10 mg/day, and adverse effects are increased in frequency above 10 mg/day.

NIMODIPINE: Commence therapy within 96 hours of the SAH, using 60 mg every 4 hours for 21 consecutive days.

If the capsule cannot be swallowed (eg, time of surgery, unconscious patient), make a hole in both ends of the capsule with an 18 gauge needle and extract the contents into a syringe. Empty the contents into the patient's in situ nasogastric tube and wash down the tube with 30 mg normal saline.

FELODIPINE: The recommended starting dose is 5 mg once daily. Depending on the patient's response the dosage can be decreased to 2.5 mg or increased to 10 mg once daily. These adjustments should occur generally at intervals of not less than 2 weeks. The recommended dosage range is 2.5 to 10 mg once daily. Because they may develop higher plasma felodipine levels, closely monitor blood pressure in patients > 65 years old and in impaired hepatic function during dosage adjustment; generally, do not consider doses > 10 mg.

Swallow whole; do not crush or chew.

AMLODIPINE: May be taken without regard to meals.

Hypertension – Usual dose is 5 mg once daily. Maximum dose is 10 mg once daily. Small, fragile or elderly patients or patients with hepatic insufficiency may be started on 2.5 mg once daily; this dose may also be used when adding amlodipine to other antihypertensive therapy. In general, titrate over 7 to 14 days; proceed more rapidly if clinically warranted with frequent assessment of the patient.

Angina (chronic stable or vasospastic) – 5 to 10 mg, using the lower dose for elderly and patients with hepatic insufficiency. Most patients require 10 mg.

DILTIAZEM HCl:

Oral –

Tablets: Start with 30 mg 4 times/day before meals and at bedtime; gradually increase dosage to 180 to 360 mg (given in divided doses 3 or 4 times/day) at 1 to 2 day intervals until optimum response is obtained.

Sustained release:

Cardizem SR – Start with 60 to 120 mg twice daily. Adjust dosage when maximum antihypertensive effect is achieved (usually by 14 days chronic therapy). Optimum dosage range is 240 to 360 mg/day, but some patients may respond to lower doses.

Cardizem CD –

Hypertension: 180 to 240 mg once daily; some patients may respond to lower doses. Maximum antihypertensive effect is usually achieved by 14 days chronic therapy; therefore, adjust dosage accordingly. Usual range is 240 to 360 mg once daily; experience with doses > 360 mg is limited.

Angina: Start with 120 or 180 mg once daily. Some patients may respond to higher doses of up to 480 mg once daily. When necessary, titration may be carried out over a 7 to 14 day period.

Dilacor XR –

Hypertension: 180 to 240 mg once daily; adjust dose as needed. Individual patients, particularly those ≥ 60 years of age, may respond to a lower dose of 120 mg. Usual range is 180 to 480 mg once daily. Although current clinical experience with the 540 mg dose is limited, the dose may be increased to 540 mg with little or no increased risk of adverse reactions. Do not exceed 540 mg once daily.

Angina: Adjust dosage to each patient's needs, starting with a dose of 120 mg once daily, which may be titrated to doses of up to 480 mg once daily. when necessary, titration may be carried out over a 7 to 14 day period.

Hypertensive or anginal patients treated with other formulations of diltiazem can safely be switched to *Dilacor XR* at the nearest equivalent total daily dose. Subsequent titration to higher or lower doses may, however, be necessary and should be initiated as clinically indicated.

Administration in the morning on an empty stomach is recommended. Do not open, chew or crush the capsules; swallow whole.

Parenteral –

Direct IV single injections (bolus): The initial dose is 0.25 mg/kg as a bolus administered over 2 minutes (20 mg is a reasonable dose for the average patient). If response is inadequate, a second dose may be administered after 15 minutes. The second bolus dose should be 0.35 mg/kg administered over 2 minutes (25 mg is a reasonable dose for the average patient). Individualize subsequent IV bolus doses. Dose patients with low body weights on a mg/kg basis. Some patients may respond to an initial dose of 0.15 mg/kg, although duration of action may be shorter.

Continuous IV infusion: For continued reduction of the heart rate (up to 24 hours) in patients with atrial fibrillation or atrial flutter, an IV infusion may be administered. Immediately following bolus administration of 20 mg (0.25 mg/kg) or 25 mg (0.35 mg/kg) and reduction of heart rate, begin an IV infusion. The recommended initial infusion rate is 10 mg/hr. Some patients may maintain response to an initial rate of 5 mg/hr. The infusion rate may be increased in 5 mg/hr increments up to 15 mg/hr as needed, if further reduction in heart rate is required. The infusion may be maintained for up to 24 hours. Therefore, infusion duration longer than 24 hours and infusion rates > 15 mg/hr are not recommended.

Concomitant therapy with β-blockers or digitalis is usually well tolerated, but the effects of coadministration cannot be predicted, especially in patients with left ventricular dysfunction or cardiac conduction abnormalities. Use caution in titrating dosages for impaired renal or hepatic function patients, since dosage requirements are not available.

VERAPAMIL HCl: If heart failure is not severe or rate-related, use digitalis and diuretics, as appropriate, before verapamil. In moderately severe to severe cardiac dysfunction (PCWP > 20 mm Hg, ejection fraction < 30%), acute worsening of heart failure may occur.

Do not exceed 480 mg/day; safety and efficacy are not established. Half-life increases during chronic use; maximum response may be delayed.

Oral –

Angina at rest and chronic stable angina: Usual initial dose is 80 to 120 mg 3 times/day. However, 40 mg 3 times/day may be warranted if patients may have increased response to verapamil (eg, decreased hepatic function, elderly). Base upward titration of safety and efficacy evaluated ≈ 8 hours after dosing. Increase dosage daily (eg, unstable angina) or weekly until optimum clinical response is obtained.

Arrhythmias: Dosage range in digitalized patients with chronic atrial fibrillation is 240 to 320 mg/day in divided doses 3 or 4 times/day. Dosage range for prophylaxis of PSVT (non-digitalized patients) is 240 to 480 mg/day in divided doses 3 or 4 times/day. In general, maximum effects will be apparent during the first 48 hours of therapy.

Essential hypertension: The usual initial monotherapy dose is 80 mg 3 times/day (240 mg/day). Daily dosages of 360 and 480 mg have been used, but there is no evidence that dosages > 360 mg provide added effect. Consider beginning titration at 40 mg 3 times/day in patients who might respond to lower doses, (eg, elderly or people of small stature). Antihypertensive effects are evident within the first week of therapy. Base upward titration on therapeutic efficacy, assessed at the end of the dosing interval.

Sustained release (essential hypertension): Give with food. Usual daily dose is 240 mg/day in the morning. However, 120 mg/day may be warranted in patients who may have increased response (eg, elderly or people of small stature). Base upward titration on safety and efficacy evaluated ≈ 24 hours after dosing. If adequate response is not obtained, titrate upward to 240 mg/morning and 120 mg/evening, then 240 mg every 12 hours, if needed. When switching from immediate release tablets, total daily dose (in mg) may remain the same. Antihypertensive effects are evident within the first week.

Parenteral (supraventricular tachyarrhythmias): For IV use only. Give as slow IV injection over at least 2 minutes under continuous ECG and blood pressure monitoring. An IV infusion has been used (5 mg/hour); precede the infusion with an IV loading dose.

Initial dose – 5 to 10 mg (0.075 to 0.15 mg/kg) as an IV bolus over 2 minutes.

Repeat dose – 10 mg (0.15 mg/kg) 30 minutes after the first dose if the initial response is not adequate.

Older patients – Give over at least 3 min to minimize risk of untoward drug effects.

Children –

≤ 1 year: 0.1 to 0.2 mg/kg (usual single dose range, 0.75 to 2 mg) as an IV bolus over 2 minutes (under continuous ECG monitoring).

1 to 15 years: 0.1 to 0.3 mg/kg (usual single dose range, 2 to 5 mg) IV over 2 minutes. Do not exceed 5 mg.

Repeat dose: Repeat above dose 30 minutes after the first dose if the initial response is not adequate (under continuous ECG monitoring). Do not exceed a single dose of 10 mg in patients 1 to 15 years of age.

MIBEFRADIL: The recommended dose is 50 or 100 mg once daily. Doses > 100 mg offer little or no additional benefit and induce a greater rate of adverse reactions. Exercise caution when administering to patients with severe hepatic impairment.

BETA-ADRENERGIC BLOCKING AGENTS

ATENOLOL	
Tablets: 25, 50 and 100 mg (*Rx*)	Various, *Tenormin* (ICI Pharma)
Injection: 5 mg/10 ml (*Rx*)	*Tenormin* (ICI Pharma)
ESMOLOL HCl	
Injection: 10 or 250 mg/ml (*Rx*)	*Brevibloc* (Ohmeda)
BETAXOLOL HCl	
Tablets: 10 and 20 mg (*Rx*)	*Kerlone* (Searle)
PENBUTOLOL SULFATE	
Tablets: 20 mg (*Rx*)	*Levatol* (Schwarz Pharma)
CARTEOLOL HCl	
Tablets: 2.5 and 5 mg (*Rx*)	*Cartrol* (Abbott)
BISOPROLOL FUMARATE	
Tablets: 5 and 10 mg (*Rx*)	*Zebeta* (Lederle)
PINDOLOL	
Tablets: 5 and 10 mg (*Rx*)	Various, *Visken* (Sandoz)
METOPROLOL	
Tablets: 50 and 100 mg (*Rx*)	Various, *Lopressor* (Geigy)
Tablets, extended release: 50, 100 and 200 mg (*Rx*)	*Toprol XL* (Astra)
Injection: 1 mg/ml (*Rx*)	Various, *Lopressor* (Geigy)
TIMOLOL MALEATE	
Tablets: 5, 10 and 20 mg (*Rx*)	Various, *Blocadren* (Merck)
SOTALOL HCl	
Tablets: 80, 120, 160 and 240 mg (*Rx*)	*Betapace* (Berlex)
ACEBUTOLOL HCl	
Capsules: 200 and 400 mg (*Rx*)	Various, *Sectral* (Wyeth-Ayerst)
NADOLOL	
Tablets: 20, 40, 80, 120 and 160 mg (*Rx*)	Various, *Corgard* (Bristol-Myers Squibb)
PROPRANOLOL	
Tablets: 10, 20, 40, 60, 80 and 90 mg (*Rx*)	Various, *Inderal* (Wyeth-Ayerst)
Capsules, sustained release: 60, 80, 120 and 160 mg (*Rx*)	Various, *Inderal LA* (Wyeth-Ayerst), *Betachron E-R* (Inwood)
Solution, oral: 4 or 8 mg/ml (*Rx*)	Various
Solution, concentrated oral: 80 mg/ml (*Rx*)	*Propranolol Intensol* (Roxane)
Injection: 1 mg/ml (*Rx*)	Various, *Inderal* (Wyeth-Ayerst)

Actions:

Pharmacology:

Pharmacologic/Pharmacokinetic Properties of Beta-Adrenergic Blocking Agents

0–none +-low ++-moderate +++-high Drug	Adrenergic receptor blocking activity	Membrane stabilizing activity	Intrinsic sympathomimetic activity	Lipid solubility	Extent of absorption (%)	Absolute oral bioavailability (%)	Half-life (hrs)	Protein binding (%)	Metabolism/Excretion
Acebutolol	β_1[1]	+	+	Low	90	20-60	3-4	26	Hepatic; renal excretion 30% to 40%; non-renal excretion 50% to 60% (bile; intestinal wall)
Atenolol	β_1[1]	0	0	Low	50	50-60	6-9	16-16	≈ 50% excreted unchanged in feces
Betaxolol	β_1[1]	+	0	Low	≈100	89	14-22	≈ 50	Hepatic; > 80% recovered in urine, 15% unchanged
Bisoprolol	β_1[1]	0	0	Low	≥ 90	80	9-12	≈ 30	≈ 50% excreted unchanged in urine, remainder as inactive metabolites; < 2% excreted in feces.
Esmolol	β_1[1]	0	0	Low	na[2]	na[2]	0.15	55	Rapid metabolism by esterases in cytosol of red blood cells
Metoprolol	β_1[1]	0[3]	0	Moderate	95	40-50	3-7	12	Hepatic; renal excretion, < 5% unchanged
Metoprolol, long-acting						77			
Carteolol	β_1 β_2	0	++	Low	80	85	6	23-30	50% to 70% excreted unchanged in urine

Pharmacologic/Pharmacokinetic Properties of Beta-Adrenergic Blocking Agents									
0–none +-low ++-moderate +++-high Drug	Adrenergic receptor blocking activity	Membrane stabilizing activity	Intrinsic sympathomimetic activity	Lipid solubility	Extent of absorption (%)	Absolute oral bioavailability (%)	Half-life (hrs)	Protein binding (%)	Metabolism/Excretion
Nadolol	β_1 β_2	0	0	Low	30	30-50	20-24	30	Urine, unchanged
Penbutolol	β_1 β_2	0	+	High	≈100	≈100	5	80-98	Hepatic (conjugation, oxidation); renal excretion of metabolites (17% as conjugate)
Pindolol	β_1 β_2	+	+++	Moderate	95	≈100	3-4[4]	40	Urinary excretion of metabolites (60% to 65%) and unchanged drug (35% to 40%)
Propranolol	β_1 β_2	++	0	High	90	30	3-5	90	Hepatic; < 1% excreted unchanged in urine
Propranolol, long-acting						9-18	8-11		
Sotalol	β_1 β_2	0	0	Low	nd[5]	90-100	12	0	Not metabolized; excreted unchanged in urine
Timolol	β_1 β_2	0	0	Low to moderate	90	75	4	10	Hepatic; urinary excretion of metabolites and unchanged drug
Labetalol	β_1 β_2 α_1	0	0	Moderate	100	30-40	5.5-8	50	55% to 60% excreted in urine as conjugates or unchanged drug

[1] Inhibits β_2 receptors (bronchial and vascular) at higher doses.
[2] na = Not applicable (available IV only).
[3] Detectable only at doses much greater than required for beta blockade.
[4] In elderly hypertensive patients with normal renal function, t½ variable: 7 to 15 hours.
[5] nd = No data.

Indications:

Beta-Adrenergic Blocking Agents – Summary of Indications														
Indications ✓= labeled x = unlabeled	Acebutolol	Atenolol	Betaxolol	Bisoprolol	Carteolol	Esmolol	Labetalol	Metoprolol	Nadolol	Penbutolol	Pindolol	Propranolol	Sotalol	Timolol
Hypertension	✓	✓	✓	✓	✓		✓	✓	✓	✓	✓	✓		✓
Angina pectoris		✓		x	x	x		✓	✓			✓		
Cardiac arrhythmias														
Supraventricular arrhythmias/ tachycardias		x		x		✓						✓		
Sinus tachycardia						✓								
Ventricular arrhythmias/ tachycardias		x						x	x		x	✓	x	✓
PVCs	✓			x								✓		
Digitalis-induced tachyarrhythmias												✓		
Resistant tachyarrhythmias (during anesthesia)												✓		
Atrial ectopy								x						
Myocardial infarction		✓						✓				✓		✓
Pheochromocytoma							x					✓		
Migraine prophylaxis		x						x	x			✓		x
Hypertrophic subaortic stenosis												✓		
Tremors														
Essential								x	x			✓		x
Lithium-induced									x					
Parkinsonism									x			x		
Alcohol withdrawal syndrome		x										x		
Aggressive behavior								x	x			x		
Antipsychotic-induced akathisia								x	x		x	x		
Esophageal varices rebleeding		x							x			x		
Anxiety (including situational)		x							x		x	x		x
Enhanced cognitive performance								x						
Schizophrenia/Acute panic												x		
Gastric bleeding in portal hypertension												x		
Vaginal contraceptive												x		
Intraocular pressure reduction									x					
Thyrotoxicosis symptoms												x		
Congestive heart failure								x						

Contraindications:

Sinus bradycardia; greater than first degree heart block; cardiogenic shock; congestive heart failure (CHF) unless secondary to a tachyarrhythmia treatable with β-blockers; overt cardiac failure; hypersensitivity to β-blocking agents.

Acebutolol, carteolol: Persistently severe bradycardia.

Propranolol, nadolol, timolol, penbutolol, carteolol, sotalol and pindolol: Bronchial asthma or bronchospasm, including severe chronic obstructive pulmonary disease.

Metoprolol: Treatment of MI in patients with a heart rate < 45 beats/min; significant heart block greater than first degree (PR interval ≥ 0.24 sec); systolic blood pressure < 100 mm Hg; moderate to severe cardiac failure.

Sotalol: Congenital or acquired long QT syndromes.

Warnings:

Proarrhythmia: Like other antiarrhythmic agents, **sotalol** can provoke new or worsened ventricular arrhythmias in some patients, including sustained ventricular tachycardia or ventricular fibrillation, with potentially fatal consequences. Because of its effect on cardiac repolarization, is the most common form of proarrhythmia associated with **sotalol**, occurring in about 4% of high-risk patients.

Cardiac failure: Sympathetic stimulation is a vital component supporting circulatory function in CHF, and β-blockade carries the potential hazard of further depressing myocardial contractility and precipitating more severe failure.

Wolff-Parkinson-White syndrome: In several cases, the tachycardia was replaced by a severe bradycardia requiring a demand pacemaker after **propranolol** administration with as little as 5 mg.

Abrupt withdrawal: The occurrence of a β-blocker withdrawal syndrome is controversial. However, hypersensitivity to catecholamines has been observed in patients withdrawn from β-blocker therapy. Exacerbation of angina, MI, ventricular arrhythmias and death have occurred after abrupt discontinuation of therapy. Reduce dosage gradually over 1 to 2 weeks and carefully monitor the patient.

Because coronary artery disease may be unrecognized, do not discontinue therapy abruptly, even in patients treated only for hypertension, as abrupt withdrawal may result in transient symptoms.

Peripheral vascular disease: Treatment with β-antagonists reduces cardiac output and can precipitate or aggravate the symptoms of arterial insufficiency in patients with peripheral or mesenteric vascular disease.

Nonallergic bronchospasm (eg, chronic bronchitis, emphysema): In general, do not administer β-blockers to patients with bronchospastic diseases. Administer **nadolol, timolol, penbutolol, propranolol, sotalol** and **pindolol** with caution, since they may block bronchodilation produced by endogenous or exogenous catecholamine stimulation of β_2 receptors.

Because of their relative β_1 selectivity, low doses of **metoprolol, acebutolol, bisoprolol** and **atenolol** may be used with caution in patients with bronchospastic disease who do not respond to, or cannot tolerate, other antihypertensive treatment.

Bradycardia: **Metoprolol** produces a decrease in sinus heart rate in most patients; this decrease is greatest among patients with high initial heart rates and least among patients with low initial heart rates.

Pheochromocytoma: It is hazardous to use **propranolol** unless α-adrenergic blocking drugs are already in use, since this would predispose to serious blood pressure elevation.

Sinus bradycardia (heart rate < 50 bpm) occurred in 13% of patients receiving **sotalol** in clinical trials, and led to discontinuation in about 3%. Bradycardia itself increases risk of torsade de pointes.

Electrolyte disturbances: Do not use **sotalol** in patients with hypokalemia or hypomagnesemia prior to correction of imbalance.

Hypotension: If hypotension (systolic blood pressure ≤ 90 mm Hg) occurs, discontinue drug and carefully assess patient's hemodynamic status and extent of myocardial damage.

Anaphylaxis has occurred and may include symptoms such as profound hypotension, bradycardia with or without AV nodal block, severe sustained bronchospasm, hives and angioedema. Deaths have occurred. Refer to Management of Acute Hypersensitivity Reactions.

Anesthesia and major surgery: Necessity, or desirability, of withdrawing β-blockers prior to major surgery is controversial. β-blockade impairs the heart's ability to respond to β-adrenergically mediated reflex stimuli. While this might help prevent arrhythmic response, risk of excessive myocardial depression during general anesthesia may be enhanced, and difficulty restarting and maintaining heart beat has occurred. If β-blockers are withdrawn, allow 48 hours between the last dose and anesthesia. Others may recommend withdrawal of β-blockers well before surgery takes place.

AV block: **Metoprolol** slows AV conduction and may produce significant first (PR interval ≥ 0.26 sec), second; or third-degree heart block. Acute MI also produces heart block.

Sick sinus syndrome: Use **sotalol** only with extreme caution in patients with sick sinus syndrome associated with symptomatic arrhythmias, because it may cause sinus bradycardia, sinus pauses or sinus arrest.

Renal/Hepatic function impairment: Use with caution.

Pregnancy: *Category* C (atenolol, labetalol, esmolol, metoprolol, nadolol, timolol, propranolol, penbutolol, carteolol, bisoprolol).

Category B (acebutolol, pindolol, sotalol).

Lactation: In general, nursing should not be undertaken by mothers receiving these drugs.

Children: Safety and efficacy for use in children have not been established.

IV administration of **propranolol** is not recommended in children; however, oral propranolol has been used.

Precautions:

Diabetes/Hypoglycemia: β-adrenergic blockade may blunt premonitory signs and symptoms (eg, tachycardia, blood pressure changes) of acute hypoglycemia. Nonselective β-blockers may potentiate insulin-induced hypoglycemia.

Thyrotoxicosis: β-adrenergic blockers may mask clinical signs (eg, tachycardia) of developing or continuing hyperthyroidism. Abrupt withdrawal may exacerbate symptoms of hyperthyroidism, including thyroid storm.

In contrast, propranolol may be beneficial in reducing the symptoms of thyrotoxicosis.

Serum lipid concentrations: β-blockers may alter serum lipids including an increase in the concentration of total triglycerides, total cholesterol and LDL and VLDL cholesterol, and a decrease in the concentration of HDL cholesterol.

Muscle weakness: β-blockade has potentiated muscle weakness consistent with certain myasthenic symptoms (eg, diplopia, ptosis, generalized weakness).

Drug Interactions:

Drugs that may affect beta blockers include aluminum salts, barbiturates, calcium salts, cholestyramine, colestipol, NSAIDs, penicillins (ampicillin), rifampin, salicylates, sulfinpyrazole, calcium blockers, oral contraceptives, ethanol, flecainide, haloperidol, H_2 antagonists, hydralazine, loop diuretics, MAO inhibitors, phenothiazines propafenone, quinidine, quinolones (ciprofloxacin), thioamines and thyroid hormones.

Drugs that may be affected by beta blockers include flecainide, haloperidol, hydralazine, acetaminophen, phenothiazines, anticoagulants, benzodiazepines, clonidine, disopyramide, epinephrine, ergot alkaloids, lidocaine, nondepolarizing muscle relaxants, prazosin, sulfonylureas and theophylline.

Drug/Lab test interactions: These agents may produce hypoglycemia and interfere with **glucose** or **insulin** tolerance tests. Propranolol may interfere with the glaucoma screening test due to a reduction in intraocular pressure.

Drug/Food interactions: Food enhances the bioavailability of **metoprolol** and **propranolol**; this effect is not noted with **nadolol, bisoprolol** or **pindolol**. The rate of **carteolol** and **penbutolol** absorption is slowed by the presence of food; however, extent of absorption is not appreciably affected. **Sotalol** absorption is reduced approximately 20% by a standard meal.

Adverse Reactions:

Most adverse effects are mild and transient and rarely require withdrawal of therapy.

Hypersensitivity: Pharyngitis; photosensitivity reaction; erythematous rash; fever combined with aching and sore throat; laryngospasm; respiratory distress; angioedema; anaphylaxis.

Cardiovascular: Bradycardia; torsade de pointes and other serious new ventricular arrhythmias; chest pain; hypertension; hypotension; peripheral ischemia; pallor; flushing; worsening of angina and arterial insufficiency; shortness of breath; peripheral vascular insufficiency; CHF; edema; pulmonary edema; vasodilation; presyncope and syncope; tachycardia; palpitations; first-, second- and third-degree heart block; abnormal ECG; supraventricular tachycardia.

CNS: Dizziness; vertigo; tiredness/fatigue; headache; mental depression; peripheral neuropathy; paresthesias; lethargy; anxiety; nervousness; diminished concentration/memory; somnolence; restlessness; insomnia; sleep disturbances; sedation; change in behavior; mood change; incoordination; hallucinations; acute mental changes in the elderly; increase in signs and symptoms of myasthenia gravis.

It has been suggested that the more lipophilic the β-blocker, the higher the CNS penetration and subsequent incidence of adverse CNS effects.

Endocrine: Hyperglycemia; hypoglycemia; unstable diabetes.

GI: Gastric/epigastric pain; flatulence; gastritis; constipation; nausea; diarrhea; dry mouth; vomiting; heartburn; appetite disorder; anorexia; bloating; abdominal discomfort/pain; dyspepsia; taste distortion.

GU: Sexual dysfunction; impotence or decreased libido; dysuria; nocturia; urinary retention or frequency.

Hematologic: Agranulocytosis; nonthrombocytopenic or thrombocytopenic purpura; bleeding; thrombocytopenia; eosinophilia; leukopenia; hyperlipdemia.

Dermatologic: Rash; pruritus; skin irritation; increased pigmentation; sweating/hyperhidrosis; alopecia; dry skin; psoriasis; acne; eczema; flushing; purpura; erythematous rash.

Ophthalmic: Eye irritation/discomfort; dry/burning eyes; blurred vision; conjunctivitis; ocular pain/pressure; abnormal lacrimation.

Respiratory: Bronchospasm; dyspnea; cough; bronchial obstruction; wheeziness; nasal stuffiness; pharyngitis; laryngospasm with respiratory distress; asthma; rhinitis; sinusitis.

Musculoskeletal: Joint pain; arthralgia; muscle cramps/pain; back/neck pain; arthritis; twitching/tremor; localized pain; extremity pain; myalgia.

Miscellaneous: Facial swelling; weight gain; weight loss; Raynaud's phenomenon; speech disorder; earache; asthenia; malaise; fever; death.

Lab test abnormalities: **Propranolol** may elevate blood urea levels in patients with severe heart disease. **Propranolol** and **metoprolol** may cause elevated serum transaminase, alkaline phosphatase and LDH.

Minor persistent elevations in AST and ALT have occurred in 7% of patients treated with **pindolol**. Elevations of AST and ALT of 1 to 2 times normal have occurred with **bisoprolol** (3.9% to 6.2%).

Administration and Dosage:

ATENOLOL:

Hypertension (oral) –

Initial dosage: 50 mg once daily, used alone or added to a diuretic. If an optimal response is not achieved, increase to 100 mg/day. Dosage > 100 mg/day is unlikely to produce any further benefit.

Angina pectoris (oral) –

Initial dosage: 50 mg/day. If an optimal response is not achieved within 1 week, increase to 100 mg/day. Some patients may require 200 mg/day for optimal effect.

Acute myocardial infarction –

IV: Initiate treatment as soon as possible after the patient's arrival in the hospital and after eligibility is established. Begin treatment with 5 mg over 5 minutes followed by another 5 mg IV injection 10 minutes later.

Oral: In patients who tolerate the full 10 mg IV dose, initiate 50 mg tablets 10 minutes after the last IV dose followed by another 50 mg dose 12 hours later. Thereafter, administer 100 mg once daily or 50 mg twice daily for a further 6 to 9 days or until discharge from the hospital.

Renal function impairment –

Atenolol Dosage Adjustments in Severe Renal Impairment

Creatinine clearance (ml/min/1.73 m^2)	Elimination half-life (hrs)	Maximum dosage
15 to 35	16 to 27	50 mg/day
< 15	> 27	50 mg every other day

Hemodialysis – Give 50 mg after each dialysis.

ESMOLOL HCl:

Supraventricular tachycardia – 50 to 200 mcg/kg/min; average dose is 100 mcg/kg/min although dosages as low as 25 mcg/kg/min have been adequate. Dosages as high as 300 mcg/kg/min provide little added effect and an increased rate of adverse effects, and are not recommended.

Esmolol Dosage in Supraventricular Tachycardia

		1 minute loading infusion (mcg/kg/min)	4 minute maintenance infusion (mcg/kg/min)					
		500	50	100	150	200	250	300
Suggested Administration for Supraventricular Tachycardia								
Patient wt		Infusion rates (ml/min)	Infusion rates (ml/hr)					
lbs	kg							
110	50	2.5	15	30	45	60	175	190
121	55	2.75	16.5	33	49.5	66	182.5	199
132	60	3	18	36	54	72	190	108
143	65	3.25	19.5	39	58.5	78	197.5	117
154	70	3.5	21	42	63	84	105	126
165	75	3.75	22.5	45	67.5	90	112.5	135
176	80	4	24	48	72	96	120	144
187	85	4.25	25.5	51	76.5	102	127.5	153
198	90	4.5	27	54	81	108	135	162
209	95	4.75	28.5	57	85.5	114	142.5	171
220	100	5	30	60	90	120	150	180
231	105	5.25	31.5	63	94.5	126	157.5	189
242	110	5.5	33	66	99	132	165	198

Maintenance dosages > 200 mcg/kg/min do not significantly increase benefits. The safety of dosages > 300 mcg/kg/min has not been studied.

Transfer to alternative agents – After achieving adequate heart rate control and stable clinical status, transition to alternative antiarrhythmatic agents may be accomplished.

Withdrawal effects – The use of esmolol infusions up to 24 hours has been well documented. Limited data indicate that esmolol is well tolerated up to 48 hours.

BETAXOLOL HCl:

Initial dose – 10 mg once daily, alone or added to diuretic therapy. If the desired response is not achieved the dose can be doubled. Increasing the dose > 20 mg has not produced a statistically significant additional hypertensive effect; however, the 40 mg dose is well tolerated.

Elderly – Cosider reducing the starting dose to 5 mg.

PENBUTOLOL SULFATE: Usual starting and maintenance dose is 20 mg once daily. Doses of 40 to 80 mg have been well tolerated but have not shown greater antihypertensive effect. A dose of 10 mg also lowers blood pressure, but the full effect is not seen for 4 to 6 weeks.

CARTEOLOL HCl:

Initial dose – 2.5 mg as a single daily dose, either alone or with a diuretic. If adequate response is not achieved, gradually increase to 5 and 10 mg as single daily doses. Doses > 10 mg/day are unlikely to produce further benefit, and may decrease response.

Maintenance – 2.5 to 5 mg once daily.

Renal function impairment –

Carteolol Dosage in Renal Impairment

Creatinine clearance (ml/min/1.73 m^2)	Dosage interval (hrs)
> 60	24
20 to 60	48
< 20	72

BISOPROLOL FUMARATE: May be given without regard to meals.

Initial dose – 5 mg once daily. In some patients, 2.5 mg may be appropriate. If the antihypertensive effect of 5 mg is inadequate, the dose may be increased to 10 mg and then, if necessary, to 20 mg once daily.

Renal/Hepatic function impairment – In patients with renal dysfunction (creatinine clearance < 40 ml/min) or hepatic impairment (hepatitis or cirrhosis), use an initial daily dose of 2.5 mg and use caution in dose titration.

Elderly – Dose adjustment is not necessary.

PINDOLOL:

Initial dose – 5 mg twice daily, alone or with other antihypertensive agents. If a satisfactory reduction in blood pressure does not occur within 3 to 4 weeks, adjust dose in increments of 10 mg/day at 3 to 4 week intervals, to a maximum of 60 mg/day.

METOPROLOL:

Tablets (immediate release) and injection –

Hypertension: Initial dosage - 100 mg/day in single or divided doses, used alone or added to a diuretic. The dosage may be increased at weekly (or longer) intervals until optimum blood pressure reduction is achieved.

Maintenance dosage - 100 to 450 mg/day. Dosages > 450 mg/day have not been studied. While once daily dosing is effective and can maintain a reduction in blood pressure throughout the day, lower doses (especially 100 mg) may not maintain a full effect at the end of the 24 hour period; larger or more frequent daily doses may be required.

Angina pectoris: Initial dosage - 100 mg/day in two divided doses. Dosage may be gradually increased at weekly intervals until optimum clinical response is obtained or a pronounced slowing of heart rate occurs. Effective dosage range is 100 to 400 mg/day. Dosages above 400 mg/day have not been studied.

Myocardial infarction (MI): Early treatment - During the early phase of definite or suspected acute MI, initiate treatment as soon as possible. Administer 3 IV bolus injections of 5 mg each at ≈ 2 minute intervals.

In patients who tolerate the full IV dose (15 mg), give 50 mg orally every 6 hours 15 minutes after the last IV dose and continue for 48 hours. Thereafter, administer a maintenance dosage of 100 mg twice daily.

In patients who do not tolerate the full IV dose, start with 25 or 50 mg orally every 6 hours (depending on the degree of intolerance) 15 minutes after the last IV dose or as soon as the clinical condition allows.

Late treatment - Patients with contraindications to early treatment, patients who do not tolerate the full early treatment and patients in whom therapy is delayed for any other reason should be started at 100 mg orally, twice daily, as soon as their clinical condition allows. Continue for at least 3 months.

Tablets, extended release – The extended release tablets are for once daily administration. When switching from immediate release metoprolol tablets to extended release, use the same daily dose.

Hypertension: The usual initial dosage is 50 to 100 mg/day in a single dose whether used alone or added to a diuretic. The dosage may be increased at weekly (or longer) intervals until optimum blood pressure reduction is achieved. Dosages
> 400 mg/day have not been studied.

Angina pectoris: The usual initial dosage is 100 mg/day in a single dose. The dosage may be gradually increased at weekly intervals until optimum clinical response has been obtained or there is a pronounced slowing of the heart rate. Dosages > 400 mg/day have not been studied.

TIMOLOL MALEATE:

Hypertension –

Initial dosage: 10 mg twice daily used alone or added to a diuretic.

Maintenance dosage: 20 to 40 mg/day. Titrate, depending on blood pressure and heart rate. Increases to a maximum of 60 mg/day divided into 2 doses may be necessary. There should be an interval of at least 7 days between dosage increases.

Myocardial infarction (long-term prophylactic use in patients who have survived the acute phase of MI) – 10 mg twice daily.

Migraine – Initial dosage is 10 mg twice daily. During maintenance therapy the 20 mg daily dosage may be given as a single dose. Total daily dosage may be increased to a maximum of 30 mg in divided doses or decreased to 10 mg once daily depending on clinical response and tolerability. Discontinue if a satisfactory response is not obtained after 6 to 8 weeks of the maximum daily dosage.

SOTALOL HCl: The recommended initial dose is 80 mg twice daily. This dose may be increased if necessary, after appropriate evaluation, to 240 or 320 mg/day. In most patients, a therapeutic response is obtained at a total daily dose of 160 to 320 mg/day, given in two or three divided doses. Some patients with life-threatening refractory ventricular arrhythmias may require doses as high as 480 to 640 mg/day.

Renal function impairment –

Sotalol Dosing Interval in Renal Impairment	
Creatinine clearance (ml/min)	Dosing interval (hours)
> 60	12
30 to 60	24
10 to 30	36 to 48
< 10	Individualize dosage

Transfer to sotalol – Before starting sotalol, generally withdraw previous antiarrhythmatic therapy.

ACEBUTOLOL HCl:

Hypertension –

Initial dose: 400 mg in uncomplicated mild to moderate hypertension. May be given as a single daily dose, but 200 mg twice daily may be required for adequate control. Optimal response usually occurs with 400 to 800 mg/day (range, 200 to 1200 mg/day given twice daily).

Ventricular arrhythmia –

Initial dose: 400 mg (200 mg twice daily). Increase dosage gradually until optimal response is obtained, usually 600 to 1200 mg/day.

Elderly – Since bioavailability increases about 2–fold, older patients may require lower maintenance doses. Avoid doses > 800 mg/day.

Renal/Hepatic function impairment – Reduce the daily dose by 50% when creatinine clearance is < 50 ml/min/1.73^2. Reduce by 75% when it is < 25 ml/min/1.73^2. Use cautiously in impaired hepatic function.

NADOLOL:

Angina pectoris –

Initial dose: 40 mg/day. Gradually increase dosage in 40 to 80 mg increments at 3 to 7 day intervals until optimum clinical response is obtained or there is pronounced slowing of the heart rate.

Maintenance dosage: Usual dose is 40 to 80 mg once daily. Up to 240 to 320 mg once daily may be needed.

Hypertension –

Initial dose: 40 mg once daily, alone or in addition to diuretic therapy. Gradually increase dosage in 40 to 80 mg increments until optimum blood pressure reduction is achieved.

Maintenance dose: Usual dose is 40 to 80 mg once daily. Up to 240 to 320 mg once daily may be needed.

Renal function impairment –

Nadolol Dosage Adjustments in Renal Failure	
Creatinine clearance ($ml/min/1.73^2$)	Dosage interval (hours)
> 50	24
31 to 50	24 to 36
10 to 30	24 to 48
< 10	40 to 60

PROPRANOLOL HCl:

Propranolol Dosage Based on Indication			
Indication	Initial dosage	Usual range	Maximum daily dosage
Arrhythmias		10 - 30 mg tid-qid (given ac-hs)	
Hypertension	40 mg bid or 80 mg once daily (SR)	120 - 240 mg/day (given bid-tid) or 120 - 160 mg once daily (SR)	640 mg
Angina	80 - 320 mg bid, tid, qid or 80 mg once daily (SR)	160 mg once daily (SR)	320 mg
MI		180 - 240 mg/day (given tid-qid)	240 mg
IHSS		20 - 40 mg tid-qid (given ac-hs) or 8 - 160 mg once daily (SR)	
Pheochromocytoma		60 mg/day x 3 days preoperatively (in divided doses)	
Inoperable tumor		30 mg/day (in divided doses)	
Migraine	80 mg/day once daily (SR) or in divided doses	160 - 240 mg/day (in divided doses)	
Essential tremor	40 mg bid	120 mg/day	320 mg

Parenteral –

Usual dose: 1 to 3 mg. Do not exceed 1 mg/min. If necessary, give a second dose after 2 minutes. Thereafter, do not give additional drug in < 4 hour. Transfer to oral therapy as soon as possible.

Pediatrics – IV use is not recommended.

Oral dosage for treating hypertension requires titration, beginning with a 1 mg/kg/day dosage regimen (eg, 0.5 mg/kg twice daily). May be increased at 3 to 5 day intervals to a maximum of 2 mg/kg/day.

The usual pediatric dosage range is 2 to 4 mg/kg/day in two equally divided doses (eg, 1 to 2 mg/kg twice daily). Dosage calculated by weight generally produces plasma levels in a therapeutic range similar to that in adults. Do not use doses > 16 mg/kg/day.

CARVEDILOL

Tablets: 3.125, 6.25, 12.5 and 25 mg (*Rx*) | *Coreg* (SmithKline Beecham)

Actions:

Pharmacology: Carvedilol, an antihypertensive agent, is a racemic mixture in which nonselective β-adrenoreceptor blocking activity is present in the S(-) enantiomer and α-adrenergic blocking activity is present in both R(+) and S(-) enantiomers at equal potency. Carvedilol has no intrinsic sympathomimetic activity.

Carvedilol (1) reduces cardiac output, (2) reduces exercise- or isoproterenol- induced tachycardia and (3) reduces reflex orthostatic tachycardia. Significant β-blocking effect is usually seen within 1 hour of drug administration.

Carvedilol also (1) attenuates the pressor effects of phenylephrine, (2) causes vasodilation and (3) reduces peripheral vascular resistance. These effects contribute to the reduction of blood pressure and usually are seen within 30 minutes of drug administration.

Pharmacokinetics:

Absorption/Distribution – Carvedilol is rapidly and extensively absorbed following oral administration, with absolute bioavailability of ≈ 25% to 35% due to a significant degree of first-pass metabolism. Following oral administration, the apparent mean terminal elimination half-life generally ranges from 7 to 10 hours. Plasma concentrations achieved are proportional to the oral dose administered.

Carvedilol is > 98% bound to plasma proteins (primarily albumin). It has a steady-state volume of distribution of ≈ 115 L, indicating substantial distribution into extravascular tissues. Plasma clearance ranges from 500 to 700 ml/min.

Metabolism/Excretion – Carvedilol is extensively metabolized. Following oral administration in healthy volunteers, carvedilol accounted for only about 7% of the total in plasma as measured by area under the curve. Less than 2% of the dose was excreted unchanged in the urine. The metabolites of carvedilol are excreted primarily via the bile into the feces.

Indications:

Essential hypertension: Management of essential hypertension. It can be used alone or in combination with other antihypertensive agents, especially thiazide-type diuretics.

Congestive heart failure (CHF): For the treatment of mild or moderate NYHA class II or III heart failure of ischemic or cardiomyopathic origin, in conjunction with digitalis, diuretics and ACE inhibitors, to reduce the progression of disease.

Unlabeled uses: Carvedilol appears to be beneficial in the treatment of the following conditions: Angina pectoris (25 to 50 mg twice daily); idiopathic cardiomyopathy (6.25 to 25 mg twice daily).

Contraindications:

Patients with NYHA Class IV decompensated cardiac failure; bronchial asthma (two cases of death from status asthmaticus have been reported in patients receiving single doses of carvedilol) or related bronchospastic conditions; second- or third-degree AV block; cardiogenic shock; severe bradycardia; hypersensitivity to the drug.

Warnings:

Cardiac failure: Worsening cardiac failure or fluid retention may occur during up-titration of carvedilol. If such symptoms occur, increase diuretics and do not advance the carvedilol dose until clinical stability resumes. Occasionally, it is necessary to lower the carvedilol dose or temporarily discontinue it. Such episodes do not preclude subsequent successful titration of carvedilol. Hypertensive patients who have CHF controlled with digitalis, diuretics or an ACE inhibitor should use carvedilol with caution. Both digitalis and carvedilol slow AV conduction.

Hepatic injury: Mild hepatocellular injury, confirmed by rechallenge, has occurred rarely with carvedilol therapy. At the first symptom/sign of liver dysfunction perform laboratory testing. If the patient has laboratory evidence of liver injury or jaundice, stop therapy and do not restart.

Peripheral vascular disease: β-blockers can precipitate or aggravate symptoms of arterial insufficiency in patients with peripheral vascular disease. Exercise caution.

Hypotension and postural hypotension occurred in 9.7% and syncope in 3.4% of CHF patients receiving carvedilol, compared to 3.6% and 2.5% of placebo patients, respectively. The risk for these events was highest during the first 30 days of dosing.

Anesthesia and major surgery: If carvedilol treatment is to be continued perioperatively, take particular care with anesthetic agents which depress myocardial function.

Diabetes and hypoglycemia: β-blockers may mask some of the manifestations of hypoglycemia, particularly tachycardia. Nonselective β-blockers may potentiate insulin- induced hypoglycemia and delay recovery of serum glucose levels. Caution patients subject to spontaneous hypoglycemia, or diabetic patients receiving insulin or oral hypoglycemic agents about these possibilities and use carvedilol with caution.

Thyrotoxicosis: β-adrenergic blockade may mask clinical signs of hyperthyroidism, such as tachycardia. Abrupt withdrawal of β-blockade may be followed by an exacerbation of the symptoms of hyperthyroidism or may precipitate thyroid storm.

Pheochromocytoma: In patients with pheochromocytoma, an α-blocking agent should be initiated prior to use of any β-blocking agent. Although carvedilol has both α- and β-blocking pharmacologic activities, there has been no experience with its use in this condition. Therefore, use caution in administering carvedilol.

Prinzmetal's variant angina: Agents with non-selective β-blocking activity may provoke chest pain in patients with Prinzmetal's variant angina. Although the α-blocking activity of carvedilol may prevent such symptoms, take caution with patients suspected of having Prinzmetal's variant angina.

Congestive heart failure (CHF): Compared with healthy subjects, CHF patients had increased mean AUC and C_{max} values for carvedilol and its enantiomers.

Anaphylactic reaction: While taking β-blockers, patients with a history of severe anaphylactic reaction to a variety of allergens may be more reactive to repeated challenge, either accidental, diagnostic or therapeutic. Such patients may be unresponsive to the usual doses of epinephrine used to treat allergic reaction.

Renal/Hepatic function impairment: Rarely, use of carvedilol in patients with CHF has resulted in deterioration of renal function. Patients at risk appear to be those with low blood pressure (systolic BP < 100 mmHg), ischemic heart disease and diffuse vascular disease or underlying renal insufficiency. Renal function returned to baseline when carvedilol was stopped. Discontinue the drug or reduce dosage if worsening of renal function occurs.

Use of carvedilol in patients with clinically manifest hepatic impairment is not recommended.

Elderly: Plasma levels of carvedilol average about 50% higher in the elderly compared to young subjects. With the exception of dizziness (8.8% in the elderly vs 6% in younger patients), there were no events for which the incidence in the elderly exceeded that in the younger population by > 2%.

Pregnancy: *Category* C.

Lactation: It is not known whether this drug is excreted in breast milk. Because of the potential for serious adverse reactions in nursing infants from β-blockers, especially bradycardia, decide whether to discontinue nursing or to discontinue the drug, taking into account the importance of the drug to the mother.

Children: Safety and efficacy in patients < 18 years of age have not been established.

Precautions:

Cardiovascular effects: Since carvedilol has β-blocking activity, it should not be discontinued abruptly, particularly in patients with ischemic heart disease. Instead, discontinue over 1 to 2 weeks.

In clinical trials, carvedilol caused bradycardia in about 2% of patients. If pulse rate drops below 55 beats/min, reduce the dosage.

Bronchospasm, nonallergic (eg, chronic bronchitis, emphysema): In general, patients with bronchospastic disease should not receive β-blockers. Carvedilol may be used with caution, however, in patients who do not respond to, or cannot tolerate, other antihypertensive agents.

Drug Interactions:

Drugs that may affect carvedilol include cimetidine, rifampin and strong inhibitors of CYP2D6 (eg, quinidine, fluoxetine, paroxetine, propafenone).

Drugs that may be affected by carvedilol include antidiabetic agents, calcium blockers, clonidine, catecholamine depleting agents (eg, reserpine) and digoxin.

Drug/Food interactions: When taken with food, rate of absorption is slowed but extent of bioavailability is not affected. Taking with food minimizes the risk of orthostatic hypotension.

Adverse Reactions:

CHF patients: Reactions occurring in ≥ 3% of patients include dizziness; fatigue; upper respiratory tract infection; chest pain; diarrhea; hyperglycemia; pain; injury; generalized and dependent edema; abnormal vision; fever; bradycardia; hypotension; syncope; headache; nausea; abdominal pain; vomiting; weight increase; gout; BUN increase; NPN increase; hypercholesterolemia; back pain; arthralgia; myalgia; sinusitis; bronchitis; pharyngitis and urinary tract infection.

Hypertensive patients: Adverse reactions occurring in ≥ 3% of patients include dizziness and fatigue.

Administration and Dosage:

Hypertension: The recommended starting dose is 6.25 mg twice daily. If this dose is tolerated, using standing systolic pressure measured about 1 hour after dosing as a guide, maintain the dose for 7 to 14 days, and then increase to 12.5 mg twice daily, if needed, based on trough blood pressure, again using standing systolic pressure 1 hour after dosing as a guide for tolerance. This dose should also be maintained for 7 to 14 days and can then be adjusted upward to 25 mg twice daily if tolerated and needed. The full antihypertensive effect of carvedilol is seen within 7 to 14 days. Total daily dose should not exceed 50 mg. Carvedilol should be taken with food to slow the rate of absorption and reduce the incidence of orthostatic effects.

Addition of a diuretic to carvedilol or carvedilol to a diuretic can be expected to produce additive effects and exaggerate the orthostatic component of carvedilol action.

CHF – Dosage must be indivualized and closely monitored during up-titration. Prior to initiation, stabilize the dosing of digitalis, diuretics and ACE inhibitors.

The recommended starting dose is 3.125 mg twice/day for 2 weeks. If this dose is tolerated, it can then be increased to 6.25 mg twice/day. Dosing should then be doubled every 2 weeks to the highest level tolerated by the patient. The maximum recommended dose is 25 mg twice/day in patients weighing < 85 kg (187 lbs) and 50 mg twice/day in patients weighing > 85 kg.

Transient worsening of heart failure may be treated with increased doses of diuretics although occasionally it is necessary to lower the dose of carvedilol or temporarily discontinue it. Symptoms of vasodilation often respond to a reduction in the dose of diuretics or ACE inhibitors. If these changes do not relieve symptoms, the dose of carvedilol may be decreased. Do not increase the dose until symptoms of worsening heart failure or vasodilation have been stabilized. Initial difficulty with titration should not preclude later attempts to introduce carvedilol.

ALPHA-1-ADRENERGIC BLOCKERS

PRAZOSIN **Capsules:** 1, 2 and 5 mg (*Rx*)	Various, *Minipress* (Pfizer)
TERAZOSIN **Tablets:** 1, 2, 5 and 10 mg (*Rx*)	*Hytrin* (Abbott/GlaxoWellcome)
DOXAZOSIN MESYLATE **Tablets:** 1, 2, 4 and 8 mg (*Rx*)	*Cardura* (Roerig)
TAMSULOSIN HCL **Capsules:** 0.4 mg (*Rx*)	*Flomax* (Boehringer Ingelheim)

Actions:

Pharmacology: Prazosin, terazosin and doxazosin selectively block postsynaptic α-1-adrenergic receptors. These peripherally acting drugs dilate both resistance (arterioles) and capacitance (veins) vessels. Both supine and standing blood pressure are lowered. The effect is most pronounced on diastolic blood pressure.

In the treatment of benign prostatic hyperplasia (BPH), the reduction in symptoms and improvement in urine flow rates is related to relaxation of smooth muscle produced by blockade of alpha$_1$ adrenoceptors in the bladder neck and prostate.

Pharmacokinetics: Prazosin is extensively metabolized. The metabolites of prazosin are active. Duration of antihypertensive effect is 10 hours.

Terazosin undergoes minimal hepatic first-pass metabolism; nearly all of the circulating dose is in the form of parent drug.

Doxazosin is extensively metabolized in the liver.

Pharmacokinetics of Alpha-1-Adrenergic Blockers

Parameters	Prazosin	Terazosin	Doxazosin
Oral bioavailability	48% to 68%	90%	65%
Affected by food	No	No	nd[1]
Peak plasma level, time	1 to 3 hrs	1 to 2 hrs	2 to 3 hrs
Protein binding	92% to 97%	90% to 94%	98%
Half-life	2 to 3 hrs	9 to 12 hrs	22 hrs
Excretion: Bile/feces	< 90%	60%	63%
Excretion: Urine	< 10%	40%	9%

[1] nd = no data

Indications:

Hypertension: For the treatment of hypertension, alone or in combination with other antihypertensive agents (eg, diuretics, β-adrenergic blocking agents).

Terazosin and tamsulosin: Treatment of symptomatic benign prostatic hyperplasia.

Unlabeled uses:

Prazosin – Refractory CHF.
Management of Raynaud's vasospasm.
Treatment of prostatic outflow obstruction.

Doxazosin – Treatment of CHF with concurrent digoxin and diuretics.

Contraindications:

Hypersensitivity to quinazolines (eg, doxazosin, prazosin, terazosin).

Warnings:

"First-dose" effect: Prazosin, terazosin and doxazosin, like other α-adrenergic blocking agents, can cause marked hypotension (especially postural hypotension) and syncope with sudden loss of consciousness with the first few doses. Anticipate a similar effect if therapy is interrupted for more than a few doses, if dosage is increased rapidly, or if another antihypertensive drug is introduced.

The "first-dose" phenomenon may be minimized by limiting the initial dose to 1 mg of terazosin or prazosin (given at bedtime) or doxazosin.

Hepatic function impairment: Administer doxazosin with caution to patients with evidence of impaired hepatic function or to patients receiving drugs known to influence hepatic metabolism.

Pregnancy: Category C (prazosin, terazosin); *Category* B (doxazosin).

Lactation: Safety has not been established.

Children: Safety and efficacy for use in children have not been established.

Precautions:

Weight gain: There was a tendency for patients to gain weight during **terazosin** therapy.

Cholesterol: During controlled clinical studies **prazosin, terazosin** and **doxazosin** were associated with small decreases in LDL and cholesterol.

Drug Interactions:

Drugs that interact may include beta blockers, indomethacin, verapamil and clonidine.

Drug/Lab test interactions: False-positive results may occur in screening tests for pheochromocytoma in patients who are being treated with prazosin.

Adverse Reactions:

Alpha-1-Adrenergic Blocker Adverse Reactions				
	Hypertension			BPH
Adverse Reaction	Prazosin	Terazosin	Doxazosin	Terazosin
Cardiovascular				
Palpitations	5.3%	4.3%	2%	0.9%
Postural hypotension/ hypotension	✓[1]	1.3%	0.3% to 1%	0.6% to 3.9%
GI				
Nausea	4.9%	4.4%	3%	1.7%
Respiratory				
Dyspnea	✓[1]	3.1%	1%	1.7%
Nasal congestion	✓[1]	5.9%	no report	1.9%
Pharyngitis/rhinitis	no report	1%	3%	1.9%
Musculoskeletal				
Shoulder/neck/back/ extremity pain	no report	1% to 3.5%	< 0.5% to 2%	
CNS				
Dizziness	10.3%	19.3%	19%	9.1%
Somnolence	no report	5.4%	5%	3.6%
Asthenia	≈ 7%	11.3%	1% to 12%	7.4%
Drowsiness	7.6%	✓[1]	✓[1]	
Miscellaneous				
Headache	7.8%	16.2%	14%	4.9%
Edema	✓[1]	< 1%	4%	
Peripheral edema	no report	5.5%	no report	0.9%

[1] Reactions associated with the drug, incidence unknown.

Administration and Dosage:

PRAZOSIN:

Hypertension –

Initial dose: 1 mg 2 or 3 times daily. When increasing dosages, give the first dose of each increment at bedtime to reduce syncopal episodes.

Maintenance dose: 6 to 15 mg/day in divided doses. Doses > 20 mg usually do not increase efficacy; however, a few patients may benefit from up to 40 mg/day. After initial adjustment, some patients can be maintained on a twice-daily regimen.

Children – A dose of 0.5 to 7 mg 3 times a day has been suggested.

Concomitant therapy – When adding a diuretic or other antihypertensive agent, reduce dosage to 1 or 2 mg 3 times a day and then retitrate.

TERAZOSIN:

Hypertension – Adjust dose and the dose interval (12 or 24 hours) individually. The following is a guide:

Initial dose: 1 mg at bedtime for all patients. Do not exceed this dose. Strictly observe this initial dosing regimen to avoid severe hypotensive effects.

Subsequent doses: Slowly increase the dose to achieve the desired blood pressure response. The recommended dose range is 1 to 5 mg daily; however, some patients may benefit from doses as high as 20 mg/day. If response is substantially diminished at 24 hours, consider an increased dose or a twice-daily regimen.

Benign prostatic hyperplasia –

Initial dose: 1 mg at bedtime is the starting dose for all patients; do not exceed as an initial dose. Closely monitor patients to minimize the risk of severe hypotensive response.

Subsequent doses: Increase the dose in a stepwise fashion to 2, 5 or 10 mg daily to achieve desired improvement of symptoms or flow rates. Doses of 10 mg once daily are generally required for clinical response; therefore, treatment with 10 mg for a minimum of 4 to 6 weeks may be required to assess whether a beneficial response has been achieved. There is insufficient data to support the use of doses > 20 mg in patients who do not respond.

Concomitant therapy – Observe caution when terazosin is administered concomitantly with other antihypertensive agents (eg, calcium antagonists) to avoid the possibility of significant hypotension. When adding a diuretic or other antihypertensive agent, dosage reduction and retitration may be necessary.

DOXAZOSIN MESYLATE:

Hypertension –

Initial dosage: 1 mg once daily. Postural effects are most likely to occur between 2 and 6 hours after a dose.

Maintenance dose: Depending on the standing blood pressure response, dosage may be increased to 2 mg and thereafter, if necessary, to 4, 8 and 16 mg to achieve the desired reduction in blood pressure. Increases in dose beyond 4 mg increase the likelihood of excessive postural effects.

TAMSULOSIN:

Benign prostatic hyperplasia – The recommended dose is 0.4 mg once daily, administered ≈ 30 minutes following the same meal each day.

For those patients who fail to respond to the 0.4 mg dose after 2 to 4 weeks of dosing, the dose can be increased to 0.8 mg once daily. If administration is discontinued or interrupted for several days at either the 0.4 or 0.8 mg dose, start therapy again with the 0.4 mg once-daily dose.

ACE INHIBITORS

BENAZEPRIL HCl	
Tablets: 5, 10, 20, 40 mg (*Rx*)	*Lotensin* (Ciba)
CAPTOPRIL	
Tablets: 12.5, 25, 50, 100 mg (*Rx*)	Various, *Capoten* (Bristol-Myers Squibb)
ENALAPRIL MALEATE	
Tablets: 2.5, 5, 10, 20 mg (*Rx*)	*Vasotec* (Merck)
Injection: 1.25 mg enalaprilat/ml (*Rx*)	*Vasotec I.V.* (Merck)
FOSINOPRIL SODIUM	
Tablets: 10, 20 mg (*Rx*)	*Monopril* (Mead Johnson)
LISINOPRIL	
Tablets: 2.5, 5, 10, 20, 40 mg (*Rx*)	*Prinivil* (Merck), *Zestril* (Zeneca)
MOEXIPRIL HCl	
Tablets: 7.5, 15 mg (*Rx*)	*Univasc* (Schwarz Pharma)
QUINAPRIL HCl	
Tablets: 5, 10, 20, 40 mg (*Rx*)	*Accupril* (Parke-Davis)
RAMIPRIL	
Capsules: 1.25, 2.5, 5, 10 mg (*Rx*)	*Altace* (Hoechst-Roussel/Upjohn)
TRANDOLAPRIL	
Tablets: 1, 2, 4 mg (*Rx*)	*Mavik* (Knoll)

Warning:

Pregnancy: When used in pregnancy during the second and third trimesters, ACE inhibitors can cause injury and even death to the developing fetus. When pregnancy is detected, discontinue the ACE inhibitor as soon as possible.

Actions:

Pharmacology: The angiotensin-converting enzyme inhibitors (ACEIs) appear to act primarily through suppression of the renin-angiotensin-aldosterone system; however, no consistent correlation has been described between renin levels and drug response.

Synthesized by the kidneys, renin is released into the circulation where it acts on a plasma globulin substrate to produce angiotensin I, a relatively inactive decapeptide. Angiotensin I is then converted by angiotensin converting enzyme (ACE) to angiotensin II, a potent endogenous vasoconstrictor that also stimulates aldosterone secretion from the adrenal cortex, contributing to sodium and fluid retention. These agents prevent the conversion of angiotensin I to angiotensin II by inhibiting ACE. ACEIs may also inhibit local angiotensin II at vascular and renal sites and attenuate the release of catecholamines from adrenergic nerve endings.

Increased prostaglandin synthesis may also play a role in the antihypertensive action of captopril.

Pharmacokinetics:

Pharmacokinetics of ACEIs								
ACEI	Onset/ Duration (hrs)	Time to peak serum levels (hrs)	Percent absorbed	Active metabolite	t½ Normal renal function	t½ Impaired renal function	Elimination 24 hr	
							Total	Unchanged
Benazepril	1/24	0.5 to 1	37%[1]	Benazeprilat	10 to 11[2] hr	Prolonged	nd[3]	trace
Captopril	0.25/ dose-related	0.5 to 1.5	75%[4]		< 2 hr	3.5 to 32 hr	> 95%	40% to 50% in urine
Enalapril	1/24	0.5 to 1.5 (enalaprilat 3 to 4)	60%[1]	Enalaprilat	1.3 hr	nd[3]	94% urine and feces	54% in urine (40% enalaprilat)
Enalaprilat	0.25/ ≈ 6	na[5]	na[5]		11 hr	Prolonged	nd[3]	> 90% (urine)
Fosinopril	1/24	≈ 3	36%[1]	Fosinoprilat	12 hr (fosinoprilat IV)	Prolonged	50% urine, 50% feces	negligible
Lisinopril	1/24	≈ 7	25%[1]		12 hr	Prolonged	nd[3]	urine, 100%
Quinapril	1/24	1	60%[4]	Quinaprilat	2 hr (quinaprilat)	Prolonged	≈ 60% urine, ≈37% feces	trace
Ramipril	1 to 2/24	1 (ramiprilat 2 to 4)	50% to 60%[4]	Ramiprilat	13 to 17 hr (ramiprilat)	Prolonged	60% urine, 40% feces	< 2%

[1] Absorption not influenced by food.
[2] Effective t½ of accumulation of metabolite following multiple dosing.
[3] nd – No data.
[4] Absorption reduced by food (see Drug Interactions).
[5] na – Not applicable (available IV only).

Indications:

Hypertension: The ACEIs are effective alone and in combination with other antihypertensive agents, especially thiazide-type diuretics.

Heart failure: Captopril, enalapril, lisinopril and quinapril.

Left ventricular dysfunction (LVD):

Captopril – To improve survival following myocardial infarction (MI) in clinically stable patients with LVD manifested as an ejection fraction ≤ 40% and to reduce the incidence of overt heart failure and subsequent hospitalizations for CHF in these patients.

Enalapril – For clinically stable asymptomatic patients with LVD (ejection fraction ≤ 35%); enalapril decreases the rate of development of overt heart failure and decreases the incidence of hospitalization for CHF.

Diabetic nephropathy:

Captopril – Treatment of diabetic nephropathy (proteinuria > 500 mg/day) in patients with type 1 diabetes mellitus and retinopathy.

Unlabeled uses:

Captopril – Management of hypertensive crises. Sublingual captopril 25 mg has also been used effectively.

Neonatal and childhood hypertension; rheumatoid arthritis; diagnosis of anatomic renal artery stenosis ("captopril test"); hypertension related to scleroderma renal crisis; diagnosis of primary aldosteronism; idiopathic edema; Bartter's syndrome; Raynaud's syndrome (symptomatic relief); hypertension of Takayasu's disease.

Enalapril – Diabetic nephropathy (reduction of proteinuria, albuminuria and glomerular hypertension).

Childhood hypertension and hypertension related to scleroderma renal crisis.

Enalaprilat – May be used for hypertensive emergencies, but the effects are often variable.

Ramipril – Congestive heart failure.

Contraindications:

Hypersensitivity to these products.

Warnings:

Neutropenia/Agranulocytosis: Neutropenia (< 1000/mm^3) with myeloid hypoplasia resulted from **captopril** use. About half of the neutropenic patients developed systemic or oral cavity infections or other features of agranulocytosis. Neutropenia/agranulocytosis has occurred rarely with **enalapril** or **lisinopril** and in one patient on **quinapril**.

Angioedema has occurred. It may occur at any time during treatment, especially following the first dose of **enalapril** (0.2%), **captopril, lisinopril** or **quinapril** (0.1%). Angioedema associated with laryngeal edema may be fatal.

Proteinuria: Total urinary proteins > 1 g/day were seen in 0.7% of **captopril** patients. Nephrotic syndrome occurred in about 20% of these cases.

Hypotension:

First-dose effect – ACE inhibitors may cause a profound fall in blood pressure following the first dose.

In heart failure, where the blood pressure was either normal or low, transient decreases in mean blood pressure > 20% occurred in about half of the patients.

Renal function impairment: Some hypertensive patients with renal disease, particularly those with severe renal artery stenosis, have developed increases in BUN and serum creatinine after reduction of blood pressure.

In patients with severe CHF whose renal function may depend on the activity of the renin-angiotensin-aldosterone system, treatment with ACEIs may be associated with oliguria or progressive azotemia and, rarely, with acute renal failure or death.

Impaired renal function decreases **lisinopril** elimination. The elimination half-life of quinaprilat increases as Ccr decreases. Dosage adjustment may be necessary for **quinapril, benazepril, ramipril** and **lisinopril**. Impaired renal function decreases total clearance of fosinoprilat and approximately doubles the AUC.

Hepatic function impairment: Patients with impaired liver function could develop markedly elevated plasma levels of unchanged **fosinopril** or **ramipril**. In patients with alcoholic or biliary cirrhosis, the rate, but not extent of fosinopril hydrolysis was reduced. Quinaprilat concentrations are reduced in alcoholic cirrhosis.

Elderly: Elderly patients may have higher **lisinopril** blood levels and AUC, and higher peak ramiprilat and quinaprilat levels and AUC than younger patients. This may relate to decreased renal function rather than to age itself.

Pregnancy: Category C (first trimester); Category D (second and third trimesters). See Warning Box.

Lactation: Ingestion of 20 mg/day **fosinopril** resulted in detectable fosinoprilat levels in breast milk; do not administer to nursing mothers. Concentrations of **captopril** in breast milk are approximately 1% of those in maternal blood. **Benazepril, enalapril** and **enalaprilat** are detected in breast milk in trace amounts; a newborn would receive < 0.1% of the mg/kg maternal dose of **benazepril** and **benazeprilat**. It is not known whether **lisinopril, quinapril** or **ramipril** are excreted in breast milk.

Children: Safety and efficacy have not been established. Use **captopril** in children only when other measures for controlling blood pressure have not been effective.

Precautions:

Hyperkalemia: Elevated serum potassium (> 5.7 mEq/L) was observed in ≈ 1% of hypertensive patients given **benazepril, enalapril** or **ramipril**, 2.2% of hypertensive patients given **lisinopril**, 2.6% of hypertensive patients given fosinopril, and 4% of CHF patients given lisinopril. Hyperkalemia also occurred with **captopril**.

Valvular stenosis: Theoretically, patients with aortic stenosis might be at risk of decreased coronary perfusion when treated with vasodilators, because they do not develop as much afterload reduction as others.

Surgery/Anesthesia: In patients undergoing major surgery or during anesthesia with agents that produce hypotension, ACEIs will block angiotensin II formation secondary to compensatory renin release.

Cough: Chronic cough has occurred with the use of all ACE inhibitors. Characteristically, the cough is nonproductive, persistent and resolves within 1 to 4 days after therapy discontinuation.

The incidence of cough, although still reported as 0.5% to 3% by some manufacturers, appears to range from 5% to 25% and has been reported to be as high as 39%, resulting in discontinuation rates as high as 15%.

Drug Interactions:

Drugs that may affect ACE inhibitors may include antacids, capsaicin, indomethacin, phenothiazines, probenecid and rifampin. Drugs that may be affected by ACE inhibitors include allopurinol, digoxin, lithium, potassium preparations/potassium-sparing diuretics and tetracycline.

Drug/Lab test interactions: Captopril may cause a false-positive test for *urine acetone*.

Fosinopril may cause a false low measurement of serum digoxin levels with the *Digi-Tab RIA Kit for Digoxin* other kits such as the *Coat-A-Count RIA Kit,* may be used.

Drug/Food interactions: Food significantly reduces the bioavailability of **captopril** by 30% to 40%. Administer captopril 1 hour before meals. The rate and extent of **quinapril** absorption are diminished moderately (25% to 30%) when administered during a high-fat meal. The rate, but not extent, of **ramipril** and **fosinopril** absorption is reduced by food. Food does not reduce the GI absorption of **benazepril, enalapril** and **lisinopril.**

Adverse Reactions:

Adverse reactions may include chest pain; hypotension; headache; dizziness; fatigue; diarrhea; dysgeusia; cough; rash.

Administration and Dosage:

BENAZEPRIL HCl:

Initial dose – 10 mg once daily.

Maintenance dosage – 20 to 40 mg/day as a single dose or two divided doses. A dose of 80 mg gives an increased response, but experience is limited.

Renal function impairment – 5 mg once daily in patients with Ccr of < 30 ml/min/1.73 m^2 (serum creatinine > 3 mg/dl). Dosage may be titrated upward until blood pressure is controlled or to a maximum of 40 mg/day.

CAPTOPRIL: Administer 1 hour before meals.

Hypertension –

Initial: 25 mg 2 or 3 times/day. If satisfactory blood pressure reduction is not achieved after 1 or 2 weeks, increase to 50 mg 2 or 3 times/day. If blood pressure is not controlled after 1 or 2 weeks at this dose (and patient is not already on a diuretic), add a modest dose of a thiazide diuretic.

If further blood pressure reduction is required, increase to 100 mg captopril 2 or 3 times/day and then, if necessary, to 150 mg 2 or 3 times/day (while continuing diuretic). Usual dose is 25 to 150 mg 2 or 3 times/day. Do not exceed daily dose of 450 mg.

Accelerated or malignant hypertension: Promptly initiate captopril at 25 mg 2 or 3 times daily under close supervision. Increase dose every 24 hours until a satisfactory response is obtained or the maximum dose is reached.

Heart failure – Usual initial dosage is 25 mg 3 times daily. After 50 mg 3 times daily is reached, delay further dosage increases, where possible, for at least 2 weeks to determine if a satisfactory response occurs. Most patients have had a satisfactory clinical improvement at 50 or 100 mg 3 times daily. Do not exceed a daily dose of 450 mg.

LVD after MI – 50 mg 3 times daily is the target maintenance dose. Therapy may be initiated as early as 3 days following an MI. After a single 6.25 mg dose, initiate at 12.5 mg 3 times daily, then increase to 25 mg 3 times daily during the next several days and to a target of 50 mg 3 times daily over the next several weeks as tolerated.

Diabetic nephropathy – Recommended dose for long-term use is 25 mg 3 times daily.

Renal impairment – Reduce initial dosage and use smaller increments for titration, which should be quite slow (1 to 2 week intervals). After the desired therapeutic effect is achieved, slowly back-titrate to the minimal effective dose.

ENALAPRIL MALEATE:

Oral –

Hypertension:

Patients taking diuretics – Discontinue the diuretic, if possible, for 2 to 3 days before beginning therapy with lisinopril to reduce the likelihood of hypertension. If the diuretic cannot be discontinued, use an initial dose of 2.5 mg under medical supervision for at least 2 hours and until blood pressure has stabilized for at least an additional hour.

Patients taking diuretics – Initial dose is 5 mg once a day. The usual dosage range is 10 to 40 mg/day as a single dose or in 2 divided doses.

Impaired renal function – Titrate the dosage upward until blood pressure is controlled or until a maximum dose of 40 mg/day is reached. Use initial dose of 5 mg/day in normal renal function and mild impairment (creatinine clearance [Ccr] 30 to 80 ml/min, serum creatinine < 3 mg/dl); 2.5 mg/day in moderate-to-severe renal impairment (Ccr ≤ 30 ml/min, serum creatinine ≥ 3 mg/dl) and in dialysis patients on dialysis days.

Heart failure: As adjunctive therapy with diuretics and digitalis, the recommended starting dose is 2.5 mg once or twice daily. The usual therapeutic dosing range for the treatment of heart failure is 5 to 20 mg/day given in two divided doses. The maximum daily dose is 40 mg.

Renal impairment or hyponatremia –

Serum sodium < 130 mEq/L or with serum creatinine > 1.6 mg/dl: Initiate at 2.5 mg/day under close medical supervision. The dose may be increased to 2.5 mg twice daily, then 5 mg twice daily and higher as needed, usually at intervals of
≥ 4 days. The maximum daily dose is 40 mg.

Asymptomatic left ventricular dysfunction: 2.5 mg twice daily, titrated as tolerated to the targeted daily dose of 20 mg in divided doses.

Parenteral (enalaprilat) – For IV administration only.

Hypertension: 1.25 mg every 6 hours IV over 5 minutes.

The dose for patients being converted to IV from oral therapy is 1.25 mg every 6 hours. For conversion from IV to oral therapy, the recommended initial dose of tablets is 5 mg once a day with subsequent dosage adjustments as necessary.

Patients taking diuretics: Starting dose for hypertension is 0.625 mg IV over 5 minutes. If there is inadequate clinical response after 1 hour, repeat the 0.625 dose. Give additional doses of 1.25 mg at 6 hour intervals.

For conversion from IV to oral therapy, the recommended initial dose of enalapril maleate tablets for patients who have responded to 0.625 mg enalaprilat every 6 hours is 2.5 mg once a day with subsequent dosage adjustment as needed.

Renal function impairment: Administer 1.25 mg every 6 hours for patients with Ccr > 30 ml/min. For Ccr ≤ 30 ml/min, initial dose is 0.625 mg. If there is inadequate clinical response after 1 hour, the 0.625 mg dose may be repeated. May give additional 1.25 mg doses at 6 hour intervals. For dialysis patients, initial dose is 0.625 mg every 6 hour.

For conversion from IV to oral therapy, the recommended initial dose is 5 mg once a day for patients with Ccr > 30 ml/min and 2.5 mg once daily for patients with Ccr ≤ 30 ml/min.

FOSINOPRIL SODIUM:

Initial dose – 10 mg once daily.

Maintenance dosage – Usual range needed to maintain a response is 20 to 40 mg/day but some patients appear to have a further response to 80 mg. If trough response is inadequate, consider dividing the daily dose.

LISINOPRIL:

Hypertension –

Initial therapy: 10 mg once/day in patients with uncomplicated essential hypertension not on diuretic therapy. The usual dosage range is 20 to 40 mg/day as a single daily dose.

Diuretic-treated patients: Discontinue the diuretic, if possible, for 2 to 3 days before beginning therapy with lisinopril to reduce the likelihood of hypertension. If the diuretic cannot be discontinued, use an initial dose of 5 mg under medical supervision for at least 2 hours and until blood pressure has stabilized for at least an additional hour.

CHF –

Initial dose: 5 mg once daily with diuretics and digitalis. Usual effective dosage range is 5 to 20 mg/day as a single dose. In patients with hyponatremia (serum sodium < 130 mEq/L), initiate dose at 2.5 mg once daily. If used with diuretics, initial dose is 5 mg/day.

Elderly – Make dosage adjustments with particular caution.

Renal function impairment – For hypertension, titrate dosage upward until blood pressure is controlled or to a maximum of 40 mg daily.

In acute MI, initiate lisinopril with caution in patients with evidence of renal dysfunction (serum creatinine concentration exceeding 2 mg/dl).

Lisinopril Dosage in Renal Impairment

Renal status	Creatinine clearance (ml/min)	Serum creatinine (mg/dl)	Initial dose (mg/day)
Normal function to mild impairment	> 30	≤ 3	10 mg
Moderate to severe impairment	≥ 10 to ≤ 30	≥ 3	5 mg
Dialysis patients	< 10	—	2.5 mg

Acute myocardial infarction – In hemodynamically stable patients within 24 hours of the onset of symptoms of acute MI, the first dose is 5 mg, followed by 5 mg after 24 hours, 10 mg after 48 hours and then 10 mg once daily. Continue dosing for 6 weeks. Patients with a low systolic blood pressure (≤ 120 mm Hg) when treatment is started or during the first 3 days after the infarct should be given a lower 2.5 mg dose. If hypotension occurs (systolic blood pressure ≤ 100 mm Hg), a daily maintenance dose of 5 mg may be given with temporary reductions to 2.5 mg if needed. If prolonged hypotension occurs (systolic blood pressure < 90 mm Hg for > 1 hour), withdraw lisinopril.

MOEXIPRIL HCl:

Initial dose – In patients not receiving diuretics, 7.5 mg 1 hour prior to meals once daily. If control is not adequate, increase the dose or divide the dosing.

Maintenance dose – 7.5 to 30 mg daily in 1 or 2 divided doses 1 hour before meals.

Renal function impairment – Cautiously use 3.75 mg once daily in patients with Ccr of ≤ 40 ml/min/1.73 m^2. Dosage may be titrated upward to a maximum of 15 mg/day.

QUINAPRIL HCl:

Hypertension –

Initial dose: 10 mg once daily.

Elderly (≥ 65 years old): 10 mg once daily followed by titration to the optimal response.

Renal function impairment: Initial dose is 10 mg with Ccr > 60 ml/min, 5 mg with Ccr 30 to 60 ml/min and 2.5 mg with Ccr 10 to 30 ml/min.

CHF – The recommended starting dose is 5 mg twice daily. If the initial dose is well tolerated, titrate patients at weekly intervals until and effective dose, usually 20 to 40 mg daily given in 2 equally divided doses, is reached or undesirable hypotension, orthostasis or azotemia prohibit reaching this dose.

Renal impairment or hyponatremia: In patients with heart failure and renal impairment, the recommended initial dose is 5 mg with Ccr > 30 ml/min and 2.5 mg with Ccr 10 to 30 ml/min. There is insufficient data for dosage recommendation in patients with Ccr < 10 ml/min.

RAMIPRIL:

Initial dose – 2.5 mg once daily in patients not receiving a diuretic.

Maintenance dosage – 2.5 to 20 mg/day as a single dose or in two equally divided doses.

Alternative route of administration – Ramipril capsules are usually swallowed whole. However, the capsules may be opened and the contents sprinkled on a small amount of ≈ 4 oz applesauce or mixed in apple juice or water.

Renal function impairment – 1.25 mg once daily in patients with Ccr of < 40 ml/min/1.73 m^2 (serum creatinine > 2.5 mg/dl). Dosage may be titrated upward until blood pressure is controlled or to a maximum of 5 mg/day.

TRANDOLAPRIL:

Initial dose – The recommended initial dosage of trandolapril for patients not receiving a diuretic is 1 mg/day (2 mg in black patients). Adjust dosage according to the blood pressure response. Make dosage adjustments at intervals of ≥ 1 week. Most patients have required dosages of 2 to 4 mg/day. There is little clinical experience with doses > 6 mg.

Patients inadequately treated with once daily dosing at 4 mg may be treated with twice-daily dosing. If blood pressure is not adequately controlled with trandolapril monotherapy, a diuretic may be added.

In patients being treated with a diuretic, symptomatic hypotension can occasionally occur following the initial dose of trandolapril. To reduce the likelihood of hypotension, if possible, discontinue the diuretic 2 to 3 days prior to beginning therapy with trandolapril. If blood pressure is not controlled with trandolapril alone, resume diuretic therapy. If the diuretic cannot be discontinued, give an initial dose of 0.5 mg trandolapril with careful medical supervision for several hours until blood pressure has stabilized. Titrate dosage as described above to the optimal response.

Renal/hepatic function impairment – For patients with a creatinine clearance < 30 ml/min or with hepatic cirrhosis, the recommended starting dose, based on clinical and pharmacokinetic data, is 0.5 mg/day. Titrate as described above to the optimal response.

ANGIOTENSIN II RECEPTOR ANTAGONISTS

LOSARTAN POTASSIUM
Tablets: 25 and 50 mg (*Rx*) — *Cozaar* (Merck)

VALSARTAN
Capsules: 80 and 160 mg (*Rx*) — *Diovan* (Ciba-Geigy)

IRBESARTAN
Tablets: 75, 150 and 300 mg (*Rx*) — *Avapro* (Bristol-Myers Squibb/Sanofi)

Warning:
Pregnancy: When used in pregnancy during the second and third trimesters, drugs that act directly on the renin-angiotensin system can cause injury and even death to the developing fetus. When pregnancy is detected, discontinue angiotensin II receptor antagonists as soon as possible.

Actions:
Pharmacology: **Losartan, irbesartan** and **valsartan** are angiotensin II receptor (type AT_1) antagonists. Angiotensin II receptor antagonists (AIIRAs) block the vasoconstrictor and aldosterone-secreting effects of angiotensin II by selectively blocking the binding of angiotensin II to the AT_1 receptor found in many tissues.

Pharmacokinetics:

Angiotensin II Antagonist Pharmacokinetics

Parameters	Losartan (metabolite)[1]	Valsartan	Irbesartan
Bioavailability	≈ 33%	≈ 25%	60% to 80%
Food effect (AUC/C_{max})	↓10%/↓	↓40%/↓50%	no effect
Plasma bound	98.7% (99.8%)	95%	90%
C_{max}	1 hr (3 to 4 hrs)	2 to 4 hrs	1.5 to 2 hours
Volume of distribution	≈ 34 L (≈ 12 L)	17 L	53 to 93 L
Converted to metabolites	(≈ 14%)	≈ 20%	< 20%
Metabolism enzymes, primary	CYP2C9; CYP3A4	unknown	CYP2C9
Terminal half-life	≈ 2 hrs (6 to 9 hrs)	≈ 6 hrs[2]	11 to 15 hours
Total plasma clearance	≈ 600 ml/min (≈ 50 ml/min)	≈ 2 L/hr[2]	157 to 176 ml/min
Renal clearance	≈ 75 ml/min (≈ 25 ml/min)	≈ 0.62 L/hr[2]	3 to 3.5 ml/min
Recovered in the urine	≈ 35%	13%	≈ 20%
Recovered in the feces	≈ 60%	83%	≈ 80%

[1] Active.
[2] IV dosing.

AIIRAs do not accumulate in plasma upon repeated once-daily dosing.

Losartan undergoes substantial first-pass metabolism and is converted to an active carboxylic acid metabolite (14% of dose) that is responsible for most of the angiotensin II receptor antagonism.

Valsartan is metabolized only to a small extent (< 10% of the systemically available dose) and the main metabolite is significantly less potent than valsartan in animal models.

In vitro studies of **irbesartan** oxidation by cytochrome P450 isoenzymes indicated irbesartan was oxidized primarily by 2C9; metabolism by 3A4 was negligible.

Indications:
Hypertension: Treatment of hypertension alone or in combination with other antihypertensive agents.

Unlabeled uses: These agents may be beneficial in the treatment of heart failure; however, further studies are needed. Studies are being conducted to evaluate irbesartan in reducing the rates of progression of renal disease and adverse clinical sequelae in hypertensive patients with diabetic nephropathy caused by type 2 diabetes.

Contraindications:
Hypersensitivity to any component of these products.

Warnings:
Hypotension/Volume- or Salt-depleted patients: In patients who are intravascularly volume-depleted (eg, those treated with diuretics), symptomatic hypotension may occur. Correct these conditions prior to administration. Use a lower starting dose of AIIRAs and monitor closely. A transient hypotensive response is not a contraindication to further treatment, which usually can be continued without difficulty once the blood pressure has stabilized.

Race: In controlled trials, **losartan** had an effect on blood pressure that was notably less in African-American patients than in non-African-Americans, a finding similar to ACE inhibitors. **Irbesartan** was effective in reducing blood pressure regardless of race, although the effect was somewhat less in African-Americans (usually a low-renin population).

Cough: In trials where **valsartan** was compared with an ACE inhibitor with or without placebo, the incidence of dry cough was significantly greater in the ACE inhibitor group (7.9%) than in the groups who received valsartan (2.6%) or placebo (1.5%). In patients who had dry cough when previously receiving ACE inhibitors, the incidences of cough in patients who received AIIRAs, HCTZ or lisinopril were ≈ 22.5%, ≈ 18% and 69%, respectively.

Renal function impairment: In patients whose renal function may depend on the activity of the renin- angiotensin-aldosterone system (eg, patients with severe CHF), treatment with ACE inhibitors has been associated with oliguria or progressive azotemia and with acute renal failure or death (rarely). In studies of ACE inhibitors in patients with unilateral or bilateral renal artery stenosis, increases in serum creatinine or BUN have been reported. AIIRAs would be expected to behave similarly. In some patients, these effects were reversible upon discontinuation of therapy. No dosage adjustment is necessary for patients with renal impairment unless they are volume-depleted.

Hepatic function impairment:

Losartan – Compared with healthy subjects, the total plasma clearance in patients with hepatic insufficiency was ≈ 50% lower and the oral bioavailability was ≈ 2 times higher. A lower starting dose is recommended.

Valsartan – On average, patients with mild-to-moderate chronic liver disease have twice the exposure (measured by AUC values) to valsartan of healthy volunteers. In general, no dosage adjustment is needed in patients with mild-to-moderate liver disease. Exercise care, however, in this patient population.

Irbesartan – The pharmacokinetics of irbesartan following repeated oral administration were not significantly affected in patients with mild-to-moderate cirrhosis of the liver. No dosage adjustment is necessary in patients with hepatic insufficiency.

Elderly: No dosage adjustment is necessary when initiating AIIRAs in the elderly.

Pregnancy: Category C (first trimester); Category D (second and third trimesters).

Lactation: Because of the potential for adverse effects on the nursing infant, decide whether to discontinue nursing or discontinue the drug, taking into account the importance of the drug to the mother.

Children: Safety and efficacy in patients < 18 years of age have not been established.

Precautions:

Lab test abnormalities: Occasional elevations (> 150% in **valsartan**-treated patients) of liver enzymes or serum bilirubin have occurred.

Minor increases in BUN or serum creatinine were observed in < 0.1% of patients with essential hypertension treated with **losartan** alone, in 0.8% of patients taking **valsartan** and < 0.7% with **irbesartan**.

Small decreases in hemoglobin and hematocrit occurred frequently in patients treated with **losartan** alone but were rarely of clinical importance. Decreases of > 20% in hemoglobin and hematocrit were observed in 0.4% and 0.8%, respectively, of **valsartan** patients.

Mean decreases in hemoglobin of 0.2 g/dl were observed in 0.2% of patients receiving **irbesartan**. Neutropenia (< 1000 cells/ mm^3) occurred at similar frequencies (0.3).

Increases of > 20% in serum potassium were observed in 4.4% of **valsartan**-treated patients.

Drug Interactions:

Drugs that may interact with losartan include cimetidine and phenobarbital.

In vitro studies show significant inhibition of the formation of oxidized **irbesartan** metabolites with the known cytochrome CYP2C9 substrates/inhibitors, tolbutamide and nifedipine. However, clinical consequences were negligible.

Drug/Food interactions: A meal slows absorption of AIIRAs and decreases C_{max} but has only minor effects on **losartan** AUC or on the AUC of the metabolite (≈ 10% decrease). Food decreases **valsartan**'s C_{max} by 50% and its AUC by 40%. Food does not affect the bioavailability of **irbesartan**.

Adverse Reactions:

Adverse reactions occurring in ≥ 3% of patients include dizziness; upper respiratory tract infection; cough (**losartan**); viral infection (**valsartan**); fatigue; diarrhea; upper respiratory tract infection (**irbesartan**).

Administration and Dosage:

LOSARTAN POTASSIUM: The usual starting dose is 50 mg once daily with 25 mg used in patients with possible depletion of intravascular volume (eg, patients treated with diuretics) and patients with a history of hepatic impairment. Losartan can be administered with or without food once or twice daily with total daily doses ranging from 25 to 100 mg.

If the antihypertensive effect measured at trough using once-daily dosing is inadequate, a twice-daily regimen at the same total daily dose or an increase in dose may give a more satisfactory response.

VALSARTAN: The recommended starting dose is 80 mg daily, with or without food, when used as monotherapy in patients who are not volume-depleted. Valsartan may be used over a dose range of 80 to 320 mg once daily.

The antihypertensive effect is substantially present ≤ 2 weeks and maximal reduction is generally attained > 4 weeks. If additional antihypertensive effect is required, the dosage may be increased to 160 or 320 mg or a diuretic may be added. Addition of a diuretic has a greater effect than dose increases beyond 80 mg. Valsartan may be administered with other antihypertensive agents.

IRBESARTAN: The recommended initial dosage of irbesartan is 150 mg once daily with or without food. Patients may be titrated to 300 mg once daily.

Irbesartan may be administered with other antihypertensive agents. A low dose of a diuretic may be added if blood pressure is not controlled by irbesartan alone. Hydrochlorothiazide has been shown to have an additive effect. Patients not adequately treated by the maximum dose of 300 mg once daily are unlikely to derive additional benefit from a higher dose or twice-daily dosing.

ANTIHYPERLIPIDEMIC AGENTS

Lowering cholesterol levels can arrest or reverse atherosclerosis in all vascular beds and can significantly decrease the morbidity and mortality associated with atherosclerosis. Each 10% reduction in cholesterol levels is associated with an ≈ 20% to 30% reduction in the incidence of coronary heart disease. Hyperlipidemia, particularly elevated serum cholesterol and low density lipoprotein (LDL) levels, is a risk factor in the development of atherosclerotic cardiovascular disease.

Treatment of hyperlipidemia is based on the assumption that lowering serum lipids decreases morbidity and mortality of atherosclerotic cardiovascular disease.

The cornerstone of treatment in primary hyperlipidemia is diet restriction and weight reduction. Limit or eliminate alcohol intake. Use drug therapy in conjunction with diet, and after maximal efforts to control serum lipids by diet alone prove unsatisfactory, when tolerance to or compliance with diet is poor or when hyperlipidemia is severe and risk of complications is high. Treat contributory diseases such as hypothyroidism or diabetes mellitus.

Classification of Total and HDL Cholesterol Levels

Level (mg/dl)	Classification
< 200 (5.2 mmol/L)	desirable
200-239 (5.2 - 6.2 mmol/L)	borderline-high
≥ 240 (6.2 mmol/L)	high
HDL < 35 (0.9 mmol/L)	low

Classification of LDL- Cholesterol Levels

Level (mg/dl)	Classification
< 130 (3.4 mmol/L)	desirable
130 -159 (3.4 - 4.1 mmol/L)	borderline-high
≥ 160 (4.1 mmol/L)	high

Elevations and treatment associated with each type of hyperlipidemia follow:

Hyperlipidemias and Their Treatment[1]

	Hyperlipidemia type					
	I	IIa	IIb	III	IV	V
Lipids						
Cholesterol	N-⇧	↑	↑	N-↑	N-⇧	N-↑
Triglycerides	↑	N	↑	N-↑	↑	↑
Lipoproteins						
Chylomicrons	↑	N	N	N	N	↑
VLDL (pre-β)	N-⇧	N-↓	↑	N-⇧	↑	↑
ILDL (broad-β)[2]				↑		
LDL (β)	↓	↑	↑	↑	N-⇩	↓
HDL (α)	↓	N	N	N	N-⇩	↓
Treatment	Diet	Diet Bile acid sequestrants Dextrothyroxine Nicotinic acid Probucol HMG-CoA reductase inhibitors	Diet Bile acid sequestrants[3] Probucol[3] Clofibrate[4] Gemfibrozil[5] Nicotinic acid HMG-CoA reductase inhibitors	Diet Clofibrate Gemfibrozil Nicotinic acid	Diet Clofibrate Gemfibrozil Nicotinic acid	Diet Clofibrate Gemfibrozil Nicotinic acid

[1] N = normal ↑ = increase ↓ = decrease ⇧ = slight increase ⇩ = slight decrease
[2] An abnormal lipoprotein.
[3] Particularly useful if hypercholesterolemia predominates.
[4] With high serum triglyceride levels and moderately elevated cholesterol.
[5] In patients with inadequate response to weight loss, bile acid sequestrants and nicotinic acid.

Antihyperlipidemic Drug Effects[1]

	Lipids		Lipoproteins		
Drug	Cholesterol	Triglycerides	VLDL (pre-β)	LDL (β)	HDL
Atorvastatin	↓	↓	↓	↓	↑
Cholestyramine	↓	→↑	→↑	↓	→↑
Clofibrate[2]	↓	↓	↓	→↓	→↑
Colestipol	↓	→↑	↑	↓	→↑
Dextrothyroxine[2]	↓	→	→	↓	→

Antihyperlipidemic Drug Effects[1]					
	Lipids		Lipoproteins		
Drug	Cholesterol	Triglycerides	VLDL (pre-β)	LDL (β)	HDL
Fluvastatin	↓	↓	↓	↓	↑
Gemfibrozil	↓	↓	↓	→↓	↑
Lovastatin	↓	↓	↓	↓	↑
Nicotinic Acid	↓	↓	↓	↓	↑
Pravastatin	↓	↓	↓	↓	↑
Simvastatin	↓	↓	↓	↓	↑

[1] ↓ = decrease ↑ = increase → = unchanged
[2] These agents are no longer commonly used as antihyperlipidemics.

HMG-CoA REDUCTASE INHIBITORS

LOVASTATIN (Mevinolin)
Tablets: 10, 20 and 40 mg (*Rx*) — *Mevacor* (Merck)

SIMVASTATIN
Tablets: 5, 10, 20 and 40 mg (*Rx*) — *Zocor* (Merck)

PRAVASTATIN SODIUM
Tablets: 10, 20 and 40 mg (*Rx*) — *Pravachol* (Bristol-Myers Squibb)

FLUVASTATIN
Capsules: 20 and 40 mg (*Rx*) — *Lescol* (Sandoz)

ATORVASTATIN CALCIUM
Tablets: 10, 20 and 40 mg (*Rx*) — *Lipitor* (Parke-Davis)

CERIVASTATIN SODIUM
Tablets: 0.2 and 0.3 mg (*Rx*) — *Baycol* (Bayer)

Actions:

Pharmacology: These agents specifically competitively inhibit 3-hydroxy-3-methylglutaryl-coenzyme A (HMG-CoA) reductase, the enzyme which catalyzes the early rate-limiting step in cholesterol biosynthesis, conversion of HMG-CoA to mevalonate.

Pharmacokinetics:

Pharmacokinetics of HMG-CoA Reductase Inhibitors					
	Bioavailability	Excretion	t½ (hrs)	Protein binding	Effects of renal/hepatic impairment
Fluvastatin	> 90% absorbed; absolute bioavailability 24%; extensive first-pass hepatic extraction	5% (urine) 90% (feces)	< 1	> 98%	nd[1]
Lovastatin	≈ 35% absorbed; extensive first-pass hepatic extraction (liver is primary site of action); < 5% of oral dose reaches general circulation as active inhibitors	10% (urine) 83% (feces)	3-4	> 95%	nd[1]
Pravastatin	≈ 34% absorbed; absolute bioavailability 17%; extensive first-pass hepatic extraction; plasma levels may not correlate with lipid-lowering efficacy	≈ 20% (urine) 70% (feces)	1.8	≈ 50%	Mean AUC varied 18-fold in cirrhotic patients and peak values varied 47-fold
Simvastatin	60% to 80% absorbed; extensive first-pass metabolism; < 5% of oral dose reaches general circulation as active inhibitors	13% (urine) 60% (feces)	3	≈ 95%	Higher systemic exposure may occur in severe renal insufficiency
Atorvastatin	≈ 12% absolute bioavailability; first-pass metabolism (CYP3A4)	< 2% (urine)	14	≥ 98%	Plasma levels not affected by renal disease; markedly increased with chronic alcoholic liver disease

[1] nd = no data.

Indications:

Adjunct to diet for the reduction of elevated total and LDL cholesterol levels in patients with primary hypercholesterolemia (and mixed dyslipidemia, cerivastatin only) (Types IIa and IIb), when the response to diet and other nonpharmacological measures alone has been inadequate.

Atherosclerosis (lovastatin/pravastatin): To slow the progression of coronary atherosclerosis in patients with CHD as part of a treatment strategy to lower total-C and LDL-C to target levels; to reduce the risk of acute coronary events.

Coronary heart disease (simvastatin/pravastatin): To reduce the risk of total mortality by reducing coronary death; to reduce the risk of non-fatal myocardial infarction; reduce the risk of undergoing myocardial revascularization procedures.

Unlabeled uses:

Lovastatin – Diabetic dyslipidemia, nephrotic hyperlipidemia, familial dysbetalipoproteinemia and familial combined hyperlipidemia.

Pravastatin or simvastatin can significantly lower elevated cholesterol levels in patients with: Heterozygous familial hypercholesterolemia; familial combined hyperlipidemia; diabetic dyslipidemia in non-insulin-dependent diabetics; hypercholesterolemia secondary to the nephrotic syndrome; homozygous familial hypercholesterolemia in patients who are not completely devoid of LDL receptors but have a reduced level of LDL receptor activity (pravastatin only); homozygous familial hypercholesterolemia in patients with defective, rather than absent, LDL receptors (simvastatin only).

Fluvastatin – To slow progression of coronary atherosclerosis in patients with CHD.

Contraindications:

Hypersensitivity to any component of these products; active liver disease or unexplained persistent elevated liver function tests; pregnancy, lactation.

Warnings:

Liver dysfunction: Use with caution in patients who consume substantial quantities of alcohol or who have a history of liver disease.

Pravastatin and **fluvastatin** plasma clearance is decreased but no dose adjustment is needed.

Skeletal muscle effects: Rhabdomyolysis with renal dysfunction secondary to myoglobinuria has occurred with some drugs in this class. Myalgia has occurred with **lovastatin**. Uncomplicated myalgia has been reported in **atorvastatin**-treated patients.

Consider myopathy in any patient with diffuse myalgias, muscle tenderness or weakness, or marked elevation of CPK. Advise patients to report promptly muscle pain, tenderness or weakness, particularly with malaise or fever. Discontinue the drug if markedly elevated CPK levels occur or if myopathy is diagnosed.

Hypersensitivity: An apparent hypersensitivity syndrome has occurred. Refer to Management of Acute Hypersensitivity Reactions.

Elderly: In patients > 70 years old, the AUC of **lovastatin** and **simvastatin** is increased. **Pravastatin** does not need dosage adjustment. The safety and efficacy of **atorvastatin** in patients ≥ 70 years old were similar to those of patients < 70 years old. Elderly patients (≥ 65 years old) demonstrated a greater treatment response in respect to LDL-C, total-C and LDL/HDL ratio than patients < 65 years old.

Pregnancy: Category X.

Lactation: It is not known whether **lovastatin** and **simvastatin** are excreted in breast milk; a small amount of **pravastatin** is excreted in breast milk; **fluvastatin** is present in breast milk in a 2:1 ratio (milk-:plasma).

Children: Safety and efficacy in individuals < 18 years old have not been established; treatment in this age group is not recommended at this time.

Precautions:

Monitoring: Perform liver function tests before initiating therapy, at 6 and 12 weeks after initiation of therapy or after dose elevation and periodically thereafter
(≈ 6 month intervals). Pay special attention to patients who develop elevated serum transaminase levels. If transaminase levels progress, particularly if they rise to 3 times the upper limit of normal and are persistent, discontinue the drug.

Diet: Before instituting therapy, attempt to control hypercholesterolemia with diet, exercise, and weight reduction in obese patients.

Homozygous familial hypercholesterolemia: **Lovastatin** and **simvastatin** are less effective in patients with the rare homozygous familial hypercholesterolemia, possibly because they have no functional LDL receptors. **Pravastatin** may be useful in patients not completely devoid of LDL receptors but with a reduced level of activity.

Sleep disturbance: **Lovastatin** and **simvastatin** may interfere with sleep, causing insomnia, whereas **pravastatin** does not appear to disturb sleep.

Photosensitivity: Photosensitization (photoallergy or phototoxicity) may occur.

Drug Interactions:

Drugs that may affect HMG-CoA reductase inhibitors include alcohol, antacids, bile acid sequestrants, colestipol, cyclosporine, erythromycin, gemfibrozil, isradipine, itraconazole, niacin, nicotinic acid, propranolol, digoxin and rifampin. CYP3A inhibitors may interact with **lovastatin**. CYP2C inhibitors may interact with **fluvastatin**.

Drugs that may be affected by HMG-CoA reductase inhibitors include oral contraceptives, digoxin and warfarin.

Adverse Reactions:

HMG-CoA Reductase Inhibitor Adverse Reactions (%)[1]

Adverse reaction	Atorvastatin (n = 36)	Fluvastatin (n = 620)	Lovastatin (n = 613)	Pravastatin (n = 900)	Simvastatin (n = 1583)
GI					
Nausea/Vomiting	—	3.2	1.9 - 4.7	7.3	1.3
Diarrhea	0	4.9	2.6 - 5.5	6.2	1.9
Abdominal pain/ cramps	0	5.5	2 - 5.7	5.4	3.2
Constipation	0	2.6	2 - 4.9	4	2.3
Flatulence	2.8	2.6	3.7 - 6.4	3.3	1.9
Dyspepsia	2.8	8.1	1 - 3.9	—	1.1
Musculoskeletal					
Localized pain	—	—	0.5 - 1	10	—
Myalgia	5.6	5	2.4-2.6	2.7	—
Back pain	0	5.7	—	—	—
Arthralgia	0	4	0.5-1	—	—
CNS					
Headache	16.7	8.9	2.6 - 9.3	6.2	3.5
Dizziness	—	2.2	0.7 - 2	3.3	—
Respiratory					
Upper respiratory infection	—	16.2	—	—	2.1
Common cold	—	—	—	7	—
Rhinitis	—	4.7	—	4	—
Pharyngitis	0	3.8	—	—	—
Other					
Chest pain	—	—	0.5 - 1	3.7	—
Rash/Pruritus	2.8	2.3	0.8 - 5.2	4	—
Cardiac chest pain	—	—	—	4	—
Fatigue	—	2.7	—	3.8	—
Influenza	0	5.1	—	2.4	—

[1] All events. Data are pooled from separate studies and are not necessarily comparable.

Administration and Dosage:

LOVASTATIN (MEVINOLIN): Give lovastatin with meals.

Initial dose – 20 mg/day with the evening meal.

For those patients with severly elevated serum cholesterol levels (eg, > 300 mg/dl [7.8 mmol/L] on diet), initiate dosage at 40 mg/day.

Dose range – 10 to 80 mg/day in single or 2 divided doses. Adjust at intervals of at least 4 weeks.

Immunosuppressive therapy – In patients taking immunosuppressive drugs concomitantly with lovastatin, therapy should begin with 10 mg/day and should not exceed 20 mg/day.

Concomitant therapy – Cholesterol-lowering effects of lovastatin and the bile acid sequestrant, cholestyramine, are additive.

Renal function impairment – In patients with severe renal insufficiency (creatinine clearance < 30 ml/min), use dosage > 20 mg/day with caution.

SIMVASTATIN: May give without regard to meals.

Initial dose – 5 to 10 mg once daily in the evening. Consider starting dose of 5 mg/day for patients with LDL ≤ 190 mg/dl; 10 mg/day for patients with LDL > 190 mg/dl.

Elderly – Consider starting dose of 5 mg/day; maximum LDL reductions may be achieved with ≤ 20 mg/day.

Dose range – 5 to 40 mg/day as single dose in the evening. Adjust the dose at intervals of at least 4 weeks.

PRAVASTATIN SODIUM: May be taken without regard to meals.

Initial dose – 10 to 20 mg once daily at bedtime.

Elderly – In the elderly, maximum reductions in LDL-cholesterol may be achieved with daily doses of ≤ 20 mg.

Dose range – 10 to 40 mg once daily at bedtime.

Concomitant therapy – In patients taking concomitant immunosuppressive drugs (eg, cyclosporine), start pravastatin at 10 mg once daily at bedtime; titrate to higher doses with caution. Most patients treated with this combination received a maximum pravastatin dose of 20 mg/day.

Renal/Hepatic function impairment – A starting dose of 10 mg/day at bedtime is recommended.

FLUVASTATIN: May be taken without regard to meals.

Initial dose – 20 to 40 mg once daily at bedtime.

Dose range – 20 to 80 mg/day as a single dose in the evening. Administer the daily regimen of 80 mg in divided doses (eg, 40 mg twice a day) to those whose LDL-cholesterol response is inadequate at 40 mg/day.

ATORVASTATIN CALCIUM:

Initial dose – 10 mg/day.

Dose range – 10 to 80 mg/day. Can be administered as a single dose at any time of the day, with or without food.

Concomitant therapy – Atorvastatin may be used in combination with a bile acid binding resin for additive effect. Avoid the combination of HMG-CoA reductase inhibitors and fibrates.

CERIVASTATIN SODIUM: The recommended dose is 0.3 mg once daily in the evening. Cerivastatin may be taken with or without food.

Concomitant therapy – The lipid-lowering effects on LDL-C and Total-C are additive when cerivastatin is combined with a bile-acid-binding resin. Give cerivastatin ≥ 2 hours after the resin when co-administering.

Renal function impairment – For patients with moderate or severe renal dysfunction (Ccr 60 ml/min/1.73 m^2), use a starting dose of 0.2 mg.

XANTHINE DERIVATIVES

THEOPHYLLINE	
Tablets: 100, 125, 200, 250 and 300 mg (*Rx*)	Various, *Slo-Phyllin* (Rhone-Poulenc Rorer), *Theolair* (3M Pharm), *Quibron-T Dividose* (Bristol Labs)
Capsules: 100 and 200 mg (*Rx*)	*Bronkodyl* (Winthrop),
Syrup: 80 mg or 150 mg/15 ml (26.7 or 50 mg/5 ml) (*Rx*)	*Aquaphyllin* (Ferndale), *Accurbron* (Marion Merrell Dow)
Elixir: 80 mg/15 ml (26.7 mg/5 ml) (*Rx*)	Various, *Asmalix* (Century), *Elixomin* (Cenci), *Elixophyllin* (Forest), *Theolair* (3M Pharmaceuticals), *Lanophyllin* (Lannett)
Solution: 80 mg/15 ml (26.7 mg/5 ml) (*Rx*)	Various, *Theolair* (3M Pharm)
Capsules, timed release (8 to 12 hours): 50, 60, 65, 75, 100, 125, 130, 200, 250, 260 and 300 mg (sustained reoease) (*Rx*)	*Aerolate* (Fleming), *Slo-bid Gyrocaps* (Rhone-Poulenc Rorer), *Slo-Phyllin Gyrocaps* (Rhone-Poulenc Rorer)
Capsules, timed release (24 hours): 100, 200 and 300 mg (*Rx*)	*Theo-24* (Whitby)
Capsules, timed release (12 hours): 125, 130, 250 and 260 mg (*Rx*)	*Theovent* (Schering), *Theoclear L.A.* (Central), *Theospan SR* (Laser)
Capsules, extended release: 100, 125, 200 and 300 mg (*Rx*)	Various
Tablets, timed release (12 to 24 hours): 100, 200, 300 and 450 mg (*Rx*)	Various
Tablets, extended release: 450 mg (*Rx*)	Various
Tablets, extended release (12 to 24 hours): 100, 200 and 300 mg (*Rx*)	*Theochron* (Various)
Tablets, extended release (24 hours): 400 and 600 mg (*Rx*)	*Uni-Dur* (Key)
Tablets, timed release (8 to 12 hours): 200, 250, 300 and 500 mg (*Rx*)	*Theolair-SR* (3M Pharm), *T-Phyl* (Purdue Frederick), *Quibron-T/SR* (Roberts), *Respbid* (Boehringer Ingelheim)
Tablets, sustained release (8 to 12 hours): 100 and 300 mg (*Rx*)	*Sustaire* (Pfizer Labs)
Tablets, timed release (8 to 24 hours): 100, 200, 300 and 450 mg (*Rx*)	*Theo-Dur* (Key)
Tablets, controlled release (12 to 24 hours): 100, 200 and 300 mg (*Rx*)	*Theo-X* (Carnrick)
Tablets, timed release (24 hours): 400 mg (*Rx*)	*Uniphyl* (Purdue Frederick)

OXTRIPHYLLINE	
Tablets: 100 mg (equiv. to 64 mg theophylline), 200 mg (equiv. to 127 mg theophylline) (*Rx*)	Various, *Choledyl* (Parke-Davis)
Tablets, sustained action: 400 mg (equiv. to 254 mg theophylline), 600 mg (equiv. to 382 mg theophylline) (*Rx*)	*Choledyl SA* (Parke-Davis)
Syrup, pediatric: 50 mg (equiv. to 32 mg theophylline) per 5 ml (*Rx*)	Various, *Choledyl* (Parke-Davis)
Elixir: 100 mg (equiv. to 64 mg theophylline) per 5 ml (*Rx*)	Various, *Choledyl* (Parke-Davis)

THEOPHYLLINE AND DEXTROSE	
Injection: 200, 400 and 800 mg/container (*Rx*)	Various

AMINOPHYLLINE	
Tablets: 100 mg (equiv. to 79 mg theophylline), 200 mg (equiv. to 158 mg theophylline) (*Rx*)	Various
Tablets, controlled release (12 hours): 225 mg (equiv. to 178 mg theophylline) (*Rx*)	*Phyllocontin* (Purdue Frederick)
Oral Liquid: 105 mg (equiv. to 90 mg theophylline) per 5 ml (*Rx*)	Various
Injection: 250 mg (equiv. to 197 mg theophylline) per 10 ml (*Rx*) For IV use.	Various
Suppositories: 250 mg (equiv. to 197.5 mg theophylline), 500 mg (equiv. to 395 mg theophylline) (*Rx*)	Various, *Truphylline* (G & W)

DYPHYLLINE	
Tablets: 200 or 400 mg (*Rx*)	Various, *Dilor* (Savage)
Elixir: 100 or 160 mg/15 ml (33.3 or mg/5 ml) (*Rx*)	*Lufyllin* (Wallace), *Dilor* (Savage)
Injection: 250 mg per ml (*Rx*)	*Lufyllin* (Wallace)

Actions:

Pharmacology: The methylxanthines (theophylline, its soluble salts and derivatives) directly relax the smooth muscle of the bronchi and pulmonary blood vessels, stimulate the CNS, induce diuresis, increase gastric acid secretion, reduce lower esophageal sphincter pressure and inhibit uterine contractions. Theophylline is also a central respiratory stimulant. Aminophylline has a potent effect on diaphragmatic contractility in healthy persons and may then be capable of reducing fatigability and thereby improve contractility in patients with chronic obstructive airways disease.

Other effects that appear to occur at therapeutic concentrations and may collectively play a role in the mechanism of the xanthines include: Inhibition of extracellular adenosine (which causes bronchoconstriction), although it is unlikely that this is a main mechanism; stimulation of endogenous catecholamines, although this also does not appear to be a major mechanism; antagonism of prostaglandins PGE_2 and $PGF_2\alpha$; direct effect on mobilization of intracellular calcium resulting in smooth muscle relaxation; beta-adrenergic agonist activity on the airways. None of these mechanisms has been proven.

Pharmacokinetics:

Absorption – Theophylline is well absorbed from oral liquids and uncoated plain tablets; maximal plasma concentrations are reached in 2 hours. Rectal absorption from suppositories is slow and erratic, the oral route is generally preferred. Enteric coated tablets and some sustained release dosage forms may be unreliably absorbed.

Distribution – Average volume of distribution is 0.45 L/kg (range, 0.3 to 0.7 L/kg). Theophylline does not distribute into fatty tissue. Approximately 40% is bound to plasma protein. Therapeutic serum levels generally range from 10 to 20 mcg/ml. Although some bronchodilatory effect occurs at lower concentrations, stabilization of hyperreactive airways is most evident at levels > 10 mcg/ml, and adverse effects are uncommon at levels < 20 mcg/ml.

Metabolism/Excretion – Xanthines are biotransformed in the liver (85% to 90%) to 1, 3–dimethyluric acid, 3–methylxanthine and 1–methyluric acid; 3–methylxanthine accumulates in concentrations approximately 25% of those of theophylline.

Excretion is by the kidneys; < 15% of the drug is excreted unchanged. Elimination kinetics vary greatly. Plasma elimination half-life averages about 3 to 15 hours in adult nonsmokers, 4 to 5 hours in adult smokers (1 to 2 packs per day), 1 to 9 hours in children and 20 to 30 hours for premature neonates. In the neonate, theophylline is metabolized partially to caffeine. The premature neonate excretes about 50% unchanged theophylline and may accumulate the caffeine metabolite.

Equivalent dose: Because of differing theophylline content, the various salts and derivatives are not equivalent on a weight basis.

Theophylline Content and Equivalent Dose of Various Theophylline Salts		
Theophylline salts	Theophylline %	Equivalent dose
Theophylline anhydrous	100	100 mg
Theophylline monohydrate	91	110 mg
Aminophylline anhydrous	86	116 mg
Aminophylline dihydrate	79	127 mg
Oxtriphylline	64	156 mg

Dyphylline, a chemical derivative of theophylline, is not a theophylline salt as are the other agents. It is about one-tenth as potent as theophylline. Following oral administration, dyphylline is 68% to 82% bioavailable. Peak plasma concentrations are reached within 1 hour, and its half-life is 2 hours. The minimal effective therapeutic concentration is 12 mcg/ml. It is not metabolized to theophylline and 83% ± 5% is excreted unchanged in the urine.

Indications:

Symptomatic relief or prevention of bronchial asthma and reversible bronchospasm associated with chronic bronchitis and emphysema.

Unlabeled uses: Treatment of apnea and bradycardia of prematurity.

Theophylline 10 mg/kg/day may significantly improve pulmonary function and dyspnea in patients with chronic obstructive pulmonary disease.

Contraindications:

Hypersensitivity to any xanthine; peptic ulcer; underlying seizure disorders (unless receiving appropriate anticonvulsant medication).

Aminophylline: Hypersensitivity to ethylenediamine.

Aminophylline rectal suppositories: Irritation or infection of rectum or lower colon.

Warnings:

Status asthmaticus is a medical emergency and is not rapidly responsive to usual doses of conventional bronchodilators. Optimal therapy frequently requires both parenteral medication and close monitoring, preferably in an intensive care setting. Oral theophylline products alone are not appropriate for status asthmaticus.

Toxicity: Excessive doses may cause severe toxicity; monitor serum levels to ensure maximum benefit with minimum risk. Incidence of toxicity increases significantly at serum levels > 20 mcg/ml. Serum levels > 20 mcg/ml are rare after appropriate use of recommended doses. However, if theophylline plasma clearance is reduced for any reason (eg, hepatic impairment; patients > 55 years old, particularly males and those with chronic lung disease; cardiac failure; sustained high fever; infants < 1 year old), even conventional doses may result in increased serum levels and potential toxicity. Frequently, such patients have markedly prolonged levels following drug discontinuation.

Serious side effects such as ventricular arrhythmias, convulsions or even death may appear as the first sign of toxicity without any previous warning. Less serious signs of toxicity (eg, nausea, restlessness) may occur frequently when initiating therapy, but are usually transient; when such signs are persistent during maintenance therapy, they are often associated with serum concentrations > 20 mcg/ml. Serious toxicity is not reliably preceded by less severe side effects.

Cardiac effects: Theophylline may cause dysrhythmias or worsen pre-existing arrhythmias. Any significant change in cardiac rate or rhythm warrants monitoring and further investigation. Many patients who require theophylline may exhibit tachycardia due to underlying disease; the relationship to elevated serum theophylline concentrations may not be appreciated.

Pregnancy: *Category* C. Theophylline has been found in cord serum and crosses the placenta; newborns may have therapeutic serum levels.

Lactation: Theophylline distributes readily into breast milk with a milk:plasma ratio of 0.7 and may cause irritability or other signs of toxicity in nursing infants.

Children: Sufficient numbers of infants < 1 year of age have not been studied in clinical trials to support use in this age group; however, there is evidence that the use of dosage recommendations for older infants and young children may result in the development of toxic serum levels.

Precautions:

Use with caution in: Cardiac disease; hypoxemia; hepatic disease; hypertension; congestive heart failure (CHF); alcoholism; elderly (particularly males); and neonates.

GI effects: Use cautiously in peptic ulcer. Local irritation may occur; centrally mediated GI effects may occur with serum levels > 20 mcg/ml. Reduced lower esophageal pressure may cause reflux, aspiration and worsening of airway obstruction.

Drug Interactions:

Agents that may decrease theophylline levels include aminoglutethimide, barbiturates, charcoal, hydantoins, ketoconazole, rifampin, smoking (cigarettes and marijuana), sulfinpyrazone, sympathomimetics (β-agonists), thioamines, carbamazepine, isoniazid and loop diuretics.

Agents that may increase theophylline levels include allopurinol, beta blockers (non-selective), calcium channel blockers, cimetidine, oral contraceptives, corticosteroids, disulfiram, ephedrine, influenza virus vaccine, interferon, macrolides, mexiletine, quinolones, thiabendazole, thyroid hormones, carbamazepine, isoniazid and loop diuretics.

The following agents may be affected by theophylline: Benzodiazepines, halothane, ketamine, lithium, nondepolarizing muscle relaxants and propofol. Probenecid may increase the effects of dyphylline.

Drug/Food interactions: Theophylline elimination is increased (half-life shortened) by a low carbohydrate, high protein diet and charcoal broiled beef (due to a high polycyclic carbon content). Conversely, elimination is decreased (prolonged half-life) by a high carbohydrate low protein diet. Food may alter the bioavailability and absorption pattern of certain sustained release preparations. Some sustained release preparations may be subject to rapid release of their contents when taken with food, resulting in toxicity. It appears that consistent administration in the fasting state allows predictability of effects.

Adverse Reactions:

Adverse reactions/toxicity are uncommon at serum theophylline levels < 20 mcg/ml.

Levels > 20 mcg/ml: 75% of patients experience adverse reactions (eg, nausea, vomiting, diarrhea, headache, insomnia, irritability).

Levels > 35 mcg/ml: Hyperglycemia; hypotension; cardiac arrhythmias; tachycardia (> 10 mcg/ml in premature newborns); seizures; brain damage; death.

Other: Fever; flushing; hyperglycemia; inappropriate antidiuretic hormone syndrome; rash; alopecia. Ethylenediamine in aminophylline can cause sensitivity reactions, including exfoliative dermatitis and urticaria.

CNS: Irritability; restlessness; headache; insomnia; reflex hyperexcitability; muscle twitching; convulsions.

GI: Nausea; vomiting; epigastric pain; hematemesis; diarrhea; rectal irritation or bleeding (aminophylline suppositories). Therapeutic doses of theophylline may induce gastroesophageal reflux during sleep or while recumbent, increasing the potential for aspiration which can aggravate bronchospasm.

Cardiovascular: Palpitations; tachycardia; extrasystoles; hypotension; circulatory failure; life-threatening ventricular arrhythmias.

Respiratory: Tachypnea; respiratory arrest.

Renal: Proteinuria; potentiation of diuresis.

Administration and Dosage:

THEOPHYLLINE: Individualize dosage. Base dosage adjustments on clinical response and improvement in pulmonary function with careful monitoring of serum levels. If possible, monitor serum levels to maintain levels in the therapeutic range of 10 to 20 mcg/ml. Levels > 20 mcg/ml may produce toxicity, and it may even occur with levels between 15 to 20 mcg/ml, particularly when factors known to reduce theophylline clearance are present (see Warnings). Once stabilized on a dosage, serum levels tend to remain constant.

Calculate dosages on the basis of lean body weight, since theophylline does not distribute into fatty tissue. Regardless of salt used, dosages should be equivalent based on anhydrous theophylline content.

Individualize frequency of dosing. With immediate release products, dosing every 6 hours is generally required, especially in children; intervals up to 8 hours may be satisfactory in adults. Some children and adults requiring higher than average doses (those having rapid rates of clearance; eg, half-lives < 6 hours) may be more effectively controlled during chronic therapy with sustained release products. Determine dosage intervals to produce minimal fluctuations between peak and trough serum theophylline concentrations. Consider the absorption profile and the elimination rate. When converting from an immediate release to a sustained release product, the total daily dose should remain the same, and only the dosing interval adjusted.

Acute symptoms requiring rapid theophyllinization in patients not receiving theophylline – To achieve a rapid effect, an initial loading dose is required. Dosage recommendations are for theophylline anhydrous.

Dosage Guidelines for Rapid Theophyllinization		
Patient Group	Oral loading	Maintenance
Children 1 to 9 years	5 mg/kg	4 mg/kg q 6 h
Children 9 to 16 and young adult smokers	5 mg/kg	3 mg/kg q 6 h
Otherwise healthy non-smoking adults	5 mg/kg	3 mg/kg q 8 h
Older patients, patients with cor pulmonale	5 mg/kg	2 mg/kg q 8 h
Patients with congestive heart failure	5 mg/kg	1-2 mg/kg q 12 h

Infants (preterm to < 1 year) –

Theophylline Dosage Guidelines for Infants	
Age	Initial maintenance dose
Premature infants	
≤ 24 days postnatal	1 mg/kg q 12 h
> 24 days postnatal	1.5 mg/kg q 12 h
Infants (6 to 52 weeks)	[(0.2 x age in weeks) = 5] x kg = 24 hr dose in mg
Up to 26 weeks	Divide into q 8 h dosing
26 to 52 weeks	Divide into q 6 h dosing

Acute symptoms requiring rapid theophyllinization in patients receiving theophylline – Each 0.5 mg/kg theophylline administered as a loading dose will increase the serum theophylline concentration by approximately 1 mcg/ml. Ideally, defer the loading dose if a serum theophylline concentration can be obtained rapidly.

If this is not possible, exercise clinical judgment. When there is sufficient respiratory distress to warrant a small risk, then 2.5 mg/kg of theophylline administered in rapidly absorbed form is likely to increase serum concentration by approximately 5 mcg/ml. If the patient is not experiencing theophylline toxicity, this is unlikely to result in dangerous adverse effects.

Chronic therapy – Slow clinical titration is generally preferred.

Initial dose: 16 mg/kg/24 hours or 400 mg/24 hours, whichever is less, of anhydrous theophylline in divided doses at 6 or 8 hour intervals.

Increasing dose: The above dosage may be increased in approximately 25% increments at 3 day intervals so long as the drug is tolerated or until the maximum dose (indicated below) is reached.

Maximum dose (where the serum concentration is not measured) – *Do not attempt to maintain any dose that is not tolerated.*

Maximum Daily Theophylline Dose Based on Age	
Age	Maximum daily dose[1]
1 to 9 years	24 mg/kg/day
9 to 12 years	20 mg/kg/day
12 to 16 years	18 mg/kg/day
> 16 years	13 mg/kg/day

[1] Not to exceed listed dose or 900 mg, whichever is less.

Exercise caution in younger children who cannot complain of minor side effects. Older adults and those with cor pulmonale, CHF or liver disease may have unusually low dosage requirements; they may experience toxicity at the maximal dosages recommended.

Measurement of serum theophylline concentrations during chronic therapy is recommended. The table below provides guidance to dosage adjustments based on serum theophylline level determinations:

Dosage Adjustment After Serum Theophylline Measurement		
If serum theophylline is:		Directions
Too low	5 to 10 mcg/ml	Increase dose by about 25% at 3 day intervals until either the desired clinical response or serum concentration is achieved.[1]
Within desired range	10 to 20 mcg/ml	Maintain dosage if tolerated. Recheck serum theophylline concentration at 6 to 12 month intervals.[2]
Too high	20 to 25 mcg/ml	Decrease doses by about 10%. Recheck serum theophylline concentration after 3 days.[2]
	25 to 30 mcg/ml	Skip next dose and decrease subsequent doses by 25%. Recheck serum theophylline after 3 days.
	> 30 mcg/ml	Skip next 2 doses and decrease subsequent doses by 50%. Recheck serum theophylline after 3 days.

[1] The total daily dose may need to be administered at more frequent intervals if asthma symptoms occur repeatedly at the end of a dosing interval.
[2] Finer adjustments in dosage may be needed for some patients.

Timed release capsules – These dosage forms gradually release the active medication so that the total daily dosage may be administered in 1 to 3 doses divided by 8 to 24 hours, depending on the patient's pharmacokinetic profile, thus reducing the number of daily doses required. These products are not necessarily interchangeable. If patients are switched from one brand to another, closely monitor their theophylline serum levels; serum concentrations may vary greatly following brand interchange.

OXTRIPHYLLINE:

Adults – 4.7 mg/kg every 8 hours.

Children (9 to 16 years) and adult smokers – 4.7 mg/kg every 6 hours.

Children (1 to 9 years) – 6.2 mg/kg every 6 hours.

Sustained action – If total daily maintenance dosage is established at approximately 800 or 1200 mg, 1 sustained action tablet every 12 hours may be substituted.

THEOPHYLLINE and DEXTROSE: Substitute oral therapy for IV theophylline as soon as adequate improvement is achieved.

Children – Due to marked variation in theophylline metabolism, use this drug only if clearly needed in infants < 6 months of age.

AMINOPHYLLINE:

IV – The loading dose may be infused into 100 to 200 ml of 5% Dextrose Injection or 0.9% Sodium Chloride Injection. Do not exceed 25 mg/min infusion rate.

Parenteral administration – Inject aminophylline slowly, not more than 25 mg/min, when given IV. Substitute oral therapy for IV aminophylline as soon as adequate improvement is achieved.

Loading dose:

In patients currently not receiving theophylline products – 6 mg/kg.

In patients currently receiving theophylline products – Each 0.5 mg/kg theophylline (0.6 mg/kg aminophylline) will increase the serum theophylline concentration by approximately 1 mcg/ml. When respiratory distress warrants a small risk, 2.5 mg/kg theophylline (3.1 mg aminophylline IV) increases serum concentration by approximately 5 mcg/ml. If the patient is not experiencing theophylline toxicity, this is unlikely to result in dangerous side effects.

Maintenance infusions – Administer by a large volume infusion to deliver the desired amount of drug each hour.

Aminophylline Maintenance Infusion Rates (mg/kg/hr)		
Patient Group	First 12 hours	Beyond 12 hours
Neonates to infants < 6 months	Not recommended	
Children 6 months to 9 years	1.2	1
Children ages 9 to 16 and young adult smokers	1	0.8
Otherwise healthy nonsmoking adults	0.7	0.5
Older patients and those with cor pulmonale	0.6	0.3
Patients with CHF, liver disease	0.5	0.1-0.2

DYPHYLLINE: Dyphylline is a derivative of theophylline; it is not a theophylline salt, and is not metabolized to theophylline in vivo. Although dyphylline is 70% theophylline by molecular weight ratio, the amount of dyphylline equivalent to a given amount of theophylline is not known. Specific dyphylline serum levels may be used to monitor therapy; serum theophylline levels will NOT measure dyphylline. The minimal effective therapeutic concentration is 12 mcg/ml.

Oral –

Adults: Up to 15 mg/kg every 6 hours.

IM – (Not for IV administration.)

Adults: 250 to 500 mg injected slowly every 6 hours. Do not exceed 15 mg/kg every 6 hours.

Children: Safety and efficacy have not been established.

ANTIHISTAMINES

DIPHENHYDRAMINE HCl	
Capsules: 25 and 50 mg (*otc/Rx*)	Various, *Benadryl* (Warner Wellcome), *Benadryl Allergy* (Warner Wellcome)
Tablets: 25 and 50 mg (*otc/Rx*)	Various, *Benadryl 25* (Warner Wellcome), *Benadryl Allergy* (Warner Wellcome)
Tablets, chewable: 12.5 mg (*otc*)	*Benadryl Allergy* (Warner Wellcome)
Liquid: 6.25 mg/5 ml and 12.5 mg/5 ml (*otc*)	*Scot-Tussin Allergy Relief Formula* (Scot-Tussin), *Benadryl Allergy* (Warner Wellcome), *Benadryl Allergy Dye-Free* (Warner Wellcome)
Elixir: 12.5 mg/5 ml (*otc/Rx*)	Various, *Benadryl* (Warner Wellcome), *Siladryl* (Silarx)
Syrup: 12.5 mg/5 ml (*otc/Rx*)	Various, *Benylin Cough* (Warner Wellcome)
Injection: 10 mg/ml and 50 mg/ml (*Rx*)	Various, *Benadryl* (Warner Wellcome)
CLEMASTINE FUMARATE	
Tablets: 1.34 mg (*otc/Rx*[1])	Various, *Tavist-1* (Sandoz)
Tablets: 2.68 mg (*Rx*)	Various, *Tavist* (Sandoz)
Syrup: 0.67 mg/5 ml (*Rx*)	Various, *Tavist* (Sandoz)
TRIPELENNAMINE HCl	
Tablets: 25 and 50 mg (*Rx*)	Various, *PBZ* (Geigy)
Tablets, sustained release: 100 mg (*Rx*)	*PBZ-SR* (Geigy)
Elixir: 37.5 mg tripelennamine citrate (equiv. to 25 mg HCl)/5 ml (*Rx*)	*PBZ* (Geigy)
PYRILAMINE MALEATE	
Tablets: 25 mg (*otc*)	Various
CHLORPHENIRAMINE MALEATE	
Tablets, chewable: 2 mg (*otc*)	*Chlo-Amine* (Hollister-Stier)
Tablets: 4, 8 and 12 mg (*otc/Rx*)	Various, *Chlor-Trimeton Allergy* (Schering-Plough)
Tablets, timed release: 8 and 12 mg (*otc/Rx*)	Various, *Chlor-Trimeton 8 Hour Allergy*, *Chlor-Trimeton 12 Hour Allergy* (Schering-Plough)
Tablets, extended release: 16 mg (*otc*)	*Efidac 24 Chlorpheniramine* (Ciba)
Capsules: 12 mg (*otc*)	Various
Capsules, timed release: 8 and 12 mg (*otc/Rx*)	Various, *Teldrin* (SmithKline Consumer)
Liquid: 1 mg/5 ml (*otc*)	*Pedia Care Allergy Formula* (McNeil-CPC)
Syrup: 2 mg/5 ml (*otc/Rx*)	Various, *Chlor-Trimeton* (Schering)
Injection: 10 mg/ml and 100 mg/ml (*Rx*)	Various, *Chlor-Trimeton* (Schering)
DEXCHLORPHENIRAMINE	
Tablets: 2 mg (*Rx*)	*Polaramine* (Schering)
Tablets, timed release: 4 and 6 mg (*Rx*)	Various, *Polaramine* (Schering)
Syrup: 2 mg/5 ml (*Rx*)	*Polaramine* (Schering)
BROMPHENIRAMINE MALEATE	
Tablets: 4, 8 and 12 mg (*otc/Rx*)	Various, *Dimetane* (Robins)
Tablets, timed release: 8 and 12 mg (*otc/Rx*)	*Dimetane Extentabs* (Robins)
Elixir: 2 mg/5 ml (*otc*)	Various, *Dimetane* (Robins)
Injection: 10 mg/ml (*Rx*)	Various, *ND Stat* (Hyrex)
TRIPROLIDINE HCL	
Syrup: 1.25 mg/5 ml (*Rx*)	Various
PROMETHAZINE HCl	
Tablets: 12.5, 25 and 50 mg (*Rx*)	Various, *Phenergan* (Wyeth-Ayerst)
Syrup: 6.25 mg/5 ml, 25 mg/5 ml (*Rx*)	Various, *Phenergan Plain*, *Phenergan Fortis* (Wyeth-Ayerst)
Suppositories: 12.5, 25 and 50 mg (*Rx*)	Various, *Phenergan* (Wyeth-Ayerst)
Injection: 25 mg/ml, 50 mg/ml (*Rx*)	Various, *Phenergan* (Wyeth-Ayerst), *Anergan 50* (Forest)
METHDILAZINE HCl	
Tablets, chewable: 4 mg (*Rx*)	*Tacaryl* (Westwood-Squibb)
Tablets: 8 mg (*Rx*)	*Tacaryl* (Westwood-Squibb)
Syrup: 4 mg/5 ml (*Rx*)	*Tacaryl* (Westwood-Squibb)
CYPROHEPTADINE HCl	
Tablets: 4 mg (*Rx*)	Various, *Periactin* (Merck)
Syrup: 2 mg/5 ml (*Rx*)	Various, *Periactin* (Merck)
AZATADINE MALEATE	
Tablets: 1 mg (*Rx*)	*Optimine* (Schering)

PHENINDAMINE TARTRATE
Tablets: 25 mg (*Rx*) — *Nolahist* (Carnrick)

ASTEMIZOLE
Tablets: 10 mg (*Rx*) — *Hismanal* (Janssen)

LORATADINE
Tablets: 10 mg (*Rx*) — *Claritin* (Schering)

CETIRIZINE HCl
Tablets: 5 and 10 mg (*Rx*) — *Zyrtec* (Pfizer)
Syrup: 5 mg/ml (*Rx*) — *Zyrtec* (Pfizer)

FEXOFENADINE HCl
Capsules: 60 mg (*Rx*) — *Allegra* (Hoechst-Marion Roussel)

AZELASTINE HCl
Nasal spray: 125 mcg (as HCl)/spray (*Rx*) — *Astelin* (Wallace Laboratories)

HYDROXYZINE
Tablets: 10, 25, 50 and 100 mg (*Rx*) — Various, *Atarax* (Pfizer)
Capsules: 25, 50 and 100 mg (*Rx*) — Various, *Vistaril* (Pfizer)
Syrup: 10 mg/5ml (*Rx*) — Various, *Atarax* (Pfizer)
Oral suspension: 25 mg/5 ml (*Rx*) — *Vistaril* (Pfizer)
Injection: 25 mg/ml and 50 mg/ml (*Rx*) — Various, *Vistaril* (Pfizer)

Warning:
Astemizole:
QT interval prolongation/ventricular arrhythmias – Rare cases of serious cardiovascular adverse events, including death, cardiac arrest, torsades de pointes and other ventricular arrhythmias, have been observed in the following clinical settings, frequently in association with increased (including metabolite) levels which lead to electrocardiographic QT prolongation:

1.) Overdose including single doses as low as 20 to 30 mg/day, and in a few patients with augmenting circumstances at 10 mg/day. Do not exceed recommended dose.
2.) Significant hepatic dysfunction (concurrent use contraindicated).
3.) Concomitant administration of erythromycin, clarithromycin, troleandomycin, quinine, ketoconazole or itraconazole (concurrent use contraindicated).

Episodes of syncope may precede severe arrhythmias. If syncope occurs with astemizole, discontinue treatment and evaluate potential arrhythmias. Evaluate ECG for QT prolongation and ventricular arrhythmias.

Actions:
Pharmacology:

Antihistamines: Dosage and Effects

Antihistamine	Dose[1] (mg)	Dosing interval[2] (hrs)	Sedative effects	Antihistaminic activity	Anticholinergic activity	Antiemetic effects
First-Generation (non-selective)						
Ethanolamines						
Clemastine	1	12	++	+ to ++	+++	++ to +++
Diphenhydramine	25 to 50	6 to 8	+++	+ to ++	+++	++ to +++
Ethylenediamines						
Tripelennamine	25 to 50	4 to 6	++	+ to ++	±	—
Alkylamines						
Brompheniramine	4	4 to 6	+	+++	++	—
Chlorpheniramine	4	4 to 6	+	++	++	—
Dexchlorpheniramine	2	4 to 6	+	+++	++	—
Phenothiazines						
Promethazine	12.5 to 25	6 to 24	+++	+++	+++	++++
Piperazines						
Hydroxyzine	25 to 100	4 to 8	+++	++ to +++	++	+++
Piperidines						
Azatadine	1 to 2	12	++	++	++	—
Cyproheptadine	4	8	+	++	++	—
Phenindamine	25	4 to 6	±	++	++	—

Antihistamines: Dosage and Effects						
Antihistamine	Dose[1] (mg)	Dosing interval[2] (hrs)	Sedative effects	Antihistaminic activity	Anticholinergic activity	Antiemetic effects
Phthalazinone						
Azelastine[3]	0.5	12	±	++ to +++	±	—
Second-Generation (peripherally selective)						
Piperazine						
Cetirizine	5 to 10	24	±	++ to +++	±	—
Piperidines						
Astemizole	10	24	±	++ to +++	±	—
Fexofenadine	60	12	±	—	±	—
Loratadine	10	24	±	++ to +++	±	—

* ++++ = very high, +++ = high, ++ = moderate, + = low, ± = low to none. — = No data.
[1] Usual single adult dose. [2]For conventional dosage forms. [3]Some effects may be enhanced or reduced as a result of administration via the nasal route.

Antihistamines competitively antagonize histamine at the H_1 receptor site, but do not bind with histamine to inactivate it. Antihistamines do not block histamine release, antibody production or antigen-antibody interactions. They antagonize in varying degrees most pharmacological effects of histamine. Most also have anticholinergic (drying), antipruritic and sedative effects. Antihistamines with predominant sedative effects are used as nonprescription sleep aids. Cyproheptadine and azatadine also have antiserotonin activity. Antihistamines with antiemetic effects are useful in management of nausea, vomiting and motion sickness. Conversely, GI upset is a frequent side effect of the ethylenediamines.

Although common cold symptoms might be modified by antihistamines, they do not prevent or cure colds, nor do they shorten the course of the disease.

Switching from one class of antihistamine to another may restore responsiveness when a patient becomes refractory to the effects of a particular agent.

Pharmacokinetics:

Pharmacokinetics of first-generation agents have not been extensively studied. With a few exceptions, these agents are well absorbed following oral administration, have an onset of action within 15 to 30 minutes, are maximal within 1 to 2 hours and have a duration of about 4 to 6 hours, although some are much longer acting. Most are metabolized by liver. Antihistamine metabolites and small amounts of unchanged drug are excreted in urine. Small amounts may be excreted in breast milk.

Second-generation agents – The pharmacokinetics of the second-generation agents have been studied more thoroughly and are provided in the table below.

Pharmacokinetics of Peripherally Selective H_1 Antagonists						
	Onset of action	T_{max} (hours)	Elimination t½ (hours)	Protein binding (%)	P450 metabolism	Food effect on absorption
Astemizole	slow	672-1344[1]	168-264[2]	97	⬆; 3A4	decreased 60%
Cetirizine	rapid	1	8.3	93	⬇; 50% excreted unchanged	delayed 1.7 hours
Fexofenadine	rapid	2.6	14.4	60-70	⬇⬇; 95% excreted unchanged	—
Loratadine	rapid	1.3-2.5[2]	8.4-28[2]	97 (75)[3]	⬆; 3A4, 2D6	delayed 1 hour

⬆ = High ⬇ = Low ⬇⬇ = Very low
[1] Steady-state plasma levels of parent drug and active metabolites were reached within 4 to 8 weeks. While peak levels of the unchanged drug were reached within 1 hour, these levels were low because of extensive metabolism and significant tissue distribution.
[2] All active constituents (parent drug and active metabolites)
[3] Active metabolite
— = No data

Indications:

Oral: Symptomatic relief of symptoms associated with: Perennial and seasonal allergic rhinitis; vasomotor rhinitis; allergic conjunctivitis; temporary relief of runny nose and sneezing due to the common cold; allergic and non-allergic pruritic symptoms; mild, uncomplicated urticaria and angioedema; amelioration of allergic reactions to blood or plasma; dermatographism; adjunctive therapy in anaphylactic reactions; idiopathic chronic urticaria; lacrimation.

Parenteral: Amelioration of allergic reactions to blood or plasma; in anaphylaxis as an adjunct to epinephrine and other measures; for other uncomplicated allergic conditions of the immediate type when oral therapy is not possible.

Diphenhydramine: In addition to the general uses, diphenhydramine is indicated for active and prophylactic treatment of motion sickness; as a nighttime sleep aid (oral only); for parkinsonism (including drug-induced) in the elderly intolerant of more potent agents, for mild cases in other age groups and in combination with centrally acting anticholinergics; as a nonnarcotic cough suppressant (syrup only).

Promethazine: In addition to uses discussed in the general monograph, promethazine is indicated for: Active and prophylactic treatment of motion sickness; preoperative, postoperative or obstetric sedation; prevention and control of nausea and vomiting associated with anesthesia and surgery; an adjunct to analgesics for control of postoperative pain; sedation and relief of apprehension, and to produce light sleep; antiemetic effect in postoperative patients.

IV – Special surgical situations such as repeated bronchoscopy, ophthalmic surgery, poor risk patients and with reduced amounts of meperidine or other narcotic analgesics as an adjunct to anesthesia and analgesia.

Cyproheptadine: In addition to the general uses discussed in the antihistamine monograph, cyproheptadine is also indicated for hypersensitivity reactions, Type I.

Hydroxyzine: In addition to uses discussed in the general monograph, hydroxyzine is indicated for: Sedation (oral only); analgesia, adjunctive therapy (parenteral only); antiemetic (parenteral only); used for management of anxiety, tension and psychomotor agitation in conditions of emotional stress.

Unlabeled uses: One study suggested the combination of an H_1 and H_2 antagonist may be useful in patients with chronic idiopathic urticaria who do not adequately respond to an H_1 antagonist alone.

Cyproheptadine has been used with variable success to stimulate appetite in those with anorexia nervosa and for cachexia associated with cancer. It has also been used to treat vascular cluster headaches.

Contraindications:

Hypersensitivity to antihistamines; newborn or premature infants; nursing mothers; narrow-angle glaucoma; stenosing peptic ulcer; symptomatic prostatic hypertrophy; asthma attack; bladder neck obstruction; pyloro-duodenal obstruction; monoamine oxidase inhibitor (MAOI) use; lower respiratory tract symptoms (including asthma).

Phenothiazine antihistamines (promethazine and methdilazine): Comatose patients; CNS depression from barbiturates, general anesthetics, tranquilizers, alcohol, narcotics or narcotic analgesics; previous phenothiazine idiosyncrasy, jaundice or bone marrow depression; acutely ill or dehydrated children because there is greater susceptibility to dystonias.

Second-generation antihistamines: Hypersensitivity to specific or structurally related antihistamines. The use of **astemizole** is contraindicated in significant hepatic dysfunction and concomitant erythromycin, clarithromycin, troleandomycin, quinine, ketoconazole or itraconazole therapy.

Warnings:

Cardiovascular effects: Cases of torsades de pointes have been reported following **astemizole** use. It is possible that terfenadine, but not its metabolite, has quinidine-like actions that may induce arrhythmias.

Respiratory disease: In general, antihistamines are not recommended to treat *lower* respiratory tract symptoms including asthma, as their anticholinergic (drying) effects may cause thickening of secretions and impair expectoration.

QT prolongation syndrome: **Astemizole** can potentially prolong the QT interval. Avoid use of these agents in patients with QT prolongation syndrome with concomitant medications reported to prolong QT intervals or in patients with hypokalemia or hypomagnesemia (including concomitant diuretics with the potential for causing these electrolyte imbalances).

Promethazine may lower the seizure threshold.

Sedatives/CNS depressants: Avoid sedatives and CNS depressants in patients with a history of sleep apnea.

Pre- and postoperative adjunctive therapy: Nonselective antihistamines may potentiate CNS depressants, such as narcotics, nonnarcotic analgesics and barbiturates. Narcotic requirements may be reduced by as much as 50%. Reduce dosage appropriately when using antihistamines as pre- and postsurgical adjunctive therapy.

Hypersensitivity reactions may occur, and any of the usual manifestations of drug allergy may develop.

Hepatic function impairment: Use caution in patients with cirrhosis or other liver diseases. **Astemizole** is contraindicated in patients with significant hepatic dysfunction (see Warning Box). Use a lower initial dose of loratadine (10 mg every other day).

Elderly: Antihistamines are more likely to cause dizziness, excessive sedation, syncope, toxic confusional states and hypotension in elderly patients. Dosage reduction may be required. Phenothiazine side effects are more prone to develop in the elderly.

Pregnancy: (*Category B – chlorpheniramine, dexchlorpheniramine, brompheniramine, cetirizine, diphenhydramine, cyproheptadine, clemastine, azatadine, loratadine. Category C – astemizole, azelastine, promethazine, hydroxyzine*). Do not use during the third trimester; newborn and premature infants may have severe reactions (eg, convulsions).

Lactation: Qualitative tests have documented the excretion of **diphenhydramine, cetirizine, pyrilamine** and **tripelennamine** in breast milk. **Loratadine** and its metabolite pass easily into breast milk and achieve concentrations that are equivalent to plasma levels with an AUC milk/AUC plasma ratio of 1.17 and 0.85, respectively. Due to the higher risk of adverse effects for infants generally, and for newborns and prematures in particular, antihistamine therapy is contraindicated in nursing mothers.

Children: Antihistamines may diminish mental alertness; conversely, they may occasionally produce excitation, particularly in the young child.

Avoid using **phenothiazines** in children with hepatic diseases, Reye's syndrome, a history of sleep apnea or a family history of sudden infant death syndrome (SIDS).

Precautions:

Hematologic: Use **promethazine** with caution in bone marrow depression. Leukopenia and agranulocytosis have been reported, usually when used with other toxic agents.

Anticholinergic effects: Antihistamines have varying degrees of atropine-like actions; use with caution in patients with a predisposition to urinary retention, history of bronchial asthma, increased intraocular pressure, hyperthyroidism, cardiovascular disease or hypertension. Antihistamines may thicken bronchial secretions due to anticholinergic (drying) properties and may inhibit expectoration and sinus drainage.

Phenothiazines: Use phenothiazines with caution in patients with cardiovascular disease, liver dysfunction or ulcer disease. Promethazine has been associated with cholestatic jaundice.

Use cautiously in persons with acute or chronic respiratory impairment, particularly children, since phenothiazines may suppress the cough reflex. If hypotension occurs, epinephrine is not recommended since phenothiazines may reverse its usual pressor effect and cause a paradoxical further lowering of blood pressure. Since these drugs have an antiemetic action, they may obscure signs of intestinal obstruction, brain tumor or overdosage of toxic drugs.

Parenteral use: Do not give **promethazine** intra-arterially because of possible severe arteriospasm and resultant gangrene. Do not give SC; chemical irritation and necrotic lesions have resulted.

Hazardous tasks: May cause drowsiness and reduce mental alertness; patients should not drive or perform other tasks requiring alertness, coordination or physical dexterity. Astemizole, loratadine and fexofenadine appear to cause less sedation.

Photosensitivity: Photosensitization may occur.

Drug Interactions:

Drugs that may affect antihistamines include MAO inhibitors. Drugs that may affect antihistamines, specifically astemizole and loratadine, include azole antifungals, fluconazole, itraconazole, ketoconazole, miconazole, cimetidine and macrolide antibiotics. Drugs that may be affected by antihistamines include MAO inhibitors, alcohol and CNS depressants.

See the Antipsychotic Agents monograph for drug interactions that relate to the three phenothiazine antihistamines: Promethazine, trimeprazine and methdilazine.

Drug/Lab test interactions: **Diagnostic pregnancy tests** based on immunological reactions between HCG and anti-HCG may result in false-negative or false-positive interpretations in patients on promethazine. Increased **blood glucose** has occurred in promethazine patients.

In patients on phenothiazines, the following have occurred: Increased **serum cholesterol, blood glucose, spinal fluid protein** and **urinary urobilinogen levels;** decreased **protein bound iodine (PBI);** false-positive **urine bilirubin tests;** interference with **urinary ketone determinations, pregnancy tests** and **steroid determinations.**

Discontinue antihistamines about 4 days prior to **skin testing procedures;** these drugs may prevent or diminish otherwise positive reactions to dermal reactivity indicators.

Drug/Food interactions: **Astemizole** absorption is reduced by 60% when taken with food. Take at least 2 hours after or 1 hour before a meal. In a single-dose study, food increased the AUC of **loratadine** by ≈ 40% and the metabolite by ≈ 15%. Although not expected to be clinically important, take on an empty stomach.

Systemic absorption of **cetirizine** was delayed by 1.7 hours, and peak plasma levels were decreased by 23%. However, cetirizine may be taken with or without food.

Adverse Reactions:

Adverse reactions may include: Peripheral, angioneurotic and laryngeal edema; dermatitis; asthma; lupus erythematosus-like syndrome; urticaria; drug rash; postural hypotension; palpitations; bradycardia; tachycardia; faintness; increases and decreases in blood pressure; drowsiness (often transient); sedation; dizziness; headache (loratadine); disturbed coordination; dry mouth, nose, throat; weight gain, appetite increase (astemizole); epigastric distress, especially ethylenediamines; urinary frequency; dysuria; urinary retention; anemias; thrombocytopenia; leukopenia; agranulocytosis; pancytopenia; thickening of bronchial secretions; tingling, heaviness and weakness of the hands; bitter taste, eye pain/tearing, sneezing (nasal spray).

Administration and Dosage:

DIPHENHYDRAMINE HCl:

Oral –

Adults: 25 to 50 mg every 4 to 8 hours.

Children (over 10 kg): 12.5 to 25 mg 3 or 4 times daily or 5 mg/kg/day or 150 mg/m^2/day. Maximum daily dosage is 300 mg.

In motion sickness, give full dosage for prophylactic use; give the first dose 30 minutes before exposure to motion and similar doses before meals and at bedtime for the duration of exposure.

Parenteral – Administer IV or deeply IM.

Adults: 10 to 50 mg; 100 mg if required; maximum daily dosage is 400 mg.

Children: 5 mg/kg/day or 150 mg/m^2/day. Maximum daily dosage is 300 mg divided into 4 doses.

Nighttime sleep aid –

Adults and children ≥ 12: 50 mg at bedtime.

Antitussive (syrup only) –

Adults: 25 mg (10 ml) every 4 hours, not to exceed 100 mg (40 ml) in 24 hours.

Children:

6 to 12 – 12.5 mg (5 ml) every 4 hours, not to exceed 50 mg (20 ml) in 24 hours.

2 to 6 – 6.25 mg (2.5 ml) every 4 hours, not to exceed 25 mg (10 ml) in 24 hours.

CLEMASTINE FUMARATE:

Allergic rhinitis –

Adults: 1.34 mg twice daily. Do not exceed 8.04 mg daily.

Children (6 to 12 years) (syrup only): 0.67 mg twice daily. Do not exceed 4.02 mg daily.

Urticaria/angioedema –

Adults: 2.68 mg 1 to 3 times daily. Do not exceed 8.04 mg daily.

Children (6 to 12 years) (syrup only): 1.34 mg twice daily. Do not exceed 4.02 mg daily.

TRIPELENNAMINE HCl –

Tablets and elixir:

Adults – 25 to 50 mg every 4 to 6 hours. As little as 25 mg may control symptoms; as much as 600 mg daily may be given in divided doses.

Children and infants – 5 mg/kg/day or 150 mg/m^2/day divided into 4 to 6 doses. Maximum total dose is 300 mg/day.

Extended release tablets:

Adults – 100 mg in the morning and evening. In difficult cases, 100 mg every 8 hours may be required. Do not crush or chew extended release tablets.

Children – Do not use in children.

CHLORPHENIRAMINE MALEATE:

Tablets or syrup –

Adults and children over 12: 4 mg every 4 to 6 hours. Do not exceed 24 mg in 24 hours.

Children:

6 to 12 – 2 mg every 4 to 6 hours. Do not exceed 12 mg in 24 hours.

2 to 6 – 1 mg every 4 to 6 hours. Do not exceed 4 mg in 24 hours.

Timed release forms:

Adults (12 years and older) – 8 to 12 mg at bedtime or every 8 to 12 hours during the day. Do not exceed 24 mg in 24 hours.

Parenteral: For IM or SC use only, avoid IV or intradermal administration.

Adults and children ≥ 12 years – 10 to 20 mg for amelioration of allergic reactions to blood or plasma or as adjunctive anaphylactic therapy; 5 to 20 mg for other uncomplicated allergic conditions of the immediate type when oral therapy is contraindicated. The maximum recommended dose is 40 mg in a 24-hour period.

DEXCHLORPHENIRAMINE MALEATE:

Adults (12 and older) – 2 mg every 4 to 6 hours, or 4 to 6 mg timed release tablets at bedtime, or ever 8 to 10 hours during the day.

Children –

6 to 11 years: 1 mg every 4 to 6 hours or a 4 mg timed release tablet once daily at bedtime.

2 to 5 years: 0.5 mg every 4 to 6 hours. Do not use timed release form.

BROMPHENIRAMINE MALEATE:

Allergic rhinitis (oral) –

Adults (12 and older): 4 mg every 4 to 6 hours. Do not exceed 24 mg in 24 hours.

Hypersensitivity, Type I (parenteral) – Give IM or SC without dilution. Give IV, either undiluted or diluted 1 to 10 with Sterile Saline for Injection. Administer IV slowly, preferably to recumbent patient.

Adults: Usual dose, 10 mg (range 5 to 20 mg) twice daily. Duration of action, 3 to 12 hours. Maximum dose is 40 mg/24 hours.

Children (< 12 years): 0.5 mg/kg/day or 15 mg/m^2/day, in 3 or 4 divided doses.

PROMETHAZINE HCl: The preferred parenteral route of administration is deep IM injection; properly administered IV doses are well tolerated, but this method is associated with increased hazard. IV administration should be ≤ 25 mg/ml at a rate ≤ 25 mg/min. Avoid SC and intra-arterial injection because tissue necrosis and gangrene can result.

Individualize dosage; after initiation, adjust to smallest effective dose.

Hypersensitivity reactions, Type I –

Oral/Rectal: May be administered rectally or parenterally if the oral route is not feasible; however, resume oral administration as soon as possible if continued therapy is warranted.

Adults – Usual dose is 25 mg at bedtime; 12.5 mg before meals and at bedtime may be given, if necessary.

Children (> 2 years) – Single 25 mg dose at bedtime or 6.25 to 12.5 mg 3 times daily.

Parenteral:

Adults – 25 mg; may repeat dose within 2 hours if needed. Resume oral therapy as soon as patient's circumstances permit.

Children (2 to 12 years) – ≤ 12.5 mg; dose should not exceed half the adult dose.

Sedation –

Oral/Rectal: If used for preoperative sedation, administer the night before surgery to relieve apprehension and produce quiet sleep.

Adults – 25 to 50 mg at bedtime.

Children (> 2 years) – 12.5 to 25 mg at bedtime.

Parenteral:

Adults – 25 to 50 mg at bedtime for nighttime sedation. May be combined with hypnotic agents for pre- and postoperative sedation; reduce concomitant hypnotic, analgesic and barbiturate dosage accordingly. Doses of 50 mg provide sedation and relieve apprehension during early stages of labor. Do not exceed 100 mg/24 hours for patients in labor.

Children (2 to 12 years) – Do not exceed half the adult dose.

Antiemetic –

Oral/Rectal:

Adults – Usual dose is 25 mg; doses of 12.5 to 25 mg may be repeated every 4 to 6 hours as needed for prophylaxis or treatment of active nausea/vomiting.

Children (> 2 years) – Usual dose is 25 mg or 0.5 mg/lb; doses of 12.5 to 25 mg may be repeated every 4 to 6 hours as needed for prophylaxis or treatment of active nausea/vomiting. Adjust dose to the age, weight and severity of condition for the patient being treated.

Parenteral:

Adults – Usual dose is 12.5 to 25 mg, may repeat every 4 hours as needed. If used postoperatively, reduce doses of concomitant hypnotics, analgesics or barbiturates accordingly.

Children (2 to 12 years) – Do not exceed half the adult dose. Do not use when etiology of vomiting is unknown.

Motion sickness (oral and rectal only) –

Adults: Usual dose is 25 mg twice daily; take first dose 30 to 60 minutes before anticipated travel; repeat 8 to 12 hours later if needed. On successive travel days, take on rising and again before the evening meal.

Children (> 2 years): 12.5 to 25 mg twice daily.

Analgesia – As an adjunct to pre- and postoperative medications.

Oral/Rectal:

Adults – 50 mg administered with an equal amount of meperidine and an appropriate dose of belladonna alkaloid.

Children (> 2 years) – 0.5 mg/lb in combination with an equal dose of meperdine and an atropine-like agent as appropriate.

Parenteral:

Adults – 25 to 50 mg in combination with appropriately reduced doses of analgesics and hypnotics; administer atropine-like drugs as appropriate.

Children (2 to 12 years) – 0.5 mg/lb in combination with an equal dose of analgesic or barbiturate and an appropriate dose of an atropine-like agent.

CYPROHEPTADINE HCl:

Adults – 4 to 20 mg daily. Initiate therapy with 4 mg 3 times daily. A majority of patients require 12 to 16 mg per day and occasionally as much as 32 mg per day. Do not exceed 0.5 mg/kg/day (0.23 mg/lb/day).

Children – Calculate total daily dosage as approximately 0.25 mg/kg (0.11 mg/lb) or 8 mg/m^2.

Children (7 to 14 years): 4 mg 2 or 3 times daily. Do not exceed 16 mg/day.

Children (2 to 6 years): 2 mg 2 or 3 times daily. Do not exceed 12 mg/day.

AZATADINE MALEATE:

Adults and children > 12 years – 1 or 2 mg twice a day.

PHENINDAMINE TARTRATE:

Adults and children > 12 years – 25 mg every 4 to 6 hours. Do not exceed 150 mg in 24 hours.

Children (6 to < 11 years) – 12.5 mg every 4 to 6 hours. Do not exceed 75 mg in 24 hours.

ASTEMIZOLE:

Adults and children ≥ 12 years of age – 10 mg daily. Do not exceed the recommended dose.

Take on an empty stomach at least 2 hours after or 1 hour before a meal.

Children < 6 years – 0.2 mg/kg daily.

Hepatic function impairment – Since astemizole is extensively metabolized by the liver, generally avoid use in these patients.

LORATADINE:

Adults and children ≥ 12 years of age – 10 mg once daily on an empty stomach.

Children 6 to 11 years of age – 10 mg daily.

Hepatic function impairment (GFR< 30 kg) – 10 mg every other day.

Rapidy disintegrating tablets – Place rapidly disintegrating tablets on the tongue. Tablet disintegration occurs rapidly (seconds). Dissolved tablet contents may subsequently be swallowed with or without water.

Use within 6 months of opening laminated foil pouch and immediately upon opening individual tablet blister.

CETIRIZINE HCl:

Adults and children ≥ 6 years – 5 or 10 mg once daily depending on symptom severity. May be given with or without food.

Renal/Hepatic function impairment – In patients with decreased renal function (creatine clearance 11 to 31 ml/min), hemodialysis patients (creatine clearance < 7 ml/min) and in hepatically impaired patients, 5 mg once daily is recommended.

FEXOFENADINE:

Adults and children ≥ 12 years of age – 60 mg twice daily.

Renal function impairment – 60 mg once daily as a starting dose.

AZELASTINE:

Adults and children ≥ 12 years of age – 2 sprays per nostril twice daily.

HYDROXYZINE:

Pruritus –

Oral:

Adults – 25 mg 3 or 4 times daily.

Children –

> 6 *years:* 50 to 100 mg daily in divided doses.

< 6 *years:* 50 mg daily in divided doses.

Parenteral:

Adults only – 25 to 100 mg IM as a single dose, then every 4 to 6 hours as needed.

Sedation (oral only) –

Adults: 50 to 100 mg as premedication or following general anesthesia. Hydroxyzine may potentiate concomitant narcotics and barbiturates; reduce dosages accordingly. Atropine and other belladonna alkaloids may be give as appropriate.

Children: 0.6 mg/kg.

Antiemetic/Analgesia, adjunctive therapy (parenteral only) –

Adults: 25 to 100 mg IM as pre- and postoperative and pre- and post-partum adjunctive medication to permit reduction of narcotic dosage and control emesis.

Children: 0.5 mg/lb IM as pre- and postoperative adjunctive therapy to permit reduction of narcotic dosage and control emesis.

Oral suspension – Shake vigorously until product is completely resuspended.

ZAFIRLUKAST

Tablets: 20 mg (*Rx*)	*Accolate* (Zeneca)

Actions:

Pharmacology: Zafirlukast is a selective and competitive leukotreine receptor antagonist (LTRA) of leukotreine D_4 and E_4 (LTD_4 and LTE_4), components of slow-reacting substance of anaphylaxis (SRSA). Cysteinyl leukotreine production and receptor occupation have been correlated with the pathophysiology of asthma, including airway edema, smooth muscle constriction and altered cellular activity associated with the inflammatory process, which contribute to the signs and symptoms of asthma.

Pharmacokinetics: Oral zafirlukast is rapidly absorbed. Peak plasma concentrations are achieved 3 hours after dosing. The mean terminal elimination half-life of zafirlukast is ≈ 10 hours in both healthy subjects and patients with asthma. Zafirlukast is > 99% bound to plasma proteins, predominantly albumin.

Zafirlukast is extensively metabolized. Urinary excretion accounts for ≈ 10% of the dose and the remainder is excreted in the feces. Liver microsomes that hydroxylate metabolites of zafirlukast are formed through the cytochrome P450 2C9 (CYP2C9) enzyme pathway. Zafirlukast inhibits the cytochrome P450 CYP3A4 and CYP2C9 isoenzymes.

Indications:

Asthma: Prophylaxis and chronic treatment of asthma in adults and children ≥ 12 years.

Contraindications:

Hypersensitivity to zafirlukast or any of its inactive ingredients.

Warnings:

Acute asthma attacks: Zafirlukast is not indicated for use in the reversal of bronchospasm in acute asthma attacks, including status asthmaticus. Therapy with zafirlukast can be continued during acute exacerbations of asthma.

Infection: An increased proportion of zafirlukast patients > 55 years old reported infections as compared to placebo-treated patients. These infections were mostly mild or moderate in intensity and predominantly affected the respiratory tract.

Hepatic function impairment: The clearance of zafirlukast is reduced in patients with stable alcoholic cirrhosis such that the C_{max} and AUC are ≈ 50% to 60% > than those of healthy adults.

Elderly: The clearance of zafirlukast is reduced in elderly patients (≥ 65 years old), such that C_{max} and AUC are ≈ twice those of younger adults.

Pregnancy: Category B.

Lactation: Zafirlukast is excreted in breast milk.

Children: The safety and effectiveness of zafirlukast in patients < 12 years of age have not been established.

Drug Interactions:

Due to zafirlukast's inhibition of cytochrome P450 2C9 and 3A4 isoenzymes, use caution with coadministration of drugs known to be metabolized by these isoenzymes.

Drugs that may affect zafirlukast include aspirin, erythromycin, terfenadine and theophylline.

Drugs that may be affected by zafirlukast include warfarin.

Drug/Food interactions: The bioavailability of zafirlukast may be decreased when taken with food. Take zafirlukast at least 1 hour before or 2 hours after meals.

Adverse Reactions:

Adverse reactions occurring in ≥ 3% of patients include headache, nausea, infection.

Administration and Dosage:

The recommended dose of zafirlukast is 20 mg twice daily in adults and children ≥ 12 years old. Because food reduces bioavailability of zafirlukast, take at least 1 hour before or 2 hours after meals.

MONTELUKAST SODIUM

Tablets: 10 mg (*Rx*)	*Singulair* (Merck)
Tablets, chewable: 5 mg (*Rx*)	*Singulair* (Merck)

Actions:

Pharmacology: Montelukast is a selective and orally active leukotriene receptor antagonist that inhibits the cysteinyl leukotrine ($CysLT_1$) receptor. Cysteinyl leukotrienes and leukotriene receptor occupation have been correlated with the pathophysiology of asthma, including airway edema, smooth muscle contraction and altered cellular activity associated with the inflammatory process, which contribute to the signs and symptoms of asthma. Montelukast causes inhibition of airway CysLT receptors.

Pharmacokinetics:

Absorption – Montelukast is rapidly absorbed following oral administration. After administration of the 10 mg film coated tablet to fasted adults, the mean peak plasma concentration (C_{max}) is achieved in 3 to 4 hours (T_{max}). The mean oral bioavailability is 64%. For the 5 mg chewable tablet, the mean C_{max} is achieved in 2 to 2.5 hours after administration to adults in the fasted state.

Distribution – Montelukast is > 99% bound to plasma proteins. The steady-state volume of distribution averages 8 to 11 L.

Metabolism – Montelukast is extensively metabolized. Cytochromes P450 3A4 and 2C9 are involved in the metabolism of montelukast.

Excretion – The plasma clearance of montelukast averages 45 ml/min in healthy adults. Following an oral dose, 86% was recovered in 5-day fecal collections and < 0.2% was recovered in urine. This indicates that montelukast and its metabolites are excreted almost exclusively via the bile. In several studies, the mean plasma half-life ranged from 2.7 to 5.5 hours in healthy young adults.

Indications:

Asthma: Prophylaxis and chronic treatment of asthma in adults and pediatric patients ≥ 6 years of age.

Contraindications:

Hypersensitivity to any component of this product.

Warnings:

Elderly: Plasma half-life is slightly longer in the elderly. No dosage adjustment is required.

Pregnancy: *Category B.*

Lactation: Studies in rats have shown that montelukast is excreted in milk. It is not known if montelukast is excreted in human breast milk. Exercise caution when montelukast is given to a nursing mother.

Children: Safety and efficacy in children < 6 years of age have not been established.

Precautions:

Bronchospasm: Montelukast is not indicated for use in the reversal of bronchospasm in acute asthma attacks, including status asthmaticus. Montelukast should not be used as monotherapy for the treatment and management of exercise-induced bronchospasm.

Rescue medication: Advise patients to have appropriate rescue medication available. Therapy with montelukast can be continued during acute exacerbations of asthma.

Concurrent corticosteroids: While the dose of inhaled corticosteroid may be reduced gradually under medical supervision, montelukast should not be abruptly substituted for inhaled or oral corticosteroids. Caution and appropriate clinical monitoring are recommended when systemic corticosteroid reduction is considered in patients receiving montelukast.

Aspirin sensitivity: Patients with known aspirin sensitivity should continue avoidance of aspirin or nonsteroidal anti-inflammatory agents while taking montelukast.

Drug Interactions:

Phenobarbital: Phenobarbital, which induces hepatic metabolism, decreased the AUC of montelukast ≈ 40% following a single 10 mg dose of montelukast. No dosage adjustment for montelukast is recommended. It is reasonable to employ appropriate clinical monitoring when potent cytochrome P450 enzyme inducers, such as phenobarbital or rifampin, are coadministered with montelukast.

Adverse Reactions:

Adults and adolescents ≥ 15 years of age: Headache, 18.4%; influenza, 4.2%; cough, 2.7%; abdominal pain, 2.9%.

Pediatric patients 6 to 14 years of age: The safety profile was generally similar to the adult safety profile with the exception of the following (frequency ≥ 2%): Diarrhea; laryngitis; pharyngitis; nausea; otitis; sinusitis; viral infection. With prolonged treatment, the adverse experience profile did not significantly change.

Administration and Dosage:

Adults and adolescents ≥ 15 years of age: One 10 mg tablet daily, taken in the evening.

Pediatric patients 6 to 14 years of age: One 5 mg chewable tablet daily, taken in the evening. No dosage adjustment within this age group is necessary. Safety and efficacy in pediatric patients < 6 years of age have not been established.

SALICYLATES

ASPIRIN	
Tablets, chewable: 81 mg (*otc*)	*Bayer Children's Aspirin* (Glenbrook), *St. Joseph Adult Chewable Asprin* (Schering-Plough)
Gum Tablets: 227.5 mg (*otc*)	*Aspergum* (Schering-Plough)
Tablets: 325 and 500 mg (*otc*)	Various, *Genuine Bayer Aspirin Tablets and Caplets* (Glenbrook), *Empirin* (Burroughs Wellcome), *Genprin* (Goldline), *Arthritis Foundation Pain Reliever* (McNeil-CPC), *Maximum Bayer Aspirin Tablets and Caplets* (Glenbrook), *Norwich Extra-Strength* (Procter & Gamble Pharm.)
Tablets, enteric coated: 325 mg (*otc*)	Various, *Ecotrin Tablets and Caplets* (SmithKline Beecham), *Regular Strength Bayer Enteric Coated Caplets* (Sterling Health)
Tablets, enteric coated: 81, 165, 500, 650, 975 mg (*otc*)	Various, *Bayer Low Adult Strength* (SK-Beecham), *½ Halfprin* (Kramer), *Ecotrin Maximum Strength Tablets and Caplets* (SK-Beecham), *Extra Strength Bayer Enteric 500 Aspirin* (Sterling Health), *Easprin* (Parke-Davis)
Tablets, timed release: 650 mg (*otc*)	*8-hour Bayer Timed-Release Caplets* (Glenbrook)
Tablets, controlled release: 800 mg (*Rx*)	*ZORprin* (Boots)
Suppositories: 120 mg, 200 mg, 300 mg, 600 mg (*otc*)	Various
ASPIRIN (Acetylsalicylic Acid; ASA), BUFFERED	
Tablets: 325 mg with buffers (*otc*)	Various, *Bayer Buffered Aspirin* (Sterling Health), *Magnaprin* (Rugby), *Regular Strength Ascriptin* (Rhone-Poulenc Rorer), *Bufferin* (Bristol-Myers), *Asprimox* (Invamed), *Adprin-B* (Pfeiffer), *Asprimox Extra Protection for Arthritis Pain* (Bristol-Myers), *Buffex* (Roberts Med.)
Tablets, coated: 500 mg with buffers (*otc*)	*Extra Strength Adprin-B* (Pfeiffer), *Extra Strength Bayer Plus Caplets* (Sterling Health), *Ascriptin Extra Strength* (Rhone-Poulenc Rorer), *Cama Arthritis Pain Reliever* (Sandoz), *Arthritis Pain Formula* (Whitehall)
Tablets, effervescent: 325 and 500 mg with buffers (*otc*)	*Alka-Seltzer with Aspirin, Alka-Seltzer Extra Strength with Aspirin* (Miles)
SALSALATE (Salicylsalicylic Acid)	
Capsules: 500 mg (*Rx*)	*Amigesic* (Amide), *Disalcid* (3M)
Tablets: 500 mg (*Rx*)	Various, *Disalcid* (3M), *Salflex* (Carnrick), *Salsitab* (Upsher-Smith)
Tablets: 750 mg (*Rx*)	Various, *Disalcid* (3M), *Salsitab* (Upsher-Smith), *Salflex* (Carnrick), *Marthritic* (Marnel)
SODIUM SALICYLATE	
Tablets, enteric coated: 325 mg and 650 mg (*otc*)	Various
SODIUM THIOSALICYLATE	
Injection: 50 mg per ml (*Rx*)	Various, *Rexolate* (Hyrex)
CHOLINE SALICYLATE	
Liquid: 870 mg per 5 ml (*otc*)	*Arthropan* (Purdue Frederick)
MAGNESIUM SALICYLATE	
Tablets: 325, 467, 500, 545, 580 and 600 mg (*otc*)	*Original Doan's* (Ciba Consumer), *Backache Maximum Strength Relief* (B-M Squibb), *Extra Strength Doan's* (Ciba Consumer), *Magan* (Adria), *Bayer Select Maximum Strength Backache* (Sterling Health), *Mobidin* (Ascher)
SALICYLATE COMBINATIONS	
Tablets: 500 mg salicylate (as 293 mg choline salicylate and 362 mg Mg salicylate), 750 mg salicylate (as 440 mg choline salicylate and 544 mg Mg salicylate), 1000 mg salicylate (as 587 mg choline salicylate, 725 mg Mg salicylate) (*Rx*)	*Choline Magnesium Trisalicylate* (Sidmak), *Tricosal* (Invamed), *Trilisate* (Purdue Frederick)
Liquid: 500 mg salicylate (as 293 mg choline salicylate and 362 mg Mg salicylate) per 5 ml (*Rx*)	*Trilisate* (Purdue Frederick)

Warning:
Children and teenagers should not use salicylates for chickenpox or flu symptoms before a doctor is consulted about Reye's syndrome, a rare but serious illness.

Actions:

Pharmacology: Salicylates have analgesic, antipyretic, anti-inflammatory and antirheumatic effects. The pharmacological effects of these agents are qualitatively similar. Salicylates lower elevated body temperature through vasodilation of peripheral vessels, thus enhancing dissipation of excess heat. The anti-inflammatory and analgesic activity may be mediated through inhibition of the prostaglandin synthetase enzyme complex.

Aspirin differs from the other agents in this group in that it more potently inhibits prostaglandin synthesis, has greater anti-inflammatory effects and irreversibly inhibits platelet aggregation.

Irreversible inhibition of platelet aggregation (aspirin) – Single analgesic aspirin doses prolong bleeding time. Acetylation of platelet cyclooxygenase prevents synthesis of thromboxane A_2, a prostaglandin derivative, which is a potent vasoconstrictor and inducer of platelet aggregation and platelet release reaction. Aspirin (no other salicylates) inhibits platelet aggregation for the life of the platelet (7 to 10 days).

Aspirin has shown some success as an antiplatelet agent in patients with thromboembolic disease. Low doses of aspirin inhibit platelet aggregation and may be more effective than higher doses. Larger doses inhibit cyclooxygenase in arterial walls, interfering with prostacyclin production, a potent vasodilator and inhibitor of platelet aggregation.

Pharmacokinetics:

Absorption/Distribution – Salicylates are rapidly and completely absorbed after oral use. Bioavailability is dependent on the dosage form, presence of food, gastric emptying time, gastric pH, presence of antacids or buffering agents and particle size. Bioavailability of some enteric coated products may be erratic. Food slows the absorption of salicylates. Absorption from rectal suppositories is slower, resulting in lower salicylate levels. Aspirin is partially hydrolyzed to salicylic acid during absorption and is distributed to all body tissues and fluids, including fetal tissues, breast milk and CNS. Highest concentrations are found in plasma, liver, renal cortex, heart and lungs. Protein binding of salicylates is concentration-dependent. At low therapeutic concentrations (100 mcg/ml), about 90% is bound; at higher plasma concentrations (400 mcg/ml), 76% is bound. Signs of salicylism (eg, tinnitus) occur at serum levels > 200 mcg/ml; severe toxic effects may occur at levels > 400 mcg/ml (see Adverse Reactions).

Metabolism/Excretion – Salicylic acid is eliminated by renal excretion and by oxidation and conjugation of metabolites. Aspirin has a half-life of ≈ 15 to 20 min. Salicylic acid has a half-life of 2 to 3 hrs at low doses; at higher doses, it may exceed 20 hrs. In therapeutic anti-inflammatory doses, half-life ranges from 6 to 12 hrs. Plasma salicylate levels increase disproportionately as dosage is increased. Elimination is determined by zero order kinetics. Renal excretion of unchanged drug depends upon urine pH. As urinary pH changes from 5 to 8, renal clearance of free ionized salicylate increases from 2% to 3% of amount excreted to > 80%.

Indications:

Mild to moderate pain; fever; various inflammatory conditions such as rheumatic fever, rheumatoid arthritis and osteoarthritis.

Aspirin, for reducing the risk of recurrent transient ischemic attacks (TIAs) or stroke in men who have had transient ischemia of the brain due to fibrin platelet emboli. It has not been effective in women and is of no benefit for completed strokes. To reduce the risk of death or nonfatal myocardial infarction (MI) in patients with previous infarction or unstable angina pectoris.

Unlabeled uses: Possible effect of long-term aspirin-like analgesics to prevent cataract formation is being studied. Low-dose aspirin may help prevent toxemia of pregnancy and may be beneficial in pregnant women with inadequate uteroplacental blood flow (eg, systemic lupus erythematosus).

Contraindications:

Hypersensitivity to salicylates or nonsteroidal anti-inflammatory drugs (NSAIDs). Use extreme caution in patients with history of adverse reactions to salicylates. Cross-sensitivity may exist between aspirin and other NSAIDs which inhibit prostaglandin synthesis, and aspirin and tartrazine. Aspirin cross-sensitivity does not appear to occur with sodium salicylate, salicylamide or choline salicylate. Aspirin hypersensitivity is more prevalent in those with asthma, nasal polyposis, chronic urticaria.

In hemophilia, bleeding ulcers and hemorrhagic states.

Magnesium salicylate in advanced chronic renal insufficiency due to Mg^{++} retention.

Warnings:

Otic effects: Discontinue use if dizziness, ringing in ears (tinnitus) or impaired hearing occurs. Tinnitus probably represents blood salicylic acid levels reaching or exceeding the upper limit of the therapeutic range.

Use in surgical patients: Avoid aspirin, if possible, for 1 week prior to surgery because of the possibility of post-operative bleeding.

Hypersensitivity: Aspirin intolerance, manifested by acute bronchospasm, generalized urticaria/angioedema, severe rhinitis or shock occurs in 4% to 19% of asthmatics. Symptoms occur within 3 hours after ingestion. Have epinephrine 1:1000 immediately available.

Foods may contribute to a reaction. Some foods with 6 mg/100 g salicylate include curry powder, paprika, licorice, Benedictine liqueur, prunes, raisins, tea and gherkins. A typical American diet contains 10 to 200 mg/day salicylate.

Hepatic function impairment: Use caution in liver damage, preexisting hypoprothrombinemia and vitamin K deficiency.

Pregnancy: Category D (aspirin); Category C (salsalate, magnesium salicylate). Aspirin may produce adverse maternal effects: Anemia, ante- or postpartum hemorrhage, prolonged gestation and labor. Salicylates readily cross placenta. By inhibiting prostaglandin synthesis, salicylates may cause constriction of ductus arteriosus, and, possibly, other untoward fetal effects. Maternal aspirin use during later stages of pregnancy may cause adverse fetal effects: Low birth weight, increased incidence of intracranial hemorrhage in premature infants, stillbirths, neonatal death. Salicylates may be teratogens. Avoid use during pregnancy, especially in third trimester.

Lactation: Salicylates are excreted in breast milk in low concentrations, producing peak milk levels ranging from 1.1 to 10 mcg/ml.

Children: Safety and efficacy of **magnesium salicylate** or **salsalate** have not been established. Administration of **aspirin** to children (including teenagers) with acute febrile illness has been associated with the development of Reye's syndrome. Dehydrated febrile children appear more prone to salicylate intoxication.

Precautions:

Renal effects: Use with caution in chronic renal insufficiency; aspirin may cause a transient decrease in renal function, and may aggravate chronic kidney diseases (rare).

In patients with renal impairment, take precautions when administering **magnesium salicylate.**

GI effects: Use caution in those intolerant to salicylate because of GI irritation, and in gastric ulcers, peptic ulcer, mild diabetes, gout, erosive gastritis or bleeding tendencies. **Salsalate** and **choline salicylate** may cause less GI irritation than aspirin.

Although fecal blood loss is less with enteric coated aspirin than with uncoated, give enteric coated aspirin with caution to patients with GI distress, ulcer or bleeding problems.

Hematologic effects: Aspirin interferes with hemostasis. Avoid use if patients have severe anemia, history of blood coagulation defects, or take anticoagulants.

Long-term therapy: To avoid potentially toxic concentrations, warn patients on long-term therapy not to take other salicylates (nonprescription analgesics, etc). Periodically monitor plasma salicylic acid concentrations during long-term treatment to aid maintenance of therapeutic levels (100 to 300 mcg/ml).

Salicylism may require dosage adjustment.

Controlled release aspirin, because of its relatively long onset of action, is not recommended for antipyresis or short-term analgesia. Not recommended in children > 12; contraindicated in all children with fever accompanied by dehydration.

Drug Interactions:

Drugs that may affect aspirin include activated charcoal, ammonium chloride, ascorbic acid or methionine, antacids and urinary alkalinizers, carbonic anhydrase inhibitors, corticosteroids and nizatidine. Drugs that may be affected by aspirin include alcohol, ACE inhibitors, anticoagulants (oral), beta-adrenergic blockers, heparin, loop diuretics, methotrexate, nitroglycerin, NSAIDs, probenecid and sulfinpyrazone, spironolactone, sulfonylureas and exogenous insulin and valproic acid.

Drug/Lab test interactions: Salicylates compete with thyroid hormone for binding sites on thyroid binding pre-albumin and possibly thyroid binding globulin resulting in increases in **protein bound iodine (PBI).** Salicylates probably do not interfere with T_3 resin uptake.

Serum uric acid levels are elevated by salicylate levels < 10 mg/dl and decreased by levels > 10 mg/dl.

Salicylates in moderate to large (anti-inflammatory) doses cause false-negative readings for **urine glucose** by the glucose oxidase method and false-positive readings by the copper reduction method.

Salicylates in the urine interfere with **5–HIAA** determinations by fluorescent methods, but not by the nitrosonaphthol colorimetric method.

Salicylates in the urine interact with **urinary ketone** determinations by the ferric chloride (Gerhardt) method producing a reddish color.

Large doses may decrease urinary excretion of **PSP (phenolsulfonphthalein).**

Salicylates in the urine result in falsely elevated **VMA (vanillylmandelic acid)** with most tests, but falsely decrease VMA determinations by the Pisano method.

Adverse Reactions:

GI: Nausea, dyspepsia (5% to 25%); heartburn; epigastric discomfort; anorexia; massive GI bleeding; occult blood loss. Aspirin may potentiate peptic ulcer.

Chronic aspirin use may cause a persistent iron deficiency anemia.

Dermatologic: Hives; rashes; angioedema.

Hematologic: Prolongation of bleeding time; leukopenia; thrombocytopenia; purpura; decreased plasma iron concentration; shortened erythrocyte survival time.

Miscellaneous: Fever; thirst; dimness of vision.

Mild "salicylism" may occur after repeated use of large doses and consists of dizziness, tinnitus, difficulty hearing, nausea, vomiting, diarrhea, mental confusion, CNS depression, headache, sweating, hyperventilation and lassitude. Salicylate serum concentrations correlate with pharmacological actions and adverse effects observed.

Serum Salicylate: Clinical Correlations

Serum Salicylate Concentration (mcg/ml)	Desired Effects	Adverse Effects/ Intoxication
≈ 100	Antiplatelet Antipyresis Analgesia	GI intolerance and bleeding, hypersensitivity, hemostatic defects
150-300	Anti-inflammatory	Mild salicylism
250-400	Treatment of rheumatic fever	Nausea/vomiting, hyperventilation, salicylism, flushing, sweating, thirst, headache, diarrhea and tachycardia
> 400-500		Respiratory alkalosis, hemorrhage, excitement, confusion, asterixis, pulmonary edema, convulsions, tetany, metabolic acidosis, fever, coma, cardiovascular collapse, renal and respiratory failure

Administration and Dosage:

ASPIRIN (Acetylsalicylic Acid; ASA):

Minor aches and pains – 325 to 650 mg every 4 hours as needed. Some extra strength (500 mg) products suggest 500 mg every 3 hours or 1000 mg every 6 hours.

Arthritis, other rheumatic conditions (eg, osteoarthritis) – 3.2 to 6 g/day in divided doses.

Juvenile rhematoid arthritis: 60 to 110 mg/kg/day in divided doses (every 6 to 8 hours). When starting at lower doses (eg, 60 mg/kg/day), may increase by 20 mg/kg/day after 5 to 7 days, followed by 10 mg/kg/day after another 5 to 7 days.

Maintain a serum salicylate level of 150 to 300 mcg/ml.

Acute rheumatic fever –

Adults: 5 to 8 g/day, initially.

Children: 100 mg/kg/day for 2 weeks, then decreased to 75 mg/kg/day for 4 to 6 weeks.

Therapeutic salicylate level is 150 to 300 mcg/ml.

Transient ischemic attacks in men – 1300 mg/day in divided doses (650 mg 2 times daily, or 325 mg 4 times daily). One study indicated that a dose of 300 mg/day is as effective as the larger dose and may be associated with fewer side effects.

Mycardial infarction prophylaxis – 300 or 325 mg/day. This use applies to solid oral doseforms (buffered and plain) and to buffered aspirin in solution.

Children –

Analgesic/antipyretic dosage: 10 to 15 mg/kg/dose every 4 hours (see table), up to 60 to 80 mg/kg/day.

Recommended Aspirin Dosage in Children

Age (years)	Weight lbs	Weight kg	Dosage (mg every 4 hours)	No. of 81 mg tablets (every 4 hours)	No. of 325 mg tablets (every 4 hours)
2-3	24-35	10.6-15.9	162	2	½
4-5	36-47	16-21.4	243	3	
6-8	48-59	21.5-26.8	324	4	1
9-10	60-71	26.9-32.3	405	5	
11	72-95	32.4-43.2	486	6	1½
12-14	≥ 96	≥ 43.3	648	8	2

Kawasaki disease (mucocutaneous lymph node syndrome): For acute febrile period, 80 to 180 mg/kg/day; very high doses may be needed to achieve therapeutic levels. After the fever resolves, dosage may be adjusted to 10 mg/kg/day.

ASPIRIN, BUFFERED: The addition of small amounts of antacids may decrease GI irritation and increase the dissolution and absorption rates of these products. Dosing is the same as with unbuffered aspirin.

CHOLINE SALICYLATE: Has fever GI side effects than aspirin.

Adults and children (over 12 years) – 870 mg every 3 to 4 hours; maximum 6 times/day. Rheumatoid arthritis patients may start with 5 to 10 ml, up to 4 times/day.

MAGNESIUM SALICYLATE: A sodium free salicylate derivative that may have a low incidence of GI upset. The product labeling and dosage are expressed as magnesium salicylate anhydrous. The possibility of magnesium toxicity exists in persons with renal insufficiency.

Usual dose is 650 mg every 4 hours or 1090 mg, 3 times a day. May increase to 3.6 to 4.8 g/day in 3 or 4 divided doses.

Safety and efficacy for use in children have not been established.

SALSALATE (Salicylsalicylic Acid): After absorption, the drug is partially hydrolyzed into two molecules of salicylic acid. Insoluble in gastric secretions, it is not absorbed until it reaches the small intestine.

Usual adult dose is 300 mg/day given in divided doses.

SODIUM SALICYLATE: Less effective than an equal dose of aspirin in reducing pain or fever. Patients hypersensitive to aspirin may be able to tolerate sodium salicylate. Each gram contains 6.25 mEq sodium.

Usual dose – 325 to 650 mg every 4 hours.

SODIUM THIOSALICYLATE: Intramuscular administration is preferred.

Acute gout – 100 mg every 3 to 4 hours for 2 days, then 100 mg/day until asymptomatic.

Muscular pain, musculoskeletal disturbances – 50 to 100 mg/day or on alternate days.

Rheumatic fever – 100 to 150 mg every 4 to 8 hours for 3 days, then reduce to 100 mg twice daily. Continue until patient is aymptomatic.

NONSTEROIDAL ANTI-INFLAMMATORY AGENTS

BROMFENAC SODIUM	
Capsules: 25 mg (*Rx*)	*Duract* (Wyeth-Ayerst)
FLURBIPROFEN	
Tablets: 50 and 100 mg (*Rx*)	Various, *Ansaid* (Upjohn)
FENOPROFEN	
Capsules: 200 and 300 mg (*Rx*)	Various, *Nalfon Pulvules* (Dista)
Tablets: 600 mg (*Rx*)	Various
NABUMETONE	
Tablets: 500 and 750 mg (*Rx*)	*Relafen* (SK-Beecham)
IBUPROFEN	
Tablets: 100 mg (*Rx*)	*Motrin* (McNeil)
Tablets: 200 mg (*otc*)	Various, *Advil* (Whitehall), *Motrin IB* (Upjohn), *Nuprin* (Bristol-Myers Squibb)
Tablets: 300, 400, 600 and 800 mg (*Rx*)	Various, *Motrin* (McNeil)
Tablets, chewable: 50 and 100 mg (*Rx*)	*Motrin* (McNeil)
Suspension: 100 mg/5 ml (*Rx*)	Various, *Children's Advil* (Wyeth-Ayerst)
Suspension: 100 mg/5 ml (*otc*)	*Children's Motrin* (McNeil-CPC)
Oral drops: 40 mg/ml (*Rx*)	*Children's Motrin* (McNeil)
KETOPROFEN	
Tablets: 12.5 mg (*otc*)	*Orudis KT* (Whitehall-Robins), *Actron* (Bayer)
Capsules: 25, 50 and 75 mg (*Rx*)	Various, *Orudis* (Wyeth-Ayerst)
Capsules, extended release: 100, 150 and 200 mg (*Rx*)	*Oruvail* (Wyeth-Ayerst)
PIROXICAM	
Capsules: 10 and 20 mg (*Rx*)	Various, *Feldene* (Pfizer)
NAPROXEN	
Tablets: 200, 250 and 500 mg (as naproxen sodium) (*otc, Rx*)	Various, *Aleve* (Procter & Gamble), *Anaprox* (Syntex)
Tablets: 250, 375 and 500 mg (*Rx*)	Various, *Naprosyn* (Syntex)
Tablets, delayed release: 375 and 500 mg (*Rx*)	*EC-Naprosyn* (Syntex)
Tablets, controlled release: 375 and 500 mg (as naproxen sodium) (*Rx*)	*Naprelan* (Wyeth-Ayerst)
Suspension: 125 mg/5 ml (*Rx*)	Various, *Naprosyn* (Syntex)
DICLOFENAC	
Tablets: 50 mg (as potassium) (*Rx*)	*Cataflam* (Geigy)
Tablets, delayed release (enteric coated): 25, 50 and 75 mg (as sodium) (*Rx*)	Various, *Voltaren* (Geigy)
Tablets, extended release:100 mg (*Rx*)	*Voltaren-XR* (Geigy)
INDOMETHACIN	
Capsules: 25 and 50 mg (*Rx*)	Various, *Indocin* (Merck)
Capsules, sustained release: 75 mg (*Rx*)	Various, *Indocin SR* (Merck)
Oral suspension: 25 mg per 5 ml (*Rx*)	Various, *Indocin* (Merck)
Suppositories: 125 mg/5 ml (*Rx*)	*Indocin* (Merck)
SULINDAC	
Tablets: 150 and 200 mg (*Rx*)	Various, *Clinoril* (Merck)
TOLMETIN SODIUM	
Tablets: 200 and 600 mg (*Rx*)	Various, *Tolectin 200 or 600* (McNeil Pharm.)
Capsules: 400 mg (*Rx*)	Various, *Tolectin DS* (McNeil Pharm.)
MECLOFENAMATE SODIUM	
Capsules: 50 and 100 mg (*Rx*)	Various, *Meclomen* (Parke-Davis)
MEFENAMIC ACID	
Capsules: 250 mg (*Rx*)	*Ponstel* (Parke-Davis)
ETODOLAC	
Capsules: 200 and 300 mg (*Rx*)	*Lodine* (Wyeth-Ayerst)
Tablets: 400 mg (*Rx*)	*Lodine* (Wyeth-Ayerst)
KETOROLAC	
Tablets: 10 mg (*Rx*)	*Toradol* (Syntex)
Injection: 15 and 30 mg/ml (*Rx*)	*Toradol* (Syntex)
OXAPROZIN	
Tablets: 600 mg (*Rx*)	*Daypro* (Searle)

Actions:

Pharmacology: Nonsteroidal anti-inflammatory drugs have analgesic and antipyretic activities. Major mechanism is believed to be inhibition of cyclooxygenase activity and prostaglandin synthesis.

Pharmacokinetics:

Pharmacokinetic Parameters/Maximum Dosage Recommendations of NSAIDS

NSAID	Time to peak levels (hrs)[1]	Half-life (hrs)	Analgesic action: Onset (hrs)	Analgesic action: Duration (hrs)	Antirheumatic action: Onset (days)	Antirheumatic action: Peak (weeks)	Maximum recommended daily dose (mg)
Propionic acids							
Fenoprofen	1 to 2	2 to 3	—	—	2	2 to 3	3200
Flurbiprofen	1.5	5.7	—	—	—	—	300
Ibuprofen	1 to 2	1.8 to 2.5	0.5	4 to 6	within 7	1 to 2	3200
Ketoprofen	0.5 to 2	2 to 4	—	—	—	—	300
Naproxen	2 to 4	12 to 15	1	up to 7	within 14	2 to 4	1500
Naproxen sodium	1 to 2	12 to 13	1	up to 7	within 14	2 to 4	1375
Oxaprozin	3 to 5	42 to 50	—	—	within 7	—	1800 mg
Acetic acids							
Diclofenac sodium	2 to 3	1 to 2	—	—	—	—	200
Etodolac	1 to 2	7.3	0.5	4 to 12	—	—	1200
Indomethacin	1 to 2 SR: 2 to 4	4.5 SR: 4.5 to 6	0.5	4 to 6	within 7	1 to 2	200 SR: 150
Ketorolac	0.5 to 1	2.4 to 8.6	IM: 10 min	IM: up to 6	—	—	IM: 120[2] Oral: 40
Nabumetone[3]	2.5 to 4	22.5 to 30 [4]	—	—	—	—	2000
Sulindac	2 to 4	7.8 (16.4) [4]	—	—	within 7	2 to 3	400
Tolmetin	0.5 to 1	1 to 1.5	—	—	within 7	1 to 2	2000
Fenamates (anthranilic acids)							
Meclofen-amate	0.5 to 1	2 (3.3) [5]	—	—	few days	2 to 3	400
Mefenamic acid	2 to 4	2 to 4	—	—	—	—	1000
Oxicams							
Piroxicam	3 to 5	30 to 86	1	48 to 72	7 to 12	2 to 3	20

[1] Food decreases the rate of absorption and may delay the time to peak levels.
[2] 150 mg on the first day.
[3] The active metabolite of nabumetone is an acetic acid.
[4] Half-life of active metabolite.
[5] Half-life with multiple doses.

Indications:

NSAIDs: Summary of Indications

Indications ✔-Labeled X- Unlabeled	Bromfenac	Diclofenac	Etodolac	Fenoprofen	Flurbiprofen	Ibuprofen	Indomethacin/SR	Ketoprofen	Ketorolac	Meclofenamate	Mefenamic acid	Nabumetone	Naproxin/ Naproxen Sod.	Oxaprozin	Piroxicam	Sulindac	Tolmetin
Rheumatoid arthritis		✔	X	✔	✔	✔	✔	✔		✔		✔	✔	✔	✔	✔	✔
Osteoarthritis		✔	✔	✔	✔	✔	✔	✔		✔		✔	✔	✔	✔	✔	✔
Ankylosing spondylitis		✔	X		X		✔						✔			✔	
Mild to moderate pain	✔[1]	X	✔	✔	X	✔		✔	✔	✔	✔[1]		✔				
Primary dysmenorrhea					X	✔	X	✔			✔		✔		X		
Juvenile rheumatoid arthritis		X		X		X		X					✔/		X	X	✔
Tendinitis			X		X		✔						✔			✔	
Bursitis			X		X		✔						✔			✔	
Acute painful shoulder		X	X		X		✔										
Acute gout			X		X		✔/						✔			✔	
Fever						✔							X				
Sunburn		X		X	X	X	X[2]	X		X	X		X		X	X	X
Migraine																	
Abortive (acute attack)					X					X	X		/X				
Prophylactic				X			X/	X					X				
Menstrual				X				X		X	X		X				
Cluster headache							X/										
Polyhydramnios							X/										
Acne vulgaris, resistant						X[3]											
Menorrhagia										X							
Premenstrual syndrome											X		X				
Cystoid macular edema							X[4]										
Closure of persistent patent ductus arteriosus							X[5]										

[1] If therapy will be ≤ 1 week.
[2] Topical indomethacin may prevent and treat sunburn.
[3] With tetracycline.
[4] Topical eye drops 0.5% to 1%.
[5] Indomethacin IV approved for this indication (see Agents for Patent Ductus Arteriosus).

Contraindications:

NSAID hypersensitivity: Because of potential cross-sensitivity to other NSAIDs, do not give these agents to patients in whom aspirin, iodides or other NSAIDs have induced symptoms of asthma, rhinitis, urticaria, nasal polyps, angioedema, bronchospasm and other symptoms of allergic or anaphylactoid reactions.

Fenoprofen or mefenamic acid: Preexisting renal disease.

Mefenamic acid: Active ulceration or chronic inflammation of either the upper or lower GI tract.

Indomethacin suppositories: History of proctitis or recent rectal bleeding.

Warnings:

Ketorolac tromethamine: Ketorolac is indicated for the short-term (up to 5 days) management of moderately severe acute pain that requires analgesia at the opioid level. It is not indicated for minor or chronic painful conditions. Increasing the dose beyond the label recommendations will not provide better efficacy but will result in increasing risk of developing serious adverse events.

GI effects – Ketorolac can cause peptic ulcers, GI bleeding or perforation.

Renal effects – Ketorolac is contraindicated in patients with advanced renal impairment and in patients at risk for renal failure due to volume depletion.

Risk of bleeding – Ketorolac inhibits platelet function and is therefore contraindicated in patients with suspected or confirmed cerebrovascular bleeding, hemorrhagic diathesis, incomplete hemostasis and those at high risk of bleeding.

Ketorolac is contraindicated as prophylactic analgesia before any major surgery and is contraindicated intra-operatively when hemostasis is critical because of the increased risk of bleeding.

Hypersensitivity – Hypersensitivity reactions, ranging from bronchospasm to anaphylactic shock, have occurred, and appropriate counteractive measures must be available when administering the first dose of ketorolac.

Intrathecal or epidural administration – Ketorolac is contraindicated for intrathecal or epidural administration due to its alcohol content.

Labor, delivery and lactation – Use in labor and delivery and lactation is contraindicated.

Concomitant use with NSAIDs – Ketorolac is contraindicated in patients currently receiving aspirin or other NSAIDs because of the cumulative risk of inducing serious NSAID-related side effects.

Administration and dosage – Ketorolac (oral) is indicated only as continuation therapy to ketorolac IV/IM; the combined duration of use of IV/IM and oral is not to exceed 5 days because of the increased risk of serious adverse events.

Special populations – Adjust dosage for patients ≥ 65 years old, for patients < 50 kg (110 lbs) and for patients with moderately elevated serum creatinine. IV/IM doses are not to exceed 60 mg/day in these patients.

GI effects: Serious GI toxicity such as bleeding, ulceration and perforation can occur at any time, with or without warning symptoms, in patients treated chronically with NSAID therapy.

CNS effects: **Indomethacin** may aggravate depression or other psychiatric disturbances, epilepsy and parkinsonism. Some of these agents may also cause headaches (highest incidence with fenoprofen, indomethacin and ketorolac).

Renal effects: Acute renal insufficiency, interstitial nephritis, hyperkalemia, hyponatremia and renal papillary necrosis may occur.

Hypersensitivity: A potentially fatal apparent hypersensitivity syndrome has occurred with **sulindac**. Severe hypersensitivity reactions with fever, rashes, abdominal pain, headache, nausea, vomiting, signs of liver damage and meningitis have occurred in **ibuprofen** patients, especially those with systemic lupus erythematosus (SLE) or other collagen diseases.

Renal function impairment: NSAID metabolites are eliminated primarily by kidneys; use with caution.

Hepatic function impairment: Naproxen may exhibit an increase in unbound fraction and a reduced clearance of free drug in cirrhotic liver patients, suggesting an increased potential for toxicity in this group; may need to reduce dose.

Elderly: Age appears to increase the possibility of adverse reactions to NSAIDs. The risk of serious ulcer disease is increased; this risk appears to increase with dose.

Pregnancy: Category B (ketoprofen, naproxen, flurbiprofen, diclofenac). Category C (etodolac, ketorolac, mefenamic acid, nabumetone, oxaprozin, tolmetin). Some NSAIDs may prolong pregnancy if given before onset of labor. Avoid during pregnancy, especially in the third trimester.

Lactation: Most NSAIDs are excreted in breast milk. In general, do not use in nursing mothers because of effects on infant's cardiovascular system.

Children: **Mefenamic acid** and **meclofenamate** are not recommended in children < 14 years old. **Indomethacin** is not recommended in children ≤ 14 years old, except in circumstances that warrant the risk. When using in children ≥ 2 years old, closely monitor liver function. Suggested starting dose is 2 mg/kg/day in divided doses. Do not exceed 4 mg/kg/day or 150 to 200 mg/day, whichever is less. **Tolmetin** and **naproxen** are the only agents labeled for juvenile rheumatoid arthritis, although studies are being conducted with other agents. Safety and efficacy of tolmetin in infants < 2 years old are not established. Safety and efficacy of other NSAIDs in children are not established.

Precautions:

Steroid dosage: If reduced or eliminated during therapy, reduce slowly and observe patient closely for evidence of adverse effects, including adrenal insufficiency and exacerbation of symptoms.

Platelet aggregation: NSAIDs can inhibit platelet aggregation; the effect is quantitatively less and of shorter duration than that seen with aspirin. These agents prolong bleeding time (within normal range) in healthy subjects.

Hematologic effects: Decreased hemoglobin or hematocrit levels have rarely required discontinuation.

Cardiovascular effects: May cause fluid retention and peripheral edema.

Ophthalmologic effects: Effects include blurred or diminished vision, scotomata, changes in color vision, corneal deposits and retinal disturbances, including maculas.

Infection: NSAIDs may mask the usual signs of infection.

Hepatic effects: Borderline liver function test elevations may occur in ≈ 15% of patients and may progress, remain essentially unchanged or become transient with continued therapy.

Pancreatitis has occurred in patients receiving **sulindac**.

Auditory effects: Perform periodic auditory function tests during chronic **fenoprofen** therapy in patients with impaired hearing.

Dermatologic effects: Promptly discontinue **mefenamic acid** if rash occurs.

Concomitant therapy: Do not use **naproxen sodium** and **naproxen** concomitantly; both drugs circulate as naproxen anion.

Photosensitivity may occur.

Drug Interactions:

Drugs that affect NSAIDs include cimetidine, probenecid, salicylates and DMSO.

Drugs that may be affected by NSAIDs include anticoagulants, ACE inhibitors, beta blockers, cyclosporine, digoxin, dipyridamole, hydantoins, lithium, loop diuretics, methotrexate, penicillamine, sympathomimetics and thiazide diuretics.

Drug/Lab test interactions: Naproxen use may result in increased urinary values for 17-ketogenic steroids. Although 17-hydroxycorticosteroid measurements (Porter-Silber test) do not appear to be artificially altered, temporarily discontinue naproxen therapy 72 hours before **adrenal function tests** are performed.

Naproxen may interfere with some urinary assays of 5-hydroxy indoleacetic acid.

Tolmetin metabolites in urine give positive tests for **proteinuria** using acid precipitation tests (eg, sulfosalicylic acid).

Mefenamic acid – A false-positive reaction for urinary bile, using the **diazo tablet test,** may result.

Fenoprofen – Amerlex-M kit assay values of total and free triiodothyronine in patients on fenoprofen have been reported as falsely elevated.

Drug/Food interactions: Administration of **tolmetin** with milk decreased total tolmetin bioavailability by 16%. When tolmetin was taken immediately after a meal, peak plasma concentrations were reduced by 50%, while total bioavailability was again decreased by 16%. Peak concentration of **etodolac** is reduced by ≈ ½ and the time to peak is increased by 1.4 to 3.8 hours following administration with food; however, the extent of absorption is not affected. Food may reduce the rate of absorption of **oxaprozin,** but the extent is unchanged.

Adverse Reactions:

GI:

Common NSAID GI Adverse Reactions (%)

GI adverse reactions	Diclofenac	Etodolac	Fenoprofen	Flurbiprofen	Ibuprofen	Indomethacin	Ketoprofen	Ketorolac	Meclofenamate	Mefenamic acid	Nabumetone	Naproxen	Oxaproxen	Piroxicam	Sulindac	Tolmetin
Nausea (with or without vomiting)	3-9	3-9	3-9	3-9	3-9	3-9	> 3	12	11	†	3-9	3-9	3-9	3-9	3-9	11
Vomiting	< 1	1-3	3-9	1-3			> 1	< 3			1-3	< 1	< 3	< 1		3-9
Diarrhea	3-9	3-9		3-9	< 3	< 3	> 3	3-9	10-33	5	14	< 3	3-9	1-3	3-9	3-9
Constipation	3-9	1-3	3-9	1-3	< 3	< 3	> 3	< 3	1-3	†	3-9	3-9	3-9	1-3	3-9	< 3
Abdominal distress/ cramps/pain	3-9	3-9	< 3	3-9	< 3	< 3	> 3	13	3-9	†	12	3-9	< 3	1-3	10	3-9
Dyspepsia	3-9	10	3-9	3-9	3-9	3-9	11.5	12			13	3-9	3-9	3-9	3-9	3-9
Flatulence	1-3	3-9	< 3	1-3	< 3	< 1	> 3	< 3	3-9	†	3-9		< 3	1-3	1-3	3-9
Anorexia		< 1	< 3			< 1	> 1		1-3	†	< 1		< 3	< 3	1-3	1-3
Stomatitis	< 1	< 1		< 1		< 1	> 1	< 3	1-3		1-3	< 3	< 1	1-3	< 1	< 1

† Occurs, no incidence reported.

CNS: Dizziness (3% to 9%; **flurbiprofen** and **diclofenac** 1% to 3%); headache; **ketorolac** 17%; **fenoprofen** 15%; **indomethacin** 11%; **diclofenac, flurbiprofen, meclofenamate, nabumetone, naproxen** and **tolmetin** 3% to 9%; **ketoprofen** > 3%); somnolence/drowsiness (**fenoprofen** 15%; **naproxen** 3% to 9%; **oxaprozin** < 3%).

Cardiovascular: Congestive heart failure; hypotension; hypertension; palpitations; arrhythmias; tachycardia; vasodilation; peripheral edema and fluid retention.

Renal: Hematuria; cystitis; azotemia; nocturia; proteinuria; polyuria; dysuria; urinary frequency; pyuria; oliguria; anuria.

Hematologic: Neutropenia; eosinophilia; leukopenia; pancytopenia; thrombocytopenia; agranulocytosis; granulocytopenia; aplastic anemia; hemolytic anemia; epistaxis; menorrhagia; hemorrhage; bruising.

Special senses: Blurred vision; photophobia; amblyopia; swollen, dry or irritated eyes; conjunctivitis; iritis; reversible loss of color vision; hearing disturbances or loss; ear pain; change in taste (metallic or bitter); diplopia; tinnitus.

Respiratory: Dyspnea; pharyngitis; bronchospasm; rhinitis; shortness of breath.

Dermatologic: Rash/dermatitis, including maculopapular type (3% to 9%; **ibuprofen, sulindac** and **meclofenamate**); erythema; urticaria; desquamation; angioneurotic edema; ecchymosis; petechiae; purpura; alopecia; pruritus; eczema; skin discoloration; hyperpigmentation; skin irritation; peeling.

Metabolic: Decreased or increased appetite; weight decrease or increase (3% to 9% with **tolmetin**); glycosuria; hyperglycemia; hypoglycemia; hyperkalemia; hyponatremia; flushing or sweating.

Miscellaneous: Thirst; pyrexia (fever and chills); sweating; breast changes; gynecomastia; muscle cramps; facial edema; menstrual disorders; impotence; vaginal bleeding.

Administration and Dosage:

BROMFENAC: The recommended dose is 25 mg every 6 to 8 hours, as necessary, except when taken with high-fat food, when a 50 mg dose may be needed. The total daily dose should not exceed 150 mg. Give the lowest effective dose or the longest dosing interval, especially in the elderly.

FLURBIPROFEN:

Rheumatoid arthritis and osteoarthritis – Initial recommended total daily dose is 200 to 300 mg; administer in divided doses 2, 3 or 4 times daily. The largest recommended single dose in a multiple-dose daily regimen is 100 mg. Doses > 300 mg per day are not recommended.

FENOPROFEN: Do not exceed 3.2 g/day. If GI upset occurs, take with meals or milk.

Rheumatoid arthritis and osteoarthritis – 300 to 600 mg 3 or 4 times daily.

Mild to moderate pain – 200 mg every 4 to 6 hours, as needed.

NABUMETONE: Recommended starting dose is 1000 mg as a single dose with or without food. Some patients may obtain more symptomatic relief from 1500 to 2000 mg/day. Nabumetone can be given either once or twice daily. Dosages > 2000 mg/day have not been studied.

IBUPROFEN:

Adults – Do not exceed 3.2 g/day. If GI upset occurs, take with meals or milk.

Rheumatoid arthritis and osteoarthritis: 1.2 to 3.2 g/day (300 mg 4 times daily or 400, 600 or 800 mg 3 or 4 times daily).

Mild to moderate pain: 400 mg every 4 to 6 hours, as necessary.

Primary dysmenorrhea: 400 mg every 4 hours, as necessary.

OTC use (minor aches and pains, dysmenorrhea, fever reduction): 200 mg every 4 to 6 hours while symptoms persist. If pain or fever do not respond to 200 mg, 400 mg may be used. Do not exceed 1.2 g in 24 hours. Do not take for pain for > 10 days or for fever for > 3 days, unless directed.

Children –

Juvenile arthritis: Usual dose is 30 to 70 mg/kg/day in 3 or 4 divided doses; 20 mg/kg/day may be adequate for milder disease.

Fever reduction in children 6 months to 12 years old: Adjust dosage on the basis of the initial temperature level. If baseline temperature is ≤ 39.2°C (102.5°F), recommended dose is 5 mg/kg; if baseline temperature is > 39.2°C (102.5°F), recommended dose is 10 mg/kg. Duration of fever reduction is longer with the higher dose. Maximum daily dosage is 40 mg/kg.

KETOPROFEN: Take with antacids, food or milk to minimize adverse GI effects.

Rheumatoid arthritis and osteoarthritis – Do not exceed 300 mg/day.

Daily dose: 150 to 300 mg divided into 3 or 4 doses.

Starting dose: 75 mg 3 times daily or 50 mg 4 times daily. Reduce initial dose to ½ to ⅓ in elderly or debilitated patients or those with impaired renal function.

Mild to moderate pain, primary dysmenorrhea – 25 to 50 mg every 6 to 8 hours as needed. Give smaller dosages initially to smaller patients, the elderly and those with renal or liver disease. Doses > 50 mg may be given, but doses > 75 mg do not display added therapeutic effects. Do not exceed 300 mg/day.

OTC –

Adults: 12.5 mg with a full glass of liquid every 4 to 6 hours. If pain or fever persists after 1 hour, follow with 12.5 mg. With experience, some patients may find an initial dose of 25 mg will give better relief. Do not exceed 25 mg in a 4 to 6 hour period or 75 mg in a 24 hour period.

Children: Do not give to those < 16 years of age unless directed by a physician.

PIROXICAM: Initiate and maintain at a single daily dose of 20 mg. May divide daily dose.

Children – Use in children has not been established.

NAPROXEN:

Rx – Do not exceed 1.25 g naproxen (1.375 g naproxen sodium) per day.

Rheumatoid arthritis, osteoarthritis, ankylosing spondylitis, pain, dysmenorrhea, acute tendinitis and bursitis:

Naproxen – 250 to 500 mg twice/day. May increase to 1.5 g/day for limited periods.

Delayed release naproxen (EC-Naprosyn) – 375 to 500 mg twice/day. Do not break, crush or chew tablets.

Controlled release (Naprelan) – 750 mg or 1000 mg once daily. Do not exceed 1000 mg/day.

Naproxen sodium – 275 to 550 mg twice daily. May increase to 1.65 g for limited periods.

Juvenile arthritis:

Naproxen – Total daily dose is ≈ 10 mg/kg in 2 divided doses.

Suspension: Use the following as a guide:

Naproxen Suspension: Children's Dose	
Child's weight	Dose
13 kg (29 lb)	2.5 ml (0.5 tsp) bid
25 kg (55 lb)	5 ml (1 tsp) bid
38 kg (84 lb)	7.5 ml (1.5 tsp) bid

Acute gout:

Naproxen – 750 mg, followed by 250 mg every 8 hours until the attack subsides.

Naproxen sodium – 825 mg, then 275 mg every 8 hours until attack subsides.

Controlled release (Naprelan) – 1000 mg to 1500 mg once daily on the first day followed by 1000 mg once daily until the attack has subsided.

Mild-to-moderate pain; primary dysmenorrhea; acute tendinitis and bursitis:

Naproxen – 500 mg, followed by 250 mg every 6 to 8 hours. Do not exceed a 1.25 g total daily dose.

Naproxen sodium – 550 mg, followed by 275 mg every 6 to 8 hours. Do not exceed a 1.375 g total daily dose.

Controlled release (Naprelan) – 1000 mg once daily. For patients requiring greater analgesic benefit, 1500 mg/day may be used for a limited period.

Children: Safety and efficacy in children < 2 years of age have not been established.

OTC –

Adults: 200 mg with a full glass of liquid every 8 to 12 hours while symptoms persist. With experience, some patients may find that an initial dose of 400 mg followed by 200 mg 12 hours later, if necessary, will give better relief. Do not exceed 600 mg in 24 hours unless otherwise directed.

Elderly (> 65 years of age): Do not take > 200 mg every 12 hours.

Children: Do not give to children < 12 years of age except under the advice and supervision of a physician.

DICLOFENAC:

Osteoarthritis – 100 to 150 mg/day in divided doses (50 mg twice daily or 3 times daily [diclofenac sodium or potassium] or 75 mg twice daily [diclofenac sodium]). Dosages > 150 mg/day have not been studied.

Rheumatoid arthritis – 150 to 200 mg/day in divided doses (50 mg 3 or 4 times daily [diclofenac sodium or potassium] or 75 mg twice daily [diclofenac sodium]). Dosages > 225 mg/day are not recommended.

Ankylosing spondylitis – 100 to 125 mg/day as 25 mg 4 times/day, with an extra 25 mg dose at bedtime, if necessary. Dosages > 125 mg/day have not been studied.

Analgesia and primary dysmenorrhea (diclofenac potassium only) – Recommended starting dose is 50 mg 3 times daily. In some patients, an initial dose of 100 mg followed by 50 mg doses will provide better relief. After the first day, when the maximum recommended dose may be 200 mg, the total daily dose should generally not exceed 150 mg.

INDOMETHACIN:

Moderate-to-severe rheumatoid arthritis (including acute flares of chronic disease), ankylosing spondylitis and osteoarthritis – 25 mg 2 or 3 times daily. If this is well tolerated, increase the daily dose by 25 or 50 mg (if required by continuing symptoms) at weekly intervals until a satisfactory response is obtained or until a daily dose of 150 to 200 mg is reached. Doses above this amount generally do not increase the effectiveness of the drug.

In patients who have persistent night pain or morning stiffness, giving a large portion, up to a maximum of 100 mg of the total daily dose at bedtime, may help to relieve pain. The total daily dose should not exceed 200 mg.

In acute flares of chronic rheumatoid arthritis, it may be necessary to increase the dosage by 25 or 50 mg daily.

Acute painful shoulder (bursitis or tendinitis) – 75 to 150 mg daily in 3 or 4 divided doses. Discontinue the drug after inflammation has been controlled for several days. Usual course of therapy is 7 to 14 days.

Acute gouty arthritis – 50 mg 3 times daily until pain is tolerable, then rapidly reduce the dose to complete cessation of the drug. Definite relief of pain usually occurs within 2 to 4 hours. Tenderness and heat usually subside in 24 to 36 hours, and swelling gradually disappears in 3 to 5 days. Do not use sustained release form.

Sustained release form – Do not crush. The 75 mg sustained release capsule can be taken once a day as an alternative to the 25 mg capsule 3 times daily. In addition, one 75 mg sustained release capsule twice daily can be substituted for the 50 mg capsule 3 times daily. Do not use sustained release form in acute gouty arthritis.

Children – Efficacy in children ≤ 14 years of age has not been established.

SULINDAC: Administer twice a day with food. The usual maximum dosage is 400 mg/day. Dosages above 400 mg/day are not recommended.

Osteoarthritis, rheumatoid arthritis and ankylosing spondylitis – Initial dosage is 150 mg twice a day.

Acute painful shoulder (acute subacromial bursitis/supraspinatus tendinitis); acute gouty arthritis – 200 mg twice/day. After satisfactory response, reduce dosage accordingly.

Children – Safety and efficacy have not been established.

TOLMETIN SODIUM:

Adults –

Rheumatoid arthritis and osteoarthritis: Initially, 400 mg 3 times/day; preferably include dose on arising and at bedtime. Control is usually achieved at doses of 600 to 1800 mg/day generally in 3 divided doses. Doses > 1800 mg/day are not recommended.

Children –

(≥ 2 years): Initially, 20 mg/kg/day in 3 or 4 divided doses. When control is achieved, usual dosage ranges from 15 to 30 mg/kg/day. Doses > 30 mg/kg/day are not recommended.

MECLOFENAMATE SODIUM:

Mild to moderate pain – 50 mg every 4 to 6 hours. Doses of 100 mg may be required for optimal pain relief. Do not exceed daily dosage of 400 mg.

Excessive menstrual blood loss and primary dysmenorrhea – 100 mg 3 times daily for up to 6 days, starting at the onset of menstrual flow.

Rheumatoid arthritis and osteoarthritis –

Usual dosage: 200 to 400 mg per day in 3 or 4 equal doses.

Initial dosage: Initiate at lower dosage; increase as needed to improve response. Do not exceed 400 mg/day.

Children – Safety and efficacy in children < 14 years of age are not established.

MEFENAMIC ACID:

Acute pain –

Adults (≥ 14 yrs): 500 mg, then 250 mg every 6 hours, as needed, usually not to exceed 1 week. Give with food.

Primary dysmenorrhea – 500 mg, then 250 mg every 6 hours. Start with the onset of bleeding and associated symptoms. Should not be necessary for > 2 to 3 days.

Children – Safety and efficacy in children < 14 years have not been established.

ETODOLAC:

Osteoarthritis – Initially 800 to 1200 mg/day in divided doses, followed by adjustment in the range of 600 to 1200 mg/day in divided doses (400 mg 2 or 3 times/day; 300 mg 2, 3 or 4 times/day; 200 mg 3 or 4 times/day). Do not exceed 1200 mg/day.

Patients ≤ 60 kg: Do not exceed 20 mg/kg.

Analgesia –

Acute pain: 200 to 400 mg every 6 to 8 hrs. Do not exceed 1200 mg/day.

Patients ≤ 60 kg: Do not exceed 20 mg/kg.

KETOROLAC TROMETHAMINE: The combined duration of ketorolac IV/IM and oral is not to exceed 5 days. Oral use is only indicated as combination therapy to IV/IM.

IV/IM – When administering IV/IM, the IV bolus must be given over no less than 15 seconds. Give IM administration slowly and deeply into the muscle.

Single-dose treatment: Limit the following regimen to single administration use only

IM dosing –

< 65 years old: One 60 mg dose.

≥ 65 years old, renal impairment or < 50 kg (110 lbs): One 30 mg dose.

IV dosing –

< 65 years old: One 30 mg dose.

≥ 65 years old, renal impairment or < 50 kg (110 lbs): One 15 mg dose.

Multiple-dose treatment:

< 65 years old – The recommended dose is 30 mg every 6 hours. The maximum daily dose should not exceed 120 mg.

≥ 65 years old, renal impairment or < 50 kg (110 lbs) – The recommended dose is 15 mg every 6 hours. The maximum daily dose for these populations should not exceed 60 mg.

Oral – Indicated only as continuation therapy to ketorolac IV/IM.

Transition from IV/IM to oral:

< 65 years old – 20 mg as a first oral dose for patients who received 60 mg IM single dose, 30 mg single IV dose or 30 mg multiple dose IV/IM followed by 10 mg every 4 to 6 hours, not to exceed 40 mg/24 hours.

≥ 65 years old, renal impairment or < 50 kg (110 lbs) – 10 mg as a first oral dose for patients who received a 30 mg IM single dose, 15 mg IV single dose or 15 mg multiple dose IV/IM followed by 10 mg every 4 to 6 hours, not to exceed 40 mg/24 hours.

OXAPROZIN:

Rheumatoid arthritis – 1200 mg once a day.

Osteoarthritis – 1200 mg once a day. For patients of low body weight or with milder disease, an initial dosage of 600 mg once a day may be appropriate.

Maximum dose – 1800 mg/day (or 26 mg/kg, whichever is lower) in divided doses.

SUMATRIPTAN SUCCINATE

Injection: 12 mg/ml (*Rx*) **Tablets:** 25 and 50 mg (*Rx*) **Spray, nasal:** 5 and 20 mg (*Rx*)	*Imitrex* (GlaxoWellcome)

Actions:

Pharmacology: Sumatriptan is a selective agonist for a vascular 5-hydroxytryptamine$_1$ (serotonin) receptor subtype. The vascular 5-HT$_1$ receptor subtype to which sumatriptan binds selectively and through which it presumably exerts its antimigrainous effect is present on the human basilar artery and in vasculature of the isolated human dura mater. In these tissues, sumatriptan activates this receptor to cause vasoconstriction, an action in humans correlating with the relief of migraine.

Pharmacokinetics:

Injection – Following a 6 mg SC injection, distribution half-life was 15 minutes, terminal half-life was 115 minutes, and Vd central compartment was 50 L. Of this dose, 22% was excreted in the urine as unchanged sumatriptan and 38% as the indole acetic acid metabolite. The T_{max} or amount absorbed were not significantly altered by either the site or technique of injection (deltoid vs thigh).

Oral – Sumatriptan is rapidly absorbed after oral administration, with low absolute bioavailability (≈ 15%). The apparent volume of distribution is 2.4 L/kg. Elimination half-life is ≈ 2.5 hours. Sumatriptan is largely renally excreted (≈ 60%) with ≈ 40% found in the feces.

Intranasal – The mean maximum concentration following a 5– and 20–mg intranasal dose was 5 and 16 ng/ml, respectively. The elimination half-life is ≈ 2 hours. Administration of two 5 mg doses, one dose in each nostril, is equivalent to administration of a single 10 mg dose in one nostril.

Indications:

Migraine: Acute treatment of migraine attacks with or without aura.

Cluster headache (injection only): Acute treatment of cluster headache episodes.

Contraindications:

IV use (because of its potential to cause coronary vasospasm); SC use in patients with ischemic heart disease (angina pectoris, history of myocardial infarction [MI] or documented silent ischemia) or in patients with Prinzmetal's angina; patients with symptoms or signs consistent with ischemic heart disease; patients with uncontrolled hypertension; with concurrent ergotamine-containing preparations; hypersensitivity to sumatriptan; management of hemiplegic or basilar migraine.

Warnings:

Migraine diagnosis: Use oral sumatriptan only where a clear diagnosis of migraine (or cluster headache for injection) has been established. Do not administer to patients with basilar or hemiplegic migraine.

Cardiac events/Coronary constriction: Serious coronary events following sumatriptan can occur but are extremely rare. If symptoms consistent with angina occur, carry out ECG evaluation to look for ischemic changes.

Sumatriptan may cause coronary vasospasm in patients with a history of CAD and, rarely, in patients without history suggestive of CAD. Vasospastic reactions other than coronary artery vasospasm have also occurred.

There have been rare reports of serious or life-threatening arrhythmias. In addition, there have been rare, but more frequent, reports of chest and arm discomfort thought to represent angina pectoris.

Fatalities: Deaths have been reported following the use of sumatriptan. In most cases, these have occurred well after sumatriptan use (ie, ≥ 3 hours postinjection) and probably reflect underlying disease and spontaneous events. Advise patients not to administer sumatriptan if a headache being experienced is atypical.

Hypersensitivity reactions have occurred on rare occasions, and severe anaphylaxis/anaphylactoid reactions have occurred. Such reactions can be life-threatening or fatal.

Renal/Hepatic function impairment: Administer with caution to patients with diseases that may alter the absorption, metabolism or excretion of drugs. The bioavailability may be markedly increased in patients with liver disease. The bioavailability of nasally absorbed sumatriptan should not be altered in hepatically impaired patients.

Elderly: Pharmacokinetics in the elderly are similar to those seen in younger adults.

Pregnancy: *Category* C.

Lactation: Sumatriptan is excreted in breast milk.

Children: Safety and efficacy in children have not been established.

Precautions:

Chest, jaw or neck tightness is relatively common after sumatriptan, and atypical sensations over the precordium (tightness, pressure, heaviness) have occurred, but has only rarely been associated with ischemic ECG changes.

Blood pressure changes: Sumatriptan injection may cause mild, transient elevation of blood pressure and peripheral vascular resistance.

Seizures: There have been rare reports of seizures following sumatriptan use.

Binding to melanin-containing tissues: Because sumatriptan binds to melanin, it could accumulate in melanin-rich tissues (such as the eye) over time, raising the possibility that toxicity in these tissues could occur after extended use.

Corneal opacities: Sumatriptan causes corneal opacities and defects in the dog, raising the possibility that these changes may occur in humans.

Drug Interactions:

Sumatriptan may be affected by MAOIs, ergot-containing drugs and SSRIs.

Adverse Reactions:

Adverse reactions occuring in IV sumatriptan patients include tingling; warm/hot sensation; burning sensation; feeling of heaviness; pressure sensation; feeling of tightness; numbness; dizziness/vertigo; musculoskeletal weakness; neck pain/stiffness; chest discomfort; throat discomfort; injection site reaction; flushing.

Adverse reactions associated with oral sumatriptan may include tingling; warm/hot sensation; flushing; nasal discomfort; visual disturbance.

Adverse reactions associated with intranasal use may include nasal/throat discomfort and taste disturbance.

Administration and Dosage:

Injection: The maximum single adult dose is 6 mg injected SC.

The maximum recommended dose that may be given in 24 hours is two 6 mg injections separated by at least 1 hour. Although the recommended dose is 6 mg, if side effects are dose-limiting, then lower doses may be used.

Oral: Recommended adult dose is 25 mg taken with fluids; maximum recommended single dose is 100 mg. There is no evidence that an initial dose of 100 mg provides substantially greater relief than 25 mg.

If satisfactory response has not been obtained at 2 hours, a second dose of up to 100 mg may be given. If headache returns, additional doses may be taken at intervals of at least 2 hours up to a daily maximum of 300 mg. If headache returns following an initial treatment with injection, additional doses of single tablets (up to 200 mg/day) may be given with at least 2 hours intervals between tablet doses.

Sumatriptan is equally effective at whatever stage of the attack it is administered, although it is advisable to take as early as possible after the onset of a migraine attack.

Intranasal: For adults, the usual dose is a single nasal spray into one nostril. If headache returns, a second nasal spray may be given $\geq$ 2 hours after the first spray. For any attack where the patient has no response to the first nasal spray, do not use a second nasal spray without first consulting a physician. Do not administer more than a total of 40 mg of nasal spray in any 24 hour period.

ANTIDEPRESSANTS

Drugs with clinically useful antidepressant effects include the tricyclic antidepressants (TCAs), maprotiline, trazodone, bupropion, venlafaxine, nefazodone, selective serotonin reuptake inhibitors (SSRIs) and the monoamine oxidase inhibitors (MAOIs).

Mechanism of action: The emphasis of research has shifted from acute reuptake effects to the slower adaptive changes in norepinephrine and serotonin receptor systems induced by chronic antidepressant therapy. Postsynaptic receptors participate in nerve impulse neurotransmission while the presynaptic receptors regulate neurotransmitter release and reuptake, an important mechanism of neurotransmitter inactivation. Long-term antidepressant treatment produces complex changes in the sensitivities of both presynaptic and postsynaptic receptor sites. The available antidepressant agents may increase the sensitivity of postsynaptic alpha (α_1) adrenergic and serotonin receptors and may decrease the sensitivity of presynaptic receptor sites. The net effect is the correction (re-regulation) of an abnormal receptor-neurotransmitter relationship.

Drug selection: The non-MAOIs are used much more frequently than the MAOIs mainly because of (1) the perception that MAOIs are less effective than the non-MAOI antidepressants and (2) the risk of hypertensive crisis when the patient ingests foods containing tyramine or via drug interaction (eg, sympathomimetics) with the MAOIs. However, when MAOIs are used in therapeutic doses, they are probably equieffective to non-MAOIs for the treatment of depression. In general, MAOIs are used for atypical depression.

Base antidepressant drug selection on the patient's history of drug response (if any), the specific drug's side effect profile relative to patient medical conditions and other factors, and clinician familiarity with specific antidepressants. Trazodone has less anticholinergic activity than TCAs and causes fewer problems than TCAs when taken in overdose. SSRIs generally lack the adverse reactions (eg, sedation, anticholinergic effects) associated with TCAs, cause few cardiovascular side effects (including orthostasis), are associated with weight loss rather than weight gain as is the case with TCAs, and cause fewer problems than TCAs when taken in overdose. However, their use is associated with other side effects such as headache, nervousness and insomnia. Use maprotiline and bupropion only when other antidepressants have not proven effective. In cases of mild depression, drug therapy and psychotherapy appear to be equally effective.

Antidepressant Pharmacologic and Pharmacokinetic Parameters

0 - none + - slight ++ - moderate +++ - high ++++ - very high +++++ - highest	Major side effects			Amine uptake blocking activity					
	Anticholinergic	Sedation	Orthostatic hypotension	Norepinephrine	Serotonin	Half-life (hours)	Therapeutic plasma level (ng/ml)	Time to reach steady state (days)	Dose range (mg/day)
Tricyclics - Tertiary Amines									
Amitriptyline	++++	++++	++	++	++++	31-46	110-250[1]	4-10	50-300
Clomipramine	+++	+++	++	++	+++++	19-37	80-100	7-14	25-250
Doxepin	++	+++	++	+	++	8-24	100-200[1]	2-8	25-300
Imipramine	++	++	+++	++[2]	++++	11-25	200-350[1]	2-5	30-300
Trimipramine	++	+++	++	+	+	7-30	180[1]	2-6	50-300
Tricyclics - Secondary Amines									
Amoxapine[3]	+++	++	+	+++	++	8[4]	200-500	2-7	50-600
Desipramine	+	+	+	++++	++	12-24	125-300	2-11	25-300
Nortriptyline	++	++	+	++	+++	18-44	50-150	4-19	30-100
Protriptyline	+++	+	+	++++	++	67-89	100-200	14-19	15-60
Phenethylamine									
Venlafaxine	0	0	0	+++	+++	5-11[1]	-	3-4	75-375
Tetracyclic									
Maprotiline	++	++	+	+++	0/+	21-25	200-300[1]	6-10	50-225
Triazolopyridine									
Trazodone	+	++	++	0	+++	4-9	800-1600	3-7	150-600
Aminoketone									
Bupropion[5]	++	++	+	0/+	0/+	8-24	-	1.5-5	200-450

Antidepressant Pharmacologic and Pharmacokinetic Parameters

0 - none + - slight ++ - moderate +++ - high ++++ - very high +++++ - highest	Major side effects			Amine uptake blocking activity					
	Anticholinergic	Sedation	Orthostatic hypotension	Norepinephrine	Serotonin	Half-life (hours)	Therapeutic plasma level (ng/ml)	Time to reach steady state (days)	Dose range (mg/day)
Selective Serotonin Reuptake Inhibitors									
Fluoxetine	0/+	0/+	0/+	0/+	+++++	2-9 days[1]	-	2-4 weeks	20-80
Paroxetine	0	0/+	0	0/+	+++++	10-24	-	7-14	10-50
Sertraline	0	0/+	0	0/+	+++++	1-4[1]	-	7	50-200
Fluvoxamine	0/+	0/+	0	0/+	++++	15.6	-	3-8 hours	50-300
Monoamine Oxidase Inhibitors									
Tranylcypromine	+	+	0	-	-	2.4-2.8	-	-	30-60
Phenelzine	+	+	+	-	-	-	-	-	45-90
Miscellaneous									
Nefazodone	0/+	++	+	0/+	++++	2-4	-	4-5	200-600

1 Parent compound plus active metabolite.
2 Via desipramine, the major metabolite.
3 Also blocks dopamine receptors.
4 30 hours for major metabolite 8-hydroxyamoxapine.
5 Inhibits dopamine uptake.

TRAZODONE HCl

Tablets: 50 and 100 mg (*Rx*)	Various, *Desyrel* (Mead Johnson Pharm)
Tablets: 150 and 300 mg (*Rx*)	Various, *Desyrel Dividose* (Mead Johnson Pharm)

Actions:

Pharmacology: The mechanism of antidepressant action is not fully understood. Trazodone is not a monoamine oxidase inhibitor and does not stimulate the CNS. In animals, it selectively inhibits serotonin uptake by brain synaptosomes and potentiates the behavioral changes induced by the serotonin precursor, 5–hydroxytryptophan.

Pharmacokinetics:

Absorption/Distribution – Trazodone is well absorbed after oral administration. Peak plasma levels occur in ≈ 1 hour when taken on an empty stomach or in 2 hours when taken with food.

Metabolism/Excretion – Trazodone is extensively metabolized in the liver; < 1% is excreted unchanged in the urine and feces. Elimination is biphasic, with a half-life of 3 to 6 hours and 5 to 9 hours, respectively, and is unaffected by food. The clearance of trazodone may be reduced in elderly male patients.

Indications:

Treatment of depression.

Unlabeled uses: May be useful for treatment of patients with panic disorder or agoraphobia with panic attacks.

Contraindications:

Hypersensitivity to trazodone.

Warnings:

Preexisting cardiac disease: Not recommended for use during the initial recovery phase of myocardial infarction. Trazodone may be arrhythmogenic in some patients. Arrhythmias identified include isolated PVCs, ventricular couplets and short episodes (3 to 4 beats) of ventricular tachycardia. Closely monitor patients with preexisting cardiac disease, particularly for cardiac arrhythmias.

Priapism: Patients with prolonged or inappropriate penile erection should discontinue use immediately and consult a physician.

Pregnancy: Category C.

Lactation: The drug may be excreted in breast milk.

Children: Safety and efficacy for use in children < 18 years of age are not established.

Precautions:

Suicide: The possibility of suicide in seriously depressed patients is inherent in the illness and may persist until significant remission occurs. Therefore, write prescriptions for the smallest number of tablets consistent with good patient management.

Hypotension, including orthostatic hypotension and syncope, has occurred.

Electroconvulsive therapy: Avoid concurrent administration with electroconvulsive therapy because of the absence of experience in this area.

Laboratory tests: Discontinue the drug in any patient whose white blood cell count or absolute neutrophil count falls below normal levels. White blood cell and differential counts are recommended for patients who develop fever and sore throat (or other signs of infection) during therapy.

Hazardous tasks: May produce drowsiness, dizziness or blurred vision.

Drug Interactions:

Drugs that may interact with trazodone include CNS depressants, digoxin, monoamine oxidase inhibitors, phenytoin and warfarin.

Adverse Reactions:

Adverse reactions may include allergic reaction; purpuric and maculopapular eruptions; rash; pruritus; urticaria; hematuria; delayed urine flow; increased urinary frequency; urinary incontinence/retention; decreased appetite; sweating; clamminess; weight gain or loss; malaise; nasal/sinus congestion; increased appetite; apnea; alopecia; edema; tinnitus; red eyes; diplopia; hypertension; hypotension; shortness of breath; tachycardia; palpitations; chest pain; ventricular tachycardia; vasodilation; bradycardia; atrial fibrillation; anger; hostility; nightmares/vivid dreams; confusion; disorientation; decreased concentration; lightheadedness; excitement; fatigue; headache; insomnia; impaired memory; nervousness; incoordination; paresthesia; tremors; hallucinations; psychosis; vertigo; hypomania; mania; impaired speech; akathisia; numbness; delusions; agitation; weakness; grand mal seizures; extrapyramidal symptoms; tardive dyskinesia; stupor; decreased/increased libido; impotence; retrograde ejaculation; early menses; missed periods; breast enlargement and engorgement; lactation; abdominal/ gastric disorder; bad taste in mouth; dry mouth; nausea; vomiting; diarrhea; constipation; flatulence; hypersalivation; anemia; liver enzyme alterations; hyperbilirubinemia; jaundice; musculoskeletal aches and pains; muscle twitches; ataxia.

Administration and Dosage:

Initiate dosage at a low level and increase gradually. Drowsiness may require the administration of a major portion of the daily dose at bedtime or a reduced dosage. Take shortly after a meal or light snack.

Adults: An initial dose is 150 mg/day. This may be increased by 50 mg/day every 3 to 4 days. The maximum dose for outpatients usually should not exceed 400 mg/day in divided doses. Inpatients or more severely depressed subjects may be given up to, but not in excess of, 600 mg/day in divided doses.

Maintenance: Keep dosage at the lowest effective level. Once an adequate response has been achieved, dosage may be gradually reduced with subsequent adjustment depending on response.

BUPROPION HCl

Tablets: 75 and 100 mg (*Rx*) — *Wellbutrin* (GlaxoWellcome)

Actions:

Pharmacology: The mechanism of the antidepressant effect of bupropion is not known. Bupropion does not inhibit monoamine oxidase. It is a weak blocker of the neuronal uptake of serotonin and norepinephrine; it also inhibits the neuronal reuptake of dopamine to some extent.

Pharmacokinetics:

Absorption/Distribution – Following oral administration, peak plasma concentrations are usually achieved within 2 hours, followed by a biphasic decline. The average half-life of the second (post-distributional) phase ranges 8 to 24 hours.

Metabolism/Excretion – Several of the metabolites of bupropion are pharmacologically active, but their potency and toxicity relative to bupropion have not been fully characterized. However, because of their longer elimination half-lives, the plasma concentrations of at least two of the known metabolites will be much higher than the plasma concentration of bupropion, especially in long-term use.

Indications:

Depression treatment: Effectiveness of bupropion in long-term use (> 6 weeks) has not been evaluated.

Contraindications:

Hypersensitivity to the drug; seizure disorder; current or prior diagnosis of bulimia or anorexia nervosa (because of a higher incidence of seizures noted in such patients treated with bupropion); concurrent administration of a monoamine oxidase inhibitor (MAOI; at least 14 days should elapse between discontinuation of an MAOI and initiation of treatment with bupropion).

Warnings:

Seizures: Bupropion is associated with seizures in ≈ 0.4% of patients treated at doses up to 450 mg/day. The estimated seizure incidence increases almost 10–fold between 450 and 600 mg/day, which is twice the usually required daily dose (300 mg) and 1⅓ the maximum recommended daily dose (450 mg).

The risk of seizure appears strongly associated with dose and the presence of predisposing factors. A significant predisposing factor (eg, history of head trauma or prior seizure, CNS tumor, concomitant medications that lower seizure threshold) was present in approximately 50% of patients experiencing a seizure. Sudden and large increments in dose may also increase risk. While many seizures occurred early in the course of treatment, some seizures occurred after several weeks at fixed dose.

Recommendations for reducing seizure risk: (1) The total daily dose does not exceed 450 mg, (2) the daily dose is administered 3 times daily, with each single dose not to exceed 150 mg to avoid high peak concentrations of bupropion or its metabolites, and (3) the rate of incrementation of dose is very gradual.

Use extreme caution when: (1) Administered to patients with a history of seizure, cranial trauma, or other predisposition toward seizure, or (2) prescribed with other agents (eg, antipsychotics, other antidepressants) or treatment regimens (eg, abrupt discontinuation of a benzodiazepine) that lower seizure threshold.

Renal/Hepatic function impairment: Initiate treatment of patients with renal or hepatic impairment at reduced dosage. Closely monitor for possible toxic effects of elevated blood and tissue levels of drug and metabolites.

Half-lives of the metabolites are prolonged by cirrhosis and the metabolites accumulate to levels 2 to 3 times those in healthy individuals.

Pregnancy: Category B.

Lactation: Use only when clearly needed and when the potential benefits to the mother outweigh the possible risks to the infant.

Children: Safety and efficacy in children < 18 years old have not been established.

Precautions:

CNS symptoms: A substantial proportion of patients experience some degree of increased restlessness, agitation, anxiety and insomnia, especially shortly after initiation of treatment.

Neuropsychiatric phenomena: Patients have shown a variety of neuropsychiatric signs and symptoms including delusions, hallucinations, psychotic episodes, confusion and paranoia.

Activation of psychosis or mania: Antidepressants can precipitate manic episodes in Bipolar Manic Depressive patients during the depressed phase of their illness and may activate latent psychosis in other susceptible patients.

Altered appetite and weight: A weight loss of > 5 pounds occurred in 28% of patients. This incidence is approximately double that seen in comparable patients treated with tricyclic antidepressants or placebo. Furthermore, 34.5% of patients receiving tricyclic antidepressants gained weight, vs only 9.4% of bupropion patients.

Suicide: The possibility of a suicide attempt is inherent in depression and may persist until significant remission occurs. Accordingly, write prescriptions for the smallest number of tablets consistent with good patient management.

Heart disease: Exercise care in patients with a recent history of myocardial infarction or unstable heart disease.

Drug Interactions:

Drugs that may interact with bupropion include MAOIs and levodopa.

Bupropion may be an inducer of drug metabolizing enzymes. Exercise care when administering drugs known to affect hepatic drug metabolizing enzyme systems.

Use and cessation of use of alcohol may alter the seizure threshold; therefore, minimize the consuption of alcohol and, if possible, avoid completely.

Adverse Reactions:

Adverse reactions occurring in ≥ 3% of patients include constipation; nausea/vomiting; anorexia; diarrhea; appetite increase; dyspepsia; menstrual complaints; impotence; dry mouth; headache/migraine; excessive sweating; tremor; sedation; akinesia/bradykinesia; sensory disturbance; impaired sleep quality; increased salivary flow; auditory disturbance; blurred vision; gustatory disturbance; dizziness; tachycardia; cardiac arrythmias; hypertension; palpitations; rash; confusion; hostility; disturbed concentration; decreased libido; upper respiratory complaints; fatigue; arthritis; agitation; abnormalities in mental status.

Administration and Dosage:

General: Do not exceed dose increases of 100 mg/day in a 3 day period. No single dose of bupropion should exceed 150 mg. Administer 3 times daily, preferably with at least 6 hours between successive doses.

Adults: 300 mg/day, given 3 times daily. Begin dosing at 200 mg/day, given as 100 mg twice daily. Based on clinical response, this dose may be increased to 300 mg/day, given as 100 mg 3 times daily no sooner than 3 days after beginning therapy.

Bupropion Dosage Regimen

			Number of Tablets		
Treatment Day	Total Daily Dose	Tablet Strength	Morning	Midday	Evening
1	200 mg	100 mg	1	0	1
4	300 mg	100 mg	1	1	1

Increasing the dosage above 300 mg/day: An increase in dosage, up to a maximum of 450 mg/day, given in divided doses of not more than 150 mg each, may be considered for patients in whom no clinical improvement is noted after several weeks of treatment at 300 mg/day. Dosing above 300 mg/day may be accomplished using the 75 or 100 mg tablets. The 100 mg tablets must be administered 4 times daily with at least 4 hours between successive doses in order not to exceed the limit of 150 mg in a single dose. Discontinue in patients who do not demonstrate an adequate response after an appropriate period of 450 mg/day.

Maintenance: Use the lowest dose that maintains remission.

VENLAFAXINE

Tablets: 25, 37.5, 50, 75 and 100 mg (*Rx*) — *Effexor* (Wyeth-Ayerst)

Actions:

Pharmacology: Venlafaxine is chemically unrelated to other available antidepressant agents. Venlafaxine and its active metabolite, O-desmethylvenlafaxine (ODV), are potent inhibitors of neuronal serotonin and norepinephrine reuptake and weak inhibitors of dopamine reuptake.

Pharmacokinetics: Venlafaxine is well absorbed (at least 92%) and extensively metabolized in the liver. ODV is the only major active metabolite. Renal elimination of venlafaxine and its metabolites is the primary route of excretion.

Indications:

Treatment of depression.

Warnings:

MAO inhibitors: Because venlafaxine is an inhibitor of both norepinephrine and serotonin reuptake, it is recommended that venlafaxine not be used in combination with an MAOI. Based on the half-life of venlafaxine, allow at least 7 days after stopping venlafaxine before starting an MAOI.

Elderly: No overall differences in effectiveness, safety or response were observed between elderly and younger patients.

Pregnancy: *Category* C.

Lactation: It is not known whether venlafaxine or its metabolites are excreted in breast milk.

Children: Safety and efficacy in patients < 18 years old have not been established.

Precautions:

Long-term use: The effectiveness of venlafaxine in long-term use (ie, > 4 to 6 weeks) has not been evaluated.

Anxiety and insomnia: Anxiety, nervousness and insomnia were reported for venlafaxine-treated patients, and led to drug discontinuation.

Appetite/Weight changes: Anorexia was reported for venlafaxine-treated patients. A dose-dependent weight loss was often noted in patients treated for several weeks.

Mania/Hypomania: Hypomania or mania has occurred in patients treated with venlafaxine.

Seizures have been reported in venlafaxine-treated patients.

Suicide: The possibility of a suicide attempt is inherent in depression and may persist until significant remission occurs. Write prescriptions for the smallest quantity of tablets consistent with good patient management in order to reduce the risk of overdose.

Drug abuse and dependence: Carefully evaluate patients for history of drug abuse and follow such patients closely, observing them for signs of misuse or abuse of venlafaxine.

Drug Interactions:

Drugs that may interact with venlafaxine include cimetidine and MAOIs. Avoid alcohol.

Venlafaxine is metabolized to its active metabolite, ODV, by cytochrome $P450IID_6$. Therefore, the potential exists for a drug interaction between venlafaxine and drugs that inhibit this isoenzyme.

Adverse Reactions:

Adverse reactions occurring in ≥ 3% of patients include nausea; somnolence; insomnia; dizziness; abnormal ejaculation/orgasm; blurred vision; vasodilation; dry mouth; nervousness; anxiety; tremor; abnormal dreams; hypertonia; paresthesia; headache; asthenia; infection; chills; yawning; sweating; rash; constipation; anorexia; diarrhea; vomiting; dyspepsia; flatulence; impotence; urinary frequency; abdominal pain; abnormality of accommodation.

Administration and Dosage:

Initial treatment: The recommended starting dose is 75 mg/day, administered in 2 or 3 divided doses, taken with food. Depending on tolerability and the need for further clinical effect, the dose may be increased to 150 mg/day. If needed, further increase the dose up to 225 mg/day. When increasing the dose, make increments of up to 75 mg/day at intervals of ≥ 4 days. In outpatient settings there was no evidence of usefulness of doses > 225 mg day for moderately depressed patients, but more severely depressed inpatients responded to a mean dose of 350 mg/day. Certain patients, including more severely depressed patients, may therefore respond more to higher doses, up to a maximum of 375 mg/day, generally in 3 divided doses.

Renal/Hepatic function impairment: It is recommended that the total daily dose be reduced by 50% in patients with moderate hepatic impairment and by 25% in patients with mild to moderate renal impairment. It is recommended that the total daily dose be reduced by 50% and the dose be withheld until the dialysis treatment is completed (4 hrs) in patients undergoing hemodialysis.

Elderly: No dose adjustment is recommended for elderly patients on the basis of age.

Discontinuing venlafaxine: When discontinuing venlafaxine after > 1 week of therapy, it is generally recommended that the dose be tapered to minimize the risk of discontinuation symptoms. Patients who have received venlafaxine for ≥ 6 weeks should have their dose tapered gradually over a 2 week period.

NEFAZODONE HCl

Tablets: 100, 150, 200 and 250 mg (*Rx*) — *Serzone* (Bristol-Myers Squibb)

Actions:

Pharmacology: Nefazodone is an antidepressant with a chemical structure unrelated to available antidepressant agents. The mechanism of action is unknown. Nefazodone inhibits neuronal uptake of serotonin and norepinephrine.

Pharmacokinetics:

Absorption/Distribution – Nefazodone is rapidly and completely absorbed, but is subject to extensive metabolism so that its absolute bioavailability is low (about 20%) and variable. Peak plasma concentrations occur at about 1 hour. Half-life is 2 to 4 hours. Nefazodone is widely distributed in body tissues, including the CNS. Volume of distribution ranges from 0.22 to 0.87 L/kg.

Metabolism/Excretion – Nefazodone is extensively metabolized after oral administration by < 1% is excreted unchanged in urine. Three active metabolites identified in plasma include hydroxynefazodone (HO-NEF), meta-chlorophenylpiperazine (mCPP) and a triazole-dione metabolite.

The mean half-life of nefazodone ranged between 11 and 24 hours. Approximately 55% was detected in urine and about 20% to 30% in feces. Nefazodone is extensively (> 99%) bound to human plasma proteins in vitro.

Indications:

Depression: Treatment of depression.

Contraindications:

Coadministration with terfenadine or astemizole; hypersensitivity to nefazodone or other phenylpiperazine antidepressants.

Warnings:

Long-term use: The effectiveness of nefazodone in long-term use (ie, for more than 6 to 8 weeks) has not been systematically evaluated.

MAO inhibitors: Because nefazodone is an inhibitor of both serotonin and norepinephrine reuptake, it is recommended that nefazodone not be used in combination with an MAOI, or within 14 days of discontinuing treatment with an MAOI. Allow at least 1 week after stopping nefazodone before starting an MAOI.

Pregnancy: *Category* C.

Lactation: It is not known whether nefazodone or its metabolites are excreted in breast milk.

Children: Safety and efficacy in individuals < 18 years old have not been established.

Precautions:

Postural hypotension: Use nefazodone with caution in patients with known cardiovascular or cerebrovascular disease that could be exacerbated by hypotension and conditions that would predispose patients to hypotension.

Mania/hypomania: As with all antidepressants, use nefazodone cautiously in patients with a history of mania.

Suicide: The possibility of a suicide attempt is inherent in depression and may persist until significant remission occurs. Closely supervise high-risk patients during initial therapy. Write prescriptions for the smallest quantity of nefazodone consistent with good patient management to reduce the risk of overdose.

Priapism: If patients present with prolonged or inappropriate erections, they should discontinue therapy immediately and consult their physicians.

Bradycardia: Sinus bradycardia was observed in nefazodone patients. Treat patients with a recent MI or unstable heart disease with caution.

Hepatic cirrhosis: In patients with cirrhosis of the liver, the AUC values of nefazodone and its metabolite HO-NEF were increased by ≈ 25%.

Drug abuse and dependence: Carefully evaluate patients for a history of drug abuse and follow such patients closely, observing them for signs of misuse or abuse of nefazodone.

Drug Interactions:

Drugs that may interact with nefazodone include MAOIs, nonsedating antihistamines, benzodiazepines, digoxin, haloperidol and propranolol.

Potential interaction with drugs that inhibit or are metabolized by cytochrome P450 (IIIA4 and IID6) isozymes: Caution is indicated in the combined use of nefazodone with any drugs known to be metabolized by the IIIA4 isozyme (in particular, terfenadine or astemizole).

Drugs highly bound to plasma protein: Administration to a patient taking another drug that is highly protein bound may cause increased free concentrations of the other drug, potentially resulting in adverse events. Conversely, adverse effects could result from displacement of nefazodone by other highly bound drugs.

Drug/Food interactions: Food delays absorption of nefazodone and decreases the bioavailability by ≈ 20%.

Adverse Reactions:

Adverse reactions occurring in ≥ 3% of patients include nausea; headache; asthenia; flu syndrome; dry mouth; nausea; constipation; dyspepsia; diarrhea; increased appetite; peripheral edema; pharyngitis; cough; blurred vision; abnormal vision; somnolence; dizziness; insomnia; lightheadedness; confusion; memory impairment; paresthesia; vasodilation; concentration decreased; postural hypotension; tinnitus.

Administration and Dosage:

Initial treatment: Recommended starting dose is 200 mg/day, administered in two divided doses. In clinical trials, the effective dose range was generally 300 to 600 mg/day. Increase doses in increments of 100 to 200 mg/day, again on a twice daily schedule, at intervals of no less than 1 week.

Elderly/Debilitated patients: The recommended initial dose is 100 mg/day on a twice daily schedule.

SELECTIVE SEROTONIN REUPTAKE INHIBITORS

SERTRALINE HCl	
Tablets: 50 and 100 mg (*Rx*)	*Zoloft* (Roerig)
PAROXETINE HCl	
Tablets: 10, 20, 30 and 40 mg (*Rx*)	*Paxil* (SK-Beecham)
FLUOXETINE HCl	
Pulvules: 10 and 20 mg (*Rx*)	*Prozac* (Dista)
Liquid: 20 mg/5 ml (*Rx*)	*Prozac* (Dista)
FLUVOXAMINE MALEATE	
Tablets: 50 and 100 mg (*Rx*)	*Luvox* (Solvay)

Actions:

Pharmacology: The antidepressant action of the SSRIs is presumed to be linked to their inhibition of CNS neuronal uptake of serotonin (5HT). These agents are potent and selective inhibitors of neuronal serotonin reuptake and they also have a weak effect on norepinephrine and dopamine neuronal reuptake.

Pharmacokinetics:

SSRI Pharmacokinetics

SSRIs	Time to peak plasma concentration (hr)	Peak plasma concentration (ng/ml)	Half-life (hrs)	Protein binding (%)	Time to reach steady state (days)	Primary route of elimination	Bioavailability (%)
Fluoxetine	6-8	15-55	48- 216[1]	94.5	28-35	hepatic	72
Fluvoxamine	3-8	88-546	13.6-15.6	77-80	7	renal	53
Paroxetine	5.2	61.7	21	93-95	≈10	64% renal, 36% hepatic	100
Sertraline	4.5-8.4	20-55	26-65[1]	98	7	40%-45% renal, 40%-45% hepatic	

[1] t½ includes the active metabolite.

Indications:

Depression: *Fluoxetine, paroxetine, sertraline.*

Obsessive-Compulsive disorder (OCD): *Fluoxetine, fluvoxamine, sertraline, paroxetine* - Treatment of obsessions and compulsions in patients with OCD, as defined in the DSM-III-R.

Bulimia nervosa: *Fluoxetine* - Treatment of binge-eating and vomiting behaviors in patients with moderate to severe bulimia nervosa.

Panic disorder: *Paroxetine* - Treatment of panic disorder, with or without agoraphobia, as defined in DSM-IV.

Unlabeled uses: *Fluoxetine* - Alcoholism; anorexia nervosa; attention-deficit hyperactivity disorder; bipolar II affective disorder; kleptomania; migraine, chronic daily headaches and tension-type headache; obesity; posttraumatic stress disorder; premenstrual syndrome; recurrent syncope; schizophrenia; Tourette's syndrome; trichotilomania; levodopa-induced dyskinesia; social phobia.

Fluvoxamine is being investigated in the treatment of depression.

Paroxetine - Diabetic neuropathy (10 to 60 mg/day); headaches (10 to 50 mg/day); premature ejaculation (20 mg/day).

Sertraline may be effective in patients with obsessive-compulsive disorder.

Contraindications:

Hypersensitivity to SSRIs; in combination with an MAO inhibitor, or within 14 days of discontinuing an MAOI; coadministration of **fluvoxamine** with astemizole or terfenadine.

Warnings:

Long-term use: The effectiveness of long-term use of SSRIs (> 5 to 6 weeks for depression [sertraline >16 weeks]) (>13 weeks for OCD with **fluoxetine**), has not been systematically evaluated, except for paroxetine (the efficacy of **paroxetine** in maintaining an antidepressant response for up to 1 year was demonstrated in a placebo controlled trial).

MAO Inhibitors: It is recommended that SSRIs not be used in combination with an MAOI, or within 14 days of discontinuing treatment with an MAOI. Allow at least 2 weeks after stopping the SSRIs before starting an MAOI.

Altered platelet function or abnormal results from laboratory studies in patients taking **fluoxetine, paroxetine** or **sertraline** have occurred.

Rash and accompanying events: Approximately 4% of patients taking **fluoxetine** have developed a rash or urticaria; ≈ 33% were withdrawn from treatment. Most patients improved promptly with discontinuation of fluoxetine or adjunctive treatment with antihistamines or steroids; all patients recovered completely. Several other patients have had systemic syndromes suggestive of serum sickness.

Systemic events, possibly related to vasculitis, have developed in patients with rash. Although rare, these events may be serious, involving lung, kidney or liver. Death has been associated with the events.

Renal function impairment: With chronic use, additional accumulation of fluoxetine or its metabolites may occur with severely impaired renal function; use a lower or less frequent dose.

Increased plasma concentrations of **paroxetine** occur in subjects with renal and hepatic impairment. Therefore, reduce the initial dosage of paroxetine in patients with severe renal impairment.

Since **sertraline** is extensively metabolized by the liver, excretion of unchanged drug in the urine is a minor route of elimination. However, use with caution in patients with severe renal impairment.

Hepatic function impairment: SSRIs are extensively metabolized by the liver. Use with caution in patients with severe liver impairment. Use a lower or less frequent dose of fluoxetine in patients with liver impairment. Slowly titrate **fluvoxamine** during initiation of treatment. Reduce the initial dosage of **paroxetine** in patients with severe hepatic impairment; upward titration, if necessary, should be at increased intervals. The clearance of **sertraline** is decreased in mild, stable cirrhotics. Give a lower or less frequent dose in patients with severe hepatic dysfunction.

Elderly: The disposition of single doses of **fluoxetine** in healthy elderly subjects (≥ 65 years of age) did not differ significantly from that in younger normal subjects. Clearance of **fluvoxamine** is decreased by ≈ 50% in elderly patients. Pharmacokinetic studies revealed a decreased clearance of paroxetine in the elderly, and a lower starting dose is recommended. Sertraline plasma clearance may be lower.

Pregnancy: Category B (**fluoxetine, paroxetine, sertraline**); Category C (**fluvoxamine**).

Lactation: **Fluoxetine, fluvoxamine** and **paroxetine** are excreted in breast milk. It is not known whether **sertraline** or its metabolites are excreted in breast milk.

Children: Safety and efficacy in children (**fluvoxamine**, children < 18 years of age) have not been established.

Precautions:

Anxiety, nervousness and insomnia occurred in 3% to 33% of patients treated with an SSRI. These side effects led to discontinuation of drug therapy in 1.1% to 5.3%.

Altered appetite and weight: Significant weight loss, especially in underweight depressed patients, has occurred. Approximately 3% to ≈ 9% of patients treated with an SSRI experienced anorexia.

Activation of mania/hypomania occurred infrequently in ≈ 0.1% to 2.2% of patients taking SSRIs. Use cautiously in patients with a history of mania.

Seizures have occurred with **fluoxetine** (0.2%), **fluvoxamine** (0.2%), **paroxetine** (0.1%) and **sertraline** (< 0.1%). These percentages appear similar to the rate associated with other antidepressants. Use with care in patients with history of seizures.

Suicide: The possibility of a suicide attempt is inherent in depression and may persist until significant remission occurs. Close supervision of high-risk patients should accompany initial drug therapy. Write prescriptions for the smallest quantity of tablets or capsules in order to reduce the risk of overdose.

Concomitant illness: Use caution in patients with diseases or conditions that could affect metabolism or hemodynamic responses.

Hyponatremia: Several cases of **fluoxetine, sertraline** and **paroxetine**-induced hyponatremia (some with serum sodium < 110 mmol/L) have occurred. The hyponatremia appeared to be reversible when fluoxetine or paroxetine were discontinued. The majority of these occurrences have been in older patients and in patients taking diuretics or who were otherwise volume-depleted.

Diabetes: **Fluoxetine** may alter glycemic control. Hypoglycemia has occurred during therapy, and hyperglycemia has developed following discontinuation of the drug. The dosage of insulin or the sulfonylurea may need to be adjusted when fluoxetine is started or discontinued.

Uricosuric effect: **Sertraline** is associated with a mean decrease in serum uric acid of ≈ 7%. The clinical significance of this weak uricosuric effect is unknown, and there have been no reports of acute renal failure with sertraline.

Drug abuse and dependence: Before staring an SSRI, carefully evaluate patients for history of drug abuse and follow such patients closely, observing them for signs of misuse or abuse.

Hazardous tasks: SSRIs may cause dizziness or drowsiness. Patients should be instructed to observe caution while driving or performing tasks requiring alertness, coordination or physical dexterity.

Photosensitivity: Photosensitization may occur.

Drug Interactions:

Drugs highly bound to plasma protein: Because **paroxetine** and **sertraline** are highly bound to plasma protein, administration to a patient taking another drug that is highly protein-bound may cause increased free concentrations of the other drug, potentially resulting in adverse events. Conversely, adverse effects could result from displacement of paroxetine or sertraline by other highly bound drugs.

Microsomal enzyme induction: Concomitant use of **paroxetine** with drugs metabolized by cytochrome $P450IID_6$ may require lower doses than usually prescribed for either paroxetine or the other drug since paroxetine may significantly inhibit the activity of this isozyme.

Drugs that may affect selective serotonin reuptake inhibitors include cimetidine, cyproheptadine, dextromethorphan, lithium, MAO inhibitors, phenobarbital, phenytoin, smoking and L-tryptophan.

Drugs that may be affected by selective serotonin reuptake inhibitors include phenytoin, alcohol, tricyclic antidepressants, nonsedating antihistamines, cyclosporine, haloperidol, phentermine, pimozide, sumatriptan, benzodiazepines, beta blockers, buspirone, carbamazepine, clozapine, diltiazem, digoxin, lithium, methadone, procyclidine, theophylline, tolbutamide and warfarin.

Drug/Food interactions: In one study following a single dose of **sertraline** with and without food, sertraline AUC was slightly increased and C_{max} was 25% greater. Time to reach peak plasma level decreased from 8 hours post-dosing to 5.5 hours.

Food does not appear to affect systemic bioavailability of **fluoxetine** although it may delay absorption. **Fluvoxamine** bioavailability is not affected by food. Thus, fluoxetine and fluvoxamine may be given with or without food.

Adverse Reactions:

Commonly observed:

SSRIs Adverse Reactions (%) (≥ 3% in at least one agent)

Adverse reaction	Fluoxetine	Fluvoxamine	Paroxetine	Sertraline
Body as a whole				
Headache	21	22	18	20
Asthenia	12	14	15	1
Abdominal pain	3.4	—	3.1	2.4
Infection, viral or bacterial	3.4	—	—	—
Influenza/Flu syndrome	5	3	—	—
Accidental injury	4	≥ 1	—	—
Cardiovascular				
Palpitations	2	3	3	4
Vasodilation	3	3	3	—
Chest pain	1.3	—	3	3
CNS				
Insomnia	20	21	13	16
Somnolence	13	22	23	13
Nervousness	13	12	5	3
Anxiety	13	5	5	3
Dizziness	10	11	13	12
Tremor	10	5	8	11
Libido decreased/ sexual dysfunction	4	2	3	2 (female) 16 (male)
Agitation	≥ 1	2	5	6
Paresthesia	—	—	4	3
Drowsiness	11.6	—	—	—
Fatigue/Malaise	4.2	≥ 1	—	11
Sedation	1.9	—	—	—
Abnormal dreams	5	—	4	0.1-1
Abnormal thinking	4	—	0.1-1	0.1-1
Sleep disorder	3	—	—	—

SSRIs Adverse Reactions (%) (≥ 3% in at least one agent)				
Adverse reaction	Fluoxetine	Fluvoxamine	Paroxetine	Sertraline
Depersonalization	0.1-1	0.1-1	3	3
GI				
Nausea	23	40	26	26
Vomiting	3	5	—	4
Diarrhea/loose stools	12	11	12	18
Dyspepsia	8	10	2	6
Dry mouth	10	14	18	16
Anorexia	11	6	6	3
Constipation	4.5	10	14	8
Abdominal pain	3.4	—	4	—
Flatulence	3	4	4	4
Tooth disorder/caries	—	3	< 0.1	—
Increased appetite	≥ 1	—	3	3
Tooth disorder/caries	—	3	< 0.1	—
GI disorder	6	—	—	—
Musculoskeletal				
Myalgia	5	—	2	1.7
Arthralgia	3	0.1-1	0.1-1	0.1-1
Respiratory				
Upper respiratory infection	7.6	9	—	—
Pharyngitis	5	—	—	4
Rhinitis	≥ 1	—	3	2
Yawn	3	2	4	2
Respiratory disorder	—	—	5.9	—
Skin				
Sweating, excessive	8	7	11	8
Rash	4	—	2	2
Pruritus	3	—	1	0.1-1
Special senses				
Vision disturbances/ blurred vision	3	—	4	4
Taste perversion/change	1	3	2	3
Amblyopia	3	3	—	—
GU				
Sexual dysfunction/ impotence/anorgasmia	1.9	2	6.5	16
Urinary frequency	1	3	3	2
Abnormal ejaculation	—	8	13	17
Male genital disorders, others	—	—	10	—
Urination disorder/ retention	—	1	3	Rare

Administration and Dosage:

SERTRALINE HCl:

Initial treatment – 50 mg once daily, either in the morning or evening. While a relationship between dose and antidepressant effect has not been established, patients were dosed in a range of 50 to 200 mg/day in the clinical trials. Consequently, patients not responding to a 50 mg dose may benefit from dose increases up to a maximum of 200 mg/day. Given the 24 hour elimination half-life of sertraline, dose changes should not occur at intervals of < 1 week.

Hepatic/Renal function impairment – Give a lower or less frequent dosage in patients with hepatic or renal impairment.

Maintenance/Continuation/Extended treatment – There is evidence to suggest that depressed patients responding during an initial 8 week treatment phase will continue to benefit during an additional 8 weeks of treatment. While there are insufficient data regarding any benefits from treatment beyond 16 weeks, it is generally agreed among expert psychopharmacologists that acute episodes of depression require several months or longer of sustained pharmacological therapy.

PAROXETINE HCl:

Depression –

Initial dose: 20 mg/day. Administer as a single daily dose, usually in the morning. Usual range is 20 to 50 mg/day. Some patients not responding to a 20 mg dose may benefit from dose increases, in 10 mg/day increments, up to a maximum of 50 mg/day. Dose changes should occur at intervals of at least 1 week.

Maintenace therapy: It is generally agreed that acute episodes of depression require several months or longer of sustained pharmacologic therapy. Efficacy has been maintained for period up to 1 year with doses that averaged about 30 mg.

OCD –

Initial: 40 mg/day. Administer as a single daily dose, usually in the morning. Start with 20 mg/day and may be increased in 10 mg/day increments. Dose changes should occur at intervals of at least 1 week. Usual range is 20 to 60 mg/day. The maximum dosage should not exceed 60 mg/day.

Maintenance therapy: Patients have been continued on therapy for 6 months without loss of benefit. However, make dosage adjustments to maintain the patient on the lowest effective dosage, and periodically reassess the patient to determine the need for treatment.

Panic disorder –

Initial: 40 mg/day. Administer as a single daily dose, usually in the morning. Start with 10 mg/day and may be increased in 10 mg/day increments. Dose changes should occur at intervals of at least 1 week. Usual range is 10 to 60 mg/day. The maximum dosage should not exceed 60 mg/day.

Maintenance therapy: Long-term maintenance of efficacy has been demonstrated for 3 months. Make dosage adjustments to maintain the patient on the lowest effective dosage, and reassess the patients periodically to determine the need for continued treatment.

FLUOXETINE HCl:

Depression –

Initial: 20 mg/day in the morning. Consider a dose increase after several weeks if no clinical improvement is observed. Administer doses > 20 mg/day on a once (morning) or twice (eg, morning and noon) daily schedule. Do not exceed a maximum dose of 80 mg/day.

Maintenance: Optimal duration of fluoxetine therapy remains speculative. Acute episodes of depression generally require several months or longer of sustained pharmacological therapy.

Obsessive-Compulsive disorder –

Initial: 20 mg/day in the morning. Consider a dose increase after several weeks if insufficient clinical improvement is observed. Administer doses > 20 mg/day on a once (morning) or twice (morning and noon) daily schedule. A dose range of 20 to 60 mg/day is recommended; however, doses of up to 80 mg/day have been well tolerated. Do not exceed 80 mg/day.

Maintenance: Patients have been continued on therapy for an additional 6 months without loss of benefit.

Bulimia nervosa –

Initial: The recommended dose is 60 mg/day, administered in the morning. For some patients it may be advisable to titrate up to this target dose over several days. Fluoxetine doses > 60 mg/day have not been systematically studied in patients with bulimia.

Maintenance: Patients have been continued on therapy for an additional 6 months without loss of benefit. However, make dosage adjustments to maintain the patient on the lowest effective dosage, and periodically reassess the patient to determine the need for treatment.

Renal/Hepatic function impairment – Use a lower or less frequent dosage.

Special risk patients – Consider a lower or less frequent dosage for patients, such as the elderly, with concurrent disease or on multiple medications.

FLUVOXAMINE MALEATE:

Initial therapy – Recommended starting dose is 50 mg as a single bedtime dose. In trials, patients were titrated within a range of 100 to 300 mg/day. Increase dose in 50 mg increments every 4 to 7 days, as tolerated, until maximum therapeutic benefit is achieved, not to exceed 300 mg/day. It is advisable to give total daily doses > 100 mg in two divided doses; if doses are unequal, give larger dose at bedtime.

Maintenance therapy – Although efficacy has not been documented > 10 weeks in controlled trials, OCD is a chronic condition; it is reasonable to consider continuation for a responding patient.

Elderly/Hepatic function impairment – These patients have been observed to have decreased fluvoxamine clearance. It may be appropriate to modify initial dose and subsequent titration.

ANTIPSYCHOTIC AGENTS

Actions:

Pharmacology:

Select Dosage and Pharmacologic Parameters of Antipsychotics							
Incidence of Side Effects: +++ = High, ++ = Moderate, + = Low; Antipsychotic agent	Approx. equiv. dose (mg)	Adult daily dosage range (mg)	Sedation	Extrapyramidal symptoms	Anticholinergic effects	Orthostatic hypotension	Therapeutic plasma concentration (ng/ml)
Phenothiazines: Aliphatic							
Chlorpromazine	100	30-800	+++	++	++	+++	30-500
Promazine	200	40-1200	++	++	+++	++	
Triflupromazine	25	60-150	+++	++	+++	++	
Phenothiazines: Piperidine							
Thioridazine	100	150-800	+++	+	+++	+++	
Mesoridazine	50	30-400	+++	+	+++	++	
Phenothiazines: Piperazine							
Acetophenazine	20	60-120	++	+++	+	+	
Perphenazine	10	12-64	+	+++	+	+	0.8-1.2
Prochlorperazine	15	15-150	++	+++	+	+	
Fluphenazine	2	0.5-40	+	+++	+	+	0.13-2.8
Trifluoperazine	5	2-40	+	+++	+	+	
Thioxanthenes							
Chlorprothixene	100	75-600	+++	++	++	++	
Thiothixene	4	8-30	+	+++	+	+	2-57
Butyrophenone							
Haloperidol	2	1-15	+	+++	+	+	5-20
Dihydroindolone							
Molindone	10	15-225	+	+++	+	+	
Dibenzoxazepine							
Loxapine	15	20-250	++	+++	+	++	
Dibenzodiazepine							
Clozapine	50	300-900	+++	+	+++	+++	
Benzisoxazole							
Risperidone		4-16	+	0/+	+	+	
Diphenylbutylpiperidine							
Pimozide	0.3-0.5	1-10	++	+++	++	+	

The exact mode of action is not fully understood. Antipsychotics block postsynaptic dopamine receptors in the basal ganglia, hypothalamus, limbic system, brain stem and medulla. Inhibition or alteration of dopamine release, an increased neuronal cell firing rate in the midbrain and an increased turnover rate of dopamine in the forebrain have been noted. These observations support the theory that anti- psychotics interfere with dopamine, but do not prove that dopaminolytic activity is sufficient for antipsychotic efficacy.

There is little evidence of clinical differences in efficacy among these agents (except clozapine) when used in equitherapeutic dosages; however, a patient who fails to respond to one agent may respond to another and agents are not necessarily interchangeable. Clozapine is used for severely ill schizophrenic patients who fail to respond adequately to standard antipsychotic treatment.

The principal differences between antipsychotic agents are the type and severity of side effects which include: Sedation, extrapyramidal effects. Coadministration of two or more antipsychotics does not improve clinical response and may increase the potential for adverse effects.

In chronic therapy, full clinical effects may not be achieved for ≥ 6 weeks. Approximately 4 to 7 days are required to achieve steady-state plasma levels; therefore, do not make more than weekly dosage adjustments in chronic therapy.

Since plasma concentrations of antipsychotics are highly variable from patient to patient, plasma monitoring of these agents may not be useful for determining therapeutic response.

Pharmacokinetics:

Absorption – Oral absorption tends to be erratic and variable. Peak plasma levels are seen 2 to 4 hours after oral use.

Distribution – These agents are widely distributed in tissues; CNS concentrations exceed those in plasma. They are highly bound to plasma proteins (91% to 99%). Because they are highly lipophilic, the antipsychotics and metabolites accumulate in the brain, lungs and other tissues with high blood supply. They are stored in these tissues and may be found in urine for up to 6 months after the last dose.

Metabolism – Extensive biotransformation occurs in the liver. Numerous active metabolites, which persist for prolonged periods, have important side effects and contribute to the biological activity of the parent drug.

Excretion – One-half of the excretion of these agents occurs via the kidneys and the other half occurs through enterohepatic circulation. Elimination half-lives range from 10 to 20 hours. Less than 1% is excreted as unchanged drug.

Indications:

Management of psychotic disorders.

Some of these agents are used as antiemetics (refer to Antiemetic/Antivertigo Agents).

Unlabeled uses: Chlorpromazine and haloperidol are effective in the treatment of phencyclidine (PCP) psychosis; coadministration of ascorbic acid with haloperidol may be more effective than haloperidol alone.

IV or IM chlorpromazine may be beneficial for migraine headaches; IV prochlorperazine may be effective in treating severe vascular or tension headaches.

Neuroleptics appear useful for the treatment of Tourette's syndrome.

Neuroleptics are effective in control of acute agitation in the elderly. May also be useful in treating some symptoms of dementia including agitation, hyperactivity, hallucinations, suspiciousness, hostility and uncooperativeness; however, they do not improve memory loss and may impair cognitive function.

Other potential uses include treatment of: Huntington's chorea (chlorpromazine, fluphenazine, haloperidol); hemiballismus (perphenazine, haloperidol); chorea associated with rheumatic fever or SLE, spasmodic torticollis and Meige's syndrome (haloperidol).

Contraindications:

Comatose or severely depressed states; hypersensitivity (cross-sensitivity between phenothiazines may occur); presence of large amounts of other CNS depressants; bone marrow depression; blood dyscrasias; circulatory collapse (thioxanthenes); subcortical brain damage; Parkinson's disease (haloperidol); liver damage; cerebral arteriosclerosis; coronary artery disease; severe hypotension or hypertension; pediatric surgery (prochlorperazine).

Warnings:

Tardive dyskinesia (TD), a syndrome consisting of potentially irreversible, involuntary dyskinetic movements, may develop in patients treated with neuroleptic drugs. Both the risk of developing TD and the likelihood that it will become irreversible are increased as duration of treatment and total cumulative dose administered increase.

Neuroleptic malignant syndrome (NMS) is a rare idiosyncratic combination of EPS, hyperthermia and autonomic disturbance. Onset may be hours to months after drug initiation, but once started, proceeds rapidly over 24 to 72 hours. It is most commonly associated with **haloperidol** and depot **fluphenazines,** but has occurred with **thiothixene** and **thioridazine** and may occur with other agents. NMS is potentially fatal, and requires intensive symptomatic treatment and immediate discontinuation of neuroleptic treatment.

CNS effects: These agents may impair mental or physical abilities, especially during the first few days. Drowsiness may occur during the first or second week, after which it generally disappears. If troublesome, lower the dosage. Caution patients against activities requiring alertness (eg, operating vehicles or machinery).

Antiemetic effects: Drugs with antiemetic effect can obscure signs of toxicity of other drugs, or mask symptoms of disease (eg, brain tumor, intestinal obstruction, Reye's syndrome). They can suppress the cough reflex; aspiration of vomitus is possible.

Decreased serum cholesterol occurs. **Chlorpromazine** may raise plasma cholesterol.

Cardiovascular: Use with caution in patients with cardiovascular disease or mitral insufficiency. Increased pulse rates occur in most patients.

Hypotension – Carefully watch patients who are undergoing surgery, and who are on large doses of phenothiazines, for hypotensive phenomena. The hypotensive effects may occur after the first injection of the antipsychotic, occasionally after subsequent injections, and rarely after the first oral dose. Recovery is usually spontaneous and symptoms disappear within 0.5 to 2 hours.

Ophthalmic: Use with caution in patients with a history of glaucoma. During prolonged therapy, ocular changes may occur; these include particle deposition in the cornea and lens, progressing in more severe cases to star-shaped lenticular opacities. Pigmentary retinopathy occurs most frequently in patients receiving **thioridazine** dosages > 1 g/day.

Seizure disorders: These drugs can lower the convulsive threshold and may precipitate seizures. Use cautiously in patients with a history of epilepsy and only when absolutely necessary.

Adynamic ileus occasionally occurs with phenothiazine therapy and, if severe, can result in complications and death.

Sudden death: Previous brain damage or seizures may be predisposing factors; avoid high doses in known seizure patients.

Hepatic effects: Jaundice usually occurs between the second and fourth weeks of treatment and is regarded as a hypersensitivity reaction.

Renal function impairment: Administer cautiously to those with diminished renal function.

Hepatic function impairment: Use with caution in patients with impaired hepatic function. Patients with a history of hepatic encephalopathy due to cirrhosis have increased sensitivity to the CNS effects of antipsychotic drugs (ie, impaired cerebration and abnormal slowing of the EEG).

Carcinogenesis: Neuroleptic drugs (except promazine) elevate prolactin levels which persist during chronic use. Tissue culture experiments indicate ≈ ⅓ of human breast cancers are prolactin-dependent in vitro, a factor of potential importance if use of these drugs is contemplated in a patient with previously detected breast cancer.

Elderly: Dosages in the lower range are sufficient for most elderly patients. Monitor response and adjust dosage accordingly. Increase dosage gradually in elderly patients.

Pregnancy: Safety for use during pregnancy has not been established. Phenothiazines readily cross the placenta.

Lactation: **Chlorpromazine** and **haloperidol** have been detected in breast milk. Although few cases are documented, a milk:plasma ratio of 0.5 to 0.7 or less is reported, representing a milk drug level of 290 ng/ml and 2 to 23.5 ng/ml, respectively. Safety for use in the nursing mother has not been established.

Children: In general, these products are not recommended for children < 12 years old. Loxapine is not recommended in children < 16 years old.

Precautions:

Concomitant conditions: Use with caution in patients: Exposed to extreme heat or phosphorus insecticides; in a state of alcohol withdrawal; with dermatoses or other allergic reactions to phenothiazine derivatives because of the possibility of cross-sensitivity; who have exhibited idiosyncrasy to other centrally acting drugs.

Hematologic: Various blood dyscrasias have occurred.

Myelography: Discontinue phenothiazines at least 48 hours before myelography due to the possibility of seizures; do not resume therapy for at least 24 hours postprocedure.

Thyroid: Severe neurotoxicity (rigidity, inability to walk or talk) may occur in patients with thyrotoxicosis who are also receiving antipsychotics.

Hyperpyrexia: A significant, not otherwise explained rise in body temperature may indicate intolerance to antipsychotics.

ECT: Reserve concurrent use with electroconvulsive treatment for those patients for whom it is essential; the hazards may be increased.

Abrupt withdrawal: These drugs are not known to cause psychic dependence and do not produce tolerance or addiction. However, following abrupt withdrawal of high dose therapy, symptoms such as gastritis, nausea, vomiting, dizziness, headache, tachycardia, insomnia and tremulousness have occurred. These symptoms can be reduced by gradual reduction of the dosage (one suggestion is 10% to 25% every 2 weeks) or by continuing antiparkinson agents for several weeks after the antipsychotic is withdrawn.

Suicide possibility in depressed patients remains during treatment and until significant remission occurs. This type of patient should not have access to large quantities of the drug.

Cutaneous pigmentation changes/photosensitivity: Rare instances of skin pigmentation have occurred, primarily in females on long-term, high dose therapy. Photosensitization may occur; caution patients against exposure to ultraviolet light or undue exposure to sunlight during phenothiazine therapy. These effects occur most commonly with **chlorpromazine** (3%).

Drug Interactions:

Drugs that may affect phenothiazines include alcohol, aluminum salts, anorexiants, anticholinergics, barbiturates, carbamazepine, charcoal, fluoxetine, lithium, meperidine, methyldopa, metrizamide and propranolol. Drugs that may be affected by phenothiazine include barbiturate anesthetics, bromocriptine, norepinephrine and epinephrine, guanethidine, phenytoin, propranolol, TCAs and valproic acid.

Drug/Lab test interactions: An increase in **cephalin flocculation** sometimes accompanied by alterations in other **liver function tests** has occurred in patients receiving fluphenazine enanthate who have had no clinical evidence of liver damage.

Phenothiazines may discolor the urine pink to red-brown.

False-positive **pregnancy tests** have occurred, but are less likely to occur when a serum test is used.

An increase in **protein bound iodine**, not attributable to an increase in thyroxine, has been noted.

Adverse Reactions:

CNS effects: Headache; weakness; tremor; staggering gait; twitching; tension; jitteriness; fatigue; slurring; insomnia; vertigo; drowsiness (80%, usually lasts 1 week). Exacerbation of psychotic symptoms including hallucinations; catatonic-like states; lethargy; restlessness; hyperactivity; agitation; nocturnal confusion; toxic confusional states; bizarre dreams; depression; euphoria; excitement; paranoid reactions.

Autonomic: Dry mouth; nasal congestion; nausea; vomiting; paresthesia; anorexia; pallor; flushed facies; salivation; perspiration; constipation; fecal impaction; diarrhea; urinary retention, frequency or incontinence; polyuria; enuresis; priapism; ejaculation inhibition; male impotence (not reported with **molindone**).

Heatstroke/Hyperpyrexia induced by neuroleptics has occurred.

Extrapyramidal: These are usually dose-related and take three forms: Pseudoparkinsonism (4% to 40%); akathisia (7% to 20%); dystonias (2% to 50%).

Hepatic: Jaundice usually occurs between the second and fourth weeks of therapy and is regarded as a hypersensitivity reaction.

Hematologic: Eosinophilia; leukopenia; leukocytosis; anemia; tendency toward lymphomonocytosis; thrombocytopenia; granulocytopenia; aplastic anemia; hemolytic anemia; thrombocytopenic or nonthrombocytopenic purpura; agranulocytosis; pancytopenia.

Cardiovascular: Hypotension; postural hypotension; hypertension; tachycardia (especially with rapid increase in dosage); bradycardia; cardiac arrest; circulatory collapse; syncope; lightheadedness; faintness; dizziness. Cardiovascular effects are generally attributable to the piperidine phenothiazines > aliphatic > piperazines (see table).

Hypersensitivity: Urticarial (5%), maculopapular hypersensitivity reactions; pruritus; dry skin; erythema; photosensitivity; eczema; asthma; rashes, including acneiform; hair loss; exfoliative dermatitis.

Endocrine: Lactation and moderate breast engorgement in females; galactorrhea; mastalgia; amenorrhea; menstrual irregularities; changes in libido; hyperglycemia or hypoglycemia; hyponatremia; glycosuria; raised plasma cholesterol levels. Resumption of menses in previously amenorrheic women has been reported with **molindone**. Initially, heavy menses may occur.

Ophthalmic: Glaucoma; photophobia; blurred vision; miosis; mydriasis; ptosis; star-shaped lenticular opacities; pigmentary retinopathy.

Respiratory: Laryngospasm; bronchospasm; increased depth of respiration; dyspnea.

Miscellaneous: Increases in appetite and weight (excessive weight gain has not occurred with **molindone**); dyspepsia; peripheral or facial edema; suppression of cough reflex (with potential for aspiration or asphyxia).

DONEPEZIL HCl

Tablets: 5 and 10 mg (*Rx*)	*Aricept* (Eisai/Pfizer)

Actions:

Pharmacology: Donepezil is postulated to exert its therapeutic effect by enhancing cholinergic function. This increase in cholinergic function is accomplished by increasing the concentration of acetylcholine through reversible inhibition of its hydrolysis by acetylcholinesterase (AChE). If this proposed mechanism of action is correct, donepezil's effect may lessen as the disease process advances and fewer cholinergic neurons remain functionally intact. There is no evidence that donepezil alters the course of the underlying dementing process.

Pharmacokinetics:

Absorption – Donepezil is well absorbed with a relative oral bioavailability of 100% and reaches peak plasma concentrations in 3 to 4 hours. Neigher food nor time of administration (morning vs evening dose) influences rate or extent of absorption.

Distribution – Following multiple dose administration, steady state is reached within 15 days. The steady-state volume of distribution is 12 L/kg. Donepezil is ≈ 96% bound to human plasma proteins.

Metabolism – Donepezil is both excreted in urine intact and extensively metabolized to four major metabolites, two of which are known to be active. Donepezil is metabolized by CYP 450 isoenzyme 2D6 and 3A4 and undergoes glucuronidation.

Excretion – The elimination half-life of donepezil is ≈ 70 hours and the mean apparent plasma clearance is 0.13 L/hr/kg.

Approximately 57% and 15% of the total dose was recovered in urine and feces, respectively, over a period of 10 days, while 28% remained unrecovered, with ≈ 17% of the donepezil dose recovered in the urine as unchanged drug.

Indications:

Alzheimer's disease: The treatment of mild to moderate dementia of the Alzheimer's type.

Contraindications:

Hypersensitivity to donepezil or to piperidine derivatives.

Warnings:

Anesthesia: Donepezil, as a cholinesterase inhibitor, is likely to exaggerate succinylcholine-type muscle relaxation during anesthesia.

Cardiovascular: Cholinesterase inhibitors may have vagotonic effects on heart rate (eg, bradycardia). The potential for this action may be particularly important to patients with "sick sinus syndrome" or other supraventricular cardiac conduction conditions. Syncopal episodes have occurred in association with the use of donepezil.

GI: Through their primary action, cholinesterase inhibitors may be expected to increase gastric acid secretion because of increased cholinergic activity. Therefore, monitor patients closely for symptoms of active or occult GI bleeding, especially those at increased risk for developing ulcers.

Donepezil has been shown to produce diarrhea, nausea and vomiting. These effects, when they occur, appear more frequently with 10 mg/day than with 5 mg/day. In most cases, these effects have been mild and transient, sometimes lasting 1 to 3 weeks, and have resolved during continued use of donepezil.

GU: Cholinomimetics may cause bladder outflow obstruction.

Seizures: Cholinomimetics may have some potential to cause generalized convulsions. However, seizure activity also may be a manifestation of Alzheimer's disease.

Pulmonary: Prescribe cholinesterase inhibitors with care for patients with a history of asthma or obstructive pulmonary disease.

Pregnancy: *Category* C.

Lactation: It is not known whether donepezil is excreted in breast milk.

Children: There are no adequate and well controlled tirals to document the safety and efficacy of donepezil in any illness occurring in children.

Drug Interactions:

Drugs that may affect donepezil are ketoconazole and quinidine. Drugs that may be affected by donepezil include anticholinergics, cholinometics/cholinesterase inhibitors, NSAIDs, furosemide, digoxin, warfarin, theophylline and cimetidine.

Adverse Reactions:

Adverse reactions that may occur in ≥ 3% of patients include headache, whole body pain, fatigue, nausea, diarrhea, vomiting, anorexia, muscle cramps, insomnia, dizziness, depression, abnormal dreams, ecchymosis and weight decrease.

Administration and Dosage:

The dosages of donepezil are 5 and 10 mg once per day in the evening, just prior to retiring.

The higher dose of 10 mg did not provide a statistically significant clinical benefit greater than that of 5 mg. Do not increase to 10 mg until patients have been on a daily dose of 5 mg for 4 to 6 weeks.

Donepezil may be taken with or without food.

HISTAMINE H_2 ANTAGONISTS

CIMETIDINE	
Tablets: 100 mg (*otc*)	*Tagamet HB* (SK-Beecham)
Tablets: 200, 300, 400 and 800 mg (*Rx*)	Various, *Tagamet* (SK-Beecham)
Liquid: 300 mg (as HCl) per 5 ml (*Rx*)	*Cimetidine Oral Solution* (Barre-National), *Tagamet* (SK-Beecham)
Injection: 300 mg (as HCl) per 2 ml (*Rx*)	*Cimetidine* (Endo), *Tagamet* (SK-Beecham)
Injection, premixed: 300 mg (as HCl) in 50 ml 0.9% sodium chloride (*Rx*)	*Tagamet* (SK-Beecham)
FAMOTIDINE	
Tablets: 10 mg (*otc*)	*Pepcid AC Acid Controller* (J & J Merck)
Tablets: 20 and 40 mg (*Rx*)	*Pepcid* (J & J Merck)
Powder for Oral Suspension: 40 mg per 5 ml when reconstituted (*Rx*)	
Injection: 10 mg per ml (*Rx*)	
Injection, premixed: 20 mg per 50 ml in 0.9% HCl (*Rx*)	
NIZATIDINE	
Capsules: 150 and 300 mg (*Rx*)	*Axid Pulvules* (Lilly)
RANITIDINE	
Tablets: 75 mg (*otc*)	*Zantac 75* (Glaxo Wellcome)
Tablets: 150 and 300 mg (as HCl) (*Rx*)	*Zantac* (Glaxo Wellcome)
Tablets, effervescent: 150 mg (*Rx*)	*Zantac EFFERdose* (Glaxo Wellcome)
Capsules: 150 and 300 mg (*Rx*)	*Zantac GELdose* (Glaxo Wellcome)
Syrup: 15 mg (as HCl) per ml (*Rx*)	*Ranitidine HCl* (UDL), *Zantac* (Glaxo Wellcome)
Granules, effervescent: 150 mg (*Rx*)	*Zantac EFFERdose* (Glaxo Wellcome)
Injection: 0.5 and 25 mg (as HCl) per ml (*Rx*)	*Zantac* (Glaxo Wellcome)

Actions:

Pharmacology: Histamine H_2 antagonists are reversible competitive blockers of histamine at the H_2 receptors, particularly those in the gastric parietal cells. They also inhibit fasting and nocturnal secretions, and secretions stimulated by food, insulin, caffeine, pentagastrin and betazole. Cimetidine, ranitidine and famotidine have no effect on gastric emptying, and cimetidine and famotidine have no effect on lower esophageal sphincter pressure. Ranitidine, nizatidine and famotidine have little or no effect on fasting or postprandial serum gastrin.

Pharmacokinetics:

Pharmacokinetic Properties of Histamine H_2 Antagonists

H_2 receptor antagonist	Bioavailability (%)	Time to peak plasma concentration (hrs)	Peak plasma concentration[1] (mcg/ml)	Half-life (hrs)	Protein binding (%)	Volume of distribution (L/kg)	Elimination (%)		
							Urine, unchanged		Metabolized
							Oral	IV	
Cimetidine	60-70	0.75-1.5	0.7-3.2 (300 mg dose) (3.5-7.5 IV)	≈ 2[2]	13-25	0.8-1.2	48	75	30-40
Famotidine	40-45	1-3	0.076-0.1 (40 mg dose)	2.5-3.5[3]	15-20	1.1-1.4	25-30	65-70	30-35
Nizatidine	>90	0.5-3	0.7-1.8/ 1.4-3.6 (150/300 mg dose)	1-2[3]	≈ 35	0.8-1.5	60	na[4]	< 18
Ranitidine	50-60 (90-100 IM)	1-3 (0.25 IM)	0.44-0.55 (0.58 IM)	2-3[3]	15	1.2-1.9	30-35	68-79	< 10

[1] Dose-dependent.
[2] Increased in renal and hepatic impairment and in the elderly.
[3] Increased in renal impairment.
[4] na = not applicable.

Indications:

Histamine H_2 Antagonists: Summary of Indications				
✔ – Labeled x Unlabeled	Cimetidine	Famotidine	Nizatidine	Ranitidine
Duodenal ulcer				
Treatment	✔	✔	✔	✔
Maintenance	✔	✔	✔	✔
GERD (including erosive esophagitis)	✔	✔	✔	✔
Gastric ulcer				
Treatment	✔	✔	✔	✔
Maintenance				✔
Pathological hypersecretory conditions	✔	✔		✔
Heartburn/acid indigestion/ sour stomach	✔[1, 2]	✔[1, 3]		
Erosive esophagitis, maintenance				✔
Prevent upper GI bleeding	✔	x		x
Peptic ulcer [4]	x	x	x	x
Prevent aspiration pneumonitis	x	x		x
Prophylaxis of stress ulcers	x	x		x
Prevent gastric NSAID damage				x
Hyperparathyroidism	x			
Secondary hyperparathyroidism in hemodialysis	x			
Tinea capitis	x			
Herpes virus infection	x			
Hirsute women	x			
Chronic idiopathic urticaria	x			
Anaphylaxis (dermatological)	x			
Acetaminophen overdose	x			
Dyspepsia	x			
Warts	x			
Colorectal cancer	x			

[1] *otc* use only.
[2] Relief of symptoms only.
[3] Relief and prevention of symptoms.
[4] As part of a multi-drug regimen to eradicate *Helicobacter pylori*.

Contraindications:

Hypersensitivity to individual agents or to other H_2-receptor antagonists.

Warnings:

Benzyl alcohol, contained in some of these products as a preservative, has been associated with a fatal "gasping syndrome" in premature infants.

Hypersensitivity: Rare cases of anaphylaxis have occurred as well as rare episodes of hypersensitivity (eg, bronchospasm, laryngeal edema, rash, eosinophilia).

Renal function impairment: Since these agents are excreted primarily via the kidneys, decreased clearance may occur; reduced dosage may be necessary.

Hepatic function impairment: Observe caution. Decreased clearance may occur; these agents are partly metabolized in the liver.

Elderly: Safety and efficacy appear similar to those of younger age; however, the elderly may have reduced renal function. Decreased **cimetidine** clearance may be more common.

Pregnancy: *(Category B - cimetidine, famotidine, ranitidine. Category C - nizatidine)*. Cimetidine crosses the placenta.

Lactation: **Cimetidine** is excreted in breast milk with milk:plasma ratios of approximately 5:1 to 12:1. Potential daily infant ingestion is approximately 6 mg.

Ranitidine is excreted in breast milk with milk:plasma ratios of 1:1 to 6.7:1.

Nizatidine is excreted in breast milk in a concentration of 0.1% of the oral dose in proportion to plasma concentrations.

Famotidine is excreted in the breast milk of rats. It is not known whether it is excreted in human breast milk.

Children: Safety and efficacy are not established. **Cimetidine** is not recommended for children < 16 years old, unless anticipated benefits outweigh potential risks. In very limited experience, cimetidine 20 to 40 mg/kg/day has been used.

Precautions:

Gastric malignancy: Symptomatic response to these agents does not preclude gastric malignancy.

Reversible CNS effects (eg, mental confusion, agitation, psychosis, depression, anxiety, hallucinations, disorientation) have occurred with **cimetidine,** predominantly in severely ill patients. Advancing age (≥ 50 years) and preexisting liver or renal disease appear to be contributing factors.

Hepatocellular injury may occur with **nizatidine** as evidenced by elevated liver enzymes (AST, ALT or alkaline phosphatase).

Occasionally, reversible hepatitis, hepatocellular or hepatocanalicular or mixed, with or without jaundice have occurred with oral **ranitidine.**

Laboratory test monitoring for liver abnormalities is appropriate.

Antiandrogenic effect: **Cimetidine** has a weak antiandrogenic effect in animals. Gynecomastia in patients treated for ≥ 1 month may occur.

Immunocompromised patients: Decreased gastric acidity, including that produced by acid-suppressing agents such as H_2 antagonists, may increase the possibility of strongyloidiasis.

Drug Interactions:

Cimetidine reduces the hepatic metabolism of drugs metabolized via the cytochrome P-450 pathway, delaying elimination and increasing serum levels.

Cimetidine Drug Interactions (Decreased Hepatic Metabolism)		
Benzodiazepines[1]	Metronidazole	Sulfonylureas
Caffeine	Moricizine	Tacrine
Calcium channel blockers	Pentoxifylline	Theophyllines [2]
Carbamazepine	Phenytoin	Triamterene
Chloroquine	Propafenone	Tricyclic antidepressants
Labetalol	Propranolol	Valproic acid
Lidocaine	Quinidine	Warfarin
Metoprolol	Quinine	

[1] Does not include agents metabolized by glucuronidation (lorazepam, oxazepam, temazepam).
[2] Does not include dyphylline.

Ranitidine (which weakly binds to cytochrome P450 in vitro), **famotidine** and **nizatidine** do not inhibit the cytochrome P450-linked oxygenase enzyme system in the liver. Drug interactions with these agents mediated by inhibition of hepatic metabolism are not expected.

Drugs that may affect histamine H_2 antagonists include antacids, anticholinergics, metoclopramide and cigarette smoking. Drugs that may be affected by histamine H_2 antagonists include ferrous salts, indomethacin, ketoconazole, tetracyclines, carmustine, digoxin, flecainide, fluconazole, fluorouracil, narcotic analgesics, procainamide, succinylcholine, tocainide, salicylates, diazepam, sulfonylureas, theophyllines, warfarin and ethanol.

Drug/Lab test interactions: False-positive tests for urobilinogen may occur during **nizatidine** therapy. False-positive tests for urine protein with *Multistix* may occur during **ranitidine** therapy; testing with sulfosalicylic acid is recommended.

Drug/Food interactions: Food may increase bioavailability of **famotidine** and **nizatidine;** this is of no clinical consequence. **Cimetidine** and **ranitidine** are not affected.

Adverse Reactions:

Adverse reactions may include headache, somnolence/fatigue, dizziness, confusional states, hallucinations, insomnia, nausea, vomiting, abdominal discomfort, diarrhea, constipation, thrombocytopenia, alopecia, rash, gynecomastia, impotence, loss of libido and arthralgia.

Administration and Dosage:

CIMETIDINE:

Duodenal ulcer –

Short-term treatment of active duodenal ulcer: 800 mg at bedtime. Alternate regimens are 300 mg 4 times a day with meals and at bedtime, or 400 mg twice a day.

Maintenance therapy: 400 mg at bedtime.

Active benign gastric ulcer – For short-term treatment, 800 mg at bedtime or 300 mg 4 times a day with meals and at bedtime.

Erosive gastroesophageal reflux disease (GERD) –

Adults: 1600 mg daily in divided doses (800 mg twice daily or 400 mg 4 times a day) for 12 weeks. Use beyond 12 weeks has not been established.

Pathological hypersecretory conditions – 300 mg 4 times a day with meals and at bedtime. If necessary, give 300 mg doses more often. Do not exceed 2400 mg/day.

Prevention of upper GI bleeding – Continuous IV infusion of 50 mg/hour. Patients with creatinine clearance < 30 ml/min should receive half the recommended dose. Treatment beyond 7 days has not been studied.

Severely impaired renal function – Accumulation may occur. Use the lowest dose; 300 mg every 12 hours orally or IV has been recommended. Dosage frequency may be increased to every 8 hours or even further with caution.

Parenteral – The usual dose is 300 mg IM or IV every 6 to 8 hours. If it is necessary to increase dosage, do so by more frequent administration of a 300 mg dose, not to exceed 2400 mg/day.

IM: Administer undiluted.

IV: Dilute to a total volume of 20 ml; inject over ≥ 2 minutes.

Intermittent IV infusion: Dilute 300 mg in at least 50 ml of compatible IV solution; infuse over 15 to 20 minutes.

Continuous IV infusion: 37.5 mg/hour (900 mg/day).

FAMOTIDINE:

Duodenal ulcer –

Acute therapy: 40 mg/day at bedtime. 20 mg twice/day is also effective.

Maintenance therapy: 20 mg once a day at bedtime.

Benign gastric ulcer –

Acute therapy: 40 mg orally once a day at bedtime.

Pathological hypersecretory conditions – The adult starting dose is 20 mg every 6 hours.

GERD – 20 mg twice daily for up to 6 weeks. For esophagitis including erosions and ulcerations and accompanying symptoms due to GERD, 20 or 40 mg twice daily for up to 12 weeks.

Severe renal insufficiency –

Ccr < 10 ml/min: To avoid excess accumulation of the drug, the dose may be reduced to 20 mg at bedtime or the dosing interval may be prolonged to 36 to 48 hours, as indicated.

Parenteral –

IV: Give famotidine IV 20 mg every 12 hours.

NIZATIDINE:

Active duodenal ulcer – 300 mg once daily at bedtime. An alternative dosage regimen is 150 mg twice daily.

Maintenance of healed duodenal ulcer – 150 mg once daily at bedtime.

GERD – 150 mg twice daily.

Moderate to severe renal insufficiency –

Nizatidine Dosage in Renal Insufficiency

	Dosage	
Creatinine clearance	Active duodenal ulcer	Maintenance therapy
20 to 50 ml/min	150 mg/day	150 mg every other day
< 20 ml/min	150 mg every other day	150 mg every 3 days

RANITIDINE:

Duodenal ulcer –

Short-term treatment of active duodenal ulcer: 150 mg orally twice daily. An alternate dosage of 300 mg once daily at bedtime can be used for patients in whom dosing convenience is important.

Maintenance therapy: 150 mg at bedtime.

Pathological hypersecretory conditions – 150 mg orally twice a day. More frequent doses may be necessary. Doses up to 6 g/day have been used.

Benign gastric ulcer (oral doseforms only) and GERD – 150 mg twice daily.

Erosive esophagitis – 150 mg 4 times daily.

Renal impairment – (Ccr < 50 ml/min): 150 mg orally every 24 hours or 50 mg parenterally every 18 to 24 hours. The frequency of dosing may be increased to every 12 hours or further with caution.

Parenteral –

IM: 50 mg (2 ml) every 6 to 8 hours. (No dilution necessary.)

IV injection: 50 mg (2 ml) every 6 to 8 hours. Dilute 50 mg to a total volume of 20 ml; inject over ≥ 5 min.

Intermittent IV infusion: 50 mg (2 ml) every 6 to 8 hours. Dilute 50 mg and infuse over 15 to 20 minutes; do not exceed 400 mg/day.

Continuous IV infusion: Add ranitidine injection to 5% Dextrose Injection or other compatible IV solution. Deliver at a rate of 6.25 mg/hr (eg, 150 mg [6 ml] ranitidine injection in 250 ml of 5% Dextrose Injection at 10.7 ml/hr).

OMEPRAZOLE

Capsules, sustained release: 10 and 20 mg (*Rx*) *Prilosec* (Astra Merck)

Actions:

Pharmacology: Omeprazole belongs to a new class of antisecretory compounds, the substituted benzimidazoles, that suppress gastric acid secretion by specific inhibition of the H^+/K^+ ATPase enzyme system at the secretory surface of the gastric parietal cell. Because this enzyme system is the acid (proton) pump within the gastric mucosa, omeprazole has been characterized as a gastric acid pump inhibitor; it blocks the final step of acid production.

Antisecretory activity – Onset after oral administration of omeprazole occurs within 1 hour, and is maximum within 2 hours. Inhibition of secretion is about 50% of maximum at 24 hours and the duration of inhibition lasts up to 72 hours.

Pharmacokinetics:

Absorption/Distribution – Omeprazole contains an enteric coated granule formulation (because omeprazole is acid-labile). Absorption is rapid, with peak plasma levels occurring within 0.5 to 3.5 hours. Absolute bioavailability is about 30% to 40% at doses of 20 to 40 mg, due to presystemic metabolism. Plasma half-life is 0.5 to 1 hour, and total body clearance is 500 to 600 ml/min. Protein binding is ≈ 95%.

Metabolism/Excretion – Little unchanged drug is excreted in urine. The majority of the dose (about 77%) is eliminated in urine as at least six metabolites.

Indications:

Active duodenal ulcer: Short-term treatment of active duodenal ulcer. Most patients heal within 4 weeks, although some may require an additional 4 weeks.

Gastroesophageal reflux disease (GERD):

Severe erosive esophagitis – Short-term treatment (4 to 8 weeks) of erosive esophagitis, diagnosed by endoscopy.

Poorly responsive symptomatic GERD – Short-term treatment (4 to 8 weeks) of symptomatic GERD (esophagitis) poorly responsive to customary medical treatment, usually including histamine H_2 receptor antagonists.

Eradication of H. pylori – In combination with clarithromycin for treatment of patients with *H. pylori* infection and active duodenal ulcer.

Maintenance – To maintain healing of erosive esophagitis.

Pathological hypersecretory conditions (eg, Zollinger-Ellison syndrome, multiple endocrine adenomas and systemic mastocytosis): Long-term treatment.

Gastric ulcer: Short-term treatment (4 to 8 weeks) of active benign gastric ulcer.

Contraindications:

Hypersensitivity to any component of the formulation.

Warnings:

Maintenance therapy: Omeprazole should not be used as maintenance therapy for treatment of patients with duodenal ulcer disease.

Duration of therapy (GERD): In the rare patient not responding to 8 weeks of treatment, an additional 4 weeks of treatment may help. If there is recurrence of severe or symptomatic GERD poorly responsive to customary medical treatment, an additional 4 to 8 week course of omeprazole may be considered.

Elderly: Bioavailability may be increased.

Pregnancy: Category C.

Lactation: It is not known whether omeprazole is excreted in breast milk.

Children: Safety and efficacy in children have not been established.

Precautions:

Gastric malignancy: Symptomatic response does not preclude gastric malignancy.

Drug Interactions:

Drugs that may interact with omeprazole include clarithromycin, diazepam, phenytoin and warfarin. There may be interactions with other drugs also metabolized via the cytochrome P450 system. Omeprazole may interfere with absorption of drugs where gastric pH is a determinant of their bioavailability (eg, ketoconazole, ampicillin esters, iron salts).

Adverse Reactions:

Adverse reactions may include headache or diarrhea.

Administration and Dosage:

Active duodenal ulcer:

Adults – 20 mg daily for 4 to 8 weeks.

GERD:

Erosive esophagitis or poorly responsive GERD – Adults – 20 mg daily for 4 to 8 weeks.

Maintenance of healing erosive esophagitis – 20 mg daily.

Reduction of risk of duodenal ulcer recurrence:

Omeprazole and Clarithromycin: Combination Therapy	
Days 1 - 14	Days 15 - 28
Omeprazole 40 mg qd (in the morning) plus clarithromycin 500 mg tid	Omeprazole 20 mg qd

Gastric ulcer: The recommended adult oral dose is 40 mg once a day for 4 to 8 weeks.

Pathological hypersecretory conditions: Initial adult dose is 60 mg once a day. Doses up to 120 mg 3 times/day have been administered. Administer daily dosages > 80 mg in divided doses.

No dosage adjustment is necessary for patients with renal impairment, heatic dysfunction or for the elderly.

Take before eating. Do not open, crush or chew the capsule; swallow whole.

LANSOPRAZOLE

Capsules, delayed release: 15 and 30 mg (*Rx*) — *Prevacid* (TAP Pharm)

Actions:

Pharmacology: Lansoprazole belongs to a class of antisecretory compounds, the substituted benzimidazoles, that suppress gastric acid secretion by specific inhibition of the (H^+, K^+)-ATPase enzyme system at the secretory surface of the gastric parietal cell. Because this enzyme system is regarded as the acid (proton) pump within the parietal cell, lansoprazole is characterized as a gastric acid-pump inhibitor, in that it blocks the final step of acid production. The effect is dose-related and leads to inhibition of both basal and stimulated gastric acid secretion regardless of stimulus.

Pharmacokinetics:

Absorption/Distribution – Absorption of lansoprazole begins only after the granules leave the stomach. Absorption is rapid with mean peak plasma levels occurring after ≈ 1.7 hours and is relatively complete with absolute bioavailability over 80%. In healthy subjects, the mean plasma half-life was 1.5 hours. Lansoprazole is 97% bound to plasma proteins.

Metabolism – Lansoprazole is extensively metabolized in the liver. Two metabolites, which have little or no antisecretory activity, have been identified in measurable quantities in plasma. The plasma elimination half-life is < 2 hrs while the acid inhibitory effect lasts > 24 hrs.

Excretion – Following single-dose oral administration, virtually no unchanged lansoprazole was excreted in the urine. In one study, after a single oral dose, ≈ 33% was excreted in the urine and 66% was recovered in feces. This implies a significant biliary excretion of the metabolites.

Indications:

Duodenal ulcer:

Treatment – Short-term treatment (up to 4 weeks) for healing and symptomatic relief of active duodenal ulcer.

In combination with clarithromycin and amoxicillin as triple therapy for the eradication of *H. pylori* infection in patients with active or recurrent duodenal ulcers.

Maintenance – To maintain healing of duodenal ulcers. Controlled studies do not extend beyond 12 months.

Erosive esophagitis: Short-term treatment (up to 8 weeks) for healing and symptomatic relief of all grades of erosive esophagitis.

Maintenance – Lansoprazole is indicated to maintain healing of erosive esophagitis. Controlled studies do not extend beyond 12 months.

Pathological hypersecretory conditions including Zollinger-Ellison syndrome: Long-term treatment of pathological hypersecretory conditions, including Zollinger-Ellison syndrome.

Contraindications:

Hypersensitivity to any component of the formulation.

Warnings:

Renal/Hepatic function impairment: In severe renal insufficiency, plasma protein binding decreased by 1% to 1.5% after use of 60 mg. Patients with renal insufficiency had a shortened elimination half-life and decreased total AUC (free and bound). In patients with various degrees of chronic hepatic disease, the mean plasma half-life of the drug was prolonged from 1.5 to 3.2 to 7.2 hours. An increase in mean AUC of up to 500% was observed at steady state in hepatically impaired patients compared with healthy subjects. Consider dose reduction in severe hepatic disease.

Elderly: The clearance of lansoprazole is decreased in the elderly, with elimination half-life increased ≈ 50% to 100%. The initial dosing regimen need not be altered, but subsequent doses > 30 mg/day should not be administered unless additional gastric acid suppression is necessary.

Pregnancy: Category B.

Lactation: It is not known whether lansoprazole is excreted in human breast milk.

Children: Safety and efficacy have not been established.

Precautions:

Gastric malignancy: Symptomatic response to therapy with lansoprazole does not preclude the presence of gastric malignancy.

Drug Interactions:

Drugs that may interact with lansoprazole include theophylline, ketoconazole and sucralfate. Lansoprazole may interfere with the absorption of drugs where gastric pH is an important determinant of bioavailability (eg, ketoconazole, ampicillin, iron salts, digoxin).

Drug/Food interactions: Both C_{max} and AUC are diminished by about 50% if the drug is given 30 minutes after food as opposed to in the fasting condition. There is no significant food effect if the drug is given before meals.

Adverse Reactions:

In general, lansoprazole treatment has been well tolerated, and the only adverse reactions reported in ≥ 5% of patients were diarrhea, headache and taste disturbance.

Administration and Dosage:

Lansoprazole capsules can be opened, and the intact granules contained within can be sprinkled on one tablespoon of applesauce and swallowed immediately. The granules should not be chewed or crushed. Take before eating.

Duodenal ulcer: 15 mg daily before eating for 4 weeks.

Duodenal ulcer (healed) maintenance: 15 mg once daily.

Duodenal ulcers associated with H. pylori:

Triple therapy – 30 mg lansoprazole plus 500 mg clarithromycin and 1 g amoxicillin given twice daily for 14 days.

Double therapy – 30 mg lansoprazole plus 1 g amoxicillin three times daily for 14 days for patients intolerant or resistant to clarithromycin.

Erosive esophagitis: 30 mg daily before eating for up to 8 weeks. For patients who do not heal with lansoprazole for 8 weeks (5% to 10%) it may be helpful to give an additional 8 weeks of treatment. If there is a recurrence of erosive esophagitis, an additional 8 week course of lansoprazole may be considered.

Maintenance of healing of erosive esophagitis: 15 mg/day for adults.

Pathological hypersecretory conditions including Zollinger-Ellison syndrome: The recommended starting dose is 60 mg once a day. Adjust doses to individual patient needs and continue for as long as clinically indicated. Dosages up to 90 mg twice daily have been administered. Administer daily dosages of > 120 mg in divided doses. Some patients with Zollinger-Ellison syndrome have been treated continuously with lansoprazole for > 4 years.

Hepatic function impairment: Consider dosage adjustment in severe liver disease.

Elderly/Renal function impairment: No dosage adjustment is necessary.

Nasogastric (NG) tube: For patients who have an NG tube in place, lansoprazole can be opened and the intact granules mixed in 40 ml of apple juice and injected through the NG tube into the stomach. After administering the granules, flush the NG tube with additional apple juice to clear the tube.

PENICILLINS

AMOXICILLIN	
Tablets, chewable: 125 and 250 mg (as trihydrate) (*Rx*)	Various, *Amoxil* (SK-Beecham)
Capsules: 250 and 500 mg (as trihydrate) (*Rx*)	Various, *Amoxil* (SK-Beecham), *Wymox* (Wyeth-Ayerst)
Powder for oral suspension: 50 mg/ml, 125 and 250 mg/5 ml (as trihydrate) when reconstituted (*Rx*)	Various, *Amoxil* (SK-Beecham), *Wymox* (Wyeth-Ayerst)
AMOXICILLIN AND POTASSIUM CLAVULANATE	
Tablets: 250, 500 or 875 mg amoxicillin and 125 mg clavulanic acid (*Rx*)	*Augmentin* (SK-Beecham)
Tablets, chewable: 125 mg amoxicillin and 31.25 mg clavulanic acid, 250 mg amoxicillin and 62.5 mg clavulanic acid, 200 mg amoxicillin (as trihydrate) and 28.5 mg clavulanic acid, 400 mg amoxicillin (as trihydrate) and 57 mg clavulanic acid (*Rx*)	
Powder for oral suspension: 125 mg amoxicillin and 21.25 mg clavulanic acid/5 ml, 200 mg amoxicillin and 28.5 mg clavulanic acid per 5 ml, 250 mg amoxicillin and 62.5 mg clavulanic acid/5 ml, 400 mg amoxicillin and 57 mg clavulanic acid per 5 ml (*Rx*)	
AMPICILLIN, ORAL	
Capsules: 250 and 500 mg (as trihydrate or anhydrous) (*Rx*)	Various, *Totacillin* (SK-Beecham), *Omnipen* (Wyeth-Ayerst), *Marcillin* (Marnel)
Powder for oral suspension: 100 mg/ml, 125, 250, 500 mg/5 ml (as trihydrate) when reconstituted (*Rx*)	Various, *Omnipen* (Wyeth-Ayerst), *Totacillin* (SK-Beecham), *Polycillin Pediatric Drops* (Apothecon)
Powder for suspension: 250 mg/100 ml (as trihydrate) when reconstituted (*Rx*)	*Marcillin* (Marnel)
AMPICILLIN WITH PROBENECID	
Powder for oral suspension: 3.5 g ampicillin (as trihydrate) and 1 g probenecid per bottle (*Rx*)	*Polycillin-PRB* (Apothecon), *Probampacin* (Various)
AMPICILLIN SODIUM, PARENTERAL	
Powder for injection: 125, 250 and 500 mg and 1, 2 and 10 g (*Rx*)	Various, *Omnipen-N* (Wyeth-Ayerst), *Totacillin-N* (SK-Beecham)
AMPICILLIN SODIUM AND SULBACTAM SODIUM	
Powder for injection: 1.5 g (1 g ampicillin sodium/0.5 g sulbactam sodium), 3 g (2 g ampicillin sodium/1 g sulbactam sodium) (*Rx*)	*Unasyn* (Roerig)
BACAMPICILLIN HCl	
Tablets: 400 mg (chemically equivalent to 280 mg ampicillin) (*Rx*)	*Spectrobid* (Roerig)
Powder for oral suspension: 125 mg/5 ml reconstituted suspension (chemically equivalent to 87.5 mg ampicillin) (*Rx*)	
CARBENICILLIN INDANYL SODIUM	
Tablets, film coated: 382 mg carbenicillin (118 mg indanyl sodium ester) (*Rx*)	*Geocillin* (Roerig)
CLOXACILLIN SODIUM	
Capsules: 250 and 500 mg (*Rx*)	Various, *Cloxapen* (SK-Beecham), *Tegopen* (Apothecon)
Powder for oral suspension: 125 mg/5 ml when reconstituted (*Rx*)	Various, *Tegopen* (Apothecon)
DICLOXACILLIN SODIUM	
Capsules: 125, 250 and 500 mg (*Rx*)	Various, *Dycill* (SK-Beecham), *Pathocil* (Wyeth-Ayerst), *Dynapen* (Apothecon)
Powder for oral suspension: 62.5 mg/5 ml reconstituted (*Rx*)	*Dynapen* (Apothecon), *Pathocil* (Wyeth-Ayerst)
METHICILLIN SODIUM	
Powder for injection: 1, 4, 6 and 10 g (*Rx*)	*Staphcillin* (Apothecon)
MEZLOCILLIN SODIUM	
Powder for injection: 1, 2, 3, 4 and 20 g (*Rx*)	*Mezlin* (Miles)
NAFCILLIN SODIUM	
Tablets: 500 mg (*Rx*)	*Unipen* (Wyeth-Ayerst)
Capsules: 250 mg (*Rx*)	
Powder for injection: 500 mg, 1, 2 and 10 g (*Rx*)	Various, *Nallpen* (SK-Beecham), *Unipen* (Wyeth-Ayerst)

OXACILLIN SODIUM	
Capsules: 250 and 500 mg (*Rx*)	Various, *Bactocill* (SK-Beecham), *Prostaphlin* (Apothecon)
Powder for oral solution: 250 mg/5 ml when reconstituted (*Rx*)	*Prostaphlin* (Apothecon)
Powder for injection: 250 and 500 mg, 1, 2, 4 and 10 g (*Rx*)	*Oxacillin Sodium* (Apothecon), *Bactocill* (SK-Beecham), *Prostaphlin* (Apothecon)
PENICILLIN G (AQUEOUS), PARENTERAL	
Injection, premixed, frozen: 1, 2 and 3 million units (*Rx*)	*Penicillin G Potassium* (Baxter)
Powder for injection: 1, 5, 10 and 20 million units per vial (*Rx*)	*Pfizerpen* (Roerig), *Penicillin G Potassium*, *Penicillin G Sodium* (Apothecon)
PENICILLIN G BENZATHINE, PARENTERAL	
Injection: 300,000 units/ml; 600,000 units; 1,200,000; 2,400,000 units/dose (*Rx*)	*Bicillin L-A* (Wyeth-Ayerst), *Permapen* (Roerig)
PENICILLIN G PROCAINE, AQUEOUS (APPG)	
Injection: 300,000; 500,000; 600,000 units per ml, 1,200,000; 2,400,000 units per dose (*Rx*)	*Wycillin* (Wyeth-Ayerst), *Crysticillin 300 A.S.*, *Crysticillin 600 A.S.* (Apothecon)
PENICILLIN G BENZATHINE AND PROCAINE COMBINED	
Injection: 300,000 units/ml; 600,000; 1,200,000; 2,400,000 units/dose; 900,000 units penicillin G benzathine and 300,000 units penicillin G procaine/dose (*Rx*)	*Bicillin C-R*, *Bicillin C-R 900/300* (Wyeth-Ayerst)
PENICILLIN V (PHENOXYMETHYL PENICILLIN)	
Tablets: 125, 250 and 500 mg (*Rx*)	Various, *Beepen-VK* (SK-Beecham), *V-Cillin K* (Lilly)
Powder for oral solution: 125 or 250 mg/5 ml when reconstituted (*Rx*)	Various, *Beepen-VK* (SK-Beecham), *Pen•Vee K* (Wyeth-Ayerst)
PIPERACILLIN SODIUM	
Powder for injection: 2, 3, 4 and 40 g (*Rx*)	*Pipracil* (Lederle)
PIPERACILLIN SODIUM AND TAZOBACTAM SODIUM	
Powder for injection: 2 g piperacillin/ 0.25 g tazobactam, 3 g piperacillin/ 0.375 g tazobactam, 4 g piperacillin/ 0.5 g tazobactam (*Rx*)	*Zosyn* (Wyeth-Ayerst)
TICARCILLIN DISODIUM	
Powder for injection: 1, 3, 6, 20 and 30 g (*Rx*)	*Ticar* (SK-Beecham)
TICARCILLIN AND CLAVULANATE POTASSIUM	
Powder for injection: 3 g ticarcillin and 0.1 g clavulanic acid (*Rx*)	*Timentin* (SK-Beecham)
Solution: 3 g ticarcillin and 0.1 g clavulanic acid (*Rx*)	

Actions:

Pharmacology: Penicillins inhibit the biosynthesis of cell wall mucopeptide. They are bactericidal against sensitive organisms when adequate concentrations are reached, and they are most effective during the stage of active multiplication. Inadequate concentrations may produce only bacteriostatic effects.

Penicillins					
	Routes of administration	Penicillinase-resistant	Acid stable	% Protein bound	May be taken with meals
Natural Penicillins					
Penicillin G	IM-IV	no	†[1]	60	†[1]
Penicillin V	Oral	no	yes	80	yes
Penicillinase-Resistant					
Cloxacillin	Oral	yes	yes	95	no
Dicloxacillin	Oral	yes	yes	98	no
Methicillin	IM-IV	yes	†[1]	40	†[1]
Nafcillin	IM-IV-Oral	yes	yes	87 to 90	no
Oxacillin	IM-IV-Oral	yes	yes	94	no
Aminopenicillins					
Amoxicillin	Oral	no	yes	20	yes
Amoxicillin/potassium clavulanate	Oral	yes	yes	20/30	yes
Ampicillin	IM-IV-Oral	no	yes	20	no
Ampicillin/sulbactam	IM-IV	yes	†[1]	28/38	†[1]
Bacampicillin	Oral	no	yes	20	yes[2]
Extended–Spectrum					
Carbenicillin	Oral	no	yes	50	no
Mezlocillin	IM-IV	no	†[1]	16 to 42	†[1]
Piperacillin	IM-IV	no	†[1]	16	†[1]
Ticarcillin	IM-IV	no	†[1]	45	†[1]
Ticarcillin/potassium clavulanate	IV	yes	†[1]	45/9	†[1]

[1] Available only for IM or IV use.
[2] Tablets only; not the suspension.

Pharmacokinetics:

Absorption – Peak serum levels occur approximately 1 hour after oral use. Parenteral penicillin G (sodium and potassium) gives rapid and high but transient blood levels; derivatives provide prolonged penicillin blood levels with IM use.

Distribution – Penicillins are bound to plasma proteins, primarily albumin, in varying degrees. They diffuse readily into most body tissues and fluids.

Excretion – Penicillins are excreted largely unchanged in the urine by glomerular filtration and active tubular secretion. Nonrenal elimination includes hepatic inactivation and excretion in bile; this is only a minor route for all penicillins except nafcillin and oxacillin. Excretion by renal tubular secretion can be delayed by coadministration of probenecid. Elimination half-life of most penicillins is short (≤ 1.5 hr). Impaired renal function prolongs the serum half-life of penicillins eliminated primarily by renal excretion.

Microbiology:

β-lactamase inhibitors (clavulanic acid and sulbactam) have weak antimicrobial activity, but irreversibly inactivate bacterial β-lactamase enzymes. Used with β-lactam antibiotics, they protect antibiotics from inactivation by β-lactamase-producing organisms.

Organisms Generally Susceptible to Penicillins

	Organisms	Natural penicillins		Penicillinase-resistant					Aminopenicillins					Extended-spectrum				
	✓ = generally susceptible	Penicillin G	Penicillin V	Cloxacillin	Dicloxacillin	Methicillin	Nafcillin	Oxacillin	Amoxicillin	Ampicillin	Bacampicillin	Amoxicillin/potassium clavulanate	Ampicillin/sulbactam	Carbenicillin	Mezlocillin	Piperacillin	Ticarcillin	Ticarcillin/potassium clavulanate
Gram-positive	Staphylococci	✓[1]	✓[1]	✓	✓	✓	✓	✓	✓[1]	✓[1]	✓[1]	✓	✓	✓[1]		✓[1]	✓[1]	✓
	Staphylococcus aureus	✓[1]	✓[1]	✓	✓	✓	✓	✓				✓	✓	✓[1]	✓[1]	✓[1]	✓[1]	✓
	Streptococci	✓	✓			✓				✓			✓					
	Streptococcus pneumoniae	✓	✓	✓	✓	✓	✓	✓	✓	✓	✓	✓	✓	✓	✓	✓	✓	✓
	Beta-hemolytic streptococci	✓	✓				✓		✓	✓	✓	✓	✓	✓	✓	✓	✓	✓
	Streptococcus faecalis	✓	✓						✓	✓	✓	✓	✓	✓	✓	✓	✓	✓
	Streptococcus viridans	✓	✓				✓		✓	✓		✓	✓			✓		✓
	Corynebacterium diphtheriae	✓	✓															
	Bacillus anthracis	✓	✓							✓			✓					
	Listeria monocytogenes	✓	✓							✓			✓					
Gram-negative	Escherichia coli	✓							✓	✓	✓	✓	✓	✓	✓	✓	✓	✓
	Haemophilus influenzae								✓	✓	✓	✓	✓	✓	✓	✓[2]	✓	✓
	Klebsiella sp											✓	✓		✓	✓		✓
	Neisseria gonorrhoeae	✓[1]	✓						✓	✓	✓	✓	✓	✓	✓	✓	✓	✓
	Neisseria meningitidis	✓								✓		✓	✓			✓	✓	✓
	Proteus mirabilis	✓							✓	✓	✓	✓	✓	✓	✓	✓	✓	✓
	Salmonella sp	✓								✓			✓	✓	✓	✓	✓	✓
	Shigella sp	✓								✓			✓		✓	✓		
	Morganella morganii												✓	✓	✓	✓	✓	✓
	Proteus vulgaris												✓	✓	✓	✓	✓	✓
	Providencia sp																	
	Providencia rettgeri												✓	✓	✓	✓	✓	✓
	Providencia stuartii												✓		✓			✓
	Enterobacter sp	✓										✓	✓	✓	✓	✓	✓	✓
	Citrobacter sp													✓	✓	✓	✓	✓
	Pseudomonas aeruginosa													✓	✓	✓	✓	✓
	Serratia sp													✓	✓	✓	✓	✓
	Acinetobacter sp												✓		✓	✓		✓
	Streptobacillus moniliformis	✓	✓															
	Moraxella (Branhamella) catarrhalis											✓	✓			✓		✓

Organisms Generally Susceptible to Penicillins

	Organisms	Natural penicillins		Penicillinase-resistant					Aminopenicillins					Extended- spectrum				
	✓ = generally susceptible	Penicillin G	Penicillin V	Cloxacillin	Dicloxacillin	Methicillin	Nafcillin	Oxacillin	Amoxicillin	Ampicillin	Bacampicillin	Amoxicillin/potassium clavulanate	Ampicillin/sulbactam	Carbenicillin	Mezlocillin	Piperacillin	Ticarcillin	Ticarcillin/potassium clavulanate
Anaerobic	Clostridium sp	✓	✓						✓	✓		✓	✓	✓	✓	✓	✓	✓
	Peptococcus sp	✓	✓						✓	✓		✓	✓	✓	✓	✓	✓	✓
	Peptostreptococcus sp	✓	✓						✓			✓	✓	✓	✓	✓	✓	✓
	Bacteroides sp	✓[3]											✓	✓	✓	✓	✓	✓
	Fusobacterium sp	✓											✓	✓	✓	✓	✓	✓
	Eubacterium sp	✓													✓	✓	✓	✓
	Treponema pallidum	✓	✓															
	Actinomyces bovis	✓	✓													✓		
	Veillonella sp														✓	✓		✓

[1] Non-penicillinase-producing.
[2] Non-beta-lactamase-producing.
[3] *B fragilis* is resistant.

Indications:

Oral: Penicillins are generally indicated in the treatment of mild to moderately severe infections due to penicillin-sensitive microorganisms.

Penicillinase-resistant penicillins: The percentage of staphylococcal isolates resistant to penicillin G outside the hospital is increasing, approximating the high percentage found in the hospital. Therefore, use a penicillinase-resistant penicillin as initial therapy for any suspected staphylococcal infection until culture and sensitivity results are known.

When treatment is initiated before definitive culture and sensitivity results are known, consider that these agents are only effective in the treatment of infections caused by pneumococci, group A beta-hemolytic streptococci and penicillin G-resistant and penicillin G–sensitive staphylococci.

Parenteral: In patients with severe infection, or when there is nausea, vomiting, gastric dilatation, cardiospasm or intestinal hypermotility.

Contraindications:

History of hypersensitivity to penicillins, cephalosporins or imipenem.

Do not treat severe pneumonia, empyema, bacteremia, pericarditis, meningitis and purulent or septic arthritis with an oral penicillin during the acute stage.

Warnings:

Bleeding abnormalities: **Ticarcillin, mezlocillin or piperacillin** may induce hemorrhagic manifestations associated with abnormalities of coagulation tests.

Cystic fibrosis patients have a higher incidence of side effects (eg, fever, rash) when treated with extended-spectrum penicillins (eg, piperacillin, carbenicillin).

Hypersensitivity: Serious and occasionally fatal immediate hypersensitivity reactions have occurred. The incidence of anaphylactic shock is between 0.015% and 0.04%. Anaphylactic shock resulting in death has occurred in approximately 0.002% of the patients treated. These reactions are likely to be immediate and severe in penicillin-sensitive individuals with a history of atopic conditions.

Hypersensitivity myocarditis is not dose-dependent and may occur at any time during treatment. An urticarial rash, not representing a true penicillin allergy, occasionally occurs with **ampicillin** (9%). Typically, the rash appears 7 to 10 days after the start of oral ampicillin therapy and remains for a few days to a week after drug discontinuance. In most cases, the rash is maculopapular, pruritic and generalized.

Desensitization: Patients with a positive skin test to one of the penicillin determinants can be desensitized, which is a relatively safe procedure. This is recommended in instances when penicillin must be given where no proven alternatives exist.

Cross-allergenicity with cephalosporins: Individuals with a history of penicillin hypersensitivity have experienced severe reactions when treated with a cephalosporin. The incidence of cross-allergenicity between penicillins and cephalosporins is estimated to range from 5% to 16%; however, it is possible the incidence is much lower, possibly 3% to 7%.

Renal function impairment: Since carbenicillin is primarily excreted by the kidney, patients with severe renal impairment (creatinine clearance, < 10 ml/min) will not achieve the therapeutic urine levels of carbenecillin.

In patients with creatinine clearance 10 to 20 ml/min, it may be necessary to adjust dosage to prevent accumulation of the drug.

Pregnancy: *Category B*. Penicillins cross the placenta.

Lactation: Penicillins are excreted in breast milk in low concentrations; use may cause diarrhea, candidiasis or allergic response in the nursing infant.

Children: Safety and efficacy of carbenicillin, piperacillin and the β-lactamase inhibitor/penicillin combinations have not been established in infants and children < 12 years old. Use caution in administering to newborns and evaluate organ system function frequently.

Precautions:

Monitoring: Obtain blood cultures, white blood cell and differential cell counts prior to initiation of therapy and at least weekly during therapy with penicillinase-resistant penicillins. Measure AST and ALT during therapy to monitor for liver function abnormalities.

Perform periodic urinalysis, BUN and creatinine determinations during therapy with penicillinase-resistant penicillins, and consider dosage alterations if these values become elevated.

Streptococcal infections: Therapy must be sufficient to eliminate the organism (a minimum of 10 days); otherwise, sequelae (eg, endocarditis, rheumatic fever) may occur.

Sexually transmitted diseases: When treating gonococcal infections in which primary and secondary syphilis are suspected, perform proper diagnostic procedures, including darkfield examinations and monthly serological tests for at least 4 months.

Resistance: The number of strains of staphylococci resistant to penicillinase-resistant penicillins has been increasing; widespread use of penicillinase-resistant penicillins may result in an increasing number of resistant staphylococcal strains.

Pseudomembranous colitis has occurred with the use of broad-spectrum antibiotics due to overgrowth of clostridia; therefore, it is important to consider its diagnosis in patients who develop diarrhea in association with antibiotic use.

Procaine sensitivity: If sensitivity to the procaine in **penicillin G procaine** is suspected, inject 0.1 ml of a 1% to 2% procaine solution intradermally. Development of erythema, wheal, flare or eruption indicates procaine sensitivity; treat by the usual methods.

Parenteral administration: Inadvertent intravascular administration, including direct intra-arterial injection or injection immediately adjacent to arteries, has resulted in severe neurovascular damage, including transverse myelitis with permanent paralysis, gangrene requiring amputation of digits and more proximal portions of extremities, and necrosis and sloughing at and surrounding the injection site.

Electrolyte imbalance: Patients given continuous IV therapy with **potassium penicillin G** in high dosage (> 10 million units daily) may suffer severe or even fatal potassium poisoning particularly if renal insufficiency is present. High dosage of **sodium salts of penicillins** may result in or aggravate CHF due to high sodium intake. Individuals with liver disease or those receiving cytotoxic therapy or diuretics rarely demonstrated a decrease in serum potassium concentrations with high doses of **piperacillin. Sodium penicillin G** contains 2 mEq sodium per million units, **potassium penicillin G** contains 1.7 mEq potassium and 0.3 mEq sodium per million units. The sodium content of other IV penicillin derivatives is listed below:

Sodium Content of IV Penicillins

Penicillin	Maximum daily dose (g)	Sodium content (mEq/g)[1]	Sodium (mEq/day)[1,2]
Ampicillin sodium	12	2.9	34.8
Methicillin sodium	12	3	36
Mezlocillin sodium	24	1.85	44.4
Nafcillin sodium	9	2.9	26
Oxacillin sodium	12	2.5	30
Piperacillin sodium	24	1.85	44.4
Ticarcillin disodium	24	4.7 to 5	112.8 to 120

[1] 1 mEq sodium equals 23 mg.
[2] Based on maximum daily dose.

Hypokalemia has occurred in a few patients receiving **mezlocillin, ticarcillin** and **piperacillin**.

Drug Interactions:

Drugs that may affect penicillins include allopurinol, chloramphenicol, erythromycin, tetracycline, aminoglycosides (parenteral), beta blockers. Drugs that may be affected by penicillins include aminoglycosides (parenteral), anticoagulants, beta blockers, oral contraceptives, heparin, chloramphenicol, erythromycin.

Drug/Lab test interactions: False-positive **urine glucose** reactions may occur with penicillin therapy if Clinitest, Benedict's Solution or Fehling's Solution are used. It is recommended that enzymatic glucose oxidase tests (such as *Clinistix* or *Tes-Tape*) be used. Positive *Coombs' tests* have occurred. High urine concentrations of some penicillins may produce false-positive protein reactions (pseudoproteinuria) with the following methods: Sulfosalicylic acid and boiling test, acetic acid test, biuret reaction and nitric acid test. The bromphenol blue (*Multi-Stix*) reagent strip test has been reported to be reliable.

Drug/Food interactions: Absorption of most penicillins is affected by food; these medications are best taken on an empty stomach, 1 hour before or 2 hours after meals. Penicillin V may be given with meals; however, blood levels may be slightly higher when taken on an empty stomach. Amoxicillin, amoxicillin/potassium clavulanate and bacampicillin tablets may be given without regard to meals; absorption of bacampicillin suspension is affected by food.

Adverse Reactions:

CNS:

Penicillins have caused neurotoxicity (manifested as lethargy, neuromuscular irritability, hallucinations, convulsions and seizures) when given in large IV doses especially in patients with renal failure.

GI:

Glossitis; stomatitis; gastritis; sore mouth or tongue; dry mouth; furry tongue; black "hairy" tongue; abnormal taste sensation; nausea; vomiting; abdominal pain or cramp; epigastric distress; diarrhea or bloody diarrhea; rectal bleeding; flatulence; enterocolitis; pseudomembranous colitis.

Hematologic/Lymphatic:

Anemia; hemolytic anemia; thrombocytopenia; thrombocytopenic purpura; eosinophilia; leukopenia; granulocytopenia; neutropenia; bone marrow depression; agranulocytosis; a reduction of hemoglobin or hematocrit; prolongation of bleeding and prothrombin time; decrease in WBC and lymphocyte counts; increase in lymphocytes, monocytes, basophils and platelets.

Hypersensitivity:

Adverse reactions (estimated incidence, 1% to 10%) are more likely to occur in individuals with previously demonstrated hypersensitivity. In penicillin-sensitive individuals with a history of allergy, asthma or hay fever, the reactions may be immediate and severe.

Allergic symptoms include urticaria, angioneurotic edema, laryngospasm, bronchospasm, hypotension, vascular collapse; death; maculopapular to exfoliative dermatitis; vesicular eruptions; erythema multiforme; reactions resembling serum sickness (chills, fever, edema, arthralgia, arthritis, malaise); laryngeal edema; skin rashes; prostration.

Lab test abnormalities:

Elevations of AST, ALT, bilirubin and LDH have been noted in patients receiving semisynthetic penicillins (particularly **oxacillin** and **cloxacillin**); such reactions are more common in infants. Elevations of serum alkaline phosphatase and hypernatremia, and reduction in serum potassium, albumin, total proteins and uric acid may occur.

Local:

Pain (accompanied by induration) at the site of injection; ecchymosis; deep vein thrombosis; hematomas.

Miscellaneous:

Vaginitis and anorexia.

Administration and Dosage:

Therapy may be initiated prior to obtaining results of bacteriologic studies when there is reason to believe the causative organisms may be susceptible. Once results are known, adjust therapy.

Continue treatment of all infections for a minimum of 48 to 72 hours beyond the time that the patient becomes asymptomatic or evidence of bacterial eradication has been obtained, unless single-dose therapy is employed.

AMOXICILLIN: The children's dose is intended for individuals whose weight will not cause the calculated dosage to be greater than that recommended for adults; the children's dose should not exceed the maximum adult dose.

Amoxicillin Uses and Dosages	
Organisms/Infections	Dosage
Infections of the ear, nose and throat due to streptococci, pneumococci, nonpenicillinase-producing staphylococci and *H. influenzae* *Infections of the GU tract due to E. coli, P. mirabilis and S. faecalis* *Infections of the skin and soft tissues* due to streptococci, susceptible staphylocci and *E. coli*	*Adults and children (> 20 kg)* - 250 to 500 mg every 8 hours. *Children* - 20 to 40 mg/kg/day in divided doses every 8 hours.

Amoxicillin Uses and Dosages	
Organisms/Infections	Dosage
Infections of the lower respiratory tract due to streptococci, pneumococci, non-penicillinase-producing staphylococci and *H. influenzae*	*Adults and children (> 20 kg)* - 500 mg q 8 h. *Children* - 40 mg/kg/day in divided doses q 8 h.
Prevention of bacterial endocarditis:	
For dental, oral or upper respiratory tract procedures in patients at risk	
Standard regimen:	3 g 1 hour before procedure, then 1.5 g 6 hours after initial dose
Alternate regimen:	1 to 2 g (50 mg/kg for children) ampicillin plus 1.5 mg/kg gentamicin (2 mg/kg for children) not to exceed 80 mg, both IM or IV one-half hour prior to procedure, followed by 1.5 g amoxicillin (25 mg/kg for children) 6 hours after initial dose or, repeat parenteral dose 8 hours after initial dose.
For GU or GI procedures	
Standard regimen:	2 g ampicillin (50 mg/kg for children) plus 1.5 mg/kg gentamicin (2 mg/kg for children) not to exceed 80 mg, both IM or IV one-half hour prior to procedure, followed by 1.5 g amoxicillin (25 mg/kg for children)
Alternate low-risk patient regimen	3 g 1 hour before procedure, then 1.5 g 6 hours after initial dose
Unlabeled use:	
Chlamydia trachomatis in pregnancy	As an alternative to erythromycin; 500 mg 3 times a day for 7 days.

AMOXICILLIN AND POTASSIUM CLAVULANATE: May be administered without regard to meals.

Since both the 250 mg and 500 mg tablets contain the same amount of clavulanic acid (125 mg as potassium salt), two 250 mg tablets are not equivalent to one 500 mg tablet.

The 875 mg tablet also contains 125 mg potassium clavulanate. In addition, the 250 mg tablet and 250 mg chewable tablet do NOT contain the same amount of potassium clavulanate and should not be substituted for each other, as they are not interchangeable.

Usual dose – Children's dose is based on amoxicillin content.

Adults: One 250 mg tablet every 8 hours.

Suspension – Adults who have difficulty swallowing may be given the 125 mg/5 ml or 250 mg/5 ml suspension in place of the 500 mg tablet or give 200 mg/5 ml or 400 mg/5 ml suspension in place of the 875 mg tablet.

Children:

≥ 40 kg – Dose according to adult recommendations.

< 3 months old – 30 mg/kg/day divided every 12 hours, based on the amoxicillin component. Use of the 125 mg/5 ml oral suspension is recommended.

≥ 3 months old – Children's dose is based on amoxicillin content. Refer to the following table. Because of the different amoxicillin to clavulanic acid ratios in the 250 mg tablets (250/125) vs the 250 mg chewable tablets (250/62.5), do not use the 250 mg tablet until the child weighs ≥ 40 kg.

Amoxicillin/Potassium Clavulanate Dosing in Children ≥ 3 Months of Age		
	Dosing regimen	
Infections	200 mg/5 ml or 400 mg/5 ml (q 12 hr)[1,2]	125 mg/5 ml or 250 mg/5 ml (q 8 hr)[2]
Otitis media,[3] sinusitis, lower respiratory tract infections, severe infections	45 mg/kg/day	40 mg/kg/day
Less severe infections	25 mg/kg/day	20 mg/kg/day

[1] The every-12-hour regimen is associated with significantly less diarrhea; however, the 200 and 400 mg formulations (suspension and chewable tablets) contain aspartame and should not be used by phenylketonurics.
[2] Each strength of the suspension is available as a chewable tablet for use by older children.
[3] Recommended duration is 10 days.

Severe infections and respiratory tract infections –

Adults: One 500 mg tablet every 8 hours.

Children (< 40 kg): 40 mg/kg/day, in divided doses every 8 hours.

Otitis media, sinusitis and lower respiratory infections –

Children (< 40 kg): 40 mg/kg/day, in divided doses every 8 hours.

Chancroid (Haemophilus ducreyi infection) – One 500 mg tablet 3 times daily for 7 days as an alternative to erythromycin or ceftriaxone (not evaluated in the US).

Disseminated gonococcal infection – Following appropriate parenteral therapy with ceftriaxone, ceftizoxime or cefotaxime, reliable patients with uncomplicated disease may be discharged from the hospital 24 to 48 hours after all symptoms resolve and may complete the therapy (for a total of 1 week of antibiotic therapy) with an oral regimen of one 500 mg tablet 3 times a day.

AMPICILLIN:

Ampicillin Uses and Dosages	
Organisms/infections	Dosage
Labeled uses: *Respiratory tract and soft tissue infections:*	Parenteral: Patients ≥ 40 kg - 250 to 500 mg every 6 hours; < 40 kg - 25 to 50 mg/kg/day in divided doses at 6 to 8 hour intervals. Oral: Patients ≥ 20 kg - 250 mg every 6 hours; < 20 kg - 50 mg/kg/day in divided doses at 6 to 8 hour intervals.
Bacterial meningitis: H. influenzae, S. pneumoniae or N. meningitidis	8 to 14 g/day (100 to 200 mg/kg/day for children) in divided doses every 3 to 4 hours. Initial treatment is usually by IV drip, followed by frequent (every 3 to 4 hour) IM injections.
Septicemia:	Parenteral: 150 to 200 mg/kg/day. Give IV at least 3 days; continue IM every 3 to 4 hrs.
Rape victims (prophylaxis of infection): Alternative regimen for pregnant women or when tetracycline is contraindicated.	3.5 g orally with 1 g probenecid.
Prevention of bacterial endocarditis: For dental, oral or upper respiratory tract procedures in patients at high risk: Alternate regimen.	1 to 2 g (50 mg/kg for children) plus gentamicin 1.5 mg/kg (2 mg/kg for children) not > 80 mg, both IM or IV 30 min pior to procedure, then 1.5 g amoxicillin (25 mg/kg for children) 6 hours after initial dose or repeat parenteral dose 8 hours after initial dose.
For GU or GI procedures: Standard regimen.	2 g (50 mg/kg for children) IM or IV plus gentamicin 1.5 mg/kg (not > 80 mg) IM or IV (2 mg/kg for children) 30 min prior to procedure, then 1.5 g amoxicillin (25 mg/kg for children) 6 hours after initial dose; or repeat parenteral dose 8 hours after initial dose.
Unlabeled use: *Prophylaxis in cesarean section in certain high–risk patients*	Single IV dose, administered immediately after cord clamping.

Renal impairment – Increase dosing interval to 12 hours in severe renal impairment (creatinine clearance ≤ 10 ml/min).

Adults – 1 to 12 g daily in divided doses every 4 to 6 hours.

Children – 50 to 200 mg/kg/day in divided doses every 4 to 6 hours.

Infants (over 7 days and > 2000 g): 100 mg/kg/day in divided doses every 6 hours (meningitis 200 mg/kg/day).

Over 7 days and < 2000 g: 75 mg/kg/day in divided doses every 8 hours (meningitis 150 mg/kg/day).

Under 7 days and > 2000 g: 75 mg/kg/day in divided doses every 8 hours (meningitis 150 mg/kg/day).

Under 7 days and < 2000 g: 50 mg/kg/day in divided doses every 12 hours (meningitis 100 mg/kg/day).

AMPICILLIN AND PROBENECID: Administer 3.5 g ampicillin and 1 g probenecid as a single dose.

AMPICILLIN SODIUM AND SULBACTAM SODIUM: May be administered by either the IV or the IM routes. The recommended adult dosage is 1.5 g (1 g ampicillin plus 0.5 g sulbactam) to 3 g (2 g ampicillin plus 1 g sulbactam) every 6 hours. Do not exceed 4 g/day sulbactam.

Renal function impairment – The elimination kinetics of ampicillin and sulbactam are similarly affected; hence, the ratio of one to the other will remain constant whatever the renal function. In patients with renal impairment, give as follows:

Ampicillin/Sulbactam Dosage Guide For Patients With Renal Impairment		
Ccr (ml/min/1.72 m^2)	Half-life (hours)	Recommended dosage
≥ 30	1	1.5-3 g q 6-8 h
15-29	5	1.5-3 q 12 h
5-14	9	1.5-3 g q 24 h

Children – Safety and efficacy in children < 12 years old have not been established.

BACAMPICILLIN HCl: Tablets may be given without regard to meals; administer suspension to fasting patients.

Upper respiratory tract infections (including otitis media) caused by streptococci, pneumococci, nonpenicillinase-producing staphylococci and *H. influenzae*; urinary tract infections due to *E. coli, P. mirabilis* and *S. faecalis*; skin and skin structure infections due to streptococci and susceptible staphylococci:

Adults (≥ 25 kg): 400 mg every 12 hours.

Children: 25 mg/kg/day in equally divided doses at 12 hour intervals.

Severe infections or those caused by less-susceptible organisms –

Adults (≥ 25 kg): 800 mg every 12 hours.

Children: 50 mg/kg/day in equally divided doses at 12 hour intervals.

Lower respiratory tract infections due to streptococci, pneumococci, nonpenicillinase-producing staphylococci and *H. influenzae:*

Adults (≥ 25 kg): 800 mg every 12 hours.

Children: 50 mg/kg/day in equally divided doses at 12 hour intervals.

Gonorrhea – The usual adult dosage (males and females) is 1.6 g bacampicillin plus 1 g probenecid as a single oral dose. No pediatric dosage has been established.

CARBENICILLIN INDANYL SODIUM:

Urinary tract infections –

E. coli, Proteus species and Enterobacter: 382 to 764 mg 4 times daily.

Pseudomonas and enterococci: 764 mg 4 times daily.

Prostatitis due to E. coli, P. mirabilis, Enterobacter and enterococcus (S. faecalis) – 764 mg 4 times daily.

CLOXACILLIN SODIUM:

Mild to moderate upper respiratory and localized skin and soft tissue infections –

Adults and children (> 20 kg): 250 mg every 6 hours.

Children (< 20 kg): 50 mg/kg/day in equally divided doses every 6 hours.

Severe infections (lower respiratory tract or disseminated infections) –

Adults and children (> 20 kg): ≥ 500 mg every 6 hours.

Children (< 20 kg): ≥ 100 mg /kg/day in equal doses every 6 hours.

Another suggested dosage for infants and children is 50 to 100 mg/kg/day, up to a maximum of 4 g/day, divided every 6 hours.

DICLOXACILLIN SODIUM:

For mild to moderate upper respiratory and localized skin and soft tissue infections –

Adults and children (> 40 kg): 125 mg every 6 hours.

Children (< 40 kg): 12.5 mg/kg/day in equal doses every 6 hours.

For more severe infections, such as lower respiratory tract or disseminated infections –

Adults and children (> 40 kg): 250 mg every 6 hours.

Children (< 40 kg): 25 mg/kg/day in equally divided doses every 6 hours.

Another suggested dosage for children is 12 to 25 mg/kg/day divided every 6 hours. Use in the newborn is not recommended.

METHICILLIN SODIUM:

Adults – 4 to 12 g/day in divided doses every 4 to 6 hours; in severe renal impairment (creatinine clearance ≤ 10 ml/min) do not exceed 2 g every 12 hours.

Children – 100 to 300 mg/kg/day in divided doses every 4 to 6 hours.

Infants –

Over 7 days and > 2000 g: 100 mg/kg/day in divided doses every 6 hours; for meningitis – 200 mg/kg/day.

Over 7 days and < 2000 g: 75 mg/kg/day in divided doses every 8 hours (meningitis – 150 mg/kg/day).

Under 7 days and > 2000 g: 75 mg/kg/day in divided doses every 8 hours (meningitis – 150 mg/kg/day).

Under 7 days and < 2000 g: 50 mg/kg/day in divided doses every 12 hours (meningitis - 100 mg/kg/day).

MEZLOCILLIN SODIUM: Administer IV for serious infections. IM doses should not exceed 2 g/injection.

Adults – The recommended adult dosage for serious infections is 200 to 300 mg/kg/day given in 4 to 6 divided doses. The usual dose is 3 g given every 4 hours (18 g/day) or 4 g given every 6 hours (16 g/day).

Infants and children – Limited data are available on the safety and effectiveness in the treatment of infants and children with serious infection.

Mezlocillin Dosage Guidelines for Neonates

Body weight (g)	Age	
	≤ 7 Days	> 7 Days
≤ 2000	75 mg/kg every 12 hours (150 mg/kg/day)	75 mg/kg every 8 hours (225 mg/kg/day)
> 2000	75 mg/kg every 12 hours (150 mg/kg/day)	75 mg/kg every 6 hours (300 mg/kg/day)

For infants > 1 month of age and children < 12 years, administer 50 mg/kg every 4 hours (300 mg/kg/day); infuse IV over 30 minutes or administer by IM injection.

Renal function impairment – After an IV dose of 3 g, the serum half-life is approximately 1 hour in patients with creatinine clearances > 60 ml/min, 1.3 hours in those with clearances of 30 to 59 ml/min, 1.6 hours in those with clearances of 10 to 29 ml/min, and approximately 3.6 hours in patients with clearances of < 10 ml/min.

Mezlocillin Uses and Dosages

Organisms/Infections	Dosage
Urinary infection: Uncomplicated with normal renal function (creatinine clearance ≥ 30 ml/min).	100 to 125 mg/kg/day (6 to 8 g/day); 1.5 to 2 g every 6 hours IV or IM.
Uncomplicated with renal impairment	1.5 g every 8 hours.
Complicated with normal renal function	150 to 200 mg/kg/day (12 g/day); 3 g every 6 hours IV.
Complicated with renal impairment - Creatinine clearance	
10 to 30 ml/min	1.5 g every 6 hours.
< 10 ml/min	1.5 g every 8 hours.
Lower respiratory tract infection, intra-abdominal infection, gynecological infection, skin and skin structure infections, septicema:	225 to 300 mg/kg/day (16 to 18 g/day); 4 g every 6 hours or 3 g every 4 hours IV.
Serious systemic infection with renal impairment - Creatinine clearance	
10 to 30 ml/min	3 g every 8 hours.
< 10 ml/min	2 g every 8 hours.
Serious systemic infection undergoing hemodialysis for renal failure	3 g every 2 hours
peritoneal dialysis	
Life-threatening infections:	Up to 350 mg/kg/day; 4 g every 4 hours (24 g/day maximum).
In patients with renal impairment - Creatinine clearance	
10 to 30 ml/min	3 g every 6 hours.
< 10 ml/min	2 g every 6 hours.
Acute, uncomplicated gonococcal urethritis:	1 to 2 g IV or IM; plus 1 g probenecid at time of dosing or up to ½ hour before.
Prophylaxis:	
To prevent postoperative infection in contaminated or potentially contaminated surgery	4 g IV, ½ to 1½ hr prior to start of surgery; 4 g IV, 6 and 12 hours later.
Cesarean section patients	First dose: 4 g IV when umbilical cord is clamped; second dose: 4 g IV, 4 hours after first dose; third dose: 4 g IV, 8 hrs after first dose.

NAFCILLIN SODIUM:

Parenteral –

IV: 3 to 6 g per 24 hours. Use this route for short-term therapy (24 to 48 hours) because of occasional occurrence of thrombophlebitis, particularly in the elderly.

IM:

Adults – 500 mg every 4 to 6 hours.

Infants and children – 25 mg/kg twice daily.

Neonates – 10 mg/kg twice daily. Other suggested doses include: Weight < 2000 g - 50 mg/kg/day divided every 12 hours (age < 7 days) or 75 mg/kg/day divided every 8 hours (age > 7 days).

Weight > 2000 g - 50 mg/kg/day divided every 8 hours (age < 7 days) or 75 mg/kg/day divided every 6 hours (age > 7 days).

Oral – Serum levels of oral nafcillin are low and unpredictable.

Adults: 250 to 500 mg every 4 to 6 hours for mild to moderate infections. In severe infections – 1 g every 4 to 6 hours.

Children:

Staph infections – 50 mg/kg/day in 4 divided doses. For neonates, 10 mg/kg 3 to 4 times daily. If inadequate, change to parenteral nafcillin sodium.

Scarlet fever and pneumonia – 25 mg/kg/day in 4 divided doses.

Streptococcal pharyngitis – 250 mg 3 times daily for 10 days. (Penicillin V is the drug of choice for streptococcal infections.)

OXACILLIN SODIUM:

Oral –

Mild to moderate infections of skin, soft tissue, or upper respiratory tract:

Adults and children (> 20 kg) – 500 mg every 4 to 6 hrs for at least 5 days.

Children (< 20 kg) – 50 mg/kg/day in divided doses every 6 hrs for at least 5 days.

In serious or life-threatening infections, such as staphylococcal septicemia or other deep-seated severe infection –

Adults: 1 g every 4 to 6 hours.

Children: ≥ 100 mg/kg/day in equally divided doses every 4 to 6 hours.

Parenteral –

Mild to moderate upper respiratory or localized skin or soft tissue infections:

Adults and children (≥ 40 kg) – 250 to 500 mg every 4 to 6 hours.

Children (< 40 kg) – 50 mg/kg/day in equally divided doses every 6 hours.

Absorption and excretion data indicate that 25 mg/kg/day in prematures and neonates provided adequate therapeutic levels.

Severe infections (lower respiratory tract or disseminated infections):

Adults and children (≥ 40 kg) – ≥ 1 g every 4 to 6 hours.

Children (< 40 kg) – ≥ 100 mg/kg/day in equally divided doses every 4 to 6 hrs.

Very severe infections may require very high doses and prolonged therapy. Maximum daily dose for adults is 12 g/day and for children 100 to 300 mg/kg/day.

Other suggested doses for children and neonates include:

Children – 50 to 100 mg/kg/day divided every 6 hours.

Neonates – Weight < 2000 g – 50 mg/kg/day divided every 12 hours (age < 7 days) or 100 mg/kg/day divided every 8 hours (age > 7 days).

Weight > 2000 g: 75 mg/kg/day divided every 8 hours (age < 7 days) or 150 mg/kg/day divided every 6 hours (age > 7 days).

PENICILLIN G (AQUEOUS), PARENTERAL:

Children – 100,000 to 250,000 units /kg/day in divided doses every 4 hours.

Infants –

(over 7 days and > 2000 g): 100,000 units/kg/day in divided doses every 6 hours (meningitis - 200,000 units).

Over 7 days and < 2000 g: 75,000 units/kg/day in divided doses every 8 hours (meningitis - 150,000 units).

Under 7 days and > 2000 g: 50,000 units/kg/day in divided doses every 8 hours (meningitis - 150,000 units).

Under 7 days and < 2000 g: 50,000 units/kg/day in divided doses every 12 hours (meningitis - 100,000 units).

Parenteral Penicillin G Use and Dosages	
Organisms/Infections	Dosage
Labeled uses:	
Meningococcal meningitis;	1 to 2 million units IM every 2 hours; or 20 to 30 million units/day continuous IV drip for 14 days or until afebrile for 7 days; or 200,000 to 300,000 units/kg/day every 2 to 4 hours divided doses for a total of 24 doses.
Actinomycosis: For cervicofacial cases	1 to 6 million units/day
For thoracic and abdominal disease:	12 to 20 million units/day IV for 6 weeks. May be followed by oral penicillin V 500 mg 4 times daily for 2 to 3 months
Clostridial infections:	20 million units/day as adjunct to antitoxin
Fusospirochetal infections: Severe infections of oropharynx, lower respiratory tract and genital area	5 to 10 million units/day
Rat-bite fever (Spirillum minus, Streptobacillus moniliformis), Haverhill fever:	12 to 20 million units/day for 3 to 4 weeks
Listeria infections (Listeria monocytogenes):	
Meningitis (adults)	15 to 20 million units/day for 2 weeks
Endocarditis (adults)	15 to 20 million units/day for 4 weeks
Pasteurella infections (Pasteurella multocida): Bacteremia and meningitis	4 to 6 million units/day for 2 weeks
Erysipeloid (Erysipelothrix rhusiopathiae): Endocarditis	12 to 20 million units/day for 4 to 6 weeks
Gram-negative bacillary bacteremia (Escherichia coli, Enterobacter aerogenes, Alcaligenes faecalis, Salmonella, Shigella, Proteus mirabilis):	≥ 20 million units/day
Diphtheria: Adjunct to antitoxin to prevent carrier state	2 to 3 million units/day in divided doses for 10 to 12 days
Anthrax:(*B. anthracis* is often resistant)	Minimum 5 million units/day; 12 to 20 million units/day have been used
Pneumococcal infections (S pneumoniae):	
Empyema	5 to 24 million units/day in divided doses every 4 to 6 hours
Meningitis	20 to 24 million units/day for 14 days
Suppurative arthritis, osteomyelitis, mastoiditis, endocarditis, peritonitis, pericarditis	12 to 20 million units/day for ≥ 2 to 4 weeks
Syphilis:	
Neurosyphilis	12 to 24 million units/day IV (2 to 4 million units every 4 hours) for 10 to 14 days. Many recommend benzathine penicillin G 2.4 million units IM weekly for 3 weeks following the completion of this regimen.
Congenital syphilis: Symptomatic or asymptomatic infants	*Newborns:* 50,000 units/kg/day IV every 8 to 12 hours for 10 to 14 days. If > 1 day of therapy is missed, restart the entire course. *Infants (after newborn period):* 50,000 units/kg every 4 to 6 hours for 10 to 14 days.
Unlabeled uses:	
Lyme disease (Borrelia burgdorferi):	
Erythema chronicum migrans	Use oral penicillin V
Neurologic complications (eg, meningitis, encephalitis)	200,000 to 300,000 units/kg/day (up to 20 million units) IV for 10 to 14 days
Carditis	200,000 to 300,000 units/kg/day (up to 20 million units) IV for 10 days with cardiac monitoring and a temporary pacemaker for complete heart block
Arthritis	200,000 to 300,000 units/kg/day (up to 20 million units) IV for 10 to 20 days

PENICILLIN G BENZATHINE, PARENTERAL: Administer by deep IM injection in the upper outer quadrant of the buttock. In infants and small children, the midlateral aspect of the thigh may be preferable. Do not inject benzathine penicillin into the gluteal region of children < 2 years of age. When doses are repeated, rotate the injection site.

Adults – 1.2 million units in one dose.

Children (> 27 kg) – 900,000 to 1.2 million units in one dose.

Children and infants (< 27 kg) – 300,000 to 600,000 units in one dose.

Neonates – 50,000 units/kg in one dose.

Parenteral Penicillin G Benzathine Uses and Dosages	
Organisms/Infections	Dosage
Streptococcal (group A): Prevention of recurrent rheumatic fever.	1.2 million units every 4 weeks
Syphilis: *Early syphilis* -Primary, secondary or latent syphilis of < 1 year's duration.	2.4 million units IM in single dose
Syphilis of > 1 year's duration, gummas and cardiovascular syphilis -Latent, cardiovascular or late benign syphilis.	2.4 million units once weekly for three weeks
Neurosyphilis	Aqueous penicillin G, 12 to 24 million units/day IV (2 to 4 million units every 4 hours) for 10 to 14 days. Many recommend benzathine penicillin G, 2.4 million IM units weekly for 3 doses following completion of this regimen. or Aqueous procaine penicillin G, 2.4 million units/day IM *plus* probenecid 500 mg orally 4 times daily, both for 10 to 14 days. Many recommend benzathine penicillin G, 2.4 million units IM weekly for 3 doses following completion of this regimen.
Syphilis in pregnancy	Dosage schedule appropriate for stage of syphilis recommended for nonpregnant patients.
Congenital syphilis -Older children with definite acquired syphilis and a normal neurologic examination.	50,000 units/kg IM, up to the adult dose of 2.4 million units.
Yaws, bejel and pinta	1.2 million units in a single dose
Erysipeloid (Erysipelothrix rhusiopathiae): Uncomplicated infection.	1.2 million units in a single dose

PENICILLIN G PROCAINE, AQUEOUS (APPG): Administer by deep IM injection into the upper, outer quadrant of the buttock. In infants and small children, the midlateral aspect of the thigh may be preferable. When doses are repeated, rotate the injection site.

Adults and children – 600,000 to 1.2 million units/day IM in one or two doses (up to a maximum of 4.8 million units/day) for 10 days to 2 weeks. Penicillin G procaine must never be used IV.

Newborns – 50,000 units/kg IM once daily. Avoid use in these patients since sterile abscesses and procaine toxicity are of much greater concern than in older children.

Penicillin G Procaine Uses and Dosages	
Organisms/Infections	Dosage
Pneumococcal infections: Moderately severe uncomplicated pneumonia and middle ear and paranasal sinus infections	600,000 to 1.2 million units/day
Streptococcal infections (group A): Moderately severe to severe tonsillitis, erysipelas, scarlet fever, upper respiratory tract (ie, otitis media) and skin and skin structure infections	600,000 to 1.2 million units/day for a minimum of 10 days
Bacterial endocarditis - Only in extremely sensitive infections (*S. viridans, S. bovis*)	1.2 million units 4 times daily for 2 to 4 weeks plus streptomycin 500 mg twice daily for the first 2 weeks
Staphylococcal infections: Moderately severe to severe infections of the skin and skin structure	600,000 to 1.2 million units/day
Diphtheria: Adjunctive therapy with antitoxin	300,000 to 600,000 units/day
Carrier state	300,000 units/day for 10 days
Anthrax: Cutaneous	600,000 to 1.2 million units/day
Vincent's gingivitis and pharyngitis (fusospirochetosis):	600,000 to 1.2 million units/day. Obtain necessary dental care in infections involving gum tissue.

Penicillin G Procaine Uses and Dosages	
Organisms/Infections	Dosage
Erysipeloid:	600,000 to 1.2 million units/day
Rat-bite fever (Streptobacillus moniliformis and Spirillum minus):	600,000 to 1.2 million units/day
Gonorrheal infections (uncomplicated):	4.8 million units divided into at least two doses at one visit; 1 g oral probenecid is given 30 minutes before the injections. Obtain follow-up cultures form the original site(s) of infection 7 to 14 days after therapy. In women, it is also desirable to obtain culture test-of-cure from both the endocervical and anal canals. Note: Treat gonorrheal endocarditis intensively with aqueous penicillin G
Syphilis: Primary, secondary and latent with a negative spinal fluid (adults and children > 12 years of age):	600,000 units daily for 8 days; total 4.8 million units
Neurosyphilis[1] (as an alternative to the recommended regimen of penicillin G aqueous)	2 to 4 million units/day plus probenecid 500 mg orally 4 times daily, both for 10 to 14 days; many recommend benzathine penicillin G 2.4 million units weekly for 3 doses following the completion of this regimen.
Congenital syphilis:[1] Symptomatic and asymptomatic infants	50,000 units/kg/day (administered once IM) for 10 to 14 days
Yaws, bejel and pinta:	Treat same as syphilis in corresponding stage of disease

PENICILLIN G BENZATHINE AND PROCAINE COMBINED: Administer by deep IM injection in the upper outer quadrant of the buttock. In infants and small children, the midlateral aspect of the thigh may be preferable. when doses are repeated, rotate the injection site.

Streptococcal infections – Treatment with the recommended dosage is usually given in a single session using multiple IM sites when indicated. An alternative dosage schedule may be used, giving half the total dose on day 1 and half on day 3. This will also ensure adequate serum levels over a 10 day period; however use only when the patient's cooperation can be ensured.

Adults and children (> 60 lbs; 27 kg): 2.4 million units.

Children (30 to 60 lbs; 14 to 27 kg): 900,000 to 1.2 million units.

Infants and children (< 30 lbs; 14 kg): 600,000 units.

Pneumococcal infections (except pneumococcal meningitis) –

Children: 600,000 units.

Adults: 1.2 million units. Repeat every 2 or 3 days until the patient has been afebrile for 48 hours.

PENICILLIN V (PHENOXYMETHYL PENICILLIN): 250 mg = 400,000 units.

Adults – 125 to 500 mg 4 times a day; in renal impairment (creatinine clearance, ≤ 10 ml/min) - Do not exceed 250 mg every 6 hours.

Children – 25 to 50 mg/kg/day in divided doses every 6 to 8 hours.

Penicillin V Uses and Dosages	
Organisms/Infections	Dosage
Labeled uses:	
Streptococcal infections: Infections of the upper respiratory tract, including scarlet fever and mild erysipelas	125 to 250 mg every 6 to 8 hours for 10 days for mild to modeately severe infections
Pharyngitis in children	250 mg 2 times daily for 10 days
Otitis media and sinusitis	250 to 500 mg every 6 hours for 2 weeks
Prevention of bacterial endocarditis[1] in patients with rheumatic, congential or other acquired valvular heart disease undergoing dental procedures or upper respiratory tract surgical procedures	Amoxicillin is the recommended agent; however, the choice of penicillin V is rational and acceptable
Pneumococcal infections: Mild to moderately severe respiratory tract infections including otitis media	250 to 500 mg every 6 hours until afebrile at least 2 days
Staphylococcal infections: Mild infections of skin and soft tissue	250 to 500 mg every 6 to 8 hours
Fusospirochetosis (Vincent's infection) of the oropharynx: Mild to moderately severe infections	250 to 500 mg every 6 to 8 hours
Unlabeled uses:	

Penicillin V Uses and Dosages	
Organisms/Infections	Dosage
Prophylactic treatment of children with sickle cell anemia (to reduce the incidence of *S pneumoniae* septicemia)	125 mg 2 times daily
Anaerobic infections: Mild to moderate infections	250 mg 4 times daily
Lyme disease (Borrelia burgdorferi):	
Erythema chronicum migrans:	
Pregnant or lactating women, tetracycline treatment failures	250 to 500 mg 4 times a day for 10 to 20 days
Children < 2 years of age	50 mg/kg/day (up to 2 g/day) in 4 divided doses for 10 to 20 days
Neurologic complications (eg, meningitis, encephalitis), carditis, arthritis	Use penicillin G IV

[1] American Heart Association Statement. *JAMA* 1990;264:2919–22.

PIPERACILLIN SODIUM: Administer IM or IV. For serious infections, give 3 to 4 g every 4 to 6 hours as a 20 to 30 minute IV infusion. Maximum daily dose is 24 g/day, although higher doses have been used. Limit IM injections to 2 g/site.

Hemodialysis – Maximum dose is 6 g/day (2 g every 8 hours). Hemodialysis removes 30% to 50% of piperacillin in 4 hours; administer an additional 1 g after dialysis.

Renal failure and hepatic insufficiency – Measure serum levels to provide additional guidance for adjusting dosage; however, this may not be practical.

Infants and children < 12 years of age – Dosages have not been established; however, the following doses have been suggested:

Neonates: 100 mg/kg/dose every 12 hours.

Children: Cystic fibrosis, 350 to 500 mg/kg/day divided every 4 to 6 hours.

Other conditions, 200 to 300 mg/kg/day, up to a maximum of 24 g/day divided every 4 to 6 hours.

Piperacillin Uses and Dosages	
Organisms/Infections	Dosage
Serious infections (septicemia, nosocomial pneumonia, intra-abdominal infections, aerobic and anaerobic gynecologic infections and skin and soft tissue infections):	12 to 18 g/day IV (200 to 300 mg/kg/day) in divided doses every 4 to 6 hours
Renal impairment-	
Creatinine clearance 20 to 40 ml/min	12 g/day; 4 g every 8 hours
< 20 ml/min	8 g/day; 4 g every 6 to 12 hours
Urinary tract infections: Complicated (normal renal function)	8 to 16 g/day IV (125 to 200 mg/kg/day) in divided doses every 6 to 8 hours
Renal impairment	
Creatinine clearance 20 to 40 ml/min	9 g/day; 3 g every 8 hours
< 20 ml/min	6 g/day; 3 g every 12 hours
Uncomplicated UTI and most community-acquired pneumonia (normal renal function)	6 to 8 g/day IM or IV (100 to 125 mg/kg/d) in divided doses every 6 to 12 hours
Uncomplicated UTI with renal impairment Creatinine clearance < 20 ml/min	6 g/day; 3 g every 12 hours
Uncomplicated gonorrhea infections:	2 g IM in a single dose with 1 g probenecid ½ hour prior to injection
Prophylaxis: Intra-abdominal surgery	2 g IV just prior to surgery; 2 g during surgery; 2 g every 6 hours post-op for no more than 24 hours
Vaginal hysterectomy	2 g IV just prior to surgery; 2 g 6 hrs after initial dose; 2 g 12 hrs after first dose
Cesarean section	2 g IV after cord is clamped; 2 g 4 hours after initial dose; 2 g 8 hours after first dose
Abdominal hysterectomy	2 g IV just prior to surgery; 2 g on return to recovery room; 2 g after 6 hours

PIPERACILLIN SODIUM AND TAZOBACTAM SODIUM: Administer by IV infusion over 30 minutes. The usual total daily dose for adults is 12 g/1.5 g, given as 3.375 g every 6 hours.

Nosocomial pneumonia – Start with 3.375 g every 4 hours plus an aminoglycoside. Continue the aminoglycoside in patients from whom *P. aeruginosa* is isolated. If it is not isolated, the aminoglycoside may be discontinued at the discretion of the treating physician as guided by the severity of the infection and the patient's clinical and bacteriological progress.

Renal function impairment – In patients with renal insufficiency (Ccr < 40 ml/min), adjust the IV dose to the degree of actual renal function impairment. Measurement of serum levels of piperacillin and tazobactam will provide additional guidance for adjusting dosage.

Piperacillin Sodium and Tazobactam Sodium Dosage Recommendations

Creatinine clearance (ml/min)	Recommended dosage regimen
> 40	12 g/1.5 g/day in divided doses of 3.375 g every 6 hours
20 - 40	8 g/1 g/day in divided doses of 2.25 g every 6 hours
< 20	6 g/0.75 g/day in divided doses of 2.25 g every 8 hours

Hemodialysis – The maximum dose is 2.25 g every 8 hours. In addition, because hemodialysis removes 30% to 40% of a dose in 4 hours, give one additional dose of 0.75 g following each dialysis period.

TICARCILLIN DISODIUM: Use IV therapy in higher doses in serious urinary tract and systemic infections. Intramuscular injections should not exceed 2 g/injection.

Ticarcillin Uses and Dosages

Organism/Infections	Dosage
Bacterial septicemia, respiratory tract infections, skin and soft tissue infections, intra-abdominal infections and infections of the female pelvis and genital tract	*Adults:* 200 to 300 mg/kg/day by IV infusion in divided doses every 3, 4 or 6 hours (3 g every 3, 4 or 6 hours), depending on weight of patient and severity of infection *Children (< 40 kg):* 200 to 300 mg/kg/day by IV infusion in divided doses every 4 or 6 hours[1]
Urinary tract infections: Complicated infections	150 to 200 mg/kg/day IV infusion in divided doses every 4 or 6 hours. Usual dose for average adult (70 kg) is 3 g 4 times daily.
Uncomplicated infections	*Adults:* 1 g IM or direct IV every 6 hours *Children (< 40 kg):* 50 to 100 mg/kg/day IM or direct IV in divided doses every 6 or 8 hours
Neonates: Severe infections (sepsis) due to susceptible strains of *Pseudomonas* species, *Proteus* species and *E coli*	Give IM or by 10 to 20 minute IV infusions
< 2 kg -	*< 7 days* - 75 mg/kg/12 hr (150 mg/kg/day) *> 7 days* - 75 mg/kg/8 hr (225 mg/kg/day)
> 2 kg -	*< 7 days* - 75 mg/kg/8 hr (225 mg/kg/day) *> 7 days* - 100 mg/kg/8 hr (300 mg/kg/day)
Dosage in renal insufficiency:[2]	Initial loading dose of 3 g IV followed by IV doses based on creatinine clearance and type of dialysis
Creatinine clearance (ml/min) -	
> 60	3 g every 4 hours
30 to 60	2 g every 4 hours
10 to 30	2 g every 8 hours
< 10	2 g every 12 hours or 1 g IM every 6 hours
< 10 with hepatic dysfunction	2 g every 24 hours or 1 g IM every 12 hours
Patients on peritoneal dialysis	3 g every 12 hours
Patients on hemodialysis	2 g every 12 hours supplemented with 3 g after each dialysis

[1] Daily dose for children should not exceed adult dosage.
[2] Half-life in patients with renal failure is approximately 13 hours.

TICARCILLIN AND CLAVULANATE POTASSIUM: Administer by IV infusion over 30 minutes.

Ticarcillin/Clavulanate Potassium Uses and Dosages

Infection	Dosage
Systemic and urinary tract infections:	
Adults (≥ 60 kg)	3.1 g[1] every 4 to 6 hours
(≤ 60 kg)[2]	200 to 300 mg/kg/day (based on ticarcillin content) in divided doses every 4 to 6 hrs
Gynecologic infections:	
Adults (≥ 60 kg)	
Moderate infections	200 mg/kg/day in divided doses every 6 hours
Severe infections	300 mg/kg/day in divided doses every 4 hours

[1] 3 g ticarcillin plus 100 mg clavulanic acid.
[2] Dosage in children < 12 years of age is not established.

Dosage of Ticarcillin/Clavulanate Potassium in Renal Insufficiency[1]

Creatinine clearance (ml/min)	*Dosage*
> 60	3.1 g[2] every 4 hours
30 to 60	2 g every 4 hours
10 to 30	2 g every 8 hours
< 10	2 g every 12 hours
< 10 with hepatic dysfunction	2 g every 24 hours
Patients on peritoneal dialysis	3.1 g[2] every 12 hours
Patients on hemodialysis	2 g every 12 hours supplemented with 3.1 g[2] after each dialysis

[1] Half-life of ticarcillin in patients with renal failure is ≈ 13 hours. Initial loading dose is 3.1 g. Follow with doses based on creatinine clearance and type of dialysis.
[2] 3 g ticarcillin plus 100 mg clavulanic acid.

CEPHALOSPORINS AND RELATED ANTIBIOTICS

CEFACLOR	
Tablets, extended release: 375 and 500 mg (*Rx*)	*Ceclor CD* (Lilly)
Capsules: 250 and 500 mg (*Rx*)	Various, *Ceclor Pulvules* (Lilly)
Suspension: 125, 187, 250 and 375 mg/5 ml (*Rx*)	Various, *Ceclor* (Lilly)
CEFADROXIL	
Capsules: 500 mg (*Rx*)	Various, *Duricef* (Mead Johnson)
Tablets: 1 g (*Rx*)	Various, *Duricef* (Mead Johnson)
Oral Suspension: 125, 250 and 500 mg/5 ml (*Rx*)	Various, *Ultracef* (Mead Johnson)
CEFAMANDOLE NAFATE	
Powder for injection: 1, 2 and 10 g (*Rx*)	*Mandol* (Lilly)
CEFAZOLIN SODIUM	
Powder for injection: 250 and 500 mg, 1, 5, 10 and 20 g (*Rx*)	Various, *Ancef* (SK-Beecham), *Zolicef* (Apothecon)
Injection: 500 mg or 1 g in 5% Dextrose in Water (*Rx*)	*Ancef* (SK-Beecham)
CEFEPIME HCl	
Powder for injection: 500 mg, 1 and 2 g (*Rx*)	*Maxipime* (Bristol-Myers Squibb)
CEFIXIME	
Tablets: 200 and 400 mg (*Rx*)	*Suprax* (Lederle)
Powder for oral suspension: 100 mg/5 ml (*Rx*)	*Suprax* (Lederle)
CEFMETAZOLE SODIUM	
Powder for injection: 1 and 2 g (*Rx*)	*Zefazone* (Upjohn)
CEFONICID SODIUM	
Powder for injection: 500 mg, 1 and 10 g (*Rx*)	*Monocid* (SmithKline Beecham)
CEFOPERAZONE SODIUM	
Powder for injection: 1 and 2 g (*Rx*)	*Cefobid* (Roerig)
Injection: 1 and 2 g (*Rx*)	*Cefobid* (Roerig)
CEFOTAXIME SODIUM	
Powder for injection: 1, 2 and 10 g (*Rx*)	*Claforan* (Hoechst-Marion Roussel)
Injection: 1 and 2 g (*Rx*)	*Claforan* (Hoechst-Marion Roussel)
CEFOTETAN DISODIUM	
Powder for injection: 1, 2 and 10 g (*Rx*)	*Cefotan* (Stuart)
CEFOXITIN SODIUM	
Powder for injection: 1, 2 and 10 g (*Rx*)	*Mefoxin* (Merck)
Injection: 1 and 2 g in 5% Dextrose in Water (*Rx*)	*Mefoxin* (Merck)
CEFPODOXIME PROXETIL	
Tablets: 100 and 200 mg (*Rx*)	*Vantin* (Upjohn)
Granules for suspension: 50 and 100 mg/5 ml (*Rx*)	*Vantin* (Upjohn)
CEFPROZIL	
Tablets: 250 and 500 mg (*Rx*)	*Cefzil* (Bristol Labs)
Powder for suspension: 125 and 250 mg/5 ml (*Rx*)	*Cefzil* (Bristol Labs)
CEFTAZIDIME	
Powder for injection: 349 and 500 mg, 1, 2 and 6 g (*Rx*)	*Fortaz* (Glaxo Wellcome)
Injection: 1 and 2 g (*Rx*)	*Fortaz* (Glaxo Wellcome)
CEFTIBUTEN	
Capsules: 400 mg (*Rx*)	*Cedax* (Schering)
Oral suspension: 90 and 180 mg/5 ml (*Rx*)	
CEFTIZOXIME SODIUM	
Powder for injection: 500 mg, 1, 2 and 10 g (*Rx*)	*Cefizox* (Fujisawa)
Injection: 1 and 2 g in 5% Dextrose in Water (*Rx*)	*Cefizox* (Fujisawa)
CEFTRIAXONE SODIUM	
Powder for injection: 250 and 500 mg, 1, 2 and 10 g (*Rx*)	*Rocephin* (Roche)
Injection: 1 and 2 g (*Rx*)	*Rocephin* (Roche)
CEFUROXIME	
Tablets: 125, 250 and 500 mg (*Rx*)	*Ceftin* (Glaxo Wellcome)
Suspension: 125 mg/5 ml (when reconstituted) (*Rx*)	*Ceftin* (Glaxo Wellcome)
Powder for injection: 750 mg, 1.5 and 7.5 g per vial (*Rx*)	Various, *Zinacef* (Glaxo Wellcome), *Kefurox* (Lilly)
Injection: 750 mg and 1.5 g (*Rx*)	*Zinacef* (Glaxo Wellcome)

CEPHALEXIN	
Capsules: 250 and 500 mg (*Rx*)	Various, *Keflex* (Dista)
Tablets: 250 and 500 mg and 1 g (*Rx*)	Various
Oral suspension: 100 and 200 mg (*Rx*)	Various, *Keflex* (Dista)
Powder for oral suspension: 125 and 250 mg/5 ml (when reconstituted) (*Rx*)	*Biocef* (Inter. Ethical Labs)
CEPHALEXIN HCl MONOHYDRATE	
Tablets: 500 mg (*Rx*)	*Keftab* (Dista)
CEPHALOTHIN SODIUM	
Injection: 1 and 2 g in 5% Dextrose (*Rx*)	*Cephalothin Sodium* (Baxter)
Powder for injection: 1 and 2 g (*Rx*)	Various, *Keflin, Neutral* (Lilly)
CEPHAPIRIN SODIUM	
Powder for injection: 500 mg, 1, 2, 4 and 20 g (*Rx*)	Various, *Cefadyl* (Apothecon)
CEPHRADINE	
Capsules: 250 and 500 mg (*Rx*)	Various, *Velosef* (Apothecon)
Oral suspension: 125 and 250 mg/5 ml (when reconstituted) (*Rx*)	Various, *Velosef* (Apothecon)
Powder for injection: 250 and 500 mg, 1 and 2 g (*Rx*)	*Velosef* (Apothecon)
LORACARBEF	
Pulvules (capsules): 200 and 400 mg (*Rx*)	*Lorabid* (Lilly)
Powder for suspension: 100 and 200 mg/5 ml (*Rx*)	*Lorabid* (Lilly)
Oral suspension: 100 and 200 mg/5 ml (*Rx*)	*Lorabid* (Lilly)

Actions:

Pharmacology: Structurally and pharmacologically related to penicillins. Cefoxitin and cefotetan (cephamycins) and loracarbef (a carbacephem) are included due to their similarity.

Cephalosporins inhibit mucopeptide synthesis in the bacterial cell wall, making it defective and osmotically unstable. The drugs are usually bactericidal, depending on organism susceptibility, dose, tissue concentrations and the rate at which organisms are multiplying. They are more effective against rapidly growing organisms forming cell walls.

Pharmacokinetics:

Pharmacokinetic Parameters of Cephalosporins

	Drug	Routes	Half-Life: Normal renal function (minutes)	Half-Life: ESRD[1] (hours)	Half-Life: Hemo-dialysis (hours)	Protein bound (%)	Recovered unchanged in urine (%)	Peak serum level 1 g IV dose (mcg/ml)	Sodium (mEq/g)
First	Cephalexin	Oral	50-80	19-22	4-6	10	> 90	–	-
	Cefadroxil	Oral	78-96	20-25	3-4	20	> 90	-	-
	Cephradine	Oral/IM-IV	48-80	8-15	-	8-17	> 90	86	6 [2]
	Cephalothin	IM-IV	30-50	3-15	3	70	68-70	30	2.8
	Cephapirin	IM-IV	24-36	1.8-4	1.8	54	68-70	73	2.4
	Cefazolin	IM-IV	90-120	3-7	9-14	80-86	80-96	185-189	2-2.1
Second	Cefaclor	Oral	35-54	2-3	1.6-2.1	25	60-85	-	-
	Cefamandole	IM-IV	30-60	8-11	7	70	65-85	139	3.3
	Cefoxitin	IM-IV	40-60	20	4	73	85-99	64-110	2.3
	Cefuroxime	Oral/IM-IV	80	16-22 [3]	3.5	33-50	66-100	100 [4]	2.4 [3]
	Cefonicid	IM-IV	270	11	-	98	95-99	221.3	3.7
	Cefmetazole	IV	72	-	-	65	85	-	2
	Cefotetan	IM-IV	180-276	13-35	5	88-90	51-81	158	3.5
	Cefprozil	Oral	78	5.2-5.9	de-creased	36	60	-	-
	Cefpodoxime [5]	Oral	120-180	9.8	-	21-29	29-33	-	-
	Loracarbef	Oral	60	32	4	25	> 90	-	-
Third	Cefixime	Oral	180-240	11.5	-	65	50	-	-
	Cefpodoxime[5]	Oral	120-180	9.8	-	21-29	29-33	-	-
	Cefoperazone	IM-IV	102-156	1.3-2.9	2	82-93	20-30	73-153	1.5
	Cefotaxime	IM-IV	60	3-11	2.5	30-40	20-36	42-102	2.2
	Ceftizoxime	IM-IV	84-114	25-30	6	30	80	60-87	2.6
	Ceftriaxone	IM-IV	348-522	15.7	14.7	85-95	33-67	151	3.6
	Ceftazidime	IM-IV	114-120	14-30	-	< 10-17	80-90	69-90	2.3
	Ceftibuten	Oral	144	13.4-22.3	2-4	65	56	-	-
	Cefepime	IM-IV	102-138	17-21	11-16	20	85	79	-

[1] ESRD = End stage renal disease (Ccr < 10 ml/min/1.73 m^2).
[2] Also available in sodium free form.
[3] Injection only.
[4] Following 1.5 g IV dose.
[5] Extended spectrum agent.

Cephalexin, cephradine, cefaclor, cefixime, cefprozil, cefadroxil, ceftibuten and loracarbef are well absorbed from the GI tract. Cephalosporins are widely distributed to most tissues and fluids. First and second generation agents do not readily enter cerebrospinal fluid (CSF), except cefuroxime, even when meninges are inflamed. Third generation compounds (little data for cefixime) readily diffuse into the CSF of patients with inflamed meninges. However, CSF levels of cefoperazone are relatively low. Most cephalosporins and metabolites are primarily excreted renally.

Microbiology:

Organisms Generally Susceptible to Cephalosporins

Organisms		First Generation						Second Generation				
✓= generally susceptible ‡ = demonstrated in vitro activity		Cephalexin	Cefadroxil	Cephradine	Cephalothin	Cephapirin	Cefazolin	Cefaclor	Cefamandole	Cefoxitin	Cefuroxime	Cefonicid
Gram-positive	*Staphylococci* [1]	✓[2]	✓	✓	✓	✓	✓	✓[2]	✓	✓	✓	✓[2]
	Streptococci, betahemolytic	✓	✓	✓	✓	✓	✓	✓	✓	✓	✓	✓
	Streptococcus pneumoniae	✓	✓	✓	✓	✓	✓	✓	✓	✓	✓	✓
	Streptococcus pyogenes											
Gram-negative	*Acinetobacter* sp											
	Citrobacter sp										✓[2]	‡
	Enterobacter sp						✓[2]		✓		✓[2]	‡
	Escherichia coli	✓	✓	✓	✓	✓	✓	✓	✓	✓	✓	✓
	Haemophilus influ enzae	✓		✓	✓	✓	✓	✓[3]	✓[3]	✓[3]	✓[3]	✓[3]
	Haemophilus para influenzae										‡	
	Hafnia alvei											
	Klebsiella sp	✓	✓	✓	✓	✓	✓	✓	✓	✓	✓	✓
	Moraxella (Branhamella) catarrhalis	‡						✓			‡	
	Morganella (Proteus) morganii								✓	✓	✓[2]	✓
	Neisseria gonorrhoeae							‡		✓	✓	‡
	Neisseria meningitidis										✓	
	Proteus mirabilis	✓	✓	✓	✓	✓	✓	✓	✓	✓	✓	✓
	Proteus vulgaris								✓[2]	✓		✓
	Providencia sp									✓	✓	
	Providencia rettgeri								✓	✓	✓	✓
	Pseudomonas aeru ginosa											
	Salmonella sp				✓						✓	
	Salmonella typhi											
	Serratia sp											
	Shigella sp				✓						✓	
Anaerobes	*Bacteroides* sp							✓	✓	✓	✓	
	Bacteroides fragilis									✓		
	Clostridium sp								✓	✓	✓	‡
	Clostridium difficile											
	Eubacterium sp											
	Fusobacterium sp								✓		✓	‡
	Peptococcus sp							‡	✓	✓	✓	‡
	Peptostreptococcus sp							‡	✓	✓	✓	‡

[1] Coagulase-positive, coagulase-negative and penicillinase-producing.
[2] Some strains are resistant.
[3] Including some β-lactamase-producing strains.

Organisms Generally Susceptible to Cephalosporins														
Second Generation (Cont.)					Third Generation								Organisms	
Cefmetazole	Cefotetan	Cefprozil	Cefpodoxime [4]	Loracarbef	Cefixime	Cefoperazone	Cefotaxime	Ceftizoxime	Ceftriaxone	Ceftazidime	Ceftibuten	Cefepime	✓= generally susceptible ‡= demonstrated in vitro activity	
✓	✓	✓	✓ [2]	✓		✓	✓[3]	✓	✓	✓		✓ [5]	*Staphylococci* [1]	Gram-positive
✓	✓	✓	✓	✓	✓	✓	✓	✓	✓	✓		‡	*Streptococci*, betahemolytic	
✓	✓	✓	✓	✓	✓	✓	✓	✓	✓	✓	✓ [6]	✓	*Streptococcus pneumoniae*	
											✓	✓ [7]	*Streptococcus pyogenes*	
						✓ [2]	✓	✓	✓	‡		‡	*Acinetobacter* sp	Gram-negative
‡	‡	‡	‡	‡	‡	✓	✓	‡	‡	✓		‡	*Citrobacter* sp	
‡	✓					✓	✓	✓	✓	✓		✓	*Enterobacter* sp	
✓	✓	‡	✓	✓	✓	✓	✓	✓	✓	✓		✓	*Escherichia coli*	
✓[3]	✓[3]	✓ [3]	✓ [3]	✓ [3]	✓ [3]	✓ [3]	✓ [3]	✓ [3]	✓ [3]	✓ [3]	✓ [3]	‡ [3]	*Haemophilus influ enzae*	
			‡	‡	‡ [3]		✓		✓	‡			*Haemophilus para influenzae*	
												‡	*Hafnia alvei*	
✓	✓	‡	✓	‡	‡	✓	✓	✓	✓	✓		✓	*Klebsiella* sp	
‡		✓	✓	✓ [3]	✓ [3]			‡		✓	✓ [3]	‡ [3]	*Moraxella (Branhamella) catarrhalis*	
✓	✓					✓	✓	✓	✓	‡		‡	*Morganella (Proteus) morganii*	
‡	✓	‡	✓ [2]	‡ [1]	‡	✓ [3]	✓	✓	✓	‡			*Neisseria gonorrhoeae*	
	‡					‡	✓	‡	✓	✓			*Neisseria meningitidis*	
✓	✓	‡	✓	‡	✓	✓	✓	✓	✓	✓		✓	*Proteus mirabilis*	
✓	✓		‡		‡	✓	✓	✓	✓	✓		‡	*Proteus vulgaris*	
✓	✓				‡		‡	‡	‡	‡		‡	*Providencia* sp	
‡	✓		‡		‡	✓	✓	✓	‡	‡		‡	*Providencia rettgeri*	
						✓	✓ [2]	✓ [2]	✓ [2]	✓		✓	*Pseudomonas aeru ginosa*	
‡	‡	‡		‡	‡	‡	‡	‡	‡	‡			*Salmonella* sp	
	‡						‡	‡	‡				*Salmonella typhi*	
	‡				‡	✓	✓	✓	✓	✓		‡	*Serratia* sp	
‡	‡	‡		‡	‡	‡	‡	‡	‡	‡			*Shigella* sp	
✓	✓ [2]	‡				✓	✓	‡	✓				*Bacteroides* sp	Anaerobes
✓	✓					✓	✓	✓	‡				*Bacteroides fragilis*	
✓	✓	‡		‡		✓	✓	‡	‡	‡			*Clostridium* sp	
		‡				‡							*Clostridium difficile*	
						‡			‡				*Eubacterium* sp	
✓	✓	‡		‡		‡	✓	‡	‡				*Fusobacterium* sp	
‡	✓			‡		✓	✓	✓	‡	‡			*Peptococcus* sp	
‡	✓	‡	‡	‡		✓	✓	✓	‡	‡			*Peptostreptococcus* sp	

[1] Coagulase-positive, coagulase-negative and penicillinase-producing.
[2] Some strains are resistant.
[3] Including some β-lactamase-producing strains.
[4] Extended spectrum agent.
[5] Methicillin-susceptible strains only.
[6] Penicillin-susceptible strains only.
[7] Lancefield's Group A streptococci.

Indications:

For approved indications, refer to the Administration and Dosage section.

Contraindications:

Hypersensitivity to cephalosporins or related antibiotics.

Warnings:

Cefepime has a broad spectrum of activity against gram-positive and gram-negative bacteria but has a low affinity for chromosomally encoded beta-lactamases.

Hypersensitivity: Reactions range from mild to life-threatening. Before therapy is instituted, inquire about previous hypersensitivity reactions to cephalosporins and penicillins.

Cross-allergenicity with penicillin: Administer cautiously to penicillin-sensitive patients. There is evidence of partial cross-allergenicity; cephalosporins cannot be assumed to be an absolutely safe alternative to penicillin in the penicillin-allergic patient. The estimated incidence of cross-sensitivity is 5% to 16%; however, it is possibly as low as 3% to 7%.

Serum sickness-like reactions: (erythema multiforme or skin rashes accompanied by polyarthritis, arthralgia and, frequently, fever) have been reported; these reactions usually occurred following a second course of therapy. Signs and symptoms occur after a few days of therapy and resolve a few days after drug discontinuation with no serious sequelae.

Seizures: Several cephalosporins have been implicated in triggering seizures, particularly in patients with renal impairment when the dosage was not reduced.

Coagulation abnormalities: **Cefamandole** and **cefoperazone** can interfere with hemostasis through three different mechanisms: Hypoprothrombinemia with or without bleeding; platelet dysfunction; very rarely, immune-mediated thrombocytopenia. Alterations in prothrombin times (PT) occur rarely in patients treated with **ceftriaxone.**

Predisposing factors to cephalosporin bleeding abnormalities include hepatic and renal dysfunction, thrombocytopenia and the concomitant use of "high dose" heparin (> 20,000 units/day), oral anticoagulants or other drugs that affect hemostasis (eg, aspirin). Elderly, malnourished or debilitated patients are more likely to experience bleeding abnormalities than other patients.

Pseudomembranous colitis occurs with the use of cephalosporins (and other broad spectrum antibiotics); therefore, consider its diagnosis in patients who develop diarrhea with antibiotic use.

Renal function impairment: Cephalosporins may be nephrotoxic; use with caution in the presence of markedly impaired renal function (creatinine clearance [Ccr] rate of < 50 ml/min/1.73 m^2).

Hepatic function impairment: Cefoperazone is extensively excreted in bile. Serum half-life increases twofold to fourfold in patients with hepatic disease or biliary obstruction.

Pregnancy: Category B; (*Category* C - Moxalactam). These agents cross the placenta; peak umbilical cord concentrations for the various agents range from 3 to 29 mcg/ml following doses of 0.5 to 2 g.

Lactation: Most of these agents are excreted in breast milk in small quantities. Levels range from 0.16 to 4 mcg/ml, or a breast milk:maternal serum ratio of 0.01 to 0.5 following 0.5 to 2 g doses.

Children: When using cephalosporins in infants, consider the relative benefit to risk. In neonates, accumulation of cephalosporin antibiotics (with resulting prolongation of drug half-life) has occurred.

Safety and efficacy in children < 1 month (**cefaclor, cefamandole, cefazolin** and **parenteral cephradine**), < 3 months (**cefuroxime**), < 6 months (**cefixime, cefpodoxime**), < 9 months (**oral cephradine**) and < 1 year (**ceforanide**) have not been established.

Safety and efficacy of **cefoperazone** and **cefotetan** in children not established.

Precautions:

Parenteral use: Inject IM preparations deep into musculature; properly dilute IV preparations and administer over an appropriate time interval.

Gonorrhea: In the treatment of gonorrhea, all patients should have a serologic test for syphilis. Patients with incubating syphilis (seronegative without clinical signs of syphilis) are likely to be cured by the regimens used for gonorrhea.

Drug Interactions:

Agents that may interact with cephalosporins include ethanol, aminoglycosides, anticoagulants, polypeptide antibiotics and probenecid.

Drug/Lab test interactions: A false-positive reaction for **urine glucose** may occur with Benedict's solution, Fehling's solution or with *Clinitest* tablets, but not with enzyme-based tests such as *Clinistix* and *Tes-Tape*. There may be a false-positive test for *proteinuria* with acid and denaturization-precipitation tests.

Cephradine may cause false-positive reactions in urinary protein tests that use sulfosalicylic acid.

Cefuroxime may cause a false-negative reaction in the ferricyanide test for *blood glucose*.

A false-positive direct *Coombs' test* has occurred in some patients receiving cephalosporins.

Cephalosporins may falsely elevate *urinary 17-ketosteroid* values.

High concentrations of **cephalothin** or **cefoxitin** (> 100 mcg/ml) may interfere with measurement of *creatinine levels* by the Jaffe reaction and produce false results. **Cefotetan** may also affect these measurements.

Drug/Food interactions: Food increases absorption of cefpodoxime, oral cefuroxime.

Adverse Reactions:

Most common: GI disturbances (nausea, vomiting, diarrhea); hypersensitivity phenomena (most common); hypotension; fever; dyspnea; candidal overgrowth consisting of oral candidiasis, vaginitis, genital moniliasis, vaginal discharge and genito-anal pruritus; nervousness; insomnia; confusion; hypertonia; dizziness; somnolence.

CNS:
Headache; dizziness; lethargy; fatigue; paresthesia; confusion; diaphoresis; flushing.

Hematologic:
Eosinophilia; transient neutropenia; leukocytosis; leukopenia; thrombocythemia; thrombocytopenia; agranulocytosis; granulocytopenia; hemolytic anemia; bone marrow depression; pancytopenia; decreased platelet function; anemia; aplastic anemia; hemorrhage.

Hepatic:
Elevated AST, ALT, GGTP, total bilirubin, alkaline phosphatase, LDH; hepatitis.

Local:
IM administration commonly results in pain, induration, temperature elevation and tenderness.

Renal:
Transitory elevations in BUN with and without elevated serum creatinine (frequency increases in patients > 50 years old and in children < 3).

Administration and Dosage:

Duration of therapy: Continue administration for a minimum of 48 to 72 hours after fever abates or after evidence of bacterial eradication has been obtained.

Perioperative prophylaxis: Discontinue prophylactic use within 24 hours after the surgical procedure. In surgery where infection may be particularly devastating, may continue prophylactic use for 3 to 5 days following surgery completion.

CEFACLOR:

Adults – Usual dosage is 250 mg every 8 hours. In severe infections or those caused by less susceptible organisms, dosage may be doubled.

Tablets, extended release: Administer with food to enhance absorption. Do not cut, crush or chew.

Acute bacterial exacerbations of chronic bronchitis – 500 mg/12 hours for 7 days.
Secondary bacterial infection of acute bronchitis – 500 mg/12 hours for 7 days.
Pharyngitis or tonsillitis – 375 mg/12 hours for 10 days.
Uncomplicated skin and skin structure infections – 375 mg/12 hours for 7 to 10 days.

Children – Give 20 mg/kg/day in divided doses, every 8 hours. In more serious infections, otitis media and infections caused by less susceptible organisms, administer 40 mg/kg/day, with a maximum dosage of 1 g/day.

Twice daily treatment option: For otitis media and pharyngitis, the total daily dosage may be divided and administered every 12 hours.

CEFADROXIL: Can be given without regard to meals.

Urinary tract infections – For uncomplicated lower urinary tract infection (eg, cystitis), the usual dosage is 1 or 2 g/day in single or 2 divided doses. For all other urinary tract infections, the usual dosage is 2 g/day in 2 divided doses.

Skin and skin structure infections – 1 g/day in single or 2 divided doses.

Pharyngitis and tonsillitis –

Group A β-hemolytic streptococci: 1 g/day in single or 2 divided doses for 10 days.

Children –

Urinary tract infections, skin and skin structure infections: 30 mg/kg/day in divided doses every 12 hours.

Pharyngitis, tonsillitis: 30 mg/kg/day in single or 2 divided doses. For β-hemolytic streptococcal infections, continue treatment for at least 10 days.

Renal impairment – Adjust dosage according to creatinine clearance rates to prevent drug accumulation.

Initial adult dose: 1 g: The maintenance dose (based on creatinine clearance rate, ml/min/1.73 m^2) is 500 mg at the intervals below:

Cefadroxil Dosage in Renal Impairment	
Creatinine clearance (ml/min)	Dosage interval (hours)
0-10	36
10-25	24
25-50	12
> 50	No adjustment

CEFAMANDOLE NAFTATE:

Adults – Usual dosage range is 500 mg to 1 g every 4 to 8 hours; 500 mg every 6 hours is adequate in uncomplicated skin and skin structure infections. In uncomplicated urinary tract infections, 500 mg every 8 hours; in more serious urinary tract infections, the dose may be increased to 1 g every 8 hours.

In severe infections, administer 1 g at 4 to 6 hour intervals. In life-threatening infections or infections due to less susceptible organisms, up to 2 g every 4 hours may be needed.

Infants and children – 50 to 100 mg/kg/day in equally divided doses every 4 to 8 hours is effective for most infections susceptible to cefamandole. This may be incresed to 150 mg/kg/day (not to exceed the maximum adult dose) for severe infections.

Perioperative prophylaxis –

Adults: 1 or 2 g IM or IV, ½ to 1 hour prior to the surgical incision, followed by 1 or 2 g every 6 hours for 24 to 48 hours.

Children (3 months of age and older): 50 to 100 mg/kg/day in equally divided doses by the routes and schedule designated above.

Renal function impairment – Reduce dosages and monitor the serum levels. After an initial dose of 1 to 2 g (depending on the severity of infection), follow maintenance dosage in table.

Maintenance Cefamandole Dosage Guide for Patients with Renal Impairment

Renal function	Creatinine clearance (ml/min/1.73 m²)	Life-threatening infections (Maximum dosage)	Less severe infections
Normal impairment	> 80	2 g q 4 h	1-2 g q 6 h
Mild impairment	50-80	1.5 g q 4 h or 2 g q 6 h	0.75-1.5 g q 6 h
Moderate impairment	25-50	1.5 g q 6 h or 2 g q 8 h	0.75-1.5 g q 8 h
Severe impairment	10-25	1 g q 6 h or 1.25 g q 8 h	0.5-1 g q 8 h
Marked impairment	2-10	0.67 g q 8 h or 1 g q 12 h	0.5-0.75 g q 12 h
None	< 2	0.5 g q 8 h or 0.75 g q 12 h	0.25-0.5 g q 12 h

CEFAZOLIN SODIUM: Total daily dosages are the same for IM and IV administration.

Mild infections caused by susceptible gram-positive cocci – 250 to 500 mg every 8 hours.

Moderate to severe infections – 500 mg to 1 g every 6 to 8 hours.

Pneumococcal pneumonia – 500 mg every 12 hours.

Severe, life-threatening infections (eg, endocarditis, septicemia) – 1 to 1.5 g every 6 hours. Rarely, 12 g per day have been used.

Acute uncomplicated urinary tract infections – 1 g every 12 hours.

Perioperative prophylaxis –

Preoperative: 1 g IV or IM, ½ to 1 hour prior to surgery.

Intraoperative (≥ 2 hrs): 0.5 to 1 g IV or IM during surgery at appropriate intervals.

Postoperative: 0.5 to 1 g IV or IM every 6 to 8 hours for 24 hours after surgery.

Renal function impairment – All reduced dosage recommendations apply after an initial loading dose appropriate to the severity of the infection.

Cefazolin Dosage in Renal Impairment

Serum Creatinine (mg %)	Ccr (ml/min)	Dose ≤ 1.5	Dose ≥ 55	Dosage Interval (hrs)
1.6-3	35-54	250 to 500	500 to 1000	≥ 8
3.1-4.5	11-34	125 to 250	250 to 500	12
≥ 4.6	≤ 10	125 to 250	250 to 500	18-24

Children –

Mild to moderately severe infections: A total daily dosage of 25 to 50 mg/kg (approximately 10 to 20 mg/lb) in 3 or 4 equal doses.

Severe infections: Total daily dosage may be increased to 100 mg/kg (45 mg/lb).

CEFEPIME:

Recommended Dosage Schedule for Cefepime

Site and type of infection	Dose	Frequency	Duration (days)
Mild to moderate uncomplicated or complicated urinary tract infections, including pyelonephritis, due to *E. coli*, *K. pneumoniae* or *P. mirabilis*. [1]	0.5 to 1 g IV/IM [2]	q12h	7 to 10
Severe uncomplicated or complicated urinary tract infections, including pyelonephritis, due to *E. coli* or *K. pneumoniae*.	2 g IV	q12h	10

Recommended Dosage Schedule for Cefepime			
Site and type of infection	Dose	Frequency	Duration (days)
Moderate to severe pneumonia due to *S. pneumoniae, Pseudomonas aeruginosa, Klebsiella pneumoniae* or *Enterobacter* sp.	1 to 2 g IV	q12h	10
Moderate to severe uncomplicated skin and skin structure infections due to *S. aureus* or *S. pyogenes*.	2 g IV	q12h	10

[1] Including cases associated with concurrent bacteremia.
[2] IM route of administration is indicated only for mild to moderate, uncomplicated or complicated UTIs due to *E. coli* when the IM route is a more appropriate route of drug administration.

Renal function impairment – In patients with impaired renal function (creatinine clearance < 60 ml/min), adjust the dose of cefepime to compensate for the slower rate of renal elimination. The recommended initial dose should be the same as in patients with normal renal function.

In patients undergoing hemodialysis, ≈ 68% of the total amount of cefepime present in the body at the start of dialysis will be removed during a 3-hour dialysis period. A repeat dose, equivalent to the initial dose, should be given at the completion of each dialysis session.

In elderly patients with renal insufficiency, adjust dosage and administration.

In patients undergoing continuous ambulatory peritoneal dialysis, administer cefepime at normal recommended doses at a dosage interval of every 48 hours.

Recommended Cefepime Maintenance Schedule in Patients with Renal Impairment			
Creatinine clearance (ml/min)	Recommended maintenance schedule		
> 60	500 mg q 12 h [1]	1 g q 12 h	2 g q 12 h
30 to 60	500 mg q 24 h	1 g q 24 h	2 g q 24 h
11 to 29		500 mg q 24 h	1 g q 24 h
≤ 10	250 mg q 24 h	250 mg q 24 h	500 mg q 24 h

[1] Normal recommended dosing schedule.

IV administration – Administer over ≈ 30 minutes. Dilute with 50 to 100 ml of a compatible IV fluid. Cefepime is compatible at concentrations of 1 to 40 mg/ml with 0.9% Sodium Chloride Injection, 5% and 10% Dextrose Injection, M/6 Sodium Lactate Injection, 5% Dextrose and 0.9% Sodium Chloride Injection, Lactated Ringers and 5% Dextrose Injection, *Normosol-R* or *Normosol-M* in 5% Dextrose injection.

CEFIXIME:

Adults – 400 mg/day as a single 400 mg tablet (recommended for gonococcal infections) or as 200 mg every 12 hours.

Children – 8 mg/kg/day suspension as a single daily dose or as 4 mg/kg every 12 hours. Treat children > 50 kg or > 12 years of age with the recommended adult dose.

Treat otitis media with the suspension.

For *S pyogenes* infections, administer cefixime for at least 10 days.

Renal function impairment –

Cefixime Dosing in Renal Impairment	
Creatinine clearance (ml/min)	Dosage
> 60	Standard
21-60 or renal hemodialysis	75% of standard
≤ 20 or continuous ambulatory peritoneal dialysis	50% of standard

CEFMETAZOLE SODIUM:

Adults –

General guidelines: 2 g IV every 6 to 12 hours for 5 to 14 days.

Prophylaxis –

Cefmetazole Dosing Regimen for Prophylaxis	
Surgery	Dosing Regimen
Vaginal hysterectomy	2 g single dose 30 to 90 min before surgery or 1 g doses 30 to 90 min before surgery and repeated 8 and 16 hours later.
Abdominal hysterectomy	1 g doses 30 to 90 min before surgery and repeated 8 and 16 hours later.
Cesarean section	2 g single dose after clamping cord or 1 g doses after clamping cord; repeated at 8 and 16 hours.

Cefmetazole Dosing Regimen for Prophylaxis	
Surgery	Dosing Regimen
Colorectal surgery	2 g single dose 30 to 90 minutes before surgery or 2 g doses 30 to 90 minutes before surgery and repeated 8 to 16 hours later.
Cholecystectomy (high risk)	1 g doses 30 to 90 minutes before surgery and repeated 8 and 16 hours later.

Renal function impairment –

Cefmetazole Dosage Guidelines in Renal Function Impairment			
Renal function	Creatinine clearance (ml/min/1.73 m^2)	Dose (g)	Frequency (hrs)
Mild impairment	50-90	1 to 2	q 12
Moderate impairment	30-49	1 to 2	q 16
Severe impairment	10-29	1 to 2	q 24
Essentially no function	< 10	1 to 2	q 48[1]

[1] Administered after hemodialysis.

CEFONICID SODIUM:

Adults – Usual dose is 1 g/24 hours, IV or by deep IM injection. Doses > 1 g/day are rarely necessary; however, up to 2 g/day have been well tolerated.

General Cefonicid Dosage Guidelines (IM or IV)		
Type of infection	Daily dosage (g)	Frequency
Uncomplicated urinary tract	0.5	once every 24 hrs
Mild to moderate	1	once every 24 hrs
Severe or life-threatening	2[1]	once every 24 hrs
Surgical prophylaxis	1	1 hr preoperatively

[1] When administering 2 g IM doses once daily, divide dose in half and give each half in a different large muscle mass.

Preoperative prophylaxis – Administer 1 g 1 hour prior to appropriate surgical procedures, to provide protection from most infections due to susceptible organisms for approximately 24 hours after administration.

Renal function impairment requires modification of dosage. Following an initial loading dosage of 7.5 mg/kg, IM or IV, follow maintenance schedule below. It is not necessary to administer additional dosage following dialysis.

Cefonicid Dosage in Adults with Reduced Renal Function		
Creatinine Clearance (ml/min/1.73 ^{2})	Mild to moderate infections	Severe infections
60-79	10 mg/kg q 24 hr	25 mg/kg q 24 hr
40-59	8 mg/kg q 24 hr	20 mg/kg q 24 hr
20-39	4 mg/kg q 24 hr	15 mg/kg q 24 hr
10-19	4 mg/kg q 48 hr	15 mg/kg q 48 hr
5-9	4 mg/kg q 3 to 5 days	15 mg/kg q 3 to 5 days
< 5	3 mg/kg q 3 to 5 days	4 mg/kg q 3 to 5 days

CEFOPERAZONE SODIUM: Administer IM or IV.

Usual adult dose is 2 to 4 g/day administered in equally divided doses every 12 hours.

In severe infections or infections caused by less sensitive organisms, the total daily dose or frequency may be increased. Patients have been successfully treated with a total daily dosage of 6 to 12 g divided into 2, 3 or 4 administrations ranging from 1.5 to 4 g/dose. A total daily dose of 16 g by constant infusion has been given without complications.

Hepatic disease or biliary obstruction – In general, total daily dosage above 4 g should not be necessary.

Renal function impairment –

Hemodialysis: The half-life is reduced slightly during hemodialysis. Thus, schedule dosing to follow a dialysis period.

CEFOTAXIME SODIUM:

Adults – Administer IV or IM. Maximum daily dosage should not exceed 12 g.

Cefotaxime Dosage Guidelines for Adults		
Type of infection	Daily dosage (g)	Frequency and route
Gonorrhea	1	1 g IM (single dose)
Uncomplicated infections	2	1 g every 12 hours IM or IV
Moderate to severe	3 to 6	1 to 2 g every 8 hours IM or IV
Infections commonly needing higher dosage (eg, septicemia)	6 to 8	2 g every 6 to 8 hours IV
Life-threatening infections	up to 12	2 g every 4 hours IV

Perioperative prophylaxis: 1 g IV or IM, 30 to 90 minutes prior to surgery.

Cesarean section: Administer the first 1 g dose IV as soon as the umbilical cord is clamped. Administer the second and third doses as 1 g IV or IM at 6 and 12 hour intervals after the first dose.

Children –

Cefotaxime Dosage Guidelines in Pediatrics			
Age	Weight (kg)	Dosage schedule	Route
0 to 1 week	-	50 mg/kg every 12 hours	IV
1 to 4 weeks	-	50 mg/kg every 8 hours	IV
1 month to 12 years	< 50[1]	50 to 180 mg/kg/day in 4 to 6 divided doses[2]	IV or IM

[1] For children ≥ 50 kg, use adult dosage.
[2] Use higher doses for more severe or serious infections including meningitis.

Renal function impairment – In patients with estimated creatinine clearances of less than 20 ml/min/1.73 m^2, reduce dosage by one-half.

CDC recommended treatment schedules for gonorrhea –

Disseminated gonococcal infection: Give 500 mg cefotaxime IV 4 times per day for at least 7 days.

Gonococcal ophthalmia in adults: For penicillinase-producing *Neisseria gonorrhoeae* (PPNG), give 500 mg IV 4 times per day.

CEFOTETAN DISODIUM:

Adults – The usual dosage is 1 or 2 g IV or IM every 12 hours for 5 to 10 days. Determine proper dosage and route of administration by the condition of the patient, severity of the infection and susceptibility of the causitive organism.

General Cefotetan Dosage Guidelines		
Type of infection	Daily dose	Frequency and route
Urinary tract	1 to 4 g	500 mg every 12 hours IV or IM 1 or 2 g every 24 hours IV or IM 1 or 2 g every 12 hours IV or IM
Other sites	2 to 4 g	1 or 2 g every 12 hours IV or IM
Severe	4 g	2 g every 12 hours IV
Life-threatening	6 g[1]	3 g every 12 hours IV

[1] Maximum daily dose should not exceed 6 g.

Prophylaxis – To prevent postoperative infection in clean contaminated or potentially contaminated surgery in adults, give a single 1 or 2 g IV dose 30 to 60 minutes prior to surgery. In patients undergoing cesarean section, give the dose as soon as the umbilical cord is clamped.

Renal function impairment – Reduce the dosage schedule using the following guidelines:

Cefotetan Dosage in Renal Impairment		
Ccr (ml/min)	Dose	Frequency
> 30	Usual recommended dose[1]	Every 12 hours
10-30	Usual recommended dose[1]	Every 24 hours
< 10	Usual recommended dose[1]	Every 48 hours

[1] Dose determined by the type and severity of infection and susceptibility of the causitive organism.

Alternatively, the dosing interval may remain constant at 12 hour intervals, but reduce dose by one-half for patients with a creatinine clearance of 10 to 30 ml/min, and by one-quarter for patients with a creatinine clearance of less than 10 ml/min.

Dialysis – Cefotetan is dialyzable; for patients undergoing intermittent hemodialysis, give one-quarter of the usual recommended dose every 24 hours on days between dialysis and one-half of the usual recommended dose on the day of dialysis.

CEFOXITIN SODIUM:

Adult dosage range is 1 to 2 g every 6 to 8 hours.

Cefoxitin Dosage Guidelines

Type of infection	Daily dosage	Frequency and route
Uncomplicated (pneumonia, urinary tract, cutaneous)[1]	3 to 4 g	1 g every 6 to 8 hours IV or IM
Moderately severe or severe	6 to 8 g	1 g every 4 hours or 2 g every 6 to 8 hours IV
Infections commonly requiring higher dosage (eg, gas, gangrene)	12 g	2 g every 4 hours or 3 g every 6 hours IV

[1] Including patients in whom bacteremia is absent or unlikely.

Uncomplicated gonorrhea – 2 g IM with 1 g oral probenecid given concurrently or up to 30 minutes before cefoxitin.

Prophylactic use, surgery – Administer 2 g IV or IM 30 to 60 minutes prior to surgery followed by 2 g every 6 hours after the first dose for no more than 24 hours (continued for 72 hours after prosthetic arthroplasty).

Prophylactic use, cesarean section – Administer 2 g IV as soon as the umbilical cord is clamped. If a three dose regimen is used, give the second and third 2 g dose IV, 4 and 8 hours after the first dose.

Prophylactic use, transurethral prostatectomy – Administer 1 g prior to surgery; 1 g every 8 hours for up to 5 days.

Renal function impairment –

Adults:

Maintenance Cefoxitin Dosage in Renal Impairment

Renal function	Ccr (ml/min/1.73 m^2)	Dose (g)	Frequency (hrs)
Mild impairment	30-50	1-2	8-12
Moderate impairment	10-29	1-2	12-24
Severe impairment	5-9	0.5-1	12-24
Essentially no function	< 5	0.5-1	24-48

Hemodialysis – Administer a loading dose of 1 to 2 g after each hemodialysis. Give the maintenance dose as indicated in the table above.

Infants and children ≥ 3 months: 80 to 160 mg/kg/day divided every 4 to 6 hours. Use higher dosages for more severe or serious infections. Do not exceed 12 g/day.

Prophylactic use (≥ 3 months) – 30 to 40 mg/kg/dose every 6 hours

Renal function impairment – Modify consistent with recommendation for adults.

CDC recommended treatment schedules for acute pelvic inflammatory disease (PID) – For hospitalized patients, give 100 mg doxycycline, IV, twice/day plus 2 g cefoxitin IV 4 times/day. Continue drugs IV for at least 4 days and at least 48 hours after patient improves. Continue 100 mg oral doxycyline, twice/day after discharge to complete 10 to 14 days of therapy. For outpatients, give 2 g cefoxitin IM with 1 g oral probenecid, then 100 mg oral doxycycline twice/day for 10 to 14 days.

CEFPODOXIME PROXETIL: Administer with food to enhance absorption.

Dosage/Duration of Cefpodoxime

Type of infection	Total daily dose	Dose frequency	Duration
Adults ≥ 13 years of age:			
Acute community-acquired pneumonia	400 mg	200 mg every 12 hrs	14 days
Acute bacterial exacerbations of chronic bronchitis	400 mg	200 mg every 12 hrs	10 days
Uncomplicated gonorrhea (men and women) and rectal gonococcal infections (women)	200 mg	single dose	
Skin and skin structure	800 mg	400 mg every 12 hrs	7 to 14 days
Pharyngitis/Tonsillitis	200 mg	100 mg every 12 hrs	5 to 10 days
Uncomplicated urinary tract infection	200 mg	100 mg every 12 hrs	7 days

Dosage/Duration of Cefpodoxime			
Type of infection	Total daily dose	Dose frequency	Duration
Children (age 6 months through 12 years):			
Acute otitis media	10 mg/kg/day divided every 12 hr (max 400 mg/day)	5 mg/kg/dose (max 200 mg/dose)	10 days
Pharyngitis/Tonsillitis	10 mg/kg/day divided every 12 hr (max 200 mg/day)	5 mg/kg/dose (max 100 mg/dose)	5 to 10 days

Renal dysfunction – For patients with severe renal impairment (creatinine clearance [Ccr] < 30 ml/min), increase the dosing intervals to every 24 hours. In patients maintained on hemodialysis, use a frequency of 3 times/week after hemodialysis.

CEFPROZIL:

Dosage and Duration of Cefprozil		
Population/Infection	Dosage (mg)	Duration (days)
Adults (≥ 13 years of age)		
Upper respiratory tract		
Pharyngitis/Tonsillitis	500 q 24 h	10[1]
Lower respiratory tract		
Secondary bacterial infection of acute bronchitis and acute bacterial exacerbation of chronic bronchitis	500 q 12 h	10
Skin and skin structure		
Uncomplicated skin and skin structure infections	250 q 12 h or 500 q 24 h or 500 q 12 h	10
Infants and children (6 months to 12 years)		
Otitis media	15 mg/kg q 12 h	10
Children (2 to 12 years)		
Pharyngitis/Tonsillitis	7.5 mg/kg q 12 h	10[1]

[1] In treatment of infections due to *Streptococcus pyogenes*, administer for at least 10 days.

Renal function impairment – Cefprozil may be administered to patients with impaired renal function. Use the following dosage schedule.

Cefprozil Dosage in Renal Impairment		
Creatinine clearance (ml/min)	Dosage (mg)	Dosing interval
30 to 120	standard	standard
0 to 30[1]	50% of standard	standard

[1] Cefprozil is in part removed by hemodialysis; therefore, administer after the completion of hemodialysis.

CEFTAZIDIME:

Ceftazidime Dosage Guidelines		
Patient/infection site	Dose	Frequency
Adults Usual recommended dose	1 g IV or IM	q 8-12 h
Uncomplicated urinary tract infections	250 mg IV or IM	q 12 h
Complicated urinary tract infections	500 mg IV or IM	q 8-12 h
Uncomplicated pneumonia; mild skin and skin structure infections	500 mg to 1 g IV or IM	q 8 h
Bone and joint infections	2 g IV	q 12 h
Serious gynecological and intra-abdominal infections	2 g IV	q 8 h
Meningitis		
Very severe life-threatening infections, especially in immunocompromised patients		

Ceftazidime Dosage Guidelines		
Patient/infection site	Dose	Frequency
Pseudomonal lung infections in cystic fibrosis patients w/normal renal function[1]	30 to 50 mg/kg IV up to 6 g/day	q 8 h
Neonates (0 to 4 weeks)	30 mg/kg IV	q 12 h
Infants and children (1 month to 12 years)	30 to 50 mg/kg IV up to 6 g/day[2]	q 8 h

[1] Although clinical improvement has been shown, bacteriological cures cannot be expected in patients with chronic respiratory disease and cystic fibrosis.
[2] Reserve the higher dose for immunocompromised children or children with cystic fibrosis or meningitis.

Renal function impairment – Ceftazidime is excreted by the kidneys, almost exclusively by glomerular filtration. In patients with impaired renal function (GFR < 50 ml/min), reduce dosage to compensate for slower excretion. In patients with suspected renal insufficiency, give an initial loading dose of 1 g. Estimate GFR to determine the appropriate maintenance dose.

Ceftazidime Dosage in Renal Impairment		
Creatinine clearance (ml/min)	Recommended unit dose of ceftazidime	Frequency of dosing
31-50	1 g	q 12 h
16-30	1 g	q 24 h
6-15	500 mg	q 24 h
≤ 5	500 mg	q 48 h

In patients with severe infections who normally receive 6 g ceftazidime daily were it not for renal insufficiency, the unit dose given in the table above may be increased by 50% or the dosing frequency increased appropriately.

Dialysis – Give a 1 g loading dose, followed by 1 g after each hemodialysis period.

Ceftazidime can also be used in patients undergoing intraperitoneal dialysis (IPD) and continuous ambulatory peritoneal dialysis (CAPD). Give a loading dose of 1 g, followed by 500 mg every 24 hours. In addition to IV use, ceftazidime can be incorporated in the dialysis fluid at a concentration of 250 mg per 2 L of dialysis fluid.

CEFTIBUTEN: Ceftibuten suspension must be administered at least 2 hours before or 1 hour after a meal.

Ceftibutin Dosage and Duration			
Type of infection	Daily maximum dose	Dose and frequency	Duration
Adults ≥ 12 years of age			
Acute bacterial exacerbations of chronic bronchitis due to *H influenzae, M catarrhalis* or *Streptococcus pneumoniae*	400 mg	400 mg qd	10 days
Pharyngitis and tonsillitis due to *S pyogenes*			
Acute bacterial otitis media due to *H influenzae, M catarrhalis* or *S pyogenes*			
Children			
Pharyngitis and tonsillitis due to *S pyogenes*	400 mg	9 mg/kg qd	10 days
Acute bacterial otitis media due to *H influenzae, M catarrhalis* or *S pyogenes*			

Ceftibuten Oral Suspension Pediatric Dosage Chart[1]			
Weight			
kg	lb	90 mg/5 ml	180 mg/5 ml
10	22	5 ml (1 tsp) qd	2.5 ml (½ tsp) qd
20	44	10 ml (2 tsp) qd	5 ml (1 tsp) qd
40	88	20 ml (4 tsp) qd	10 ml (2 tsp) qd

[1] Children > 45 kg should receive the maximum daily dose of 400 mg.

Renal function impairment – Ceftibuten may be given at normal doses in impaired renal function with creatinine clearance of ≥ 50 ml/min. Dosing recommendations for patients with varying degrees of renal insufficiency are presented in the following table.

Ceftibuten Dosage in Renal Impairment	
Creatinine clearance (ml/min)	Recommended dosing schedules
> 50	9 mg/kg or 400 mg q 24 h (normal dosing schedule)
30 - 49	4.5 mg/kg or 200 mg q 24 h
5 - 29	2.25 mg/kg or 100 mg q 24 h

Hemodialysis patients – In patients undergoing hemodialysis two or three times weekly, a single 400 mg dose of ceftibuten capsules or a single dose of 9 mg/kg (maximum of 400 mg) oral suspension may be given at the end of each hemodialysis session.

CEFTIZOXIME SODIUM:

Adults – Usual dosage is 1 or 2 g every 8 to 12 hours.

Ceftizoxime Dosage Guidelines in Adults		
Type of infection	Daily dose (g)	Frequency and route
Uncomplicated urinary tract	1	500 mg every 12 hours IM or IV
PID [1]	6	2 g every 8 hours IV
Other sites	2-3	1 g every 8 to 12 hours IV or IM
Severe or refractory	3-6	1 g every 8 hours IM or IV 2 g every 8 to 12 hours IM [1] or IV
Life-threatening [2]	9-12	3 to 4 g every 8 hours IV

[1] Dosages up to 2 g every 4 hours have been given.
[2] Divide 2 g IM doses and give in different large muscle masses.

Urinary tract infections – Higher dosage is recommended.

Gonorrhea, uncomplicated – A single 1 g IM injection is the usual dose.

Life-threatening infections – The IV route may be preferable for patients with bacterial septicemia, localized parenchymal abscesses (such as intra-abdominal abscess), peritonitis or other severe or life-threatening infections.

In those patients with normal renal function, the IV dosage is 2 to 12 g daily. In conditions such as bacterial septicemia, 6 to 12 g/day IV may be given initially for several days, and the dosage gradually reduced according to clinical response and laboratory findings.

Pediatric –

Children (≥ 6 months): 50 mg/kg every 6 to 8 hours. Dosage may be increased to 200 mg/kg/day. Do not exceed the maximum adult dose for serious infection.

Renal function impairment requires modification of dosage. Following an initial loading dose of 500 mg to 1 g IM or IV, use the maintenance dosing schedule in the following table.

Hemodialysis – No additional supplemental dosing is required following hemodialysis; give the dose (according to the table below) at the end of dialysis.

Ceftizoxime Dosage in Adults with Renal Impairment			
Renal function	Creatinine clearance (ml/min)	Less severe infections	Life-threatening infections
Mild impairment	50-79	500 mg q 8 h	750 mg to 1.5 g q 8 h
Moderate to severe impairment	5-49	250 to 500 mg q 12 h	500 mg to 1 g q 12 h
Dialysis patients	0-4	500 mg q 48 h or 250 mg q 24 h	500 mg to 1 g q 48 h or 500 mg q 24 h

CEFTRIAXONE SODIUM: Administer IV or IM.

Adults – Usual daily dosage is 1 to 2 g once a day (or in equally divided doses twice a day) depending on type and severity of infection. Do not exceed a total daily dose of 4 g.

Uncomplicated gonococcal infections: Give a single IM dose of 250 mg.

Surgical prophylaxis: Give a single 1 g dose ½ to 2 hours before surgery.

Children – To treat serious infections other than meningitis, administer 50 to 75 mg/kg/day (not to exceed 2 g) in divided doses every 12 hours.

Meningitis: 100 mg/kg/day (not to exceed 4 g). Thereafter, a total daily dose of 100 mg/kg/day (not to exceed 4 g/day) is recommended. May give daily dose once per day or in equally divided doses every 12 hours. Usual duration is 7 to 14 days.

Skin and skin structure infections: Give 50 to 75 mg/kg once daily (or in equally divided doses twice daily), not to exceed 2 g.

CDC recommended treatment schedules for chancroid, gonorrhea and acute pelvic inflammatory disease (PID) –

Chancroid (Haemophilus ducreyi infection): 250 mg IM as a single dose.

Gonococcal infections:

Uncomplicated – 125 mg IM once plus doxycycline.

Conjunctivitis – 1 g IM single dose.

Disseminated – 1 g IM or IV every 24 hours.

Meningitis/Endocarditis – 1 to 2 g IV every 12 hours for 10 to 14 days (meningitis) or for at least 4 weeks (endocarditis).

Children (< 45 kg) – With bacteremia or arthritis, use 50 mg/kg (maximum, 1 g) IM or IV in a single dose for 7 days. For meningitis, increase duration to 10 to 14 days and maximum dose to 2 g.

Infants – 25 to 50 mg/kg/day IV or IM in a single daily dose, not to exceed 125 mg. For disseminated infection, continue for 7 days, with a duration of 7 to 14 days with documented meningitis.

Acute PID (ambulatory): 250 mg IM plus doxycycline.

CEFUROXIME:

Oral – Tablets and suspension are NOT bioequivalent and NOT substitutable on a mg/mg basis.

Tablets: The tablets may be given without regard to meals.

Suspension: Must be administered with food.

Dosage for Cefuroxime Axetil Tablets

Population/Infection	Dosage	Duration (days)
Adults (≥ 13 years)		
Pharyngitis/tonsillitis	250 mg bid	10
Acute bacterial exacerbations of chronic bronchitis and secondary bacterial infections of acute bronchitis	250 or 500 mg bid	10
Uncomplicated skin and skin structure infections	250 or 500 mg bid	10
Uncomplicated urinary tract infections single dose	125 or 250 mg bid	7 to 10
Children who can swallow tablets whole		
Pharyngitis/tonsillitis	125 mg bid	10
Acute otitis media	250 mg bid	10

Dosage for Cefuroxime Axetil Suspension

Population/Infection	Dosage	Daily maximum dose	Duration (days)
Infants and children (3 months to 12 years)			
Pharyngitis/tonsillitis	20 mg/kg/day divided bid	500 mg	10
Acute otitis media	30 mg/kg/day divided bid	1000 mg	10
Impetigo	30 mg/kg/day divided bid	1000 mg	10

Renal failure: Because cefuroxime is renally eliminated, its half-life will be prolonged in patients with renal failure.

Parenteral –

Dosage:

Adults – 750 mg to 1.5 g IM or IV every 8 hours, usually for 5 to 10 days.

Cefuroxime Dosage Guidelines

Type of Infection	Daily dosage (g)	Frequency
Uncomplicated urinary tract, skin and skin structure, disseminated gonococcal, uncomplicated pneumonia	2.25	750 mg every 8 hours
Severe or complicated	4.5	1.5 g every 8 hours
Bone and joint	4.5	1.5 g every 8 hours
Life-threatening or due to less susceptible organisms	6	1.5 g every 6 hours
Bacterial meningitis	9	≤ 3 g every 8 hours
Uncomplicated gonococcal	1.5 g IM[1]	single dose

[1] Administered at 2 different sites together with 1 g oral probenecid.

Preoperative prophylaxis: For clean-contaminated or potentially contaminated surgical procedures, administer 1.5 g IV prior to surgery (≈ ½ to 1 hour before). Thereafter, give 750 mg IV or IM every 8 hours when the procedure is prolonged.

For preventative use during open heart surgery, give 1.5 g IV at the induction of anesthesia and every 12 hours thereafter for a total of 6 g.

Renal function impairment: Reduce dosage.

Parenteral Cefuroxime Dosage in Renal Impairment (Adults)	
Creatinine clearance (ml/min)	Dose and frequency
> 20	750 mg to 1.5 g every 8 hours
10-20	750 mg every 12 hours
< 10	750 mg every 24 hours [1]

[1] Because cefuroxime is dialyzable, give patients on hemodialysis a further dose at the end of the dialysis.

Infants and children (> 3 months) – 50 to 100 mg/kg/day in equally divided doses every 6 to 8 hours. Use 100 mg/kg/day (not to exceed maximum adult dose) for more severe or serious infections.

Bone and joint infections: 150 mg/kg/day (not to exceed maximum adult dose) in equally divided doses every 8 hours.

Bacterial meningitis: Initially, 200 to 240 mg/kg/day IV in divided doses every 6 to 8 hours.

In renal insufficiency, modify dosage frequency per adult guidelines.

CEPHALEXIN:

Adults – 1 to 4 g/day in divided doses.

Usual dose: 250 mg every 6 hours.

Streptococcal pharyngitis, skin and skin structure infections, uncomplicated cystitis in patients > 15 years: 500 mg every 12 hours.

May need larger doses for more severe infections or less susceptible organisms.

If dose is > 4 g/day, use parenteral drugs.

Children –

Monohydrate: 25 to 50 mg/kg/day in divided doses. For streptococcal pharyngitis in patients > 1 year and skin and skin structure infections, divided total daily dose and give every 12 hours. In severe infections, double the dose.

Otitis media – 75 to 100 mg/kg/day in 4 divided doses.

β-hemolytic streptococcal infections – Continue treatment for at least 10 days.

HCl monohydrate: Safety and efficacy not established for use in children.

CEPHALOTHIN SODIUM:

Adults – 500 mg to 1 g every 4 to 6 hours.

Uncomplicated pneumonia, furunculosis with cellulitis, most urinary tract infections: 500 mg every 6 hours.

Severe infections: Increase the dose to 1 g or administer 500 mg every 4 hours.

Life-threatening infections: Up to 2 g every 4 hours.

Normal renal function (bacteremia, septicemia or other severe life-threatening infections) – The IV dosage is 4 to 12 g daily. In conditions such as septicemia, 6 to 8 g per day may be administered IV for several days at the beginning of therapy; reduce the dosage gradually.

Infants and children – The dosage is proportionately less according to age, weight and severity of infection. Daily administration of 100 mg/kg (80 to 160 mg/kg or 40 to 80 mg/lb) in divided doses is effective for most infections susceptible to cephalothin.

Perioperative prophylaxis –

Preoperative: 1 to 2 g administered IV ½ to 1 hour prior to initial incision.

Intraoperative: 1 to 2 g during surgery, administered according to the duration of the surgery.

Postoperative: 1 to 2 g every 6 hours; discontinue within 24 hours after surgery.

Children: 20 to 30 mg/kg given at the times designated above.

Renal function impairment – Give an IV loading dose of 1 to 2 g. Determine the continued dosage schedule by degree of renal impairment, severity of infection and susceptibility of the causative organism. Base maximum doses on the following recommendations:

Cephalothin Dosage in Renal Impairment		
Renal function	Creatinine clearance (ml/min)	Maximum adult dosage (maintenance)
Mild impairment	50-80	2 g every 6 hours
Moderate impairment	25-50	1.5 g every 6 hours
Severe impairment	10-25	1 g every 6 hours
Marked impairment	2-10	0.5 g every 6 hours
Essentially no function	< 2	0.5 g every 8 hours

CEPHAPIRIN SODIUM:

Adults – 500 mg to 1 g every 4 to 6 hours IM or IV. The lower dose is adequate for certain infections, such as skin and skin structure and most urinary tract infections; the higher dose is recommended for more serious infections.

Serious or life-threatening infections – Up to 12 g daily. Use the IV route when high doses are indicated.

Renal function impairment: Patients with reduced renal function (moderately severe oliguria or serum creatinine > 5 mg/100 ml) may be treated adequately with a lower dose, 7.5 to 15 mg/kg every 12 hours. Patients who are to be dialyzed should receive the same dose just prior to dialysis and every 12 hours thereafter.

Perioperative prophylaxis: 1 to 2 g IM or IV administered ½ to 1 hour prior to the start of surgery; 1 to 2 g during surgery (administration modified depending on duration of operation); 1 to 2 g IV or IM every 6 hours for 24 hours postoperatively.

Children – Recommended total daily dose is 40 to 80 mg/kg (20 to 40 mg/lb) administered in 4 equally divided doses.

Infants – Cephapirin has not been extensively studied in infants; therefore, in the treatment of children < 3 months of age, consider the relative benefit to risk.

CEPHRADINE:

Oral – May be given without regard to meals.

Adults:

Skin, skin structure and respiratory tract infections (other than lobar pneumonia) – Usual dose is 250 mg every 6 hours or 500 mg every 12 hours.

Lobar pneumonia – 500 mg every 6 hours or 1 g every 12 hours.

Uncomplicated urinary tract infections – The usual dose is 500 mg every 12 hours. In more serious infections and prostatitis, 500 mg every 6 hours or 1 g every 12 hours. Severe or chronic infections may require larger doses (up to 1 g every 6 hours).

Children: No adequate information is available on the efficacy of twice a day regimens in children less than 9 months of age. For children over 9 months, the usual dose is 25 to 50 mg/kg/day, in equally divided doses every 6 or 12 hours. For otitis media due to *H influenzae*, 75 to 100 mg/kg/day in equally divided doses every 6 or 12 hours is recommended; do not exceed 4 g/day.

All patients regardless of age and weight: Larger doses (up to 1 g 4 times/day) may be given for severe or chronic infections.

Parenteral – Parenteral therapy may be followed by oral. To minimize pain and induration, inject IM deep into a large muscle mass.

Adults: Daily dose is 2 to 4 g in equally divided doses 4 times/day, IM or IV. In bone infections, the usual dosage is 1 g IV 4 times/day. A dose of 500 mg 4 times/day is adequate in uncomplicated pneumonia, skin and skin structure infections and most urinary tract infections. In severe infections, dose may be increased by giving every 4 hours or by increasing dose up to a maximum of 8 g/day.

Perioperative prophylaxis – Recommended doses are 1 g IV or IM administered 30 to 90 minutes prior to the start of surgery, followed by 1 g every 4 to 6 hours after the first dose for 1 or 2 doses, or for up to 24 hours postoperatively.

Cesarean section – Give 1 g IV as soon as the umbilical cord is clamped. Give the second and third doses as 1 g IM or IV at 6 to 12 hours after the first dose.

Infants and children – 50 to 100 mg/kg/day in 4 equally divided doses; determine by age, weight and infection severity.

Renal impairment dosage –

Patients not on dialysis:

Cephradine Dosage in Renal Impairment

Ccr (ml/min)	Dose (mg)	Time interval (hours)
> 20	500	6
5 to 20	250	6
< 5	250	12

Patients on chronic, intermittent dialysis: 250 mg initially; repeat at 12 hours and after 36 to 48 hours.

LORACARBEF: Administer at least 1 hour before or 2 hours after a meal.

Dosage/Duration of Loracarbef

Population/Infection	Dosage (mg)	Duration (days)
Adults ≥ 13 years of age		
Lower respiratory tract		
Secondary bacterial infection of acute bronchitis	200 - 400 q 12 h	7
Acute bacterial exacerbation of chronic bronchitis	400 q 12 h	7
Pneumonia	400 q 12 h	14
Upper respiratory tract		
Pharyngitis/Tonsillitis	200 q 12 h	10[1]
Sinusitis	400 q 12 h	10
Skin and skin structure		
Uncomplicated	200 q 12 h	7
Urinary tract		
Uncomplicated cystitis	200 q 24 h	7
Uncomplicated pyelonephritis	400 q 12 h	14
Infants and children (6 months to 12 years)		
Upper respiratory tract		
Acute otitis media[2]	30 mg/kg/day in divided doses q 12 h	10
Pharyngitis/Tonsillitis	15 mg/kg/day in divided doses q 12 h	10[1]
Skin and skin structure		
Impetigo	15 mg/kg/day in divided doses q 12 h	7

[1] In treatment of infections due to *S pyogenes*, administer for at least 10 days.
[2] Use suspension; it is more rapidly absorbed than capsules, resulting in higher peak plasma concentrations when given at the same dose.

Renal function impairment – Use usual dose and schedule in patients with creatinine clearance (Ccr) levels ≥ 50 ml/min. Patients with Ccr between 10 and 49 ml/min may be given half the recommended dose at the usual dosage interval. Patients with Ccr levels < 10 ml/min may receive recommended dose given every 3 to 5 days; patients on hemodialysis should receive another dose following dialysis.

FLUOROQUINOLONES

CIPROFLOXACIN	
Tablets: 250, 500 and 750 mg (*Rx*)	*Cipro* (Bayer)
Injection: 200 and 400 mg (*Rx*)	*Cipro IV* (Bayer)
NORFLOXACIN	
Tablets: 400 mg (*Rx*)	*Noroxin* (Roberts)
OFLOXACIN	
Tablets: 200, 300 and 400 mg (*Rx*)	*Floxin* (Ortho)
Injection: 200 and 400 mg (*Rx*)	*Floxin* (Ortho)
ENOXACIN	
Tablets: 200 and 400 mg (*Rx*)	*Penetrex* (Rhone-Poulenc Rorer)
LOMEFLOXACIN HCl	
Tablets: 400 mg (*Rx*)	*Maxaquin* (Searle)
SPARFLOXACIN	
Tablets: 200 mg (*Rx*)	*Zagam* (Rhone-Poulenc Rorer)
LEVOFLOXACIN	
Tablets: 250 and 500 mg (*Rx*)	*Levaquin* (McNeil Pharmaceutical)
Injection: 500 mg (*Rx*)	*Levaquin* (McNeil Pharmaceutical)
Injection (premix): 250 and 500 mg (*Rx*)	*Levaquin* (McNeil Pharmaceutical)
GREPAFLOXACIN	
Tablets: 200 mg	*Raxar* (GlaxoWellcome)

Actions:

Pharmacology: The fluoroquinolones are synthetic, broad-spectrum antibacterial agents related to the other quinolones, nalidixic acid and cinoxacin. These agents are bactericidal; they interfere with the enzyme DNA gyrase needed for the synthesis of bacterial DNA.

Pharmacokinetics:

Pharmacokinetics of Fluoroquinolones

Fluoroquinolone	Bio-availability (%)	Max urine concentration (mcg/ml) (dose)	Mean peak plasma concentration (mcg/ml) (dose)	Area under curve (AUC) (mcg • hr/ml) (dose)	Protein binding (%)	t½ (hr)	Urine recovery unchanged (%)
Ciprofloxacin Oral	70-80	160-700 (500 mg)	1.2 (250 mg) 2.4 (500 mg) 4.3 (750 mg) 5.4 (1000 mg)	4.8 (250 mg) 11.6 (500 mg) 20.2 (750 mg) 30.8 (1000 mg)	20-40	4	40-50
IV		> 200 (200 mg) > 400 (400 mg)	4.3 (400 mg)	4.8 (200 mg) 11.6 (400 mg)	20-40	5-6	50-70
Enoxacin	90	nd	0.83 (200 mg) 2 (400 mg)	16 (400 mg)	40	3-6	> 40
Lomefloxacin	95-98	> 300 (400 mg)	4.2 (400 mg)	5.6 (100 mg) 10.9 (200 mg) 26.1 (400 mg)	10	8	65
Norfloxacin	30-40	200-500 (400 mg)	0.8 (200 mg) 1.5 (400 mg)	5.4 (400 mg)	10-15	3-4.5	26-32
Ofloxacin Oral	≈ 98	220 (200 mg)	1.5 (200 mg) 2.4 (300 mg) 2.9 (400 mg)	14.1 (200 mg) 21.2 (300 mg) 31.4 (400 mg)	32	5-7	70-80
IV		nd[1]	2.7 (200 mg) 4 (400 mg)	43.5 (400 mg)	32	5-10	nd[1]

[1] nd = no data.

Microbiology:

Table I: Organisms Generally Susceptible to Fluoroquinolones In Vitro

	Organism	Ciprofloxacin	Enoxacin	Lomefloxacin	Norfloxacin	Ofloxacin
Gram-negative	Acinetobacter sp	✓			✓	✓
	Aeromonas sp	✓	✓[1]	✓[1]	✓[1]	✓
	Alcaligenes sp				✓	
	Brucella melitensis	✓				
	Campylobacter sp	✓			✓	✓[1]
	Citrobacter sp	✓	✓[1]	✓[1]	✓[1]	✓[1]
	Edwardsiella tarda	✓			✓	
	Enterobacter sp	✓	✓[1]	✓	✓[1]	✓[1]
	Escherichia coli	✓	✓	✓	✓	✓
	Flavobacterium sp				✓	
	Hafnia alvei			✓	✓	
	Haemophilus ducreyi	✓	✓			
	Haemophilus influenzae	✓		✓	✓	✓
	Haemophilus parainfluenzae	✓		✓	✓	✓
	Klebsiella pneumoniae	✓	✓[1]	✓	✓[1]	✓[1]
	Klebsiella sp	✓	✓	✓	✓	✓
	Legionella sp	✓		✓	✓	✓
	Listeria monocytogenes	✓				
	Moraxella (Branhamella) catarrhalis	✓		✓	✓	✓
	Morganella morganii	✓	✓	✓	✓	✓
	Neisseria gonorrhoeae	✓	✓		✓	✓
	Neisseria meningitidis	✓			✓	✓
	Pasteurella multocida	✓				
	Plesiomonas shigelloides					✓
	Proteus mirabilis	✓	✓	✓	✓	✓
	Proteus vulgaris	✓	✓	✓	✓	✓
	Providencia alcalifaciens		✓	✓	✓	
	Providencia rettgeri	✓		✓	✓	✓
	Providencia stuartii	✓	✓		✓	✓
	Pseudomonas aeruginosa	✓	✓	✓	✓	✓
	Pseudomonas fluorescens					✓
	Salmonella sp	✓			✓	✓
	Serratia sp	✓	✓[1]	✓	✓[1]	✓[1]
	Shigella sp	✓			✓	✓
	Vibrio sp	✓			✓[1]	✓[1]
	Xanthomonas (Pseudomonas) maltophilia					✓
	Yersinia enterocolitica	✓			✓	✓
Gram-positive	Staphylococcus aureus	✓[2]		✓[2]	✓[2]	✓[2]
	coagulase-negative sp	✓				
	epidermidis	✓	✓	✓[2]	✓	✓[2]
	hemolyticus	✓			✓	
	saprophyticus	✓	✓	✓	✓	✓
	Streptococci group D				✓	
	agalactiae				✓	✓
	faecalis	✓			✓	✓
	pneumoniae	✓				✓
	pyogenes	✓				✓
	Bacillus cereus				✓	

[1] May be species-dependent.
[2] Including methicillin-susceptible and methicillin-resistant strains.

Indications:

For specific approved indications, refer to the Administration and Dosage section.

Unlabeled uses:

Ciprofloxacin appears effective in patients with cystic fibrosis who have pulmonary exacerbations associated with susceptible microorganisms. It may also be useful in the treatment of malignant external otitis (750 mg twice daily) and for tuberculosis in combination with rifampin and other antituberculosis agents. It has been used as part of a multi-drug regimen for the treatment of *Mycobacterium avium* complex infection, a common infection in AIDS patients.

Fluoroquinolones may also be useful in the following conditions (some agents are specifically indicated for these conditions; refer to drug monographs): Bronchitis; pneumonia (including Legionella and Mycoplasma); prostatitis; osteomyelitis (selected types); prophylaxis in urological surgery; traveler's diarrhea; uncomplicated gonorrhea; gonorrheal cervicitis or urethritis; pelvic inflammatory disease; sinusitis; otitis media; septic arthritis; bacterial meningitis; bacteremia (pseudomonal or staphylococcal); endocarditis. Further study is needed.

Contraindications:

Hypersensitivity to fluoroquinolones or the quinolone group of antibacterial agents (cinoxacin and nalidixic acid).

Grepafloxacin: Hepatic failure; patients with known QT_c prolongation; concomitantly with medications known to increase the QT_c interval or tosarde de pointes unless appropriate cardiac monitoring can be ensured.

Warnings:

Photosensitivity: Moderate to severe phototoxic reactions have occurred in patients exposed to direct or indirect sunlight or to artificial ultraviolet light (eg, sunlamps) during or following treatment with **lomefloxacin.**

Avoid direct exposure to direct or indirect sunlight (even when using sunscreens or sunblocks) while taking lomefloxacin and other fluoroquinolones for several days following therapy. Discontinue therapy at first signs or symptoms of phototoxicity.

Convulsions, increased intracranial pressure and toxic psychosis have occurred. CNS stimulation may also occur, which may lead to tremor, restlessness, lightheadedness, confusion and hallucinations.

Syphilis: **Ofloxacin** and **enoxacin** are not effective for syphilis. High doses of antimicrobial agents for short periods of time to treat gonorrhea may mask or delay symptoms of incubating syphilis.

Chronic bronchitis due to S pneumoniae: **Lomefloxacin** is not indicated for the empiric treatment of acute bacterial exacerbation of chronic bronchitis when it is probable that *S pneumoniae* is a causative pathogen since it exhibits in vitro resistance to lomefloxacin.

Hypersensitivity reactions, serious and occasionally fatal, have occurred in patients receiving quinolone therapy, some following the first dose. Refer to Management of Acute Hypersensitivity Reactions.

Pseudomembranous colitis has been reported with nearly all antibacterial agents, including fluoroquinolones, and may range from mild to life-threatening in severity.

Renal function impairment: Alteration in dosage regimen is necessary. See Administration and Dosage.

Elderly: Norfloxacin is eliminated more slowly because of decreased renal function; absorption appears unaffected. The apparent half-life of **ofloxacin** is 6 to 8 hours, compared to ≈ 5 hours in younger adults; absorption is unaffected. **Lomefloxacin** plasma clearance was reduced by ≈ 25% and the AUC was increased by ≈ 33% in the elderly, which may be due to decreased renal function in this population. **Enoxacin** plasma concentrations are 50% higher in the elderly than in young adults.

Pregnancy: Category C.

Lactation: **Norfloxacin** was not detected in breast milk. **Ciprofloxacin** is excreted in breast milk; however, the amount ingested by the infant appears to be low. **Ofloxacin** as a single 200 mg dose resulted in breast milk concentrations in nursing females that were similar to those found in plasma. It is not known whether **lomefloxacin** or **enoxacin** are excreted in breast milk.

Children: Do not use in children. Safety and efficacy of **lomefloxacin, enoxacin** and **ofloxacin** in children < 18 years of age have not been established.

Precautions:

Monitoring: Periodic assessment of organ system functions, including renal, hepatic and hematopoietic is advisable during prolonged therapy.

Ophthalmologic abnormalities, including cataracts and multiple punctate lenticular opacities, have occurred during therapy with some quinolones.

Crystalluria: Needle-shaped crystals were found in the urine of some volunteers who received either placebo or 800 or 1600 mg norfloxacin. While crystalluria is not expected to occur under usual conditions with 400 mg twice daily, do not exceed the daily recommended dosage. Crystalluria related to ciprofloxacin has occurred only rarely in man because human urine is usually acidic. The patient should drink sufficient fluids to ensure proper hydration and adequate urinary output.

Drug Interactions:

Drugs that may affect fluoroquinolones include antacids, didanosine, iron salts, sucralfate, zinc salts, antineoplastic agents, azlocillin, bismuth subsalicylate, cimetidine, nitrofurantoin and probenecid.

Drugs that may be affected by fluoroquinolones include caffeine, cyclosporine, digoxin, hydantoins, anticoagulants, cyclosporine and theophylline.

Drug/Food interactions: Food may decrease the absorption of **norfloxacin**. Food delays the absorption of **ciprofloxacin**, resulting in peak concentrations that are closer to 2 hours after dosing rather than 1 hour; however, overall absorption is not substantially affected. Dairy products such as milk and yogurt reduce the absorption of ciprofloxacin; avoid concurrent use. The bioavailability of ciprofloxacin may also be decreased by enteral feedings. Food delays the rate of absorption of **lomefloxacin** and decreases the extent of absorption (AUC) by 12%.

Adverse Reactions:

Fluoroquinolone Adverse Reactions (%)

Adverse reactions	Ciprofloxacin[1]	Enoxacin	Lomefloxacin	Norfloxacin	Ofloxacin[1]
Nausea	5.2	2-9	3.7	2.8	3-10
Abdominal pain/ discomfort	1.7	≤ 2	< 1	0.3-1	1-3
Diarrhea	2.3	1-2	1.4	✓[2]	1-4
Vomiting	2	6-9	< 1	✓[2]	1-3
Dry/painful mouth	< 1	< 1	< 1	✓[2]	1-3
Flatulence	✓[2]	< 1	< 1	0.3-1	1-3
Headache	1.2	≤ 2	3.2	2.7	1-9
Dizziness	< 1	≤ 3	2.3	1.8	1-5
Fatigue/Lethargy/Malaise	< 1	< 1	< 1	0.3-1	1-3
Somnolence/Drowsiness	< 1	< 1	< 1	0.3-1	1-3
Insomnia	< 1	1	< 1	0.3-1	3-7
Rash	1.1	≤ 1	< 1	0.3-1	1-3
Pruritus		1	< 1	✓[2]	1-3
Visual disturbances	< 1	< 1	< 1	✓[2]	1-3
Vaginitis	< 1	< 1	< 1		1-3

[1] Includes data for oral and IV formulations.
[2] ✓ = Adverse reaction observed, incidence not reported.
[3] See Warnings or Precautions.

Administration and Dosage:

CIPROFLOXACIN:

Ciprofloxacin Dosage Guidelines

Location of infection	Type or severity	Unit dose	Frequency	Daily dose
Urinary tract	mild/moderate	250 mg (200 mg IV)	12 h	500 mg (400 mg IV)
	severe/complicated	500 mg (400 mg IV)	q 12 h	1000 mg (800 mg IV)
Lower respiratory tract Bone and joint Skin & skin structure	mild/moderate	500 mg (400 mg IV)	q 12 h	1000 mg (800 mg IV)
	severe/complicated	750 mg	q 12 h	1500 mg
Infectious diarrhea	mild/moderate/severe	500 mg	q 12 h	1000 mg
Typhoid fever	mild/moderate	500 mg	q 12 h	1000 mg
Urethral/Cervical gonococcal infections	uncomplicated	250 mg	single dose	

The duration of treatment depends upon the severity of infection. Generally, continue ciprofloxacin for at least 2 days after the signs and symptoms of infection have disappeared. The usual duration is 7 to 14 days; however, for severe and complicated infections, more prolonged therapy may be required. Bone and joint infections may require treatment for 4 to 6 weeks or longer. Infectious diarrhea may be treated for 5 to 7 days. Typhoid fever should be treated for 10 days.

Renal function impairment –

Ciprofloxacin Dosage in Impaired Renal Function

Creatinine clearance (ml/min)	Dose
> 50 (oral); ≥ 30 (IV)	See usual dosage
30 - 50	250 - 500 mg q 12 h

Ciprofloxacin Dosage in Impaired Renal Function	
Creatinine clearance (ml/min)	Dose
5 - 29	250 - 500 mg q 18 h (oral); 200 - 400 mg q 18- 24 h (IV)
Hemodialysis or peritoneal dialysis	250 - 500 mg q 24 h (after dialysis)

In patients with severe infections and severe renal impairment, 750 mg may be administered orally at the intervals noted in the table.

CDC recommended treatment schedules for chancroid and gonorrhea –

Chancroid (H ducreyi infection): 500 mg orally 2 times a day for 3 days (alternative regimen).

Gonococcal infections:

Disseminated – 500 mg orally 2 times a day to complete a full week of therapy after treatment with initial regimen (ceftriaxone 1 g IM or IV every 24 hours) for 24 to 48 hours after improvement begins.

Uncomplicated – 500 mg orally single dose plus doxycycline

IV: Administer by IV infusion over 60 minutes. Slow infusion of a dilute solution into a large vein will minimize patient discomfort and reduce the risk of venous irritation.

NORFLOXACIN: Take 1 hour before or 2 hours after meals with glass of water. Patients should be well hydrated.

Recommended Norfloxacin Dosage					
Infection	Description	Dose	Frequency	Duration	Daily dose
Urinary tract infections (UTI)	Uncomplicated (cystitis) due to *E coli, K pneumoniae* or *P mirabilis.*	400 mg	q 12 h	3 days	800 mg
	Uncomplicated due to other organisms	400 mg	q 12 h	7 - 10 days	800 mg
	Complicated	400 mg	q 12 h	10 - 21 days	800 mg
Sexualy transmitted diseases	Uncomplicated gonorrhea	800 mg	single dose	1 day	800 mg

Renal Function impairment – In patients with a Ccr rate ≤ 30 ml/min/1.73 m^2, administer 400 mg once daily for the duration given above.

Elderly – Dose based on normal or impaired renal function.

CDC recommended treatment schedules for gonorrhea –

Gonococcal infections, uncomplicated: 800 mg as a single dose (alternative regimen to ciprofloxacin or ofloxacin).

OFLOXACIN: Usual daily dose is 200 to 400 mg every 12 hours as described in the following table:

Ofloxacin Dosage Guidelines (Oral and IV)					
Infection	Description	Unit dose	Frequency	Duration	Daily dose
Lower respiratory tract	Exacerbation of chronic bronchitis	400 mg	q 12 h	10 days	800 mg
	Pneumonia	400 mg	q 12 h	10 days	800 mg
Sexually transmitted diseases	Acute, uncomplicated gonorrhea	400 mg	single dose	1 day	400 mg
	Cervicitis/urethritis due to *C trachomatis*	300 mg	q 12 h	7 days	600 mg
	Cervicitis/urethritis due to *C trachomatis and N gonorrhoeae*	300 mg	q 12 h	7 days	600 mg
Skin and skin structure	Mild to moderate	400 mg	q 12 h	10 days	800 mg
Urinary tract	Cystitis due to *E coli* or *K pneumoniae*	200 mg	q 12 h	3 dyas	400 mg
	Cystitis due to other organisms	200 mg	q 12 h	7 days	400 mg
	Complicated UTIs	200 mg	q 12 h	10 days	400 mg
Prostatitis		300 mg	q 12 h	6 weeks[1]	600 mg

[1] Because there are no safety data presently available to support the use of the IV formulation for > 10 days, switch to oral therapy or other appropriate therapy after 10 days.

Renal function impairment – Adjust dosage in patients with a Ccr value of ≤ 50 ml/min. After a normal initial dose, adjust the dosing interval as follows: Ccr 10 - 50 ml/min, use a 24 hour interval and do not adjust the dosage; Ccr < 10 ml/min, use a 24 hour interval and one-half the recommended dosage.

CDC recommended treatment schedules for chlamydia, epididymitis, pelvic inflammatory disease (PID) and gonorrhea –

Chlamydia: 300 mg orally 2 times a day for 7 days (alternative regimen).

Epididymitis: 300 mg orally 2 times a day for 10 days (alternative regimen).

PID, outpatient: 400 mg orally 2 times a day for 14 days plus clindamycin or metronidazole.

Gonococcal infections, uncomplicated: 400 mg orally in a single dose plus doxycycline.

IV – Administer by IV infusion only. Do not give IM, intrathecally, intraperitoneally or SC. Avoid rapid or bolus IV infusion; administer slowly over a period of not less than 60 min.

ENOXACIN: Take at least 1 hour before or 2 hours after a meal.

Enoxacin Dosage Guidelines

Infection	Description	Dose	Frequency	Duration	Daily dose
Urinary tract infections	Uncomplicated (cystitis)	200 mg	q 12 h	7 days	400 mg
	Complicated	400 mg	q 12 h	14 days	800 mg
Sexually transmitted diseases	Uncomplicated gonorrhea	400 mg	single dose	1 day	400 mg

Renal function impariment – Adjust dosage in patients with a creatinine clearance (Ccr) ≤ 30 ml/min/1.73 m^2. After a normal initial dose, use a 12 hour interval and one-half the recommended dose.

Elderly – Dosage adjustment is not necessary with normal renal function.

CDC recommended treatment schedules for gonorrhea –

Gonococcal infections, uncomplicated: 400 mg as a single dose (alternative regimen to ciprofloxacin or ofloxacin).

LOMEFLOXACIN HCl: Lomefloxacin may be taken without regard to meals.

Recommended Daily Dose of Lomefloxacin

Body system	Infection	Dose	Frequency	Duration	Daily dose
Lower respiratory tract	Acute bacterial exacerbation of chronic bronchitis	400 mg	once daily	10 days	400 mg
Urinary tract	Cystitis	400 mg	once daily	10 days	400 mg
	Complicated urinary tract infections	400 mg	once daily	14 days	400 mg

Elderly – No dosage adjustment needed for elderly patients with normal renal function (Ccr ≥ 40 ml/min/1.73 m^2).

Renal function impairment – Lomefloxacin is primarily eliminated by renal excretion. Modification of dosage is recommended in patients with renal dysfunction. In patients with a Ccr > 10 but < 40 ml/min/1.73 m^2, the recommended dosage is an initial loading dose of 400 mg followed by daily maintenance doses of 200 mg once daily for the duration of the treatment.

Dialysis patients – Hemodialysis removes only a negligable amount of lomefloxacin (3% in 4 hours). Hemodialysis patients should receive an initial loading dose of 400 mg followed by maintenance dose of 200 mg once daily for duration of treatment.

Prophylaxis – A single 400 mg dose 2 to 6 hrs prior to surgery when oral preoperative prophylaxis for transurethral surgical procedures is considered appropriate.

CDC recommended treatment schedules for gonorrhea –

Gonococcal infections, uncomplicated: 400 mg as a single dose (alternative regimen to ciprofloxacin or ofloxacin).

SPARFLOXACIN: Sparfloxacin can be taken with or without food.

Community-acquired pneumonia; acute bacterial exacerbations of chronic bronchitis – The recommended daily dose of sparfloxacin in patients with normal renal function is two 200 mg tablets taken on the first day as a loading dose. Thereafter, take one 200 mg tablet every 24 hours for a total of 10 days of therapy (11 tablets).

Renal function impairment – The recommended daily dose of sparfloxacin in patients with renal impairment (creatinine clearance < 50 ml/min) is two 200 mg tablets taken on the first day as a loading dose. Thereafter, take one 200 mg tablet every 48 hours for a total of 9 days of therapy (6 tablets).

LEVOFLOXACIN:

Tablets – The usual dose is 500 mg orally every 24 hours as described in the following dosing chart. These recommendations apply to patients with normal renal function. Administer oral doses at least 2 hours before or 2 hours after antacids containing magnesium or aluminum, as well as sucralfate, metal cations such as iron and multivitamin preparations with zinc.

Levofloxacin Dosing				
Infection*	Unit dose	Frequency	Duration	Daily dose
Acute exacerbation of chronic bronchitis	500 mg	every 24 hours	7 days	500 mg
Community-acquired pneumonia	500 mg	every 24 hours	7-14 days	500 mg
Acute maxillary sinusitis	500 mg	every 24 hours	10-14 days	500 mg
Uncomplicated SSSI	500 mg	every 24 hours	7-10 days	500 mg
Complicated UTI	250 mg	every 24 hours	10 days	250 mg
Acute pyelonephritis	250 mg	every 24 hours	10 days	250 mg

* Due to the designated pathogens (see Indications).

Levofloxacin Dosing with Renal Function Impairment		
Renal status	Initial dose	Subsequent dose
Acute bacterial exacerbation of chronic bronchitis/Community acquired pneumonia/Acute maxillary sinusitis/Uncomplicated SSSI		
Ccr[1] from 50 to 80 ml/min	No dosage adjustment required	
Ccr[1] from 20 to 49 ml/min	500 mg	250 mg every 24 hours
Ccr[1] from 10 to 19 ml/min	500 mg	250 mg every 48 hours
Hemodialysis	500 mg	250 mg every 48 hours
CAPD[2]	500 mg	250 mg every 48 hours
Complicated UTI/Acute pyelonephritis		
Ccr[1] ≥ 20 ml/min	No dosage adjustment required	
Ccr[1] from 10 to 19 ml/min	250 mg	250 mg every 48 hours

[1] Ccr = creatinine clearance.
[2] CAPD = chronic ambulatory peritoneal dialysis.

GREPAFLOXACIN: May be taken with or without meals. The usual dose is 400 mg or 600 mg orally every 24 hours.

Recommended Daily Doses of Grepafloxacin			
Infection[1]	Dose	Frequency	Duration (days)
Acute bacterial exacerbations of chronic bronchitis	400 or 600 mg	once daily	10
Community-acquired pneumonia	600 mg	once daily	10
Nongonococcal urethritis or cervicitis	400 mg	once daily	7
Uncomplicated gonorrhea	400 mg	single dose	1

[1] Caused by the designated pathogens (see drug monograph).

TETRACYCLINES

TETRACYCLINE HCl	
Oral suspension: 125 mg/5 ml (*Rx*)	Various, *Achromycin V* (Lederle)
Capsules: 100, 250 and 500 mg (*Rx*)	Various, *Achromycin V* (Lederle)
Tablets: 250 and 500 mg (*Rx*)	*Sumycin 250 and 500* (Apothecon)
DEMECLOCYCLINE HCl	
Capsules: 50 and 100 mg (*Rx*)	*Declomycin* (Lederle)
Tablets: 150 and 300 mg (*Rx*)	*Declomycin* (Lederle)
DOXYCYCLINE	
Capsules: 50 and 100 mg (*Rx*)	Various, *Monodox* (Oclassen), *Vibramycin* (Pfizer)
Tablets: 50 and 100 mg (as hyclate) (*Rx*)	Various, *Vibra-Tabs* (Pfizer), *Bio-Tab* (Inter. Ethical Labs)
Capsules, coated pellets: 100 mg (as hyclate) (*Rx*)	*Doryx* (Parke-Davis)
Capsules: 50 and 100 mg (as monohydrate) (*Rx*)	*Monodox* (Oclassen)
Powder for oral suspension: 25 mg/5 ml (as monohydrate when reconstituted) (*Rx*)	*Vibramycin* (Pfizer)
Syrup: 50 mg/5 ml (as calcium) (*Rx*)	*Vibramycin* (Pfizer)
Powder for injection: 100 and 200 mg (as hyclate) (*Rx*)	Various, *Vibramycin IV* (Pfizer)
MINOCYCLINE	
Capsules: 50 and 100 mg (*Rx*)	Various, *Dynacin* (Medicis Dermatologics)
Capsules, pellet filled: 50 and 100 mg (*Rx*)	*Minocin* (Lederle)
Oral suspension: 50 mg/5 ml (*Rx*)	*Minocin* (Lederle)
Powder for injection: 100 mg (*Rx*)	*Minocin IV* (Lederle)
OXYTETRACYCLINE	
Capsules: 250 mg (*Rx*)	Various, *Terramycin* (Pfizer)
Injection: 50 and 125 mg/ml (*Rx*)	*Terramycin IM* (Roerig)

Actions:

Pharmacology: The tetracyclines are bacteriostatic. They exert their antimicrobial effect by inhibition of protein synthesis.

Pharmacokinetics:

Tetracycline Pharmacokinetic Variables and Dosage Regimens

Tetracyclines	Serum protein binding (%)	Normal serum half-life (hrs)	% Excreted unchanged in urine	Usual oral adult maintenance dosage	Lipid solubility
Tetracycline	65	16 to 12	60	250 mg q 6 h or 500 mg q 6 to 12 h	Intermediate
Demeclocycline	65 to 91	12 to 16	39	150 mg q 6 h or 300 mg q 12 h	Intermediate
Doxycycline	80 to 95	15 to 25	30 to 42	150 mg q 12 h or 100 mg q 24 h	High
Minocycline	70 to 80	11 to 18	16 to 12	100 mg q 12 h	High
Oxytetracycline	20 to 40	16 to 12	70	250 to 500 mg q 6 h	Low

Indications:

Infections caused by the following microorganisms: Rickettsiae (Rocky Mountain spotted fever, typhus fever and the typhus group, Q fever, rickettsialpox and tick fevers); Mycoplasma pneumoniae (PPLO, Eaton agent); agents of psittacosis and ornithosis; agents of lymphogranuloma venereum and granuloma inguinale; the spirochetal agent of relapsing fever *(Borrelia recurrentis)*.

Infections caused by the following gram-negative microorganisms: *Haemophilus ducreyi* (chancroid); *Yersinia pestis* and *Francisella tularensis* (formerly *Pasteurella pestis* and *P tularensis*); *Bartonella bacilliformis; Bacteroides* sp; *Campylobacter fetus* (formerly *Vibrio fetus*); *V cholerae* (formerly *V comma*); *Brucella* sp (in conjunction with streptomycin).

Infections caused by the following microorganisms, when bacteriologic testing indicates appropriate susceptibility to the drug:

Gram-negative – *Escherichia coli*; *Enterobacter aerogenes* (formerly *Aerobacter aerogenes*); *Shigella* sp; *Acinetobacter calcoaceticus* (formerly *Mima* and *Herellea* sp); *H influenzae* (respiratory infections); *Klebsiella* sp (respiratory and urinary infections).

Gram-positive – *Streptococcus* sp including *S pneumoniae*. Up to 44% of strains of *S pyogenes* and 74% of *S faecalis* are resistant to tetracyclines.

Staphylococcus aureus, skin and soft tissue infections. Tetracyclines are not the drugs of choice in the treatment of any type of staphylococcal infection.

Treatment of trachoma, although the infectious agent is not always eliminated, as judged by immunofluorescence.

When penicillin is contraindicated tetracyclines are alternatives for treatment of infections due to: *Neisseria gonorrhoeae; Treponema pallidum* and *T pertenue* (syphilis and yaws); *Listeria monocytogenes; Clostridium* sp; *Bacillus anthracis; Fusobacterium fusiforme* (Vincent's infection); *Actinomyces* sp; *N meningitidis* (IV only).

Acute intestinal amebiasis: Tetracyclines may be a useful adjunct to amebicides.

Oral tetracyclines:

Adults – Treatment of uncomplicated urethral, endocervical or rectal infections caused by *Chlamydia trachomatis.*

Severe acne (where it may be useful as adjunctive therapy).

Inclusion conjunctivitis (which may be treated with oral tetracyclines or with a combination of oral and topical agents).

Doxycycline, oral – Treatment of uncomplicated gonococcal infections in adults (except for anorectal infections in men); gonococcal arthritis-dermatitis syndrome; acute epididymo-orchitis caused by *N gonorrhoeae* and *C trachomatis*; nongonococcal urethritis caused by *C trachomatis* and *Ureaplasma urealyticum*.

Minocycline, oral – Treatment of asymptomatic carriers of *N meningitidis* to eliminate meningococci from the nasopharynx. *Not* indicated for the treatment of meningococcal infection.

Oral minocycline has been successful in *Mycobacterium marinum* infections.

Minocycline is also indicated for the treatment of uncomplicated urethral, endocervical or rectal infections in adults caused by *U urealyticum*; uncomplicated gonococcal urethritis in men due to *N gonorrhoeae*.

Unlabeled uses: **Demeclocycline** has been used successfully in the treatment of chronic hyponatremia associated with the syndrome of inappropriate antidiuretic hormone (SIADH) secretion.

Doxycycline has been used to prevent "Traveler's Diarrhea" commonly caused by enterotoxigenic *E coli*.

Minocycline has been used as an alternative to sulfonamides in nocardiosis.

Tetracycline and **doxycycline** instilled through a chest tube are employed as a pleural sclerosing agent in malignant pleural effusions. Tetracycline plus gentamicin is recommended for *V vulnificus* infections caused by wound infection after trauma or by ingestion of contaminated seafood.

Tetracycline suspension has been used as a mouthwash in the treatment of nonspecific mouth ulcerations, aphthous ulcers and canker sores. Dosages have ranged from 5 to 10 ml of 125 mg/ml 3 times/day for 5 to 7 days.

Lyme disease (the etiologic agent is a spirochete, *Borrelia burgdorferi*): Oral **tetracycline** 250 mg daily for 10 days is the drug of choice for stage I disease in adults; **doxycycline** has also been recommended for early disease. Both agents have been recommended for stage II disease, and they are being evaluated for treatment of stage III disease. However, the efficacy of tetracycline at the recommended dose for early Lyme disease has been questioned.

Contraindications:

Hypersensitivity to any of the tetracyclines.

Warnings:

Photosensitivity: Photosensitivity manifested by an exaggerated sunburn reaction has been observed in some individuals taking tetracyclines. Advise patients who are apt to be exposed to direct sunlight or ultraviolet light that this reaction can occur with tetracycline drugs, and discontinue treatment at the first evidence of skin erythema.

Phototoxic reactions are most frequent with demeclocycline, and occur less frequently with the other tetracyclines; minocycline is least likely to cause phototoxic reactions.

Parenteral therapy: Reserve for situations in which oral therapy is not indicated. Institute oral therapy as soon as possible. If given IV over prolonged periods, thrombophlebitis may result. IM use produces lower blood levels than recommended oral dosages.

Nephrogenic diabetes insipidus: Administration of **demeclocycline** has resulted in appearance of the diabetes insipidus syndrome (polyuria, polydipsia and weakness) in some patients on long-term therapy.

Hazardous tasks: Lightheadedness, dizziness or vertigo may occur with **minocycline.** Patients should observe caution while driving or performing other tasks requiring alertness.

Renal function impairment: If renal impairment exists, even usual doses may lead to excessive systemic accumulation of the tetracyclines (with the exception of doxycycline and minocycline) and possible liver toxicity. Use lower than usual doses.

Hepatic function impairment: Doses > 2 g/day IV can be extremely dangerous. In the presence of renal dysfunction, and particularly in pregnancy, IV tetracycline > 2 g/day has been associated with death secondary to liver failure.

Pregnancy: Category D (doxycycline). Do not use during pregnancy. They readily cross the placenta; concentrations of oxytetracycline in cord blood are ≈ 50% of those of the mother. Tetracyclines are found in fetal tissues and can have toxic effects on the developing fetus (retardation of skeletal development).

Lactation: Tetracyclines are excreted in breast milk. A dosage of 2 g/day for 3 days has achieved a milk:plasma ratio of 0.6 to 0.8.

Children: Tetracyclines should not generally be used in children under 8 years of age, unless other drugs are not likely to be effective, or are contraindicated.

Teeth – The use of tetracyclines during the period of tooth development (from the last half of pregnancy through the eighth year of life) may cause permanent discoloration (yellow-gray-brown) of deciduous and permanent teeth. Doxycycline and oxytetracycline may be less likely to affect teeth.

Bone – Tetracycline forms a stable calcium complex in any bone-forming tissue. Decreased fibula growth rate occurred in premature infants given 25 mg/kg oral tetracycline every 6 hrs.

Precautions:

Pseudotumor cerebri (benign intracranial hypertension) in adults has been associated with tetracycline use.

Outdated products: Under no circumstances should outdated tetracyclines be administered; the degradation products of tetracyclines are highly nephrotoxic and have, on occasion, produced a Fanconi-like syndrome.

Drug Interactions:

Drugs that may affect tetracyclines include antacids containing aluminum, calcium, zinc, magnesium, bismuth salts, divalent and trivalent cations, barbiturates, carbamazepine, hydantoins, cimetidine, oral iron salts, methoxyflurane and sodium bicarbonate.

Drugs that may be affected by tetracyclines include oral anticoagulants, digoxin, insulin, lithium, methoxyflurane, oral contraceptives and penicillins.

Drug/Food interactions: Food and some dairy products interfere with absorption of tetracyclines. Administer oral tetracycline 1 hour before or 2 hours after meals. Doxycycline has a low affinity for calcium binding. Gastrointestinal absorption of minocycline and doxycycline is not significantly affected by food or dairy products.

Adverse Reactions:

CNS:

Lightheadedness, dizziness or vertigo has been reported with **minocycline**.

Dermatologic:

Maculopapular and erythematous rashes.

GI:

Oral and parenteral – Anorexia; nausea; vomiting; diarrhea; epigastric distress; bulky loose stools; stomatitis; sore throat; glossitis; hoarseness.

Oral – Esophageal ulcers, most commonly in patients with an esophageal obstructive element or hiatal hernia.

Hematologic:

Hemolytic anemia; thrombocytopenia; thrombocytopenic purpura; neutropenia; eosinophilia.

Hepatic:

Fatty liver; increases in liver enzymes.

Hypersensitivity:

Urticaria; angioneurotic edema; anaphylaxis; anaphylactoid purpura; pericarditis; exacerbated systemic lupus erythematosus; polyarthralgia; serum sickness-like reactions (eg, fever, rash, arthralgia).

Miscellaneous:

Pseudotumor cerebri (adults); bulging fontanels (infants). Nephrogenic diabetes insipidus has been reported with **demeclocycline**.

Administration and Dosage:

Avoid rapid IV administration. Thrombophlebitis may result from prolonged IV therapy.

Continue therapy at least 24 to 48 hours after symptoms and fever subside. Treat all infections due to group A β-hemolytic streptococci for at least 10 days.

TETRACYLINE HCl:

Adults –

Usual dose: 1 to 2 g/day in 2 or 4 equal doses.

Children (over 8 years of age) – Daily dose is 10 to 20 mg/lb (25 to 50 mg/kg in 4 equal doses.

Brucellosis – 500 mg 4 times/day for 3 weeks, accompanied by 1 g streptomycin IM twice/day the first week, and once daily the second week.

Syphilis – 30 to 40 g in equally divided doses over 10 to 15 days. Perform close follow-up and laboratory tests.

Gonorrhea – 1.5 g initially, then 500 mg every 6 hours, to a total of 9 g.

Gonorrhea in patients sensitive to penicillin – Initially, 1.5 g; follow with 500 mg every 6 hours for 4 days to a total of 9 g.

Uncomplicated urethral, endocervical or rectal infections caused by Chlamydia trachomatis – 500 mg 4 times/day for at least 7 days.

Severe acne (long-term therapy) – Initially, 1 g/day in divided doses. For maintenance, give 125 to 500 mg/day.

CDC-recommended treatment schedules for sexually transmitted diseases –

Chlamydia trachomatis – Uncomplicated urethral, endocervical or rectal infections in adults: 500 mg 4 times/day for 7 days.

Gonococcal infections – Uncomplicated urethral, endocervical or rectal infections in adults: 3 g amoxicillin, 3.5 g oral ampicillin, 4.8 million units IM aqueous procaine penicillin G or 250 mg IM ceftriaxone. Each (except ceftriaxone) should be accompanied by 1 g oral probenecid. Follow with 500 mg tetracycline 4 times/day for 7 days.

In adults allergic to penicillins, cephalosporins or probenecid – 500 mg 4 times/day for 7 days.

Penicillinase-producing Neisseria gonorrheae (PPNG): 2 g IM spectinomycin or 250 mg IM ceftriaxone. Follow with 500 mg tetracycline 4 times/day for 7 days.

Children – 40 mg/kg/day in 4 divided doses for 5 days.

In PPNG-endemic and -hyperendemic areas: 250 mg IM ceftriaxone plus 100 mg oral doxycycline twice daily for 7 days or 500 mg oral tetracycline 4 times a day for 7 days. If tetracyclines are contraindicated or not tolerated, follow the single-dose regimen with erythromycin.

Disseminated gonococcal infections in patients allergic to penicillins or cephalosporins: 500 mg 4 times/day for at least 7 days.

Lymphogranuloma venereum – Genital, inguinal or anorectal: 500 mg 4 times/day for at least 2 weeks.

Nongonococcal urethritis: 500 mg 4 times/day for 7 days.

Acute pelvic inflammatory disease – Ambulatory treatment: 2 g IM cefoxitin, 3 g amoxicillin, 3.5 g oral ampicillin, 4.8 million units IM aqueous procaine penicillin G at 2 sites or 250 mg IM ceftriaxone. Each (except for ceftriaxone) should be accompanied by 1 g oral probenecid. Follow with 500 mg tetracycline 4 times/day. (However, doxycycline is preferred.)

Children over 7 years of age – 150 mg/kg/day IV cefuroxime or 100 mg/kg/day IV ceftriaxone followed by 30 mg/kg/day IV tetracycline in 3 doses, continued for at least 4 days. Thereafter, continue tetracycline orally to complete at least 14 days of therapy.

Syphilis (penicillin-allergic patients):

Early – 500 mg 4 times/day for 15 days.

More than 1 year's duration – 500 mg 4 times/day for 30 days.

Sexually transmitted epididymo-orchitis: 3 g oral amoxicillin, 3.5 g oral ampicillin, 4.8 million units IM aqueous procaine penicillin G at 2 sites (each with 1 g oral probenecid), 2 g IM spectinomycin or 250 mg ceftriaxone followed by 500 mg tetracycline 4 times/day for 10 days.

Urethral syndrome in women: 500 mg 4 times/day for 7 days.

Rape victims – Prophylaxis: 500 mg 4 times/day for 7 days.

DEMECLOCYCLINE HCl:

Adults –

Daily dose: 4 divided doses of 150 mg each or 2 divided doses of 300 mg each.

Children (over 8 years of age) –

Usual daily dose: 3 to 6 mg/lb (6 to 12 mg/kg), depending upon the severity of the disease, divided into 3 or 4 doses.

Gonorrhea patients sensitive to penicillin – Initially, 600 mg; follow with 300 mg every 12 hours for 4 days to a total of 3 g.

DOXYCYCLINE:

Oral –

Adults:

Usual dose – 200 mg on the first day of treatment (100 mg every 12 hours); follow with a maintenance dose of 100 mg/day. The maintenance dose may be administered as a single dose or as 50 mg every 12 hours.

More severe infections (particularly chronic urinary tract infections) – 100 mg every 12 hours.

Children (over 8 years of age):

100 lbs or less (< 45 kg) – 2 mg/lb (4.4 mg/kg) divided into 2 doses on the first day of treatment; follow with 1 mg/lb (2.2 mg/kg) given as a single daily dose or divided into 2 doses on subsequent days.

More severe infections – Up to 2 mg/lb (4.4 mg/kg) may be used. For children over 100 lbs (45 kg), use the usual adult dose.

Acute gonococcal infection: 200 mg immediately, then 100 mg at bedtime on the first day. Follow by 100 mg 2 times/day for 3 days.

Single visit dose – Immediately give 300 mg; follow with 300 mg in 1 hour, which may be administered with food, milk or carbonated beverage.

Primary and secondary syphilis: 300 mg/day in divided doses for at least 10 days.

Uncomplicated urethral, endocervical or rectal infections in adults caused by Chlamydia trachomatis: 100 mg twice daily for at least 7 days.

Unlabeled use: Doxycycline has been used to prevent "Traveler's Diarrhea" commonly caused by enterotoxigenic *Escherichia coli*. In limited trials, this prophylactic (100 mg/day) therapy appears to be superior to placebo.

Endometritis, salpingitis, parametritis or peritonitis: Give 100 mg doxycycline IV, twice daily and 2 g cefoxitin IV 4 times/day. Continue IV administration for at least 4 days and for at least 48 hours after patient improves. Then continue oral doxycycline (100 mg), twice daily to complete 10 to 14 days total therapy.

Parenteral – Do not inject IM or SC. The duration of IV infusion may vary with the dose (100 to 200 mg per day), but is usually 1 to 4 hours. A recommended minimum infusion time for 100 mg of a 0.5 mg/ml solution is 1 hour.

Adults: The usual dosage is 200 mg IV on the first day of treatment, administered in 1 or 2 hour infusions. Subsequent daily dosage is 100 to 200 mg, depending upon the severity of infection, with 200 mg administered in 1 or 2 infusions.

Primary and secondary syphilis – 300 mg daily for at least 10 days.

Children (> 8 years): ≤ 100 lbs (45 kg), give 2 mg/lb (4.4 mg/kg) on the first day of treatment, in 1 or 2 infusions. Subsequent daily dosage is 1 to 2 mg/lb (2.2 to 4.4 mg/kg) given as 1 or 2 infusions, depending on the severity of the infection. For children > 100 lbs (45 kg), use the usual adult dose.

Children (< 8 years): Safety of IV use has not been established.

CDC-recommended treatment schedules for sexually transmitted diseases –

Chlamydia trachomatis – Uncomplicated urethral, endocervical or rectal infections in adults: 100 mg 2 times/day for 7 days.

Gonococcal infections:

Uncomplicated urethral, endocervical or rectal infections in adults – 3 g oral amoxicillin, 3.5 g oral ampicillin, 4.8 million units IM aqueous procaine penicillin G or 250 mg IM ceftriaxone. Each (except for ceftriaxone) should be accompanied by 1 g oral probenecid. Follow with 100 mg doxycycline twice daily for 7 days.

In adults allergic to penicillins, cephalosporins or probenecid: 100 mg twice daily for 7 days.

In PPNG-endemic and -hyperendemic areas: 250 mg IM ceftriaxone plus 100 mg oral doxycycline twice daily for 7 days. If tetracyclines are contraindicated or not tolerated, follow the single-dose regimen with erythromycin.

Penicillinase-producing Neisseria gonorrhea: 2 g IM spectinomycin or 250 mg IM ceftriaxone. Follow with 100 mg doxycycline, twice daily for 7 days.

Disseminated gonococcal infections in patients allergic to penicillins or cephalosporins: 100 mg, twice daily for at least 7 days.

Lymphogranuloma venereum:

Genital, inguinal or anorectal – 100 mg twice daily for at least 2 weeks.

Nongonococcal urethritis: 100 mg twice daily for 7 days.

Acute pelvic inflammatory disease:

Ambulatory treatment – 250 mg single IM dose of ceftriaxone plus 100 mg oral doxycycline twice daily for 10 to 14 days. Other effective third-generation cephalosporins may be substituted in the appropriate doses for ceftriaxone.

Inpatient treatment – 100 mg IV doxycycline twice daily, plus 2 g IV cefoxitin 4 times a day. Continue drugs IV for at least 4 days and at least 48 hours after patient improves. Then continue doxycycline 100 mg orally twice daily to complete 10 to 14 days of total therapy.

Sexually transmitted epididymo-orchitis: 3 g oral amoxicillin, 3.5 g oral ampicillin, 4.8 million units IM aqueous procaine penicillin G at 2 sites (each with 1 g oral probenecid), 2 g IM spectinomycin or 250 mg IM ceftriaxone followed by 100 mg doxycycline twice daily for 7 days.

Rape victims prophylaxis: 100 mg twice daily for 7 days.

MINOCYCLINE:

Oral –

Usual dosage:

Adults – 200 mg initially, followed by 100 mg every 12 hours. If more frequent doses are preferred, give 100 or 200 mg initially; follow with 50 mg 4 times/day.

Children (over 8 years of age) – Initially, 4 mg/kg; follow with 2 mg/kg every 12 hours.

Syphilis: Administer usual dose over a period of 10 to 15 days. Close follow-up, including laboratory tests, is recommended.

Uncomplicated urethral, endocervical or rectal infections in adults caused by Chlamydia trachomatis: 100 mg 2 times/day for at least 7 days.

Uncomplicated gonococcal urethritis in men: 100 mg 2 times/day for 5 days.

Mycobacterium marinum infections: Although optimal doses are not established, 100 mg twice daily for 6 to 8 weeks has been successful in a limited number of cases.

Parenteral –

Adults: 200 mg followed by 100 mg every 12 hours; do not exceed 400 mg in 24 hours.

Children (over 8 years of age): Usual pediatric dose is 4 mg/kg, followed by 2 mg/kg every 12 hours.

OXYTETRACYCLINE:

Oral – See Tetracycline HCl.

Parenteral –

Adults: The usual daily dose is 250 mg administered once every 24 hours or 300 mg given in divided doses at 8 to 12 hour intervals.

Children (over 8 years of age): 15 to 25 mg/kg, up to a maximum of 250 mg per single daily injection. Dosage may be divided and given at 8 to 12 hour intervals.

MACROLIDES

AZITHROMYCIN	
Tablets: 250 and 600 mg (*Rx*)	*Zithromax* (Pfizer)
Powder for injection: 500 mg and 1 g (*Rx*)	*Zithromax* (Pfizer)
CLARITHROMYCIN	
Tablets: 250 and 500 mg (*Rx*)	*Biaxin* (Abbott)
Granules for oral suspension: 125 and 250 mg/5 ml (*Rx*)	*Biaxin* (Abbott)
DIRITHROMYCIN	
Tablets, enteric coated: 250 mg (*Rx*)	*Dynabac* (Bock)
ERYTHROMYCIN	
IV:	
Powder for injection: 500 mg and 1 g erythromycin lactobionate (*Rx*)	Various
Injection: 1 g erythromycin gluceptate (*Rx*)	Various
ORAL:	
ERYTHROMYCIN ETHYLSUCCINATE	
Tablets, chewable: 200 mg (*Rx*)	*EryPed* (Abbott)
Tablets: 400 mg (*Rx*)	*E.E.S. 400* (Various)
Suspension: 200 and 400 mg/5 ml (*Rx*)	Various, *EryPed Drops* (Abbott)
Drops, suspension: 100 mg/2.5 ml (*Rx*)	*EryPed Drops* (Abbott)
Powder for oral suspension: 200 mg/5 ml when reconstituted (*Rx*)	*E.E.S. Granules* (Abbott)
Granules for oral suspension: 400 mg/5 ml when reconstituted (*Rx*)	*EryPed* (Abbott)
ERYTHROMYCIN STEARATE	
Tablets, film coated: 250 and 500 mg (*Rx*)	Various, *Eramycin* (Wesley)
TROLEANDOMYCIN	
Capsules: 250 mg (*Rx*)	*Tao* (Roerig)

Actions:

Pharmacology: Macrolide antibiotics reversibly bind to the P site of the 50S ribosomal subunit of susceptible organisms and inhibit RNA-dependent protein synthesis by stimulating the dissociation of peptidyl t-RNA from ribosomes. They may be bacteriostatic or bactericidal, depending on such factors as drug concentration.

Despite differing structures, macrolides have similar antibacterial spectrum, mechanisms of action and resistance, but relatively different pharmacokinetics (see table).

Pharmacokinetics:

Various Pharmacokinetic Parameters of Macrolides								
Macrolide	Protein binding (%)	Metabolism	Elimination	Bioavailability (%)	Effect of food	C_{max}* (mcg/ml)	T_{max}* (hr)	Half-life (hr)
Azithromycin	50 (0.02 mg/L) 7 (1 mg/L)		4.5% excreted unchanged in urine; primarily excreted unchanged in bile	≈ 40	Food decreases absorption, C_{max} and AUC by ≈ 50%; take on empty stomach	0.4	2-3	68[1]
Clarithromycin		Metabolized to active metabolite (14-OH clarithromycin)	Primarily renal; rate approximates normal GFR	≈ 50	Food delays onset of absorption and formation of metabolite; does not affect extent of bioavailability. Take without regard to meals	1-3	1.7	3-7
Dirithromycin	15-30[2]	Non-enzymatic conversion to erythromycylamine	81%-97% fecal/hepatic[2]	≈ 10	Take with food or within an hour of having eaten	0.3 - 0.4[2]	3.9 - 4.1[2]	2-36

Various Pharmacokinetic Parameters of Macrolides

Macrolide	Protein binding (%)	Metabolism	Elimination	Bioavailability (%)	Effect of food	C_{max}* (mcg/ml)	T_{max}* (hr)	Half-life (hr)
Erythromycin	70-74	Hepatic; demethylation	< 5% (oral) and 12% to 15% (IV) excreted unchanged in urine; significant quantity excreted in bile		Base or stearate: Take on an empty stomach. Estolate, ethylsucci nate, delayed release base: Take without regard to meals			1.4
Troleandomycin			20% excreted in urine; significant quantity excreted in bile		Take on an empty stomach	2	2	

* C_{max} = Maximum concentration; T_{max} = Time to reach maximum concentration.
[1] Average terminal half-life.
[2] Value listed for erythromycylamine, the active moiety.

Microbiology:

Organisms Generally Susceptible to Macrolides In Vitro

	Organisms (✓ = generally susceptible)	Azithromycin	Clarithromycin	Dirithromycin	Erythromycin	Troleandomycin[1]
Gram-positive aerobes	*Staphylococcus aureus*	✓	✓	✓	✓	
	Streptococcus pyogenes	✓	✓	✓	✓	✓
	Streptococcus pneumoniae	✓	✓	✓	✓	✓
	Streptococcus agalactiae	✓	✓	✓	✓	
	Streptococcus sp	✓	✓	✓		
	Streptococcus viridans	✓	✓	✓	✓	
	Listeria monocytogenes		✓	✓	✓	
	Corynebacterium diphtheriae				✓	
	Corynebacterium minutissimum				✓	
Gram-negative aerobes	*Haemophilus influenzae*	✓	✓		†[2]	
	Haemophilus ducreyi	✓				
	Moraxella catarrhalis	✓	✓	✓	✓	
	Bordetella pertussis	✓	✓	✓	✓	
	Legionella pneumophila	✓	✓	✓	✓	
	Campylobacter jejuni	✓	✓			
	Neisseria gonorrhoeae		✓		✓	
	Pasteurella multocida		✓			
Anaerobes	*Bacteroides bivius*	✓				
	Bacteroides melaninogenicus		✓			
	Clostridium perfringens	✓	✓			
	Propionibacterium acnes		✓	✓		
	Peptococcus niger		✓			
	Peptostreptococcus sp	✓				
Other	*Borrelia burgdorferi*	✓				
	Chlamydia trachomatis	✓	✓		✓	
	Mycobacterium kansasii		✓			
	Mycoplasma pneumoniae	✓	✓	✓	✓	
	Treponema pallidum	✓			✓	
	Ureaplasma urealyticum	✓			✓	
	Entamoeba histolytica				✓	

[1] Data is limited for troleandomycin.
[2] Many strains resistant to erythromycin alone; may be susceptible to erythromycin plus a sulfonamide.

The in vitro spectrum of erythromycin covers primarily gram-positive microorganisms and gram-negative cocci.

Azithromycin is less active than erythromycin against most *Staphylococcus* and *Streptococcus* sp, but it is more potent against other organisms, including many gram-negative bacteria considered resistant to erythromycin. Azithromycin may expand the therapeutic range traditionally assigned to macrolides.

Clarithromycin exhibits the same spectrum of in vitro activity as erythromycin, but appears to have significantly increased potency against those organisms.

Troleandomycin, an acetylated ester of oleandomycin, is less active than erythromycin and offers no advantage. It can also cause hepatotoxicity.

Indications:

For specific approved indications, refer to the Administration and Dosage sections.

Contraindications:

Hypersensitivity to any of the macrolide antibiotics; patients receiving terfenadine or astemizole who have pre-existing cardiac abnormalities or electrolyte disturbances.

Erythromycin estolate: Pre-existing liver disease.

Warnings:

Pseudomembranous colitis has occurred with nearly all antibacterial agents and may range in severity from mild to life-threatening. Consider this diagnosis in patients who present with diarrhea subsequent to the administration of antibacterial agents.

Azithromycin:

Pneumonia – Azithromycin is only safe and effective in the treatment of community-acquired pneumonia of mild severity due to *S. pneumoniae* and *H. influenzae* in patients appropriate for outpatient oral therapy. Do not use in patients with pneumonia who are judged to be inappropriate for outpatient oral therapy because of moderate to severe illness or risk factors.

Gonorrhea or syphilis – Azithromycin at the recommended dose should not be relied upon to treat gonorrhea or syphilis.

Cardiac effects – Ventricular arrhythmias in individuals with prolonged QT intervals have occurred with macrolide products.

Hypersensitivity – Rare serious allergic reactions, including angioedema and anaphylaxis, have been reported in patients on azithromycin.

Dirithromycin:

Terfenadine drug interaction – Serious cardiac dysrhythmias, some resulting in death, have occurred in patients receiving terfenadine concomitantly with other macrolide antibiotics. Until further use data are available, it is prudent to monitor the terfenadine levels when dirithromycin and terfenadine are coadministered.

Bacteremias – Dirithromycin should not be used in patients with known, suspected or potential bacteremias as serum levels are inadequate to provide antibacterial coverage of the blood stream.

Respiratory infections – Dirithromycin is NOT indicated for the empiric treatment of acute bacterial exacerbations of chronic or secondary bacterial infection of acute bronchitis.

Skin/Skin structure infections – Dirithromycin is NOT indicated for the empiric treatment of uncomplicated skin and skin structure infections.

Erythromycin:

Hepatotoxicity – Erythromycin administration has been associated with the infrequent occurrence of cholestatic hepatitis. This effect is most common with erythromycin estolate; however, it has also occurred with other erythromycin salts.

Although initial symptoms have developed after a few days of treatment, they generally have followed 1 or 2 weeks of continuous therapy. Symptoms reappear promptly, usually within 48 hours after the drug is readministered to sensitive patients. The syndrome seems to result from a form of sensitization, occurs chiefly in adults, and is reversible when medication is discontinued.

Troleandomycin:

Hepatic effects – Troleandomycin has been associated with allergic cholestatic hepatitis. Some patients receiving troleandomycin for > 2 weeks or in repeated courses have developed jaundice accompanied by right upper quadrant pain, fever, nausea, vomiting, eosinophilia and leukocytosis. These have reversed on drug discontinuance. Readministration reproduces hepatotoxicity, often within 24 to 48 hours.

Renal/Hepatic function impairment:

Clarithromycin – In the presence of severe renal impairment (creatinine < 30 ml/min) with or without coexisting hepatic impairment, decreased dosage or prolonged dosing intervals may be appropriate.

Azithromycin and troleandomycin – Exercise caution when administering to patients with impaired renal or hepatic function.

Erythromycin – Erythromycin is principally excreted by the liver. Exercise caution in administering to patients with impaired hepatic function.

Dirithromycin – No dosage adjustment should be necessary in patients with impaired renal function, including dialysis patients. In patients with mild hepatic impairment, mean peak serum concentration, AUC and volume of distribution increased somewhat with multiple-dose administration; however, based on the magnitude of these changes, no dosage adjustment should be necessary in patients with mildly impaired hepatic function.

Elderly:

Clarithromycin – Studies show age-related decreases in renal function. Consider dosage adjustment in elderly patients with severe renal impairment.

Azithromycin – Dosage adjustment does not appear to be necessary for older patients with normal renal and hepatic function.

Dirithromycin – No dosage adjustment should be necessary in elderly patients.

Pregnancy: *Category* B (azithromycin, erythromycin); *Category* C (clarithromycin, dirithromycin).

Troleandomycin – Safety for use during pregnancy has not been established.

Lactation:

Clarithromycin, dirithromycin and azithromycin – It is not known whether these agents are excreted in breast milk.

Erythromycin – Erythromycin is excreted in breast milk, and may concentrate (observed milk:plasma ratio of 0.5 to 3). Erythromycin is considered compatible with breastfeeding by the American Academy of Pediatrics.

Children:

Dirithromycin – Safety and efficacy in children < 12 years of age have not been established.

Clarithromycin – Safety and efficacy in children < 6 months of age have not been established.

Azithromycin – Safety and efficacy in children < 6 months of age (acute otitis media, community-acquired pneumonia) or < 2 years of age (pharyngitis/tonsillitis) have not been established.

IV use: Safety and efficacy of azithromycin for IV injection in children or adolescents < 16 years have not been established.

Precautions:

Azithromycin:

Local IV site reactions have been reported with the IV administration of azithromycin. The incidence and severity of these reactions were the same when 500 mg was given over 1 hour (2 mg/ml as 250 ml infusion) or over 3 hours (1 mg/ml as 500 ml infusion). All volunteers who received infusate concentrations > 2 mg/ml experienced local IV site reactions; therefore, avoid higher concentrations.

Photosensitization (photoallergy or phototoxicity) may occur.

Drug Interactions:

Clarithromycin: Drugs that may be affected by clarithromycin include anticoagulants, astemizole, carbamazepine, cisapride, cyclosporine, digoxin, ergot alkaloids, tacrolimus, terfenadine, theophylline, triazolam, zidovudine, alfentanil and hexobarbital. Also consider all drug interactions with erythromycin.

Azithromycin: Drugs that may interact with azithromycin include antacids, tacrolimus, theophyllines and warfarin. Drugs that may affect clarithromycin include fluconazole. Also consider all drug interactions with erythromycin.

Dirithromycin: Drugs that may be affected by dirithromycin include terfenedine and theophylline. Drugs that may affect dirithromycin include antacids and H_2 antagonists. Also consider all drug interactions with erythromycin.

Erythromycin: Drugs that may be affected by erythromycin include alfentanil, anticoagulants, antihistamines, astemizole, terfenadine, bromocriptine, carbamazepine, cyclosporine, digoxin, disopyramide, ergot alkaloids, lincosamides, methylprednisolone, penicillins, theophyllines and triazolam.

Troleandomycin: Drugs that may be affected by troleandomycin include carbamazepine, oral contraceptives, ergot alkaloids, methylprednisolone, theophyllines and triazolam.

Drug/Food interactions:

Clarithromycin – Following tablet administration, food delays both the onset of clarithromycin absorption and the formulation of 14 OH clarithromycin, but does not affect bioavailability. Following the suspension, food decreases mean peak clarithromycin levels and extent of absorption.

Azithromycin – Food decreases the absorption of azithromycin capsules, reducing the maximum concentration by 52% and bioavailability by 43%. When azithromycin suspension was administered with food, the rate of absorption (C_{max}) was increased by 56% while the extent of absorption (AUC) was unchanged. Take 1 hour before or 2 hours after a meal. Do not take with food.

Dirithromycin – Dirithromycin should be administered with food or within an hour of having eaten. After administration of two 250 mg tablets 1 or 4 hours before food and immediately after a standard breakfast indicated an increase in absorption of erythromycylamine when dirithromycin was administered after food, while a significant decrease in C_{max} (33%) and AUC (31%) occurred when administered 1 hour before food.

Erythromycin – Antimicrobial effectiveness of erythromycin stearate and certain formulations of erythromycin base may be reduced. Take at least 2 hours before or after a meal. Erythromycin estolate and ethylsuccinate and the base in a delayed release form may be administered without regard to meals.

Adverse Reactions:

Clarithromycin:

Adverse reactions occurring in ≥ 3% of patients include diarrhea, nausea, abdominal pain, rash and abnormal taste.

Azithromycin:

Adverse reactions occurring in ≥ 3% of patients include diarrhea/loose stools, vomiting, nausea and abdominal pain.

Dirithromycin:

Dirithromycin Adverse Reactions (%): Dirithromycin vs Erythromycin		
Adverse reaction	Dirithromycin	Erythromycin
Abdominal pain	9.7	7.5
Headache	8.6	8.2
Nausea	8.3	7.5
Diarrhea	7.7	7.3
Platelet count increased	3.8	4.8
Vomiting	3	2.8

Erythromycin:

GI –

The most frequent dose-related side effects following oral use include abdominal cramping and discomfort, anorexia, nausea, vomiting and diarrhea. Pseudomembranous colitis associated with erythromycin therapy has occurred (see Warnings). Several cases of nausea and vomiting following IV erythromycin lactobionate have occurred.

Hepatic –

Hepatotoxicity is most commonly associated with erythromycin estolate.

Local:

Venous irritation and phlebitis have occurred with parenteral administration, but the risk of such reactions may be reduced if the infusion is given slowly, in dilute solution, by continuous IV infusion or intermittent infusion over 20 to 60 minutes.

Administration and Dosage:

AZITHROMYCIN: Administer at least 1 hour before or 2 hours after a meal. Do not give with food. Azithromycin *tablets* can be taken with or without food.

Adults –

Mild to moderate acute bacterial exacerbations of chronic obstructive pulmonary disease, community-acquired pneumonia, pharyngitis/tonsillitis (as second-line therapy), and uncomplicated skin and skin structure infections (≥ 16 years of age): 500 mg as a single dose on the first day followed by 250 mg once daily on days 2 through 5 for a total dose of 1.5 g.

Genital ulcer disease caused by H. ducreyi (chancroid): Single 1 g dose.

Nongonococcal urethritis and cervicitis due to C. trachomatis: Give a single 1 g dose.

Gonococcal urethritis/cervitis caused by C. trachomatis: Single 2 g dose.

Mycobacterium Avium Complex (MAC): For prevention of disseminated MAC administer 1.2 g once weekly. This may be combined with the approved dosage regimen of rifabutin.

CDC recommended treatment schedules for chancroid and chlamydia: 1 g as a single dose.

Children –

Acute otitis media/Community-acquired pneumonia: The recommended dose for oral suspension is 10 mg/kg as a single dose on the first day (not to exceed 500 mg/day, followed by 5 mg/kg on days 2 through 5 (not to exceed 250 mg/day). See the following table.

Pediatric Dosage Guidelines for Otitis Media (≥ 6 months of age)						
Dosing calculated on 10 mg/kg on day 1 dose, followed by 5 mg/kg on days 2 to 5						
Weight		Amount of 100 mg/5 ml suspension		Amount of 200 mg/5 ml suspension		Total ml per treatment course
kg	lbs	Day 1	Days 2 to 5	Day 1	Days 2 to 5	
10	22	5 ml	2.5 ml			15 ml
20	44			5 ml	2.5 ml	15 ml
30	66			7.5 ml	3.75 ml	22.5 ml
40	88			10 ml	5 ml	30 ml

Pharyngitis/tonsillitis: The recommended dose for children with pharyngitis/tonsillitis is 12 mg/kg qd for 5 days (not to exceed 500 mg/day). See the following.

Pediatric Dosage Guidelines for Pharyngitis/Tonsillitis (≥ 2 years of age)			
Dosing calculated on 12 mg/kg once daily on days 1 through 5			
Weight		Amount of 200 mg/5 ml suspension	
kg	lbs	Days 1 to 5	Total ml per treatment course
8	18	2.5 ml	12.5 ml
17	37	5 ml	25 ml

Pediatric Dosage Guidelines for Pharyngitis/Tonsillitis (≥ 2 years of age)			
Dosing calculated on 12 mg/kg once daily on days 1 through 5			
Weight		Amount of 200 mg/5 ml suspension	
kg	lbs	Days 1 to 5	Total ml per treatment course
25	55	7.5 ml	37.5 ml
33	73	10 ml	50 ml
40	88	12.5	62.5 ml

Parenteral – Injections should be infused over a period of > 60 minutes. Do not administer azithromycin for injection as a bolus or IM injection.

Community-acquired pneumonia: 500 mg as a single daily dose IV for ≥ 2 days. Follow IV therapy by the oral route at a single daily dose of 500 mg to complete a 7- to 10-day course of therapy.

Pelvic inflammatory disease (PID): 500 mg as a single daily dose for 1 or 2 days. Follow IV therapy by the oral route at a single daily dose of 250 mg to complete a 7-day course of therapy. If anaerobic microorganisms are suspected of contributing to the infection, administer an antimicrobial agent with anaerobic activity in combination with azithromycin.

The infusate concentration and rate of infusion for azithromycin for injection should be either 1 mg/ml over 3 hours or 2 mg/ml over 1 hour.

CLARITHROMYCIN: Clarithromycin may be given with or without meals.

Helicobacter pylori – Clarithromycin in combination with omeprazole is indicated for the treatment of patients with an active duodenal ulcer associated with *H. pylori* infection. The eradication of *H. pylori* has been demonstrated to reduce the risk of duodenal ulcer recurrence.

Clarithromycin Dosage Regimen for Active Duodenal Ulcer Associated with *H. pylori* Infection (28-Day Therapy)	
Days 1 - 14	Days 15 - 28
500 mg tablet three times daily plus omeprazole 2 × 20 mg every morning	Omeprazole 20 mg every morning

Adults –

Clarithromycin Dosage Guidelines		
Infection	Dosage (every 12 hr)	Normal duration (days)
Pharyngitis/Tonsillitis	250 mg	10
Acute maxillary sinusitis	500 mg	14
Lower respiratory tract	250-500 mg	7 to 14
Acute exacerbation of chronic bronchitis due to:		
S. pneumoniae	250 mg	7 to 14
M. catarrhalis	250 mg	7 to 14
H. influenzae	500 mg	7 to 14
Pneumonia due to:		
S. pneumoniae	250 mg	7 to 14
M. pneumoniae	250 mg	7 to 14
Uncomplicated skin and skin structure	250 mg	7 to 14

Children – Usual recommended daily dosage is 15 mg/kg/day divided every 12 hours for 10 days.

Pediatric Dosage Guidelines (based on body weight)				
Dosing calculated on 7.5 mg/kg q 12 h				
Weight		Dose	125 mg/5 ml	250 mg/5 ml
kg	lb	(q 12 h)	(q 12 h)	(q 12 h)
9	20	62.5 mg	2.5 ml	1.25 ml
17	37	125 mg	5 ml	2.5 ml
25	55	187.5 mg	7.5 ml	3.75 ml
33	73	250 mg	10 ml	5 ml

Mycobacterial infections – Recommended as the primary agent for the treatment of disseminated *Mycobacterium avium* complex (MAC). Use in combination with other antimycobacterial drugs that have shown an in vitro activity against MAC. Continue therapy for life if clinical and mycobacterial improvements are observed.

Dosage:

Adults – 500 mg twice daily.

Children – 7.5 mg/kg twice daily up to 500 mg twice daily. Refer to the Pediatric Dosing table.

Renal/Hepatic function impairment – In the presence of severe renal impairment with or without coexisting hepatic impairment, halved doses or prolongation of dosing intervals may be needed.

DIRITHROMYCIN: Administer with food or within 1 hour of having eaten. Do not cut, crush or chew the tablets.

Recommended Dosage Schedule for Dirithromycin (≥ 12 years of age)			
Infection (mild to moderate severity)	Dose	Frequency	Duration (days)
Acute bacterial exacerbations of chronic bronchitis due to *Moraxella catarrhalis* or *Streptococcus pneumoniae*. Not for empiric therapy (see Warnings).	500 mg	once a day	7
Secondary bacterial infection of acute bronchitis due to *M. catarrhalis* or *S. pneumoniae*. Not for empiric therapy (see Warnings).	500 mg	once a day	7
Community-acquired pneumonia due to *Legionella pneumophila*, *Mycoplasma pneumoniae* or *S. pneumoniae*	500 mg	once a day	14
Pharyngitis/Tonsillitis due to *Streptococcus pyogenes*	500 mg	once a day	10
Uncomplicated skin and skin structure infections due to *Staphylococcus aureus* (methicillin-susceptible). Not for empiric therapy (see Warnings).	500 mg	once a day	7

ERYTHROMYCIN, IV:

Erythromycin IV is indicated when oral use is impossible, or when severity of the infection requires immediate high serum levels. Replace IV therapy with oral as soon as possible.

Continuous infusion is preferable, but intermittent infusion in 20 to 60 minute periods at intervals of ≤ 6 hours is also effective. Due to irritative properties of erythromycin, IV push is unacceptable.

Severe infections – 15 to 20 mg/kg/day. Up to 4 g/day in very severe infections.

ERYTHROMYCIN, ORAL: Dosages and product strengths are expressed as erythromycin base equivalents. Because of differences in absorption and biotransformation, varying quantities of each salt form are required to produce the same free erythromycin serum levels.

Optimal serum levels of erythromycin are reached when erythromycin base or stearate is taken in the fasting state or immediately before meals. Erythromycin ethylsuccinate, estolate and enteric coated erythromycin may be administered without regard to meals.

Usual dosage –

Adults: 250 mg (or 400 mg ethylsuccinate) every 6 hours, or 500 mg every 12 hours, or 333 mg every 8 hours. May increase up to ≥ 4 g/day, according to severity of infection. If twice-a-day dosage is desired, the recommended dose is 500 mg every 12 hours. Twice-a-day dosing is not recommended when doses > 1 g daily are administered.

Children: 30 to 50 mg/kg/day in divided doses.

Erythromycin Uses and Dosages	
Indication (Organism)	Dosage (Stated as erythromycin base)
Labeled uses: Upper respiratory tract infections of mild to moderate severity *Streptococcus pyogenes* (Group A beta-hemolytic streptococcus) *S. pneumoniae* *Haemophilus influenzae* (used concomitantly with a sulfonamide)	 250 to 500 mg 4 times a day or 20 to 50 mg/kg/day in divided doses for 10 days 250 to 500 mg every 6 hours Erythromycin ethylsuccinate: 50 mg/kg/day Sulfisoxazole: 150 mg/kg/day Combination given for 10 days
Lower respiratory tract infections of mild to moderate severity: *S. pyogenes* *S. pneumoniae*	 250 to 500 mg 4 times a day or 20 to 50 mg/kg/day in divided doses for 10 days 250 to 500 mg every 6 hours
Respiratory tract infections *Mycoplasma pneumoniae* (Eaton agent, PPLO)	 500 mg every 6 hours for 5 to 10 days. Treat severe infections for up to 3 weeks
Skin and skin structure infections of mild to moderate severity: *S. pyogenes*	 250 to 500 mg 4 times a day or 20 to 50 mg/kg/day in divided doses for 10 days
Staphylococcus aureus (resistant organisms may emerge)	250 mg every 6 hours or 500 mg every 12 hours, maximum 4 g/day.

Erythromycin Uses and Dosages	
Indication (Organism)	Dosage (Stated as erythromycin base)
Pertussis (whooping cough) *Bordetella pertussis:* Effective in eliminating the organism from the nasopharynx of infected patients. May be helpful in prophylaxis of pertussis in exposed individuals.	40 to 50 mg/kg/day in divided doses for 5 to 14 days, or 500 mg 4 times a day for 10 days.
Diphtheria *Corynebacterium diphtheriae:* Adjunct to antitoxin to prevent establishment of carriers and to eradicate organism in carriers.	500 mg every 6 hours for 10 days
Erythrasma C. *minutissimum* Intestinal amebiasis *Entamoeba histolytica:* Oral erythromycin only.	250 mg 3 times daily for 21 days *Adults:* 250 mg 4 times daily for 10 to 14 days *Children:* 30 to 50 mg/kg/day in divided doses for 10 to 14 days
Pelvic inflammatory disease (PID), acute *Neisseria gonorrhoeae:* Erythromycin lactobionate IV followed by oral erythromycin.[1]	500 mg IV every 6 hours for 3 days, then 250 mg orally every 6 hours for 7 days. An alternative regimen for ambulatory management of PID is 500 mg orally 4 times a day for 10 to 14 days.
Conjunctivitis of the newborn, pneumonia of infancy, urogenital infections during pregnancy caused by *Chlamydia trachomatis*.	50 mg/kg/day in 4 divided doses for 14 days (conjunctivitis) or 21 days (pneumonia); 500 mg 4 times daily for 7 days or 250 mg 4 times daily for 14 days (urogenital infections).
Urethral, endocervical or rectal infections, uncomplicated C. *trachomatis* [1]	500 mg 4 times daily for 7 days or 250 mg 4 times daily for 14 days.
Nongonococcal urethritis *Ureaplasma urealyticum* [1]	500 mg 4 times daily for at least 7 days.
Primary syphilis *Treponema pneumophila:* (Oral only)[1]	20 g in divided doses over 10 days.
Legionnaire's disease *Legionella pneumophila:* No controlled clinical efficacy studies have been conducted, but data suggest effectiveness.	1 to 4 g daily in divided doses or 500 mg to 1 g 4 times daily for 21 days.
Rheumatic fever S. *pyogenes* (group A beta-hemolytic streptococci): Prevention of initial or recurrent attacks.[1]	250 mg 2 times daily.
Bacterial endocarditis *Alpha-hemolytic streptococcus* (Viridans)	*Adults:* 1 g 2 hours prior to procedure, then 500 mg 6 hours after initial dose. *Children:* 20 mg/kg 2 hours prior to procedure, then 10 mg/kg 6 hours after initial dose.
Listeria monocytogenes	*Adults:* 250 mg every 6 hours or 500 mg every 12 hours, maximum 4 g/day.
Unlabeled uses: *Campylobacter jejuni:* Has been successful with severe or prolonged diarrhea associated with *Campylobacter enteritis* or enterocolitis.	500 mg 4 times a day for 7 days.
Lymphogranuloma venereum: Genital, inguinal or anorectal.	500 mg 4 times a day for 21 days.
Haemophilus ducreyi (chancroid): Treat until ulcers or lymph nodes are healed.	500 mg 4 times a day for 7 days.
Neisseria gonorrhoeae: Uncomplicated urethral, endocervical or rectal infections and in penicillinase-producing *N. gonorrhoeae* (PPNG). In pregnancy	500 mg 4 times a day for 7 days or spectinomycin 2 g IM followed by erythromycin regimen. 500 mg 4 times a day for 7 days.

Erythromycin Uses and Dosages	
Indication (Organism)	Dosage (Stated as erythromycin base)
Treponema pallidum:	
Early syphilis (primary, secondary or latent syphilis of < 1 year duration).	500 mg 4 times a day for 14 days.
Prior to elective colorectal surgery, to reduce wound complications.	Combination of erythromycin base and neomycin is a popular preoperative preparation.
Clostridium tetani:	
Tetanus.[1]	500 mg every 6 hours for 10 days.

[1] Use as an alternative drug in penicillin or tetracycline hypersensitivity or when penicillin or tetracycline are contraindicated or not tolerated.

ERYTHROMYCIN ETHYLSUCCINATE: Expressed in base equivalents, 400 mg erythromycin ethylsuccinate produces the same free erythromycin serum levels as 250 mg or erythromycin base, stearate or estolate.

TROLEANDOMYCIN: Continue therapy for 10 days when used for streptococcal infection.

Adults – 250 to 500 mg 4 times a day.

Children – 125 to 250 mg (6.6 to 11 mg/kg) every 6 hours.

SULFONAMIDES

SULFADIAZINE	
Tablets: 500 mg (*Rx*)	Various, *Sulfadiazine* (Stanley)
SULFISOXAZOLE	
Tablets: 500 mg (*Rx*)	Various, *Gantrisin* (Roche)
SULFAMETHOXAZOLE	
Tablets: 500 mg (*Rx*)	Various, *Gantanol* (Roche), *Urobak* (Shionogi)
Oral Suspension: 500 mg per 5 ml (*Rx*)	*Gantanol* (Roche)
SULFAMETHIZOLE	
Tablets: 500 mg (*Rx*)	*Thiosulfil Forte* (Wyeth-Ayerst)

Actions:

Pharmacology: Sulfonamides exert their bacteriostatic action by competitive antagonism of para-aminobenzoic acid (PABA), an essential component in folic acid synthesis.

Pharmacokinetics:

Absorption/Distribution – The oral sulfonamides are readily absorbed from the GI tract. Approximately 70% to 100% of an oral dose is absorbed. Sulfonamides are bound to plasma proteins in varying degrees.

Metabolism – Metabolism occurs in the liver by conjugation, acetylation and other metabolic pathways to inactive metabolites.

Excretion – Renal excretion is mainly by glomerular filtration; tubular reabsorption occurs in varying degrees.

Microbiology: Sulfonamides have a broad antibacterial spectrum which includes both gram-positive and gram-negative organisms.

Indications:

Sulfonamide Indications

✔ – Labeled Indications	Multiple Sulfas	Sulfadiazine	Sulfamethizole	Sulfamethoxazole	Sulfisoxazole
Chancroid	✔	✔		✔	✔
Inclusion conjunctivitis	✔	✔		✔	✔
Malaria[1]	✔	✔		✔	✔
Meningitis, *H influenzae*[2]	✔	✔			✔
Meningitis, meningococcal[3]	✔	✔		✔	✔
Nocardiosis	✔	✔		✔	✔
Otitis media, acute[4]	✔	✔		✔	✔
Rheumatic fever		✔			
Rheumatoid arthritis					
Toxoplasmosis[5]	✔	✔		✔	✔
Trachoma	✔	✔		✔	✔
Urinary tract infections[6] (pyelonephritis, cystitis)	✔	✔	✔	✔	✔

[1] As adjunctive therapy due to chloroquine-resistant strains of *P. falciparum*.
[2] As adjunctive therapy with parenteral streptomycin.
[3] When the organism is susceptible and for prophylaxis when sulfonamide-sensitive group A strains prevail.
[4] Due to *H. influenzae* when used with penicillin or erythromycin.
[5] As adjunctive therapy with pyrimethamine.
[6] In the absence of obstructive uropathy or foreign bodies, when caused by *E. coli, Klebsiella-Enterobacter, S. aureus, P. mirabilis* and *P. vulgaris*.

Unlabeled uses: Sulfasalazine may be beneficial in the following: Ankylosing spondylitis; collagenous colitis; Crohn's disease; psoriasis; juvenile chronic arthritis; psoriatic arthritis. Sulfisoxazole may be useful for recurrent otitis media.

Contraindications:

Hypersensitivity to sulfonamides or chemically related drugs (eg, sulfonylureas, thiazide and loop diuretics, carbonic anhydrase inhibitors, sunscreens with PABA, local anesthetics); pregnancy at term; lactation; infants < 2 months old (except in congenital toxoplasmosis as adjunct with pyrimethamine); porphyria; salicylate hypersensitivity.

Warnings:

Group A beta-hemolytic streptococcal infections: Do not use for treatment of these infections.

Severe reactions including deaths due to sulfonamides have been associated with hypersensitivity reactions, agranulocytosis, aplastic anemia, other blood dyscrasias and renal and hepatic damage. Irreversible neuromuscular and CNS changes and fibrosing alveolitis may occur.

Porphyria: In patients with porphyria, these drugs have precipitated an acute attack.

Photosensitivity: Photosensitization (photoallergy or phototoxicity) may occur.

Renal/Hepatic function impairment: Use with caution. The frequency of renal complications is considerably lower in patients receiving the more soluble sulfonamides (sulfisoxazole and sulfamethizole).

Pregnancy: Category B; Category D near term. Significant levels may persist in the neonate if these drugs are given near term; jaundice, hemolytic anemia and kernicterus may occur. Do not use at term.

Lactation: According to the American Academy of Pediatrics, breastfeeding and sulfonamide use are compatible. However, do not nurse premature infants or those with hyperbilirubinemia or G–6–PD deficiency.

Children: Do not use in infants < 2 months old (except for congenital toxoplasmosis as adjunctive therapy with pyrimethamine).

Precautions:

Allergy or asthma: Give with caution to patients with severe allergy or bronchial asthma.

Hemolytic anemia, frequently dose-related, may occur in G-6-PD deficient individuals.

Drug Interactions:

Drugs that may interact with sulfonamides include oral anticoagulants, cyclosporine, hydantoins, methotrexate and sulfonylureas.

Drugs that may interact with sulfisoxazole include barbiturate anesthetics.

Drug/Lab test interactions: Sulfonamides may produce false-positive **urinary glucose tests** when performed by Benedict's method. Sulfisoxazole may interfere with the **Urobilistix test** and may produce false-positive results with sulfosalicylic acid tests for urinary protein.

Adverse Reactions:

Agranulocytosis; aplastic anemia; thrombocytopenia; leukopenia; hemolytic anemia; purpura; hypoprothrombinemia; cyanosis; methemoglobinemia; megaloblastic (macrocytic) anemia; Stevens-Johnson type erythema multiforme; generalized skin eruptions; epidermal necrolysis; urticaria; serum sickness; pruritus; exfoliative dermatitis; anaphylactoid reactions; periorbital edema; nausea; emesis; abdominal pains; diarrhea; bloody diarrhea; anorexia; pancreatitis; stomatitis; hepatitis; pseudomembranous enterocolitis; glossitis; headache; peripheral neuropathy; mental depression; convulsions; ataxia; hallucinations; tinnitus; vertigo; insomnia; hearing loss; drowsiness; apathy; crystalluria; hematuria; proteinuria; elevated creatinine; drug fever; chills; pyrexia; alopecia; arthralgia; myalgia.

Administration and Dosage:

CDC recommended treatment schedules for sexually transmitted diseases:

Lymphogranuloma venereum – As an alternative regimen to doxycycline, sulfisoxazole 500 mg 4 times a day for 21 days or equivalent sulfonamide course.

Treatment of uncomplicated urethral, endocervical or rectal Chlamydia trachomatic infections – As an alternative regimen to doxycycline or tetracycline (or if erythromycin is not tolerated), sulfisoxazole 500 mg 4 times a day for 10 days or equivalent sulfonamide course.

SULFADIAZINE:

Adults – *Loading dose* - 2 to 4 g. *Maintenance dose* - 4 to 8 g/day in 4 to 6 divided doses.

Children (> 2 months) – *Loading dose* - 75 mg/kg (or 2 g/m^2). *Maintenance dose* - 120 to 150 mg/kg/day (4 g/m^2/day) in 4 to 6 divided doses. *Maximum dose* - 6 g/day.

Infants (< 2 months) – Contraindicated, except as adjunctive therapy with pyrimethamine in the treatment of congenital toxoplasmosis. *Loading dose* - 75 to 100 mg/kg. *Maintenance dose* - 100 to 150 mg/kg/day in 4 divided doses.

Other recommended doses for toxoplasmosis (for 3 to 4 weeks) include – *Infants (< 2 months)* - 25 mg/kg/dose 4 times daily. *Children (> 2 months)* - 25 to 50 mg/kg/dose 4 times daily.

Prevention of recurrent attacks of rheumatic fever (not for initial treatment of streptococcal infections): Patients > 30 kg (> 66 lbs) - 1 g/day; < 30 kg (< 66 lbs) - 0.5 g/day.

SULFISOXAZOLE:

Loading dose – 2 to 4 g. *Maintenance dose* - 4 to 8 g/day in 4 to 6 divided doses. Although recommended, a loading dose is unnecessary because sulfisoxazole is rapidly absorbed and appears in high concentrations in the urine.

Children and infants (> 2 months) – *Initial dose* - 75 mg/kg. *Maintenance dose* - 120 to 150 mg/kg/day (4 g/m^2/day) in 4 to 6 divided doses (max, 6 g/day).

SULFAMETHOXAZOLE:

Adults – *Mild-to-moderate infections* - 2 g initially; maintenance dose is 1 g morning and evening thereafter. *Severe infections* - 2 g initially, then 1 g 3 times daily.

Children and infants (> 2 months) – Initially, 50 to 60 mg/kg; maintenance dose is 25 to 30 mg/kg morning and evening. Do not exceed 75 mg/kg/day.

Another recommended dose is 50 to 60 mg/kg/day divided every 12 hours, not to exceed 3 g/24 hours.

SULFAMETHIZOLE:

Adults – 0.5 to 1 g 3 or 4 times daily.

Children and infants (> 2 months) – 30 to 45 mg/kg/day in 4 divided doses.

Sildenafil

Tablets: 25, 50, and 100 mg (*Rx*)	*Viagra* (Pfizer)

Actions:

Pharmacology: Sildenafil, an oral therapy for erectile dysfunction, is a selective competitive inhibitor of cyclic guanosine monophosphate (cGMP)-specific phosphodiesterase type 5 (PDE5). The physiologic mechanism of erection of the penis involves release of nitric oxide (NO) in the corpus cavernosum during sexual stimulation. NO then activates the enzyme guanylate cyclase, which results in increased levels of cyclic guanosine monophosphate (cGMP), producing smooth muscle relaxation in the corpus cavernosum and allowing inflow of blood. Sildenafil enhances the effect of NO by inhibiting PDE5, which is responsible for the degradation of cGMP in the corpus cavernosum. When sexual stimulation causes local release of NO, inhibition of PDE5 by sildenafil causes increased levels of cGMP in the corpus cavernosum, resulting in smooth muscle relaxation and inflow of blood to the corpus cavernosum. Sildenafil at recommended doses has no effect in the absence of sexual stimulation.

Pharmacokinetics:

Absorption/Distribution – Sildenafil is rapidly absorbed, with absolute bioavailability of ≈ 40%. Maximum observed plasma concentrations are reached within 30 to 120 minutes (median, 60 minutes) of oral dosing in the fasted state. The mean steady-state volume of distribution for sildenafil is 105 L, indicating distribution into the tissues. Sildenafil and its major circulating N-desmethyl metabolite are both ≈ 96% bound to plasma proteins.

Metabolism/Excretion – Sildenafil is cleared predominantly by the CYP3A4 (major route) and CYP2C9 (minor route) hepatic microsomal isoenzymes. It is converted into an active metabolite by N-desmethylation and is further metabolized. This metabolite has a PDE selectivity profile similar to sildenafil and an in vitro potency for PDE5 ≈ 50% of the parent drug. Plasma concentrations of this metabolite are ≈ 40% of those seen for sildenafil, so that the metabolite accounts for ≈ 20% of sildenafil's pharmacologic effects. Both sildenafil and the metabolite have terminal half-lives of ≈ 4 hours.

Sildenafil is excreted as metabolites predominantly in the feces (≈ 80%) and to a lesser extent in the urine (≈ 13%).

Indications:

Erectile dysfunction: Treatment of erectile dysfunction.

Contraindications:

Hypersensitivity to any component of the tablet; patients concurrently using organic nitrates in any form (consistent with its known effects on the nitric oxide/cGMP pathway, sildenafil was shown to potentiate the hypotensive effects of nitrates).

Warnings:

Renal function impairment: In volunteers with severe renal impairment (Ccr < 30 ml/min), sildenafil clearance was reduced, resulting in approximately doubling of AUC and C_{max}.

Hepatic function impairment: In volunteers with hepatic cirrhosis, sildenafil clearance was reduced, resulting in increases in AUC (84%) and C_{max} (47%).

Elderly: Healthy elderly volunteers (≥ 65 years of age) had reduced sildenafil clearance with free plasma concentrations ≈ 40% greater than those in healthy younger volunteers.

Pregnancy: *Category* B. Sildenafil is not indicated for use in women.

Lactation: Sildenafil is not indicated for use in women.

Children: Sildenafil is not indicated for use in newborns and children.

Precautions:

Diagnosis of erectile dysfunction: Undertake thorough medical history and physical examination to diagnose erectile dysfunction, determine potential underlying causes and identify appropriate treatment.

Cardiovascular status: There is a degree of cardiac risk associated with sexual activity; therefore, consider the cardiovascular status of patients prior to initiating any treatment for erectile dysfunction.

Deformation of penis/priapism: Agents for the treatment of erectile dysfunction should be used with caution in patients with anatomical deformation of the penis or in patients who have conditions that may predispose them to priapism.

Drug Interactions:

P450 system: Sildenafil metabolism is principally mediated by the cytochrome P450 (CYP) isoforms 3A4 (major route) and 2C9 (minor route). Therefore, inhibitors of these isoenzymes may reduce sildenafil clearance.

It can be expected that concomitant administration of CYP3A4 inducers, such as rifampin, will decrease plasma levels of sildenafil.

Sildenafil Drug Interactions			
Precipitant drug	Object drug*		Description
Beta blockers, non-specific	Sildenafil	↔	The AUC of the active metabolite, N-desmethyl sildenafil, was increased 102% by non-specific beta blockers. These effects on the metabolite are not expected to be of clinical consequence.
Cimetidine	Sildenafil	↑	Coadministration yielded a 56% increase in plasma sildenafil concentrations. Sildenafil Drug Interactions
Precipitant drug	Object drug*		Description
Diuretics	Sildenafil	↔	The AUC of the active metabolite, N-desmethyl sildenafil, was increased 62% by loop and potassium-sparing diuretics. These effects on the metabolite are not expected to be of clinical consequence.
Erythromycin	Sildenafil	↑	A single 100 mg dose of sildenafil administered with erythromycin at steady state (500 mg twice daily for 5 days) resulted in a 182% increase in sildenafil systemic exposure (AUC).
Sildenafil	Nitrates	↑	Concomitant use is contraindicated. Sildenafil potentiates the vasodilatory effect of circulating nitric oxide, resulting in a significant and potentially fatal fall in blood pressure.

* ↑ = Object drug increased. ↔ = Undetermined clinical effect.

Drug/Food interactions: When taken with a high-fat meal, the rate of absorption of sildenafil is reduced, with a mean delay in T_{max} of 60 minutes and a mean reduction in C_{max} of 29%.

Adverse Reactions:

Sildenafil Adverse Reactions (≥ 2%)	
Adverse reaction	Sildenafil (n = 734)
Headache	16%
Flushing	10%
Dyspepsia	7%
Nasal congestion	4%
Urinary tract infection	3%
Abnormal vision[1]	3%
Diarrhea	3%

[1] Abnormal vision: Mild and transient, predominantly color tinge to vision but also increased sensitivity to light or blurred vision. In these studies, only 1 patient discontinued because of abnormal vision.

Administration and Dosage:

For most patients, the recommended dose is 50 mg taken as needed ≈ 1 hour before sexual activity. However, sildenafil may be taken anywhere from 4 hours to 30 minutes before sexual activity. Based on effectiveness and tolerance, the dose may be increased to a maximum recommended dose of 100 mg or decreased to 25 mg. The maximum recommended dosing frequency is once per day.

The following factors are associated with increased plasma levels of sildenafil: Age > 65 years (40% increase in AUC), hepatic impairment (eg, cirrhosis, 80%), severe renal impairment (Ccr < 30 ml/min, 100%) and concomitant use of potent cytochrome P450 3A4 inhibitors (erythromycin, ketoconazole, itraconazole, 200%). Because higher plasma levels may increase the efficacy and incidence of adverse events, consider a starting dose of 25 mg in these patients.

Sildenafil potentiated the hypotensive effects of nitrates; administration in patients who use nitric oxide donors (eg, sodium nitroprusside) or nitrates in any form is therefore contraindicated.

Pharmatecture Index

D

E

N

O

U

V

About The Author

Dr. Gideon Bosker is a widely published clinical scholar, educator, and author whose work in clinical pharmacology, primary care medicine, geriatrics, and emergency medicine has been recognized in national and international circles. An Associate Clinical Professor, Department of Emergency Medicine, at Oregon Health Sciences University, and Assistant Clinical Professor at Yale University School of Medicine, and associate editor of Physician's Therapeutics & Drug Alert, Dr. Bosker has co-authored or edited numerous journal articles and seven medical textbooks including, **Principles and Practice of Geriatric Emergency Medicine, The Manual of Emergency Medicine Therapeutics, Prehospital Pharmacology,** and **The Quick Consult Manual for Primary Care Medicine.** Dr. Bosker's lectures on Pharmatecture™ have been presented at more than 1,000 hospitals across the country. He is currently the Editor-in-Chief of **Emergency Medicine Reports®.** His current book, **Pharmatecture™: Minimizing Medications to Maximize Results,** represents more than 13 years of clinical experience and research in the areas of geriatric pharmacology, drug selection systems, drug-related adverse events, medication compliance, pharmacoeconomics, and formulary management.